D1568056

Spine and Spinal Cord Trauma

Evidence-Based Management

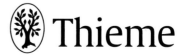

Spine and Spinal Cord Trauma
Evidence-Based Management

Alexander R. Vaccaro, MD, PhD
Professor
Departments of Orthopaedics and Neurosurgery
The Rothman Institute at Jefferson
Division of Orthopaedics
Thomas Jefferson University Hospital
Philadelphia, Pennsylvania

Michael G. Fehlings, MD, PhD, FRCSC
Professor
Department of Surgery
University of Toronto Faculty of Medicine
Division of Neurosurgery
Toronto Western Hospital
Toronto, Canada

Marcel F. Dvorak, MD, FRCSC
Professor
Department of Pediatrics
University of British Columbia
Head
Spine Program
Vancouver General Hospital
Vancouver, Canada

Thieme
New York • Stuttgart

Thieme Medical Publishers, Inc.
333 Seventh Ave.
New York, NY 10001

Editorial Director: Michael Wachinger
Executive Editor: Kay Conerly
Managing Editor: J. Owen Zurhellen
International Production Director: Andreas Schabert
Production Editor: Richard Rothschild
Vice President, International Sales and Marketing: Cornelia Schulze
Chief Financial Officer: James W. Mitos
President: Brian D. Scanlan
Compositor: Thomson Digital
Printer: Replika Press
Medical Illustrator: Andy Evansen
DVD Designed and Produced by Multi-Media Interactive Technology, Inc.
Historic cover image courtesy of Dr. James Tait Goodrich

Library of Congress Cataloging-in-Publication Data

Spine and spinal cord trauma : evidence-based management / [edited by]
Alexander R. Vaccaro, Michael G. Fehlings, Marcel F. Dvorak.
    p. ; cm.
  Includes bibliographical references and index.
  ISBN 978-1-60406-221-2 (alk. paper)
  1. Spine—Wounds and injuries. 2. Spinal cord—Wounds and injuries. 3. Evidence-based medicine. I. Vaccaro, Alexander R.
II. Fehlings, Michael. III. Dvorak, Marcel F.
  [DNLM: 1. Spinal Injuries—therapy. 2. Evidence-Based Medicine.
3. Spinal Cord Injuries—diagnosis. 4. Spinal Cord Injuries—therapy.
5. Spinal Injuries—diagnosis. WE 725 S759115 2010]
  RD533.S685 2010
  617.4'82044—dc22
                        2009040381

Important note: Medical knowledge is ever-changing. As new research and clinical experience broaden our knowledge, changes in treatment and drug therapy may be required. The authors and editors of the material herein have consulted sources believed to be reliable in their efforts to provide information that is complete and in accord with the standards accepted at the time of publication. However, in view of the possibility of human error by the authors, editors, or publisher of the work herein or changes in medical knowledge, neither the authors, editors, nor publisher, nor any other party who has been involved in the preparation of this work, warrants that the information contained herein is in every respect accurate or complete, and they are not responsible for any errors or omissions or for the results obtained from use of such information. Readers are encouraged to confirm the information contained herein with other sources. For example, readers are advised to check the product information sheet included in the package of each drug they plan to administer to be certain that the information contained in this publication is accurate and that changes have not been made in the recommended dose or in the contraindications for administration. This recommendation is of particular importance in connection with new or infrequently used drugs.

Some of the product names, patents, and registered designs referred to in this book are in fact registered trademarks or proprietary names even though specific reference to this fact is not always made in the text. Therefore, the appearance of a name without designation as proprietary is not to be construed as a representation by the publisher that it is in the public domain.

Printed in India

5 4 3 2 1

ISBN 978-1-60406-221-2

I dedicate this book to my family, and to the tireless efforts and dedicated work ethic
of the members of the Spine Trauma Study Group.

—Alexander R. Vaccaro

I dedicate this book to my beloved wife Darcy, to my family, my teachers,
and my friends and colleagues at the University of Toronto and the Toronto Western Hospital.

—Michael G. Fehlings

I dedicate this book to all the patients whom I have had the privilege of treating
and learning from over the years. This book would not have been possible without the support
and dedication of my loving and understanding wife, Sue, and our beautiful children
of whom I am so proud: Emily, Adam, Madeline, Eva, Levi, and Veronica.

—Marcel F. Dvorak

Contents

Contents

VI Subaxial Cervical Spine Injuries and Their Management

VII Thoracolumbar Spine Injuries and Their Management

DVD Contents

Foreword

This book offers unique access to the current views of experts in the field of spine and spinal cord trauma according to the principles of evidence-based medicine involving literature review, consensus agreement, and in-depth personal experience. These experts have used the most recent iterations of evidence-based medicine, including the recently announced five levels of evidence. The practice of spine medicine and spine surgery has changed markedly, and so have the principles of evidence-based medicine; thus this distillation of material on spine trauma offers the reader previously unavailable material and very valuable recommendations for practice. In the relatively circumscribed field of spine and spinal cord trauma, there are major inherent problems with data evaluation due to the acuteness of the condition, the dispersal of cases among centers and practitioners, and the highly variable mix of spinal injuries and spinal cord injuries, all of which have produced a literature of underpowered, and in some cases controversial, studies. To counteract these problems, this book provides practice recommendations according to consensus among experts who have thoroughly examined the literature and have amassed personal experience through focused practice and scholarship. Pooling the experience of spine surgeons has had most salutary benefits, as seen by the emergence of consortia of practitioners such as the Surgical Treatment of Acute Spinal Cord Injury Study

(STASCIS) Group that I founded in 1995. It is of interest that two of the editors of this book (AV and MF) are the current leaders of STASCIS.

The book covers a most compressive and panoramic list of spine topics, including all types of spinal and spinal cord traumatic conditions at all levels of the spine. It covers subjects ranging from intensive care to rehabilitation. Thus it will be very useful to a wide variety of clinicians, students, and researchers. Its major relevance will be for practicing neurosurgeons and orthopedic surgeons, residents and fellows in these fields, and the army of allied health professionals and their trainees who care for spinal and spinal cord injured patients, including intensivists, physiatrists, nurses, and rehabilitation therapists.

Congratulations to the editors and authors for easing the burden on practitioners, students, and researchers in spine trauma who wish to make their practice decisions and evaluations based on currently available best evidence.

Charles H. Tator, CM, MD, PhD, FRCSC, FACS
Professor of Neurosurgery
University of Toronto and Toronto Western Hospital
Toronto, Canada
Former Chair of Neurosurgery
University of Toronto

Preface

Traumatic injury to the spine and spinal cord is common and carries with it significant morbidity and mortality. This book, *Spine and Spinal Cord Trauma: Evidence-Based Management*, represents the collective efforts of members of the Spine Trauma Study Group (STSG), a multidisciplinary and multi-national group of spinal neurosurgeons and orthopedic surgeons to generate state-of-the-art, evidence-based reviews of the key issues facing clinicians when they are managing these unfortunate patients. This book is relevant to neurosurgeons, orthopedic surgeons, residents and fellows in training, and allied health professionals who care for spinal injured patients, including intensivists, physiatrists, and other professionals such as nurses and therapists. In addition, this book is of value to translationally oriented researchers who wish to learn about the key clinical and research issues in the field of spine and spinal cord injury.

The management of spinal trauma has often been relegated to academic training facilities throughout the world, with care being determined through experience and common practice. Innovations in spinal care are usually first pioneered and developed in the management of elective procedures; specifically geared around the management of symptomatic degenerative disk disease. Spinal fixation techniques and the biomechanics of their performance have subsequently been utilized in the management of spinal injury. Due to the paucity of patients treated at any particular trauma institution and the difficulties in performing controlled, prospective, randomized trials on patients with spinal injury, consensus statements as well as high-level evidence-based literature on the management of spinal injury were almost nonexistent. For this book, a group of experts in the field of spinal trauma throughout the world has undertaken the goal of distilling the best available evidence on this topic for the educational benefit of spinal care providers throughout the world.

A systematic review of the literature with recommended grades of treatment has been provided, illustrating the state-of-the-art recommended management protocols for pathologies ranging from cervical spinal cord injury to fractured dislocations of the sacrum. This book is only a start toward our understanding the value of evidence-based analysis in the care of spinal injury. We hope our project will stimulate further research and methods to develop multi-institutional trials to better understand means of improving the quality of lives of those inflicted with this unfortunate dilemma.

The vast majority of textbooks, reviews, and guidelines that attempt to synthesize the literature seem to conclude that further research is needed, and no conclusive recommendations can be made. The treating physician or surgeon, however, is faced with the necessity of making a therapeutic decision now, regardless of the quality of the literature. The decisions that we as spine trauma caregivers make each day include choices about the pharmaceutical management of spinal cord injury, when to operate, the timing of intervention, and the surgical approach and other technical issues. These decisions are made by many surgeons on a daily basis, and there can be remarkable agreement on the "best approach" for certain cases even when the quality of the literature may be graded as low or very low.

The editors of and contributors to this book have attempted to consider all aspects of what is known as evidence-based medicine in producing these chapters. When appropriate for the topic, authors have produced a comprehensive systematic review and then presented the results of the review to the membership of the Spine Trauma Study Group. This group of experts in spine trauma care has added their years of clinical experience as well as their appreciation of what approaches patients tend to prefer in order to create recommendations that we hope and expect will be helpful in assisting those who try to provide the best treatment available to their spine injured patients. We also hope that the compilation of this evidence and these recommendations will serve as background and encouragement to advance the spine literature with relevant, high-quality studies that will facilitate evidence-based treatment decisions.

Contributors

Bizhan Aarabi, MD, FRCSC, FACS
Professor
Department of Neurosurgery
University of Maryland School of Medicine
Director, Neurotrama
Division of Neurosurgery
University of Maryland Medical Center
Baltimore, Maryland

Amit O. Agarwala, MD
Orthopaedic Surgery
Panorama Orthopedics and Spine Center
Golden, Colorado

Ahmet Alanay, MD
Professor
Orthopeadics and Spine Unit
Istanbul Bilim University School of Medicine
Spine Unit
Avrupa Florence Nightingale Hospital
Istanbul, Turkey

Neel Anand, MD, Mch Orth.
Director
Orthopaedic Spine Surgery
Cedars-Sinai Spine Center
Los Angeles, California

Karen K. Anderson, BSc
Research Assistant
Department of Neurological Surgery
University of Kansas Medical Center
Kansas City, Kansas

Paul A. Anderson, MD
Professor
Department of Orthopaedics and Rehabilitation
University of Wisconsin School of Medicine and Public Health
Spine Medicine Clinic
University of Wisconsin Hospital and Clinics
Madison, Wisconsin

Paul M. Arnold, MD
Professor
Department of Neurological Surgery
University of Kansas School of Medicine
Kansas City, Kansas

Stephane Aunoble, MCU, PH
Orthopedic Surgeon
Pellegrin Group Hospital
Bordeaux, France

Eli M. Baron, MD
Neurosurgeon, Spinal Surgeon
Cedars-Sinai Spine Center
Cedars-Sinai Medical Center
Los Angeles, California

S. Samuel Bederman, MD, MSc, FRCSC
Visiting Assistant Professor
Department of Orthopaedic Surgery
University of California School of Medicine–San Francisco
San Francisco, California

Carlo Bellabarba, MD
Associate Professor
Department of Orthopaedics and Sports Medicine
University of Washington School of Medicine
Department of Orthopaedic Surgery
Harborview Medical Center
Seattle, Washington

David M. Benglis Jr., MD
Resident
Department of Neurosurgery
University of Miami, Miller School of Medicine
Miami, Florida

Christopher M. Bono, MD
Department of Orthopaedics
Brigham & Women's Hospital
Boston, Massachusetts

Richard J. Bransford, MD
Assistant Professor
Departments of Orthopaedics and Sports Medicine
University of Washington School of Medicine
Harborview Medical Center
Seattle, Washington

C. F. M. Buckens, MD
Department of Orthopaedics
University Hospital Utrecht
Utrecht, The Netherlands

Daniel J. Burval, MD
Department of Orthopaedic Surgery
Skyline Medical Center
Nashville, Tennessee

Peter G. Campbell, MD
Resident
Department of Neurological Surgery
Thomas Jefferson University, Jefferson School
   of Medicine
Philadelphia, Pennsylvania

Leah Y. Carreon, MD, MSc
Clinical Research Director
Kenton D. Leatherman Spine Center
Louisville, Kentucky

Jens R. Chapman, MD
Professor
Departments of Orthopaedics and Sports Medicine
University of Washington School of Medicine
Harborview Medical Center
Seattle, Washington

Ampar Cuxart, MD, PhD
Chief of Physical Medicine and Rehabilitation
Spine Unit
Vall d'Hebron University Hospital
Barcelona, Spain

Andrew T. Dailey, MD
Associate Professor
Department of Neurosurgery
University of Utah School of Medicine
Salt Lake City, Utah

Mark B. Dekutoski, MD
Associate Professor of Orthopaedics
Department of Orthopaedic Surgery
Mayo Clinic
St. Mary's Hospital–Mayo Foundation
Rochester, Minnesota

John R. Dimar, MD
Professor
Department of Orthopaedic Surgery
University of Louisville School of Medicine
Chief
Kenton D. Leatherman Spine Center
Louisville, Kentucky

Christian P. DiPaola, MD
Division of Spine Surgery
UMass Memorial Medical Center
Worcester, Massachusetts

Marcel F. Dvorak, MD, FRCSC
Professor
Department of Pediatrics
University of British Columbia
Head
Spine Program
Vancouver General Hospital
Vancouver, Canada

Daniel R. Fassett, MD
Assistant Professor
Department of Neurosurgery
Illinois Neurological Institute
Peoria, Illinois

Michael G. Fehlings, MD, PhD, FRCSC
Professor
Department of Surgery
University of Toronto Faculty of Medicine
Division of Neurosurgery
Toronto Western Hospital
Toronto, Canada

Charles G. Fisher, MD, MHSc, FRCSC
Associate Professor
Department of Orthopaedics
University of British Columbia Faculty of Medicine
Division of Neurosurgery and Orthopaedics
Spine Program
Vancouver General Hospital
Vancouver, Canada

Kathy Flint, RN, MSN
Indiana Orthopaedic Hospital
Indianapolis, Indiana

John C. France, MD
Professor
Department of Orthopaedics
West Virginia University School of Medicine
Chief
Spine Service
Robert Byrd Health Sciences Center
Morgantown, West Virginia

Ralf H. Gahr, MD, PhD
Department of Trauma and Orthopaedic Surgery
Trauma Center
Saint George Clinic
Leipzig, Germany

M. A. González-Viejo, MD, PhD
Associate Professor
Department of Physical Medicine and Rehabilitation
Universitat Autonoma de Barcelona
Department of Rehabilitation
Vall d'Hebron University Hospital
Barcelona, Spain

Jonathan N. Grauer, MD
Associate Professor
Department of Orthopaedics and Rehabilitation
Yale University School of Medicine
New Haven, Connecticut

Zbigniew Gugala, MD
Assistant Professor
Clinical Research
The Department of Orthopaedic Surgery and Rehabilitation
The University of Texas Medical Branch
Galveston, Texas

Eric B. Harris, MD
Department of Orthopaedics
Naval Medical Center San Diego
San Diego, California

Mitchel B. Harris, MD, FACS
Associate Professor
Department of Orthopaedic Surgery
Harvard Medical School
Chief
Division of Orthopaedic Trauma
Department of Orthopaedic Surgery
Brigham and Women's Hospital
Boston, Massachusetts

James S. Harrop, MD
Associate Professor
Department of Neurosurgery
Thomas Jefferson University, Jefferson Medical College
Philadelphia, Pennsylvania

Gregory W. J. Hawryluk, MD
Senior Resident and PhD Candidate
Division of Neurosurgery
Department of Surgery
University of Toronto Faculty of Medicine
Division of Genetics and Development
Toronto Western Research Institute
Toronto, Canada

Neal G. Haynes, MD
Department of Neurosurgery
University of Kansas Medical Center
Kansas City, Kansas

Rune Hedlund, MD
Department of Orthopaedics
Huddinge University Hospital
Karolinska Institute
Stockholm, Sweden

R. John Hurlbert, MD, PhD, FRCSC, FACS
Associate Professor
Division of Neurology
Department of Clinical Neurosciences
University of Calgary Faculty of Medicine
Division of Neurosurgery
Foothills Hospital and Medical Centre
Calgary, Canada

Jacqueline E. Karp, MD
Resident
Department of Orthopaedics
University of Maryland Medical System
Baltimore, Maryland

Ory Keynan, MD
Department of Orthopaedics B
The Tel Aviv Sourasky Medical Center and Tel Aviv University
Tel Aviv, Israel

Ahmad Khaldi, MD
Department of Neurological Surgery
Loyola University Medical Center
Maywood, Illinois

Stephen P. Kingwell, MD, FRCSC
Division of Orthopaedics
University of Ottowa Faculty of Medicine
Orthopaedic Surgery
Ottawa Hospital–Civic Campus
Ottawa, Canada

Brian K. Kwon, MD, PhD, FRSCS
Assistant Professor
Department of Orthopaedics
University of British Columbia Faculty of Medicine
Combined Neurosurgical and Orthopedic Spine Program
Vancouver General Hospital
Vancouver, Canada

James P. Lawrence, MD, MBA
Assistant Professor
Department of Surgery
Division of Orthopaedics
Albany Medical College
Albany, New York

Darren R. Lebl, MD
Chief Resident
Department of Orthopaedic Surgery
Harvard Medical School
Division of Spine Surgery
Massachusetts General Hospital
Boston, Massachusetts

Jean-Charles Le Huec, MD, PhD
Professor
Department of Orthopaedics, Spine Unit
Bordeaux 2 University School of Medicine
Deterca Laboratory
CHU Bordeaux
Bordeaux, France

Allan D. Levi, MD, PhD, FACS
Professor
Department of Neurological Surgery
University of Miami, Miller School of Medicine
Chief of Neurosurgery
University of Miami Hospital
Miami, Florida

Ronald W. Lindsey, MD
Department of Orthopaedics and Rehabilitation
The University of Texas Medical Branch–Galveston
Galveston, Texas

Steven C. Ludwig, MD
Associate Professor
Department of Orthopaedics
University of Maryland Medical System
Baltimore, Maryland

Ignacio Madrazo, MD, PhD, MSc, FACS
Department of Neuroscience
Hospital Ángeles del Pedregal
Research Unit
Department of Neurological Diseases
Hospital de Especialidades Cento Medio Siglo XXI-IMS
Mexico City, Mexico

Peter H. Maughan, MD
Division of Neurological Surgery
Barrow Neurological Institute
St. Joseph's Hospital and Medical Center
Phoenix, Arizona

Todd McCall, MD
Department of Neurosurgery
Illinois Neurological Institute
Saint Francis Medical Center
Peoria, Illinois

Richard Meyrat, MD
Department of Neurosurgery
Methodist Dallas Medical Center
Methodist Neurosurgical Associates
Dallas, Texas

Timothy A. Moore, MD
Assistant Professor
Department of Orthopaedic Surgery
Case Western Reserve University School of Medicine
Department of Orthopaedic Surgery
MetroHealth Medical Center
Cleveland, Ohio

Robert A. Morgan, MD
Assistant Professor
Department of Orthopaedic Surgery
University of Minnesota
Minneapolis, Minnesota
Department of Orthopaedics
Regions Hospital
St. Paul, Minnesota

Russ P. Nockels, MD
Associate Professor/Vice Chair
Department of Neurological Surgery
Loyola University–Chicago Stritch School of Medicine
Maywood, Illinois

Vanessa K. Noonan, PhD, PT
Department of Orthopaedics
University of British Columbia Faculty of Medicine
Division of Spine
Vancouver General Hospital
Vancouver, Canada

David O. Okonkwo, MD, PhD
Assistant Professor
Department of Neurological Surgery
University of Pittsburgh Medical Center
Pittsburgh, Pennsylvania

Z. Deniz Olgun, MD
Department of Orthopaedics and Traumatology
Hacettepe University School of Medicine
Sihhiye, Turkey

F. C. Oner, MD
Department of Orthopaedics
University Hospital Utrecht
Utrecht, The Netherlands

Alpesh A. Patel, MD
Assistant Professor
Department of Orthopaedics
University of Utah School of Medicine
Salt Lake City, Utah

Joseph L. Petfield, MD
Medical Student
Thomas Jefferson University, Jefferson Medical College
Philadelphia, Pennsylvania

Y. Raja Rampersaud, MD
Associate Professor
Department of Surgery
University of Toronto, Faculty of Medicine
Department of Surgery
Division of Orthopaedic Surgery
Toronto Western Hospital
Toronto, Canada

Glenn R. Rechtine II, MD
Professor
Department of Orthopaedics and Rehabilitation
University of Rochester Medical Center
Rochester, New York

Jeremy Reynolds
The Old Bakery
Oxford, United Kingdom

Jeffrey Rihn, MD
The Rothman Institute at Jefferson
Thomas Jefferson University Hospital
Philadelphia, Pennsylvania

Joseph Riina, MD
Orthopaedic Research Foundation
Division of Spinal Surgery
Indiana Orthopaedic Hospital
Indianapolis, Indiana

Yohan Robinson, MD
Institute for Surgical Sciences
Department of Orthopaedics
Uppsala University Hospital
Uppsala, Sweden

James W. Rowland, BScH
Graduate Student
University of Toronto Faculty of Medicine
Division of Genetics and Development
Toronto Western Research Institute
Toronto, Canada

Rick C. Sasso, MD
Professor and Chief of Spine Surgery
Department of Clinical Orthopaedic Surgery
Indiana University School of Medicine
President
Indiana Spine Group
Indianapolis, Indiana

Thomas A. Schildhauer, MD, PhD
Professor and Chairman
Universitatsklinik fur Unfallchirurgie
  und Sporttraumatologie
Medizinische Universitat–Graz
Graz, Austria

Oliver I. Schmidt, MD
Fellow
Department of Trauma and Orthopaedic Surgery
Trauma Center
Saint George Clinic
Leipzig, Germany

Miguel A. Schmitz, MD
Orthopaedic and Spine Surgery
Providence Holy Family Hospital
Spokane Orthopaedics
Deaconess Medical Center
Spokane, Washington

David G. Schwartz, MD
Assistant Clinical Professor
Department of Orthopaedic Surgery
Indiana University School of Medicine
Orthopaedic Surgeon
Division of Spinal Surgery
Indiana Orthopaedic Hospital
Indianapolis, Indiana

Lali H. S. Sekhon, MD, PhD, MB, BS, FRACS, FACS
Adjunct Associate Professor
Department of Physiology and Cell Biology
Faculty of Medicine, University of Nevada–Reno
Neurological Surgeon
Spine Nevada
Reno, Nevada

Christopher I. Shaffrey, MD
Harrison Distinguished Teaching Professor
Department of Neurological Surgery
Director
Spine Division
University of Virginia School of Medicine
Charlottesville, Virginia

Jason E. Smith, MD
Clinical Assistant Professor
Department of Orthopaedics
Louisiana State University School of Medicine
Spine Institute
Baton Rouge Orthopaedic Clinic
Baton Rouge, Louisiana

Justin S. Smith, MD
Assistant Professor
Departments of Neurosurgery and Orthopaedic Surgery
University of Virginia School of Medicine
Charlottesville, Virginia

Nicholas Theodore, MD
Director, Neurotrauma
Associate Director, Neurosurgery Resident Program
Barrow Neurological Institute
Neurological Surgery
St. Joseph's Hospital and Medical Center
Phoenix, Arizona

Marcus M. Timlin, MB, BCH, BAO, LRCP, MCH, FRCSI
Consultant
Orthopaedic Spine Surgeon
Department of Orthopaedic Surgery
Mater Private Healthcare
Dublin, Ireland

Stavropoula I. Tjoumakaris, MD
Department of Neurological Surgery
Thomas Jefferson University, Jefferson Medical College
Philadelphia, Pennsylvania

Jared A. Toman, MD, USAF
Chief Resident
Boston Medical Center
Boston, Massachusetts

Nestor D. Tomycz, MD
Resident
Department of Neurological Surgery
University of Pittsburgh Medical Center
Department of Neurological Surgery
Presbyterian Hospital
Pittsburgh, Pennsylvania

Andrew J. Tsung, MD
Assistant Professor
Department of Neurosurgery
Illinois Neurological Institute
University of Illinois College of Medicine
Peoria, Illinois

Alexander R. Vaccaro, MD, PhD
Professor
Departments of Orthopaedics and Neurosurgery
The Rothman Institute at Jefferson
Division of Orthopaedics
Thomas Jefferson University Hospital
Philadelphia, Pennsylvania

Jorrit-Jan Verlaan, MD
Division of Orthopaedics
University Hospital Utrecht
Utrecht, The Netherlands

Carlos Villanueva, MD, PhD
Departments of Anesthesiology and Spine Surgery
Traumatology and Rehabilitation Area
Vall d'Hebron University Hospital
Barcelona, Spain

Michael M. Vosbikian, MD
Robert Wood Johnson Medical School
Cooper University Hospital
Camden, New Jersey

Peter G. Whang, MD
Assistant Professor
Department of Orthopaedics and Rehabilitation
Yale University School of Medicine
Yale New Haven Hospital
New Haven, Connecticut

Allister R. Williams, MD
Head of Spine Surgery
Mountain Valley Orthopedics, PC
East Stroudsburg, Pennsylvania

Kirkham B. Wood, MD
Department of Orthopaedics
Massachusetts General Hospital
Boston, Massachusetts

Cao Yang, MD
Associate Professor
Department of Orthopaedic Surgery
Huazhong University of Science and Technology
Department of Orthopeadic Surgery
Union Hospital
Wuhan, China

Yasutsugu Yukawa, MD, DMSc
Director
Department of Orthopedic Surgery
Division of Spine Surgery
Chubu Rosai Hospital
Nagoya, Japan

Usman Zahir, MD
Resident
Department of Orthopaedics
University of Maryland School of Medicine
Baltimore, Maryland

Carlos Zamorano, MD
Professor
Department of Neurosurgery
Hospital de Especialidades Cento Medio Siglo XXI-IMS
Department of Neurosurgery
Hospital Ángeles del Pedregal
Mexico City, Mexico

DVD Contributors

Tierney Holmes, BS
Jefferson Medical College
Thomas Jefferson University
Philadelphia, Pennsylvania

Kornelis A. Poelstra, MD, PhD
The Spine Institute at Orthopaedic Associates
Fort Walton Beach, Florida

Todd Rubin, BS
Jefferson Medical College
Thomas Jefferson University
Philadelphia, Pennsylvania

Adam L. Shimer, MD
Assistant Professor
Department of Orthopaedic Surgery
University of Virginia
Charlottesville, Virginia

James Zaslavsky, DO
Orthopaedic Surgery Resident
The Rothman Institute
Thomas Jefferson University
Philadelphia, Pennsylvania

DVD Editor

Harvey E. Smith, MD
Houston, TX

I

Evidence-Based Medicine: Outcomes Assessment

1

Principles of Evidence-Based Medicine in Spine Trauma

Charles G. Fisher and Ory Keynan

Confronted with a rapidly growing body of scientific literature, the spine surgeon wishing to administer optimal evidence-based care to the patient is faced with an ever growing challenge. Given the fact that the volume of medical papers published doubles every 10 to 15 years,[1] and the time resources of the average surgeon do not expand at the same rate, it would seem necessary to find a tool that would help the busy clinician sift through the plethora of published medical literature for high-quality, useful evidence.

The concept of critically weighing the evidence for efficacy is not new, but the techniques for doing so have dramatically evolved over the last 2 decades. Building on the foundation laid out by Cochrane in 1972,[2] the explicit methodologies needed to extract "best evidence" were first published less than 2 decades ago,[3–5] providing for the first time a powerful tool for critically appraising the evidence for quality and applicability to patient care.

Evidence-based medicine (EBM), then, can be defined as an approach to health care that promotes the collection, interpretation, and integration of valid, important, and applicable patient-reported, clinician-observed, and research-derived evidence. The best available evidence, moderated by patient circumstances and preferences, is applied to improve the quality of clinical judgments.[6]

The idea of evidence-based practice thus conveys the idea of a rigorous and critical approach to the development and evaluation of clinical expertise while maintaining a strong commitment to patient-centered and humanistic values.[5]

EBM can be practiced at an organizational level by a multidisciplinary panel of experts assessing the literature, distilling it into clinically useful recommendations for the surgeon to use in patient management. Alternatively, it can be performed at an individual level—by the surgeon reviewing the pertinent literature to answer a clinically relevant question.

Either way, the scientific evidence component of EBM involves five steps: formulating a clinically relevant question, collecting the evidence, critically appraising it, applying the results to clinical practice, and assessing the outcome of applying those results to clinical practice. Understanding and assimilating the techniques of EBM into the everyday practice of spine surgeons has become fundamental to sound and responsible clinical practice and is the subject of this chapter. Assessing clinically relevant spine trauma topics, employing EBM techniques at an organizational level is the essence of this book.

◆ History of the Scientific Basis of Patient Management

The scientific basis for patient management in spine trauma, not unlike the rest of orthopedics, was traditionally based on tenuous evidence typically obtained through retrospective reviews, frequent use of analytical methods lacking clinical and biostatistical integration, as well as reliance on nonvalidated clinical outcome measures. In fact, the choice of outcome measures in clinical studies represents a classic example of the limitations of the research that has shaped clinical practice for years. It was well accepted for years that the outcome of patient management should be assessed through the eyes of the treating surgeon. Consequently, purported objective outcome measures such as radiographic appearance, complication rate, and fusion or union rates were generally used to gauge success of treatment and guide future interventions, as opposed to more patient-oriented outcome measures. This dependence on what might be called surrogate outcome measures to formulate recommendations regarding patient care, however, has eventually proven to be problematic. There is often little correlation between surgeon-oriented outcome measures and the functional outcome of the patient, as has been shown in the spine trauma and orthopedic literature.[7–13]

It eventually became apparent that if the ultimate focus of management of trauma patients is the patient, and not the management process, it should be reflected in the evaluation and reporting of the success of management. This should be accomplished through the use of more objective patient-oriented outcome measures that reflect the concerns of the patient and society, as has been shown in the general and orthopedic trauma literature in recent years,[14–24] and to a much lesser extent in the spine trauma literature.[7–10,25] This use of patient-focused outcomes as the primary study objective has led to improved study quality and thus better evidence.

As important as the outcome of a surgical or medical intervention is, even more fundamental to the EBM process is the *initial question of interest that sparks the need for evaluation of a treatment method*. This initial spark is that burning question encountered by the busy clinician in everyday practice, which drives him or her to take time out of a hectic schedule to critically appraise the existing literature for the answer, or better yet, locate a clinical practice recommendation or guideline addressing that question, the latter formulated by a panel of experts who already reviewed the evidence using EBM techniques.

◆ Evidence-Based Medicine Process

Formulating the Question

Although biostatistics plays a prominent role, especially in research, its significance is often overemphasized, particularly relative to issues of study design and methodology. In any research study, the clinician scientist must first develop a question. This question can be the basis for performing a study, or a clinical question raised by the clinician practicing EBM, and setting out to answer the question based on existing studies. On the surface, formulating a question may seem simple, but clearly defining the primary study question is indeed difficult. For example: What are the outcomes of patients with thoracolumbar burst fractures treated conservatively with a brace or without a brace? This question may appear adequate, but on further inspection what does one mean by outcome? Is the outcome pain, function, or return to work? Studies can usually only be designed to answer one question precisely and provide probable or possible answers to other secondary questions. Generally speaking, an adequate question should comprise four parts. First, it should clearly define the population under scrutiny. Second, it should specify the intervention the researcher is interested in evaluating. Third, it should identify any comparative interventions. Finally, it should identify the outcome measure we intend to use to assess the success of the intervention. So a better question for the foregoing example might be: For patients with acute AO type A3 thoracolumbar burst fractures treated with either a thoracolumbosacral orthosis (TLSO) or without a brace, what is the general health-related quality of life (HRQoL) at 1 year posttreatment? Once a researcher has a clearly defined question the assessment of the literature and study design becomes more focused and straightforward.

The optimal study design also flows directly from the primary question. For example, to answer the question of the thoracolumbar burst fracture mentioned above, the prospective randomized controlled trial (RCT) is ideal because bracing techniques are standardized with a short learning curve, there is equipoise within the surgeon and patient, selection and observer bias is minimized, and a component of blinding is even possible.

On the other hand, looking at the HRQoL 10 years out from injury in patients who suffered from thoracolumbar burst fractures and were treated either surgically or nonsurgically is more suitable for a prospective cohort design or even retrospective with cross-sectional outcome at 10 years. Multiple surgical options, poor generalizability, technological advancement, patient complexity, variability, and preference and selection bias make an RCT all but impossible.

Just as developing a research question is the first step in clinical research, it is similarly the first and most important step in practicing EBM as a clinician. Identifying the clinical problem and developing the question to ensure an appropriate literature search are critical. Exceedingly vague questions will bring a flood of irrelevant papers, whereas too narrow or specific a question may yield no or very little literature.

Collecting the Evidence

With a well-defined question in hand, the next task is to look for the published literature relevant to our question. Before embarking on a potentially costly and time-consuming project, it is vital to have a good grasp of the past and current literature on the subject of interest by performing a literature search. This will often help refine or modify the primary research question and will frequently spawn secondary questions.

There are various techniques for searching for articles in the medical literature, and more comprehensive tutorials are available in print,[26] online, or in libraries. Some general searching strategies are worth mentioning. First, it is a good tactic to use multiple databases simultaneously to assure a comprehensive survey of the literature. The best known and most comprehensive medical literature database is MEDLINE (Medical Literature, Analysis, and Retrieval System Online), which is the U.S. National Library of Medicine's (NLM's) premier bibliographic database containing over 12 million references to journal articles in the life sciences with a concentration on biomedicine, dating back to 1966. It is widely accessible from several institutional and commercial providers on the Internet (http://www.ncbi.nlm.nih.gov/entrez/query.fcgi), or on CD-ROM. Other important databases are EMBASE (the electronic version of the *Excerpta Medica* database), which is a comprehensive bibliographic database covering the worldwide literature on biomedical and pharmaceutical fields, with strong European content and little overlap with MEDLINE in terms of journals covered. Sources for evidence-based literature include the Cochrane Library (which contains more than 1100 systematic reviews in its Database of Systematic Reviews, prepared by the Cochrane Collaboration), Clinical Evidence (http://www.clinicalevidence.org), and Best Evidence (the electronic version of ACP Journal Club and Evidence-Based Medicine).

The search itself can generally be performed using keywords, author, or both; or by using MeSH (medical subject headings) terms in addition to keywords. MeSH terms make up a hierarchical vocabulary that is used for indexing articles in MEDLINE, with more specific terms organized underneath more general terms. Terms are updated annually, and each article indexed is assigned the most specific terms applicable, usually an average of 10 terms per article.[27] The advantage of searching with MeSH terms is that the search is done according to the subject content of the article, rather than the authors' wording in the article.

In the case of the systematic review or meta-analysis, the reproducibility and pervasiveness of a literature search are especially important and should include reliance on the aforementioned databases, as well as experts in the field, personal files, registries, meeting abstracts, and hand searching of references in retrieved articles. Furthermore, the retrieved abstracts should then be subjected to predetermined inclusion and exclusion criteria, preferably by two blinded reviewers, and only for those abstracts that according to both reviewers meet the criteria are the full articles retrieved. This should then be followed by applying the same inclusion and exclusion criteria to the full articles, until the final eligible articles are reached and constitute the basis for the systematic review or meta-analysis.[28-30]

Because a systematic review is the gold standard for determining best available evidence it has been adopted for this book.

Critical Appraisal of the Evidence

In this step of the process, the surgeon is compelled to sort out the evidence and grade the quality of its methodology and consequent relevance to clinical practice. In general, studies can be categorized in several different ways. One way would be to characterize a study according to the type of data analyzed. Thus clinical studies can be classified into one of two broad types: those that collect and analyze primary data and those that analyze secondary data. The former include case reports and series, case control, cross-sectional, cohort—both prospective and retrospective, and the RCT. The latter comprise systematic reviews or meta-analyses. Another way to broadly characterize studies is according to the use of an intervention. Viewed in this way, an experimental study is one in which an intervention is introduced to subjects and is under the control of the researcher and the outcome recorded, whereas an observational study is one in which no intervention is actively introduced but rather the outcome of one or more therapeutic options is observed and compared. Finally, studies can be categorized according to the direction of data gathering, being either retrospective, in which data recorded in the past are analyzed; or prospective, where the gathering of the data is begun after the initiation of the study and is thus under more rigorous control and is planned a priori.

The fundamental idea behind grading the quality of clinical evidence based on the study methodology is the assumption that as you ascend the study design hierarchy, there is greater likelihood that the results accurately represent the true or real outcome. It is important to keep in mind, however, that choosing the highest level of methodology for the study does not guarantee flawless execution of the study or proper analysis of its results. Indeed it is the question that determines the study design; not all questions need to be answered by an RCT.

Clinical evidence is graded in hierarchical order based on study design. Class I evidence is awarded to the systematic review of prospective randomized clinical trials and is considered the highest form of clinical evidence, whereas class V is considered the lowest evidence and represents expert opinion (**Table 1.1**).[5,31]

Study Design

Observational Studies

Traditionally criticized for having unrecognized and unpredictable confounding factors that may distort the results, observational studies have been regarded with caution in the medical literature. Some authors have even gone as far as recommending that "If you find that a study was not randomized,

Table 1.1 Levels of Evidence for Primary Research Question

	Types of Studies			
	Therapeutic Studies: Investigating the Results of Treatment	**Prognostic Studies: Investigating the Outcome of Disease**	**Diagnostic Studies: Investigating a Diagnostic Test**	**Economic and Decision Analyses: Developing an Economic or Decision Model**
Level I	1. Randomized, controlled trial a. Significant difference b. No significant difference but confidence intervals 2. Systematic review[2] of level I randomized, controlled trials (studies were homogeneous)	1. Prospective study[1] 2. Systematic review[2] of level I studies	1. Testing of previously developed diagnostic criteria in series of consecutive patients (with universally applied reference "gold" standard) 2. Systematic review[2] of level I studies	1. Clinically sensible costs and alternatives; values obtained from many studies; multiway sensitivity analyses 2. Systematic review[2] of Level-I studies
Level II	1. Prospective cohort study[5] 2. Poor-quality randomized, controlled trial (e.g., < 80% follow-up) 3. Systematic review[2] a. Level II studies b. Nonhomogeneous level I studies	1. Retrospective study[4] 2. Study of untreated controls from a previous randomized, controlled trial 3. Systematic review[2] of Level II studies	1. Development of diagnostic criteria on basis of consecutive patients (no consistently applied reference "gold" standard) 2. Systematic review[2] of level III studies	1. Clinically sensible costs and alternatives; values obtained from limited studies; multiway sensitivity analyses 2. Systematic review[2] of Level-II studies
Level III	1. Case-control study[5] 2. Retrospective cohort study[4] 3. Systematic review[2] of level III studies		1. Study of nonconsecutive patients (no consistently applied reference "gold" standard) 2. Systematic review[2] of level III studies	1. Limited alternatives and costs; poor estimates 2. Systematic review[2] of level III studies

(Continued on page 6)

Table 1.1 Levels of Evidence for Primary Research Question *(Continued)*

	Types of Studies			
	Therapeutic Studies: Investigating the Results of Treatment	**Prognostic Studies: Investigating the Outcome of Disease**	**Diagnostic Studies: Investigating a Diagnostic Test**	**Economic and Decision Analyses: Developing an Economic or Decision Model**
Level IV	Case series (non-, or historical, control groups)	Case series	1. Case control study 2. Poor reference standard	No sensitivity analyses
Level V	Expert opinion	Expert opinion	Expert opinion	Expert opinion

[1] All patients were enrolled at the same point in their disease course (inception cohort) with ≥ 80% follow-up of enrolled patients.

[2] A study of results from two or more studies.

[3] Patients were compared with a control group of patients treated at the same time and institution.

[4] The study was initiated after treatment was performed.

[5] Patients with a particular outcome ("cases" with, for example, a failed arthroplasty) were compared with those who did not have the outcome ("controls" with, for example, a total hip arthroplasty that did not fail).

Source: From Wright JG, Swiontkowski MF, Heckman JD. Introducing levels of evidence to the journal. J Bone Joint Surg Am 2003;85-A:2. Reprinted with permission.

we'd suggest that you stop reading it and go on to the next article."[32] This is due in large part to several high-impact, comparative studies published 2 and 3 decades ago, which suggested that observational studies significantly overestimate the positive effect of a therapeutic intervention when compared with RCTs.[33-37]

More recent systematic reviews, however, challenge that conventional wisdom.[38-40] Benson and Hartz[38] searched the general and internal medical literature for observational comparative studies published between 1985 and 1998 that compared two or more treatments or interventions for the same condition. For each paper that met their inclusion criteria, they then performed an additional search to identify all the RCTs and observational studies, comparing the same treatments, using the same outcome measure and inclusion criteria, but this time spanning more than 30 years, from 1966 to 1998. They found 19 treatment comparisons that were the subject of at least one observational study and at least one RCT, resulting in a systematic review of 53 observational studies and 83 RCTs. They ultimately found that in all but two of the 19 treatment comparisons the estimates of treatment effects from observational studies and RCTs were similar.

Concato et al[39] set out to evaluate the modern-day role of the observational study within the framework of the commonly accepted level of evidence for clinical trials. They looked at meta-analyses of RCTs and of observational studies that assessed the same clinical topic and published in one of five high impact journals from 1991 to 1995. They, too, found remarkable similarity between the average results of the observational studies and those of the RCTs.

Unfortunately for the spine surgeon-reader, things are not as encouraging, as evidenced by a systematic review looking at observational studies evaluating the surgical management of lumbar disk herniation, showing the vast majority of studies failed to used statistical methods to adjust for confounding, with only a handful pointing them out at all as a limitation, thus casting a great shadow on their validity.[40]

So, although the observational study can rival the RCT with the exception of controlling for unknown bias, its conduct is critical to validity. With current objective outcome measures and sophisticated statistical methods, high quality observational studies can be done and are starting to appear regularly in the spine literature.[41-47] Following is an overview of the various types of observational studies commonly encountered in the literature.

Case Reports

Case reports are valuable in rare conditions or if they provide compelling findings that can be hypothesis generating for further studies. Small sample size, no control group, and nonobjective outcome measures limit them. The natural extension of a case report is a case series, which allows for a more valid assessment of a clinical course or response to an intervention. Few conclusions can be made because of the selection bias, subjective assessment, a small often ill-defined number of subjects (n), and lack of a comparison group. Case series can be improved by addressing some of these limitations such as using objective outcome measures and clearly defining their inclusion criteria, which makes them very similar to cohort studies.

Case Control Studies

Case control studies usually involve a cross-sectional analysis on similar subjects and classically compare cases with controls for the presence of risk factors. This design is ideal for assessing etiologic or risk factors for rare diseases and is useful in studies of prognosis. Although these studies are efficient from a time and cost perspective there are limitations. Finding appropriately matched controls and defining inclusion and exclusion criteria that are similar for both cases and controls are steps taken to control for confounding variables. Because both the exposure and the disease have already occurred and there is different recall bias between cases and controls, proving causation is difficult. An example of a surgical case control study would be comparing patients who have all had cervical facet dislocations treated by anterior fusion and developed the complication of postoperative kyphosis (cases), to patients treated the same way who did not develop postoperative focal kyphosis (controls). The results may allow the identification of risk factors for developing sagittal malalignment following anterior fusion for cervical facet dislocations.[48] Ideally the control:case ratio should be 1:1, up to a maximum of 4:1.

Cohort Studies

Cohort studies can be retrospective or prospective, with the latter providing better scientific evidence. Cohort studies are similar to case series but more tightly controlled. They require a time zero, strict inclusion/exclusion criteria, standardized follow-up at regular time intervals, and efforts to optimize follow-up and reduce dropouts. For these reasons prospective cohort studies are expensive and time consuming. Cohort designs are ideal for identifying risk factors for disease, determining the outcome of an intervention, and examining the natural history of a disease. The Framingham cohort study examining cardiovascular disease is one of the more famous cohort studies. It was begun in 1948 with the primary goal of evaluating risk factors for heart disease. A total of 5209 men and women who ranged in age from 28 to 62 years were recruited from a sample of two thirds of the residences in Framingham, Massachusetts, and have been examined biennially for more than 50 years.[49]

Prospective cohorts can be compared with historical controls but problems with data quality, selection bias, outcome parameters, and temporal trends make this less desirable than a nonrandomized, prospective outcomes study.

Retrospective Studies

Retrospective studies have the advantage of being less expensive and time consuming. The records (usually charts) are made out without knowledge of exposure or disease, and therefore recall bias is not an issue. However, because the records used for data are collected for other reasons and in a nonstandardized manner critical information such as confounders is almost always missing. The incorporation of a cross-sectional outcome analysis to a retrospective cohort study provides a standardized outcome, but many subjects maybe deceased or lost to follow-up leading to poor response rates.

Randomized, Controlled Trials

RCTs are justifiably recognized as the gold standard in clinical evidence; however, they have well-recognized disadvantages, including high costs, administrative complexity, prolonged time to completion, and difficulty ensuring methodological vision. Furthermore, RCTs in surgery are complicated by difficulties in blinding, randomization, technique standardization, and generalizability. Nevertheless, the ability to control for known and unknown bias outweighs these disadvantages. Randomization is unrivaled in ensuring the balancing of the experimental and control groups for unknown confounders. Known confounders are also well balanced if the group sizes are large enough; however, if the sample sizes are small the balancing of known confounders can easily be performed through stratification. Blinding is designed to induce comparability in the handling and evaluation of the participants,

it preserves the integrity of the randomization, and it allows for objective collection and analysis of data. Surgical RCTs are difficult to do, and hence there is a paucity of them in the surgical literature. Practical and ethical issues limit their use in surgery, but above all they are extremely difficult, time consuming, and expensive to do. This should not deter clinical scientists from pursuing this study design so that needed answers to important questions can be obtained.

Systematic Reviews

A systematic review provides a rational synopsis of the available literature. By summarizing all relevant literature on a particular topic, the systematic review tends to be a tremendous asset to the busy clinician. A systematic review attempts to overcome the bias that is associated with the majority of "traditional," or more appropriately termed "narrative," reviews. Through the application of rigorous methodology, potential bias is minimized. A properly conducted systematic review will ensure all published and unpublished literature is considered, will evaluate each study for its relevance and quality through independent assessment, and will then synthesize the remaining studies in a fair and unbiased manner. A good systematic review is transparent. Transparency implies openness by the authors so that the reader can determine the validity of the conclusions for themselves. A properly conducted systematic review should allow a second group of authors using the same methodology to arrive at the same conclusion(s).

Component studies of a systematic review may be combined qualitatively or, in the case of RCTs, quantitatively. When a quantitative synthesis is performed it is termed a meta-analysis. Meta-analysis is the statistical technique used for combining independent studies. A meta-analysis is particularly useful when combining several small studies whose results may be inconclusive due to low power. Meta-analyses have a greater ability to detect uncommon but clinically relevant end points such as mortality.

Knowing the immense importance of the question being asked in a study, and having an overview of the types of studies utilized in clinical research to answer a particular question, the next step is to look at data analysis, which validates the answer to the question.

Grades of Recommendation

Through evaluation of study design and methodology, studies can be graded, with the grade helping to determine the strength of recommendation for a particular intervention. Numerous systems have been developed to categorize the levels of evidence, and most provide grades of recommendation based solely on the level of evidence.[50] In January 2003, the editorial board of the American edition of the *Journal of Bone and Joint Surgery* adopted a level of evidence rating system[51,52] based only on study design (**Table 1.1**). Then, in 2005, grades of recommendation were introduced, and in 2006 they were revised based on levels of evidence and consistency.[53] Despite these modifications, the recommendation remained focused on study quality and did not include the clinical expertise and patient preference components of EBM.

The most recent and compelling method of grading evidence is the one proposed by Guyatt and others in several articles[54–58] as part of the GRADE (Grading of Recommendations, Assessment, Development, and Evaluation) Working Group, and is used throughout this textbook. It is based on a sequential assessment of the quality of evidence, followed by assessment of the balance between benefits versus downsides and subsequent judgment about the strength of recommendations. This process thus separates the evaluation of evidence from the evaluation of the recommendation, thereby empowering clinical expertise to be part of the recommendation process.

The quality of evidence designates the extent to which one can be confident that an estimate of effect is correct. The strength of a recommendation indicates the extent to which one can be confident that adherence to the recommendation will do more good than harm.[56–58]

When assessing the quality of evidence, reviewers should consider four key elements in their evaluation of the evidence: study design, study quality, consistency, and directness. The issues of study design and study quality were discussed in detail earlier in the chapter. Study consistency refers to the similarity of estimates of effect across studies. If there is important unexplained inconsistency in the results, our confidence in the estimate of effect for that outcome diminishes. Directness or generalizability refers to the extent to which the study population, interventions, and outcome measures are similar to the patient population of interest. For example, there may be uncertainty about the directness of the evidence if the population of interest is older, sicker, or has more comorbidity than the populations studied.[56] Definitions of the different grades of evidence are summarized in **Table 1.2**.

Formulating the strength of recommendations based on the evidence is performed at an organizational level by a group of experts in the field and, if applicable, involves patients. The strength of the recommendation is given priority over the quality of the evidence, thus separating the judgments regarding the quality of evidence from judgments about the strength of recommendations. The strength of a recommendation reflects the degree of confidence that the desirable effects of adherence to a recommendation outweigh the undesirable effects. Although the degree of confidence is a continuum, this approach classifies recommendations for or against treatments into two simple grades, strong and weak.

If the risk:benefit ratio is clear nearly all the patients and clinicians would choose the treatment; therefore a strong recommendation is made. If the magnitude of the ratio is less certain in support of variation in patient and/or clinician values, then a majority of patients and clinicians would choose the treatment, but many would not; this constitutes a weak recommendation (**Table 1.3**).

The uniqueness of this approach to grading the evidence and subsequent formulation of recommendations is that, despite lower-quality evidence, a strong recommendation can

still be made based on the risk:benefit ratio and whether the question being asked is appropriate for the study design.

It must be remembered, however, that current concepts around levels of evidence and critical appraisal are based on a medical model, and surgical studies have unique issues that may be better dealt with in an evidence-based surgical model.[59] The nature of a surgical intervention introduces challenges around selection and observer bias, blinding, standardization of the technique, learning curve, generalizability, prevalence of the problem, and patient and surgeon equipoise.[59] Surgical research is complex, so the research question framed by the foregoing surgical considerations determines the best study design. In other words, strong recommendations can be based on lower levels of evidence if the question and circumstances dictate it.[60]

Applying the Results and Assessing the Outcome

Having gone through the first three steps of the process, the surgeon, or more likely, the expert panel, should arrive at a clinically useful recommendation. The final steps are then application of the recommendation and critically assessing the outcome. Outcome assessment should be performed using validated outcome instruments or measures. Patient-oriented outcome measures can be generally classified into two broad categories: generic health-related quality of life outcome instruments, and disease-specific outcome instruments.

Generic outcome instruments allow for a comparison of people with disabilities to the general population in which they live, as well as for comparison across disease states. These generic measures also provide an overall assessment of the quality of care in a given health care environment.

Disease-specific outcome measures offer the advantage of being tailored to assess a particular condition and can therefore be useful for longitudinal assessment of a specific condition or disability over time. They are less useful for cross-sectional analysis of the overall patient quality of life for a range of different conditions.

It has therefore been suggested that a combination of a disease-specific outcome instrument with a generic HRQoL outcome instrument, probably constitute the optimal method for assessing functional patient outcome for a given condition.[61] Theoretically, utilizing this approach affords the best of both worlds: an in-depth longitudinal assessment of the patients' condition over time, coupled with a cross-sectional comparison of the study patient population, with the normal population, as well as other disabled patient populations.

There are three general psychometric criteria that should be established in HRQoL measures before they are endorsed. Reliability is the ability of the tool to be reproducible and

Table 1.2 Grades of Evidence

Grade	Definition
High	Further research is very unlikely to change our confidence in the estimate of effect
Moderate	Further research is likely to have an important impact on our confidence in the estimate of effect and may change the estimate
Low	Further research is very likely to have an important impact on our confidence in the estimate of effect and is likely to change the estimate
Very low	Any estimate of effect is very uncertain

Source: Adapted from Atkins D, Best D, Briss PA, et al; Grade Working Group. Grading quality of evidence and strength of recommendations. BMJ. 2004;328:1490A. Adapted with permission.

Table 1.3 Examples of Implications of Strong and Weak Recommendations for Different Groups of Guideline User

Recommendation	Patients	Clinicians	Policy Makers
Strong	Most individuals in this situation would want the recommended course of action and only a small proportion would not	Most individuals should receive the intervention Adherence to this recommendation according to the guideline could be used as a quality criterion or performance indicator	The recommendation can be adapted as policy in most situations
Weak	The majority of individuals in this situation would want the suggested course of action, but many would not	Decision aids may be useful in helping individuals make decisions consistent with their values and preferences Examine the evidence or a summary of the evidence yourself	Policy making will require substantial debates and involvement of many stakeholders

Source: Adapted from Schünemann HJ, Jaeschke R, Cook DJ, et al; ATS Documents Development and Implementation Committee. An official ATS statement: grading the quality of evidence and strength of recommendations in ATS guidelines and recommendations. Am J Respir Crit Care Med 2006;174:607. Adapted with permission.

internally consistent over time. Validity ensures that the instrument is accurately measuring what it is supposed to be measuring. Finally, responsiveness is the ability of the questionnaire to detect clinically relevant change or differences. Responsiveness will vary depending on the type of HRQoL questionnaire and the patient population and intervention being evaluated. For example, if an outcome tool is designed for the functional assessment of spinal cord injury patients, and it is given to patients with mild radiculopathy, it would probably produce all perfect scores, the so-called ceiling effect. Likewise, a questionnaire developed for the general population would not discriminate among severely impaired patients in a rehab setting because all patients would end up with the worst possible score (floor effect).

Although there are not enough data to establish "evidence-based" guidelines for HRQoL assessments in spine trauma patients, based on reported outcomes and their application in the general and head trauma patient population, the Glasgow Outcome Scale and the SF-36 stand out as the most appropriate generic tools for HRQoL assessment across all trauma patients.[62]

Indeed, the usefulness of the SF-36 in assessing HRQoL is illustrated in over 1000 publications, with articles describing more than 130 diseases and conditions, making it the most widely used generic health outcome instrument.[61] It has also been translated into more than 50 languages,[61] making it useful for international multicenter collaborative studies.

Finally, because cost effectiveness of treatment interventions is attracting more interest, the use of preference-based measures, such as the EQ-5D[64] and the Health Utilities Index,[65] are being incorporated into clinical trials to allow for cost utility analysis. There is also a trend toward applying economic methods to health measures, such as the SF-36 and the development of new preference-based measures, such as the SF-6D.[66] This has the advantage of being able to obtain quality-adjusted life-years from existing or prospective SF-36 data.[66]

◆ Summary

In the current era of increasing accountability for health care services, the issues of quality and access to health care are of paramount importance. A major focus to date has been on efficiency of care, with a view to maximizing productivity and optimizing resource utilization. Thus improvements in accountability must clearly include indicators of efficiency. Accountability requires that increased emphasis be placed on

bringing patterns of clinical practice into line with current scientific evidence and that we determine the effectiveness of current health services at producing desirable health outcomes.

To continually improve the quality of care, the modern clinician should be able to formulate a clinically relevant research question and search the literature for an answer to that question by personally performing a systematic review of the relevant literature or by relying on a clinical recommendation or guideline from an expert panel. Finally, the clinician should be able to critically appraise the outcome of applying that recommendation to patient care.

The true spirit of EBM is integrating sound scientific evidence with clinical expertise and patient-informed preference. The notion of equating EBM with the RCT should give way to the understanding that levels of evidence are just part of the criteria constituting the decision regarding integrating new evidence into clinical practice. It should be clear to the clinician that the clinical circumstances and the question being asked will most often dictate a study design, and that the RCT is not the panacea of EBM. Useful recommendations in the realm of cost utility, risk:benefit ratio, and ultimately patient care can frequently be gained from such evidence if sound methodology was used. The ability to critically appraise the quality and applicability of the scientific evidence to the specific patient under the clinician's care is at the heart of evidence-based practice. By ensuring that the evidence on which we base our care is sound, we will be able to remain ethical advocates of effective care for our patients.

References

1. Höök O. Scientific communications: history, electronic journals and impact factors. Scand J Rehabil Med 1999;31:3–7
2. Cochrane AL. Effectiveness and efficiency: random reflections on health services. London: Nuffield Provinicial Hospitals Trust; 1972
3. Eddy DM. Practice policies: where do they come from? JAMA 1990; 263:1265–1272, 1269, 1272
4. Guyatt G, Cairns J, Churchill D, et al; Evidence-Based Medicine Working Group. Evidence-based medicine: a new approach to teaching the practice of medicine. JAMA 1992;268:2420–2425
5. Sackett DL, Rosenberg WM, Gray JA, Haynes RB, Richardson WS. Evidence based medicine: what it is and what it isn't. BMJ 1996;312:71–72
6. McKibbon K, Wilczynski N, Hayward R, Walker-Dilks C, Haynes R. The medical literature as a resource for health care practice. J Am Soc Inf Sci 1995;46:737–742
7. McEvoy RD, Bradford DS. The management of burst fractures of the thoracic and lumbar spine: experience in 53 patients. Spine 1985;10: 631–637

8. Weinstein JN, Collalto P, Lehmann TR. Thoracolumbar "burst" fractures treated conservatively: a long-term follow-up. Spine 1988;13:33–38

9. Kraemer WJ, Schemitsch EH, Lever J, McBroom RJ, McKee MD, Waddell JP. Functional outcome of thoracolumbar burst fractures without neurological deficit. J Orthop Trauma 1996;10:541–544

10. Wood K, Buttermann G, Mehbod A, et al. Operative compared with nonoperative treatment of a thoracolumbar burst fracture without neurological deficit: a prospective, randomized study. J Bone Joint Surg Am 2003;85-A:773–781

11. Sledge CB. Crisis, challenge, and credibility. J Bone Joint Surg Am 1985; 67:658–662

12. Gartland JJ. Orthopaedic clinical research: deficiencies in experimental design and determinations of outcome. J Bone Joint Surg Am 1988; 70:1357–1364

13. Howe J, Frymoyer JW. The effects of questionnaire design on the determination of end results in lumbar spinal surgery. Spine 1985;10:804–805

14. Randell AG, Nguyen TV, Bhalerao N, Silverman SL, Sambrook PN, Eisman JA. Deterioration in quality of life following hip fracture: a prospective study. Osteoporos Int 2000;11:460–466

15. McCarthy ML, MacKenzie EJ, Bosse MJ, Copeland CE, Hash CS, Burgess AR. Functional status following orthopedic trauma in young women. J Trauma 1995;39:828–836, discussion 836–837

16. MacKenzie EJ, McCarthy ML, Ditunno JF, et al; Pennsylvania Study Group on Functional Outcomes Following Trauma. Using the SF-36 for characterizing outcome after multiple trauma involving head injury. J Trauma 2002;52:527–534

17. Peterson MG, Allegrante JP, Cornell CN, et al. Measuring recovery after a hip fracture using the SF-36 and Cummings scales. Osteoporos Int 2002;13:296–302

18. Stannard JP, Harris HW, Volgas DA, Alonso JE. Functional outcome of patients with femoral head fractures associated with hip dislocations. Clin Orthop Relat Res 2000; (377):44–56

19. Stannard JP, Harris HW, McGwin G Jr, Volgas DA, Alonso JE. Intramedullary nailing of humeral shaft fractures with a locking flexible nail. J Bone Joint Surg Am 2003;85-A:2103–2110

20. Bailey CS, MacDermid J, Patterson SD, King GJ. Outcome of plate fixation of olecranon fractures. J Orthop Trauma 2001;15:542–548

21. Kerr-Valentic MA, Arthur M, Mullins RJ, Pearson TE, Mayberry JC. Rib fracture pain and disability: can we do better? J Trauma 2003; 54:1058–1063, discussion 1063–1064

22. Gofton WT, Macdermid JC, Patterson SD, Faber KJ, King GJ. Functional outcome of AO type C distal humeral fractures. J Hand Surg [Am] 2003; 28:294–308

23. Pollak AN, McCarthy ML, Bess RS, Agel J, Swiontkowski MF. Outcomes after treatment of high-energy tibial plafond fractures. J Bone Joint Surg Am 2003;85-A:1893–1900

24. Stevens DG, Beharry R, McKee MD, Waddell JP, Schemitsch EH. The long-term functional outcome of operatively treated tibial plateau fractures. J Orthop Trauma 2001;15:312–320

25. Boucher M, Bhandari M, Kwok D. Health-related quality of life after short segment instrumentation of lumbar burst fractures. J Spinal Disord 2001;14:417–426

26. Ebbert JO, Dupras DM, Erwin PJ. Searching the medical literature using PubMed: a tutorial. Mayo Clin Proc 2003;78:87–91

27. Lowe HJ, Barnett GO. Understanding and using the medical subject headings (MeSH) vocabulary to perform literature searches. JAMA 1994;271:1103–1108

28. Bhandari M, Guyatt GH, Montori V, Devereaux PJ, Swiontkowski MF. User's guide to the orthopaedic literature: how to use a systematic literature review. J Bone Joint Surg Am 2002;84-A:1672–1682

29. Bhandari M, Morrow F, Kulkarni AV, Tornetta P III. Meta-analyses in orthopaedic surgery: a systematic review of their methodologies. J Bone Joint Surg Am 2001;83-A:15–24

30. Bhandari M, Schemitsch EH. Randomized trials: a brief history and modern perspective. Tech Orthop 2004;19:54–56

31. Bhandari M, Tornetta P III. Evidence-based orthopaedics: a paradigm shift. Clin Orthop Relat Res 2003;413:9–10

32. Sackett DL, Richardson WS, Rosenberg W, Haynes RB. Evidence-based medicine: how to practice and teach EBM. New York: Churchill Livingstone; 1997

33. Chalmers TC, Matta RJ, Smith H Jr, Kunzler AM. Evidence favoring the use of anticoagulants in the hospital phase of acute myocardial infarction. N Engl J Med 1977;297:1091–1096

34. Chalmers TC, Celano P, Sacks HS, Smith H Jr. Bias in treatment assignment in controlled clinical trials. N Engl J Med 1983;309:1358–1361

35. Sacks H, Chalmers TC, Smith H Jr. Randomized versus historical controls for clinical trials. Am J Med 1982;72:233–240

36. Miller JN, Colditz GA, Mosteller F. How study design affects outcomes in comparisons of therapy, II: Surgical. Stat Med 1989;8:455–466

37. Colditz GA, Miller JN, Mosteller F. How study design affects outcomes in comparisons of therapy, I: Medical. Stat Med 1989;8:441–454

38. Benson K, Hartz AJ. A comparison of observational studies and randomized, controlled trials. N Engl J Med 2000;342:1878–1886

39. Concato J, Shah N, Horwitz RI. Randomized, controlled trials, observational studies, and the hierarchy of research designs. N Engl J Med 2000;342:1887–1892

40. Hartz A, Benson K, Glaser J, Bentler S, Bhandari M. Assessing observational studies of spinal fusion and chemonucleolysis. Spine 2003; 28:2268–2275

41. Atlas SJ, Keller RB, Wu YA, Deyo RA, Singer DE. Long-term outcomes of surgical and nonsurgical management of lumbar spinal stenosis: 8 to 10 year results from the Maine Lumbar Spine Study. Spine 2005;30:936–943

42. Atlas SJ, Keller RB, Wu YA, Deyo RA, Singer DE. Long-term outcomes of surgical and nonsurgical management of sciatica secondary to a lumbar disc herniation: 10 year results from the Maine Lumbar Spine Study. Spine 2005;30:927–935

43. Atlas SJ, Keller RB, Robson D, Deyo RA, Singer DE. Surgical and nonsurgical management of lumbar spinal stenosis: four-year outcomes from the Maine Lumbar Spine Study. Spine 2000;25:556–562

44. Dvorak MFS, Fisher CG, Aarabi B, et al. Clinical outcomes of 90 isolated unilateral facet fractures, subluxations, and dislocations treated surgically and nonoperatively. Spine 2007;32:3007–3013

45. Fanuele JC, Abdu WA, Hanscom B, Weinstein JN. Association between obesity and functional status in patients with spine disease. Spine 2002;27:306–312

46. Slover J, Abdu WA, Hanscom B, Weinstein JN. The impact of comorbidities on the change in short-form 36 and Oswestry scores following lumbar spine surgery. Spine 2006;31:1974–1980

47. Weinstein JN, Lurie JD, Tosteson TD, et al. Surgical versus nonsurgical treatment for lumbar degenerative spondylolisthesis. N Engl J Med 2007;356:2257–2270

48. Johnson MG, Fisher CG, Boyd M, Pitzen T, Oxland TR, Dvorak MF. The radiographic failure of single segment anterior cervical plate fixation in traumatic cervical flexion distraction injuries. Spine 2004;29:2815–2820

49. Dawber TR, Meadors GF, Moore FE Jr. Epidemiological approaches to heart disease: the Framingham Study. Am J Public Health Nations Health 1951;41:279–281

50. Atkins D, Eccles M, Flottorp S, et al; GRADE Working Group. Systems for grading the quality of evidence and the strength of recommendations, I: Critical appraisal of existing approaches The GRADE Working Group. BMC Health Serv Res 2004;4:38

51. Wright JG, Swiontkowski MF, Heckman JD. Introducing levels of evidence to the journal. J Bone Joint Surg Am 2003;85-A:1–3

52. Obremskey WT, Pappas N, Attallah-Wasif E, Tornetta P III, Bhandari M. Level of evidence in orthopaedic journals. J Bone Joint Surg Am 2005; 87:2632–2638

53. Wright JG, Einhorn TA, Heckman JD. Grades of recommendation. J Bone Joint Surg Am 2005;87:1909–1910

54. Guyatt G, Schunemann H, Cook D, Jaeschke R, Pauker S, Bucher H; American College of Chest Physicians. Grades of recommendation for antithrombotic agents. Chest 2001;119(1, Suppl):3S–7S

55. Canadian Task Force on the Periodic Health Examination. The periodic health examination. Can Med Assoc J 1979;121:1193–1254

56. Guyatt G, Vist G, Falck-Ytter Y, Kunz R, Magrini N, Schunemann H. An emerging consensus on grading recommendations? Evid Based Med 2006;11:2–4

57. Atkins D, Best D, Briss PA, et al; GRADE Working Group. Grading quality of evidence and strength of recommendations. BMJ 2004;328:1490

58. Schünemann HJ, Jaeschke R, Cook DJ, et al; ATS Documents Development and Implementation Committee. An official ATS statement: grading the quality of evidence and strength of recommendations in ATS guidelines and recommendations. Am J Respir Crit Care Med 2006;174: 605–614

59. Meakins JL. Innovation in surgery: the rules of evidence. Am J Surg 2002;183:399–405

60. Stein PD, Collins JJ Jr, Kantrowitz A. Antithrombotic therapy in mechanical and biological prosthetic heart valves and saphenous vein bypass grafts. Chest 1986;89(2, Suppl):46S–53S

61. Ware JE Jr. SF-36 health survey update. Spine 2000;25:3130–3139

62. Neugebauer E, Bouillon B, Bullinger M, Wood-Dauphinée S. Quality of life after multiple trauma—summary and recommendations of the consensus conference. Restor Neurol Neurosci 2002;20:161–167

63. Garratt A, Schmidt L, Mackintosh A, Fitzpatrick R. Quality of life measurement: bibliographic study of patient assessed health outcome measures. BMJ 2002;324:1417

64. Brooks R. EuroQol: the current state of play. Health Policy 1996; 37:53–72

65. Feeny D, Furlong W, Boyle M, Torrance GW. Multi-attribute health status classification systems. Health Utilities Index. Pharmacoeconomics 1995;7:490–502

66. Brazier J, Roberts J, Deverill M. The estimation of a preference-based measure of health from the SF-36. J Health Econ 2002;21:271–292

2

Outcome Assessment Tools for Spinal Trauma Patients

F. C. Oner and C. F. M. Buckens

In the broadest sense, clinical practice is intervention in the complex process of a disorder of a human being with the aim of changing the natural course of that process in a favorable way. This implies that to assess whether this intervention is successful we have to know what the course of this process would be without intervention and how we can measure the difference between the results with or without the intervention. Any attempt to find evidence for the effectiveness of our practices should start by asking these two basic questions. This means that we should find a way to measure in a meaningful and reproducible way the outcome of these complex processes. It is also important to realize that outcome can be approached from different perspectives: from the standpoint of the patient, of the physician, of the care-payer, or of the society. Of course the simplest and objectively measurable outcome is the mortality, which has been a historical model for all outcome measurement instruments. In all nonmortality outcome measurements, however, the task becomes increasingly difficult and subjective. In this area two different approaches can be developed: general health or disease-specific measurement tools. General health or generic measurement tools provide normative data that allow for demographically adjusted approximations and comparisons between populations. Disease-specific tools, on the other hand, are specifically designed to measure the progression of certain parameters that are considered important for a specific condition with a reasonably well-known natural history.

For trauma victims, defining and measuring the outcome is becoming an urgent task as greater numbers of these patients survive serious trauma and their life expectancies have increased dramatically in the last 2 decades.[1,2] The strain on medical services caused by trauma patients is making evidence-based justification of the costly interventions and treatment strategies imperative. Among survivors of major trauma, those with spinal trauma make up a significant fraction. In a recent consecutive series in the Netherlands, spinal injuries occurred in 24% of all high-energy trauma survivors, and 6% had concurrent spinal cord injury.[3]

Little work has been done on developing and validating outcome assessments in spinal trauma patients. Most studies have assessed spine-injured patients from the acute care medicine perspective, or they have focused solely on injury to the spinal cord from the perspective of rehabilitation medicine.[4] Studies investigating outcomes in (spinal) trauma patients typically use a combination of several outcome measures or improvise their own measures.[5,6]

The spinal cord injury (SCI) group, which usually includes only patients with serious injury to the spinal cord and not patients with transient or subtle neurological involvement, represents a minority of all spinal trauma patients.[3,7,8] Concomitantly, between 75% and 85% of SCIs are caused by trauma.[4,9] This makes it very difficult to extrapolate work done on outcomes from these populations to a spinal trauma population.

Spinal trauma patients are also evidently dissimilar to the patients with chronic spinal disorders at which all of the existing back/neck/spinal outcome measures have been directed.[10] Valid outcome assessment tools specific to the characteristics of this population are necessary to establish the efficacy of the interventions in the acute phase.

This chapter evaluates the outcome measurements commonly used in spinal trauma patients. It reviews a select number of widely used outcome measures deemed most significant and discusses their applicability to spinal trauma outcome.

◆ Materials and Methods

A literature search was performed on PubMed and Embase using the MeSH terms *outcome assessment*, *trauma*, and *spine* and the keywords *trauma*, *spine*, *spinal trauma*, *outcome*, *assessment*, *measurement*, *psychometrics*, *SCI*, and *fracture*. The abstracts were reviewed and if deemed relevant the full-length article was retrieved. The references of the resulting papers were manually screened for other potentially relevant articles, as were the related article lists as generated by PubMed.

◆ Results

There is no consensus on which instruments to use when measuring nonmortality trauma outcomes in general.[11] Commonly used outcome measures that are recommended for use in trauma patients include the Functional Independence Measure (FIM), Glasgow Outcome Scale (GOS), the Short Form-36 (SF-36), the EuroQoL-5D, the Musculoskeletal Function Assessment (MFA), and the Health Utilities Index Mark 3 (HUI 3).[6,12,13] The only trauma-specific measure found is the Functional Capacity Index (FCI).[14]

The population of SCI patients with or without traumatic causes is largely treated as a separate population in the literature. Similar to the trauma outcomes field, there is no consensus about which outcome assessments are to be used in SCI patients.[9,15] Several frequently used outcome measures used in SCI populations include the walking index for spinal cord injury (WISCI), the Spinal Cord Independence Measure (SCIM), the FIM, the SF-36, and the GOS.

The psychological outcome assessments recommended for use in both trauma and SCI populations such as the Hospital Anxiety and Depression Scale and the Hamilton Depression Index will not be discussed here in detail. Components of generic health-related quality of life (HRQoL) tools (such as the SF-36) also measure psychological well-being. These instruments seem to be psychometrically sound, at least in SCI patients.[16]

Research into the psychometrics of outcome measures that are applied to spinal trauma patients have typically been conducted on the larger and more heterogeneous population of multiple trauma patients, or on the smaller subset of SCI patients. This makes it difficult to draw any firm conclusions about the psychometric properties of these outcome measures in spinal trauma patients as a population. For this reason the current state of outcome research in these two overlapping groups will be assessed here in an effort to extract meaningful information about the current knowledge and limitations concerning outcome measurement in spinal trauma patients. A discussion of all outcome measures designed for and used in trauma and SCI patient populations is beyond the scope of this review. Here a select number are presented to provide context for further discussion.

Outcome Measures and Measurement Tools

Generic (General Health) Instruments

The SF-36 is a widely applied generic measure consisting of 36 items including eight dimensions that has been validated in numerous patient populations.[17,18] It is not designed for measuring any disability and suffers from limitations such as inappropriate items for SCI patients.[12] Additionally, the psychometrics of the SF-36 have not been extensively tested in SCI populations.[16]

The EQ-5D is a self-administered generic quality of life (QoL) measure with five dimensions (mobility, self-care, activities, pain, anxiety/depression) and a general health state visual analogue scale (VAS) item. It was developed by the interdisciplinary EuroQoL group.[19] Although initially intended to complement condition-specific measures such as spine-specific instruments, it is being used increasingly as a stand-alone measure in spine research.[18] The EQ-5D has the added benefit of being able to generate utilities allowing for economic evaluations such as the calculation of quality-adjusted life years (QALYs).

Although these generic measures provide normative data that allow for demographically adjusted approximations of pretrauma scores and comparisons between populations, they were not designed for any specific population. This "one-size-fits-all" approach is a source of methodological limitations (i.e., ceiling and floor effects, large minimally clinically important difference, and low responsiveness) if they are relied on too heavily as primary measures in spinal trauma populations. Indeed, the applicability of generic QoL assessments as primary outcome measures in SCI studies has come under question recently as measures of function might be more meaningful and sensitive in discriminating between different treatment modalities.[20]

The HUI 3 is a "generic multiattribute preference-based measure of health status and health-related quality of life."[21] It encompasses both physical and emotional dimensions of health and emphasizes the functional potential over actual performance, to avoid the assumption that patients always choose to realize their full functional potential and directly measure impairment. The HUI also allows for economic evaluation. The applicability of the HUI in trauma populations has yet to be tested.[2]

Other generic outcome instruments such as the sickness impact profile (SIP), World Health Organization Disability Assessment Schedule III (WHODAS III), and GOS are not discussed here because they are either comparable to the generic instruments already discussed or are not directly applicable to spinal trauma.

Spine-Specific Instruments

The Oswestry Disability Index (ODI) and the Roland-Morris Disability Questionnaire (RMDQ) are two widely used condition-specific instruments for chronic back pain patients to assess disability.[10,22] Many adaptations have been proposed and used especially for the low-back and neck pain patients, sometimes in combination with a generic measurement tool. The ODI and RMDQ are discussed here because they are illustrative of the outcome measures commonly employed in this related population. The RMDQ was derived from the sickness impact profile (SIP), a widely used generic measure, which assesses pain and daily function. It has been extensively validated and demonstrates good reliability and consistency in low back pain patients. It is slightly more sensitive to changes over time than the ODI. The ODI is a self-administered tool consisting of sections assessing activities of daily living (ADL). It seems slightly more sensitive to improvements in condition than the RMDQ.

Both of these instruments are designed and mainly used to assess disability in chronic low back pain patients. A similar instrument, the Neck Disability Index is used for similar purposes in patients with cervical spine disorders. As such they have limited applicability to spinal trauma patients in the sense that the domains they measure and the relative weighting of each in the scoring does not correspond to the domains perceived to be important in the fundamentally different population of spinal trauma patients. For instance, chronic pain is less of an issue in trauma patients, including spinal trauma victims, than in chronic cervical or lumbar pain syndromes.[23] Although pain may be relevant for SCI patients, the lower incidence and lower pain scores in spinal trauma patients after the acute phase render the emphasis on pain measures in the instruments used in chronic patients misplaced in the spinal trauma population.[20] Additionally, the high psychometric quality of the ODI and RMDQ in lower back pain (LBP) patients might not apply to the very different spinal trauma patient group (e.g., ceiling and floor effects and responsiveness).

Trauma-Specific Instruments

The FCI has been validated in major trauma populations.[1] It is a preference-based, multiattribute functional outcome measure that provides 10 dimension-specific scores and one overall score that summarizes function across these dimensions. The dimensions include "eating, excretory function, sexual function, ambulation, hand/arm movement, bending/lifting, vision, hearing, speech and cognitive function."[14] It does not assess psychosocial outcomes and is targeted mainly toward measuring outcome in general trauma patients, reflecting the domains relevant in that group. At 12-month follow-up FCI does not correlate with initial FCI or initial trauma severity, indicating that FCI may not be a suitable tracker of outcome progression over time. Although never yet reported for spinal trauma patients it is the only outcome measure designed specifically for trauma populations.[24]

The WISCI is a measure of mobility designed for SCI, with demonstrated high sensitivity.[25] Although outcome measures like the WISCI might be useful in populations with serious spinal cord injury, they are too narrow to form the basis of evidence-based decisions in spinal trauma patients in general with a wide spectrum of neurological involvement.

More comprehensive functional outcome measures such as the FIM and SCIM incorporate a mobility domain. The FIM is a well-established functional outcome assessment score that also relies on the patient's ability to perform ADL.[26] Although initially designed for stroke patients, it has been extensively used in trauma outcome and is likely the most widely used functional outcome measure for the SCI population, with demonstrated validity and reliability in that specific population.[2,9,27]

A recent article that has performed outcomes research directly on acute trauma patients as a single population used the FIM.[8] It was found that FIM scores improved significantly in survivors in 12 months posttrauma. Additionally no correlation was found between FIM administered on admission and at 1-year postinjury. The authors also found no significant correlation with Injury Severity Score (ISS) and 1-year FIM outcome; although a different article that also employed the FIM in spinal trauma patients with polytrauma did find a correlation with the ISS to 1- and 2-year FIM scores.[28] This discrepancy is possibly related to the study population selected and/or the differing statistical methods applied. The study investigating spine patients with polytrauma further found that the severity of spinal injuries was the most important predictor of disability as measured by the FIM, although they acknowledge that this finding may partly result for the spine-bias of the FIM.[28] Nonetheless, this result again emphasizes the importance of spinal trauma in mid- to long-term disability in polytrauma patients.

Although the use of the FIM has merit in spinal trauma patients, it is not free of limitations.[29] Briefly, the FIM scoring aggregation creates a masking effect in that unequal ordinal items are simply summed (apples and oranges, so to speak).

Additionally the FIM measures a narrow set of domains reflecting mainly impairments, and focusing on SCI-specific domains.[29,30] Another limitation is that it is not a patient-directed questionnaire.

Nonetheless, the research discussed above represents one of the few attempts to perform outcomes research in spinal trauma patients. The limitations and challenges faced by these studies with regard to outcome measurement mirror those of the field as a whole.

The SCIM is a recently developed disability measure designed and validated for patients with spinal cord lesions.[6] It measures patients' ability to perform daily tasks and demonstrates good reliability and validity in the SCI population subset. Because it is designed specifically for patients with substantial neurological damage it would not be suitable for use in a spinal trauma population with no or varying degrees of neurological involvement. Nevertheless, it still warrants mention given that it is an excellent tool for assessing the spinal cord–related functional outcome component of spinal injury.[31]

Indirect Outcome Measures

Besides the generic and functional outcome measures, the practice of measuring a single meaningful parameter of outcome has also been implemented as a way to expedite the outcome assessment process. Measures of work status or mobility are often included in the commonly used generic and functional outcome measures but they are also applied independently. Two of these constructs are discussed here to illustrate the usefulness of this approach and its limitations.

Return to work (RTW) represents an interesting construct in that it is a meaningful outcome from a societal as well as an individual point of view, and it can serve as an indirect proxy for the domain of participation. Of course it also reflects the other domains of impairment and activities, making it a complex as well as a useful construct.[32,33] RTW has been used as a primary outcome in a patient population that underwent surgery for spinal fractures resulting from high-energy trauma.[34] It is found that the presence of neurological symptoms was a major predictor of RTW status at follow-up.

A similarly complex but useful and important measure of injury outcome is the measure of health service use (HSU). The complexity and multifactorial nature of this measure have been established but not adequately explored in trauma patients, let alone spinal trauma patients.[35] Like RTW it is an important measure from a societal point of view. These two single-item outcomes are interesting in that they produce a single measure directly dependent on multiple parameters spread over all the World Health Organization (WHO) International Classification of Functioning (ICF) health domains.

Domains Relevant for Spinal Trauma Populations

The WHO ICF, disability and health, provides a useful and expansive theoretical underpinning for newly developed measures targeting, among others, trauma patients.[36] It describes domains to consider when comparing instruments and assessing their validity: body structures/impairments, activities/activity limitations, and participation/participation restrictions.

This framework reflects a biopsychosocial model of health and functioning. It is generic in nature and not designed with any particular patient group in mind. As such, the practice of selecting a subset of ICF domains and constructs to generate condition-specific "ICF core-sets" has emerged to better take advantage of the ICF in specific patient groups.[37] This approach has been applied both to the SCI population and to acute and postacute musculoskeletal populations.[38–41] A separate consensus conference identified physical, psychological, social, and functional domains as key domains in trauma patients, largely mirroring the main ICF criteria but working independently of it.[12]

For acute musculoskeletal patients a consensus conference selected 47 ICF categories for inclusion into a core set for acute musculoskeletal injuries.[40] The ICF categories for acute musculoskeletal patients were selected from the ICF components body functions, body structures, activities/participation, and environmental factors, emphasizing the integrity and function of musculoskeletal structures.[37,40] By comparison, for postacute musculoskeletal patients 70 categories were selected from the same components, with additional emphasis placed on activities/participation.[41]

The patient population did not include SCI trauma patients, who were lumped into a different core set, namely that of acute and postacute neurological patients.[42,43] This population includes patients with head injury, cerebrovascular diseases, and central nervous system neoplasms. As can be expected, a large number of the categories selected for this population would be unsuitable for a spinal trauma population.

The postacute core sets as they are described in the literature reviewed earlier seem to be more applicable to outcome assessment because the acute core sets include assessments of the current state of patients in the acute settings (e.g., temperature or electrolytes). These categories are not meant as outcomes but rather as classification aids.

Domains Specific for Spinal Trauma Patients

Before discussing the relevant domains, several distinguishing characteristics of spinal trauma patients need to be considered. First, the ideal outcome is, in contrast to many other subacute or chronic ailments, recovery of previous function/HRQoL. An acute trauma patient generally goes suddenly and violently from a high to a low level of functioning. This is in contrast to the typical chronic spine patient, who is supposed to gain function after intervention and whose baseline is relatively low. For spinal trauma patients themselves the most important outcome parameter is probably the extent of functional loss. This is reflected in the empirical observation that the first order of business for trauma patients upon discharge is to assay which prior activities are impaired and to what extent. Additionally, pain, which is central to the pathology and hence outcome of chronic spinal disorders, is probably not in and of itself as important to traumatic spinal patients, although it may be an issue in certain aspects of functioning.

Another methodological obstacle specific to trauma outcome is the absence of individualized preinjury baseline data. Using populationwide normative data (collected by survey) assumes that trauma patients are a representative sample of their society, an assumption that empirical evidence usually contradicts. At any rate, the relatively high amount of interpersonal variability in normative functioning and HRQoL scores makes individualized baseline data preferable.

One possible way to generate normative data is to ask trauma survivors to recall their preinjury levels of functioning.

This creates the possibility of individualized baseline data.[2,4] Although recall of preinjury functioning is commonly used, this introduces recall bias, which may adversely influence the quality of these baseline data. One way to attenuate this bias would be to replace the previously pursued recall format in which a recalled baseline is generated with one that seeks purely to compare the posttraumatic present with the pretraumatic baseline. For example, instead of asking a patient to recall pretrauma mobility, a patient could be asked to estimate the extent of loss in mobility. Because this is what patients commonly do after the acute phase of trauma it can eliminate some of the recall bias by being more congruent with the psychological processes.

Second, it is to be expected that some degree of recovery of functioning/HRQoL would take place even in the absence of any intervention. Consequently, any outcome instrument would need to be sensitive and responsive enough to detect relatively subtle differences in study populations over a range of disability severities and time points.

Third, the influence of pretrauma capabilities and psychosocial coping capacity and style on outcome cannot be understated. For this reason baseline demographic indicators need to be considered as well as the inclusion of a psychosocial component. Additionally, psychopathology such as posttraumatic stress disorders constitutes an important part of the posttrauma disability for patients. For example the incidence of depression in the orthopedic trauma population is elevated, validating the inclusion of a psychological domain in spinal trauma assessment.[44] Psychological distress also occurs in a significant minority of SCI patients.[45,46]

From a societal and familial perspective the most important outcome factor after trauma is the eventual burden of the injuries in terms of required care, lost productivity, and earning capacity. In recognition of this the inclusion of such domains is warranted in any spinal trauma outcome measure.

Using the considerations above and working on previous efforts in related patient populations, it is possible to select several ICF criteria from the four ICF sections that would be relevant to measuring outcome in the spinal trauma population. This is summarized in **Table 2.1**. An overview of ICF criteria measured in frequently used outcome instruments is presented in **Table 2.2**.

◆ Discussion

This review sought to assess the current state of outcome measurement in spinal trauma patients and to address the question whether this group is adequately served by currently used measurement instruments. Little work was found that directly pertains to outcomes analysis of spinal trauma patients as a specific group. It appeared that most of the outcomes analysis was being performed on the general (multi)trauma population and/or the SCI population. The spinal trauma group sometimes appeared as a subset in the trauma studies. In SCI outcome studies a large portion of the group was often of traumatic etiology, representing a subset of spinal trauma patients.

Chronic lumbar or cervical pain patients constitute a related population in which much outcomes research is being directed. Although many studies use these outcome measurements for spinal trauma patients, there is actually very little overlap between these chronic pain patients and the patients with acute spinal trauma. The question is whether these

Table 2.1 Overview of Spine Trauma–Relevant International Classification of Functioning Chapters

Body functions	Chapter 1: mental functions
	Chapter 2: sensory and pain
	Chapter 6: genitourinary and reproductive
	Chapter 7: neuromusculoskeletal
Body structures	Chapter 1: nervous system
	Chapter 7: movement structures
Activities and participation	Chapter 4: mobility
	Chapter 5: self-care
	Chapter 6: domestic life
	Chapter 7: interpersonal relationships
	Chapter 8: major life areas
	Chapter 9: community, social and civic life
Environmental factors	Chapter 3: support and relationships
	Chapter 5: services systems and policies
Other	Comorbidity

measurement instruments have any relevance at all for the fundamentally different category of trauma patients.

Recent work in outcomes research was assessed in the trauma and SCI fields in an attempt to extract and synthesize relevant conclusions about the state of outcome research in the spinal trauma group. This approach was necessitated by the paucity of research performed directly on spinal trauma patients as a group. This is an indication that outcomes in spinal trauma patients might not be adequately measured with existing instruments.

Identifying those ICF criteria relevant to spinal trauma and summarily evaluating which domains were measured in the outcome tools are important issues in the discussion on this subject. The domains we identified as relevant for this specific population include those dealing with the function and structure of directly damaged body regions, as well as indirectly affected mental functions and the presence of pain, domains pertaining to limitations in the daily activities, leisure activities, work activities, and interpersonal relationships and domains dealing with the "environmental" factors by which we envision factors such as social support utilization and health services utilization. In this way we hope to generate a conceptual list of domains, which can serve as a basis for further discussion.

After reviewing both the most commonly used outcome measures and current consensus on the underlying domains we have come to the conclusion that the outcome tools in current use are not adequate for assessing spinal trauma patients as a specific population. It seems that the ICF criteria pertinent to the spinal trauma group could be more or less completely covered by a combination of generic and condition-specific trauma and SCI outcome assessments, but there would be significant redundancy and psychometric limitations to taking this approach.

The lack of tools designed specifically for the spinal trauma population and the lack of research into the applicability and validity of existing tools to the spinal trauma population produce a situation in which the efficacy of interventions targeting this group cannot be adequately evaluated. The status quo, in which spinal trauma patients are effectively split between trauma patients and SCI patients, is suboptimal for

Table 2.2 Overview of International Classification of Functioning Criteria Measured in Selected Outcome Instruments[a]

Inclusion of putative spinal trauma domains in selected outcome measures	SF-36	EQ-50	HUI	ODI	RMQD	FCI	WISCI	FIM	SCIM	RTW	HSU
Mental functions	+	+	+			+		+			
Sensory and pain	+	+	++	+		+					
Genitourinary and reproductive						+		+	+		
Neuromusculoskeletal						+	+		+		
Nervous system											
Movement structures											
Mobility	+	+	+	+	+	+	++	++	++		
Self-care	+	+		+		+		++	++		
Domestic life	+			−/+	−/+						
Interpersonal relationships	+			+	−/+	+		+			
Major life areas	+	−/+								++	
Community, social and civic life	+			+	−/+						
Support and relationship					−/+						+
Services systems and polices											++

Abbreviations: EQ-5D, EuroQol 5D; FCI, Functional Capacity Index; FIM, Functional Independence Measure; HSU, health services use; HUI 3, Health Utilities Index Mark 3; ODI, Oswestry Disability Index; RMQO, Roland Morris Disability Questionnaire; SCIM, Spinal Cord Independence Measure; RTW, return to work; SF-36, Short Form-36; WISCI, walking index for spinal cord injury.

[a]This is a rough indication of which spinal trauma relevant chapters are addressed in the instruments. This indicates only their presence or absence and does not implicate the quality of these items in the measurement instruments.

this reason. Additionally it would be desirable to treat spinal trauma patients as a single unified group because of the common factors found within this group.

There is much activity in the field of outcome assessments, and the cacophony of new instruments discourages the development of even more measures. Merely administering a combination of existing measures when conducting studies is suboptimal, however, leading to psychometric limitations and overlap. Additionally, no measurement tools were identified that would potentially succeed in capturing all the domains pertinent to spinal trauma patients.

Therefore, it is important to consider the design and implementation of an outcome measure designed specifically for spinal trauma patients. Such an outcome measure could draw upon the ICF as a theoretical framework and implement lessons learned in outcomes research in related patient populations.

One difficulty facing trauma outcome is the lack of individualized baseline data. Retrospective instruments could provide these data but inevitably suffer from recall bias. A potential approach to this issue could be to administer a "loss of function" VAS scale, as opposed to two separate VAS items: recalled prior functioning and current functioning. Intuitively, this approach would also be more valid from the perspective of the patients—directly measuring the perceived loss of function and eventual recovery. The use of VAS scales has been shown to be a valid option in measuring recalled baseline data in trauma patient groups.[48]

A possible danger facing any comprehensive outcome measure designed for spinal trauma patients is the problem of the large divide in scores and domains between SCI and non-SCI spinal trauma patients. Usually, only serious spinal cord injury has been included in the studies on neurological and functional outcome so far. However, spinal trauma patients show a wide spectrum of neurological involvement patterns varying from no involvement to subtle dysfunction to (partially) recovering incomplete neurological injury to permanent SCI. This spectrum cannot be captured in the simple dichotomy of SCI/no-SCI. The new instruments should be able to capture this whole spectrum but also be able to overcome the large divide between the far ends of the spectrum.

A second potential obstacle is the incongruence between the priorities and concerns of the immediate postacute patient and the late follow-up patient. Empirically, the same patients undergo large changes in functional capacities and outlook during a typical follow-up period. Attempting to track the same patient from the early postacute setting to late follow-up might conceivably blunt the sensitivity and responsiveness of the putative instrument but is crucial in finding the differences between various interventions with potential socioeconomic and financial consequences.

In summary, widespread outcome measures currently in use fail to capture the domains most relevant to spinal trauma patients. There is currently very little work that deals with them directly as a single, specific patient population.

◆ Summary and Recommendations

Unfortunately there is no condition-specific outcome measurement tool available that is appropriate for the whole spinal column trauma population. Based on the evidence and the expert opinion of a specialist body of spinal trauma surgeons, the Spinal Trauma Study Group (STSG), we can only make the following recommendations:

- Specifically for the spinal cord injury population FIM and SCIM tools should be used (strong recommendation).
- For trauma patients in general generic tools such as SF-36 and EQ-5D together with FCI can be used (weak recommendation).
- The spine-specific measurement tools such as ODI, RMDQ, and their derivatives are not appropriate for spinal trauma patients and should not be used (weak recommendation).
- Efforts should be directed to the development of validated, condition-specific tools for the spinal column trauma population.

References

1. MacKenzie EJ, Sacco WJ, Luchter S, et al; Pennsylvania Study Group on Functional Outcomes Following Trauma. Validating the Functional Capacity Index as a measure of outcome following blunt multiple trauma. Qual Life Res 2002;11:797–808

2. van Beeck EF, Looman CW, Mackenbach JP. Mortality due to unintentional injuries in the Netherlands, 1950-1995. Public Health Rep 1998; 113:427–439

3. Holtslag HR, Post MW, Lindeman E, Van der Werken C. Long-term functional health status of severely injured patients. Injury 2007;38:280–289

4. Thomas KC, Fisher CG, Noonan V. Recalled pre-injury health related quality of life in patients who have sustained spine trauma. 2007. Annual Meeting of the American Spinal Injury Association, Dallas. 13/5/2005

5. Butler JS, Fitzpatrick P, Ni Mhaolain AM, Synnott K, O'Byrne JM. The management and functional outcome of isolated burst fractures of the fifth lumbar vertebra. Spine 2007;32:443–447

6. Van Beeck EF, Larsen CF, Lyons RA, Meerding WJ, Mulder S, Essink-Bot ML. Guidelines for the conduction of follow-up studies measuring injury-related disability. J Trauma 2007;62:534–550

7. Hu R, Mustard CA, Burns C. Epidemiology of incident spinal fracture in a complete population. Spine 1996;21:492–499

8. Akmal M, Trivedi R, Sutcliffe J. Functional outcome in trauma patients with spinal injury. Spine 2003;28:180–185

9. Wood-Dauphinée S, Exner G, Bostanci B, et al; SCI Consensus Group. Quality of life in patients with spinal cord injury—basic issues, assessment, and recommendations. Restor Neurol Neurosci 2002;20:135–149

10. Müller U, Röder C, Greenough CG. Back related outcome assessment instruments. Eur Spine J 2006;15(Suppl 1):S25–S31

11. Gabbe BJ, Williamson OD, Cameron PA, Dowrick AS. Choosing outcome assessment instruments for trauma registries. Acad Emerg Med 2005; 12:751–758

12. Neugebauer E, Bouillon B, Bullinger M, Wood-Dauphinée S. Quality of life after multiple trauma—summary and recommendations of the consensus conference. Restor Neurol Neurosci 2002;20:161–167

13. Cameron PA, Gabbe BJ, McNeil JJ. The importance of quality of survival as an outcome measure for an integrated trauma system. Injury 2006;37:1178–1184

14. MacKenzie EJ, Damiano A, Miller T, Luchter S. The development of the Functional Capacity Index. J Trauma 1996;41:799–807

15. Fisher CG, Noonan VK, Dvorak MF. Changing face of spine trauma care in North America. Spine 2006;31(11, Suppl):S2–S8, discussion S36

16. Hallin P, Sullivan M, Kreuter M. Spinal cord injury and quality of life measures: a review of instrument psychometric quality. Spinal Cord 2000;38:509–523

17. Hays RD, Morales LS, Reise SP. Item response theory and health outcomes measurement in the 21st century. Med Care 2000;38(9, Suppl): II28–II42

18. Németh G. Health related quality of life outcome instruments. Eur Spine J 2006;15(Suppl 1):S44–S51

19. The EuroQol Group. EuroQol—a new facility for the measurement of health-related quality of life. The EuroQol Group. Health Policy 1990; 16:199–208

20. Steeves JD, Lammertse D, Curt A, et al; International Campaign for Cures of Spinal Cord Injury Paralysis. Guidelines for the conduct of clinical trials for spinal cord injury (SCI) as developed by the ICCP panel: clinical trial outcome measures. Spinal Cord 2007;45:206–221

21. Feeny D, Furlong W, Torrance GW, et al. Multiattribute and single-attribute utility functions for the Health Utilities Index Mark 3 system. Med Care 2002;40:113–128

22. Resnik L, Dobrykowski E. Outcomes measurement for patients with low back pain. Orthop Nurs 2005;24:14–24

23. Anagnostis C, Gatchel RJ, Mayer TG. The pain disability questionnaire: a new psychometrically sound measure for chronic musculoskeletal disorders. Spine 2004;29:2290–2302, discussion 2303

24. Schluter PJ, Neale R, Scott D, Luchter S, McClure RJ. Validating the functional capacity index: a comparison of predicted versus observed total body scores. J Trauma 2005;58:259–263

25. Morganti B, Scivoletto G, Ditunno P, Ditunno JF, Molinari M. Walking index for spinal cord injury (WISCI): criterion validation. Spinal Cord 2005;43:27–33

26. Stineman MG, Shea JA, Jette A, et al. The Functional Independence Measure: tests of scaling assumptions, structure, and reliability across 20 diverse impairment categories. Arch Phys Med Rehabil 1996;77:1101–1108

27. Scheuringer M, Grill E, Boldt C, Mittrach R, Müllner P, Stucki G. Systematic review of measures and their concepts used in published studies focusing on rehabilitation in the acute hospital and in early post-acute rehabilitation facilities. Disabil Rehabil 2005;27:419–429

28. Hebert JS, Burnham RS. The effect of polytrauma in persons with traumatic spine injury: a prospective database of spine fractures. Spine 2000;25(1):55–60

29. Matheson LN. Functional outcome in trauma patients with spinal injury. Spine 2003;28:105–106

30. Hetherington H, Earlam RJ. Measurement of disability after multiple injuries: the functional independence measure: clinical review. Eur J Surg 1995;161:549–555

31. Catz A, Itzkovich M, Tesio L, et al. A multicenter international study on the Spinal Cord Independence Measure, version III: Rasch psychometric validation. Spinal Cord 2007;45:275–291

32. Brenneman FD, Redelmeier DA, Boulanger BR, McLellan BA, Culhane JP. Long-term outcomes in blunt trauma: who goes back to work? J Trauma 1997;42:778–781

33. Soberg HL, Finset A, Bautz-Holter E, Sandvik L, Roise O. Return to work after severe multiple injuries: a multidimensional approach on status 1 and 2 years postinjury. J Trauma 2007;62:471–481

34. McLain RF. Functional outcomes after surgery for spinal fractures: return to work and activity. Spine 2004;29:470–477, discussion Z6

35. Schluter PJ, Cameron CM, Purdie DM, Kliewer EV, McClure RJ. How well do anatomical-based injury severity scores predict health service use in the 12 months after injury? Int J Inj Contr Saf Promot 2005;12:241–246

36. World Health Organization. World Health Organization International Classification of Functioning, Disabilities and Health (ICF). Geneva: WHO; 2001

37. Biering-Sørensen F, Scheuringer M, Baumberger M, et al. Developing core sets for persons with spinal cord injuries based on the International Classification of Functioning, Disability and Health as a way to specify functioning. Spinal Cord 2006;44:541–546

38. Biering-Sørensen F, Charlifue S, DeVivo M, et al. International Spinal Cord Injury Data Sets. Spinal Cord 2006;44:530–534

39. DeVivo M, Biering-Sørensen F, Charlifue S, et al; Executive Committee for the International SCI Data Sets Committees. International Spinal Cord Injury Core Data Set. Spinal Cord 2006;44:535–540

40. Stoll T, Brach M, Huber EO, et al. ICF Core Set for patients with musculoskeletal conditions in the acute hospital. Disabil Rehabil 2005;27: 381–387

41. Scheuringer M, Stucki G, Huber EO, et al. ICF Core Set for patients with musculoskeletal conditions in early post-acute rehabilitation facilities. Disabil Rehabil 2005;27:405–410

42. Ewert T, Grill E, Bartholomeyczik S, et al. ICF Core Set for patients with neurological conditions in the acute hospital. Disabil Rehabil 2005;27: 367–373

43. Stier-Jarmer M, Grill E, Ewert T, et al. ICF Core Set for patients with neurological conditions in early post-acute rehabilitation facilities. Disabil Rehabil 2005;27:389–395

44. Crichlow RJ, Andres PL, Morrison SM, Haley SM, Vrahas MS. Depression in orthopaedic trauma patients: prevalence and severity. J Bone Joint Surg Am 2006;88:1927–1933

45. Craig AR, Hancock KM, Dickson HG. A longitudinal investigation into anxiety and depression in the first 2 years following a spinal cord injury. Paraplegia 1994;32:675–679

46. Scivoletto G, Petrelli A, Di Lucente L, Castellano V. Psychological investigation of spinal cord injury patients. Spinal Cord 1997;35:516–520

47. Holtslag HR, van Beeck EF, Lindeman E, Leenen LP. Determinants of long-term functional consequences after major trauma. J Trauma 2007;62: 919–927

48. Knop C, Oeser M, Bastian L, Lange U, Zdichavsky M, Blauth M. [Development and validation of the Visual Analogue Scale (VAS) Spine Score]. Unfallchirurg 2001;104:488–497

3

The Impact of Evidence-Based Medicine in Cervical Trauma

Paul A. Anderson and Michael M. Vosbikian

The primary goals in the management of patients with cervical spine injuries are to protect the spinal cord from further injury, stabilize the spine, minimize long-term disability, and create an environment for maximum neurological recovery. These tenets were authored 6 decades ago by Rogers, and they have not changed.[1] Despite many basic scientific advances, few proven changes in the management of spinal cord injuries have occurred since this foundation was established.

In the past 2 decades, major strides have been made in the overall medical care of the injured patient. These advances have started at the trauma scene and include more advanced spinal stabilization, basic life support, transportation to either trauma or spinal centers of excellence, improved diagnostic capabilities with the more widespread use of computed tomography (CT) and magnetic resonance imaging (MRI), which provide superb discrimination of injury patterns, and more attention to respiratory support with early intubation or tracheostomy or both if needed (**Table 3.1**).[2–4] However, the role of surgery and its timing remain unclear. Early reduction of cervical fracture dislocations is being performed less commonly and is more often substituted with immediate surgery. The surgical techniques of decompression and arthrodesis of unstable spinal segments with rigid constructs are well established, but still show limited proof that patients are actually benefiting. Finally, neural protection using pharmacological agents that decrease or prevent the secondary cascade of spinal cord injury are well established in animal models but are yet without validation in human clinical trials.[5] Despite the excitement after the publication of the Second National Acute Spinal Cord Injury Study (NASCIS 2) trial on high-dose methylprednisolone, little functional improvement after its use has been reported to date.[6] Regeneration of the injured spinal cord still remains a hope for the future.

This chapter examines the overall effect of the theoretical improvement in the medical care of patients with spinal cord injuries. It reviews the medical evidence documenting improvements in the care of the spinal cord injured over time. As a gauge to measure the effectiveness of medical advances, the chapter examines mortality and changes in neurological function on admission to spinal cord injury rehabilitation centers over time.

Table 3.1 Theoretical Improvements in Overall Medical Care

On scene stabilization
Advanced life support
Stabilization techniques
Transportation advances
Spinal and trauma centers
Respiratory support
Hemodynamic support
Rapid diagnostic testing with computed tomography and/or magnetic resonance imaging
Neural protection
Availability of trained spinal surgeons
Rehabilitation centers of excellence

◆ Mortality

Advances in medical care close to the time of injury would be expected to result in decreased mortality. The benchmark to be examined will be mortality within the first year, which reflects the majority of the initial management and early rehabilitation of the injured patient. The Model Spinal Cord Injury Care Systems has prospectively monitored epidemiological as well as prognostic data of patients with spinal cord injuries at 16 centers throughout the United States.[7] This effort has been funded by the National Institutes of Health and has resulted in numerous publications.

Important trends have occurred with respect to the time of admission to rehabilitation centers as well as the duration of hospital stay. The mean number of days from injury to admission to a spinal cord center has decreased from 23 days in 1975 to 7 days within the last 5 years.[8] Acute hospitalization stays have decreased from 28 days in 1973 to 9 days in 2006. Similarly, the lengths of stay at rehabilitation centers have decreased significantly from a high of 145 days in 1974 to only 26 days in 2006.[8] Although these changes could be classified as positive, the trends may indicate improvements in medical care as well as changes in reimbursement, practice patterns, and insurance coverage.

Life expectancy in the first year following injury from the years 1973 through 1999 was evaluated in 9805 patients enrolled in the Model Systems Program and at Shriners Hospital.[9] A 67% drop in the first year mortality was seen over those years. This significant decline was affirmation of an overall improvement in general medical care.

◆ Changes in Neurological Functions

Neurological Deterioration

Neurological deterioration is a catastrophic event and thought to be preventable in the majority of cases because one of the primary goals in the management of spinal injured patients is to prevent further neural injury. This is best accomplished by resuscitation, spinal immobilization, and transportation to centers with experience in managing spinal injury patients. Expedient diagnosis, reduction of displaced fractures and dislocations, and correctly indicated surgery have all minimized the potential for neurological decline following cervical trauma. Multiple retrospective studies and one prospective study have reported the incidence and factors associated with deterioration.

Frankel reported the experience at Stoke Mandeville rehabilitation in 692 patients treated from 1951 to 1968.[10] Their treatment was largely nonoperative but included advanced methods to achieve postural reduction and long-term cervical traction. Only 2% of cervical spine patients deteriorated. Bohlman retrospectively reviewed 300 cervical spine injury patients treated between 1950 and 1972.[11] Only 200 of the patients had a diagnosis of spinal injury made in the emergency department. The most common etiologies for the delay in diagnosis were intoxication and traumatic brain injury. In the majority of these cases, no radiographic examination was performed. Overall, 11 patients (3.6%) had spinal cord injury or significant worsening after hospital admission.

Heiden et al reviewed the experience of 199 complete spinal cord injury patients treated in Southern California from 1963 to 1972.[12] Neurological deterioration was seen in 1.5% of those treated with anterior decompression, whereas none of the patients treated nonoperatively or by laminectomy deteriorated. Also noteworthy was the finding that neurological deterioration was not seen in patients with incomplete lesions. Colterjohn and Bednar retrospectively reviewed 281 patients with spinal cord injury who were treated at a regional center from 1987 to 1992.[13] They found that 19 patients (5%) deteriorated following admission. Risk factors included fractures in ankylosed spines, flexural injuries, and low energy fractures (which occur more commonly in the elderly). Farmer et al reported a 1.8% incidence of neurological deterioration in 1031 patients treated at a regional spinal cord injury center between 1977

and 1993.[14] Risk factors in this study included sepsis, intubation, and vertebral artery injury. Additionally, timing of surgical intervention was shown to be a statistical factor. Eight patients deteriorated postoperatively, all of whom had surgery within 4 days, whereas only one who had surgery later showed deterioration.

Marshall also reported a significant association between early surgery and deterioration. In a prospective multicenter study, 14 of 283 patients had neurological deterioration. The associated factors were thought to be surgery (four patients), halo-vest immobilization (two patients), turning frames (three patients), and traction (three patients).[15] The timing of surgery was an important factor confirming the observation of Farmer in that all deterioration occurred in patients having surgery within the first 5 days of injury. However, the incidence of deterioration during closed treatment was similar to that occurring after surgery.

Conclusions from these studies are somewhat limited because the surgical treatment was not standardized and likely included laminectomy, which has been shown to be harmful in many cases. Other factors limiting conclusions in these studies were the lack of modern imaging studies such as MRI and failure to adequately resuscitate patients before and during surgery.

Not infrequently, preventable delays in diagnosis may result in neurological deterioration. Levi et al reported a retrospective multicenter study of cases of neurological deterioration at a level 1 trauma thought to be secondary to delayed or missed diagnosis in 24 of 44,520 (0.025%) patients admitted to eight level 1 trauma centers over a 2- to 8-year period.[16] This accounted for 0.21% of all spinal injured patients. The common causes associated with delay in diagnoses were inadequate radiological studies (58%), incorrect reading (33%), and poor quality (18%). In this study, 16 patients developed or had worsened their spinal cord injury, whereas three patients died as a result of the neurological deterioration. Notably, traumatic brain injury was present in 25% of cases.

In summary, improvements in overall care compared with the report by Bohlman appear to show decreasing incidence of neurological deterioration once a patient is admitted to an emergency department. However, even at level 1 trauma centers, delays in diagnosis still occur, which may result in spinal cord injury or even death.

Neurological Recovery

An important goal of treatment is to maximize neurological recovery and overall function. In cervical injuries, these outcomes are measured by the modified Frankel Impairment Scale, Functional Independence Measure (FIM), and Craig Handicap Assessment and Reporting Technique (CHART), which reflects social integration. According to reports by the Model Systems, the overall modified Frankel Impairment Score at discharge from rehabilitation centers has improved each decade form 1970 to 2000–2006.[8] The functional impairment measure, however, has decreased, thus reflecting less independence at discharge. This was felt to be secondary to the shortened duration of rehabilitation, which has decreased over time, as already noted. On a per day average, the FIM improvement has shown an increase since the 1980s. The CHART scores show a 5 to 10% improvement from 1992 to 2006 in function and occupational independence, social integration, as well as economic self-sufficiency.

Neurological Extent of Injury at Admission

Improper or neglected treatment of spinal cord injury was common due to the fact that many practitioners believed that little could be done and that the prognosis was poor. As we have shown, neurological deterioration was not uncommon. Efforts at early management with the goal of further preventing neurological injury have resulted in improvement in the severity of spinal cord injury over time by preventing the change from incomplete to complete cord injuries. During the years from 1973 through 1979, 45.9% of patients were incomplete injuries compared with 55.6% from 2000 through 2006.[17] This change is an important statistic because it validates, to some degree, that improvements in overall medical care have occurred.

◆ Summary

The overall medical care of spinal cord injury patients is improving over time. Level 1 evidence exists demonstrating that patients currently have lower mortality in the first year after injury as well as improved neurological recovery. Unfortunately, the functional independence measures show a decrease in function at discharge from rehabilitation centers. However, this is most likely a result of a shortened rehabilitation time. Despite this decrease, an improvement in social integration and economic viability has definitely occurred in the last decade. Weak evidence, which is based on retrospective studies, has shown improvements in the early diagnosis of spinal cord injuries along with a lesser chance of neurological deterioration. Correspondingly, there has been an improvement in controlling the extent of cord injury, which is illustrated by more frequent incomplete injuries seen upon admission to rehabilitation centers.

References

1. Rogers WA. Treatment of fracture-dislocation of the cervical spine. J Bone Joint Surg Am 2007;24:245–258
2. Cervical spine immobilization before admission to the hospital. Neurosurgery 2002;50(3, Suppl):S7–S17
3. Transportation of patients with acute traumatic cervical spine injuries. Neurosurgery 2002;50(3, Suppl):S18–S20
4. Clinical assessment after acute cervical spinal cord injury. Neurosurgery 2002;50(3, Suppl):S21–S29
5. Fehlings MG, Perrin RG. The timing of surgical intervention in the treatment of spinal cord injury: a systematic review of recent clinical evidence. Spine 2006;31(11, Suppl):S28–S35, discussion S36
6. Bracken MB, Shepard MJ, Collins WF, et al. A randomized, controlled trial of methylprednisolone or naloxone in the treatment of acute spinal-cord injury. Results of the Second National Acute Spinal Cord Injury Study. N Engl J Med 1990;322:1405–1411
7. Richards JS. Collaborative research in the model spinal cord injury systems: process and outcomes. J Spinal Cord Med 2002;25:331–334
8. National Spinal Cord Injury Statistical Center. The 2006 Annual Statistical Report for the Model Spinal Cord Injury Care Systems. Birmingham, AL: National Spinal Cord Injury Statistical Center; 2006
9. DeVivo MJ, Krause JS, Lammertse DP. Recent trends in mortality and causes of death among persons with spinal cord injury. Arch Phys Med Rehabil 1999;80:1411–1419
10. Frankel HL, Hancock DO, Hyslop G, et al. The value of postural reduction in the initial management of closed injuries of the spine with paraplegia and tetraplegia, I. Paraplegia 1969;7:179–192
11. Bohlman HH. Acute fractures and dislocations of the cervical spine: an analysis of three hundred hospitalized patients and review of the literature. J Bone Joint Surg Am 1979;61:1119–1142
12. Heiden JS, Weiss MH, Rosenberg AW, Apuzzo ML, Kurze T. Management of cervical spinal cord trauma in Southern California. J Neurosurg 1975;43:732–736
13. Colterjohn NR, Bednar DA. Identifiable risk factors for secondary neurologic deterioration in the cervical spine-injured patient. Spine 1995;20:2293–2297
14. Farmer J, Vaccaro A, Albert TJ, Malone S, Balderston RA, Cotler JM. Neurologic deterioration after cervical spinal cord injury. J Spinal Disord 1998;11:192–196
15. Marshall LF, Knowlton S, Garfin SR, et al. Deterioration following spinal cord injury: a multicenter study. J Neurosurg 1987;66:400–404
16. Levi AD, Hurlbert RJ, Anderson P, et al. Neurologic deterioration secondary to unrecognized spinal instability following trauma: a multicenter study. Spine 2006;31:451–458
17. Becker BE, DeLisa JA. Model Spinal Cord Injury System trends, and implications for the future. Arch Phys Med Rehabil 1999;80:1514–1521

4

The Impact of Evidence-Based Medicine in Thoracolumbar Trauma

Joseph L. Petfield, James P. Lawrence, Jeffrey Rihn, Eric B. Harris, Alexander R. Vaccaro, and Christopher M. Bono

The past few decades have seen remarkable advancement in the evaluation, treatment, and rehabilitation of injuries to the spine and spinal cord. The development of new surgical techniques, imaging modalities, diagnostic classification systems, and biological materials gives cause for hope of improved patient outcomes following spinal trauma. Despite this progress in the understanding and treatment of thoracolumbar trauma, the topic remains one of considerable controversy.

Historically, advances in spine surgical care were introduced to clinical practice without definitive empirical proof of improved clinical outcomes.[1] Evidence-based approaches to the treatment of thoracolumbar spinal trauma are becoming increasingly prevalent as physicians, patients, and policy makers seek scientifically grounded data of improved and cost-effective patient care. Evidence-based medicine (EBM) is defined as "the conscientious, explicit, and judicious use of current best evidence in making decisions about the care of individual patients."[2]

Evidence-based medicine is not merely the use of the latest clinical evidence, but rather the integration of this information with clinical expertise, critical judgment, and the patient's individual needs.[3] Such a realistic evidence-based approach is currently being applied to answer important clinical questions, such as the effect of early versus late surgical decompression on neurological recovery, as well as the comparison of operative versus nonoperative treatment in thoracolumbar fractures.[4] Moreover, evidence-based techniques are also being utilized to validate the development of new surgical interventions. Large, multicenter clinical trials are under way to definitively address the important questions regarding thoracolumbar spine trauma, a field whose research has been characterized as persistently lacking statistical power.[4,5] This chapter addresses the contributions of EBM over the last few decades on a variety of treatment aspects of thoracolumbar trauma.

◆ Initial Treatment and Examination of Thoracolumbar Trauma

The acute treatment of trauma and potential spine injuries has undergone a radical transformation over the last 30 years. Prior to the 1970s, the specifics and organization of trauma care varied widely by location and provider. Most initial care was not based on evidence of efficacy, but rather upon local expert opinion. Landmark studies in the 1960s and '70s recognized accidental death and injury as a long neglected cause of preventable death that lacked a body of strong empirical data.[6–8] As trauma care grew to become an issue of national importance in the United States, states developed uniformly organized, regionally based trauma care systems that showed definitive evidence of improved outcomes.[9,10] This widespread reorganization of trauma care has resulted in more efficient resource utilization, more targeted clinical care, and improved patient outcomes.

Regional trauma care decreases patient mortality by minimizing the duration of prehospital treatment, directing the transport of patients to designated, accredited specialty trauma centers, and allowing the pooling of resources to provide more cost-effective, efficient treatment (**Fig. 4.1**).[11] Specifically regarding spinal cord injury (SCI), clinical evidence has demonstrated that patients sustaining an SCI demonstrate fewer complications and improved outcomes when cared for by a specialist management system.[12,13] Regionalization of spine trauma care to designated centers has also facilitated the organization of much-needed large, multicenter, randomized trials investigating spine injury. There are currently 13 designated centers for the treatment of spinal cord injury in the United States.

The acute, prehospital care of potential SCIs is currently under reevaluation. Spinal immobilization following primary spine trauma, although widely recommended, has not been definitively proven to prevent subsequent secondary spine injuries.[14,15] Moreover, spine immobilization is painful and can

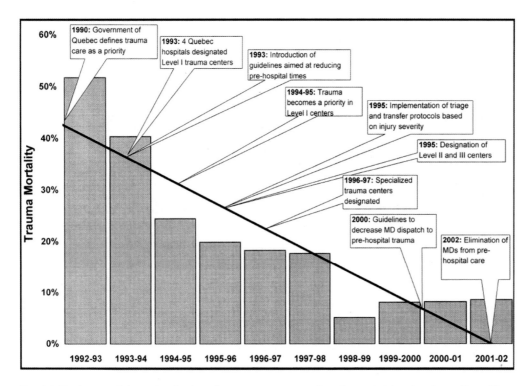

Fig. 4.1 The impact of the regionalization of trauma care on mortality of severely injured patients. (From Liberman M, Mulder DS, Lavoie A, Sampalis JS. Implementation of a trauma care system: evolution through evaluation. J Trauma 2004;56:1330–1335. Reprinted with permission.)

result in several potentially unnecessary complications in the trauma patient.[16] Definitive research, if feasible, is indicated to identify trauma patients appropriate for immobilization, as well as when and how this immobilization is applied. Clearly, distinguishing between stable and unstable injuries requiring immobilization in a field setting is quite challenging.

There has been a near quantum leap in diagnostic imaging over the past 30 years. The radiographic diagnosis of acute spine trauma has evolved in similar fashion, as sophisticated imaging technology has become more available, more rapid, and less costly.[4,17] In many centers, helical computed tomographic scanning has replaced plain radiography in the initial evaluation of the spine in the blunt trauma patient because of its greater sensitivity as a screening tool, decreased overall cost, and potentially decreased total radiation exposure to the patient.[18] Magnetic resonance imaging (MRI) has also become an essential tool in the evaluation of the spine-injured patient because it allows for sensitive visualization of injuries to the intervertebral disk, the bony structures, the posterior ligamentous structures, and the neural elements themselves.

A lack of standardization of radiographic measurement parameters used to assess thoracolumbar fractures has complicated both patient evaluation and the reporting of clinical outcomes in the spine literature. A recent systematic review of the literature was conducted by the Spine Trauma Study Group with the purpose of standardizing radiographic interpretation and reducing observer variability (**Fig. 4.2**).[19]

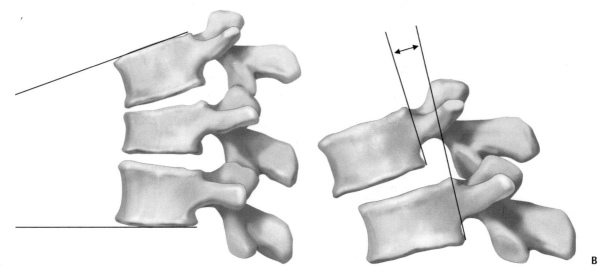

A   B

Fig. 4.2 The recommended radiographic parameters to depict the properties of the injured spinal column. **(A)** The Cobb angle to assess sagittal alignment. **(B)** The vertebral body translation percentage to express traumatic anterolisthesis.

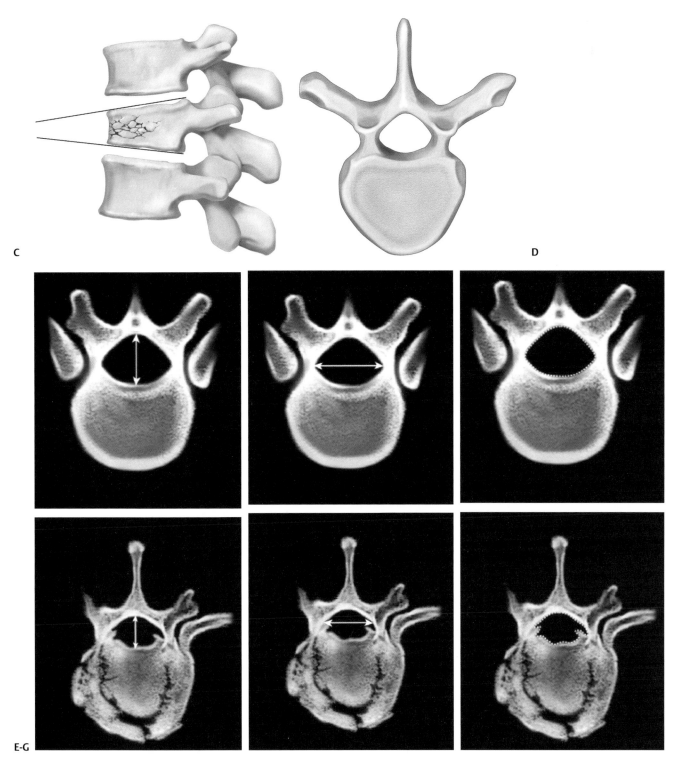

C   D

E-G

Fig. 4.2 (*Continued*) **(C,D)** Anterior vertebral body compression percentage to assess vertebral body compression. **(E,F)** The sagittal to transverse canal diameter ratio. **(G)** Canal total cross-sectional area (measured or calculated). (From Keynan O, Fisher CG, Vaccaro A, et al. Radiographic measurement parameters in thoracolumbar fractures: a systematic review and consensus statement of the Spine Trauma Study Group. Spine 2006;31:E162–E163. Reprinted with permission.)

◆ Evidence-Based Classification Systems of Thoracolumbar Injury

Clinical classification systems can serve several purposes. Ideally, they facilitate accurate communication between treatment providers, provide insight into injury severity and morphology, guide treatment, and promote consistency in clinical research. In the field of thoracolumbar spinal trauma, several classification systems have been developed with these goals in mind. However, there is not currently a definitive classification system that has been clinically proven to be consistently valid and reliable.[20,21] The Thoracolumbar Injury

Classification and Severity Score (TLICS) represents the first attempt at validating a thoracolumbar fracture classification system in a scientific manner.[22]

Beginning with Böhler's research of spine fractures in the 1930s, no less than six thoracolumbar injury classification systems have been devised.[23–29] The most popular classification system used currently in North America is the Denis system, based on his model of the three-column spine.[27] This system defines four major categories of injury with 16 subgroupings and relies mainly on the condition of the middle column to define fracture severity and predict neurological risk. Recently, the intraobserver and interobserver reliability of the Denis system has been shown to be relatively low.[20,21] Evidence has also shown that the stability of the middle column of the spine is not the most integral factor of injury severity.

The alternative system currently in use is the AO system proposed by Magerl and colleagues.[28] This so-called comprehensive system uses a large number of classification steps to precisely define the injury in question. It is perhaps this complexity that contributes to the limited intra- and interobserver reliability cited for the AO system.[20–22]

The Spine Trauma Study Group's (STSG's) TLICS is the most recent attempt at devising a clinically reliable and valid system. Originally proposed as the Thoracolumbar Injury Severity Score (TLISS),[30] and modified to become the TLICS,[22,31,32] this classification system presents a scoring mechanism to be used by care providers to assist in the decision between operative and nonoperative treatment. This scoring system is based on three variables corresponding to the spinal injury: the morphological appearance of the fracture, the integrity of the posterior ligamentous complex, and the patient's neurological status (**Fig. 4.3**). Follow-up studies have found this classification system to have a moderate degree of reliability in classifying thoracolumbar fractures, but a high degree of intra- and interobserver reliability when predicting physician's treatment decisions.[33–35] Audigé and colleagues recently outlined a three-phase process by which classification systems can be clinically validated.[36] To date, the TLICS has completed the first two phases, which consist of development and initial multisurgeon studies.[22] The third phase consists of large, multicenter clinical studies, which are currently in development.

◆ Influences of Evidence-Based Medicine on Surgical Decision Making and Surgical Treatment of Thoracolumbar Trauma

Surgery or Conservative Treatment

Immediate thoracolumbar spinal surgical treatment is indicated in patients with unstable fractures, spinal cord compression, and the presence of neurological deficit.[37–40] Surgical versus nonsurgical treatment of thoracolumbar burst fractures, however, remains a controversial issue because several well-designed studies exhibit conflicting results.[41–44]

In a prospective, randomized trial of 53 patients with a thoracolumbar fracture without neurological deficit, Wood et al[43] found no difference in functional outcome between patients managed operatively or nonoperatively with a body cast or orthosis. In a second prospective, randomized trial on this issue, Siebenga et al[42] reported significantly better results when treating AO type A3 spine fractures with posterior short-segment transpedicular screw fixation when compared with bed rest and an orthotic device.

Although both of these studies represent a step toward evidence-based clinical decision-making for the treatment of thoracolumbar burst fractures, larger studies with greater statistical power are needed to provide definitive treatment guidelines. However, the execution of such trials is complicated by the difficulty of randomizing injured patients to conservative care in what constitutes a complex ethical scenario. More importantly, the key factor in the stability of thoracolumbar burst fractures appears to be the integrity of the posterior ligamentous complex (PLC).[41] Thus clinical equipoise exists only for those patients believed to have an intact PLC complex, which is the group that can be ethically randomized to operative versus nonoperative treatment.

Timing of Decompression and Stabilization

The timing of decompression or fixation following traumatic thoracolumbar injury has been a subject of considerable debate. Experimental evidence in animals indicates that immediate surgical decompression following fracture can be effective in minimizing secondary injury to the spinal cord resulting from inflammatory mechanisms and ischemia.[45,46] A recent meta-analysis of both cervical and thoracolumbar spine injuries has suggested that surgical decompression performed within 24 hours of initial injury demonstrates better neurological outcome in patients with incomplete spinal cord injury when compared with late operative or conservative management.[47] Although a definitive, high-quality, multicenter, randomized trial is yet to be published regarding early versus late decompression, a recent evidence-based review of the literature by Fehlings and Perrin reviewing cervical spinal cord injuries suggests that surgical decompression should be performed as soon as possible, preferably within 24 hours of injury.[46] Similar evidence for decompression in the setting of thoracolumbar trauma with neurological deficits is lacking.

Yet clinical studies have not shown that early stabilization or fixation (within 72 hours of injury) demonstrates any benefit regarding neurological outcome. Despite this, nonneurological outcomes have been shown to improve. Various studies have shown that early thoracic and lumbar spine stabilization is associated with significant decreases in intensive care unit (ICU) and hospital length of stays, shorter use of a mechanical ventilator, as well as a decreased incidence postoperative pneumonia and deep venous thrombosis.[40,48–51] Ideally, a prospective, randomized, controlled trial would be necessary to provide definitive recommendations for early surgical interventions in thoracolumbar fractures.

Advancements in Surgical Instrumentation

Great advancements have been made in the surgical treatment of thoracolumbar trauma over the past 30 years. Increasingly sensitive and specific imaging modalities have allowed for an improved ability to identify and localize the patterns of injury to the spinal column and the neural axis. This allows a more complete understanding of the morphology of the injury and more detailed preoperative planning.

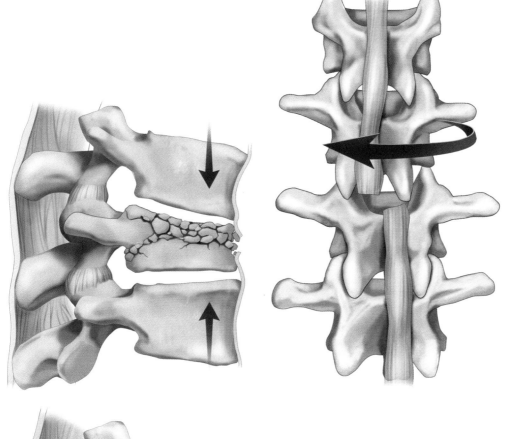

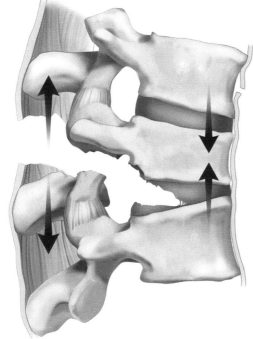

Fig. 4.3 The three major morphological descriptors in the Thoracolumbar Injury Classification and Severity Score include **(A)** compression, **(B)** translation/rotation, and **(C)** distraction. These are determined from a combination of plain film, computed tomographic images, and magnetic resonance imaging. **(A)** Compression: in this description, the vertebral body buckles under load to produce a compression or burst fracture. **(B)** Translation/rotation: the vertebral column is subjected to shear or torsional forces that cause the rostral part of the spinal column to translate or rotate with respect to the caudal part. **(C)** Distraction: the rostral spinal column becomes separated from the caudal segment because of distractive forces. Combinations of these morphological patterns may occur.

When surgery is required, continually evolving operative techniques and the availability of specialized instrumentation, such as pedicle rod and screw fixation systems, have enabled surgeons to more aggressively pursue the goal of stability to the injured spine.

A systematic review conducted in 2004 by Verlaan et al represents one of the first major evidence-based attempts to directly compare the various surgical treatment options for thoracic and lumbar spine fractures.[52] The review analyzed studies of five major surgical techniques: posterior short-segment instrumentation, posterior long-segment instrumentation, posterior short- or long-segment instrumentation, anterior instrumentation, and combined anterior and posterior instrumentation. Inequalities of the preoperative condition for prospective surgical therapies rendered their direct comparison impossible. However, it was found that no currently used surgical technique was able to maintain the corrected angle of spinal kyphosis. Partial neurological deficit had similar potential to resolve irrespective of the choice of operative treatment. The surgical treatment of thoracic and lumbar traumatic fractures was found to be safe and effective, with a low rate of serious complications.

Vertebroplasty and Kyphoplasty

Vertebroplasty and kyphoplasty for thoracolumbar fractures have recently drawn considerable attention regarding outcomes, potential complications, and indications. The increasing mean age at injury of spinal fractures, higher proportion of patients over 60 years of age, and rising prevalence of osteoporosis in women strongly suggest that scrutiny of these procedures will only increase over time.[4,53]

A prospective study published in 2006 by Álvarez et al[54] found that, compared to a nonrandomized, nonoperative cohort, percutaneous vertebroplasty (PV) was shown to be more effective at rapidly reducing pain and improving quality of life of patients suffering from osteoporotic vertebral fractures. However, these differences disappear after 6 months. Similarly, a recent systematic review[55] found that vertebroplasty and kyphoplasty provide short-term pain reduction effectiveness and have a relatively low rate of complications. Leakage of polymethylmethacrylate was found to be the most commonly occurring complication. Though this is usually asymptomatic, its potential neurological consequences are cause for further research.[56]

More recently in 2009, two prospective randomized controlled trials[57,58] found that in the treatment of painful osteoporotic vertebral fractures, vertebroplasty demonstrated no beneficial effect in comparison to a sham procedure when assessed at multiple time intervals after treatment. Surprisingly, the data from these high level studies conflicts with much of the previous literature which had cited encouraging results. Both of these trials, however, confirm that pain from osteoporotic compression fractures substantially diminishes over a period of months. Future research will hopefully delineate which patients benefit from these procedures. Spine care providers should carefully consider all of the literature when considering the appropriate use of vertebroplasty and kyphoplasty.

Minimally Invasive Surgical Techniques

Most current surgical techniques for the treatment of thoracolumbar trauma involve conventional open anterior or posterior exposures. These can be associated with postoperative complications such as infection, blood loss,[52] scarring, adjacent segment, degeneration, or paraspinal muscle injury.[59,60] Gejo and coworkers[61] have demonstrated that the amount of injury to lumbar musculature is directly related to the duration of muscle retraction during posterior lumbar surgery. Patients undergoing long retraction times also reported postoperative lower back pain more frequently.

Minimally invasive surgical (MIS) techniques are increasingly being applied to the field of spine trauma in an attempt to minimize these negative consequences of conventional surgical techniques. Recent studies using MIS techniques to treat thoracolumbar fractures have suggested equivalent or favorable clinical outcomes when compared with open techniques.[60,62] Potential drawbacks of MIS as a treatment choice include the substantial learning curve

required to master the operative techniques, the longer operative times routinely associated with their utilization, as well as the necessity of intraoperative imaging with potentially increased radiation exposure to both the patient and the surgeon.

Over the past decade, several operative treatments for spine trauma have been applied using minimally invasive techniques. Anterior endoscopic decompression and stabilization has been reported as a safe and feasible treatment alternative to a conventional thoracotomy or thoracolumbar approach with the benefit of reduced approach-related morbidity, postoperative pain, and recovery time.[62,63] Percutaneous tension band restoration or augmentation has been reported as a feasible technique for the treatment of stable burst or flexion-distraction injuries.[60] A preliminary short-term study of 57 patients has demonstrated that reconstruction of the anterior column in thoracolumbar trauma using cages and minimally invasive techniques is a safe treatment.[64] Unfortunately, definitive, multicenter, randomized trials have not been performed for any of the MIS treatments discussed to demonstrate superior clinical outcomes. The future of minimally invasive spine surgery appears promising as a means to minimize approach-related morbidity, iatrogenic muscle injury, blood loss, and postoperative pain. Definitive, long-term studies will clearly define its evidence-based use as a treatment for thoracolumbar trauma in the future.

◆ Rehabilitation of Thoracolumbar Trauma

Only a limited number of studies to date have provided evidence-based recommendations regarding the rehabilitative treatment of thoracolumbar spine trauma. The need for rigid bracing of anterior column compression fractures is currently a matter of debate. A retrospective study by Ohana and colleagues[65] compared treating compression fractures by early ambulation with or without a Genuine Jewett Hyperextension brace (Florida Brace Corporation, Winter Park, FL). They found that thoracolumbar fractures with up to 30% height loss can be treated by early ambulation without a brace. In regard to postoperative bracing, it has been hypothesized that rigid braces do little to further stabilize the spine following thoracolumbar fixation.[66] Apple and Perez[67] have recently demonstrated that the discontinuation of a Jewett brace or thoracic lumbar sacral orthosis at 4 weeks following operative fixation does not alter clinical outcome if the patient had a healthy spine prior to suffering a fracture. Moreover, the addition of a muscle-strengthening exercise program to the postoperative rehabilitation of thoracolumbar fractures has been shown to induce hypertrophy of the paraspinal musculature but has not been shown to correlate with pain relief.[68] More comprehensive, randomized trials are needed to further refine the necessity of bracing and muscle strengthening following a thoracolumbar injury.

◆ Summary

The management of thoracolumbar trauma is a controversial, rapidly evolving field. Many new diagnostic modalities and surgical treatments have been introduced in the past few decades, yet, until recently, most have not been scientifically validated using evidence-based protocols. The increasing importance of scientific and fiscal accountability will serve as an impetus for the organization of definitive, multicenter, randomized trials to provide quality evidence-based treatment recommendations in a field with historically underpowered research methodology.

References

1. Carr AJ. Evidence-based orthopaedic surgery: what type of research will best improve clinical practice? J Bone Joint Surg Br 2005;87:1593–1594
2. Sackett DL, Rosenberg WM, Gray JA, Haynes RB, Richardson WS. Evidence based medicine: what it is and what it isn't. BMJ 1996;312:71–72
3. Fisher CG, Wood KB. Introduction to and techniques of evidence-based medicine. Spine 2007;32(19, Suppl):S66–S72
4. Fisher CG, Noonan VK, Dvorak MF. Changing face of spine trauma care in North America. Spine 2006;31(11, Suppl):S2–S8, discussion S36
5. Bailey CS, Fisher CG, Dvorak MF. Type II error in the spine surgical literature. Spine 2004;29(10):1146–1149
6. Committee on Trauma, and Committee on Shock, Division of Medical Sciences, National Academy of Sciences/National Research Countil (US). Accidental Death and Disability: The Neglected Disease of Modern Society. Washington: National Academy of Sciences; 1966
7. West JG, Trunkey DD, Lim RC. Systems of trauma care: a study of two counties. Arch Surg 1979;114:455–460
8. Mullins RJ. A historical perspective of trauma system development in the United States. J Trauma 1999;47(3, Suppl):S8–S14
9. Cowley RA, Hudson F, Scanlan E, et al. An economical and proved helicopter program for transporting the emergency critically ill and injured patient in Maryland. J Trauma 1973;13(12):1029–1038
10. West JG, Cales RH, Gazzaniga AB. Impact of regionalization. The Orange County experience. Arch Surg 1983;118:740–744
11. Liberman M, Mulder DS, Lavoie A, Sampalis JS. Implementation of a trauma care system: evolution through evaluation. J Trauma 2004;56:1330–1335
12. DeVivo MJ, Kartus PL, Stover SL, Fine PR. Benefits of early admission to an organised spinal cord injury care system. Paraplegia 1990;28:545–555
13. Smith M. Efficacy of specialist versus non-specialist management of spinal cord injury within the UK. Spinal Cord 2002;40:10–16
14. Hauswald M, Ong G, Tandberg D, Omar Z. Out-of-hospital spinal immobilization: its effect on neurologic injury. Acad Emerg Med 1998;5:214–219
15. Báez AA, Schiebel N. Evidence-based emergency medicine/systematic review abstract: is routine spinal immobilization an effective intervention for trauma patients? Ann Emerg Med 2006;47:110–112
16. Hauswald M, Braude D. Spinal immobilization in trauma patients: is it really necessary? Curr Opin Crit Care 2002;8:566–570
17. Verlaan JJ, van de Kraats EB, Dhert WJ, Oner FC. The role of 3-D rotational x-ray imaging in spinal trauma. Injury 2005;36(Suppl 2):B98–B103
18. Sheridan R, Peralta R, Rhea J, Ptak T, Novelline R. Reformatted visceral protocol helical computed tomographic scanning allows conventional radiographs of the thoracic and lumbar spine to be eliminated in the evaluation of blunt trauma patients. J Trauma 2003;55:665–669
19. Keynan O, Fisher CG, Vaccaro A, et al. Radiographic measurement parameters in thoracolumbar fractures: a systematic review and consensus statement of the Spine Trauma Study Group. Spine 2006;31:E156–E165
20. Oner FC, Ramos LM, Simmermacher RK, et al. Classification of thoracic and lumbar spine fractures: problems of reproducibility: a study of 53 patients using CT and MRI. Eur Spine J 2002;11:235–245
21. Wood KB, Khanna G, Vaccaro AR, Arnold PM, Harris MB, Mehbod AA. Assessment of two thoracolumbar fracture classification systems as used by multiple surgeons. J Bone Joint Surg Am 2005;87:1423–1429
22. Bono CM, Vaccaro AR, Hurlbert RJ, et al. Validating a newly proposed classification system for thoracolumbar spine trauma: looking to the future of the thoracolumbar injury classification and severity score. J Orthop Trauma 2006;20:567–572
23. Böhler L. Die Techniek Deknochenbruchbehandlung im Grieden und im Kreigen. Vienna: Verlag von Wilhem Maudrich;1930
24. Nicoll EA. Fractures of the dorso-lumbar spine. J Bone Joint Surg Am 1949;31:376–394
25. Holdsworth F. Fractures, dislocations, and fracture-dislocations of the spine. J Bone Joint Surg Am 1970;52:1534–1551
26. Louis R. Unstable fractures of the spine, III: Instability, A: Theories concerning instability. Rev Chir Orthop Repar Appar Mot 1977;63:423–425
27. Denis F. The three column spine and its significance in the classification of acute thoracolumbar spinal injuries. Spine 1983;8:817–831
28. Magerl F, Aebi M, Gertzbein SD, Harms J, Nazarian S. A comprehensive classification of thoracic and lumbar injuries. Eur Spine J 1994;3:184–201
29. McCormack T, Karaikovic E, Gaines RW. The load sharing classification of spine fractures. Spine 1994;19:1741–1744
30. Vaccaro AR, Zeiller SC, Hulbert RJ, et al. The thoracolumbar injury severity score: a proposed treatment algorithm. J Spinal Disord Tech 2005;18:209–215
31. Vaccaro AR, Lehman RA Jr, Hurlbert RJ, et al. A new classification of thoracolumbar injuries: the importance of injury morphology, the integrity of the posterior ligamentous complex, and neurologic status. Spine 2005;30:2325–2333
32. Fassett DR, Politi R, Patel A, Brown Z, Vaccaro AR. Classification systems for acute thoracolumbar trauma. Curr Opin Orthop 2007;18:253–258
33. Harrop JS, Vaccaro AR, Hurlbert RJ, et al; Spine Trauma Study Group. Intrarater and interrater reliability and validity in the assessment of the mechanism of injury and integrity of the posterior ligamentous complex: a novel injury severity scoring system for thoracolumbar injuries. Invited submission from the Joint Section Meeting On Disorders of the Spine and Peripheral Nerves, March 2005. J Neurosurg Spine 2006;4:118–122
34. Vaccaro AR, Baron EM, Sanfilippo J, et al. Reliability of a novel classification system for thoracolumbar injuries: the Thoracolumbar Injury Severity Score. Spine 2006;31(11, Suppl):S62–S69, discussion S104
35. Patel AA, Vaccaro AR, Albert TJ, et al. The adoption of a new classification system: time-dependent variation in interobserver reliability of the thoracolumbar injury severity score classification system. Spine 2007;32:E105–E110
36. Audigé L, Bhandari M, Hanson B, Kellam J. A concept for the validation of fracture classifications. J Orthop Trauma 2005;19:401–406
37. McLain RF. Functional outcomes after surgery for spinal fractures: return to work and activity. Spine 2004;29:470–477, discussion Z6
38. Trivedi JM. Spinal trauma: therapy—options and outcomes. Eur J Radiol 2002;42:127–134
39. Hierholzer C, Buhren V, Woltmann A. Operative timing and management of spinal injuries in multiply injured patients. European Journal of Trauma and Emergency Surgery 2007;33:488–500
40. Rutges JPHJ, Oner FC, Leenen LPH. Timing of thoracic and lumbar fracture fixation in spinal injuries: a systematic review of neurological and clinical outcome. Eur Spine J 2007;16:579–587
41. Rechtine GR II. Nonoperative management and treatment of spinal injuries. Spine 2006;31(11, Suppl):S22–S27, discussion S36
42. Siebenga J, Leferink VJ, Segers MJ, et al. Treatment of traumatic thoracolumbar spine fractures: a multicenter prospective randomized study of operative versus nonsurgical treatment. Spine 2006;31:2881–2890
43. Wood K, Buttermann G, Mehbod A, et al. Operative compared with nonoperative treatment of a thoracolumbar burst fracture without neurological deficit: a prospective, randomized study. J Bone Joint Surg Am 2003;85-A:773–781
44. Yi L, Jingping B, Gele J, Baoleri X, Taixiang W. Operative versus non-operative treatment for thoracolumbar burst fractures without neurological deficit. Cochrane Database Syst Rev 2006;(4):CD005079
45. Amar AP, Levy ML. Pathogenesis and pharmacological strategies for mitigating secondary damage in acute spinal cord injury. Neurosurgery 1999;44:1027–1039, discussion 1039–1040
46. Fehlings MG, Perrin RG. The timing of surgical intervention in the treatment of spinal cord injury: a systematic review of recent clinical evidence. Spine 2006;31(11, Suppl):S28–S35, discussion S36
47. La Rosa G, Conti A, Cardali S, Cacciola F, Tomasello F. Does early decompression improve neurological outcome of spinal cord injured patients? Appraisal of the literature using a meta-analytical approach. Spinal Cord 2004;42:503–512
48. Croce MA, Bee TK, Pritchard E, Miller PR, Fabian TC. Does optimal timing for spine fracture fixation exist? Ann Surg 2001;233:851–858
49. Kerwin AJ, Frykberg ER, Schinco MA, Griffen MM, Murphy T, Tepas JJ. The effect of early spine fixation on non-neurologic outcome. J Trauma 2005;58:15–21
50. Schinkel C, Frangen TM, Kmetic A, Andress HJ, Muhr G; German Trauma Registry. Timing of thoracic spine stabilization in trauma patients: impact on clinical course and outcome. J Trauma 2006;61:156–160, discussion 160
51. Albert TJ, Kim DH. Timing of surgical stabilization after cervical and thoracic trauma. Invited submission from the Joint Section Meeting on Disorders of the Spine and Peripheral Nerves, March 2004. J Neurosurg Spine 2005;3:182–190
52. Verlaan JJ, Diekerhof CH, Buskens E, et al. Surgical treatment of traumatic fractures of the thoracic and lumbar spine: a systematic review of the literature on techniques, complications, and outcome. Spine 2004;29:803–814
53. Truumees E, Hilibrand A, Vaccaro AR. Percutaneous vertebral augmentation. Spine J 2004;4:218–229

54. Alvarez L, Alcaraz M, Pérez-Higueras A, et al. Percutaneous vertebroplasty: functional improvement in patients with osteoporotic compression fractures. Spine 2006;31:1113–1118

55. Hulme PA, Krebs J, Ferguson SJ, Berlemann U. Vertebroplasty and kyphoplasty: a systematic review of 69 clinical studies. Spine 2006;31:1983–2001

56. Patel AA, Vaccaro AR, Martyak GG, et al. Neurologic deficit following percutaneous vertebral stabilization. Spine 2007;32:1728–1734

57. Buchbinder R, Osborne RH, Ebeling PR, et al. A randomized trial of vertebroplasty for painful osteoporotic vertebral fractures. N Engl J Med 2009;361:557–568

58. Kallmes DF, Comstock BA, Haegerty PJ, et al. A randomized trial of vertebroplasty for osteoporotic spinal fractures. N Engl J Med 2009;361:269–279

59. Kawaguchi Y, Matsui H, Tsuji H. Back muscle injury after posterior lumbar spine surgery: a histologic and enzymatic analysis. Spine 1996;21:941–944

60. Rampersaud YR, Annand N, Dekutoski MB. Use of minimally invasive surgical techniques in the management of thoracolumbar trauma: current concepts. Spine 2006;31:S96–102; discussion S104.

61. Gejo R, Matsui H, Kawaguchi Y, Ishihara H, Tsuji H. Serial changes in trunk muscle performance after posterior lumbar surgery. Spine 1999;24:1023–1028

62. Schultheiss M, Kinzl L, Claes L, Wilke HJ, Hartwig E. Minimally invasive ventral spondylodesis for thoracolumbar fracture treatment: surgical technique and first clinical outcome. Eur Spine J 2003;12:618–624

63. Khoo LT, Beisse R, Potulski M. Thoracoscopic-assisted treatment of thoracic and lumbar fractures: a series of 371 consecutive cases. Neurosurgery 2002;51(5, Suppl):S104–S117

64. Kossmann T, Rancan M, Jacobi D, Trentz O. Minimally invasive vertebral replacement with cages in thoracic and lumbar spine. Eur J Trauma 2001;27:292–300

65. Ohana N, Sheinis D, Rath E, Sasson A, Atar D. Is there a need for lumbar orthosis in mild compression fractures of the thoracolumbar spine?: A retrospective study comparing the radiographic results between early ambulation with and without lumbar orthosis. J Spinal Disord 2000;13:305–308

66. Connolly PJ, Grob D. Bracing of patients after fusion for degenerative problems of the lumbar spine—yes or no? Spine 1998;23:1426–1428

67. Apple DF Jr, Perez M. Prospective study of orthotic use after operative stabilization of traumatic thoracic and lumbar fractures. Top Spinal Cord Inj Rehabil 2006;12:77–82

68. Kramer M, Dehner C, Katzmaier P, et al. Device-assisted muscle strengthening in the rehabilitation of patients after surgically stabilized vertebral fractures. Arch Phys Med Rehabil 2005;86:558–564

II

Fundamental Principles and Clinical Assessment

5

The Changing Face of Spinal Trauma Throughout the World

Charles G. Fisher, Jeremy Reynolds, and Vanessa K. Noonan

Changes in technology and demographics in the latter half of the twentieth century have generated new challenges and enormous opportunity to the spine trauma surgeon and allied professionals. Treatment-related decisions are affected by geography, resources, and culture. Industrialized nations demonstrate a seemingly inexhaustible demand for biomechanical and biomaterial science to overcome complex problems that have previously been beyond the scope of traditional management. In concert with innovative instrumentation new, less invasive techniques are being developed to reduce the deleterious effects of the open surgical insult. In the developing world access to these techniques is limited. In the present medical and economic environment the aim of low- and medium-income nations should be injury prevention and practical, affordable, effective intervention.

This chapter summarizes available data regarding evolving areas of spine trauma and some of the pertinent controversial issues. It gives an overview of the main challenges faced by developing economies. Finally, it places some of the epidemiological, clinical, and research issues influencing spine trauma in a longitudinal and, where possible, global perspective and provides guidance to ensure that philosophies around the betterment of spine trauma care are understood and supported.

◆ Evolving Global Issues and Evidence in Spinal Trauma

The seductive nature of new technology is powerful. The risk of embracing surgical practices without rigorous evaluation remains very real even today. However, now more than ever a trend exists toward adopting new concepts only in the presence of sound evidence. This trend is a product not only of the desire to maintain a more scientific approach on behalf of the surgeon, but is also due to more stringent levels of fiscal accountability enforced by health care purchasers. The answers that we seek, however, are often hidden by the lack of adequately powered studies,[1] a symptom of both the idiosyncrasies of spinal trauma and the difficulty in expressing the impact of an intervention on an individual. This is especially so when considering patients with spinal cord injury (SCI) where changes in population outcome scores or neurological grade may be small. Even in large studies where planning and execution seem well conceived results can be unclear and conclusions overstated with an outcome where controversy remains the rule rather than the exception despite millions of dollars spent (e.g., Third National Acute Spinal Cord Injury Study [NASCIS 3]).[2-7]

Recently there has been recognition that most hypothesis-driven clinical research cannot be generated by one center or institution, but rather must be executed through collaboration at a national and often international level involving experts in study design and the treatment of the condition under study. This approach allows for pooling of patient data to address the hitherto chronically underpowered spine literature.

The successful development of national arthroplasty registers in Scandinavia has shown how powerful large multicenter databases are at recognizing trends, enabling health care planning, and establishing acceptable standards.[8] The National SCI Statistics Centre, founded in 1983, provides an overview of the experience from the Model SCI Care Systems, a large multicenter American database dedicated to the spinal cord injured population. It publishes yearly statistical reports available to the general public in modified form. It is the largest of its kind with data on nearly 24,000 patients included in the most recent report.[9] Along with similar national and multinational databases elsewhere, this center produces a wealth of basic data on the patient with SCI. Even in their best form, however, data measured by traditional means (such as American Spinal Injury Association [ASIA] scores) provide only a blunt tool from which to base large-scale conclusions. Continued development of disease-specific outcome measures will improve the responsiveness and generalizability of databases to specific interventions. As the momentum builds for contribution to these large databases, the selection of mutually acceptable scoring systems will become paramount.

Currently, much of the available data comes from North America with a population of 334 million[10] and Europe (the EU 25) with a population 460 million.[11] Collectively this represents only a small proportion of the world population (6.6 billion). In contrast India (1.13 billion) and China (1.32 billion)[10] together represent one third of the global population, a proportion likely to expand even more as the Indian and Chinese populations continue to grow (while Western populations have largely stabilized). These demographics underscore the need to involve highly populated nations in multinational databases to gain a truly global perspective.

As has already been alluded to, the relevance of new technologies for the majority of the 2.5 billion people in India and China is questionable, at least in the foreseeable future. This is not to say that these technologies are not already available in select centers, but on the whole there remains a large gap in health care provision on a population basis in comparison with modernized nations. The World Health Organization concluded in 2002 that low and middle-income countries accounted for ~85% of the deaths and 90% of the annual disability-adjusted life-years (DALYs) lost due to road traffic injury.[12] Certainly a paramount area of concern should therefore focus on prevention. An aspect, although less glamorous in appeal, that remains fundamental to the key issue is reducing the number of people with disabilities and the severity of their disability.

India and China are both experiencing unparalleled economic growth, with GDP increases of 9.4% and 11.1%, respectively, in 2006.[13] Although both populations continue to expand, India is growing more rapidly (1.6% compared with 0.6%) and is expected to match China by 2025 at almost 1.5 billion.[10] The most marked transformation is the rapid progress of urbanization. The urban population rose in China from 178 million in 1978 to 524 million in 2003,[14] and in India from 160 million in 1981 to 285 million in 2001.[15] Increased demand for casual unskilled labor has created a large transient population from rural communities swelling these figures further.[16]

Particularly in China, economic growth has improved per capita wealth resulting in a reciprocal rise in private vehicle ownership.[17] Increases in heavy industry and construction in conjunction with higher vehicle utilization also raise the likelihood of increasing volumes of spinal trauma. Injury statistics are even further magnified by, among other things, inadequate seatbelt compliance, more prominent than might otherwise be predicted due to a lack of health and safety legislation and failure to regulate such legislation where it exists.[12,18] This is particularly the case for the large volumes of relatively unprotected, unskilled, migratory workers who drift into the large cities from rural communities.[19] Accordingly there is a far greater risk of work-related injury in these modernized cities than is seen in the other large centers.[20,21] One study has reported construction fatality rates, predominantly from falls, of up to 120/100,000 per year (1995) in the construction industry during the peak of expansion in one of China's economic zones.[22] Although this rate fell over the duration of the study, it remained more than eight times the figure for the US construction industry (4/100,000).[23]

Vehicle expansion in both India and China has been estimated to progress from 1992 figures of 0.006 vehicles per head of population to 0.02 and 0.06, respectively. Risk of death from a road traffic accident in India has tripled.[17] In China, injuries are the leading cause of death from age 1 to 44 years, accounting for ~750,000 deaths and 3.5 million hospitalizations each year.[24] There has been a fivefold increase in the number of road traffic accidents in China over the last 3 decades, an ongoing trend that has tracked vehicle ownership

and economic growth. In both countries, the absolute accuracy of such figures is unknown because China's data are released through traditionally guarded government sources and India's data collection has been called into question.[25]

Urbanization carries obvious risks in terms of high population concentrations, vehicle use, heavy industry, and construction but provides opportunities to introduce legislation in a more controlled environment than exists in the vast expanses of rural hinterland. It is vital that developing countries learn from the successes and failures of nearly 150 years of health and safety legislation in established industrial nations. This may require continued pressure and monitoring where possible from international health and labor organizations. Projects such as the China Seat Belt Intervention Study being sponsored by the George Institute for International Health in Guangzhou[26] will help determine the feasibility of traffic legislation enforcement and population education. Encouraging the development of spinal injury databases at least in the large urban areas of developing countries should be considered a priority. These will be the building blocks that will enable future versions of this chapter to have a truly global epidemiological component.

◆ Epidemiology of Spinal Column Injury

Spinal column injury encompasses clinical diagnoses ranging from soft tissue cervical spine injuries, through low-energy insufficiency fractures, high-energy fracture dislocations, and ultimately complete cord injury. The apparent explosion in incidence of whiplash-associated disorders coincides with factors including increased seatbelt use, traffic congestion, and an increasingly litigious culture in the West. These cases consume considerable resources with up to a million lawsuits in the United States per year and with related litigation costs in the United Kingdom standing at 3 billion pounds (or US$6 billion) annually.[27] However, they make up a negligible component of a spine surgeon's practice and therefore will not be discussed further.

Vertebral compression fractures (VCFs) from osteoporosis are extremely common. Twenty-five percent of women over the age of fifty sustain at least one osteoporotic VCF in their lifetime. The reported US incidence is 700,000 new cases per year.[28] These figures have been the basis of pharmaceutical industry advocacy in the widespread use of medications that preserve bone mineral density. The incidence and prevalence have also contributed to the development of vertebral augmentation techniques. Yet long-term morbidity from these fractures is low, with up to two thirds being identified only incidentally on unrelated radiographs. The vast majority of low-energy, symptomatic fractures are self-limiting and respond well to nonoperative measures.[28] Although a role may exist for vertebral augmentation the obvious indications pertain much more definitively toward symptomatic vertebral column metastatic disease.[29] Osteoporotic VCFs become more challenging to address in the setting of instability requiring more aggressive operative stabilization. With the advent of fit, mobile, adventure-seeking septa- and octogenarians a greater degree of surgical cases can be expected.

To the author's knowledge only one population-based study has attempted to examine the epidemiology of spinal column injuries.[30] Further population-based studies are needed to gain a full appreciation of epidemiology, eliminating selection bias that largely skews the results of current observational or experimental studies. The devastating and emotive consequences of SCI will most certainly continue to stimulate research. However, because spinal column injuries without neurological deficit affect a greater proportion of the population there is optimism that future research will provide the answers that are lacking. For now though, much of the available detailed epidemiological information is specific to SCI.

Incidence

The incidence of SCI worldwide is estimated to be 10.4 to 83 cases per million population and has been stable over the past 30 years.[31] North American estimates are lower at 27 to 47 cases per million population.[30,32–36] There has been a significant increase in the number of individuals with SCI who survive. In North America 38% of individuals with SCI died prior to hospitalization in 1970–1971,[37] and this decreased to 15.8% in 1997–2000.[34] Improvements in automobile design, legislation that requires passengers to wear seatbelts, as well as improved care at the scene of the injury[38] are most likely responsible for this increase in survival. Presently though, epidemiological data like these tend to be fragmented and geographically isolated in nature. Regionalization of spine trauma care and standards such as the International Core Data Set for SCI[39] will make it possible to compare SCI data internationally in the future. Multinational focus groups such as the Spine Trauma Study Group (STSG) will also provide a more global perspective on the epidemiology of spinal cord and spinal column injuries.

Prevention strategies have had a significant impact on the incidence of SCI. Tremendous progress has been made preventing injuries in sports such as diving[40–42] and rugby[43] as a result of educational injury prevention programs. However, in new thrill-seeking sports such as snowboarding[44,45] and mountain biking[46] there has been a rising number of spinal injuries, and future studies must determine the epidemiology of these injuries and the effect of protective equipment so that injury prevention programs can be targeted. Fall-induced injuries represent a major health problem highlighting a need for fall prevention measures and proactive treatments for osteoporosis.

Demographics

The average age at the time of SCI worldwide is reported to be the early thirties, with the exception of Taiwan and Portugal, which report late forties and early fifties.[31] Presumably related to an aging population, the mean age at the time of injury has increased in North America from 28.6 years in the 1970s to 38.0 years in 2000. Concordantly there has been an increase in the proportion of individuals with SCI over the age of 60 rising from 4.7% prior to 1980 to 10.9% in 2000.[47] There has also been a shift in the ratio of men to women with SCI. In earlier studies the ratio was 4.8:1, and more recent studies report 3.8:1.[31] This shift toward more women sustaining SCIs is expected to continue due to changes in the workplace, increased participation in high-risk sporting activities, and a higher incidence of osteoporosis in women.[4]

As the population continues to age, the role of comorbidities and their impact on patient outcome will need to be assessed. In the trauma literature it is estimated that between 5 and 37%[32,48] of patients have comorbidities at the time of injury. The sequelae that develop following injury are also receiving more attention in the literature. Problems with spasticity, neuropathic pain, and bowel, bladder, and sexual dysfunction are common following SCI and have been identified as priority research areas by this patient population.[49,50] Future care must incorporate patient education and ensure appropriate follow-up by health care providers to ameliorate the impact of these conditions.

Etiology

In North America motor vehicle crashes have remained the number one cause of SCI, accounting for ~50% of all injuries followed by falls (21%), violence (11%), sports/recreation (10%), and other causes (8%).[36,40,47,51–53] There are some differences among countries in the etiology of SCI. According to American statistics from the year 2000 violence accounted for 11% of all SCI cases, whereas in Canada violence was the cause in only 4% from 1997 to 2001.[34,54] One of the most noticeable trends in causation seems to be the increasing number of spinal injuries due to falls in the elderly of industrialized countries. For example, in Finland, the incidence of SCI due to falls increased from 5.2 per 100,000 in 1970 to 12.0 in 2004 and could not be explained by demographics alone.[55]

Types of Injuries

The cervical spine has remained the most common anatomical region for SCI, accounting for 55% of injuries.[56] Due to advances in critical care medicine there are fewer deaths resulting from high cervical lesions. Unsurprisingly, the number of patients discharged from hospital on a ventilator has increased from 2.3 to 6.8%.[40] A study in Australia forecast a 143% increase in the number of individuals sustaining incomplete tetraplegia, rising from 88 cases per year in 1997 to 214 cases in 2021 due to an aging population and a higher incidence of SCI in the elderly.[57]

Life Expectancy and Mortality

Although survival has significantly improved after SCI, life expectancy is still lower when compared with the general population.[47,48,58] An Australian study reported the 1-year survival from SCI to be 95% of the general population based on age and gender and 92% at 10 years. Similar trends in survival are being reported in other industrialized countries such as Denmark and the United States.[58,59] Very little information is available in developing countries; it is generally unknown whether they have benefited from advances in medical care.[60] In industrialized countries causes of mortality have changed, with respiratory infections now the primary cause of death instead of genitourinary disease.[47,48,58] Factors such as age at injury, gender, neurological level, and type of injury are important determinants of survival.[60]

A concerted effort is needed to promote health and reduce the burden of chronic disease in the SCI population. Heart disease now ranks second as a cause of death in individuals living with SCI in both the United States and Norway.[47,61] The rising epidemic of obesity, particularly in the United States, will have a dramatic impact on mortality of the spine trauma population. A recent study of severely injured blunt trauma patients reported a higher number of deaths in obese compared with nonobese patients (32% vs 16%, $p = 0.008$). This concerning trend has resulted in new research developing evidence-based physical activity for individuals with SCI such as the Study of Health and Activity in People with SCI (SHAPE SCI).[62]

◆ Changes in the Management of Spine and Spinal Cord Injuries

Spine Trauma Care Systems

Trauma care in industrialized nations has evolved from local to regional care systems. Such programs deliver treatment pathways that span the continuum from prevention, through acute care, and to reintegration into the community.[63,64] These changes have resulted in a 10% reduction in mortality.[65–71]

Dedicated SCI units were first introduced to treat injured soldiers during the Second World War.[72] These specialized units have since been shown to improve patient outcome and have led to a reduction in complications and length of stay.[37,41,73–75] Common sense suggests that we will see similar trends through the provision of regionalized specialist care for spinal column injuries. For the spine trauma community regionalization has tremendous advantages, including enhancing standardized care, accessing patients for clinical trials, developing benchmarks for national spinal trauma outcomes facilitating population-based studies through registries, and having the ability to intervene in a timely fashion with new repair and regeneration interventions should these become available.

Spine trauma registries have become highly sophisticated and can now provide information important to understanding and improving patient care. Statistics are slowly becoming available detailing the number of prehospital deaths, survival following hospital discharge (i.e., 30-day survival),[65,67,76] and measures of functional status, utility, and health-related quality of life (HRQoL) as opposed to the more traditional method of mortality as a measure of interventional effectiveness.[67,77] With measured interpretation such a wealth of data will facilitate directed development of the care pathways.

Prehospital Care

When considering spinal trauma in a global context the extreme variability of prehospital care is striking. Absence of organized prehospital care in some developing countries is in sharp contrast to advanced systems in some industrialized countries where a trained physician can be rapidly placed at the scene of the injury enabling optimized acute management.[76] Tremendous variability in patient mix, process of care, and performance seen in systems worldwide[76,78] demand a minimum dataset with standard definitions for the prehospital phase of care to compare countries and facilitate international studies.

The benefits of prehospital care have been documented in the spine trauma population. Advances in prehospital screening have reduced the incidence of misdiagnosis in the field from 19 to 5%,[36,43] resulting in less neurological deterioration.[33,47] Recently there has been an interest in determining the role of immobilization at the scene of injury. Further research is needed to determine which patients need to be immobilized and how they should be immobilized.[79]

Acute Diagnostics

Advances in the speed and accuracy of diagnostic imaging such as computed tomography (CT) and magnetic resonance imaging (MRI) in concert with evidence-based guidelines for the use of imaging in suspected and established spine trauma have revolutionized assessment of acute spinal injury over the last decade. Two questions in this field that remain difficult to answer involve imaging of the cervical spine (1) in the patient with minor trauma, and (2) in the unconscious polytrauma patient. The Canadian C Spine Rules, a prospective study that developed guidelines for when to obtain plain radiographs in the alert trauma patient, has addressed the former problem.[80] Supplementary guidelines are required for geriatric and pediatric patients.[81]

Despite extensive research it has been more challenging to develop a protocol for cervical spine clearance in the obtunded patient. To facilitate nursing and medical care of these patients it is beneficial to declare the cervical spine as being stable. The process balances this benefit against the risk of failing to identify an unstable injury that may lead to SCI. In the hands of experienced personnel flexion/extension views can probably exclude frank instability in adults; however, some soft tissue injuries (notably herniated cervical disk) and SCIs may not be identified.[82] MRI provides the answers to these questions with the obvious, though receding, issue surrounding availability. CT is now the first-line evaluation of the cervical and thoracolumbar spine in the polytrauma patient.[82–84] CT is quicker, more cost-effective, and more diagnostically accurate than plain x-rays.[85] The lateral C spine x-ray with its inherent difficulties in obtaining radiographic adequacy has largely been made obsolete.

Despite these quantum leaps in imaging, clinical acumen remains fundamental to determining pretest likelihood and thus achieving the highest diagnostic accuracy. In the acute trauma phase one must decide whether the risk of delaying treatment to obtain further imaging is outweighed by the benefit of additional information. This quandary is illustrated by the patient with an incomplete neurological deficit resulting from a cervical facet injury requiring reduction and the risk of a damaged disk causing further neurological insult on manipulation. It may be prudent to proceed directly to anterior diskectomy, reduction, and fusion given the established utility of the procedure,[86] rather than accept the risks associated with delay and immobilization to perform an MRI.

Surgical Treatment

Instrumentation

There has been an exponential growth over the last 15 to 20 years in the surgical options and technologies available to spinal surgeons, significantly changing the face of surgical intervention for spinal injuries. Diagnostic imaging has enabled accurate spinal cord and column visualization, not only enhancing preoperative planning for implant placement but also directing the choice of surgical approach to enable adequate decompression. As a result of advances in biomaterial properties and new surgical techniques restoration of spinal column alignment has become relatively easy compared with the challenges faced by previous generations of spinal surgeons. Examples of this evolution can be found in anterior cervical locking plates and posterior segmental rigid fixation systems, which arguably render the halo vest somewhat obsolete.[87] C1–C2 transarticular, C1 lateral mass, C2 pars/laminar, and various anterior C1–C2 fixation techniques[88,89] are addressing previously daunting anatomical and biomechanical challenges at the occipitocervical junction. Halo vest immobilization remains a gold standard for reduction and stabilization of odontoid fractures; however, anterior odontoid fixation has gained widespread popularity. Nonetheless, proof of theoretical and perceived superiority must await the results of appropriately powered prospective, randomized studies now in progress.

Safe, minimally invasive surgery is currently not feasible in cervical trauma. However, with improvements in intraoperative CT and MRI, spinal surgeons will soon be able to accurately identify anatomical landmarks and pathology that will make it possible. A synergy between new image guidance technologies and percutaneous/endoscopic techniques currently used in elective spinal surgery will spawn a raft of new procedures. These should enable the rapid realignment, decompression, precise localization of instrumentation, and thus improved care with less local and systemic morbidity. It is important though that the seemingly obvious and intuitive utility of these techniques not be allowed to overwhelm the fundamental anatomical, biomechanical, and clinical relationships and knowledge that are paramount to optimal surgical care.

Thoracic pedicle screws have enabled appropriately trained surgeons to attain better alignment and more rigid fixation in the thoracic spine without compromising safety and accuracy.[90] The superiority of screws over hooks, or other conventional forms of fixation or treatment, such as bed rest, is yet to be determined. Stiffer and more rigid constructs with fewer points of fixation should, however, lead to shorter constructs sparing adjacent motion segments and allowing more aggressive postoperative mobilization without orthoses. Circumferential spinal column reconstruction has been aided by a spectrum of prosthetic devices. These include fixed and expandable cages, allograft, and new anterior instrumentation systems that can be placed with open or minimally invasive techniques such as endoscopic surgery.[91,92] The hypothetical advantages of endoscopic surgery are tempered by a noticeable surgical learning curve. Issues with respect to applicability of these techniques in the setting of trauma to the thoracic and lumbar spine have not yet been determined.[93]

Surgical decision making in thoracolumbar trauma continues to be one of the most controversial areas in the subspecialty of spinal surgery, particularly as it pertains to burst fractures. Most of the evidence is based on retrospective case series and is insufficient to develop evidence-based guidelines for the treatment of these fractures. Two well-designed systematic reviews have summarized this controversy, one addressing surgical technique[94] and the second examining operative versus nonoperative treatment for thoracolumbar burst fractures.[95] Siebenga's randomized, controlled clinical trial suggested surgery to be more effective than nonoperative management.[96] Higher levels of evidence are often contradictory with regard to the treatment of so-called stable burst fractures based on health-related quality of life (HRQoL),[97] the Roland Morris Disability Questionnaire (RMDQ)-24,[96] and visual analogue scale (VAS). On balance, the weight of evidence suggests that functional outcomes progress satisfactorily regardless of treatment modalities, with the caveat that one well-constructed recent study challenges this premise, acknowledging its small sample size.[96] Future studies must consider outcomes more relevant to cost

issues and early functional recovery and be appropriately powered.

Despite lacking some of the essential components of a comprehensive classification system, traditional thoracolumbar trauma classification systems have contributed to more standardized treatment of thoracolumbar injuries. Work by Vaccaro and the STSG toward a reliable, valid, and clinically relevant classification method is now at the validation stage.[98]

Timing of Surgery

Timing of surgical intervention for spinal trauma continues to generate much discussion and debate as well, particularly as it relates to SCI. It has not been possible to verify the basic science studies that support the early decompression of compromised neurological tissues with similar studies in humans. The large prospective "STASCIS" observational study currently undertaken by Fehlings, Vaccaro, and the STSG is attempting to overcome the complexities of studying this subject identified in previous meta-analysis. The preliminary results of this study corroborate the basic science research suggesting that early decompression may enhance neurological recovery in the patient with SCI.[99] Certainly, in those patients who are neurologically intact there is evidence that expeditious stabilization is probably indicated (within 3 days of injury) to decrease hospital and ICU stay, while reducing complications associated with prolonged immobilization and hospital charges.[100]

Use of Biologics

Increasing utilization of biologics in elective spine surgery has not as yet translated to spine trauma surgery. As minimally invasive surgery gains momentum in the treatment of spine trauma and the cost of biologics decreases, the role for osteoconductive bone substitutes may expand, pending appropriate clinical trials and regulatory clearances.[101-103]

Bioabsorbable implants have gained some credence in orthopedic trauma fracture management. Their perceived role in spine trauma is based on overcoming the limitations of current instrumentation, namely, stress shielding, implant loosening, and image degradation.[104] These polymers are still only at the preclinical or early clinical phase. Pending appropriate clinical trials and regulatory clearances, they hold promise not only for fixation and containment but also for the delivery of bone substitutes and antimicrobials.

Without doubt the most compelling area in biologics is spinal cord regeneration and repair attempting to cure paralysis, a promise scientists have made to patients and clinicians for over 3 decades. Animal research continues to generate promising experimental therapies but has also revealed a daunting complexity of the neurobiological challenges that impede neural repair after injury.[105] Further development of therapeutic strategies will depend upon our understanding of these factors. There is guarded optimism that truly effective therapies for spinal cord injuries will emerge in our generation based on encouraging reports of axonal regeneration and the effect of novel neuroprotective agents such as minocycline and erythropoietin. It is vital that human trials commence only after sound epidemiological evaluation and utilize rigorous clinical assessments, or risk adding to the growing list of negative studies. As research into these and other therapies moves into the clinical arena, physicians with interest and expertise in research methodology will need to take an increasing share of the leadership role, currently in the realm of laboratory researchers, to ensure appropriate clinical relevance and interpretation.

◆ Changes in Assessment of Outcomes of Spine and Spinal Cord Injuries

Assessment of outcomes following spine trauma has shifted from mortality rates and x-ray findings (referred to as a bio-medical model) to more patient-derived information including expectations, personal feelings, satisfaction, and quality of life (referred to as an outcomes model).[106] Researchers and clinicians are redefining what constitutes health by considering the behavioral and social impacts that result from health conditions such as spine trauma. Increasingly, conceptual models such as the International Classification of Functioning, Disability and Health (ICF)[107] are being used worldwide. The ICF, a revised version of the International Classification of Impairments, Disabilities and Handicaps, views health from the perspective of three components: the body, the individual, and society. It recognizes the role of personal factors and environment, providing a comprehensive view of health. International work is under way to establish core sets for individuals with SCI using the ICF.[108] To date, a core set has not been established for spine trauma but datasets designed for the acute and early postacute rehabilitation facilities may prove useful.[109] The development of ICF datasets will further enhance standardization using an internationally accepted terminology and will produce new instruments that measure health in a comprehensive, clinically meaningful manner.

Currently, instruments such as the Short Form 36 (SF-36),[110] World Health Organization Disability Assessment Schedule II (WHODAS II)[111] and the World Health Organization Quality of Life Assessment Short Form (WHOQoL-BREF)[112] have been used worldwide to measure the health status and quality of life in individuals with spine trauma.[53,113–116] Because these instruments have been validated cross-culturally they will ensure that inferences from international studies are valid. The SF-36, WHODAS II, and WHOQoL-BREF are all generic instruments. With the recognition that disease-specific instruments provide unique information specific to the injury, instruments such as the Spinal Cord Independence Measure have been developed to assess functional status by interview.[56] Members of the STSG are developing a disease-specific instrument for spinal column injuries, which will ask patients to compare how they are now with respect to before their injury because it is not possible to obtain baseline data.

In the future we will see innovative psychometric methods such as item response theory used to develop appropriate outcome instruments, and dynamic assessment of patient outcomes through computerized adaptive testing.[117] With rising health care costs there will be a growing demand to incorporate economic evaluations so health planners can evaluate interventions using cost–benefit frameworks.[118] Preference-based instruments such as the Quality of Well-Being Scale,[119] EQ-5D,[120] Health Utility Index,[56] and SF-6D derived from the SF-36[121] provide several options. It is of tremendous benefit to apply economic methods to instruments such as the SF-36, which allows quality-adjusted life-years to be obtained from existing or prospective SF-36 data.[122]

◆ Summary

The twenty-first century finds the spinal community armed with an abundance of new technology and techniques. These advancements, in concert with an expanding wealth of data, should empower it to proceed in an evidence-based manner. It will be extremely important to ensure high-quality multi-center data that will provide the long-awaited answers to important questions in spine trauma. A further challenge will be to oversee practice change enabled by these results within both the industrialized and developing world. There is a clear role for established members of the spine trauma community to act in an advisory capacity to underprivileged countries, facilitating institution of local databases that blend seamlessly with their international equivalents. Additionally, there is a requirement for provision of educational opportunities to surgeons from low-income countries through established educational structures, encouraging the adoption of evidence-based techniques. Subsequent data will enhance generalizability, ensure adequate power, and prevent unconstrained use of new, but not necessarily proven, technology. In this way the changing face of spinal trauma truly takes on global proportions.

References

1. Bailey CS, Fisher CG, Dvorak MF. Type II error in the spine surgical literature. Spine 2004;29:1146–1149

2. Sayer FT, Kronvall E, Nilsson OG. Methylprednisolone treatment in acute spinal cord injury: the myth challenged through a structured analysis of published literature. Spine J 2006;6:335–343

3. Fehlings MG. Editorial: recommendations regarding the use of methyl-prednisolone in acute spinal cord injury: making sense out of the controversy. Spine 2001;26(24, Suppl):S56–S57

4. Nesathurai S. Steroids and spinal cord injury: revisiting the NASCIS 2 and NASCIS 3 trials. J Trauma 1998;45:1088–1093

5. Hurlbert RJ. Methylprednisolone for acute spinal cord injury: an inappropriate standard of care. J Neurosurg 2000;93(1, Suppl):1–7

6. Hurlbert RJ. The role of steroids in acute spinal cord injury: an evidence-based analysis. Spine 2001;26(24, Suppl):S39–S46

7. Coleman WP, Benzel D, Cahill DW, et al. A critical appraisal of the reporting of the National Acute Spinal Cord Injury Studies (II and III) of methylprednisolone in acute spinal cord injury. J Spinal Disord 2000;13:185–199

8. Malchau H, Garellick G, Eisler T, Kärrholm J, Herberts P. Presidential guest address: the Swedish Hip Registry: increasing the sensitivity by patient outcome data. Clin Orthop Relat Res 2005;441:19–29

9. US Department of Education. 2006 Annual Statistical Report for the Model Spinal Cord Injury Care Systems. Birmingham, AL: National Spinal Cord Injury Statistical Center; 2006

10. U.S. Census Bureau. International Data Base. Available at: http://www.census.gov/ipc/www/idb/. Accessed November 15, 2007

11. European Commission. Europe in figures—Eurostat yearbook 2006–07. Luxembourg: Eurostat; 2007

12. World Health Organization. World report on road traffic injury prevention, 2002. Available at: http://www.who.int/violence_injury_prevention. Accessed November 13, 2007

13. Central Intelligence Agency. The World Factbook 2007. Available at: https://www.cia.gov/library/publications/the-world-factbook/index.html. Accessed November 15, 2007

14. National Bureau of Statistics of China. China Statistical Yearbook 2003. Beijing: China Statistical Press; 2004

15. Office of the Registrar General of India. The Census of India 2001: Rural–Urban Distribution of Population in India. Available at: http://www.censusindia.gov.in/. Accessed November 15, 2007

16. World Health Organization. A Health Situation Assessment of the People's Republic of China. Beijing, China: United Nations Health Partners Group in China; 2005

17. Pucher J, Peng Z-R, Mittal N, Zhu Y, Korattyswaroopam N. Urban transport trends and policies in China and India: impacts of rapid economic growth. Transp Rev 2007;27:379–410

18. Hay D, Wei W. Development of occupational safety and health in the People's Republic of China. Ann Occup Hyg 1994;38:79–88

19. Saha A, Ramnath T, Chaudhuri RN, Saiyed HN. An accident-risk assessment study of temporary piece rated workers. Ind Health 2004;42: 240–245

20. Yu TS, Liu YM, Zhou JL, Wong TW. Occupational injuries in Shunde City—a county undergoing rapid economic change in southern China. Accid Anal Prev 1999;31:313–317

21. Sathiyasekaran BWC. Population-based cohort study of injuries. Injury 1996;27:695–698

22. Xia Z, Sorock GS, Zhu J, et al. Fatal occupational injuries in the construction industry of a new development area in East China, 1991 to 1997. AIHAJ 2000;61:733–737

23. Derr J, Forst L, Chen HY, Conroy L. Fatal falls in the US construction industry, 1990 to 1999. J Occup Environ Med 2001;43:853–860

24. Zhou Y, Baker TD, Rao K, Li G. Productivity losses from injury in China. Inj Prev 2003;9:124–127

25. Gururaj G, Thomas AA, Reddi MN. Under reporting of road traffic injuries in Bangalore: implications for road safety policies and programmes. In: Proceedings of the 5th World Conference on Injury Prevention and Control. Delhi: Macmillan India Ltd.; 2000:54–55

26. Stevenson M, Yu J, Ying Z, et al. China Seat Belt Intervention. Beijing, P.R. China; 2007

27. Galasko C, Murray P, Stephenson W. Incidence of whiplash-associated disorder. B C Med J 2002;44:237–240

28. Wu SS, Lachmann E, Nagler W. Current medical, rehabilitation, and surgical management of vertebral compression fractures. J Womens Health (Larchmt) 2003;12:17–26

29. Garfin SR, Yuan HA, Reiley MA. New technologies in spine: kyphoplasty and vertebroplasty for the treatment of painful osteoporotic compression fractures. Spine 2001;26:1511–1515

30. Hu R, Mustard CA, Burns C. Epidemiology of incident spinal fracture in a complete population. Spine 1996;21:492–499

31. Wyndaele M, Wyndaele JJ. Incidence, prevalence and epidemiology of spinal cord injury: what learns a worldwide literature survey? Spinal Cord 2006;44:523–529

32. Bracken MB, Freeman DH Jr, Hellenbrand K. Incidence of acute traumatic hospitalized spinal cord injury in the United States, 1970-1977. Am J Epidemiol 1981;113:615–622

33. Burke DA, Linden RD, Zhang YP, Maiste AC, Shields CB. Incidence rates and populations at risk for spinal cord injury: a regional study. Spinal Cord 2001;39:274–278

34. Dryden DM, Saunders LD, Rowe BH, et al. The epidemiology of traumatic spinal cord injury in Alberta, Canada. Can J Neurol Sci 2003;30:113–121

35. Pickett W, Simpson K, Walker J, Brison RJ. Traumatic spinal cord injury in Ontario, Canada. J Trauma 2003;55:1070–1076

36. Price C, Makintubee S, Herndon W, Istre GR. Epidemiology of traumatic spinal cord injury and acute hospitalization and rehabilitation charges for spinal cord injuries in Oklahoma, 1988-1990. Am J Epidemiol 1994; 139:37–47

37. Burke DC, Burley HT, Ungar GH. Data on spinal injuries, II: Outcome of the treatment of 352 consecutive admissions. Aust N Z J Surg 1985;55: 377–382

38. Kelly DF, Becker DP. Advances in management of neurosurgical trauma: USA and Canada. World J Surg 2001;25:1179–1185

39. DeVivo M, Biering-Sørensen F, Charlifue S, et al; Executive Committee for the International SCI Data Sets Committees. International spinal cord injury core data set. Spinal Cord 2006;44:535–540

40. Jackson AB, Dijkers M, Devivo MJ, Poczatek RB. A demographic profile of new traumatic spinal cord injuries: change and stability over 30 years. Arch Phys Med Rehabil 2004;85:1740–1748

41. Tator CH, Duncan EG, Edmonds VE, Lapczak LI, Andrews DF. Changes in epidemiology of acute spinal cord injury from 1947 to 1981. Surg Neurol 1993;40:207–215

42. Tator CH, Edmonds VE, New ML. Diving: a frequent and potentially preventable cause of spinal cord injury. Can Med Assoc J 1981;124:1323–1324

43. Quarrie KL, Gianotti SM, Hopkins WG, Hume PA. Effect of nationwide injury prevention programme on serious spinal injuries in New Zealand rugby union: ecological study. BMJ 2007;334:1150

44. Tarazi F, Dvorak MF, Wing PC. Spinal injuries in skiers and snowboarders. Am J Sports Med 1999;27:177–180

45. Wakahara K, Matsumoto K, Sumi H, Sumi Y, Shimizu K. Traumatic spinal cord injuries from snowboarding. Am J Sports Med 2006;34:1670–1674

46. Kim PT, Jangra D, Ritchie AH, et al. Mountain biking injuries requiring trauma center admission: a 10-year regional trauma system experience. J Trauma 2006;60:312–318

47. National Spinal Cord Injury Statistical Center. Spinal Cord Injury Facts and Figures at a Glance. 2005. Available at: http://www.spinalcord.uab.edu/show.asp?durki=21446. Accessed June 27, 2005

48. DeVivo MJ, Krause JS, Lammertse DP. Recent trends in mortality and causes of death among persons with spinal cord injury. Arch Phys Med Rehabil 1999;80:1411–1419

49. Anderson KD. Targeting recovery: priorities of the spinal cord-injured population. J Neurotrauma 2004;21:1371–1383

50. Bloemen-Vrencken JH, Post MW, Hendriks JM, De Reus EC, De Witte LP. Health problems of persons with spinal cord injury living in the Netherlands. Disabil Rehabil 2005;27:1381–1389

51. Kraus JF, Franti CE, Riggins RS, Richards D, Borhani NO. Incidence of traumatic spinal cord lesions. J Chronic Dis 1975;28:471–492

52. Thurman DJ, Burnett CL, Jeppson L, Beaudoin DE, Sniezek JE. Surveillance of spinal cord injuries in Utah, USA. Paraplegia 1994;32:665–669

53. Fisher CG, Noonan VK, Smith DE, et al. Motor recovery, functional status, and health-related quality of life in patients with complete spinal cord injuries. Spine 2005;30:2200–2207

54. Canadian Institutes of Health Information. National Trauma Registry 2003 Report. Hospital Injury Admissions 2000/2001 data. Ottawa: Canadian Institutes of Health Information; 2003

55. Kannus P, Niemi S, Parkkari J, Palvanen M, Sievänen H. Alarming rise in fall-induced severe head injuries among elderly people. Injury 2007; 38:81–83

56. Itzkovich M, Tamir A, Philo O, et al. Reliability of the Catz-Itzkovich Spinal Cord Independence Measure assessment by interview and comparison with observation. Am J Phys Med Rehabil 2003;82:267–272

57. O'Connor PJ. Forecasting of spinal cord injury annual case numbers in Australia. Arch Phys Med Rehabil 2005;86:48–51

58. Frankel HL, Coll JR, Charlifue SW, et al. Long-term survival in spinal cord injury: a fifty year investigation. Spinal Cord 1998;36:266–274

59. Davis JW, Phreaner DL, Hoyt DB, Mackersie RC. The etiology of missed cervical spine injuries. J Trauma 1993;34:342–346

60. O'Connor PJ. Survival after spinal cord injury in Australia. Arch Phys Med Rehabil 2005;86:37–47

61. Lidal IB, Huynh TK, Biering-Sørensen F. Return to work following spinal cord injury: a review. Disabil Rehabil 2007;29:1341–1375

62. Adams MM, Ginis KA, Hicks AL. The spinal cord injury spasticity evaluation tool: development and evaluation. Arch Phys Med Rehabil 2007;88(9, Issue 9):1185–1192

63. Liberman M, Mulder DS, Jurkovich GJ, Sampalis JS. The association between trauma system and trauma center components and outcome in a mature regionalized trauma system. Surgery 2005;137:647–658

64. Simons R, Kirkpatrick A. Assuring optimal trauma care: the role of trauma centre accreditation. Can J Surg 2002;45:288–295

65. Jurkovich GJ, Mock C. Systematic review of trauma system effectiveness based on registry comparisons. J Trauma 1999;47(3, Suppl):S46–S55

66. Liberman M, Mulder DS, Lavoie A, Sampalis JS. Implementation of a trauma care system: evolution through evaluation. J Trauma 2004;56: 1330–1335

67. Mann NC, Mullins RJ, MacKenzie EJ, Jurkovich GJ, Mock CN. Systematic review of published evidence regarding trauma system effectiveness. J Trauma 1999;47(3, Suppl):S25–S33

68. Mullins RJ, Mann NC. Population-based research assessing the effectiveness of trauma systems. J Trauma 1999;47(3, Suppl):S59–S66

69. Nathens AB, Jurkovich GJ, Cummings P, Rivara FP, Maier RV. The effect of organized systems of trauma care on motor vehicle crash mortality. JAMA 2000;283:1990–1994

70. Sampalis JS, Denis R, Lavoie A, et al. Trauma care regionalization: a process-outcome evaluation. J Trauma 1999;46:565–579, discussion 579–581

71. Séguin J, Garber BG, Coyle D, Hébert PC. An economic evaluation of trauma care in a Canadian lead trauma hospital. J Trauma 1999;47(3, Suppl):S99–S103

72. Guttmann L. I. Organisation of spinal units. History of the National Spinal Injuries Centre, Stoke Mandeville Hospital, Aylesbury. Paraplegia 1967;5:115–126

73. DeVivo MJ, Kartus PL, Stover SL, Fine PR. Benefits of early admission to an organised spinal cord injury care system. Paraplegia 1990;28:545–555

74. Dunn M, Love L, Ravesloot C. Subjective health in spinal cord injury after outpatient healthcare follow-up. Spinal Cord 2000;38:84–91

75. Smith M. Efficacy of specialist versus non-specialist management of spinal cord injury within the UK. Spinal Cord 2002;40:10–16

76. Roudsari BS, Nathens AB, Cameron P, et al. International comparison of prehospital trauma care systems. Injury 2007;38:993–1000

77. Mann NC, Mullins RJ. Research recommendations and proposed action items to facilitate trauma system implementation and evaluation. J Trauma 1999;47(3, Suppl):S75–S78

78. Roudsari BS, Nathens AB, Arreola-Risa C, et al. Emergency Medical Service (EMS) systems in developed and developing countries. Injury 2007; 38:1001–1013

79. Hauswald M, Braude D. Spinal immobilization in trauma patients: is it really necessary? Curr Opin Crit Care 2002;8:566–570

80. Stiell IG, Clement CM, McKnight RD, et al. The Canadian C-spine rule versus the NEXUS low-risk criteria in patients with trauma. N Engl J Med 2003;349:2510–2518

81. Bub LD, Blackmore CC, Mann FA, Lomoschitz FM. Cervical spine fractures in patients 65 years and older: a clinical prediction rule for blunt trauma. Radiology 2005;234:143–149

82. Tins BJ, Cassar-Pullicino VN. Imaging of acute cervical spine injuries: review and outlook. Clin Radiol 2004;59:865–880

83. Richards PJ. Cervical spine clearance: a review. Injury 2005;36:248–269, discussion 270

84. Sheridan R, Peralta R, Rhea J, Ptak T, Novelline R. Reformatted visceral protocol helical computed tomographic scanning allows conventional radiographs of the thoracic and lumbar spine to be eliminated in the evaluation of blunt trauma patients. J Trauma 2003;55:665–669

85. Blackmore CC, Ramsey SD, Mann FA, Deyo RA. Cervical spine screening with CT in trauma patients: a cost-effectiveness analysis. Radiology 1999;212:117–125

86. Kwon BK, Fisher CG, Boyd MC, et al. A prospective randomized controlled trial of anterior compared with posterior stabilization for unilateral facet injuries of the cervical spine. J Neurosurg Spine 2007; 7:1–12

87. Vender JR, Rekito AJ, Harrison SJ, McDonnell DE. The evolution of posterior cervical and occipitocervical fusion and instrumentation. Neurosurg Focus 2004;16:E9

88. Dvorak MF, Fisher C, Boyd M, Johnson M, Greenhow R, Oxland TR. Anterior occiput-to-axis screw fixation: part I: a case report, description of a new technique, and anatomical feasibility analysis. Spine 2003;28:E54–E60

89. Dvorak MF, Sekeramayi F, Zhu Q, et al. Anterior occiput to axis screw fixation, II: A biomechanical comparison with posterior fixation techniques. Spine 2003;28:239–245

90. Fisher C, Sahajpal V, Keynan O, et al. Accuracy and Safety of Pedicle Screw Fixation in Thoracic Trauma. J Neurosurg Spine 2006;5(6): 520–526

91. Dvorak MF, Kwon BK, Fisher CG, Eiserloh HL III, Boyd M, Wing PC. Effectiveness of titanium mesh cylindrical cages in anterior column reconstruction after thoracic and lumbar vertebral body resection. Spine 2003;28:902–908

92. Horn EM, Henn JS, Lemole GM Jr, Hott JS, Dickman CA. Thoracoscopic placement of dual-rod instrumentation in thoracic spinal trauma. Neurosurgery 2004;54:1150–1153, discussion 1153–1154

93. Wimberley DW, Goyal N, Goins ML, Zeiller SC, Yuan PS, Vaccaro AR. Advances in surgical techniques and instrumentation and their impact on the spinal cord injury rehabilitation process. Top Spinal Cord Inj Rehabil 2004;10:35–48

94. Verlaan JJ, Diekerhof CH, Buskens E, et al. Surgical treatment of traumatic fractures of the thoracic and lumbar spine: a systematic review of the literature on techniques, complications, and outcome. Spine 2004;29:803–814

95. Thomas K, Bailey C, Dvorak M, Kwon B, Fisher C. Comparison of Operative and Nonoperative Treatment for Thoracolumbar Burst Fractures in Patients without Neurologic Deficit: A Systematic Review. J Neurosurg 2006;4(5):351–358

96. Siebenga J, Leferink VJM, Segers MJM, et al. Treatment of traumatic thoracolumbar spine fractures: a multicenter prospective randomized study of operative versus nonsurgical treatment. Spine 2006;31: 2881–2890

97. Wood K, Buttermann G, Mehbod A, et al. Operative compared with nonoperative treatment of a thoracolumbar burst fracture without neurological deficit: a prospective, randomized study. J Bone Joint Surg Am 2003;85-A:773–781

98. Vaccaro AR, Zeiller SC, Hulbert RJ, et al. The thoracolumbar injury severity score: a proposed treatment algorithm. J Spinal Disord Tech 2005;18:209–215

99. La Rosa G, Conti A, Cardali S, Cacciola F, Tomasello F. Does early decompression improve neurological outcome of spinal cord injured patients? Appraisal of the literature using a meta-analytical approach. Spinal Cord 2004;42:503–512

100. Fehlings MF, Dvorak M, Fisher C, Aarabi B, Shaffrey C, Vaccaro ARA. Prospective, multicenter trial to evaluate the role and timing of decompression in patients with cervical spinal cord injury: initial one year results of the STASCIS study. Presented at the ASIA Symposium; Boston; June 24, 2006

101. Kerwin AJ, Frykberg ER, Schinco MA, Griffen MM, Murphy T, Tepas JJ. The effect of early spine fixation on non-neurologic outcome. J Trauma 2005;58:15–21

102. Verlaan JJ, Dhert WJ, Verbout AJ, Oner FC. Balloon vertebroplasty in combination with pedicle screw instrumentation: a novel technique to treat thoracic and lumbar burst fractures. Spine 2005;30:E73–E79

103. Blattert TR, Delling G, Dalal PS, Toth CA, Balling H, Weckbach A. Successful transpedicular lumbar interbody fusion by means of a composite of osteogenic protein-1 (rhBMP-7) and hydroxyapatite carrier: a comparison with autograft and hydroxyapatite in the sheep spine. Spine 2002;27:2697–2705

104. Cho DY, Lee WY, Sheu PC. Treatment of thoracolumbar burst fractures with polymethyl methacrylate vertebroplasty and short-segment pedicle screw fixation. Neurosurgery 2003;53:1354–1360, discussion 1360–1361

105. Vaccaro AR, Madigan L, Fitzhenry L, Eichenbaum M, Robbins M. Bioabsorbable instrumentation in treatment of cervical degenerative and traumatic disorders. Curr Opin Orthop 2004;15:192–195

106. Kwon BK, Fisher CG, Dvorak MF, Tetzlaff W. Strategies to promote neural repair and regeneration after spinal cord injury. Spine 2005; 30(17, Suppl):S3–S13

107. Korolija D, Wood-Dauphinee S, Pointner R. Patient-reported outcomes: how important are they? Surg Endosc 2007;21:503–507

108. World Health Organization. International Classification of Functioning, Disability and Health. Geneva: World Health Organization; 2001

109. Biering-Sørensen F, Scheuringer M, Baumberger M, et al. Developing core sets for persons with spinal cord injuries based on the International Classification of Functioning, Disability and Health as a way to specify functioning. Spinal Cord 2006;44:541–546

110. Stucki G, Ustün TB, Melvin J. Applying the ICF for the acute hospital and early post-acute rehabilitation facilities. Disabil Rehabil 2005; 27:349–352

111. Ware J Jr, Kosinski M, Gandek B. SF-36 Health Survey: Manual and Interpretation Guide. Lincoln: Quality Metric Incorporated; 2000

112. World Health Organization. WHODAS II. Available at: http://www.who.int/icidh/whodas. November 2001. Accessed March 10, 2006

113. The WHOQOL Group. Development of the World Health Organization WHOQOL-BREF quality of life assessment. Psychol Med 1998;28: 551–558

114. Dvorak MF, Johnson MG, Boyd M, Johnson G, Kwon BK, Fisher CG. Long-term health-related quality of life outcomes following Jefferson-type burst fractures of the atlas. J Neurosurg Spine 2005;2:411–417

115. Jang Y, Hsieh CL, Wang YH, Wu YH. A validity study of the WHOQOL-BREF assessment in persons with traumatic spinal cord injury. Arch Phys Med Rehabil 2004;85:1890–1895

116. Lin MR, Hwang HF, Chen CY, Chiu WT. Comparisons of the brief form of the World Health Organization Quality of Life and Short Form-36 for persons with spinal cord injuries. Am J Phys Med Rehabil 2007;86: 104–113

117. Soberg HL, Bautz-Holter E, Roise O, Finset A. Long-term multidimensional functional consequences of severe multiple injuries two years after trauma: a prospective longitudinal cohort study. J Trauma 2007; 62:461–470

118. Ware JE Jr. Conceptualization and measurement of health-related quality of life: comments on an evolving field. Arch Phys Med Rehabil 2003;84(4, Suppl 2):S43–S51

119. Robinson R. Economic evaluation and health care. What does it mean? BMJ 1993;307:670–673

120. Kaplan RM, Bush JW, Berry CC. Health status: types of validity and the index of well-being. Health Serv Res 1976;11:478–507

121. Brooks R. EuroQol: the current state of play. Health Policy 1996;37:53–72

122. Brazier J, Roberts J, Deverill M. The estimation of a preference-based measure of health from the SF-36. J Health Econ 2002;21:271–292

6

Spinal Embryology and Anatomy of the Pediatric and Adult Spine

Michael M. Vosbikian, Joseph L. Petfield, James P. Lawrence, Jeffrey Rihn, Eric B. Harris, and Alexander R. Vaccaro

◆ Embryology of the Spine

The spine and the neural axis serve to facilitate bodily motion, maintain structural integrity and erect posture, transmit complex signaling to and from the brain, and coordinate motor, sensory, and autonomic pathways. The spine and spinal cord are themselves composed of several different tissue types responsible for these varied functions. The embryological development of the human spinal column and spinal cord is a complex process resulting in the formation of sophisticated and vital body structures. Despite tremendous advancements in the molecular and biological techniques made available through decades of modern research, the embryological development of the spine and the nervous system remains incompletely understood. A complex cascade of molecular signaling events is involved in the congenital development of the spinal and neural elements. Alterations in these important developmental steps can result in congenital variations and abnormalities, some of which can compromise the integrity and function of these structures in the developing and mature human, potentially resulting in neurological dysfunction or an increased susceptibility to neurological injury from minor trauma.

Early Embryological Origins of the Spine

The formation of the spine, as well as the body's form as a whole, begins during the period of gastrulation (**Fig. 6.1**), in which the bilaminar embryonic disk transforms into the trilaminar embryonic disk. This process occurs early in the third week following fertilization and is characterized by the invagination of ectodermal cells through the primitive groove of the primitive streak, creating the embryonic mesoderm. A convergence of invaginating intraembryonic mesoderm cells at the cranial end of the primitive streak forms the primitive pit or node.[1] The continuously infolding cells at the primitive node form a conduit that is continuous with the amniotic cavity termed the notochordal tube. These invaginating cells move in a cephalad direction and attach to the embryonic endoderm to form the notochordal plate, which subsequently matures to create the notochord.[2] The migration of cells forming the notochord is controlled by the chemotactic factors fibroblast growth factor-4 and fibroblast growth factor-8.[1,3] The presence of the notochord induces the overlying ectodermal cells to proliferate and thicken to form the neural plate. At ~19 days, this neuroectodermal tissue will curl up to form the neural groove, which subsequently closes to become the neural tube.

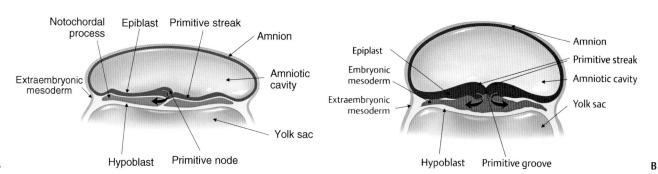

Fig. 6.1 **(A)** Gastrulation: invagination of ectodermal cells to create the embryonic mesoderm. **(B)** The creation of a trilaminar disk as a result of gastrulation.

The notochord also plays a pivotal role later in fetal development in coordinating the maturation of the vertebral column.[4]

Invaginating cells that migrate more laterally differentiate into three main regions: paraxial, intermediate, and lateral plate mesoderm.[1,5] These mesodermal precursors will develop to form the spinal column, urogenital system, and gut cavity, respectively. This close spatial developmental relationship may be the reason that there is a significant association of vertebral abnormalities occurring with genitourinary abnormalities.[6–8] The paraxial mesoderm develops into 42 to 44 pairs of somites over a period of a few days. Somites develop in a cranial-to-caudal fashion, and their number can serve as an estimate of embryonic age. These structures are perhaps the most obvious example of the embryological concept of metamers, in which multiple anatomically similar units are arranged linearly to form a sophisticated structure or organ. Each individual somite

further differentiates into two major regions. The dorsolateral area of the somite, made up of the dermatome and myotome, will mature to eventually form the spinal musculature and overlying dermis of the skin, respectively. The ventromedial region, the sclerotome of the somite, is the precursor to the vertebral column of the developing human.[1] The neural tube differentiates to form the spinal cord (**Fig. 6.2**).[2]

Development of the Vertebral Column

As gestational development continues into weeks 4 and 5, the formation of individual vertebral bodies from the metameric somites occurs. This process is best explained by the theory of resegmentation, in which each sclerotome divides into a rostral and caudal half. Individual vertebrae are formed from

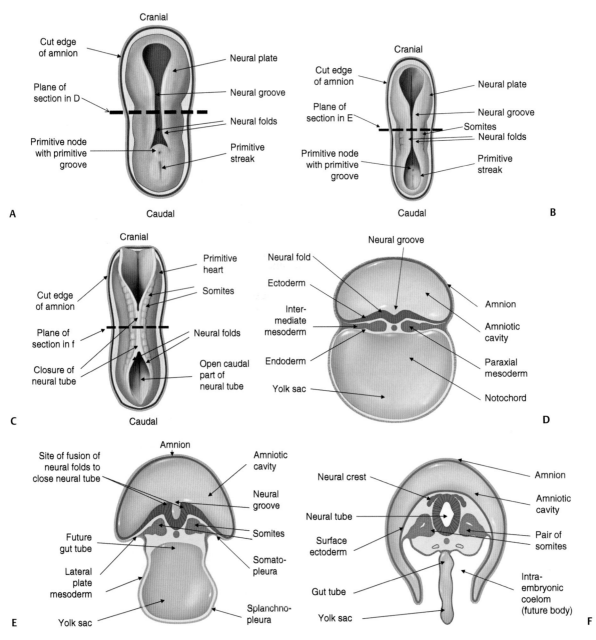

Fig. 6.2 **(A)** Dorsal view of the neural groove. **(B)** Dorsal view of the formation of somites. **(C)** Dorsal view of the closure of the neural groove. **(D)** Transverse view of the beginning of neural crest cell migration. **(E)** Transverse view of the neural groove. **(F)** Transverse view of the neural tube, neural crest, and forming somites.

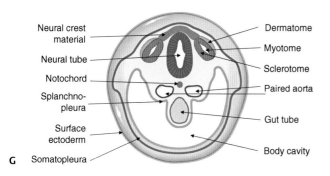

Neural crest material

Neural tube

Notochord

Splanchno-pleura

Surface ectoderm

G Somatopleura

Dermatome

Myotome

Sclerotome

Paired aorta

Gut tube

Body cavity

Fig. 6.2 *(Continued)* **(G)** Transverse view of the neural tube, notochord, paired aortae, and somites consisting of myotome and sclerotome.

the caudal half of one sclerotome and the cranial half of the adjacent sclerotome (**Fig. 6.3**). The fusion of these two sclerotomes forms the centrum, which will become an individual vertebral body.[1,9] Each vertebra formed has accompanying segmental arteries and nerves. Resegmentation theory has been proven experimentally in chick embryo models.[2,10,11] Patterning of the vertebrae during resegmentation is influenced by the *HOX* and *Pax* genes.[1,2] It has also been recently suggested that the notochord may play a role in coordinating this resegmentation.[12] Mesodermal cells adjacent to the neural tube develop into the neural arches, the lamina and pedicle, which serve to protect the structures traveling through the vertebral canal.[5]

The notochord is the central axis for the newly formed centra, and it eventually disintegrates between the vertebrae as chondrification progresses, but it enlarges at the intervertebral disk to contribute to the nucleus pulposus.[2] Cells of the sclerotome proliferate to form the surrounding anulus fibrosus. During week 6, molecular factors from the notochord and neural tube signal the initiation of vertebral chondrification. Two chondrification centers in the centrum fuse to form a single large segment of cartilage.[2,5] A single chondrification center is located on each vertebral arch, which subsequently grows to fuse with the opposing arch. Ossification of this cartilaginous precursor begins around week 9 of development. Three ossification centers can be found in each vertebra, one located in the centrum and one in each half of the vertebral arch. Ossification begins in the lower thoracic vertebrae and proceeds from this point both cranially and caudally.[4] This continual, slow process proceeds well after birth because the halves of the vertebral arch do not completely fuse until approximately 6 years of age.[5]

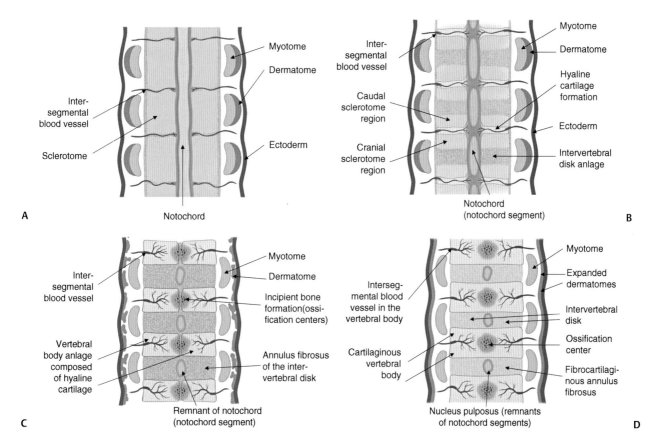

Fig. 6.3 **(A)** View of sclerotomes around the notochord separated by arteries located between segments. **(B)** Resegmentation of the sclerotomes into rostral and caudal portions. **(C)** Formation of the centrum from the fusion of adjacent sclerotomes. **(D)** Further development into the early vertebral body and intervertebral disk.

Development of the Spinal Cord

As stated, the nervous system begins as a thickened, ectodermal neural plate forming immediately overlying the notochord. As proliferation continues, the edges of the neural plate fold up and eventually fuse to form the neural tube. Failure of neural tube closure results in the congenital defect termed spina bifida cystica (myelomeningocele).[1] Around week 5 of fetal development, proliferation within the neural tube creates dorsal and ventral pairs of swellings, the alar and basal plate. These swellings are separated structurally by the sulcus limitans and will eventually become the sensory and motor tracts, respectively. The sulcus limitans disappears during week 6 because of continual proliferation. The previously divided structures, however, retain their respective functions. Dorsal and ventral horns appear as fetal growth progresses with white matter tracts beginning to appear around weeks 7 to 8.[2]

Maturation of the Spine in Childhood and Adolescence

The continued growth of the spinal column throughout childhood and adolescence provides a mechanical axis for all movement of the appendicular skeleton and also allows the safe passage of the spinal cord and nerve roots. Ossification of the spine continues after birth from the three primary ossification centers consisting of the centrum and the vertebral arches. Interestingly, humans are unlike most other vertebrates in that the centrum does not form true end plate physes and epiphyses, but rather a thin, chondroepiphyseal region at the end plates, which also contributes to circumferential growth.[13] A pair of neurocentral synchondroses at the junction of the pedicles to the vertebral body and a single posterior synchondrosis at the head of the neural arch provide for continued growth of the vertebrae and expansion of the spinal canal.[14] These synchondroses are easily visualized on conventional radiographs as radiolucent clefts and should not be mistaken for a fracture or malformation. The spinal canal reaches its adult diameter during the ages of 6 to 8 years, upon closure of the neurocentral synchondroses.[15] Early fusion or asymmetric growth of these synchondroses may result in the development of spinal stenosis or scoliosis.[14]

Initially, the neonate is born with an entirely kyphotic spine. This primary curvature remains in the thoracic region, with secondary curvatures of the spine appearing as the child develops. Cervical lordosis develops as the posterior muscles of the cervical spine enlarge and strengthen as a result of the child lifting its head upright. Lumbar lordosis develops later in maturation as the child begins to sit, stand, and walk, and does not completely stabilize until puberty (**Fig. 6.4**).[16] Secondary ossification centers appear in each vertebra at the onset of adolescence and are located at the tips of the spinous, transverse, and articulating processes and at both the superior and inferior ring epiphyses of the vertebral corpora.[17] Like the primary ossification centers, these structures can be visualized radiographically and must be visualized in context during the evaluation of traumatic injury. It must also be noted that incomplete ossification of the vertebrae results in significant differences in signal when visualized with magnetic resonance imaging.[17] Growth at these ossification sites occurs throughout young adulthood, with fusion to the vertebra occurring until ~25 years of age. Upon the cessation of growth, the upper and lower epiphyseal growth plates ossify to form the raised margin, which surrounds each vertebral body and articulates with the adjacent vertebral disk.

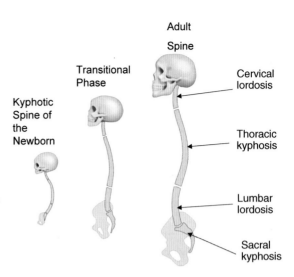

Fig. 6.4 Development of the curvatures of the adult spine.

The overwhelming majority of trauma to the pediatric spine occurs at the cervical level, particularly in younger children.[18] A relatively larger head size relative to a smaller body, considerably decreased neck muscle mass, increased flexibility of the interspinous ligaments, and more horizontally oriented facet joints can increase the potential for injury to the cervical spine.[19,20]

Congenital Malformations and Spinal Trauma

Congenital malformations of the spine can alter the normal anatomy and biomechanics of the spine, create symptomatic premature degeneration of spinal elements, and in some cases predispose the patient to traumatic neurological injury. Developmental disorders are classically defined as defects of formation and defects of segmentation. Congenital scoliosis and kyphosis are among the more common anomalies resulting from these developmental abnormalities. During embryogenesis, failures of formation are caused by the absence of a vertebral structural element. These errors can be partial or complete, resulting in a wedged vertebra or hemivertebra, respectively. Failures of segmentation are produced as the deficiency of normally occurring apoptotic events that facilitate controlled division and can be partial, causing formation of a bar, or complete, causing formation of a block vertebra.

As previously discussed, the development of the spine from paraxial mesoderm occurs in close proximity to the mesodermal precursors of other organs. Congenital abnormalities of the spinal column thus can frequently coexist with anomalies of other organ systems. These comorbid abnormalities have been found to occur in 30 to 60% of children with congenital spine deformity.[21] Vertebral defects make up part of the VACTERL association. This acronym was coined to represent a group of congenital deficiencies that commonly occur in association: vertebral anomalies (V), anal atresia (A), cardiac defects (C), tracheoesophageal fistula (TE), renal dysplasias (R), and limb malformations (L).

Klippel-Feil syndrome occurs in ~1 in 40,000 births and is characterized by congenital synostosis of one or more cervical vertebrae[22] and corresponding abnormalities of the ligamentous, disk, and vascular elements. This disorder results from abnormal segmentation of the cervical vertebrae during embryonic development. Patients with Klippel-Feil syndrome may exhibit decreased flexion, extension, axial rotation, and lateral bending of the cervical spine, as well as cervical instability causing subluxation and impingement of the neural elements.[8]

Several anatomical defects of the cervical spinal cord can result in pathology due to stenosis. Occipitocervical synostosis is defined as the partial or complete fusion of the atlas and the base of the occiput often associated with flattening of the clivus and also referred to as platybasia. Neurological symptoms can result from altered position of the odontoid process, which, because of the decreased height of the atlas, may project into the foramen magnum and apply pressure to the brainstem.[23] These symptoms commonly do not present until the third decade and may be worsened by spinal trauma. Atlanto-occipital and atlantoaxial instability can occur in several developmental disorders, such as Down syndrome,[24] Marfan syndrome,[25] and Morquio syndrome.[26] Ligamentous laxity or odontoid hypoplasia can result in upper cervical subluxation or dislocation and a concomitant higher risk of neurological compromise.[8]

Errors in the formation of the posterior arch of C1 can be associated with neck pain or neurological symptoms. Severity can range from a minor cleft in the posterior arch to near complete absence.[23] Absence of a lateral facet of C1 has also been reported, which presents with severe torticollis. This disorder may accompany Klippel-Feil syndrome or other deficits of the cervical spine. Abnormalities in blood supply to the upper cervical spine have also been noted with this disorder and may have considerable consequences during surgical intervention.

Congenital spinal stenosis of the cervical spine has been shown to predispose adults to neurological deficit. Specifically, developmental stenosis defined by a Torg ratio of 0.8 is highly sensitive to transient neuropraxia.[27,28] It is not, however, associated with increased risk of permanent, catastrophic spinal cord injury.[29]

◆ Anatomy of the Adult Spine

The normally developed human spine is composed of a column of 33 bony vertebrae that provide stability and posture to the human body. The individual vertebrae are grouped into cervical, thoracic, lumbar, sacral, and coccygeal regions. The most superior region of the vertebral column is the lordotic cervical spine, which consists of seven vertebrae that provide the structure for the neck and support for the head. The kyphotic thoracic spine is composed of 12 vertebrae that articulate with the ribs. The lordotic lumbar spine consists of five vertebrae, the most caudal of which articulates with the sacrum, which, respectively, articulates with the pelvis. The sacrum consists of four vertebrae that are typically fused. Finally, the coccyx, a similarly fused region made up of five successively smaller vertebrae and likely representing a vestigial tail, is the most caudal region of the spine. Between adjacent vertebrae, there are bilateral pathways called neuroforamina through which each of the paired 31 spinal nerves will emerge (**Fig. 6.5**).

The Vertebrae

The vertebrae have slight anatomical variation from region to region (**Fig. 6.6**). All vertebrae from C3 to L5 consist of an

anterior vertebral body connected via paired pedicles to the posterior elements, which are composed of articular processes that form the bilateral facet joints, and the posteriorly sweeping laminae, which coalesce as they near the midline to form the spinous processes. Above the superior articular process of each facet joint is the pars interarticularis, which sweeps superiorly and laterally, giving rise to the inferior articular process of the facet above before transitioning into the lateral mass in the cervical spine and the transverse process in the thoracic and lumbar spine.

The atlantoaxial complex is composed of the first and second cervical vertebra. This complex forms a base upon which the skull rests. The unique anatomy of C1, or the atlas, and C2, or the axis, allows for ~50% of total cervical rotational and 50% of total cervical sagittal plane motion. The ringlike atlas is distinguished from the subaxial vertebrae by the absence of a true vertebral body and spinous process as well as the presence of bilateral posterior and superior grooves within which the paired vertebral arteries run prior to ascending through the foramen magnum. In addition to the articulations with the skull base, a true synovial joint lies on the posterior aspect of the anterior portion of the C1 ring

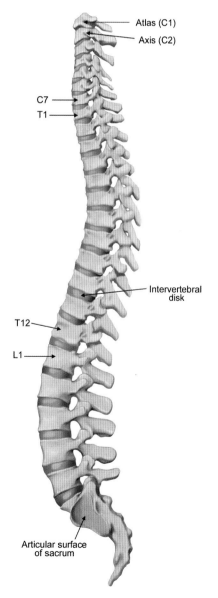

Atlas (C1)
Axis (C2)
C7
T1
Intervertebral disk
T12
L1
Articular surface of sacrum

Fig. 6.5 The bony spinal column: left lateral view.

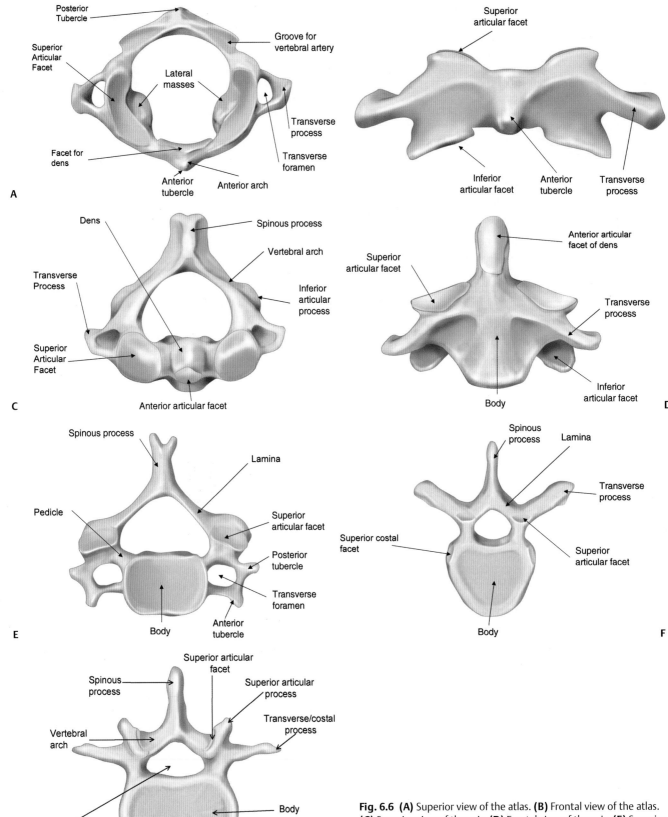

Fig. 6.6 (A) Superior view of the atlas. **(B)** Frontal view of the atlas. **(C)** Superior view of the axis. **(D)** Frontal view of the axis. **(E)** Superior view of a characteristic cervical vertebra. **(F)** Superior view of a characteristic thoracic vertebra. **(G)** Superior view of a characteristic lumbar vertebra.

where it articulates with the peglike portion of the C2 vertebrae known as the odontoid process, or dens. This articulation allows the majority of rotation of the head as well as prevents excessive anterior-posterior translation of the skull.

Stability at this joint is of paramount importance in maintaining adequate space for the spinal cord. A ligamentous complex consisting of oblique, transverse, and alar ligaments maintains stability at this articulation.

The 12 vertebrae of the thoracic spine also have characteristic features. They are larger in size than the subaxial cervical vertebrae, possess a convexity along the posterior cortical surface, and have articulations for the ribs along the lateral surface of the vertebral body.

The five lumbar vertebrae share an oval-shaped vertebral body and broad articular facets, which prevent excessive axial rotation. Notably, the structures of the lumbar vertebrae are thicker and more substantial than their counterparts in the thoracic or lumbar spine. From a mechanical standpoint, the presence of the greater surface area at the base of the spine helps augment the stability and load-bearing capacity of the vertebral column.

The sacral spine forms the posterior aspect of the pelvis via the sacral bodies and the alae and is the support for the presacral lumbar spine. The sacral spine is the largest area that does not have articulating vertebrae due to the fact that all five vertebrae are fused. The sacrum bears a large compressive load and therefore requires high strength and stability.[16] The high bone density of the sacral spine helps facilitate this mechanical role. The sacral spine also serves as a conduit for the neural elements of the lumbosacral trunk. The neuroforamina lie on the anterior and posterior surfaces of the sacrum, which reflects its solid structural form of the sacrum and the absence of a continuous distal tubular canal resulting in the exiting of the dorsal and ventral rami from their respective foramina at similar levels. The pine cone–shaped coccyx provides no supportive function but remains significant for the attachments of the gluteus maximus muscle and the musculature of the pelvic diaphragm.

Joints and Soft Tissue of the Vertebrae

The spine's ability to serve its structural and functional roles depends in part on the articulations within it. Between the vertebral bodies themselves are the intervertebral disks. These highly elastic structures provide resistance to compression while simultaneously preventing excessive rotation, flexion, and extension. The disk is best described as a flattened cylinder with a soft nucleus pulposus enclosed by a tough, fibrous, outer anulus fibrosus. The disk has no direct blood supply, but rather receives nutrition by diffusion from the adjacent vertebral articular end plates.[30]

The anulus fibrosus is composed primarily of type I collagen arranged in a series of concentric or lamellar layers at 30 degrees to one another. The nucleus pulposus is made up of a gelatinous, viscoelastic material, composed predominantly of type II collagen.[31] Proteoglycans and chondrocytes make up the remainder of the nucleus. This complex matrix serves to attract and bind water. This flow of the water within the matrix occurs in a controlled, rate-dependent fashion, which imparts the disk with its native viscoelasticity. The intervertebral disk is somewhat isolated from the adjacent vertebral bodies by a layer of hyaline cartilage covering the surfaces of the end plates and attached via the insertional fibers of the anulus.[32] These structural characteristics of intervertebral disks provide the basis for the stability and flexibility of the spinal column during motion as well as load dispersion of axial forces.

The constraints to excessive motion in the spine are provided by a series of strong, longitudinally oriented ligaments. The spinal ligaments may be categorized as either ligaments of the vertebral bodies or ligaments of the vertebral arches. The ligaments of the vertebral bodies include the anterior longitudinal ligament (ALL) and posterior longitudinal ligament (PLL), which both play an important role in guiding normal motion and providing stability against excessive motion. The ALL, as its name suggests, lies on the anterior surface of the vertebral bodies and provides resistance under tension to excessive extension of the spine. Conversely, the PLL, which is an extension of the tectorial membrane, courses continuously along the posterior surfaces of the vertebral bodies and contributes, along with other posterior structures, to the stability of the spine in flexion. Anatomically, the PLL effectively forms the anterior border of the central canal.

The vertebral arch ligaments are more complex in terms of orientation and function than the ligaments of the vertebral bodies. The ligamentum flavum, or yellow ligament, is present throughout the length of the spinal column connecting adjacent vertebral laminae behind the intervertebral foramina. This ligament possesses the protein elastin, which allows it to endure greater elastic deformation under tension. The interspinous ligament connects adjacent spinous processes and acts as a tension band maintaining stability and alignment of the spinal column during flexion. The most posteriorly located ligament, running along the tips of the spinous processes, is the supraspinous ligament running from C7 to the sacrum. This adds further stability to the spine in rotation and flexion. Above C7, the supraspinous ligament is continuous with the nuchal ligament, which widens as it approaches its origin at the occipital protuberance of the skull and is of primary importance in maintaining normal head position without fatigue. The last of the vertebral arch ligaments are the intertransverse ligaments. These ligaments connect the transverse processes of the vertebrae and serve to limit lateral bending.[16]

The zygapophyseal (facet) joints are the paired synovial joints that, in concert with the intervertebral disk, make up the three-joint complex present at each subaxial vertebral motion segment. The orientation of the facet joints varies from lying more in the coronal plane in the thoracic spine and in a sagittal orientation in the lumbar spine. This is one factor involved in the determination of the direction and degree of motion of the spine within a given segment. Within the thoracic spine, the vertebrae also articulate with their respective rib heads. The head of the rib articulates with the vertebral body, whereas the tubercle of the rib attaches to the transverse process of the thoracic vertebral arch. These articulations play an important role in adding stability to the axial skeleton (**Fig. 6.7**).

Musculature

The muscles of the back primarily lie along the posterolateral aspect of the spinal column. These facilitate ipsilateral bending (during unilateral contraction) and extension (during bilateral contraction). The muscles that mediate these actions are divided into the lateral and medial tracts. The lateral tract muscles include the iliocostalis, longissimus, splenius, intertransversarii, and levatores costarum muscles, whereas the medial tract muscles consist of the interspinalis, spinalis, rotatores breves, rotatores longi, multifidus, and semispinalis muscles. There are certain nuances that exist within these tracts that distinguish the more specific actions of certain muscles. The splenius muscles and

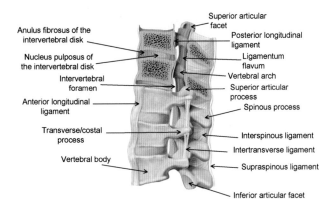

Fig. 6.7 The ligaments of the spinal column at the level of the thoracolumbar junction.

the longissimus capitis muscle have an additional function to rotate the head to the same side as flexion on unilateral contraction. The levatores costarum axially rotate the thoracic spine to the side opposite their location while lateral bending the spine ipsilaterally. Other muscles responsible for rotation contralateral to their direction of flexion include the rotatores, multifidus, and semispinalis muscles of the medial tract.

The muscles intrinsic to the cervical spine must facilitate fine movements to allow for positioning of the cranium. These are located both anteriorly and posteriorly along the cervical spine. The posterior short nuchal and craniovertebral muscles, including the rectus capitis posterior major and minor as well as the obliquus capitis superior and inferior are the constituents of this group. They all extend the head on bilateral contraction, but on unilateral contraction, they have their own specific actions. The rectus capitis posterior group and the obliquus capitis inferior rotate the head to the ipsilateral side, whereas the obliquus capitis superior rotates the head to the contralateral side while also causing ipsilateral lateral bending.

In the anterior cervical spine, the prevertebral muscles have opposing biomechanical actions to the posterior groups. The most important of these muscles is the longus capitus, which, during unilateral contraction laterally bends and ipsilaterally rotates the head. During bilateral contraction, they

flex the head. The longus colli serves a similar purpose in the cervical spine. The rectus capitis anterior and lateralis share a function of acting upon the atlanto-occipital joint. Unilaterally, these muscles mediate the lateral flexion of this joint, allowing the head to tilt to the side without much movement in the cervical region, whereas bilaterally they will cause a forward flexion at the same joint.

The spine is also acted upon by extrinsic muscles of the trunk. The abdominal muscles are divided into sections based on the directions in which the muscles run. The external and internal oblique abdominals both flex the trunk during bilateral contraction. Unilateral contraction of these muscles causes ipsilateral rotation. The external oblique muscles serve to provide contralateral axial rotation of the trunk, while the internal obliques, along with the transversus abdominis, oppose this motion through an ipsilateral axial rotation of the trunk. However, pure flexion of the lumbar spine is mostly the duty of the rectus abdominis. Moving more inferiorly into the lumbosacral region, the quadratus lumborum and iliopsoas muscles are responsible for ipsilateral truncal bending. In order for the iliopsoas to cause lateral bending of the trunk, the femur must be fixed, and when it is contracted bilaterally with the person supine, this muscle serves to lift the trunk (**Fig. 6.8**).[16]

Gross Motion of the Spine

The dynamic nature of the spine allows for significant motion, including flexion and extension in the sagittal plane, lateral bending in the coronal plane, and rotation in the axial plane. The cervical spine and thoracolumbar spine are the most mobile regions of the spinal axis.

Range of motion in the cervical spine is necessary for head movement and direction of gaze. In the frontal plane, the cervical spine undergoes ~35 degrees of lateral flexion when an angle is formed between a line extending laterally from the clavicle and another line extending downward from the lateral angle of the eye. In the sagittal plane, the cervical spine can normally flex 65 degrees, bringing the chin toward the chest, and extend 40 degrees. The normal degree of axial rotation with respect to the sagittal plane is ~50 degrees bilaterally (**Fig. 6.9**).

In the thoracolumbar spine, contributions to range of motion may be divided between the thoracic and lumbar regions.

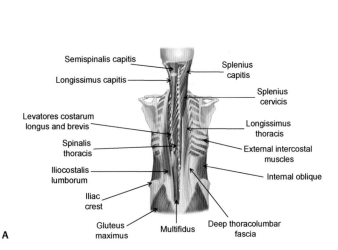

A

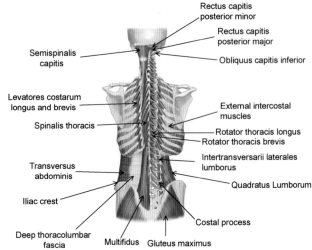

B

Fig. 6.8 (A) Superficial layer of the medial tract of the intrinsic back muscles. (B) Deep layer of the medial tract of the intrinsic back muscles.

With respect to forward flexion, 35 degrees can be attributed to the thoracic spine and 50 degrees to the lumbar spine. This produces a total thoracolumbar forward flexion of ~85 degrees using the greater trochanter of the hip as the fulcrum of motion and the acromion as the dynamic point of reference. Using the same landmarks, thoracolumbar extension is the sum of 25 degrees of extension in the thoracic spine and 35 degrees of extension in the lumbar spine. In the frontal plane, lateral bending is ~40 degrees to a given side. This motion is equally divided between thoracic and lumbar

movement, which is measured using the S1 vertebral body as the fulcrum and the L1 vertebra and the C7 vertebra as the dynamic points of reference for lumbar and thoracic lateral flexion, respectively. Axial rotation primarily occurs in the thoracic spine and is divided into ~35 degrees in the thoracic spine and 5 degrees in the lumbar spine.

Total movement of the spine during any specific action can be estimated by the addition of movements of each spinal region. For example, in a normal patient, total forward flexion = cervical (65 degrees) + thoracic (35 degrees) + lumbar

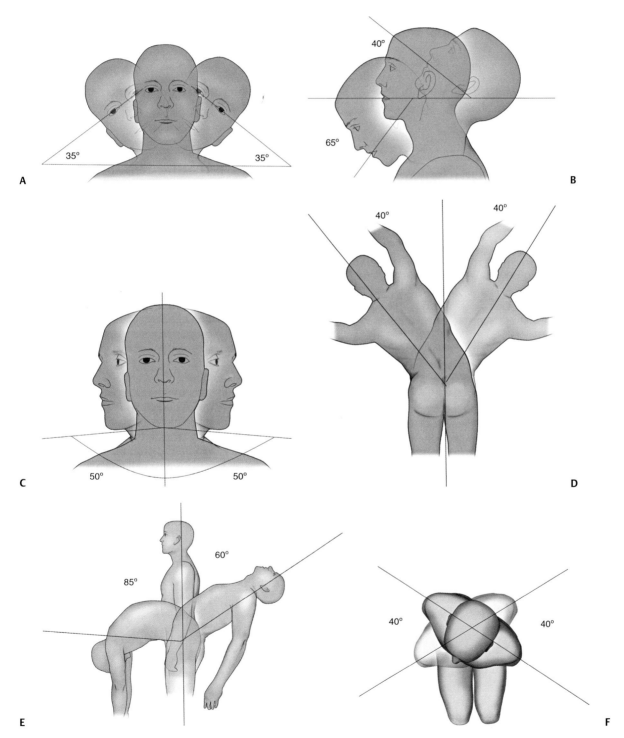

Fig. 6.9 **(A)** Lateral bending of the cervical spine. **(B)** Flexion and extension of the cervical spine. **(C)** Rotation of the cervical spine. **(D)** Lateral bending of the thoracolumbar spine. **(E)** Flexion and extension of the thoracolumbar spine. **(F)** Rotation of the thoracolumbar spine.

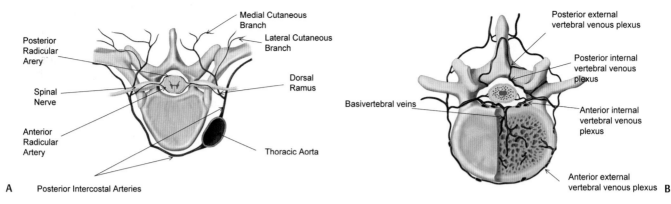

A   Posterior Intercostal Arteries   **B**

Fig. 6.10 **(A)** Superior view of the arterial supply of the vertebral canal from the thoracic aorta. **(B)** Superior view of venous drainage from a typical lumbar vertebra.

(50 degrees) = 150 degrees total. Not surprisingly, the cervical spine is the most flexible in all planes of movement.[16]

Vasculature

The blood supply to the cervical spinal column is normally derived from branches of the subclavian artery distal to the origin of the common carotid arteries. Studies show that there is variation to this vascular network. The first three cervical vertebrae most often receive their blood supply from the vertebral artery, whereas the fourth through sixth cervical vertebrae are typically supplied by the ascending cervical artery, which arises from the thyrocervical trunk. The seventh cervical vertebra is supplied by the deep cervical artery, which arises from the costocervical trunk.[33] The thoracic and lumbar spinal segments receive their blood supply from segmental arteries arising from the aorta known as the intercostal and lumbar arteries, respectively. The vessels arising from the posterior branches of these arteries are the key blood source to the bony vertebrae and parts of the spinal cord once they have penetrated the intervertebral foramina.[33] In the sacral spine, the most common origin of the blood supply is the lateral sacral artery, though other contributors include the fifth lumbar, iliolumbar, and middle sacral arteries.[34]

The segmental spinal artery, a branch of the segmental artery, enters the intervertebral foramen and travels along the course of the nerve root. This artery, in turn, divides into three parts: the anterior and posterior spinal canal branches and the radicular artery. The anterior and posterior spinal canal branches supply the vertebral structures and ligaments, whereas the radicular artery continues to travel along the nerve root and eventually enters the subarachnoid space and bifurcates into an anterior and posterior branch.[33]

The anterior spinal artery, which runs in the medial sulcus, and the two posterior spinal arteries, which run along the posterolateral sulci, share the burden of spinal cord perfusion. Both of these vessels typically arise from the vertebral arteries and descend the length of the spinal cord. In some cases, the posterior spinal arteries may also arise from the posterior inferior cerebellar artery.[33] The anterior spinal artery perfuses roughly two thirds of the spinal cord, whereas the posterior arteries perfuse the remaining one third. The radiculomedullary arteries provide collateral flow between the anterior and posterior spinal arteries and certain radicular arterial branches. These collaterals are crucial in maintaining the neurological integrity of the spinal column in the case of a vascular lesion (**Fig. 6.10**).

Neuroanatomy

The neuroanatomy of the spinal cord is consistent throughout its length from the foramen magnum to the lumbar spine where it normally terminates in the region of the first lumbar vertebra. Grossly, the spinal cord gradually becomes smaller in diameter as it descends due to progressively less afferent and efferent axons as the spinal nerves branch off through the neural foraminae. Exceptions to this rule occur at the cervical and lumbar enlargements. In these areas the spinal cord becomes larger in cross section as the numerous motor and sensory neurons along with their associated interneurons which form the brachial and lumbar plexus participate in rich synaptic networks. The preponderance of anterior horn cells also contributes to the increased spinal cord diameter seen in these regions.

Histologically, the periphery of the spinal cord is composed of myelinated white matter, whereas the central "H-shaped" area is composed of unmyelinated gray matter. The posterior funiculus of the spinal cord contains the dorsal column medial lemniscus pathway, which transmits sensory information including fine touch, vibration, and proprioception (**Fig. 6.11**). Degeneration or a lesion in this area will predictably compromise these sensory discriminations and severely impair joint and vibratory sense distal to the lesion. The other main area of sensory afferent conduction is the lateral funiculus. This region contains the spinocerebellar tracts, responsible for

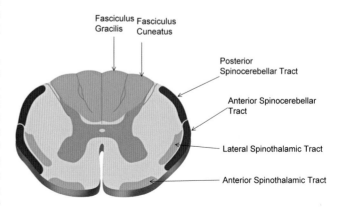

Fig. 6.11 Ascending tracts of the spinal cord.

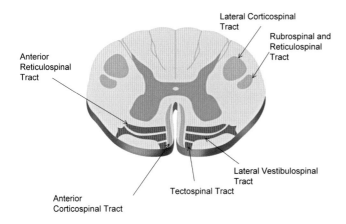

Fig. 6.12 Descending tracts of the spinal cord.

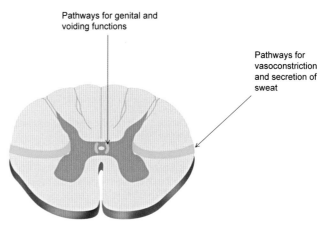

Fig. 6.13 Autonomic pathways of the spinal cord.

added joint and position sense, and the anterolateral sensory system containing the spinothalamic tract. The spinothalamic tract is divided into an anterior portion, which transmits touch signals, and a lateral portion, which transmits signals for pain and temperature. Impulses within these tracts are routed from the periphery to the thalamus for central processing and integration.

The other main function of the spinal cord is to provide distal motor innervation. The anterior funiculus and a portion of the lateral funiculus contain the pyramidal and extrapyramidal motor tracts from their origin in the brain through the cord. Both voluntary and involuntary motor impulses are transmitted through these tracts (**Fig. 6.12**). However, the more anterior pyramidal tracts are primarily responsible for the majority of the body's voluntary movements. The spinal cord also relays motor and sensory information of the autonomic nervous system to control visceral function (**Fig. 6.13**).

Within the gray matter core of the spinal cord as seen on cross-section lie anterior and posterior horns. These are composed of white matter fibers coursing in a cranial–caudal direction. The axons that have their cell bodies in the anterior horn are lower motor neurons that are synapsing with the regulatory upper motor neurons. These axons exit from the anterolateral aspect of the spinal cord segment as the ventral roots and merge with the dorsal root to make up the spinal nerve, which then exits the spinal column via the neural foramen. In the posterior horn is the tract of Lissauer, which is the first synapse of the fibers coming from the neuron in the dorsal root ganglion to transmit their signals through the secondary axons to the thalamus for central processing. This tract, along with the posterior funiculus, receives its blood supply from the posterior spinal arteries.

◆ Summary

Study of the embryology and anatomy of the spine is of great importance for practitioners caring for spine patients. Knowledge of the spine's embryological origins and understanding of the numerous congenital spinal disorders allow for correct diagnoses of spinal pathology and appropriate referral of patients for the multidisciplinary care often required in these conditions. The complex three-dimensional structure of the spine can also make diagnosis and treatment of spinal disorders quite challenging. It has often been said that knowledge of anatomy is surgical power. Nowhere is this more true than

in spinal surgery. The implications of surgical intervention in the spine must be carefully considered when planning spinal procedures, and the intricate balance of the spinal column must be preserved to whatever extent possible to provide maximum function and prevent or decrease pain. Only by remaining a vigilant student of the origin, structure, and function of the spine can one provide the best possible care for the spinal patient.

References

1. Sadler TW. Langman's Medical Embryology. 10th ed. Philadelphia: Lippincott Williams & Wilkins; 2006
2. Bono C, Parke W, Garfin S. Development of the spine. In: Herkowitz H, Garfin S, Eismont F, Bell G, Balderston R, eds. Rothman-Simeone the Spine. Vol 1. 5th ed. Philadelphia, PA: Saunders Elsevier; 2006:3
3. Yang X, Dormann D, Münsterberg AE, Weijer CJ. Cell movement patterns during gastrulation in the chick are controlled by positive and negative chemotaxis mediated by FGF4 and FGF8. Dev Cell 2002;3:425–437
4. Nolting D, Hansen BF, Keeling J, Kjaer I. Prenatal development of the normal human vertebral corpora in different segments of the spine. Spine 1998;23:2265–2271
5. Kaplan KM, Spivak JM, Bendo JA. Embryology of the spine and associated congenital abnormalities. Spine J 2005;5:564–576
6. MacEwen GD, Winter RB, Hardy JH. Evaluation of kidney anomalies in congenital scoliosis. J Bone Joint Surg Am 1972;54:1451–1454
7. Rai AS, Taylor TKF, Smith GHH, Cumming RG, Plunkett-Cole M. Congenital abnormalities of the urogenital tract in association with congenital vertebral malformations. J Bone Joint Surg Br 2002;84:891–895
8. Ferguson RL. Medical and congenital comorbidities associated with spinal deformities in the immature spine. J Bone Joint Surg Am 2007;89(Suppl 1):34–41
9. Saga Y, Takeda H. The making of the somite: molecular events in vertebrate segmentation. Nat Rev Genet 2001;2(11):835–845
10. Bagnall KM, Higgins SJ, Sanders EJ. The contribution made by a single somite to the vertebral column: experimental evidence in support of resegmentation using the chick-quail chimaera model. Development 1988;103:69–85
11. Huang R, Zhi Q, Brand-Saberi B, Christ B. New experimental evidence for somite resegmentation. Anat Embryol (Berl) 2000;202:195–200
12. Fleming A, Keynes R, Tannahill D. A central role for the notochord in vertebral patterning. Development 2004;131:873–880
13. Labrom RD. Growth and maturation of the spine from birth to adolescence. J Bone Joint Surg Am 2007;89(Suppl 1):3–7
14. Ganey TM, Ogden JA. Development and maturation of the axial skeleton. In: Weinstein SL, ed. The Pediatric Spine: Principles and Practice. 2nd ed. Philadelphia: Lippincott, Williams, and Wilkins; 2001:3–54
15. Lustrin ES, Karakas SP, Ortiz AO, et al. Pediatric cervical spine: normal anatomy, variants, and trauma. Radiographics 2003;23:539–560
16. Ross LM, Lamperti ED, eds. Thieme Atlas of Anatomy. Stuttgart: Georg Thieme Verlag; 2006
17. El-Khoury GY, Sato Y. Imaging modalities. In: Weinstein SL, ed. The Pediatric Spine: Principles and Practice. 2nd ed. Philadelphia: Lippincott, Williams and Wilkins; 2001:93

18. Cirak B, Ziegfeld S, Knight VM, Chang D, Avellino AM, Paidas CN. Spinal injuries in children. J Pediatr Surg 2004;39:607–612

19. Khanna G, El-Khoury GY. Imaging of cervical spine injuries of childhood. Skeletal Radiol 2007;36:477–494

20. Avarello JT, Cantor RM. Pediatric major trauma: an approach to evaluation and management. Emerg Med Clin North Am 2007;25:803–836, x

21. Launay F, Sponseller PD. Congenital scoliosis. In: Herkowitz H, Garfin S, Eismont F, Bell G, Balderston R, eds. Rothman Simeone the Spine. Vol 1. 5th ed. Philadelphia: Saunders Elsevier; 2006:507

22. Kusumi K, Turnpenny PD. Formation errors of the vertebral column. J Bone Joint Surg Am 2007;89(Suppl 1):64–71

23. Bedi A, Hensinger RN. Congenital abnormalities of the cervical spine. In: Herkowitz H, Garfin S, Eismont F, Bell G, Balderston R, eds. Rothman Simeone the Spine. Vol 1. 5th ed. Philadelphia: Saunders Elsevier; 2006:630

24. Uno K, Kataoka O, Shiba R. Occipitoatlantal and occipitoaxial hypermobility in Down syndrome. Spine 1996;21:1430–1434

25. Herzka A, Sponseller PD, Pyeritz RE. Atlantoaxial rotatory subluxation in patients with Marfan syndrome: a report of three cases. Spine 2000;25:524–526

26. Bostrom A, Weinzierl M, Spangenberg P, Wiesner M, Krings T. Radiographic and clinical features in Morquio's syndrome. Clinical Neuroradiology 2006;16:249–253

27. Torg JS, Pavlov H, Genuario SE, et al. Neurapraxia of the cervical spinal cord with transient quadriplegia. J Bone Joint Surg Am 1986;68:1354–1370

28. Torg JS, Guille JT, Jaffe S. Injuries to the cervical spine in American football players. J Bone Joint Surg Am 2002;84-A:112–122

29. Torg JS, Naranja RJ Jr, Pavlov H, Galinat BJ, Warren R, Stine RA. The relationship of developmental narrowing of the cervical spinal canal to reversible and irreversible injury of the cervical spinal cord in football players. J Bone Joint Surg Am 1996;78:1308–1314

30. Rajasekaran S, Naresh-Babu J, Murugan S. Review of postcontrast MRI studies on diffusion of human lumbar discs. J Magn Reson Imaging 2007;25:410–418

31. Ghosh P, Bushell GR, Taylor TF, Akeson WH. Collagens, elastin and noncollagenous protein of the intervertebral disk. Clin Orthop Relat Res 1977;(129):124–132

32. Akeson WH, Woo SL, Taylor TK, Ghosh P, Bushell GR. Biomechanics and biochemistry of the intervertebral disks: the need for correlation studies. Clin Orthop Relat Res 1977;(129):133–140

33. Brockstein B, Johns L, Gewertz BL. Blood supply to the spinal cord: anatomic and physiologic correlations. Ann Vasc Surg 1994;8:394–399

34. Dommisse GF. The blood supply of the spinal cord: a critical vascular zone in spinal surgery. J Bone Joint Surg Br 1974;56:225–235

7

Emergency Room Evaluation of the Spinal Injury Patient Including Assessment of Spinal Shock

Bizhan Aarabi and Yasutsugu Yukawa

◆ Spinal Shock and Digital Rectal Examination in the Emergency Room

How do we grade the anatomical and functional integrity of the spinal cord after an injury? Consider the four images in **Fig. 7.1**, taken within hours of an accident, depicting injury profiles ranging from contusion to transection.[1,2] In severe apparently complete cases of acute spinal cord injury (SCI) how do we verify whether residual connectivity exists between higher centers and distal sacral segments of the spinal cord? For such conclusions the *Modified Standard Classification of Spinal Cord Injury, American Spinal Injury Association (ASIA) Impairment Scale (AIS) v1.1* suggests three fields.[3] Two of these fields attempt to determine sacral sparing[4,5] and the third examines for the absence of a cutaneospinal reflex called the bulbocavernosus reflex, a sign of spinal shock.[6–9] Sacral sensory or motor sparing and/or the presence of a bulbocavernosus reflex is proposed to mitigate against an ASIA grade A categorization with inherently poor prognosis. The presence of spinal shock is also traditionally associated with a poor prognosis. Use of the digital rectal examination (DRE) to check for sacral sparing and spinal shock is currently advocated by Advanced Trauma Life Support (ATLS) guidelines in the secondary survey of trauma victims.[10,11] This chapter critically analyzes the literature for evidence supporting the usefulness of digital rectal examination (DRE) in establishing spinal shock and spinal cord injury. We will examine the evidence for the following questions:

- Can DRE establish SCI in the emergency room?
- Can DRE for the bulbocavernosus reflex predict ASIA grade?

Literature Search Criteria

The National Library of Medicine (MEDLINE/PubMed) computerized literature database was searched for evidence from 1966 to 2009. Search strategy was application of the following Medical Subject Headings (MeSH) terms:

- Spinal shock AND spinal cord injury: 386 articles found.
- Digital rectal exam AND spinal shock: no articles found
- Digital rectal examination AND spinal cord injury: 10 articles found
- Digital rectal exam AND trauma, nervous system: 4 articles found
- Digital rectal exam AND shock: no items found
- Digital rectal exam AND quadriplegia: no items found
- Digital rectal exam AND paraplegia: no items found
- Spinal cord injury/diagnosis/pathophysiology AND digital rectal exam: 3 items found
- Spinal cord injury/diagnosis AND physical examination: 67 items found, 27 related

In the general term window we also used:

- Spinal shock AND spinal cord injury AND ASIA impairment: 1 item found
- Spinal shock AND spinal cord injury AND digital rectal examination: no item found
- Rectal exam AND spinal cord injury: 1 item found
- Digital rectal exam AND trauma: 2 items found

Applying Single Citation Matchers, we selected references from printed articles to increase the quality and quantity of evidence. The titles and abstracts of the articles retrieved were reviewed and, when indicated, the entire article was reviewed for relevance. Overall 13 articles were used to compile our evidence. Known authorities in the fields of spinal cord injury and spinal shock were contacted for their expert opinion in reference to recovery of reflexes in spinal shock and their relationship with AIS scoring.

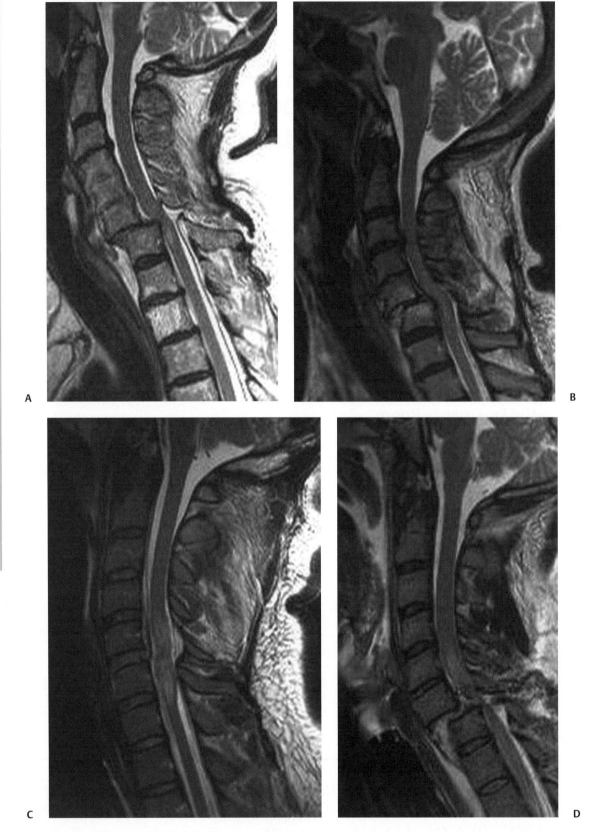

Fig. 7.1 Composite midsagittal T2-weighted images of the cervical spine belonging to four subjects with different degrees of cervical spinal cord injury severity ranging from signal change limited to **(A)** one skeletal segment, **(B)** more than one skeletal segment, **(C)** intramedullary hemorrhage, and **(D)** complete transaction.

Table 7.1 Evidentiary Table: Digital Rectal Exam and Spinal Shock

Investigator	Description	Level of Evidence of Primary Question	Topic and Conclusion
Ko et al 1999[9]	Recovery of bulbocavernosus reflex and its prognostic significance for walking 200 yards at discharge was prospectively studied within hours of emergency department (ED) admission, 5–7 days per week and for 6–8 weeks in 50 patients with spinal cord injury.	II	Bulbocavernosus reflex was elicited after 5 or after 20 hours following trauma in patients with incomplete or complete spinal cord injury, respectively. The reflex presenting rate was 100% in both groups; 86.4% of incomplete injuries (19/22) and 53.6% of complete injuries (15/28) had the bulbocavernosus reflex in the ED. Presence or absence of bulbocavernosus reflex could not be used to assign an American Spinal Injury Association (ASIA) grade in patients with spinal cord injury.

Scientific Foundation

What we now call spinal shock was first described by Whytt in 1750.[12] In 1841 Hall coined the term *shock* to describe the phenomenon.[13,14] At the turn of the century Sherrington began important scientific study of spinal shock through animal experimentation.[12,15] Spinal shock is characterized by depression or extinction of spinal reflexes such as delayed plantar response, bulbocavernosus reflex, or myotatic reflex after acute spinal cord injury.[6,8,9,12,14–23] The pathogenesis, evolution, and clinical significance of spinal shock continue to be the subjects of intense debate (**Tables 7.1, 7.2, 7.3**).[6,8,9,12,14–18,21–30] Evidence indicates that spinal shock stems from depression or blockade of monosynaptic or polysynaptic transmission in Ia sensory fibers originating from intrafusal muscle fibers and concomitant hypoactivity in gamma motor neurons secondary to presynaptic inhibition.[6,8,16] Regardless of the severity of spinal cord injury, recovery of spinal reflexes begins within hours of trauma, signifying the end of spinal shock.[8,9] What then is the relationship, if any, between spinal shock and its evolution and the severity of injury and functional outcome?

Reflexes are the simplest models of sensory–motor integration.[20,31] Muscle tone and the sensitivity and strength of myotatic reflexes, primarily organized through annulospiral (Ia) and fusimotor fibers, are modulated by either or both excitatory and inhibitory descending motor pathways from higher centers, primarily the brain stem (**Fig. 7.2**).[12,32,33] Modulation of muscle tone is necessary for balance and posture in proximal muscles (Rexed lamina VIII), so that distal limbs (Rexed lamina IX) can perform goal-directed activities with dexterity. Volitional and reflex motor integration is accomplished through coordinated function of motor cortex,

Table 7.2 Evidentiary Table: Digital Rectal Exam (DRE) as a Diagnostic Measure

Investigator	Description	Level of Evidence of Primary Question	Topic and Conclusion
Eckardt et al 1993[35]	In this prospective study, anal resting pressure and anal squeeze were checked by anorectal manometry and DRE. 64 patients complaining of either constipation (24) or fecal incontinence (40) took part in the study. The clinician performing the DRE was blinded to the results of anorectal manometry.	II	The sensitivity of DRE for diagnosing incompetent sphincters ranged from 63% to 84%, whereas specificity was calculated as 57%. The study concluded that even the experienced examiner needs to use more sophisticated methods than DRE for evaluation of anal sphincter incontinence.
Esposito et al 2005[36]	Prospective study of 512 patients undergoing DRE to diagnose gastrointestinal bleeding, spinal cord injury, or urethral disruption. Other clinical indicators were used to confirm the diagnosis.	II	The overall positive predictive value of DRE for the diagnosis of spinal cord injury was 47% and negative predictive value was 98%. The overall accuracy of DRE was 36%. The investigators concluded that when other clinical indicators are available, omission of DRE as a diagnostic tool for spinal cord injury appears permissible, safe, and advantageous.
Guldner et al 2006[37]	Retrospective review of 1032 consecutive adult patients with blunt trauma over a 2-year period. The DRE result was compared with the presence or absence of spinal cord injury at discharge.	III	The sensitivity, specificity, positive predictive value, and negative predictive values were 50%, 93%, 27%, and 97%, respectively. The DRE is insensitive in diagnosing spinal cord injury.
Shlamovitz et al 2007[38]	Retrospective review of 1401 consecutive trauma patients with documented DRE treated in the emergency department over a 3-year period.	III	The calculated sensitivity and specificity of the DRE for detecting spinal cord injury was 37% (95% CI 23–50%) and 96% (95% CI 95–97%), respectively. DRE has a poor sensitivity for the diagnosis of spinal cord injury.

Table 7.3 Evidentiary Table: Digital Rectal Exam as an Indication of Sacral Sparing

Investigator	Description	Level of Evidence of Primary Question	Topic and Conclusion
Frankel et al 1969[50]	Retrospective analysis of 33 Frankel B patients among 218 patients with spinal cord injury.	III	Following postural reduction and appropriate management, five of 33 patients had complete motor recovery and 14 improved to motor useful or Frankel D grade.
Maynard et al 1979[46]	Retrospective analysis of 123 patients with traumatic quadriplegia admitted to a California Regional Spinal Cord Injury Care System.	III	Functional outcome of 103 patients with normal cognition 1 year after spinal cord injury. Among 53 motor complete patients at 72 hours, none regained walking ability at 1 year. Among 17 in Frankel B category, 47% regained walking ability; among motor incomplete patients, 87% were ambulatory.
Foo et al 1981[45]	Retrospective study of functional outcome in 13 patients with posttraumatic acute anterior spinal cord syndrome.	III	Frankel B patients were subdivided into two groups. Frankel B1 (seven patients) had preserved light touch and Frankel B2 (six patients) had preserved pin prick sensation in addition to light touch. Frankel grade B improved to grade D in only 1 patient (14.3%) in the B1 group versus four of six (66.7%) patients in Group B2. One additional patient in Group B2 improved to Frankel grade C.
Crozier et al 1991[41]	During a 6-year period, 27 patients with motor complete and sensory incomplete [light touch 18 (B1) and light touch and pinprick 9 (B2) patients] were followed up for 200-foot ambulation.	III	Two of 18 in the B1 group versus 8 of 9 in the B2 group were ambulatory at follow-up. It was concluded that Frankel B patients with only touch preservation below the zone of injury had poor prognosis for ambulation; those with preserved pin appreciation below the zone of injury had excellent prognosis to regain functional ambulation.
Waters et al 1994[51]	Prospective examination of 50 patients with incomplete tetraplegia to quantify motor and sensory recovery.	II	None of five patients who were motor complete with the presence of sacral (S4–S5) sharp/dull touch sensation unilaterally recovered any lower extremity motor function. However, in eight motor complete subjects having bilateral sacral sharp/dull sensation preserved, the mean lower extremity motor score increased to 12.1 ± 7.8 at 1 year. In three of the eight cases, functional ($\geq 3/5$) recovery was seen in some muscles at 1 year.
Marino et al 1999[4]	Retrospective review of neurological recovery of 3585 individuals with traumatic spinal cord injury admitted to 21 Model Spinal Cord Injury systems over 10 years.	III	Individuals who were motor complete with extended zones of sensory preservation but without sacral sparing were less likely to convert to motor incomplete status than those with sacral sparing (13.3% vs 53.6%; $p < 0.001$)
Coleman et al 2004[40]	Retrospective analysis of data prospectively collected for the multicenter trial of GM-1 study from 28 centers. Injury severity and region of injury were related to marked recovery (MR), defined as improvement of at least 2 grades from ASIA Impairment Scale (AIS) at baseline to modified Benzel scale at week 26.	III	Among 760 patients, 482 were complete. AIS Groups C and D had ($p < .0001$) more MR (84%) than Group B (46.6%), which recovered more than Group A (12.8%). Conclusion: AIS severity was the strongest predictor.
Oleson et al 2005[5]	Retrospective analysis of ambulation at 26 and 52 weeks in 131 patients with motor complete and sensory incomplete spinal cord injury from 28 tertiary care centers in the United States and Canada.	III	A higher percentage of subjects with sacral pinprick preservation at baseline were ambulating at 26 (39.4% vs 28.3%) and 52 weeks (53.6% vs 41.5%) (not statistically significant). The presence of sacral pinprick preservation at 4 weeks postinjury was significant for predicting ambulation at 52 weeks postinjury (36% vs 4.4% $p < 0.01$). Conclusion: Baseline lower extremity pinprick preservation and sacral pinprick preservation at 4 weeks postinjury are associated with an improved prognosis for ambulation.

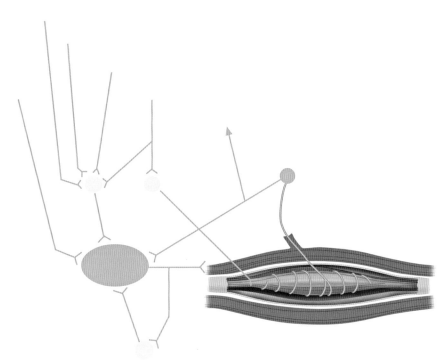

brain stem, and spinal cord.[31,32] In the anterior horn sector of the spinal cord, the medial motor cell group of spinal gray (Rexed lamina VIII) is primarily influenced by vestibulospinal, reticulospinal, and tectospinal tracts, whereas the lateral motor cell group (Rexed lamina IX) is influenced by the rubrospinal tract (**Fig. 7.3**). Pathological processes at the level of the cerebral cortex, brain stem, and spinal cord, disturbing descending lateral and medial motor pathways, may alter presentation of monosynaptic or polysynaptic reflexes. For example, when Sherrington transected cat midbrain in between the superior and inferior colliculi, stretch reflexes were exaggerated, resulting in decerebrate rigidity.[12,15,19,20,33] However, when he transected the ape spinal cord at or below the level of cervicomedullary junction, muscle tone disappeared and most of the baseline reflexes were extinct. Hence he witnessed spinal shock. In Sherrington's experiments, extinction of spinal cord reflexes was only temporary, and

within 20 minutes delayed plantar response was back.[7] Recovery of reflexes has been witnessed in human beings. In 1917, during the First World War, Barre observed recovery of delayed plantar response within 1 hour of acute spinal cord injury,[7] indicating the end of the phenomenon of spinal shock.[8,9,12,15,21,23,29,30]

It is conceivable that by the time we visit trauma victims with acute spinal cord injury, they may well be on their way to recovery from spinal shock.[7–9] In cervical spinal cord injuries, patients may retain distal sacral reflexes such as the bulbocavernosus reflex.[6] Opinion differs as when to declare the end of spinal shock.[7,28,34] Orthopedic surgeons prefer the bulbocavernosus reflex, which usually appears within the first 3 days following spinal cord injury, as an indicator of the end of spinal shock.[7] On the other hand, neurologists take deep tendon reflexes, and urologists tend to choose contractions of detrusor muscle as the first sign of the end of spinal shock. Deep tendon reflexes may not recover for 2 weeks after spinal cord injury, and recovery of detrusor contractions may take 6 weeks.[7,8] Of significance may be the evolution of the recovered spinal reflexes beyond spinal shock. As an example, persistence of delayed plantar response beyond 3 to 7 days following spinal cord injury suggests an ASIA grade A, and delayed recovery of bulbocavernosus reflex beyond 2 days suggests a lower motor neuron lesion.[7,8]

In their prospective study of the pattern of reflex recovery during spinal shock, Ko and colleagues examined on a daily basis 50 consecutive patients first seen within 24 hours of spinal cord injury (range 30 minutes to 24 hours). Reflex recovery, observed during a 6- to 8-week period, was correlated with ambulation of 200 feet at the time of discharge.[9] In this descriptive study, spinal cord injury was complete (AIS grade A) in 28 and incomplete (AIS grades B, C/D) in 22 patients. Recovery of bulbocavernosus reflex was observed as early as 5 hours after injury in incomplete patients and as late as 20 hours after injury in complete patients. The bulbocavernosus reflex was confirmed in the emergency department in 53.6% of complete and 86.4% of incomplete patients. The

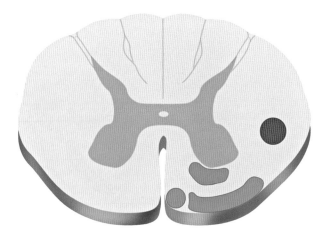

Fig. 7.3 Schematic representation of Rexed lamination at the level of the anterior horn cell layer of spinal cord and suprasegmental influence by different descending pathways. See text for explanation.

bulbocavernosus reflex presenting rate was 100% in AIS grades A to D. Thirty-four of 36 patients (95%) with persistence of delayed plantar response (DPR) for more than 1 day after admission had complete injury; 14 of 14 patients with no DPR beyond the first day following trauma had incomplete injury and were able to ambulate at discharge.

It was concluded that the presence of spinal shock, defined as the absence of all reflexes on the day of injury, was unusual in clinical practice, and evolution of reflexes rather than mere presence or absence of them should be used as a prognosticating tool.[7–9]

Digital Rectal Examination as a Measure of Spinal Cord Injury

The Advanced Trauma Life Support program mandates the DRE as a diagnostic measure during a secondary survey of trauma patients.[10,11] The DRE may help verify lower gastrointestinal bleeding, urethral injuries, anal resting pressure, anal squeeze pressure, and conscious perception of touch or nociception.[4,5,35–38]

To evaluate the reliability of the DRE for detecting anal sphincter tone, Eckardt and Kanzler[35] prospectively and blindly evaluated 64 consecutive patients referred to their center for either constipation (24 patients) or incontinence (40 patients). First, a standard pull-through manometric evaluation of anal resting and anal squeeze pressures was determined. Then, an experienced gastroenterologist performed a DRE. The strength of the internal and external anal sphincter was graded as normal (+3), mildly diminished (+2), markedly diminished (+1), or totally absent (0). When comparative analysis of the data was performed, the sensitivity of the DRE for diagnosing incompetent sphincters ranged from 63 to 84%, whereas specificity was calculated as only 57%. Digital examination appeared reliable only in extreme cases when the observer could not detect any increase in pressure during voluntary squeeze. The authors concluded that the DRE is unreliable in unbiased assessment of sphincter tone. Similarly, anal squeeze pressures may be overestimated by DRE if the patient contracts accessory muscles rather than the external sphincter.

In 2005 Esposito and colleagues reported on reasons to omit the DRE in trauma patients. These authors prospectively used other clinical indicators (OCIs) (i.e., other than DRE) to verify gastrointestinal bleeding, urethral disruption, and spinal cord injury in 512 patients.[36] Comatose and pharmacologically paralyzed patients were excluded from the study. Thirty index injuries were identified in 29 patients (6%): 17 were spinal cord injuries (3%), 11 gastrointestinal bleeding (2%), and two urethral disruption. Overall, the negative predictive values of DRE and OCIs in diagnosing spinal cord injury were virtually the same, ~99%. The positive predictive value of the DRE in diagnosing spinal cord injury was 47% versus 44% for OCIs. The authors concluded that omission of DRE in virtually all trauma patients appears permissible and safe.

In a retrospective study of 1032 patients, Guldner and Brzenski evaluated the sensitivity and specificity of the DRE for detecting spinal cord injury in adult patients with blunt trauma.[37] Fifty-four (5.2%) of these patients had diagnoses consistent with spinal cord injury. Ninety-nine patients had decreased rectal tone, 27 of whom also had spinal cord injuries. The sensitivity, specificity, positive predictive value, and negative predictive values were 50%, 93%, 27%, and 97%,

respectively. The authors concluded that DRE is insensitive to spinal cord injury and has a poor positive predictive value.

Shlamovitz et al[38] have reported poor test characteristics for the DRE in trauma patients. In their retrospective study of data from 2003 to 2005, the authors reviewed 1401 patients with trauma. The calculated sensitivity and specificity for the DRE were 27% (95% CI 23 to 50%) and 96% (95% CI 95 to 97%), respectively, for detection of spinal cord injury. The authors concluded that the DRE has poor sensitivity for the diagnosis of spinal cord injury.

Two components of the DRE, when performed repeatedly and if reproducible, can indicate residual connectivity of distal sacral segments (S2–S5) and higher centers[4,5,39–48]: These are conscious perception of touch and voluntary anal squeeze. They indicate residual connectivity in nociceptive (lateral spinothalamic) and touch (anterior spinothalamic and posterior columns) afferents and corticospinal efferents, respectively (**Fig. 7.4**).[33] We must confirm whether sensory perception is superficial touch or the patient feels the discomfort and pain of DRE and if prick sensation is intact around the saddle area. The major reason for segregating the two sensory afferents is the prognostic significance in functional outcome.[40,41,45,46,49,50]

In 1969 Frankel et al[50] reported on 33 Frankel B patients among 218 patients with spinal cord injury. Following postural reduction and appropriate management, five of 33 patients had complete motor recovery and 14 improved to motor useful or Frankel D grade.

In 1979 Maynard and his colleagues[46] reported on the functional outcome of 103 patients 1 year after spinal cord injury. All were cognitively intact. Among 53 motor complete patients at 72 hours, none regained walking ability at 1 year. Among 17 Frankel B patients, 47% regained walking ability; among motor incomplete patients, 87% were ambulatory.

Foo et al[45] (1981), reporting on posttraumatic acute anterior spinal cord syndrome in 13 patients, noticed better motor recovery in Frankel B patients with preserved prick sensation in addition to light touch. There were seven patients in group B1 (only light touch preserved) and six patients in group B2 (prick and touch preserved). In the Frankel grade B1 group only one patient (14.3%) improved to grade D; in the B2 group 4 (66.7%) did so. One additional patient in group B2 improved to Frankel grade C.

In 1991 Crozier and colleagues[41] reported on the prospects for ambulation of 27 Frankel grade B patients after spinal cord injury. They classified them on the basis of the patient's

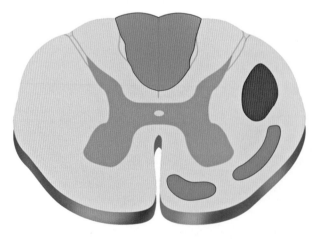

Fig. 7.4 Schematic representation of nociceptive, discriminative, and motor pathways in the spinal cord. See text for explanation.

ability to perceive only touch (B1 group) or touch and prick sensation (B2 group). Independent ambulation at discharge was noted in two of 18 patients in the B1 group and in eight of nine in the B2 group ($p < 0.0002$ by Fisher exact test).

In a study reported in 1994 by Waters et al,[51] investigators prospectively examined 50 patients with incomplete tetraplegia to quantify motor and sensory recovery. None of five patients who were motor complete with the presence of sacral (S4–S5) sharp/dull touch sensation unilaterally recovered any lower extremity motor function. However, in eight motor complete subjects having bilateral sacral sharp/dull sensation preserved, the mean lower extremity motor score increased to 12.1 ± 7.8 at 1 year. In three of the eight cases functional ($\geq 3/5$) recovery was seen in some muscles at 1 year.

When Marino et al[4] (1999) evaluated 3585 individuals from 21 Model Spinal Cord Injury Systems, they noticed better recovery of function in AIS grade B patients. Sixty of 719 (8.3%) individuals classified as AIS grade A had an extended zone of partial preservation (more than three levels). Eight (13.3%) converted to motor-incomplete by discharge, as compared with 24 of 659 (3.6%) of those without an extended zone of partial preservation ($p < 0.01$). This conversion rate was much smaller than that for AIS grade B subjects with sacral sparing (53.6%; $p < 0.01$). At 1-year follow-up 73% of 129 patients in the AIS grade B category had converted to AIS C (38.0%), D (33.3%), or E (1.5%) grades.

In their 2004 retrospective analysis of the GM-1 ganglioside database, Coleman and Geisler[40] found AIS severity to be the strongest predictor of outcome following acute spinal cord injury. Marked recovery (MR), defined as improvement of at least two grades from AIS at baseline to modified Benzel scale at week 26, was noticed in 15.5% of 317 complete cervical and 7% of 143 thoracic injuries. The rates of recovery for patients in AIS B and CD categories were 46.6% and 84.1%, respectively.

In 2005 Oleson and colleagues[5] retrospectively analyzed motor recovery (modified Benzel scale) at 6 and 12 months in 131 patients who were motor complete but sensory incomplete following spinal cord injury. Patients were from 28 tertiary care centers in the United States and Canada. The results indicated that a higher percentage of subjects with sacral pinprick preservation at baseline were ambulating at 26 (39.4% vs 28.3%) and 52 weeks (53.6% vs 41.5%). The presence of sacral sparing at 4 weeks postinjury was a significant predictor of ambulation at 52 weeks (36.0% vs 4.4%, $p < 0.01$) and approached significance at 26 weeks (15.2% vs 0.0%, $p < 0.056$). The authors concluded that baseline lower extremity pinprick preservation and sacral pinprick sparing at 4 weeks postinjury are associated with an improved prognosis for ambulation.

Summary and Recommendation

1. The presence or absence of a bulbocavernosus reflex does not correlate with ASIA grade in patients with acute spinal cord injury (strong evidence) and for this reason should not be routinely performed. If desired, the presence or absence of spinal shock can be established by more traditional means of extremity tone, deep tendon reflexes, and plantar responses. However, the presence or absence of spinal shock carries little prognostic significance in comparison with the ASIA motor exam.
2. When used in the acute trauma setting to establish the presence or absence of spinal cord injury, DRE of sphincter tone is of limited value (strong evidence) and for this reason should not be routinely performed.
3. In patients with known SCI and motor complete injuries, DRE can be used as a tool in the subacute setting (during early hospital admission) to detect sacral motor or sensory sparing. This carries considerable prognostic significance and should be performed to differentiate ASIA A from ASIA B1 and ASIA B1 from ASIA B2 patients (strong).

◆ Neurogenic Shock

Postmortem, preclinical, and clinical studies have confirmed the essential role ischemia plays in secondary central nervous system insults, predisposing the victims of trauma to neurological worsening from minutes to days after injury.[52–67] Evidence indicates that autoregulation is erratic following traumatic brain and spinal cord injury,[67–70] and neurogenic shock may aggravate biochemical cascades influential in secondary ischemic insults. There is class III evidence that maintaining adequate spinal cord blood flow may be advantageous to the trauma victim in improving outcome after spinal cord injury.[71–76] We will examine the evidence concerning the question, What is the timing and natural history of neurogenic shock in patients presenting with acute motor and sensory complete spinal cord injury?

Literature Search Criteria

A National Library of Medicine computerized literature search from 1966 to 2008 was undertaken using Medical Subject Headings in combination with "neurogenic shock: spinal cord injury, management, assessment, time, period and natural course." One hundred twenty-one citations were acquired. Non-English-language citations were deleted. Titles and abstracts of the remaining publications were reviewed, and relevant articles were selected to answer the key question. Additional references were culled from the reference lists of the selected papers. Articles describing nonhuman laboratory investigations germane to the topic, related general review articles, and relevant studies of neurogenic shock and human traumatic brain injury referenced in the Scientific Foundation are also included in the bibliography. Four articles were used to compile our evidence.

- Neurogenic shock AND spinal cord injury: 54 articles
- Neurogenic shock AND acute spinal cord injury: 14 articles
- Neurogenic shock AND management: 35 articles
- Neurogenic shock AND assessment: 5 articles
- Neurogenic shock AND time: 13 articles
- Neurogenic shock AND period: 14 articles

Four articles were relevant to our question and were used to compile evidence (**Table 7.4**).

Scientific Foundation

Although descending vasomotor pathways (VMPs) originate in the rostroventrolateral medulla, they are primarily under the influence of suprasegmental centers that form the main bulk of the autonomic nervous system. These include the limbic cortex, amygdala, ventral striatum, hypothalamus, dorsomedial

Table 7.4 Evidentiary Table for Neurogenic Shock

Investigator	Description	Level of Evidence of Primary Question	Topic and Conclusion
Piepmeier et al 1985[93]	Retrospective analysis of cardiovascular instability following isolated acute cervical spinal cord trauma within 48 hours of admission in 45 patients.	III	There was a direct correlation between the severity of the cord injury and the incidence and severity of cardiovascular problems. Twenty-nine of 45 patients maintained an average pulse rate < 55 bpm for 1 or more days during the study period. The incidence of average daily pulse < 55 was 87%, 62%, 28%, and 28% in Frankel A, B, C, and D patients, respectively. This incidence declined rapidly during the second week and was present in only Frankel grade A patients after day 9. All patients who were hypotensive (SBP < 100 mm Hg) received fluids, and nine Frankel A patients required additional support with vasopressors.
Lehmann et al 1987[97]	The frequency of cardiovascular abnormalities and their time course were evaluated in 71 consecutive patients with acute spinal cord injury. Thirty-one of 71 patients had severe cervical cord injury, 17 had milder cervical injury, and 23 had thoracolumbar injury.	III	Bradycardia (HR < 60 bpm) was universal in all 31 patients with severe cervical cord injury and was seen in six of 17 with milder cervical injury and in three of 23 with thoracolumbar injury ($p < 0.00001$). Hypotension (SBP < 90 mm Hg) was seen in 68 vs 0 and 0%, $p < 0.00001$, respectively. Bradyarrhythmias peaked on day 4, and all observed abnormalities resolved spontaneously within 2 to 6 weeks.
Bilello et al 2003[98]	Retrospective analysis of neurogenic shock in 83 patients with quadriplegia over an 8-year period (1993–2001). The level of the cervical spinal cord injury (CSCI) was high (C1–5) in 62 patients and low (C6,7) in 21. There was no significant difference between the groups in age, injury severity, base deficit or mortality. Pressors, chronotropic agents, and pacemakers were used as interventions.	III	Neurogenic shock was present in 19 (31%) of the 62 patients with high CSCI and in five (24%) of the 21 patients with low CSCI ($p = .56$). There was a marked difference in the use of a cardiovascular intervention between those with a high and those with a low CSCI: 15 (24%) of 62 patients vs one (5%) of 21 patients ($p = .02$). Two patients with C1 through C5 spinal cord injuries required cardiac pacemakers. The authors concluded there was no significant difference in the frequency of neurogenic shock by injury level. Patients with high cervical spine injury had a significantly greater requirement for a cardiovascular intervention than did patients with lower (C6-C7) injuries.
Guly et al 2008[99]	Retrospective analysis of trauma registry database from 1989 to 2003 from England and Wales. Four hundred ninety patients had sustained an isolated spinal cord injury.	III	The heart rate and systolic blood pressure were determined upon arrival at the hospital. Neurogenic shock was defined as SBP < 100 mm Hg and HR < 80 bpm. The incidence of neurogenic shock in cervical cord injuries was 19.3% (95% CI 14.8–23.7%). The incidence in thoracic and lumbar cord injuries was 7% (3–11.1%) and 3% (0–8.85%).

nucleus of thalamus, and periaqueductal gray. Vasomotor pathways eventually converge in the intermediolateral cell column located, in humans, between T1 and L2 spinal segments (Rexed lamina VII), passing through the dorsolateral funiculi.[33,77,78] These cells account for most of the preganglionic cells of the sympathetic nervous system. Disruption of the descending cardiovascular pathways results in four phenomena: initial sympathetic hypoactivity, alterations in the morphology of sympathetic preganglionic neurons, plastic changes within the spinal circuits (sprouting), and the development of changes in sympathetic neurovascular transmission and smooth muscle responsiveness.[79-81] A chronic effect of disruption of

descending VMPs is the autonomic dysreflexia associated with significant surges of blood pressure in response to afferent stimuli (**Fig. 7.5**).[78,82-84]

Animal Studies

Attempts have been made to reproduce neurogenic shock by compressing or disrupting the descending vasomotor pathways in different experimental animals.[85-92] Alexander and Kerr compressed the cervical and thoracic spinal cord by epidural balloons with pressures ranging from 50 to 250 mm Hg for

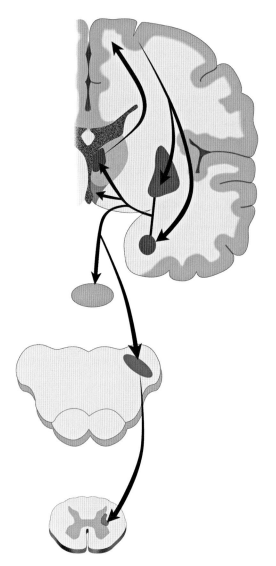

Fig. 7.5 Schematic representation of vasomotor pathways (VMPs) and their suprasegmental connections. See text for explanation.

and escape arrhythmias. Young et al and Rawe and Perot produced similar pressor responses in different models of cat cervical spinal cord injury and were able to eliminate the responses with thoracic sympathectomy, adrenalectomy, or infusion of phenoxybenzamine to oppose activation of α-adrenergic receptors.[90,92]

Clinical Investigations of Neurogenic Shock in Humans

Five clinical reports mention the presence of hypotension in their clinical cohorts, but neurogenic shock was not investigated in a focused fashion.[72,74,93–95] Evaluating hemodynamic parameters in 50 patients with acute cervical spinal cord injury, Levi et al found 9.1% of Frankel C+D versus 23.6% of Frankel A patients to be hypotensive at admission in the emergency department. Hypotension was defined as a systolic blood pressure < 90 mm Hg.[72] In the Soderstrom and Ducker study of peptic gastrointestinal complications of 408 patients with cervical spinal cord injury, 88 patients were admitted in shock. The incidence of shock (BP < 100 mm Hg) was 4.7% (5/107) in neurologically intact patients, and 20.7% and 31.6% for those with incomplete (23/111) and complete (60/190) lesions, respectively.[94] In a report by Zipnick et al, 75 patients with penetrating spinal cord injury were studied for hemodynamic derangements. In that study 23 patients were hypotensive at the time of admission, 18 from bleeding and five in neurogenic shock. Two of the five in neurogenic shock patients had incomplete cervical, two incomplete thoracic, and one complete thoracolumbar spinal cord injuries.[95] In an attempt to improve outcome following spinal cord injury, Vale et al maintained the mean arterial blood pressure of 77 patients with acute spinal cord injury at > 85 mm Hg while in neurosurgical intensive care. In this study four of 10 patients with AIS grade A cervical spine injury were in neurogenic shock. None of the 25 patients with incomplete cervical spinal cord injuries was in neurogenic shock.[74]

In 1982 Dro and colleagues reported a unique finding of a patient with necropsy-proven C1/C2 spinal cord traumatic transection and a clinical picture compatible with neurogenic shock.[96] The patient was 18 years old, and 15 minutes after admission had a blood pressure of 130 mm Hg and a heart rate of 90 bpm, indicating a sympathetic overactivity. At ~35 to 40 minutes after admission his blood pressure dropped to 40 mm Hg and he had a bradycardia of 35 to 40/min, indicating a classic case of neurogenic shock. Although comatose at the time of admission, he woke up with resuscitation and manifested a neurological level at C2. Air myelogram indicated cord transection at the C1/C2 level. The patient lived for 15 days and then died with a clinical picture compatible with autonomic dysreflexia and a temperature of 41°C. Autopsy showed complete transection of the spinal cord at the C1/C2 level.

In 1985 and 1987 two studies were reported by investigators at Yale University. In a retrospective study of 45 patients admitted within 48 hours of injury with cervical spinal cord trauma and cardiovascular instability, Piepmeier and colleagues found a direct correlation between the severity of the cervical spinal cord injury and the incidence and severity of cardiovascular problems.[93] Twenty-nine of the 45 patients maintained an average pulse rate < 55 bpm for 1 or more days during the study period. Thirty-two patients had one or more recorded episodes of pulse rate(s) < 50 bpm. The incidence rapidly declined during the second week.

5 to 120 seconds. Within 2 to 5 seconds of spinal cord compression there was a hypertensive response of up to 100 mm Hg above the resting pressure, which lasted for minutes and was associated with bradycardia. Combined thoracic sympathectomy and adrenalectomy before balloon compression of the spinal cord prevented the surge in blood pressure.[85] Greenhoot and colleagues used the weight drop technique to produce cervical spinal cord injury in dogs. Within seconds there was onset of hypertension and ventricular tachycardia that lasted 2 to 5 minutes. Sympathetic overstimulation resulted in myocardial degeneration.[88,89] Eidelberg produced hypertensive crisis in cats following cervical spinal cord injury by applying the weight drop technique. He was able to prevent the hypertensive episode by infusion of the α-adrenergic blocking agent phenoxybenzamine. He eliminated the pressor and electrocardiographic (EKG) response to compression at C3–C4 by spinal cord transection at T1.[86] A classic picture of neurogenic shock was produced in dogs by Tibbs and his colleagues following cervical spinal cord transection.[91] In this model of cervical spinal cord injury, 15 minutes following a pressor response the blood pressure dropped to 71% of normal values. This episode was also associated with bradycardia

Bradycardia < 50 bpm was present in 96%, 62%, 42%, and 28% of patients having Frankel scores of A, B, C, and D, respectively. Although the authors do not specifically mention incidence of hypotension, they do report that all hypotensive (< 100 mm Hg) patients received intravenous fluids, and nine Frankel A patients needed vasopressors to maintain adequate blood pressure.

In the 1987 report,[97] cardiovascular abnormalities were studied in 71 patients with cervical, thoracic, or lumbar injuries admitted within 12 hours of their injuries. Persistent bradycardia, < 60 bpm, was universal in all 31 patients with severe (Frankel A and B) cervical cord injury but was less common in Frankel C and D cervical patients (six of 17 patients) and in thoracolumbar patients (three of 23 patients) ($p < 0.00001$). In the same group of patients, hypotension (BP < 90 mm Hg) was noted in 68 versus 0 patients ($p < 0.00001$). The frequency of bradyarrhythmias peaked on day 4 after injury and gradually declined thereafter. All observed abnormalities resolved spontaneously within 2 to 6 weeks.

Bilello et al[98] retrospectively studied the incidence of neurogenic shock and response to treatment among 83 tetraplegic patients (62 C1–C5 and 21 C6–C7 injuries). Age and injury severity scores were similar in the two groups. Neurogenic shock was present in 19 (31%) of the 62 patients with high cervical spinal cord injury and in five (24%) of the 21 patients with low cervical spinal cord injury ($p < 0.56$). There was a marked difference in the use of a cardiovascular intervention between those with a high and those with a low cervical spinal cord injury: 24% vs 5% of patients ($p < 0.02$). Two patients with C1 through C5 spinal cord injuries required cardiac pacemakers. The authors concluded that there was no significant difference in the frequency of neurogenic shock by injury level. Patients with a high cervical spinal cord injury (C1–C5) had a significantly greater requirement for a cardiovascular intervention than did patients with lower injuries (C6–C7).

Guly et al[99] have studied the incidence of neurogenic shock in England and Wales by analyzing data collected by the Trauma Audit and Research Network (TARN) from patients seen with isolated spinal cord injury in the emergency department. During the period 1989 to 2003, 490 such patients were admitted to the emergency department. For this analysis, neurogenic shock was defined as SBP < 100 mm Hg and heart rate < 80 BPM. On that basis, the incidence of neurogenic shock in cervical cord injuries was 19.3% (95% CI 14.8 to 23.7%). The incidences in thoracic and lumbar cord injuries were 7% (95% CI 3 to 11%) and 3% (CI 0 to 8.85%), respectively.

Summary and Recommendation

Animal experimental studies and clinical investigations indicate (supported by level III evidence) that immediately following spinal cord injury, depending on the severity and spinal level, there is a vasopressor response that lasts from 2 to 15 minutes, followed by hypotension and bradycardia (neurogenic shock), from which recovery is gradual over 2 to 6 weeks. Recovery is associated with various degrees of autonomic dysreflexia typified by surges of high blood pressure, tachyarrhythmia, sweating, and hyperthermia that may be detrimental, causing intracerebral hematomas, seizures, or even death. Derangement in vasomotor activity is due to total loss of α-adrenergic activity.

References

1. Miyanji F, Furlan JC, Aarabi B, Arnold PM, Fehlings MG. Acute cervical traumatic spinal cord injury: MR imaging findings correlated with neurologic outome—prospective study with 100 consecutive patients. Radiology 2007;243(3):820–827

2. Schaefer DM, Flanders AE, Osterholm JL, Northrup BE. Prognostic significance of magnetic resonance imaging in the acute phase of cervical spine injury. J Neurosurg 1992;76:218–223

3. PhDx Systems, Inc. Modified Standard Neurological Classification of Spinal Cord Injury/ASIA Impairment Scale V1.1. Albuquerque, NM: PhDx Systems, Inc.; 2004

4. Marino RJ, Ditunno JF Jr, Donovan WH, Maynard F Jr. Neurologic recovery after traumatic spinal cord injury: data from the Model Spinal Cord Injury Systems. Arch Phys Med Rehabil 1999;80:1391–1396

5. Oleson CV, Burns AS, Ditunno JF, Geisler FH, Coleman WP. Prognostic value of pinprick preservation in motor complete, sensory incomplete spinal cord injury. Arch Phys Med Rehabil 2005;86:988–992

6. Atkinson PP, Atkinson JL. Spinal shock. Mayo Clin Proc 1996;71:384–389

7. Ditunno JF Jr, Little JW, Burns A. Spinal shock: old terms, new paradigm. Lecture at Univ. Pittsburgh, Dept. PM&R, provided by Dr. J Harrop. 2003

8. Ditunno JF, Little JW, Tessler A, Burns AS. Spinal shock revisited: a four-phase model. Spinal Cord 2004;42:383–395

9. Ko HY, Ditunno JF Jr, Graziani V, Little JW. The pattern of reflex recovery during spinal shock. Spinal Cord 1999;37:402–409

10. Alexander RH, Proctor HJ. Advanced Trauma Life Support (ATLS) Program for Physicians. 1993 Instructor Manual. Chicago: American College of Surgeons; 1993

11. American College of Surgeons. Advanced Trauma Life Support (ATLS). 7th ed. Chicago: ACS; 2004

12. Sherrington CS. The Integrative Action of the Nervous System. London: Constable & Company LTD; 1906

13. Hall M. On the diseases and derangements of the nervous system. In: Their Primary Forms and in Their Modifications by Age, Sex, Constitution, Hereditary Disposition, Excesses, General Disorder, and Organic Disease. London: H. Bailliere; 1841:256

14. Hall M. Synopsis of the Diastolic Nervous System: or the System of the Spinal Marrow, and Its Reflex Arc; as the Nervous Agent in All the Functions of Integration and of Egestion in the Animal Oeconomy. London: Mallett J; 1850

15. Sherrington CS. The mammalian spinal cord as an organ of reflex action. Croonian Lecture (1897). Philos Trans 1898;190(B):128–138

16. Ashby P, Verrier M, Lightfoot E. Segmental reflex pathways in spinal shock and spinal spasticity in man. J Neurol Neurosurg Psychiatry 1974;37:1352–1360

17. Bach-y-Rita P, Illis LS. Spinal shock: possible role of receptor plasticity and non synaptic transmission. Paraplegia 1993;31:82–87

18. Dietz V, Colombo G. Recovery from spinal cord injury—underlying mechanisms and efficacy of rehabilitation. Acta Neurochir Suppl (Wien) 2004;89:95–100

19. Ghez C, Gordon J. Muscles and muscle receptors. In Kandel ER, Schwartz JH, Jessell TM, eds. Essentials of Neural Science and Behavior. Norwalk, CT: Appleton & Lange; 1995:501–513

20. Ghez C, Gordon J. Spinal reflexes. In Kandel ER, Schwartz JH, Jessell TM, eds. Essentials of Neural Science and Behavior. Norwalk, CT: Appleton & Lange; 1995:515–527

21. Holdsworth FW. Neurological diagnosis and the indications for treatment of paraplegia and tetraplegia, associated with fractures of the spine. Manit Med Rev 1968;48:16–18

22. Nacimiento W, Noth J. What, if anything, is spinal shock? Arch Neurol 1999;56:1033–1035

23. White RJ, Likavec MJ. Spinal shock—spinal man. J Trauma 1999;46:979–980

24. Calancie B, Molano MR, Broton JG. Tendon reflexes for predicting movement recovery after acute spinal cord injury in humans. Clin Neurophysiol 2004;115:2350–2363

25. Fisher CG, Noonan VK, Smith DE, et al. Motor recovery, functional status, and health-related quality of life in patients with complete spinal cord injuries. Spine 2005;30:2200–2207

26. Guttmann L. Studies on reflex activity of the isolated cord in the spinal man. J Nerv Ment Dis 1952;116:957–972

27. Hiersemenzel LP, Curt A, Dietz V. From spinal shock to spasticity: neuronal adaptations to a spinal cord injury. Neurology 2000;54:1574–1582

28. Stauffer ES. Diagnosis and prognosis of acute cervical spinal cord injury. Clin Orthop Relat Res 1975;112:9–15

29. van Gijn J. The Babinski Sign–a Centenary. Utrecht: Universiteit Utrecht; 1996

30. Weinstein DE, Ko HY, Graziani V, Ditunno JF Jr. Prognostic significance of the delayed plantar reflex following spinal cord injury. J Spinal Cord Med 1997;20:207–211

31. Pearson K, Gordon J. Spinal reflexes. In Kandel ER, Schwartz JH, Jessell TM, eds. Principles of Neural Science. 4th ed. New York: McGraw-Hill; 2000:713–736

32. Ghez C, Gordon J. An introduction to movement. In: Kandel ER, Schwartz JH, Jessell TM, eds. Essentials of Neural Science and Behavior. Norwalk, CT: Appleton & Lange; 1995:489–500

33. Parent A, Carpenter MB. Carpenter's Human Neuroanatomy. 9th ed. Baltimore: Williams & Wilkins; 1996

34. Holdsworth FH. Fractures, common dislocations, fractures-dislocations of the spine. J Bone Joint Surg Br 1963;45:6–26

35. Eckardt VF, Kanzler G. How reliable is digital examination for the evaluation of anal sphincter tone? Int J Colorectal Dis 1993;8:95–97

36. Esposito TJ, Ingraham A, Luchette FA, et al. Reasons to omit digital rectal exam in trauma patients: no fingers, no rectum, no useful additional information. J Trauma 2005;59:1314–1319

37. Guldner GT, Brzenski AB. The sensitivity and specificity of the digital rectal examination for detecting spinal cord injury in adult patients with blunt trauma. Am J Emerg Med 2006;24:113–117

38. Shlamovitz GZ, Mower WR, Bergman J, et al. Poor test characteristics for the digital rectal examination in trauma patients. Ann Emerg Med 2007;50:25–33, 33, e1

39. American Spinal Injury Association. International Standards for Neurological and Functional Classification of Spinal Cord Injury. Chicago: ASIA/IMSOP; 1992

40. Coleman WP, Geisler FH. Injury severity as primary predictor of outcome in acute spinal cord injury: retrospective results from a large multicenter clinical trial. Spine J 2004;4:373–378

41. Crozier KS, Graziani V, Ditunno JF Jr, Herbison GJ. Spinal cord injury: prognosis for ambulation based on sensory examination in patients who are initially motor complete. Arch Phys Med Rehabil 1991;72:119–121

42. Ditunno JF Jr, Young W, Donovan WH, Creasey G; American Spinal Injury Association. The international standards booklet for neurological and functional classification of spinal cord injury. Paraplegia 1994; 32:70–80

43. Ditunno JF Jr. New spinal cord injury standards, 1992. Paraplegia 1992; 30:90–91

44. El Masry WS, Tsubo M, Katoh S, El Miligui YH, Khan A. Validation of the American Spinal Injury Association (ASIA) motor score and the National Acute Spinal Cord Injury Study (NASCIS) motor score. Spine 1996;21: 614–619

45. Foo D, Subrahmanyan TS, Rossier AB. Post-traumatic acute anterior spinal cord syndrome. Paraplegia 1981;19:201–205

46. Maynard FM, Reynolds GG, Fountain S, Wilmot C, Hamilton R. Neurological prognosis after traumatic quadriplegia: three-year experience of California Regional Spinal Cord Injury Care System. J Neurosurg 1979; 50:611–616

47. Waters RL, Adkins RH, Sie IH, Yakura JS. Motor recovery following spinal cord injury associated with cervical spondylosis: a collaborative study. Spinal Cord 1996;34:711–715

48. Waters RL, Adkins RH, Yakura JS. Definition of complete spinal cord injury. Paraplegia 1991;29:573–581

49. Bedbrook G. Recovery of spinal cord function. Paraplegia 1980;18:315–323

50. Frankel HL, Hancock DO, Hyslop G, et al. The value of postural reduction in the initial management of closed injuries of the spine with paraplegia and tetraplegia, I. Paraplegia 1969;7:179–192

51. Waters RL, Adkins RH, Yakura JS, Sie I. Motor and sensory recovery following incomplete tetraplegia. Arch Phys Med Rehabil 1994;75: 306–311

52. Anderson DK, Means ED, Waters TR, Spears CJ. Spinal cord energy metabolism following compression trauma to the feline spinal cord. J Neurosurg 1980;53:375–380

53. Bergsneider M, Wu C, Huang H, Hovda D, Becker D, Martin N. Early abnormalities of regional brain metabolism following human traumatic brain injury: FDG and O-15 PET studies of hyperglycolysis, metabolic depression, and ischemia. Presented at the 2005 Annual Scientific Meeting of the American Association of Neurological Surgeons held in New Orleans, Louisiana. April 16–21, 2005

54. Bramlett HM, Dietrich WD. Pathophysiology of cerebral ischemia and brain trauma: similarities and differences. J Cereb Blood Flow Metab 2004;24:133–150

55. Bullock R, Butcher SP, Chen MH, Kendall L, McCulloch J. Correlation of the extracellular glutamate concentration with extent of blood flow reduction after subdural hematoma in the rat. J Neurosurg 1991;74:794–802

56. Carlson G, Gorden C, Wada E, Nakazawa S, Biro C, La Manna J. Vascular re-perfusion and neurol preservation after spinal cord injury. J Neurotrauma 1998;15:860

57. Coles JP. Regional ischemia after head injury. Curr Opin Crit Care 2004; 10:120–125

58. Coles JP, Fryer TD, Smielewski P, et al. Incidence and mechanisms of cerebral ischemia in early clinical head injury. J Cereb Blood Flow Metab 2004;24:202–211

59. Fehlings MG, Tator CH, Linden RD. The relationships among the severity of spinal cord injury, motor and somatosensory evoked potentials and spinal cord blood flow. Electroencephalogr Clin Neurophysiol 1989; 74:241–259

60. Fujisawa H, Maxwell WL, Graham DI, Reasdale GM, Bullock R. Focal microvascular occlusion after acute subdural haematoma in the rat: a mechanism for ischaemic damage and brain swelling? Acta Neurochir Suppl (Wien) 1994;60:193–196

61. Graham DI, Adams JH. Ischaemic brain damage in fatal head injuries. Lancet 1971;1:265–266

62. Hoelper BM, Reinert MM, Zauner A, Doppenberg E, Bullock R. rCBF in hemorrhagic, non-hemorrhagic and mixed contusions after severe head injury and its effect on perilesional cerebral blood flow. Acta Neurochir Suppl (Wien) 2000;76:21–25

63. Hovda DA, Lee SM, Smith ML, et al. The neurochemical and metabolic cascade following brain injury: moving from animal models to man. J Neurotrauma 1995;12:903–906

64. Schröder ML, Muizelaar JP, Bullock MR, Salvant JB, Povlishock JT. Focal ischemia due to traumatic contusions documented by stable xenon-CT and ultrastructural studies. J Neurosurg 1995;82:966–971

65. Simard JM, Kent TA, Chen M, Tarasov KV, Gerzanich V. Brain oedema in focal ischaemia: molecular pathophysiology and theoretical implications. Lancet Neurol 2007;6:258–268

66. Stiefel MF, Tomita Y, Marmarou A. Secondary ischemia impairing the restoration of ion homeostasis following traumatic brain injury. J Neurosurg 2005;103:707–714

67. Tator CH, Fehlings MG. Review of the secondary injury theory of acute spinal cord trauma with emphasis on vascular mechanisms. J Neurosurg 1991;75:15–26

68. Kobrine AI, Doyle TF, Rizzoli HV. Spinal cord blood flow as affected by changes in systemic arterial blood pressure. J Neurosurg 1976;44:12–15

69. Lewelt W, Jenkins LW, Miller JD. Autoregulation of cerebral blood flow after experimental fluid percussion injury of the brain. J Neurosurg 1980;53:500–511

70. Senter HJ, Venes JL. Loss of autoregulation and posttraumatic ischemia following experimental spinal cord trauma. J Neurosurg 1979;50:198–206

71. Hadley MN, Walters BC, Grabb PA, et al. Blood pressure management after acute spinal cord injury. Neurosurgery 2002;50(3, Suppl):S58–S62

72. Levi L, Wolf A, Belzberg H. Hemodynamic parameters in patients with acute cervical cord trauma: description, intervention, and prediction of outcome. Neurosurgery 1993;33:1007–1016, discussion 1016–1017

73. Tator CH, Rowed DW, Schwartz ML, et al. Management of acute spinal cord injuries. Can J Surg 1984;27:289–293, 296

74. Vale FL, Burns J, Jackson AB, Hadley MN. Combined medical and surgical treatment after acute spinal cord injury: results of a prospective pilot study to assess the merits of aggressive medical resuscitation and blood pressure management. J Neurosurg 1997;87:239–246

75. Wolf A, Levi L, Mirvis S, et al. Operative management of bilateral facet dislocation. J Neurosurg 1991;75:883–890

76. Zäch GA, Seiler W, Dollfus P. Treatment results of spinal cord injuries in the Swiss Parplegic Centre of Basle. Paraplegia 1976;14:58–65

77. Furlan JC, Fehlings MG, Shannon P, Norenberg MD, Krassioukov AV. Descending vasomotor pathways in humans: correlation between axonal preservation and cardiovascular dysfunction after spinal cord injury. J Neurotrauma 2003;20:1351–1363

78. Krassioukov A, Claydon VE. The clinical problems in cardiovascular control following spinal cord injury: an overview. Prog Brain Res 2006; 152:223–229

79. Krassioukov AV, Bunge RP, Pucket WR, Bygrave MA. The changes in human spinal sympathetic preganglionic neurons after spinal cord injury. Spinal Cord 1999;37:6–13

80. Teasell RW, Arnold JM, Krassioukov A, Delaney GA. Cardiovascular consequences of loss of supraspinal control of the sympathetic nervous system after spinal cord injury. Arch Phys Med Rehabil 2000;81:506–516

81. Yeoh M, McLachlan EM, Brock JA. Tail arteries from chronically spinalized rats have potentiated responses to nerve stimulation in vitro. J Physiol 2004;556(Pt 2):545–555

82. Bravo G, Guízar-Sahagún G, Ibarra A, Centurión D, Villalón CM. Cardiovascular alterations after spinal cord injury: an overview. Curr Med Chem Cardiovasc Hematol Agents 2004;2:133–148

83. Helkowski WM, Ditunno JF Jr, Boninger M. Autonomic dysreflexia: incidence in persons with neurologically complete and incomplete tetraplegia. J Spinal Cord Med 2003;26:244–247

84. Naftchi NE, Wooten GF, Lowman EW, Axelrod J. Relationship between serum dopamine-beta-hydroxylase activity, catecholamine metabolism, and hemodynamic changes during paroxysmal hypertension in quadriplegia. Circ Res 1974;35:850–861

85. Alexander S, Kerr FWL. Blood pressure responses in acute compression of the spinal cord. J Neurosurg 1964;21:485–491

86. Eidelberg EE. Cardiovascular response to experimental spinal cord compression. J Neurosurg 1973;38:326–331

87. Evans DE, Kobrine AI, Rizzoli HV. Cardiac arrhythmias accompanying acute compression of the spinal cord. J Neurosurg 1980;52:52–59

88. Greenhoot JH, Shiel FO, Mauck HP Jr. Experimental spinal cord injury: electrocardiographic abnormalities and fuchsinophilic myocardial degeneration. Arch Neurol 1972;26:524–529

89. Greenhoot JH, Mauck HP Jr. The effect of cervical cord injury on cardiac rhythm and conduction. Am Heart J 1972;83:659–662

90. Rawe SE, Perot PL Jr. Pressor response resulting from experimental contusion injury to the spinal cord. J Neurosurg 1979;50:58–63

91. Tibbs PA, Young B, McAllister RG, Brooks WH, Tackett L. Studies of experimental cervical spinal cord transection, I: Hemodynamic changes after acute cervical spinal cord transection. J Neurosurg 1978;49:558–562

92. Young W, DeCrescito V, Tomasula JJ, Ho V. The role of the sympathetic nervous system in pressor responses induced by spinal injury. J Neurosurg 1980;52:473–481

93. Piepmeier JM, Lehmann KB, Lane JG. Cardiovascular instability following acute cervical spinal cord trauma. Cent Nerv Syst Trauma 1985;2:153–160

94. Soderstrom CA, Ducker TB. Increased susceptibility of patients with cervical cord lesions to peptic gastrointestinal complications. J Trauma 1985;25:1030–1038

95. Zipnick RI, Scalea TM, Trooskin SZ, et al. Hemodynamic responses to penetrating spinal cord injuries. J Trauma 1993;35:578–582, discussion 582–583

96. Dro P, Gschaedler R, Dollfus P, Komminoth R, Florange W. Clinical and anatomical observation of a patient with a complete lesion at C1 with maintenance of a normal blood pressure during 40 minutes after the accident. Paraplegia 1982;20:169–173

97. Lehmann KG, Lane JG, Piepmeier JM, Batsford WP. Cardiovascular abnormalities accompanying acute spinal cord injury in humans: incidence, time course and severity. J Am Coll Cardiol 1987;10:46–52

98. Bilello JF, Davis JW, Cunningham MA, Groom TF, Lemaster D, Sue LP. Cervical spinal cord injury and the need for cardiovascular intervention. Arch Surg 2003;138:1127–1129

99. Guly HR, Bouamra O, Lecky FE; Trauma Audit and Research Network. The incidence of neurogenic shock in patients with isolated spinal cord injury in the emergency department. Resuscitation 2008;76:57–62

8

American Spinal Injury Association Neurological Examination and Neurological Assessment of Spinal Cord Injury

Stavropoula I. Tjoumakaris and James S. Harrop

Traumatic spinal cord injury (SCI) is a devastating event with an estimated annual incidence in the United States of 40 cases per 1 million people, or ~11,000 new patients per year.[1] This heterogeneous disease process affects each patient differently, and outcomes can be influenced by the baseline neurological dysfunction, age of patient, concurrent comorbidities, and social influences. Therefore, the variability of each patient's individual neurological examination and the consequent differences in functional outcome mandate a systematic approach in the assessment of this population. A universal grading system should provide the clinician with an accurate assessment of a patient's initial neurological status, a predicting tool to a patient's functional outcome, a grading scheme for evaluation of implemented therapies, and a simple method for transmitting patient SCI severity to colleagues.

A variety of grading schemes or assessment strategies have been proposed for the neurological assessment of SCI. Unfortunately, however, there is limited evidence-based medical documentation and no class I literature to support the usage of any system or one in particular. Presently, the American Spinal Injury Association (ASIA) scale is most commonly utilized because it provides an accurate and reliable classification with a low interrater variability. This chapter outlines the components of this scheme and provides evidence for its value in the assessment of SCI.

◆ The American Spinal Injury Association Classification System

The American Spinal Injury Association, after assessing the need for a uniform grading scale for SCI patients, introduced a new classification system in 1984. Limitations of the scale and areas of improvement were identified, and it was then later revised in 1992 to incorporate the modified Frankel scale, the ASIA Impairment Scale, and the Functional Independence Measure (FIM).[2]

The ASIA neurological assessment features two main components, a motor and a sensory evaluation. The motor examination is graded utilizing a scale from 0 to 5:

- 0—Total paralysis (no movement)
- 1—Palpable or visible muscular contraction
- 2—Full range of movement with gravity eliminated
- 3—Full range of movement against gravity
- 4—Full range of movement against gravity and partial additional resistance
- 5—Normal or full motor activity

The exam separates upper and lower limbs, which are further subdivided into five major muscle groups, where each muscle group represents a specific spinal segment (**Fig. 8.1**). For example, the C7 spinal segment is represented by the elbow extensors because the primary muscle is the triceps, which is innervated by a majority of C7 nerve fibers. In addition, the left and right sides are scored separately where each limb gets a total maximum of 25, and a score of 100 represents an individual without a motor deficit.

The sensory examination utilizes a numeric scale from 0 to 2:

- 0—Absent sensation
- 1—Presence of sensation but "abnormal"
- 2—Normal or intact sensation.

The system divides the sensory examination in a total of 28 dermatomes: seven cervical, 12 thoracic, five lumbar, and four sacral (**Fig. 8.1**), and similar to the motor evaluation, the left and right sides of the body are graded individually. It further

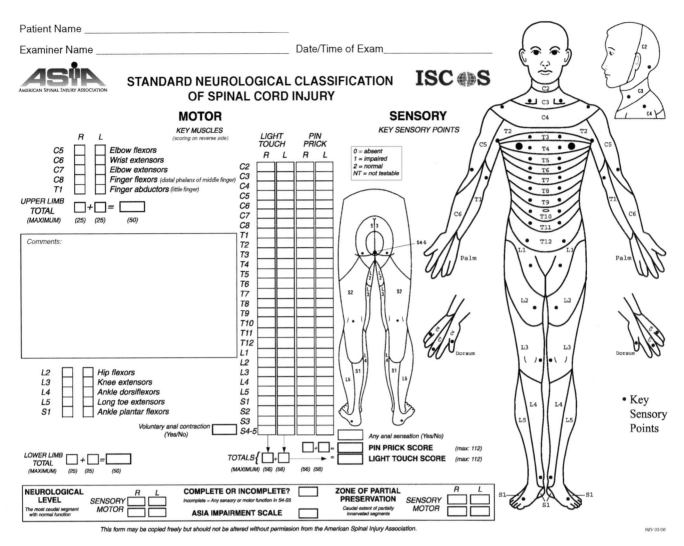

Fig. 8.1 American Spinal Injury Association neurological classification of spinal cord injury. (From American Spinal Injury Association. International Standards for Neurological Classification of Spinal Cord Injury. Revised 2000; reprinted 2008. Atlanta, GA. Reprinted with permission.)

examines two distinct sensory modalities, light touch and pinprick, thus assessing two separate spinal sensory pathways, the dorsal columns and spinothalamic systems, respectively. Each sensory modality has a maximum bilateral total of 112 points, thus making 224 for a patient without a sensory deficit.

Based on both the motor and sensory assessments, a cumulative neurological evaluation is defined. This system in addition provides the ability to identify the level of where a spinal injury occurred based on the most caudal level with normal function. An injury can be broadly classified as complete or incomplete based on the presence of any motor or sensory function distal to the area of injury. To further precisely define the location and extent of the injury the ASIA Impairment Scale is included in the final score, which is similar to the modified Frankel score. Specifically, an ASIA A patient has a complete injury without preservation of motor and sensory function below the injury and specifically at S4–S5. An ASIA B patient has an incomplete injury with some sensory preserved but no motor function below the level of injury. In addition the ASIA C and D patients are also incomplete injuries with both motor and sensory partial preservation below the injury. To differentiate between an ASIA C and ASIA D patient if the grading of half of the key muscle groups,

below the injury, is less than 3 of 5 motor strength then the injury is classified as an ASIA C, whereas if greater than 3 of 5 motor strength then the patient is classified as an ASIA D. Finally, the ASIA E classification is reserved for an individual that sustained an SCI and then has a return to a normal motor and sensory examination. The steps in the ASIA classification system are depicted in **Fig. 8.2**.[3]

History of the ASIA Classification System

The importance of a classification system for SCI is exemplified by the numerous systems that have been proposed over time. The first assessment system of acute SCI was reported by Frankel and colleagues in 1969.[4] They reviewed 682 SCI patients that presented to Stoke Mandeville Hospital over a 19-year period. Frankel et al stratified the injuries into a five-letter grade (A to E) based on decreasing severity. Grade A was described as a complete motor and sensory deficit below the level of the lesion. Grade B patients had sensory but no motor function below the level of the injury. Grades C and D had both motor and sensory functions below the level of injury; in grade C, motor function was present but not useful for the patient, as opposed to grade D.

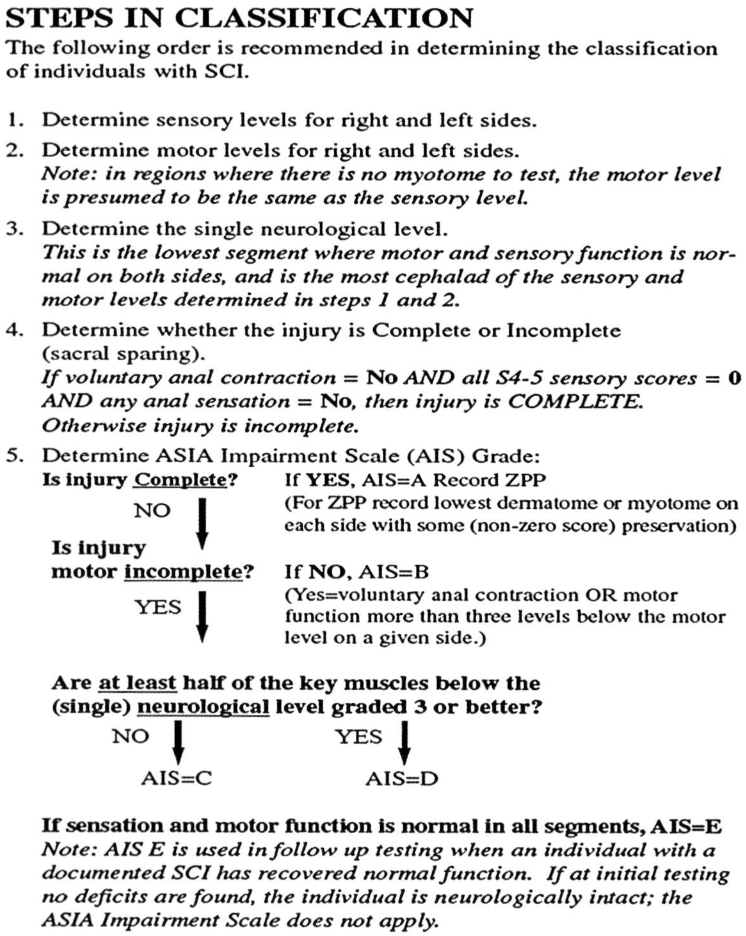

STEPS IN CLASSIFICATION

The following order is recommended in determining the classification of individuals with SCI.

1. Determine sensory levels for right and left sides.

2. Determine motor levels for right and left sides.
   Note: in regions where there is no myotome to test, the motor level is presumed to be the same as the sensory level.

3. Determine the single neurological level.
   This is the lowest segment where motor and sensory function is normal on both sides, and is the most cephalad of the sensory and motor levels determined in steps 1 and 2.

4. Determine whether the injury is Complete or Incomplete (sacral sparing).
   If voluntary anal contraction = No AND all S4-5 sensory scores = 0 AND any anal sensation = No, then injury is COMPLETE. Otherwise injury is incomplete.

5. Determine ASIA Impairment Scale (AIS) Grade:

   Is injury Complete?   If **YES**, AIS=A Record ZPP
   (For ZPP record lowest dermatome or myotome on each side with some (non-zero score) preservation)

   NO ↓

   Is injury motor incomplete?   If **NO**, AIS=B
   (Yes=voluntary anal contraction OR motor function more than three levels below the motor level on a given side.)

   YES ↓

   Are at least half of the key muscles below the (single) neurological level graded 3 or better?

   NO ↓   YES ↓

   AIS=C   AIS=D

   If sensation and motor function is normal in all segments, AIS=E
   Note: AIS E is used in follow up testing when an individual with a documented SCI has recovered normal function. If at initial testing no deficits are found, the individual is neurologically intact; the ASIA Impairment Scale does not apply.

Fig. 8.2 American Spinal Injury Association classification system algorithm. (From American Spinal Injury Association. International Standards for Neurological Classification of Spinal Cord Injury. Revised 2000; reprinted 2008. Atlanta, GA. Reprinted with permission.)

Finally, grade E patients had full neurological recovery without any motor or sensory deficits. The Frankel classification system was modified in later years in attempts to improve its sensitivity in detecting functional outcome in SCI patients and was used as a template for the ASIA classification system.[5]

In the late 1970s, Bracken and colleagues introduced a new SCI classification system based on five-scale motor and seven-scale sensory examinations.[6] However, this system did not gain wide acceptance by clinicians because it lacked an assessment of sacral function in terms of bowel and bladder exams and the further complexity of the two separate scales. Later that decade, Lucas and Ducker attempted to classify acute SCI based solely on their motor examination of 14 major muscle groups.[7] Although this system was not used widely, it did provide the basis for the motor examination of the presently utilized ASIA system. In the 1980s, the three further SCI classification systems were endorsed by separate groups in Miami, Yale, and Sunnybrook. The University of Miami Neuro-spinal Index was a very detailed system, but this resulted in it being a cumbersome rating system comprising 44 muscle groups and 30 dermatomes.[8] The Yale scale simplified the motor grading into 10 muscle categories and sensory grading into three modalities; however, it failed to assess sacral nerve function, as well as bowel and bladder functions.[9] The Sunnybrook Cord Injury Scale, in addition, also had limited assessment of the lower sacral function and did not present a reliable muscle grading system.[5]

In 1989, ASIA, in an attempt to standardize the grading and classification of SCI patients, introduced its first neurological grading system for SCI patients. This system incorporated a 0–5 motor scale on 10 representative muscle groups, a functional classification based on the older Frankel system; however, it did not provide a systematic grading system for the sensory examination.[10] These standards were reevaluated and revised in 1989 to include a more specific and detailed sensory examination.[11] Finally, in 1992, an update of the ASIA standards was proposed in association with the International Medical Society of Paraplegia (IMSOP). This version included a functional impairment scale, the Functional Independence Measure (FIM).[2] The FIM provide a systematic evaluation of a patient's functional status by grading the ability to perform activities of daily living such as eating, grooming, and dressing. Concurrently there was the completion of two National Acute SCI studies (NASCIS I and II), which utilized and introduced an alternate grading system. Specifically, the motor grading of 14 major muscle groups in scales of either 1 to 6 (NASCIS I) or 0 to 5 (NASCIS II), the sensory grading in a scale of 0 to 3.[12,13] However, both grading scales did not include a measure of the patient's functional status. The ASIA standard was last revised in 1996 by ASIA and IMSOP and has been used widely for the neurological assessment of patients with acute SCI.[14]

Comparison of ASIA and Other Classification Systems

Fortunately, the ASIA classification system has been evaluated for its reliability, accuracy, and construct validity, and it has been compared with previous assessment scales. In 1993, Bednarczyk and Sanderson compared three different scales as functional and medical assessment tools in SCI, namely, the ASIA scale, Bracken scale (BS), and wheelchair basketball (BB) Sports Test.[15] Thirty SCI patients were graded based on each of the aforementioned scales by one examiner and the results were compared. The Spearman's rho correlation coefficients revealed positive associations between the ASIA Scale and BB Sports Test to the patient's neurological examination (0.81). However, the BS did not show a positive correlation. The ASIA scale was superior in that it illustrated the greatest discrimination in grouping subjects with SCI in mixed (complete and incomplete) as well as incomplete injuries.

Wells and Nicosia published a prospective analysis on 35 patients with acute SCI based on five different grading systems (Frankel scale, Yale scale, ASIA Motor Index Score, Modified Barthel Index, and Functional Independence Measurement scores).[16] The evaluation included important clinical parameters of functional outcome. Their analysis revealed that none of these scales individually correlated with significant functional milestones, such as mobility and nutrition. They concluded that the combined use of two scales, one for neurological impairment and the other for functional disability, provides a more accurate description of the SCI population.

El Masry et al performed a retrospective review of 62 patients with acute SCI in an attempt to compare the validity of the ASIA and NASCIS motor scores.[17] The data illustrated both motor scores were representative of the conventional motor score for the evaluation of the motor deficit and the motor recovery of patients ($p < 0.0001$). Therefore, they concluded that both scales could be used interchangeably for the neurological quantification of motor deficit and motor recovery in patients with acute SCI.

The 1992 revision of the ASIA classification system was prospectively assessed by Cohen and colleagues[18] by testing 106 clinicians to assess the accuracy of the classification of two SCI patients, one complete and one incomplete, before and after an instructive presentation and video on ASIA classification. The authors found that the classification accuracy was high for the complete patient but considerably lower for the incomplete patient before and after professional education. They concluded that the 1992 ASIA standards required further revisions and clarification to ensure interrater reliability and accuracy. Jonsson et al further confirmed a weak interrater reliability in SCI classification based on the 1992 standards.[19] In this study, two physicians and two physical therapists classified 23 SCI patients according to the 1992 ASIA standards. The Kappa values varied from 0 to 0.83 (poor to very good correlation) for the pinprick, 0 to 1 (poor to excellent correlation) for the light touch, and from 0 to 0.89 for motor function (poor to excellent correlation). In 1994, ASIA and IMSOP proposed new standards for the neurological and functional classification of SCI patients, including the ASIA impairment scale, the ASIA motor index score, the ASIA sensory scale, and FIM outcome based on the finding and criticisms of clinicians.

Utilizing these current standards, Savic et al in 2007 in a prospective observational study tested the interrater reliability of motor and sensory examinations.[20] Two experienced examiners evaluated the motor and sensory ASIA scores of 45 patients with SCI. Total ASIA scores showed very strong correlation between the two examiners, with Pearson correlation coefficients greater than 0.96, and p-value < 0.01 for total motor, light touch, and pinprick scores. The two examiners were in agreement with the majority of individual muscle testing, with highest correlation coefficient for grade 0 strength and

least correlation with grade 3 motor strength. The ASIA impairment scores did not show any statistical difference between the two examiners. As a result, the authors concluded that the new ASIA standards have an excellent interrater validity and reliability in the assessment of SCI patients.

In 2006, Graves et al proposed improvement of the ASIA classification standards through the use of separate upper and lower extremity motor scales of SCI.[21] A retrospective analysis of 6116 patients with SCI assessments by ASIA motor scales showed that the use of separate upper and lower extremity motor scales had a variance of 87%, as opposed to a single motor scale with 82%. The authors concluded that the subdivision of the ASIA motor classification into two separate dimensions provides a more accurate representation of the SCI motor examination and further reflects on patient functional outcome.

With the assistance of the evidence-based classification guidelines proposed by Fisher et al and Schünemann et al,[22,23] the different articles related to the reliability of the ASIA classification system were graded and tabulated (**Table 8.1**).

◆ Outcome Assessment Based on ASIA Score

In 1989, Lazar et al evaluated the relationship between early motor score and functional outcome in 78 patients with acute SCI.[24] Within 72 hours following injury, 52 tetraplegic and 26 paraplegic patients were evaluated with the ASIA motor score in addition to the functional Modified Barthel Index (MBI). This evaluation was performed by a senior physical therapist and repeated every 30 days during rehabilitation. In tetraplegic patients, the ASIA motor score correlated with their functional outcome at admission, during rehabilitation, and at time of discharge ($p = 0.001$). However, this statistical correlation was not supported in the paraplegic subgroup. In this group, the correlation was statistically significant in the self-care functional subgroup ($p = 0.01$) but not in the mobility subgroup. The complete injured patients had a statistical significance correlation of initial ASIA motor score and functional outcome upon discharge ($p = 0.001$), which was not seen with the incomplete injured patients. Therefore, Lazar et al concluded that the ASIA motor score is a useful tool in predicting functional outcome in patients with SCI, with considerable limitations in ambulatory outcome, especially for the paraplegic patients.

Outcome analysis of SCI patients in terms of ambulation has been investigated by multiple research groups. Waters et al, in 1994, performed a prospective study in 36 patients with SCI comparing the strength of ASIA motor scores to motor scores obtained from walking biomechanics in predicting ambulation.[25] Their ambulatory assessment included measurements of strength, gait performance, and energy expenditures. The ASIA score showed a strong correlation with the percent increase in the rate of oxygen consumption above normal ($p < 0.0005$), oxygen cost per meter ($p < 0.0006$), peak axial load exerted by the arms on crutches ($p < 0.0001$), velocity ($p < 0.0001$), and cadence ($p < 0.0001$). It also showed a strong correlation with the complex biomechanical motor score system. These authors also found that patients with lower extremity ASIA scores less than or equal to 20 were limited ambulators as opposed to greater than or equal to 30 who were community ambulators. Overall, the authors concluded that the ASIA motor score is a simple yet useful tool in predicting patient walking ability following SCI.

Table 8.1 American Spinal Injury Association Scoring Reliability and Accuracy in the Neurological Exam of Spinal Cord Injury Patients

Reference	Study Design	Evidence	Level of Evidence
Savic et al[20]	Prospective observational	100% interrater reliability for total ASIA scoring; Pearson correlation coefficient of 0.9986 and 0.9999 for sensory and motor subcategories.	III
Graves et al[21]	Retrospective	Separate scales for upper and lower extremities more accurately represent motor function than the single motor scale of ASIA scoring; chi^2 (difference) of 2596; df = 1; $p < 0.0001$.	III
Cohen et al[18]	Prospective	ASIA classification accuracy compared in two professionals before and after classification education. Accuracy was high for the complete patient but considerably lower for the incomplete patient before and after education.	III
El Masry et al[17]	Retrospective	ASIA and NASCIS motor scores were both representative of the conventional motor score for the evaluation of the motor deficit percentage and the motor recovery percentage in all levels ($p < 0.0001$). They can both be used for the neurological quantification of motor deficit and motor recovery.	III
Wells and Nicosia[16]	Prospective	Analysis of the Frankel scale, Yale scale, ASIA Motor Index Score, Modified Barthel Index, and Functional Independence Measurement scores revealed that none on these scales individually correlated with significant functional milestones.	III
Bednarczyk and Sanderson[15]	Prospective	Spearman's rho correlation coefficients revealed positive associations between the ASIA scale and BB Sports Test to the patient's neurological examination (0.81). The ASIA scale was superior in that it illustrated the greatest discrimination in grouping subjects with SCI in mixed (complete and incomplete), as well as incomplete injuries.	III
Jonsson et al[19]	Prospective	Weak interrater reliability in SCI classification based on the 1992 ASIA standards. Kappa values varied from 0 to 0.83 (poor to very good correlation) for the pinprick, 0 to 1 (poor to excellent correlation) for the light touch, and from 0 to 0.89 for motor function (poor to excellent correlation) between four professionals	III

Abbreviations: ASIA, American Spinal Injury Association; BB, basketball; df, degrees of freedom; NASCIS, National Acute Spinal Cord Injury Study; SCI, spinal cord injury.

Curt et al published two articles in 1997 and 1998 on the predictive value of ASIA motor and sensory scores as they relate to ambulatory status. In the earlier study, 70 acute and 34 chronic SCI patients were studied by an initial ASIA evaluation and ambulatory capacity 6 months following rehabilitation.[26] In the acute SCI group, the initial ASIA scores showed statistical significance in the correlation with ambulatory capacity ($p < 0.001$). The authors found that the motor but not the sensory ASIA subgroup showed a significant increase ($p < 0.05$) during the 6-month rehabilitation period. An additional parameter, tibial and pudendal somatosensory evoked potentials (SSEPs), was investigated and found to have a similar predictive value. Therefore, the authors concluded that ASIA scores and SSEPs were related to the ambulatory outcome in acute SCI patients and can contribute to the selection of the appropriate therapeutic approaches during rehabilitation. In the later article, Curt investigated the ambulatory and hand function correlation to ASIA scores and motor evoked potentials (MEPs).[27] Thirty-six acute and 34 chronic SCI patients were evaluated with ASIA scores in addition to upper and lower limb MEP. The author noted that both ASIA scores and MEP recordings had statistical significance ($p < 0.001$) in predicting ambulation and hand function. In the acute SCI subgroup, for the 6 months following trauma, the ASIA motor scores increased significantly [analysis of variance (ANOVA), $p < 0.05$], whereas the ASIA sensory scores and MEP recordings

were unchanged (ANOVA, $p > 0.1$). Lastly, Dobkin et al in 2007 published a multicenter SCI locomotor trial.[28] This single-blinded, randomized study compared 12 weeks of step training with body weight support on a treadmill training (BWSTT) in 107 patients with incomplete traumatic SCI within 8 weeks of onset. The FIM for walking and lower extremity motor score (LEMS) were collected every 2 weeks. Although there were no statistical differences in ambulation between admission and discharge from rehabilitation, the ASIA levels showed correlation with walking outcome. Specifically, FIM for walking greater than or equal to 4 was achieved in less than 10% of ASIA B patients, 92% of ASIA C patients, and all of ASIA D patients. The authors concluded that time after SCI is an important variable for entering patients into a trial with mobility outcomes, and they suggested future patient inclusion at greater than 8 weeks after onset, if still graded ASIA B, and at greater than 12 weeks if still ASIA C.

The assessment of sacral function in terms of bladder function correlation with ASIA scores and SSEPs was investigated by Curt et al in 1997.[26] Seventy patients with acute traumatic SCI were evaluated with ASIA scores as well as tibial and pudendal SSEPs within 10 days following injury and after 6 months of rehabilitation. The degree of bladder function recovery was assessed by urodynamic examination. The recovery of somatic nerve function (external urethral sphincter) was correlated to both the initial ASIA scores and SSEP recordings (Spearman correlation, $p < 0.001$). However, no statistical correlation was found with the outcome of autonomic nerve function (e.g., detrusor muscle function) (Spearman correlation, $p = 0.1$). The authors concluded that initial ASIA and electrophysiological examinations are important in the assessment of the degree to which the patient will recover somatic nervous control of bladder function, but they do not have predictive value in the urodynamic recovery of the patient.

Marino et al reported on the importance of ASIA subgroups in predicting functional outcome in SCI patients.[29] The first publication in 1995 compared motor level (ML) and upper extremity motor score (UEMS) to the neurological level (NL) in predicting self-care functional status in 50 patients with traumatic motor complete tetraplegia. Following initial examination with the aforementioned ASIA subgroups, the ability to perform six feeding activities of the Quadriplegia Index of Function (QIF) was documented. The best and worst ML and UEMS were more highly correlated to the QIF feeding score than was the NL (0.74 and 0.72 vs 0.56, $p < 0.05$). Specifically, the UEMS had the highest correlation to the QIF feeding score (0.78). In conclusion the ASIA ML and UEMS have a stronger predictive value than the NL in the assessment of functional outcome of patients with complete motor tetraplegia. In the later publication (2004), Marino et al investigated the importance of ASIA motor scale subgrouping in motor FIM instrument scores. In a retrospective analysis, 4338 patients with traumatic SCI were studied upon discharge from rehabilitation programs with ASIA motor and subgroup scores and motor FIM scores. The analysis revealed that the use of distinct ASIA upper extremity and lower extremity motor scores improved prediction of motor FIM scores compared with the total ASIA motor score (R^2 for motor FIM score, 0.71 vs 0.59).

In 2004, Kirshblum et al reported several parameters to assess late neurological recovery in SCI patients.[30] The ASIA score, motor index score, and neurological level were determined in 987 patients at 1 and 5 years following traumatic SCI. The majority of subjects (94.4%) who had a neurologically complete injury at 1 year remained complete at 5 years following trauma. However, 3.5% improved to ASIA grade B and 1.05% to ASIA grades C and D. There was a statistically significant change noted for motor index score. Therefore, the authors concluded that, although small, there are a percentage of patients who will progress from a motor complete to an incomplete status up to 5 years following traumatic SCI.

The articles on the ASIA classification system as a prognostic tool for functional outcome are categorized and tabulated based on the Fisher and Schünemann proposed evidence-based guidelines (**Table 8.2**).[22,23]

◆ Summary and Recommendations

◆ *Is ASIA the most reliable and accurate neurologic examination for spinal cord injury patients?* The ASIA classification system, which includes the ASIA impairment scale, the ASIA motor index score, the ASIA sensory scale, and FIM outcome, is one of the most clinically utilized systems for traumatic SCI. It has an interrater validity and reliability that are comparable to previous scales, and a superior predictive value for functional outcome.

Table 8.2 American Spinal Injury Association Classification as a Prognostic Tool for Functional and Rehabilitative Recovery of Spinal Cord Injury Patients

Reference	Study Design	Evidence	Level of Evidence
Dobkin et al[28]	Prospective, single-blinded, randomized	Functional walking ability achieved in < 10% of ASIA B, 92% of ASIA C, and 100% of ASIA D patients.	III
Marino and Graves[29]	Retrospective analysis of prospectively collected data	Functional impairment in SCI is more accurately characterized by using separate ASIA upper and lower extremity motor scores than by using a single motor score, with a 71% vs 59% FIM variance, respectively.	III
Kirshblum et al[30]	Retrospective longitudinal	20% SCI patients improved motor level, neurological level of injury and motor impairment scale from year 1 to year 5 postinjury. Improvement was more likely to occur in ASIA levels B, C, and D as opposed to A.	III
Curt et al[27]	Prospective cohort correlation	In acute and chronic SCI, the initial ASIA score was significantly related ($p < 0.0001$) to the outcome of ambulatory capacity and hand function. Ambulatory capacity could be predicted by the ASIA motor score of the lower limbs (Spearman correlation coefficient, 0.78; $p < 0.0001$).	II
Curt et al[26]	Prospective	Recovery of somatic nerve function (external urethral sphincter function) involved in bladder function was correlated to the initial ASIA scores (Spearman correlation, $p < 0.001$). However, recovery of autonomic nerve function (e.g., detrusor vesicae function) did not show such correlation (Spearman correlation, $p = 0.1$).	III
Curt and Dietz[31]	Prospective cohort correlation	In acute SCI the initial ASIA scores are related ($p < 0.001$) to the outcome of ambulatory capacity. In acute paraplegia the ASIA motor score (Spearman correlation coefficient. 0.90; $p < 0.001$) was best related to the outcome of ambulatory capacity.	III

Table 8.2 American Spinal Injury Association Classification as a Prognostic Tool for Functional and Rehabilitative Recovery of Spinal Cord Injury Patients (*Continued*)

Reference	Study Design	Evidence	Level of Evidence
Marino et al[32]-	Prospective cohort	NL is an imprecise descriptor of the impairment in SCI and is therefore a poor predictor of the resultant disability. The ML and the UEMS better reflect the severity of impairment and disability after motor complete tetraplegia.	III
Waters et al[25]	Prospective	ASIA score showed a strong correlation with the percent increase in the rate of oxygen consumption above normal ($p < 0\ 0.0005$), oxygen cost per meter ($p < 0\ 0.0006$), peak axial load exerted by the arms on crutches ($p < 0\ 0.0001$), velocity ($p < 0.0001$), and cadence ($p < 0.0001$). It also showed a strong correlation with the complex biomechanical motor score system.	III
Lazar et al[24]	Prospective	In tetraplegic patients, the ASIA motor score correlated with their functional outcome at admission, during rehabilitation, and at time of discharge ($p = 0.001$). Complete injuries had a statistical significance correlation of initial ASIA motor score and functional outcome upon discharge ($p = 0.001$).	III

Abbreviations: ASIA, American Spinal Injury Association; FIM, Functional Independence Measure; ML, motor level; NL, neurological level; SCI, spinal cord injury; UEMS, upper extremity motor score.

◆ *Is the ASIA examination a prognostic tool for functional and rehabilitative recovery of spinal cord injury patients*? The ASIA classification system is a great prognostic tool for the rehabilitative recovery of SCI patients. Ambulatory capacity, hand function, bladder function, and feeding are some of the patient functional outcomes that have been found to have statistical correlation with initial ASIA classification scores. The subdivision of the ASIA motor score into distinct upper and lower extremity scales has shown to provide ASIA classification with an improved interrater validity and a stronger predictive value of patient functional outcome.

References

1. Spinal Cord Injury Information Network. SCI Facts and Stats. 2006. Available at:http://www.spinalcord.vab.edu/show.asp?durk;=21390. Accessed September 18, 2007
2. ASIA/IMSOP. Standards for Neurological and Functional Classification of Spinal Cord Injury. Chicago: American Spinal Injury Association/International Medical Society of Paraplegia; 1992
3. Standards for Neurological and Functional Classification of Spinal Cord Injury. Chicago: American Spinal Injury Association/International Medical Society of Paraplegia; 2006
4. Frankel HL, Hancock DO, Hyslop G, et al. The value of postural reduction in the initial management of closed injuries of the spine with paraplegia and tetraplegia, I. Paraplegia 1969;7:179–192
5. Clinical assessment after acute cervical spinal cord injury. Neurosurgery 2002;50(3, Suppl):S21–S29
6. Bracken MB, Webb SB Jr, Wagner FC. Classification of the severity of acute spinal cord injury: implications for management. Paraplegia 1978;15:319–326
7. Lucas JT, Ducker TB. Motor classification of spinal cord injuries with mobility, morbidity and recovery indices. Am Surg 1979;45:151–158
8. Klose KJ, Green BA, Smith RS, Adkins RH, MacDonald AM. University of Miami Neuro-spinal Index (UMNI): a quantitative method for determining spinal cord function. Paraplegia 1980;18:331–336
9. Chehrazi B, Wagner FC Jr, Collins WF Jr, Freeman DH Jr. A scale for evaluation of spinal cord injury. J Neurosurg 1981;54:310–315
10. ASIA. Standards for Neurological Classification of Spinal Injury Patients. Chicago: American Spinal Injury Association; 1984
11. ASIA. Standards for Neurological Classification of Spinal Injury Patients. Chicago: American Spinal Injury Association; 1989
12. Bracken MB, Shepard MJ, Collins WF Jr, et al. Methylprednisolone or naloxone treatment after acute spinal cord injury: 1-year follow-up data. Results of the second National Acute Spinal Cord Injury Study. J Neurosurg 1992;76:23–31
13. Bracken MB, Shepard MJ, Hellenbrand KG, et al. Methylprednisolone and neurological function 1 year after spinal cord injury. Results of the National Acute Spinal Cord Injury Study. J Neurosurg 1985;63:704–713
14. ASIA. Standards for Neurological and Functional Classification of Spinal Cord Injury. Chicago: American Spinal Injury Association; 1996
15. Bednarczyk JH, Sanderson DJ. Comparison of functional and medical assessment in the classification of persons with spinal cord injury. J Rehabil Res Dev 1993;30:405–411
16. Wells JD, Nicosia S. Scoring acute spinal cord injury: a study of the utility and limitations of five different grading systems. J Spinal Cord Med 1995;18:33–41
17. El Masry WS, Tsubo M, Katoh S, El Miligui YH, Khan A. Validation of the American Spinal Injury Association (ASIA) motor score and the National Acute Spinal Cord Injury Study (NASCIS) motor score. Spine 1996;21:614–619
18. Cohen ME, Ditunno JF Jr, Donovan WH, Maynard FM Jr. A test of the 1992 International Standards for Neurological and Functional Classification of Spinal Cord Injury. Spinal Cord 1998;36:554–560
19. Jonsson M, Tollbäck A, Gonzales H, Borg J. Inter-rater reliability of the 1992 international standards for neurological and functional classification of incomplete spinal cord injury. Spinal Cord 2000;38:675–679
20. Savic G, Bergström EM, Frankel HL, Jamous MA, Jones PW. Inter-rater reliability of motor and sensory examinations performed according to American Spinal Injury Association standards. Spinal Cord 2007;45:444–451
21. Graves DE, Frankiewicz RG, Donovan WH. Construct validity and dimensional structure of the ASIA motor scale. J Spinal Cord Med 2006;29:39–45
22. Fisher CG, Wood KB. Introduction to and techniques of evidence-based medicine. Spine 2007;32(19, Suppl):S66–S72
23. Schünemann HJ, Jaeschke R, Cook DJ, et al; ATS Documents Development and Implementation Committee. An official ATS statement: grading the quality of evidence and strength of recommendations in ATS guidelines and recommendations. Am J Respir Crit Care Med 2006;174:605–614
24. Lazar RB, Yarkony GM, Ortolano D, et al. Prediction of functional outcome by motor capability after spinal cord injury. Arch Phys Med Rehabil 1989;70:819–822
25. Waters RL, Adkins R, Yakura J, Vigil D. Prediction of ambulatory performance based on motor scores derived from standards of the American Spinal Injury Association. Arch Phys Med Rehabil 1994;75:756–760
26. Curt A, Rodic B, Schurch B, Dietz V. Recovery of bladder function in patients with acute spinal cord injury: significance of ASIA scores and somatosensory evoked potentials. Spinal Cord 1997;35:368–373
27. Curt A, Keck ME, Dietz V. Functional outcome following spinal cord injury: significance of motor-evoked potentials and ASIA scores. Arch Phys Med Rehabil 1998;79:81–86
28. Dobkin B, Barbeau H, Deforge D, et al; Spinal Cord Injury Locomotor Trial Group. The evolution of walking-related outcomes over the first 12 weeks of rehabilitation for incomplete traumatic spinal cord injury: the multicenter randomized Spinal Cord Injury Locomotor Trial. Neurorehabil Neural Repair 2007;21:25–35

29. Marino RJ, Graves DE. Metric properties of the ASIA motor score: subscales improve correlation with functional activities. Arch Phys Med Rehabil 2004;85:1804–1810

30. Kirshblum S, Millis S, McKinley W, Tulsky D. Late neurologic recovery after traumatic spinal cord injury. Arch Phys Med Rehabil 2004;85: 1811–1817

31. Curt A, Dietz V. Ambulatory capacity in spinal cord injury: significance of somatosensory evoked potentials and ASIA protocol in predicting outcome. Arch Phys Med Rehabil 1997;78:39–43

32. Marino RJ, Rider-Foster D, Maissel G, Ditunno JF. Superiority of motor level over single neurological level in categorizing tetraplegia. Paraplegia 1995;33:510–513

9

Emergency Nursing and Allied Health Care of the Spine and Spinal Cord Injury Patients

Joseph Riina, Jason E. Smith, and Kathy Flint

The role of nursing and allied health professionals in the care of spinal cord injury (SCI) patients is often overlooked. These members of the health care team make up the first line of defense in critical care scenarios, yet their actions remain in the background to many physicians. Nurses not only play a crucial role in the acute care of SCI patients, but are invaluable in the long-term care and outcomes of these patients. Their many roles include initial defense against skin breakdown, respiratory problems (pneumonia, acute respiratory distress syndrome, etc.), gastrointestinal (GI) and genitourinary (GU) disturbances, as well as cardiovascular problems and thromboembolic events.

The beneficial effect of current emergency nursing and paramedic interventions can be seen not only in a decrease in morbidity and mortality rates but also in reduction of global costs for the care of these critically injured SCI patients. SCI patients are in a lifelong battle with general health maintenance and long-term medical issues such as skin complications and pressure ulcers, and urologic and pulmonary complications. Early preventive measures can help minimize long-term costs and lower overall mortality rates.

The average expense of caring for SCI patients with high cervical lesions is estimated at nearly $750,000.00 in the first year and $130,000.00 each subsequent year, with an average estimated lifetime cost of $3,000,000.00 in patients who are 25 years of age at injury. The costs are less for lower lesions involving the thoracic or lumbar area but are still substantial: nearly $1,000,000.00 over a lifetime.[1] These expenses primarily represent treatment of preventable complications such as those previously mentioned. With aggressive measures initiated early in the course of treatment, annual and lifetime savings can be substantially lowered. Recent studies by Strauss (US) and Frankel (UK) examined the overall trend in life expectancy after SCI, indicating that, since World War II, survivability improvements have been made. Because of earlier interventions by paramedics, nurses, and allied health professionals there has

been a 40% reduction in mortality in the first 2 years postinjury. This trend, however, is not significantly improved following the 2-year mark, indicating that continued, focused, preventive interventions are needed to improve long-term survivability.[2,3]

Nurses have led the health care field in the incorporation of evidence-based medicine (EBM) to their literature and teaching. This chapter discusses how certain EBM guidelines have helped minimize postinjury complications in SCI patients and improved long-term survival in these patients (**Table 9.1**). Additionally, the chapter looks further at what financial benefits these interventions have upon the care of SCI patients.

◆ Acute Care of Spinal Cord Injury Patients

Upon initial evaluation of the patient with spinal injury, basic (Advanced Trauma Life Support) ATLS protocol is initiated. Nurses begin with an initial assessment and are vital in helping to maintain an airway regardless of whether intubation is indicated. They are key in immobilization of the cervical spine until clearance can be established. The goal of immobilization is prevention of further neurological injury in the presence of an unstable spine. Measures commonly used in spinal immobilization are the placement of a rigid cervical collar, transportation on a spine board, and proper logrolling of patients. Although these may be seemingly benign interventions, pain and impairment of chest wall mobility can occur in up to 70% of patients.[4] For this reason, nursing professionals have established guidelines for interventions such as logrolling. In Alberta, Canada, a multidisciplinary group of health care providers developed regional policies and procedures for logrolling with and without cervical spine injuries. Their goal was to evaluate regional practices and establish and implement consistent logrolling practices

Table 9.1 Evidence-Based Review of Resources

Reference	Description	Level of Evidence	Literature on Evidence for Effectiveness of Nursing and Allied Health Care of the Spine and Spinal Cord Injury Patient
Ball[13]	Systematic review of primarily level III studies	III	Review of published reports evaluating pathophysiology and management of the pulmonary and hemodynamic complications that occur after SCI. Concluded that careful attention to support of the pulmonary and cardiovascular systems can reduce the morbidity associated with acute SCI.
Stevens et al[4]	Review of primarily level III evidence	III	Review of critical care interventions in the perioperative period of SCI patients. The review also centered on conditions that are encountered in a critical care or perioperative setting, in particular, traumatic SCI. Concluded that survival of patients with traumatic SCI has improved over the past decades. This better prognosis is thought to reflect changes in prehospital care, rapid triage to facilities with SCI expertise, and advances in medical, surgical, and rehabilitative care.
Murphy[7]	Review article with primarily expert opinion	V	Review of rehabilitative management in the acute care setting as well as a review of the process for selecting an appropriate rehab facility. Concluded that a multidisciplinary team approach is required in the acute care setting to implement a plan of care that will ensure the SCI patient is free of complications prior to transfer to a rehab center.
Mitcho, Yanko[18]	Review of primarily level III evidence	III	Comprehensive, evidence-based review of the needs of SCI patients in the acute care setting including optimal patient outcomes, methods to prevent complications, and a plan that provides an expeditious transition to rehabilitation. Concluded that templates for SCI care in the acute, intermediate, and long-term phases can be preestablished utilizing an evidence-based approach. This template can then be altered for the individual needs of each patient.
Groeneveld et al[5]	Descriptive implementation of new practice guidelines	V	Outlined the process required to establish and implement consistent logrolling practices throughout Alberta, Canada. Described the procedure and policy development aspect as well as the process required to educate staff. Reviewed the implementation and evaluation thereafter in an evidence-based approach to improve patient safety through a single intervention. Conclusion is ongoing process of this evaluation with the trend indicating success.
Catania et al[6]	Description of protocol development and systematic review of primarily level III studies	III	Description of the implementation of a pressure ulcer prevention protocol at a single institution as well as a systematic review of literature describing the costliness of failing to prevent pressure ulcers. This literature review was used to educate staff. Concluded that within 3 months of implementation their Pressure Ulcer Prevention Protocol Interventions and educational program reduced the incidence of pressure ulcers at their institution more than one half.
Heffner[12]	Systematic review of primarily level III evidence	III	Concluded that while there is insufficient evidence to support the impression that tracheotomy provides universal benefit, patients who require long-term ventilation because of marginal respiratory mechanics may be weaned more rapidly from mechanical ventilation with conversion to tracheotomy because of the enhanced psychological well-being provided by the ability to eat orally, communicate by articulated speech, and experience enhanced mobility. Enhanced mobility may assist physical therapy and more rapid recovery of ventilatory muscle strength.
Fagon et al[11]	Retrospective cohort study	III	Retrospective review of 48 ventilated patients with nosocomial pneumonia and matched controls. Intent was to determine if nosocomial pneumonias acquired in ventilator-dependent patients increased mortality of prolonged hospitalization. Concluded that *Pseudomonas* or *Acinetobacter* pneumonias in ventilator-dependent patients are associated with considerable mortality in excess of that resulting from the underlying disease alone and significantly prolongs length of stay in ICU.
Craven[10]	Systematic review of primarily level III evidence	III	Used evidence-based techniques to review current literature on the diagnosis of ventilator-associated pneumonia caused by bacterial pathogens. Concluded that current literature highlights the limitation of existing knowledge of this disease and underscores the need for further studies to examine benefits, risks, and costs of diagnostic procedures and to measure the effectiveness in terms of outcomes rather than sensitivity and specificity.

Table 9.1 Evidence-Based Review of Resources (*Continued*)

Reference	Description	Level of Evidence	Literature on Evidence for Effectiveness of Nursing and Allied Health Care of the Spine and Spinal Cord Injury Patient
Bergstrom et al[8]	Prospective cohort study	II	Clinical trial evaluating the Braden Scale as a predictive instrument for pressure sore risk in an ICU setting. Sixty consecutive ICU patients were evaluated at admission. The patients were pressure sore free at admission and the Braden Scale was compared with the existing Norton Scale to accurately predict patients at risk for developing pressure sores. The Braden Scale compared favorably with the Norton in sensitivity, and the Norton Scale had a tendency to overpredict risk with a higher specificity, which could lead to a greater number of patients receiving unnecessary and expensive treatments using the Norton Scale.
Frankel et al[3]	Retrospective cohort study	III	Review of long-term survivorship over 50 years in SCI patients. Goal was to identify risk factors contributing to deaths and to explore trends in cause of death over the decades in SCI patients. Analyzed the records of 3179 patients and found higher mortality risk was associated with higher neurological level and completeness of SCI, older age at injury, and earlier year of injury. Over 50 years, respiratory issues were the number one cause of death followed by urinary and cardiovascular issues, but trends have changed over time.
Priebe et al[1]	Economic and decision analysis with clinically relevant costs and alternatives; values obtained from limited studies	II	Economic review of the impact of SCI, including lifelong direct costs, life care planning, and factors affecting employment. Identified current ethical issues facing the SCI community and reviewed advances made through legislation.
Strauss et al[2]	Retrospective prognostic study investigating the outcome of disease	II	Review of over 30,000 patients with SCI. The main question addressed is whether there has been improved survival in SCI patients since the 1970s in both the immediate postinjury period (1 to 2 years) and in the longer term. Concluded that with other factors being equal, over the last 3 decades there has been a 40% decline in mortality during the critical first 2 years postinjury. However, the decline in mortality over time in the post-2-year period is small and not statistically significant in this study.
Geerts et al[14]	Prospective prognostic study investigating outcome of disease	I	Prospective study of the incidence of venous thrombosis after major trauma. Goal was to determine prospectively with the use of contrast venography the frequency of DVT in a broad spectrum of trauma patients. Additional goal was to determine the incidence of thrombosis in subgroups according to site of injury or presence of a specific injury. Finally, to identify characteristics of patients with trauma that may be high risk for development of DVT. Concluded that venous thromboembolism is a common complication in patients with major trauma and safe, effective prophylactic regimens are needed. Predictive factors for development of DVT included need for surgery or blood transfusion, lower extremity or SCI, and young patients with trauma.
Velmahos et al[15]	Systematic review of primarily level III evidence	III	Evidence-based review of literature evaluating various risk factors for development of thromboembolus and assessing the role of vena caval filters in preventing PE. Summarized available evidence and intended to identify areas where evidence is lacking. Concluded that SCI, spine injuries, and age are risk factors for development of DVT. Prophylactic placement of vena caval filters in selected trauma patients may decrease incidence of PE. Further well-designed studies are necessary to provide definitive answers.
Geertz et al[16]	Systematic review of primarily level I evidence	I	Systematic review of literature related to risks of VTE and its prevention. Final recommendations are made based on results of authors' pooled data as well as major randomized trials and/or formal, published meta-analyses. For acute SCI, the recommendation is prophylaxis with LMWH (Grade 1B). Low dose unfractionated heparin, compression stockings, and intermittent pneumatic compression devices appear to be relatively ineffective when used alone and are not recommended (Grade 1C). In conjunction with LMWH or unfractionated heparin or if anticoagulation is contraindicated early after injury (Grade 2B) in the rehabilitation phase of acute SCI the recommendation is continuation of LMWH or conversion to full-dose oral anticoagulation (INR target 2.5) (Grade 1C).

9 Emergency Nursing and Allied Health Care

(Continued on page 74)

Table 9.1 Evidence-Based Review of Resources *(Continued)*

Reference	Description	Level of Evidence	Literature on Evidence for Effectiveness of Nursing and Allied Health Care of the Spine and Spinal Cord Injury Patient
Zejdlik[9]	Textbook	V	Synopsis of the management of SCI patients including urogenital and gastrointestinal regimen to help prevent common complications.
Consortium for Spinal Cord Medicine[17]	Consortium meeting	I	Guidelines and recommendations based on evidence-based approach toward preventing venous thromboembolism, utilizing various randomized trials to establish these guidelines.

Abbreviations: DVT, deep vein thrombosis; ICU, intensive care unit; LMWH, low molecular weight heparin; SCI, spinal cord injury; PE, pulmonary embolism.

throughout the area to maximize patient safety and minimize secondary neurological injury. In a 5- to 6-week period, over 1500 staff members were trained in educational sessions focusing on subjects such as "who needs spinal immobilization," "sizing and applying a hard cervical collar," and "logrolling with cervical spine control."[5] This example suggests how evidence-based medicine has been used to establish consistent practices in immobilizing and safely turning patients to minimize secondary injury.

Once an airway has been established and immobilization has occurred, a full assessment for other potential injuries must take priority. At this point, nurses assume the role of supportive caregivers. The goal in this long-term care scenario is to anticipate and prevent complications from occurring that could be devastating for the SCI patient.

◆ Long-Term Care of Spinal Cord Injury Patients

Patients with spinal injuries are at exceedingly high risk for specific complications, including skin breakdown, bowel problems, urinary tract infections, thromboembolic events, and others. An educated team with a high index of suspicion is essential in anticipating and preventing these types of events before they can occur. In the acute phase of injury, immobilization is essential, but in the long-term phase early rehabilitation and intervention are key factors in the prevention of potential complications that can occur primarily due to immobility.

Prevention or Management of Skin Complications

Prevention of pressure ulcers is of paramount importance for the SCI patient. A cognizant staff that is willing to educate patients and their families is an essential component of the multidisciplinary action plan. The National Pressure Ulcer Advisory Panel (NPUAP) reviewed studies published between 1990 and 2000 to determine the incidence rate of pressure ulcers in acute care settings. They found that between 0.4 and 38% of patients suffered from pressure ulcers with a mean hospital cost of $15,000 per patient for treatment.[6] Pressure ulcers remain a serious and costly complication with serious potential medicolegal implications. Evidence-based nursing interventions are paramount in preventing these potentially grave consequences. Proper positioning of the patient in bed as well as in a chair will reduce the risk of pressure ulcer development. The position in the bed should be changed hourly, and all bony prominences should be inspected for a breach in skin integrity. When out of bed, SCI patients need to shift their weight to reduce the risk of pressure ulcer formation. To perform a proper weight shift, the majority of the patient's weight is shifted from one hip to the other or by the patient lifting him- or herself completely off the seat for 2 minutes. These weight shifts should be performed every 15 minutes.[7]

Health care professionals at Ohio State University Medical Center developed the Pressure Ulcer Prevention Protocol Interventions, a nursing initiative that involves assessing risk and nutritional status, providing skin care, documentation, and eliciting referrals as needed. After implementation, the prevalence of pressure ulcers was reduced by more than 50% in their institution. Daily rounds determined the consistency and reliability of nursing assessments not only in patients at risk but in all patients. This intervention has helped maintain an incidence rate in pressure ulcers well below the national benchmark. Nurses utilized the Braden Scale, which focuses on six subcategories: sensory perception, moisture, activity, mobility, nutrition, and friction/shear. Points are awarded from 6 to 23 and a score of 18 or less is predictive of pressure ulcer development.[6] This scale has demonstrated both validity and reliability in predicting pressure ulcer development and was reported to have a sensitivity of 83% and a specificity of 64%.[8] Again, by utilizing a systematic, multidisciplinary approach based on available evidence to solve the problem, patient safety, care, and long-term survivability were maximized.

Splinting will also assist in proper positioning and prevent pressure ulcer development when used on a routine schedule. Splints are usually fashioned by orthotic specialists or occupational therapists. They are typically constructed of plastic or metal with lamb's wool fabric placed next to the skin. The goal of foot splinting is to prevent contractures and to prevent pressure ulcer development over bony prominences. Hand splints also prevent contractures and maximize potential recovery of hand function by maintaining a functional position of the hands.[7] Along with splinting; contractures are also prevented by early mobilization of extremities. Physical and occupational therapists play a huge role in helping to maintain the functionality of the limbs postinjury. Passive range-of-motion exercises should be utilized and the joints should be moved through a full range if possible. Exercises should take place at least every 8 hours and can be incorporated into other activities such as bathing or positioning.[7]

Management of Gastrointestinal and Genitourinary Complications

Patients with spinal cord injuries and particularly cervical spine injuries are at high risk for GI and GU complications. These complications can have devastating results, including death, resulting from systemic sepsis secondary to a urinary tract infection or from autonomic dysreflexia. Being hypersensitive to these issues and combating them prior to their presentation are the keys to success. During the long-term hospitalization, a bowel regimen is recommended. It is not unusual for patients to develop constipation and bowel incontinence. Through retraining a patient can regain control of bowel function. In the acute phase, a daily docusate sodium enema can be used. This is usually administered in the evening. A short time after the enema is administered, the patient is assisted in using a bedpan or bedside commode to evacuate the bowels. A digital exam may be performed following evacuation to assess the effectiveness of the attempt.[7]

Over the long term, a diet high in fiber including many fruits and vegetables should be encouraged. Also, a fluid intake of 2000 to 3000 mL/day is necessary to keep the stools soft and to avoid cramping constipation when high-fiber diets or stool softeners are used. Exercise, even passive movements, can help prevent sluggish bowel activity. Patients can assist with evacuation by increasing abdominal pressure. This requires strong, voluntary abdominal muscle contraction. In addition, abdominal massage can be used as an adjunct to help push feces into the rectum. Digital stimulation techniques can also be useful because these help encourage the anal sphincter to relax, allowing the stool to pass.[9]

SCI patients will inevitably have altered GU function, potentially one of the most disruptive problems an individual with SCI will face. Maintenance of bladder emptying is a major nursing responsibility requiring a combination of knowledge, skill, and patience to ensure individualized, tailor-made programs. Any voluntary control of voiding must be documented as well as any awareness the patient may have of the need to void. This may be simply a sensation of increased perspiration and does not necessarily have to be a lower abdominal sensation.[9] It is recommended that the patient have a Foley catheter initially after admission. However, the Foley catheter should be removed after 3 to 4 days. The patient can then be placed on an intermittent catheterization schedule as soon as possible to prevent urinary tract infection. Urinary volume should be maintained at approximately half of the normal bladder capacity. The intermittent catheterization schedule should be performed a minimum of every 4 to 6 hours. Modifications in the schedule can be made based on urinary volume at the time of catheterization. In conjunction with intermittent catheterization, manual techniques to elicit bladder emptying can be used such as trigger voiding, straining to void (Valsalva), and manual expression.

Trigger voiding involves using additional trigger stimuli to augment bladder contraction and effectively empty the bladder. These may include firmly tapping or pinching the abdomen and inner thigh. However, this technique can only be used if the reflex arcs to the sacral voiding center are intact. The Valsalva technique requires strong abdominal muscles and a level of injury below T6–T12 because these are the levels at which the abdominal muscles are innervated. This technique can be useful in patients with an areflexic bladder. Manual expression involves the application of external pressure over and around the bladder in an attempt to increase the pressure within the bladder and effectively overcome the resistance of the bladder neck and urinary sphincters. This technique can only be used in flaccid bladders and when a voiding cystourethrogram confirms absence of ureterovesical reflux. It should be used cautiously because it can cause

reflux in those with hyperreflexic bladders, predisposing these patients to infections.[9]

A dedicated team alert to the potential catastrophic complications of urinary sepsis and autonomic dysreflexia can make these events the exception rather than a common occurrence in SCI patients. Nurses and other allied health care workers play a role not only in assisting patients with bowel and bladder control but also in educating the patient and the family in techniques so that they can regain control over this aspect of life.

Prevention or Management of Pulmonary Complications

Respiratory complications are a leading cause of death in SCI patients, with the majority of deaths due to pneumonia. Ventilator-associated pneumonia (VAP) is a consequence of intubation and mechanical ventilation. The risk of VAP increases 1 to 3% per day of intubation.[10] The mortality attributed to VAP has been reported to be 27% overall and 43% in cases due to *Pseudomonas aeruginosa*.[11] Effective treatment of VAP and other respiratory complications is dependent not only on accurate diagnosis but also on anticipating which patients are at risk and implementing a respiratory protocol to minimize these complications.

Nursing interventions include assisted coughing, which is used to clear secretions. It is recommended that assisted coughing be performed every 2 hours. This technique should be used with any patient unable to perform a cough independently.[7] Other potentially useful interventions include aggressive pulmonary hygiene such as frequent suctioning, chest percussion, positional changes, deep breathing, and incentive spirometry. Studies have shown that early tracheostomy should be considered when the need for ventilatory support is anticipated to exceed 2 to 3 weeks. Tracheostomy has been associated with enhanced subjective tolerance, decreased dead space ventilation, reduced airway resistance, and perhaps shorter ventilator weaning when compared with orotracheal intubation.[12] Clinically, tracheostomy is typically more comfortable for the patient as the irritation of the endotracheal tube against the posterior pharyngeal wall is eliminated. A concern about tracheotomy, however, is that it carries inherent surgical risks, and the incision is proximate to a possible incision site for anterior cervical stabilization procedures. Although unclear, 2 weeks is often used as a period of time to separate these two procedures, potentially to allow adequate healing of the tissue planes.[13]

Prevention or Management of Cardiovascular Complications

Cardiovascular instability is a frequent complication of spinal cord injury, notably if the injury occurs in the upper thoracic or cervical area. Interruption of the sympathetic fibers that exit the spinal cord in the thoracic region and subsequent unopposed parasympathetic outflow can then result in cardiac arrhythmias and hypotension. The most common arrhythmia is bradycardia, although supraventricular tachycardia and ventricular tachycardia can also be seen. Arrhythmias are most common in the first 14 days after injury, and their severity is based upon significance of injury. Hypotension is due to loss of vasoconstrictor tone in the peripheral arterioles leading to subsequent pooling of blood in the peripheral vasculature. Prolonged hypotension and shock are deleterious to the injured spinal cord and will contribute to cord hypoperfusion, which can precipitate secondary injury.

The first line of treatment is volume resuscitation in the acute phase. If infusion of 1 to 2 L of intravenous fluids fails to normalize blood pressure, consideration should be given to the placement of a pulmonary artery catheter. As extra volume is infused and venous return increases, cardiac output needs to increase. With disruption of cardiac sympathetic fibers the heart is unable to increase its cardiac output by increasing the heart rate. It must then rely on increased stroke volume, which may be unattainable. The placement of a pulmonary artery catheter will allow measurement of cardiac output directly, which can allow guidance of vasopressor therapy. Vasopressors should have both α- and β-adrenergic actions, such as dopamine or norepinephrine.[13]

The supporting staff managing a patient with traumatic SCI should be attentive to all potential causes of hemodynamic instability, including neurogenic shock, bleeding, tension pneumothorax, myocardial injury, pericardial tamponade, and sepsis. Appropriate steps should then be taken to combat these factors before they occur, including careful monitoring of blood pressure, heart rate, cardiac output, and so forth.[4]

Prevention or Management of Thromboembolic Events

In a large prospective evaluation of trauma patients, SCI was the strongest independent predictor of deep vein thrombosis (DVT).[14] A recent meta-analysis indicated that patients with SCI have a more than threefold risk of sustaining a DVT compared with trauma patients without SCI.[15] Patients with acute SCI have the highest incidence of venous thromboembolic disease among all hospital admissions. The incidence of DVT in patients with SCI not receiving prophylaxis is 39 to 100%, compared with 9 to 32% in untreated patients.[16] Among patients with SCI, DVT risk is also higher in complete versus incomplete lesions, and in thoracic versus cervical level lesions. Risk is higher the first 3 months following injury.[16] The incidence of pulmonary embolus after SCI in the absence of prophylaxis is less well documented but is estimated to be 4 to 10%. Pulmonary embolus is one of the three most common causes of death after SCI.[4]

Although there is agreement that prophylaxis is necessary, uncertainty persists as to which is the best prophylactic regimen. Some of the debates focus on whether low molecular weight heparin combined with nonpharmacological means is superior to either alone, how soon after SCI it may be instituted, how long it should be continued, and the utility of vena cava filters in this high-risk population. However, in 1997 the Consortium for Spinal Cord Medicine recommended the following evidence-based guidelines for the prevention of thromboembolism based on level of risk. Compression stockings or pneumatic devices should be applied to the lower extremities for the first 2 weeks following injury. The effects of these devices may be enhanced by combining them with antithrombotic agents. In the event that thromboprophylaxis is delayed for more than 72 hours, the extremities should be tested with either noninvasive Doppler or venography for thrombi formation prior to application of these devices.[17]

The prophylactic placement of an inferior vena cava (IVC) filter is a procedure whose efficacy has yet to be proven. This is primarily because the incidence of pulmonary embolus from DVT is low and the complications from placement of an IVC filter are not inconsequential. Nevertheless, vena cava filters are recommended for SCI patients who have complete motor loss with other known risks, patients who have failed anticoagulation prophylaxis, or patients who have a contraindication for anticoagulation.[18]

Anticoagulation prophylaxis with unfractionated or low molecular weight heparin should be initiated within 72 hours following SCI and continued until discharge in patients with incomplete motor injuries. It should be continued for 8 weeks in patients with uncomplicated, complete motor injuries and it should be continued for a full 12 weeks or until discharge from rehabilitation for patients with complete injuries with other risk factors such as pneumonia, thrombosis, cancer, obesity, heart failure, or age > 70. Careful assessment should be done at least every 8 hours to properly inspect the lower extremities for swelling or edema formation, to ensure proper placement of pneumatic devices, and to evaluate for evidence of skin ecchymoses or injury from the pneumatic devices.[17]

◆ Care in a Specialized Spinal Cord Injury Rehabilitation Center

Oftentimes after the initial management of the SCI patient is complete and the patient is adequately stabilized, most tertiary centers are not equipped with the technology or staff knowledge to provide long-term care for these individuals. For this reason specialized SCI rehabilitation centers were created. The multidisciplinary team must initiate conversations regarding the future with the patient and family early in the acute care hospitalization. The timing must be right to facilitate the family's ability to make decisions about the future. The multidisciplinary team members must be sensitive to this timing when developing their communication plans.

The goal of the health care worker during the initial interview with the patient and family is to achieve a professional, trusting relationship to effectively educate and assist them in dealing with this new life-altering situation. Effective communication and listening skills are essential for the health care worker dealing with these patients. Members of the team facilitate the patient and their family's decision making regarding the selection of a rehabilitation facility for the next phase of care. Three criteria must be met for a successful transfer to a rehabilitation facility: (1) the identification of a recognized traumatic SCI program that is approved by the Commission for the Accreditation of Rehabilitation Facilities (CARF); (2) a family that is confident that they have explored adequately the rehabilitation facilities and feel comfortable with their choice; and (3) insurance coverage that is accepted by the rehab facility of choice. To provide reassurance, the family should also have the opportunity to meet the rehab facility staff and visit the facility prior to the patient's transfer.[7]

◆ Summary of Recommendations

Nurses, social workers, physical and occupational therapists, respiratory therapists, and other medical and mental health professionals all make up the multidisciplinary team that is needed to help care for the SCI patient both acutely as well as in the long term. These particular patients are at great risk for routine medical complications like infection and cardiovascular complications. They are also at increased risk for unique sets of complications secondary to their injury such as autonomic dysreflexia, ventilator-acquired pneumonia, pressure ulcers, and others. Their overall health status can make it difficult for these patients to combat these events once they have been set in motion. Thus a hypervigilant attitude toward prevention is critical for the long-term survival and function of these patients.

By establishing strict guidelines and protocols based on the best available medical evidence aimed at minimizing secondary injury, care can be standardized at facilities worldwide. We have seen how evidence-based medicine helped establish practical and safe protocols for the transfer of patients in Canada. We have also seen how a multidisciplinary initiative was established to significantly decrease the incidence of pressure ulcers and all of their complications at a facility in Ohio. A consortium was established to develop guidelines in the prophylaxis of thromboembolic events in the SCI patient. These and many other evidence-based practices have helped increase overall survivability of the SCI patient by anticipating adverse events before they occur and initiating plans of prevention.

◆ *What effect do current emergency nursing and allied health interventions have on spine trauma and SCI patients with respect to morbidity and mortality?* Recommendation (strength): Current emergency nursing and allied health interventions reduce morbidity and mortality and are cost effective according to the literature. As such, the Spine Trauma Study Group (STSG) strongly recommends current emergency nursing interventions versus no emergency nursing interventions.

References

1. Priebe MM, Chiodo AE, Scelza WM, Kirshblum SC, Wuermser LA, Ho CH. Spinal cord injury medicine, VI: Economic and societal issues in spinal cord injury. Arch Phys Med Rehabil 2007;88(3, Suppl 1):S84–S88
2. Strauss DJ, Devivo MJ, Paculdo DR, Shavelle RM. Trends in life expectancy after spinal cord injury. Arch Phys Med Rehabil 2006;87:1079–1085
3. Frankel HL, Coll JR, Charlifue SW, et al. Long-term survival in spinal cord injury: a fifty year investigation. Spinal Cord 1998;36:266–274
4. Stevens RD, Bhardwaj A, Kirsch JR, Mirski MA. Critical care and perioperative management in traumatic spinal cord injury. J Neurosurg Anesthesiol 2003;15:215–229
5. Groeneveld A, McKenzie ML, Williams D. Logrolling: establishing consistent practice. Orthop Nurs 2001;20:45–49
6. Catania K, Huang C, James P, Madison M, Moran M, Ohr M. Wound wise: PUPPI: the Pressure Ulcer Prevention Protocol Interventions. Am J Nurs 2007;107:44–52, quiz 53
7. Murphy M. Traumatic spinal cord injury: an acute care rehabilitation perspective. Crit Care Nurs Q 1999;22:51–59
8. Bergstrom N, Demuth PJ, Braden BJ. A clinical trial of the Braden Scale for Predicting Pressure Sore Risk. Nurs Clin North Am 1987;22:417–428
9. Zejdlik CP. Management of Spinal Cord Injury. 2nd ed. Boston: Jones and Bartlett; 1992
10. Craven DE. Epidemiology of ventilator-associated pneumonia. Chest 2000;117(4, Suppl 2):186S–187S
11. Fagon JY, Chastre J, Hance AJ, Montravers P, Novara A, Gibert C. Nosocomial pneumonia in ventilated patients: a cohort study evaluating attributable mortality and hospital stay. Am J Med 1993;94:281–288
12. Heffner JE. The role of tracheotomy in weaning. Chest 2001;120(6, Suppl):477S–481S
13. Ball PA. Critical care of spinal cord injury. Spine 2001;26(24, Suppl): S27–S30
14. Geerts WH, Code KI, Jay RM, Chen E, Szalai JP. A prospective study of venous thromboembolism after major trauma. N Engl J Med 1994;331: 1601–1606
15. Velmahos GC, Kern J, Chan LS, Oder D, Murray JA, Shekelle P. Prevention of venous thromboembolism after injury: an evidence-based report, II: Analysis of risk factors and evaluation of the role of vena caval filters. J Trauma 2000;49:140–144
16. Geerts WH, Heit JA, Clagett GP, et al. Prevention of venous thromboembolism. Chest 2001;119(1, Suppl):132S–175S
17. Consortium for Spinal Cord Medicine. Prevention of thromboembolism in spinal cord injury. J Spinal Cord Med 1997;20:261–283
18. Mitcho K, Yanko JR. Acute care management of spinal cord injuries. Crit Care Nurs Q 1999;22:60–79, quiz 100

10

Principles of Nonoperative and Intensive Care Unit Management of Spinal Cord Injury

Christian P. DiPaola and Glenn R. Rechtine II

Spinal cord injury (SCI) is best treated with a multidisciplinary protocol. Multiple teams should be coordinated to ensure that all of the proper medical and surgical support is available to treat the life-threatening and multiorgan system problems that an SCI presents. The spine surgeon plays a role as patient advocate to direct the teams so as to optimize spine stability, spinal cord function, and recovery. Each injury is unique; thus the specific treatment algorithm must be tailored on an individual basis according to the level and severity of the injury. However, there are standard treatments that should be considered for all SCI patients. This chapter focuses on nonoperative treatment principles that can apply to all SCI patients, with emphasis on intensive care unit (ICU) care and optimization of spinal immobilization. The chapter is organized to reflect the order of importance for patient care tasks, from life-saving to spine-stabilizing efforts. Many of these efforts occur simultaneously from the point the patient enters the trauma bay or ICU. ICU care and life saving are presented first, followed by blood pressure management (prevention of secondary SCI). Then nonorthotic, nonoperative spine immobilization is addressed, and the question of whether thoracic and thoracolumbar SCI can be treated nonoperatively is reviewed. These two topics will be the subject of the two evidence-based review questions. Finally, a treatment algorithm for thoracic and thoracolumbar SCI treatment is presented.

◆ Intensive Care Unit Management

Animal studies have shown that acute SCI results in systemic and disrupted local and vascular autoregulation.[1–3] Human studies have all shown that after SCI, bradycardia, hypotension, decreased systemic vascular resistance, and cardiac output are all common.[2,4–7] Respiratory insufficiency is also an equally serious life-threatening complication. The physiological sequelae and resultant hypoxia may lead to further secondary SCU.[8] Respiratory insufficiency is an independent risk factor for mortality and a major source of post-SCI morbidity that is also related to level of injury.[9–11] Cardiovascular and respiratory complications can be transient and episodic and may occur after periods of relative stability. Early detection and aggressive treatment reduce morbidity and mortality of cardiac and respiratory dysfunction that is common with acute SCI.[8]

A recent systematic review of the effect of ICU care on SCI outcomes was published in 2002.[12] The article included 17 studies for a systematic review. All studies were graded as level III evidence, but the specific grading criteria were not listed. The studies were mixed retrospective case series and cohorts that documented the incidence, time frame, and severity of common cardiovascular and respiratory complications associated with acute SCI.[12] Many of the studies had no control or compared historical cohorts. The majority documented the authors' experiences with ICU protocols instituted for the aggressive resuscitation and monitoring of SCI patients. Protocols were not standardized, but they commonly recommend invasive monitoring with Swan-Ganz catheters and arterial lines. These studies showed that early ICU care optimizes patient outcome due to decreased mortality and decreased cardiovascular and respiratory morbidity.[12] Vale et al performed a prospective case series which claims that neurological recovery in the setting of ICU care must have been attributed to ICU care because all of the other factors, such as selection for surgery and timing, did not have a significant effect.[13] It appears that due to the lack of control groups and lack of randomization of other treatments in the series, the authors may not be able to fully justify those claims. However, they proved that their ICU care protocol is safe and may have benefit. The final guideline set forth by the 2002 guidelines supplement is that the frequency and severity of life-threatening complications after SCI are common enough and the benefits of ICU care great enough to justify that all SCI patients initially (within 7 to 14 days of injury) should receive ICU-level care.[12]

◆ Blood Pressure Management to Prevent Secondary Spinal Cord Injury

The initial insult in spinal cord trauma is mechanical. This leads to secondary injury resulting from vascular compromise, ischemia, inflammation, edema, complex biochemical dysregulation, and, ultimately, neuronal cell death.[4–8,14] Maintenance of optimized cardiac output, blood pressure, and tissue oxygenation may also protect from secondary spinal cord injury.[2,4–7,14] The effect of hypotension and maintenance of minimum mean arterial pressure (MAP) on SCI outcomes was also extensively reviewed in 2002.[8] Many of the studies set a goal for MAP for a minimum of 85 to 90 mm Hg. These studies often employ the analogy of SCI to traumatic brain injury (TBI). In TBI hypoxia and hypotension worsen secondary neuronal injury and hinder optimal recovery.[7,15] Studies of TBI suggest that MAP < 90 or hypoxia (paO_2 < 60 mm Hg) has been shown to significantly increase morbidity and mortality.[5,7,14,15]

Animal studies suggest that avoidance of hypotension has a protective effect on the spinal cord and a beneficial effect on spinal cord recovery.[1–3] No study in human patients directly compared systemic hypotension and SCI outcome. There is a scarcity of clinical protocols presented in the review, but the general principles are to correct hypotension with volume replacement (crystalloid first followed by colloid as necessary).[8] Vasopressors may also be needed and can safely be used.[8] Occasionally, patients may necessitate cardiac pacing to maintain cardiac output. No specific evidence exists to suggest that SCI outcomes are improved with this protocol; therefore, a strong recommendation for adherence to this practice cannot be made. The final result of the review is that maintenance of MAP for SCI patients ≥ 85 to 90 mmHg is a safe clinical practice.[8]

◆ Initial Immobilization

Besides life-saving measures the main priority of SCI treatment is to prevent neurological deterioration, regain spinal stability, and possibly gain back neurological function. Once a patient is brought under the care of medical personnel there is still a real risk of neurological deterioration of 6 to 10%.[16] The SCI patient deserves special attention due to the need for "controlled mobilization." Initial immobilization for the patient with SCI often involves bed rest with "spine precautions." A rigid cervical orthosis is maintained until cervical spine injury can be ruled out. Cadaver studies on the unstable cervical spine have shown that when cervical instability exists rigid collars allow similar amounts of motion compared with cadavers with no collars, in a stretcher to bed, or bed to bed transfer situation.[17] The cervical collar thus may not protect against transfer-induced C-spine motion and thus care must be taken when transferring patients, despite the presence of a collar. The evidence does not negate the need for cervical collar application and maintenance until safe clearance, however. At the very least, the cervical collar provides a warning sign to caregivers that the patient has an unstable or potentially unstable cervical spine. The collar also aids in maintaining neutral cervical alignment and provides proprioceptive cues to patients that may be protective. Therefore, we recommend that, until cleared, strict spine precautions be adhered to and cervical collars be left in place.

Transportation of patients on spine boards as part of the prehospitalization immobilization of the trauma patient has become standard of care in North America.[18] Special attention to removal of patients from spine boards should be a priority. It is important to emphasize that use of spine boards should be for transport and transfer of patients and that they should be removed from beneath the patient as soon as clinically feasible. Patient positioning on the spine board has been associated with 21 to 33% higher rates of neck and back pain.[18] Vacuum mattresses have been successfully implemented in Europe to counteract this problem; however, they are cumbersome, costly, and fragile. Prolonged spine board immobilization may also result in respiratory compromise through a decrease in forced vital capacity (FVC) and FRC. They have also been proven to cause increased sacral and occipital pressures, which put the patient (especially those with neurological compromise) at risk for pressure sores.[18] Based on these findings we recommend use of the spine board for prehospital transport and efficient removal of the patient from the apparatus when clinically appropriate.

Previous studies have shown that the spine-injured patient who is subjected to bed rest (which is the initial form of spine immobilization in the trauma bay or ICU) is at risk for pulmonary complications, skin breakdown, deep vein thrombosis (DVT), and muscle atrophy.[19–23] Frequent patient repositioning has been shown to decrease morbidity of bed rest.[20,22,24] A mechanized version of patient repositioning has been developed by creating a laterally rotating bed, which generates "kinetic therapy" (KT). The senior author has found KT to be useful, not only as a preoperative measure of spine immobilization but also as a means of definitive thoracic and thoracolumbar spine immobilization (**Fig. 10.1**).

◆ Two Clinical Questions on Nonoperative Treatment of Spinal Cord–Injured Patients for Evidence-Based Review

A systematic evidence-based review of two questions related to SCI and nonoperative treatment was performed. PubMed and Medline search engines were used to search for abstracts and screen potential studies. Subject headings and key words including "spinal cord injury," "nonoperative treatment," "immobilization," "preoperative care" and "ICU management" were searched. All abstracts were read and screened for relevance. Reference lists of pertinent articles were also reviewed, and appropriate articles were gathered from this search as well. The level of evidence was assessed for the selected articles based on the Center for Evidence Based Medicine (www.cebm.net). The articles were reviewed, and final strength of clinical recommendation was based on the criteria proposed by Guyatt et al.[25–30]

Optimum Techniques for Immobilization and Transfer of SCI Patients in the Hospital and Intensive Care Unit

The following review addresses the optimum methods of nonorthotic spine immobilization in patients with spine instability for preoperative and/or definitive treatment. Methods

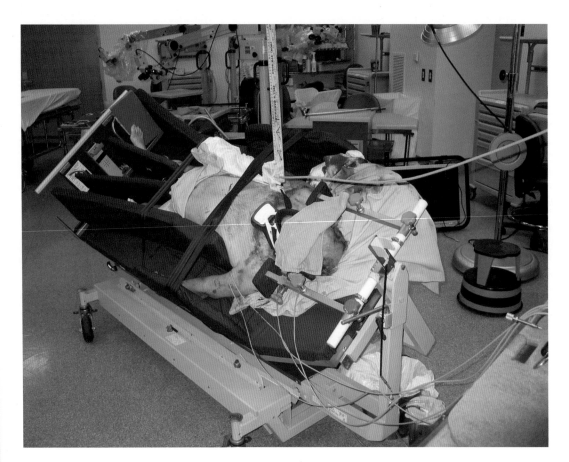

Fig. 10.1 A cadaver in a RotoRest bed undergoing biomechanical testing.

of preoperative patient prone positioning with cervical, thoracic, or lumbar instability are also reviewed. The goal for the patient with spinal instability is effective mobilization while maintaining spinal immobilization. This may be done prior to definitive surgery, or for definitive treatment of the patient's fracture. Patient transfers and positioning have the potential to confer dangerous amounts of motion to the unstable spine, which may lead to neurological deterioration.[16] Thus we consider spine immobilization as a paramount goal of nonoperative treatment whether in the ICU or not. Here we identify and discuss six studies that specifically address different types of KT and/or logrolling in relation to spine instability.

We also consider prone positioning prior to operative intervention to be a maneuver that can potentially generate neurological deterioration due to the generation of motion in the unstable spine.[16] We identified four sources that address optimum means of patient positioning. It should be noted that electrophysiological monitoring and awake intubation are important tools in the spine surgeon's armamentarium to help detect impending neurological deterioration in the setting of spine surgery.[31] These techniques are relevant but beyond the scope of this chapter.

Brackett and Condon performed a retrospective review comparing the wedge-turning frame and KTT in patients with complete cervical or thoracic spine injury. The mortality of the wedge-tuning frame group was 28.6%, and the KTT group was zero.[32] Pulmonary complications were far less frequent with KTT and much less severe. ICU stays were also less with KTT. Lack of randomization and ability to account for confounding variables and standardization of patient health status make conclusions limited. But KTT appeared to have a safety advantage. McGuire et al compared the RotoRest bed (KCI Technologies, Inc., Sparks, MD) to the Stryker frame (Stryker Medical, Portage, MI) in ability to immobilize the unstable spine in cadavers.[33] They found that the RotoRest bed was superior in immobilization of the cervical and lumbar spine with instability. A retrospective cohort study was done on patients with SCI awaiting surgery. Half were maintained in a RotoRest bed and half were treated in a Foster frame. When complications were analyzed, there were mixed results. RotoRest patients had a higher rate of skin complications. Pulmonary emboli were higher in the Foster frame group.[33] No conclusions could be drawn as to which treatment was most effective; however, both treatments appeared to provide sufficient spine immobilization. Rechtine et al performed a study on embalmed cadavers that compared logroll to KTT. They looked specifically at patient mobilization as might occur in an ICU setting. Embalmed cadavers with cervical and thoracolumbar instability were used. An electromagnetic motion tracking device was used to measure relative motion between unstable segments (**Fig. 10.1**). They found that KTT generated significantly less cervical and thoracolumbar spine motion when compared with logroll.[34] Conrad et al found similar results when fresh cadavers were studied.[35] When Rechtine et al studied hospital bed transfers in cadavers they found that the act of transferring a patient from stretcher to bed may impart potentially dangerous amounts of cervical spine motion in the unstable spine regardless of whether a rigid collar is used.[17] They emphasized that patients with true cervical instability should be handled with inline manual cervical stabilization whenever a patient transfer is performed. The presence of a rigid collar should not be a sign that one can be less attentive to the head and neck; rather, the converse is true. The collar will not protect against transfer-induced cervical motion.

Following that same theme, the cervical collar is not adequate to optimally immobilize the cervical spine in operating room supine to prone positioning. This has been demonstrated in multiple cadaver studies for C1–C2 and C5–C6 instability.[36,37] In these scenarios, the Jackson table turning technique immobilizes the cervical spine to a significantly greater degree in the majority of motion parameters for angular displacement (axial rotation, lateral bending and flexion-extension) and linear displacement (anteroposterior, axial, and medial-lateral) whether a rigid collar is used or not.[38] The Jackson table prone positioning technique involves positioning a patient supine on the flat Jackson table and then applying the carbon frame, with pads over the ventral surface of the patient. The patient is held in place with tension in the system created by the locking T-pins, and safety straps are applied around the whole setup. The patient is flipped prone by unlocking the manual lock at the head and foot of the bed and then rotating the whole system. The Jackson table turning method has also been proven to provide better spine immobilization in the setting of thoracolumbar instability when compared with a standard log roll, for supine to prone positioning (**Fig. 10.2A,B**).[36]

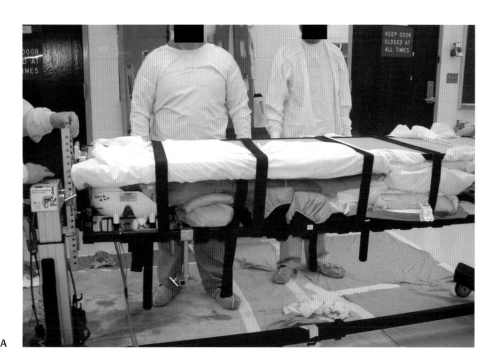

A

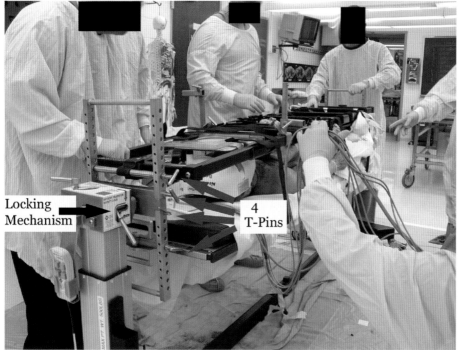

B

Fig. 10.2 (A) Jackson table setup with patient supine locked into the frame. Five safety straps are in place and the locking pins on the H-frame are noted. **(B)** Jackson table and patient in the prone position after turning.

Based on the data presented, we recommend that KT treatment be considered for initial immobilization of patients with cervical, thoracic, or lumbar instability. KT appears to allow adequate controlled mobilization of the patient while also providing optimum spine immobilization. However, based on the quality of the literature (**Table 10.1**), expert opinion, cost, and practicality, the grade of recommendation based on Guyatt et al is still weak.

The biomechanical data for patient positioning in the operating room is of high quality (**Table 10.1**). It supports the use of the Jackson table turn in the preoperative supine to prone patient transfer. The data and expert opinion offer a strong recommendation for the use of the Jackson table turn in the preoperative supine to prone patient transfer.

The Most Effective Nonoperative Treatment Options for Thoracic and Thoracolumbar Trauma with SCI Based on Outcome Measures Including Complications, LOS, Healing/Stability, Function/Pain Medication, Cost, Neurological Recovery

The majority of the studies involving thoracolumbar SCI involve surgical treatment. Most studies that address nonoperative treatment of thoracolumbar fractures involve injuries without neurological deficit. To select studies for review, Medline and PubMed searches were performed with the following search criteria: "nonoperative treatment," "thoracic trauma," "lumbar trauma," and "spinal cord injury." Abstracts were screened to

Table 10.1 Evidence-Based Review of Articles

Study	Conclusion	Level of Evidence	Grade of Recommendation
Rechtine et al[34]	Kinetic bed therapy provides superior spine immobilization to logroll. Cadaver study, significant stats/p values.	I	1A
Del Rossi et al, J Athl Training 2003	Lift-slide technique better spine immobilization than logroll. Healthy subjects, significant stats/p values.	I	1B
Del Rossi et al, Spine 2004	Logroll similar to lift-slide. Cadaver study in embalmed cadavers. Question of similarity to real patient and need for more subjects/fresh cadavers.	II	2C
Conrad et al, ASIA presentation 2007	Lift-slide technique better C-spine immobilization than logroll in the injured football player. Fresh cadaver study, significant stats/p values.	I	1A
Horodyski et al, ASIA presentation 2007	Lift-slide technique better spine immobilization than logroll for the unstable C-spine. Fresh cadaver study, significant stats/p values.	I	1A
Rechtine et al[17]	Cervical collars permit a potentially dangerous amount of motion in the unstable C-spine during bed transfers. Need to maintain strict precautions for immobilization even with collar on. Fresh cadaver study, significant stats/p values.	I	1A
Genelello et al, Critical Care Medicine 1990	Decreased pulmonary complications with use of kinetic bed therapy versus standard bed immobilized in the intensive care unit. PRCT	I	1A
Borkowski, J, Neurosci. Nursing 1989	Less pulmonary infection and ventilator time in patients treated with kinetic bed	III	2A
Rechtine et al[41]	Nonoperative treatment for thoracolumbar trauma w/SCI is superior to operative treatment due to decreased complications and infections; no difference can be determined for functional results or pain. LOS is longer for nonoperative treatment.	III	1C in favor of nonop due to no infections. 2C for function, pain, and clinical results
Hartman et al[40]	Nonoperative treatment for thoracolumbar trauma w/SCI is superior to operative treatment due to decreased complications and infections, no difference can be determined for functional results or pain. LOS is longer for nonoperative treatment.	IV	1C in favor of nonop due to no infections. 2C for function, pain, and clinical results
Dai et al[42]	Nonoperative treatment for patients w/incomplete and incomplete SCI in the setting of thoracolumbar trauma can be treated successfully nonoperatively. Nonoperative SCI patients achieved similar neuron recovery to operative treatment. Biased by nonrandomization and nonstandardization of protocols.	IV	2C operative or nonoperative treatment may be equally as good. Patient and surgeon preference appears to play a role.
Capen[39]	Nonoperative treatment is a plausible option even for SCI and fracture dislocation in thoracic fractures. These fractures can heal in a stable fashion with similar risk of neuron/functional results.	IV	2C
Seybold et al[45]	Trend toward better outcomes w/nonoperative treatment for low lumbar burst fractures	III	2C
An et al, Spine 1999	Nonoperative and operative treatment for low lumbar burst fractures are plausible options.	III	2C
Dai et al, 2008			

Abbreviations: LOS, length of stay; SCI, spinal cord injury.

include studies that involved thoracic, thoracolumbar, and lumbar trauma patients with SCI or neurological injury. These articles were reviewed and the reference lists from them were screened for further articles that may fit the criteria. There were four series that investigated the outcomes of SCI patients treated nonoperatively and thus met the appropriate criteria. Low lumbar fractures with neurological injury were also included in the review. Technically these do not involve SCI, but they fall within the realm of lumbar fractures with neurological injury. The search yielded two studies that addressed lumbar burst fractures with neurological injury that compared operative and nonoperative treatment.

Capen et al published a retrospective case series of a mixed group of 118 patients with thoracic spine fractures from T1–T8, treated operatively and nonoperatively. Forty-nine patients were treated nonoperatively. Of this group, 44 had neurological injuries (29 complete and 16 incomplete). The patients were not randomized, and the authors did not specify how patients were selected for treatment but suggested that the nonoperative group wasn't able to safely undergo surgery due to life-threatening causes in the period surrounding the injury.[39] Nonoperative treatment protocol was not standardized or fully specified, but it appeared to involve a period of bed rest from 2 to 6 weeks and then application of a custom-molded orthosis. From the nonoperatively treated group, there was one episode of neurological worsening. Two patients had so-called significant kyphosis progression of 10 and 18 degrees. All fractures healed, and no others had major deformity progression. There were eight cases of skin necrosis and 12 cases of DVT. They concluded that nonoperative treatment of thoracic spine fractures with neurological injury can be treated with bed rest and progression to orthosis, when surgery is not possible.[39]

Hartman and Rechtine published a case series that looked at 69 patients with fractures from T3–L5. Twelve had multilevel injuries.[40] Nine patients had incomplete neurological injury, and three had complete neurological injury. Thirty-two of the 69 were treated nonoperatively. The patients were not randomized to treatment groups, and the operative treatment was not standardized. Nonoperative treatment involved immobilization of patients in a RotoRest kinetic bed for 4 to 6 weeks, and then they were braced for 2 to 3 months. For all incomplete SCIs that were nonoperatively treated, patients improved at least one Frankel grade. This was similar to operatively treated patients. When outcomes were compared, patients had similar return to work, pain medication usage, kyphosis progression, and cost. The operative group had a higher infection rate (8% vs 0%). The nonoperatively treated group had a higher length of stay.[40]

A later study that compared nonoperative and operative treatment of thoracolumbar spine fractures with SCI was performed as a retrospective cohort of a nonrandomized group of patients with thoracolumbar fractures.[41] Nonoperative treatment was provided for 117 patients, and 118 were treated operatively. There was a higher number of incomplete SCIs in the operative group (39 vs 18). Twenty-two percent of the injuries were multilevel, and 85 were noncontiguous. Injuries included two- and three-column injuries with or without fracture dislocation. Purely ligamentous injuries were only given the option of surgery. Operative patients were treated according to surgeon preference. All nonoperatively treated patients were treated for 6 weeks in a kinetic bed (RotoRest), then in a brace. There were no significant differences in decubiti, DVT, pulmonary emboli, or mortality. There was no difference in neurological recovery rate for operative versus nonoperative groups. Deep wound infection rate was 8% for the operative group and 0% for the nonoperative group. Length of stay was 24 days longer for the nonoperative group. Rechtine et al concluded that operative and nonoperative treatment of thoracolumbar fractures with or without neurological injury is a reasonable option.[41]

Dai et al performed the most recent retrospective nonrandomized series of conservatively managed traumatic thoracolumbar burst fractures in 127 patients. The study assessed the relationship of the load-sharing classification to clinical outcome in conservatively managed thoracolumbar trauma. The study was not designed to compare outcomes of surgical versus nonoperative treatment. All patients underwent postural reduction of fracture and bed rest until symptoms or clinical status permitted mobilization. Treatment in a body cast or brace was then instituted for at least 3 months. Of the 22 patients (17.3%) had SCI, 1 complete and 22 incomplete. American Spinal Injury Association (ASIA) motor scores ranged from 0 to 40 on presentation, and recovery rate at final exam ($>$ 1 year) ranged from 63 to 100%. The study demonstrated one neurological deterioration and otherwise safe and clinically effective use of conservative treatment in this nonrandomized group.[42]

An et al reported on a retrospective cohort of 31 patients with low lumbar burst fracture, 13 of whom had neurological injury. Patients were not randomized and were treated in multiple ways, including body casts, Harrington rods, Luque rods, and Steffee plates. Their conclusion was that operative and nonoperative treatments were viable options.[43,44]

Seybold et al published a multicenter retrospective cohort on low lumbar burst fractures in 42 patients, 18 of whom had neurological injury. Twenty were treated nonoperatively and 22 were treated operatively.[45] Criteria for treatment choice were not specified, and treatment was not randomized. However, it appeared that the presence of neurological injury may have influenced the choice to operate because 16 of the 18 patients with neurological injury were treated operatively. Nonoperative treatment involved 1 to 7 days of bed rest and custom-molded orthosis. There was no neurological deterioration, and the majority of patients with neurological deficit had complete recovery regardless of treatment. Also, functional and radiographic outcome was not significantly different between groups, though this study was not powered to account for differences between operatively and nonoperatively treated patients.[45]

Overall, it appears that the presence of neurological injury has been an indication for operative treatment of most thoracolumbar trauma. The aforementioned studies do not achieve a level of evidence that can guide a specific recommendation as to whether operative or nonoperative treatment is better when neurological injury is present. The kinetic bed is a reasonable option for "aggressive nonoperative treatment." Potential complications to KT include disconnection of intravascular lines, patient intolerance to rotation, and cardiac arrhythmias.[46,47] However, KT appears to be an aggressive means of nonoperative spinal immobilization and a safe alternative to operative treatment in properly selected cases. Operative treatment carries with it a much higher infection rate, but shorter length of hospital stay. It has been shown that both operative and nonoperative treatment can result in neurological recovery, but no studies compare these patient cohorts head to head. Risk–benefit analysis between physician and patient needs to be considered for each case. Differences in cost, healing, pain/function, neurological improvement, and stability are difficult to assess given the level III and IV evidence

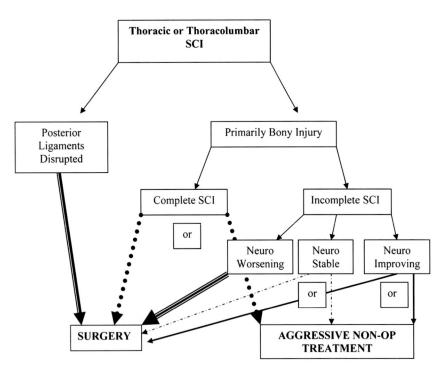

Fig. 10.3 The flow diagram depicts the senior author's preferred treatment algorithm for thoracic and thoracolumbar spinal cord injury. Risks and benefit of each decision are discussed with the patient based on the given rules. The rules are based on presence of bony versus ligamentous injury, neurological status, and decline or improvement. SCI, Spinal cord injury; Neuro, neurologically; Non-op, nonoperative.

available. No definitive recommendation can be made about which spinal injuries are best treated by KT, but based on the senior author's expert opinion, a treatment algorithm has been proposed (**Fig. 10.3**). Overall a weak recommendation can be given to use KT bed therapy for conservative management of thoracolumbar SCI based on the literature available because alternative treatments such as surgical decompression and stabilization may be equivalent or superior alternatives in properly selected cases. Refer to **Table 10.1** for an evidence-based review of articles.

◆ Nonoperative Treatment Protocol for Thoracic and Thoracolumbar Spine Fractures

For definitive treatment of suitable (nonligamentous) thoracic and thoracolumbar spine fractures, kinetic bed therapy was performed for 6 weeks for all patients regardless of age, symptoms, or severity of injury.[41] Since publication of the original study, the protocol has been adapted to allow for the bed rest duration to be determined by patient symptoms and radiographic evidence of stability. Kinetic bed therapy is performed for a minimum of 2 weeks and subsequently until patients are off narcotic pain medication. During kinetic bed therapy the bed is set at 40 degree stops and is run for a minimum of 18 hours per day. There is little convincing evidence, however, about which rotation parameters (duration, angulation, or frequency) are most effective.[47] Sequential compression devices and subcutaneous heparin or low molecular weight heparin are started 48 hours after injury. All patients with an ASIA A injury receive an inferior vena cava (IVC) filter. The Hatch care protocol is performed every shift for skin protection. It is recommended that the patient perform a daily regimen of arm- and leg-strengthening exercises with resistance bands that are

attached to the bed. Programs are tailored to each patient's motor abilities and involve as many muscle groups as possible, several times throughout the day.

When patients are off narcotic medication, recumbency is discontinued and upright x-rays are taken as tolerated. If the neurological exam remains stable and x-rays are deemed acceptable, then the patient is fit into a custom-molded plastic orthosis so that total duration of fracture treatment is 12 weeks.

Case Presentation

- 63-year-old woman, s/p 30-foot fall 3 weeks previously (**Fig. 10.4**)
- T9 burst fracture, ASIA C initially treated at an outside hospital with standard hospital bed rest and attempted mobilization in a brace, 47 degree kyphosis (**Fig. 10.5**)
- Transferred to the care of the senior author with neurological deterioration
- Immediately treated with KTT and offered anterior decompression and AP fusion
- Patient refused operative Rx and elected for continued bed rest in RotoRest bed.
- Five months postinjury: walking with walker, normal strength (ASIA E), minimal pain, 22 degree kyphosis (**Fig. 10.6**)
- 1 year postinjury: walking unassisted several miles per day, no pain medication

Recommendations

1. Weak recommendation for use of kinetic table therapy for initial immobilization prior to definitive stabilization in SCI patients. Strong recommendation for Jackson table turning method for supine to prone positioning for spine-injured patients in the operating room. Both KTT and Jackson table positioning are superior to logrolling patients.

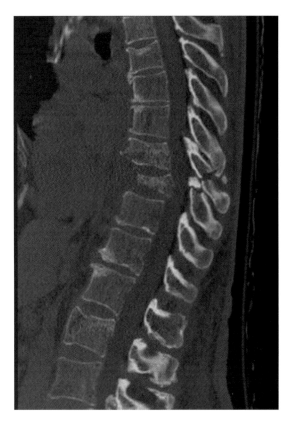

Fig. 10.4 Initial injury computed tomographic scan of the 63-year-old patient, s/p 30-foot fall, ASIA C.

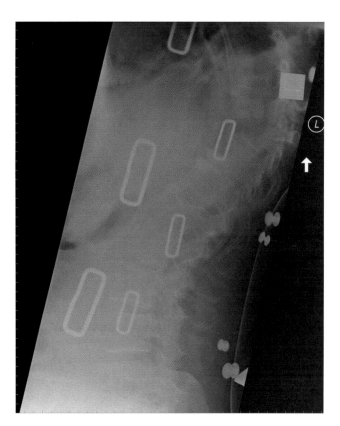

Fig. 10.5 Upright x-ray, 3 weeks s/p injury, treated w/bed rest and bracing.

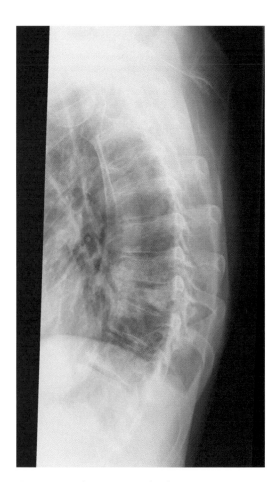

Fig. 10.6 Upright x-ray, 5 months s/p RotoRest treatment protocol, ASIA E.

2. Nonoperative treatment for thoracolumbar injury with SCI appears to be an option for treatment. A weak recommendation in favor of nonoperative treatment can be given when considering complications such as infection. Operative treatment has a much higher infection rate than nonoperative treatment. A weak recommendation can be given in favor of nonoperative treatment when considering length of hospital stay. Operatively treated patients spend significantly less time in the hospital. Nonoperative treatment also appears to be able to yield neurological recovery. No good evidence has emerged to make strong recommendations for exactly which patients with thoracolumbar SCI would benefit from nonoperative treatment over operative treatment. Patient and surgeon choice, cost, failure of treatment, and long-term results need to be considered as important decision-making factors as well.

References

1. Amar AP, Levy ML. Pathogenesis and pharmacological strategies for mitigating secondary damage in acute spinal cord injury. Neurosurgery 1999;44:1027–1039, discussion 1039–1040
2. Dolan EJ, Tator CH. The effect of blood transfusion, dopamine, and gamma hydroxybutyrate on posttraumatic ischemia of the spinal cord. J Neurosurg 1982;56:350–358
3. Ducker TB, Kindt GW, Kempf LG. Pathological findings in acute experimental spinal cord trauma. J Neurosurg 1971;35:700–708
4. Osterholm JL. The pathophysiological response to spinal cord injury: the current status of related research. J Neurosurg 1974;40:5–33
5. Tator CH. Vascular effects and blood flow in acute spinal cord injuries. J Neurosurg Sci 1984;28:115–119
6. Tator CH. Review of experimental spinal cord injury with emphasis on the local and systemic circulatory effects. Neurochirurgie 1991;37:291–302

7. Tator CH, Fehlings MG. Review of the secondary injury theory of acute spinal cord trauma with emphasis on vascular mechanisms. J Neurosurg 1991;75:15–26

8. Blood pressure management after acute spinal cord injury. Neurosurgery 2002;50(3, Suppl):S58–S62

9. Claxton AR, Wong DT, Chung F, Fehlings MG. Predictors of hospital mortality and mechanical ventilation in patients with cervical spinal cord injury. Can J Anaesth 1998;45:144–149

10. Jackson AB, Groomes TE. Incidence of respiratory complications following spinal cord injury. Arch Phys Med Rehabil 1994;75:270–275

11. Lemons VR, Wagner FC Jr. Respiratory complications after cervical spinal cord injury. Spine 1994;19:2315–2320

12. Management of acute spinal cord injuries in an intensive care unit or other monitored setting. Neurosurgery 2002;50(3, Suppl):S51–S57

13. Vale FL, Burns J, Jackson AB, Hadley MN. Combined medical and surgical treatment after acute spinal cord injury: results of a prospective pilot study to assess the merits of aggressive medical resuscitation and blood pressure management. J Neurosurg 1997;87:239–246

14. King BS, Gupta R, Narayan RK. The early assessment and intensive care unit management of patients with severe traumatic brain and spinal cord injuries. Surg Clin North Am 2000;80:855–870, viii–ix

15. Chesnut RM. The management of severe traumatic brain injury. Emerg Med Clin North Am 1997;15:581–604

16. Harrop JS, Sharan AD, Vaccaro AR, Przybylski GJ. The cause of neurologic deterioration after acute cervical spinal cord injury. Spine 2001;26:340–346

17. Rechtine GR, Del Rossi G, Conrad BP, Horodyski M. Motion generated in the unstable spine during hospital bed transfers. J Trauma 2004;57:609–611, discussion 611–612

18. Vickery D. The use of the spinal board after the pre-hospital phase of trauma management. Emerg Med J 2001;18:51–54

19. Chulay M, Brown J, Summer W. Effect of postoperative immobilization after coronary artery bypass surgery. Crit Care Med 1982;10:176–179

20. Convertino VA, Bloomfield SA, Greenleaf JE. An overview of the issues: physiological effects of bed rest and restricted physical activity. Med Sci Sports Exerc 1997;29:187–190

21. Curry K, Casady L. The relationship between extended periods of immobility and decubitus ulcer formation in the acutely spinal cord-injured individual. J Neurosci Nurs 1992;24:185–189

22. Dittmer DK, Teasell R. Complications of immobilization and bed rest, I: Musculoskeletal and cardiovascular complications. Can Fam Physician 1993;39:1428–1432, 1435–1437

23. Krishnagopalan S, Johnson EW, Low LL, Kaufman LJ. Body positioning of intensive care patients: clinical practice versus standards. Crit Care Med 2002;30:2588–2592

24. Teasell R, Dittmer DK. Complications of immobilization and bed rest, II: Other complications. Can Fam Physician 1993;39:1440–1442, 1445–1446

25. Fisher CG, Wood KB. Introduction to and techniques of evidence-based medicine. Spine 2007;32(19, Suppl):S66–S72

26. Guyatt G, Cook D, Haynes B. Evidence based medicine has come a long way. BMJ 2004;329:990–991

27. Guyatt G, Vist G, Falck-Ytter Y, Kunz R, Magrini N, Schunemann H. An emerging consensus on grading recommendations? Evid Based Med 2006;11:2–4

28. Guyatt GH, Haynes RB, McKibbon KA, Cook DJ. Evidence-based health care. Mol Diagn 1997;2:209–215

29. Guyatt GH, Naylor CD, Juniper E, Heyland DK, Jaeschke R, Cook DJ; Evidence-Based Medicine Working Group. Users' guides to the medical literature, XII: How to use articles about health-related quality of life. JAMA 1997;277:1232–1237

30. Guyatt GH, Sinclair J, Cook DJ, Glasziou P; Evidence-Based Medicine Working Group and the Cochrane Applicability Methods Working Group. Users' guides to the medical literature, XVI: How to use a treatment recommendation. JAMA 1999;281:1836–1843

31. Ofiram E, Lonstein JE, Skinner S, Perra JH. "The disappearing evoked potentials": a special problem of positioning patients with skeletal dysplasia: case report. Spine 2006;31:E464–E470

32. Brackett TO, Condon N. Comparison of the wedge turning frame and kinetic treatment table in the acute care of spinal cord injury patients. Surg Neurol 1984;22:53–56

33. McGuire RA, Green BA, Eismont FJ, Watts C. Comparison of stability provided to the unstable spine by the kinetic therapy table and the Stryker frame. Neurosurgery 1988;22:842–845

34. Rechtine GR, Conrad BP, Bearden BG, Horodyski M. Biomechanical analysis of cervical and thoracolumbar spine motion in intact and partially and completely unstable cadaver spine models with kinetic bed therapy or traditional log roll. J Trauma 2007;62:383–388, discussion 388

35. Conrad BP, Horodyski M, Wright J, Ruetz P, Rechtine GR II. Log-rolling technique producing unacceptable motion during body position changes in patients with traumatic spinal cord injury. J Neurosurg Spine 2007;6:540–543

36. DiPaola CP, DiPaola MJ, Conrad BP, et al. Comparison of thoracolumbar motion produced by manual and Jackson-table-turning methods: study of a cadaveric instability model. J Bone Joint Surg Am 2008;90:1698–1704

37. DiPaola MJ, DiPaola CP, Conrad BP, et al. Cervical spine motion in manual versus Jackson table turning methods in a cadaveric global instability model. J Spinal Disord Tech 2008;21:273–280

38. Bearden BG, Conrad BP, Horodyski M, Rechtine GR. Motion in the unstable cervical spine: comparison of manual turning and use of the Jackson table in prone positioning. J Neurosurg Spine 2007;7:161–164

39. Capen DA, Gordon ML, Zigler JE, Garland DE, Nelson RW, Nagelberg S. Nonoperative management of upper thoracic spine fractures. Orthop Rev 1994;23:818–821

40. Hartman MB, Chrin AM, Rechtine GR. Non-operative treatment of thoracolumbar fractures. Paraplegia 1995;33:73–76

41. Rechtine GR II, Cahill D, Chrin AM. Treatment of thoracolumbar trauma: comparison of complications of operative versus nonoperative treatment. J Spinal Disord 1999;12:406–409

42. Dai LY, Jiang LS, Jiang SD. Conservative treatment of thoracolumbar burst fractures: a long-term follow-up results with special reference to the load sharing classification. Spine 2008;33:2536–2544

43. An HS, Simpson JM, Ebraheim NA, Jackson WT, Moore J, O'Malley NP. Low lumbar burst fractures: comparison between conservative and surgical treatments. Orthopedics 1992;15:367–373

44. An HS, Vaccaro A, Cotler JM, Lin S. Low lumbar burst fractures: comparison among body cast, Harrington rod, Luque rod, and Steffee plate. Spine 1991;16(8, Suppl):S440–S444

45. Seybold EA, Sweeney CA, Fredrickson BE, Warhold LG, Bernini PM. Functional outcome of low lumbar burst fractures: a multicenter review of operative and nonoperative treatment of L3-L5. Spine 1999;24:2154–2161

46. Fink MP, Helsmoortel CM, Stein KL, Lee PC, Cohn SM. The efficacy of an oscillating bed in the prevention of lower respiratory tract infection in critically ill victims of blunt trauma: a prospective study. Chest 1990;97:132–137

47. Goldhill DR, Imhoff M, McLean B, Waldmann C. Rotational bed therapy to prevent and treat respiratory complications: a review and meta-analysis. Am J Crit Care 2007;16:50–61, quiz 62

11

Pharmacological Management of Acute Spinal Cord Injury

R. John Hurlbert

The previous chapters of this section have provided a comprehensive overview of traumatic spinal cord injury (SCI) from an epidemiological, anatomical, and pathophysiological point of view. It is appropriate now to consider some type of neuroprotective strategy to rescue sublethally injured neurons and glial cells, to prevent death of tissues by secondary processes adjacent to the injury epicenter, and even to promote the regeneration of tissues irreversibly damaged by the primary injury mechanism. This chapter examines the pharmacological agents that have so far been used to treat SCI in humans and the successes reported with them. After finishing this chapter the reader should have an understanding of the therapeutic agents available to treat SCI and the science behind them.

◆ Methods

A Medline search was conducted for 1996 through 2008, using the keywords "spinal cord injury." The resulting database was limited to human studies and those describing treatment protocols. Titles and abstracts were examined for suitability based on several inclusion and exclusion criteria (**Table 11.1**). Studies meeting inclusion criteria were grouped according to level of evidence defined by the American Thoracic Society.[1] Content was reviewed and analyzed for design methodology, execution, and results. Recommendations for clinical practice were based on correlation with level of evidence.[2]

Table 11.1 Study Inclusion and Exclusion Criteria

Inclusion	Exclusion
Cervical or thoracic spinal cord injury	Conus/cauda injuries
Pharmacological treatment	Animal/in vitro studies
Clinical (human) studies	Treatment not primary focus of study
English	Non-English publications

◆ Results

There are a total of 13,435 articles identified as related to SCI. Through the primary search strategy, by limiting the papers to those that were written in English, pertain to human research, and are focused on therapy for acute injuries, 123 publications were retrieved. Examination of titles and abstracts yielded 18 articles appropriate for this review (**Table 11.2**). Pharmaceutical agents tested included methylprednisolone (MP), naloxone, tirilazad, thyrotropin-releasing hormone (TRH), and GM-1 ganglioside.

Methylprednisolone (Naloxone and Tirilazad)

The most research into pharmacotherapy for SCI has been generated by investigation of the potential beneficial effects of MP administration. Certainly the most widely recognized studies are the National Acute SCI Study (NASCIS) II and III trials published between 1990 and 1998.[3–6] These trials also investigated the effects of naloxone and tirilazad (NASCIS II and III, respectively).

The original NASCIS I trial reported negative results in comparing "high dose" to "low dose" MP in 306 patients with acute SCI.[7] High-dose patients received an MP loading dose of 1000 mg followed by the same dose daily thereafter for a period of 10 days. Low-dose patients received a loading dose of 100 mg, followed by 100 mg each day for 10 days. Six-month follow-up available on 58% of patients suggested an improvement of 10 points (scale range 14 to 84) in the high-dose group compared with low-dose patients ($p = 0.59$). However, wound infection was three times more frequent in the high-dose group ($p = 0.01$), and three times as many patients receiving high-dose MP died within the first 2 weeks of treatment (6% versus 2% mortality).

NASCIS II investigated the effect of MP and naloxone administration in 487 patients with acute SCI.[3] Although the naloxone data was uniformly uninteresting, the paper claimed a mean improvement of 5 points in American Spinal Injury Association (ASIA) motor scores (total possible score = 50) and

Table 11.2 Evidence Table for Pharmacological Management of Acute Spinal Cord Injury

Reference	Agent	Description	Level of Evidence (Primary Question)	Conclusion (Primary Outcomes)
Aito et al, 2005[15]	MP	Retrospective	IV	Positive[†]
Bracken et al, 1984[7]	MP (NASCIS I)	Prospective randomized	I	Negative
Bracken et al, 1992[4]	MP, naloxone (NASCIS II)	Prospective randomized	I	Negative*
Bracken et al, 1998[6]	MP, tirilazad (NASCIS III)	Prospective randomized	I	Negative*
Edwards et al, 2005[18]	MP (head injury)	Prospective randomized	I	Harmful
Geisler et al, 1991[20]	GM-1 Ganglioside	Prospective randomized	I	Positive (pilot)
Geisler et al, 2001[21]	GM-1 Ganglioside	Prospective randomized	I	Negative
George et al, 1995[22]	MP	Retrospective	IV	Negative
Gerndt et al, 1997[23]	MP	Retrospective case control	III	Negative
Kiwerski, 1993[14]	Dexamethasone	Retrospective	IV	Positive[†]
Otani et al, 1994[24]	MP	Prospective randomized	I	Negative*
Pitts et al, 1995[19]	TRH	Prospective randomized	I	Negative
Pointillart et al, 2000[25]	MP	Prospective randomized	I	Negative
Pollard and Apple, 2003[26]	MP	Retrospective	IV	Negative
Poynton et al, 1997[27]	MP	Retrospective case control	III	Negative
Prendergast et al, 1994[28]	MP	Retrospective	IV	Negative
Quian et al, 2005[16]	MP (SCI)	Retrospective	IV	Harmful
Tsutsumi et al, 2006[29]	MP	Retrospective	IV	Positive[†]

Abbreviations: MP, methylprednisolone; NASCIS, National Acute Spinal Cord Injury Study; SCI, spinal cord injury.

*Post hoc comparisons reported positive.

[†]Methodological errors and reporting inconsistencies.

4 points in ASIA sensory scores (total possible score 58) for patients treated with MP compared with controls at 6 months, as long as they received the drug within 8 hours. Improved motor scores persisted at 1 year ($p = 0.030$) (**Fig. 11.1A**), but the difference in light touch and pinprick sensation between MP and placebo groups was lost.[4]

NASCIS III compared the effect of 24- and 48-hour MP administration after SCI, also including a third group receiving tirilazad mesylate, a potent lipid peroxidation inhibitor developed specifically for central nervous system (CNS) protection. In a manner similar to naloxone (NASCIS II), data analyses demonstrated tirilazad to be uninteresting in influencing outcome after SCI, at least compared with 24-hour MP; no placebo control group was included in this study. However, there appeared to be an enhanced effect of steroids given for 48 hours in those patients receiving treatment between 3 and 8 hours after injury. Mean motor scores were presented as significantly improved by an average of 5 points

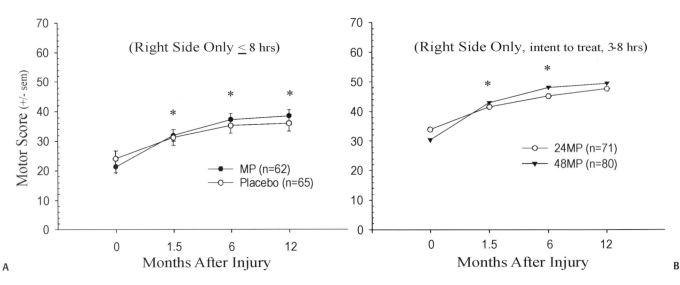

Fig. 11.1 Motor scores from post hoc analyses in **(A)** NASCIS II and **(B)** III demonstrate significant improvement in all groups with time. Although asterisks indicate statistical significance, differences between treatment groups are not compelling. All other outcome measures were also negative.

in the 48-hour group at 6 months ($p = 0.01$) and 1 year ($p = 0.053$) compared with the 24-hour group (**Fig. 11.1B**).

As a result of the NASCIS trials MP administration to patients with acute SCI became commonplace through the late 1990s and the early 21st century. However, largely arising from medicolegal and standard-of-care issues, much has been subsequently published with respect to how the NASCIS II and III results should be interpreted in day to day clinical practice.[8–13] Through the course of these critical reviews several interesting points have been made raising serious concern about the way the NASCIS results were presented and the validity of the conclusions drawn.

In designing and executing a prospective randomized clinical trial, it is important to define a priori the hypothesis to be tested as well as the primary and secondary outcome measures that will be used to enable this testing. In this sense preplanned comparisons are carefully determined during the study planning stages. Both NASCIS II and III met these criteria. However, both studies failed to show differences among treatment groups in any of their preplanned comparisons of primary or secondary outcome measures. Instead, all reported beneficial effects were based on post hoc analyses—comparisons that were made on data subsets not anticipated at the time of study design.

Although the NASCIS II cohort totaled 487 patients, beneficial effects from MP administration were discernable only after a post hoc 8-hour therapeutic window was imposed. The rationale for this 8-hour cutoff has never been substantiated.[10] Two hundred ninety one patients randomized later than 8 hours from injury were therefore excluded from the analyses, eliminating over half of the study population. Indeed, when all was said and done the observed 5-point improvement in motor score was present in only 66 MP-treated patients compared with 69 controls. Only neurological scores from the right half of the body were reported, although bilateral neurological testing was performed. As mentioned earlier sensory improvements were the same among MP- and placebo-treated patients by 1 year. No corrections were made for more than 66 statistical comparisons performed in the study. Considering the high number of negative preplanned and post hoc comparisons along with the lack of any other supporting positive outcomes, it is entirely possible if not probable that the 5-point motor improvement reported in NASCIS II arose from random chance alone.

Reporting of the NASCIS III data suffered from similar flaws. Six-week, 3-month, 6-month, and 1-year follow-up data demonstrated no difference in preplanned primary or secondary outcomes among the 24- and 48-hour MP treatment groups. Positive results were reported when a 3- to 8-hour therapeutic window was imposed from time of injury, again excluding over half of the 499 patients randomized. Even then, the five-point improvement seen in the 48-hour MP group ($n = 80$) compared with the 24-hour MP group ($n = 71$) was of questionable significance at 1 year ($p = 0.053$). In addition to ignoring left-sided neurological scores a preplanned 15th ASIA motor segment was eliminated from the reported data. Sensory improvements and Functional Independence Measure scores were no different between the 24- and 48-hour MP groups. No corrections were made for more than 100 statistical comparisons performed in the study. Hence the possibility of random chance and type I error accounting for the observed differences is very real.

When confronted with graphical representation of the data, it can be appreciated that in both NASCIS II (**Fig. 11.1A**) and NASCIS III (**Fig. 11.1B**) overall improvement from injury to 1 year was significant for all patients. However, differences in ASIA motor scores between study groups are difficult to discern and unconvincing despite their statistical significance. Because these differences arise from unplanned post hoc comparisons in a small and select group of patients, because they represent only one ASIA outcome measure (no difference in at least two types of sensory scores), because only results from right-sided motor scores are reported less one ASIA myotome, and because multiple post hoc statistical t-tests were performed without correction, the level of evidence from these two studies can reasonably be downgraded to a "very low" (IV) quality rating.[1]

The NASICS trials are not the only clinical studies investigating the effect of steroids on SCI. Ten other publications ranging from class I to class III evidence detail experience with these agents in the SCI population (**Table 11.2**). The majority of these studies report the absence of beneficial effect. Three claiming beneficial effects suffer from methodological errors and reporting inconsistencies.

In 1993, Kiwerski[14] published what is perhaps the largest retrospective review of 620 acute SCI patients treated in Poland over a 15-year period beginning in 1976. There were 290 patients who were administered MP and 330 who were not. However, the dose varied according to age, weight, medical condition, and preference of the attending physician. The usual dose was 8 mg three times a day for several days up to 1 week. Although consistently more patients in the MP group improved compared with controls, there was consistently higher mortality observed in the controls, likely indicating more severe injuries to this group and therefore less likelihood of recovery (**Fig. 11.2A,B**).

Twelve years later, Aito et al reported retrospective results in 61 patients with complete and incomplete SCI from diving accidents collected over a 24-year period.[15] In a sub-analysis they identified 30 patients in an 8-year period, 20 of whom received high-dose MP and 10 who did not. Although degree of improvement (motor vs sensory, segmental vs long-tract) was not provided, the authors reported logistic regression applied to multivariate analysis demonstrated statistical significance. Details of the multivariate or logistic variables were not provided. They concluded that "treatment with high dose methylprednisolone during the first 8 hours after trauma seemed to influence the neurological outcome positively."

In 2006, Tsutsumi and colleagues reported on a retrospective cohort of patients with acute SCI treated at their rehabilitation facility over a 5-year period. Of 278 patients admitted they restricted their report to 70 who were transferred within 7 days of injury. Thirty-seven had received MP at NASCIS II doses, whereas 33 received no drug according to the preference of the treating physician at the time of injury. Sensory function was not tested. Baseline motor scores were not provided.

Although no differences were observed in ASIA motor scores among ASIA A patients, an 18-point motor score difference was observed at 6 weeks between the incomplete patients (ASIA B, C, and D) and 26 points at 6 months. The authors acknowledge inequality of ASIA grade distribution among the groups ($p = 0.02$) but do not provide baseline motor scores. The majority of patients in the non-MP group had ASIA D injuries, whereas the majority in the MP group had ASIA B and C injuries. Hence, a ceiling effect could also account for comparatively less improvement observed in non-MP patients. After excluding patients with ASIA A injuries the

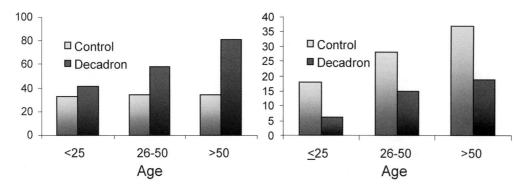

Fig. 11.2 (A) Comparison of proportion of patients improving from admission neurological assessment for those treated with Decadron and those not, stratified by age in Kiwerski's retrospective analysis of 620 Polish patients with spinal cord injury. Dosage was not standardized. It appears that more Decadron-treated patients improved than controls.

(B) Comparison of mortality between the same groups of patients demonstrates mortality in the control group to be twice as high as the Decadron group, suggesting that controls had more serious spinal cord and other systemic injuries predetermining a less favorable neurological outcome.

control group consisted of only eight patients and the MP group only 19.

Potentially harmful side effects of high-dose MP administration have been reported. In NASCIS II adverse events such as gastrointestinal hemorrhage, wound infection, and pulmonary embolus were 1.5 to 3.0 times higher in the MP-treated group, statistically inconclusive due to low power. In NASCIS III, a twofold higher incidence of severe pneumonia and a fourfold higher incidence of severe sepsis were observed in the 48-hour MP group compared with the 24-hour group. There were six times the deaths in the 48-hour group as compared with the 24-hour ($p = 0.056$). Quian et al[16] reported an association with myopathy in eight of their patients treated with MP. The CRASH trial, in which MP was randomly given to 10,008 head-injured patients in doses comparable to the NASCIS III 48-hour protocol, was closed before reaching its target population of 20,000 because interim analyses showed the relative risk of death to be 1.18 for the MP-treated patients compared with controls ($p = 0.0001$).[17,18] These results suggest that, for every 30 patients treated with 48-hour MP, one will die because of the drug.

Thyrotropin-Releasing Hormone

In 1995, Pitts et al published their prospective, randomized, double-blind, placebo-controlled study investigating the effect of TRH on clinical outcome following acute spinal cord injury in 20 patients.[19] Although at 4 months TRH-treated patients demonstrated a mean (bilateral) motor score of 59 compared with 37 in the placebo group ($n = 6$ TRH, $n = 3$ placebo), only six patients returned for follow-up in the TRH group and three patients in the placebo. Further patient dropout at 1 year led the authors to conclude their data were "not highly informative."

GM-1 Ganglioside (Sygen)

Found indigenously in cell membranes of mammalian CNS tissue, GM-1 ganglioside is a compound thought to have antiexcitotoxic activity, promote neuritic sprouting, potentiate the effects of nerve growth factor, and prevent apoptosis. In 1991, Geisler and colleagues reported promising results of a pilot study investigating its use in acute SCI.[20] The subsequent multicenter study involved 28 neurotrauma institutions and randomized 797 patients within 72 hours of injury to receive

either GM-1 ganglioside (100 or 200 mg IV/day) or placebo for 56 days.[21] Follow-up was for 1 year. Although patients with ASIA grade C and D injuries treated with Sygen demonstrated statistically significant improvements in modified Benzel grades compared with placebo-treated patients 4 and 8 weeks after injury, the advantage was lost at subsequent follow-up visits. No differences between actively treated and placebo-treated patients were noted in any of the outcome measures after 1 year. Consequently GM-1 ganglioside is not used in routine clinical practice to treat SCI at this time.

◆ Summary and Recommendations

In summary, despite several well-executed human studies there are no class I data that pharmaceutical agents are of a major benefit in the treatment of acute SCI at this time. Several drugs have been evaluated but only methylprednisolone has been widely used. However, it is important to note that *no Class I evidence illustrates MP at any dose results in neurological recovery that impacts on functional outcomes.* Small-scale neurological benefits have been reported only in post hoc or retrospective analyses. The clinician should recognize the possibility for harmful side effects of MP, including a potentially increased risk of infection, which was reported in the NASCIS III study with a 48-hour infusion protocol. Moreover, in patients with severe traumatic brain injury, there is level I evidence for an association between high-dose MP and mortality. Therefore, from an evidence-based perspective MP may be considered an option in the treatment of SCI, but only with the understanding that the evidence of harmful side effects, including the possibility of death, is stronger than the evidence of any significant neurological benefit. MP should not be considered an obligatory standard or a necessary part of routine clinical practice.

Based on the strength of evidence in the literature, further supplemented with clinical experience these statements are made based on a grade of "weak recommendation" against the use of MP in acute SCI. Considerable discussion within the Spine Trauma Study group centered on individual case examples and personal practice patterns in which some members would prescribe MP for a patient with SCI. Seventeen members voted in accordance with the guideline, whereas 10 members expressed dissent.

References

1. Schünemann HJ, Jaeschke R, Cook DJ, et al; ATS Documents Development and Implementation Committee. An official ATS statement: grading the quality of evidence and strength of recommendations in ATS guidelines and recommendations. Am J Respir Crit Care Med 2006;174:605–614

2. Wright JG, Einhorn TA, Heckman JD. Grades of recommendation. J Bone Joint Surg Am 2005;87:1909–1910

3. Bracken MB, Shepard MJ, Collins WF, et al. A randomized, controlled trial of methylprednisolone or naloxone in the treatment of acute spinal-cord injury: results of the Second National Acute Spinal Cord Injury Study. N Engl J Med 1990;322:1405–1411

4. Bracken MB, Shepard MJ, Collins WF Jr, et al. Methylprednisolone or naloxone treatment after acute spinal cord injury: 1-year follow-up data: results of the second National Acute Spinal Cord Injury Study. J Neurosurg 1992;76:23–31

5. Bracken MB, Shepard MJ, Holford TR, et al. Administration of methylprednisolone for 24 or 48 hours or tirilazad mesylate for 48 hours in the treatment of acute spinal cord injury. Results of the Third National Acute Spinal Cord Injury Randomized Controlled Trial. National Acute Spinal Cord Injury Study. JAMA 1997;277:1597–1604

6. Bracken MB, Shepard MJ, Holford TR, et al. Methylprednisolone or tirilazad mesylate administration after acute spinal cord injury: 1-year follow up: results of the third National Acute Spinal Cord Injury randomized controlled trial. J Neurosurg 1998;89:699–706

7. Bracken MB, Collins WF, Freeman DF, et al. Efficacy of methylprednisolone in acute spinal cord injury. JAMA 1984;251:45–52

8. Coleman WP, Benzel D, Cahill DW, et al. A critical appraisal of the reporting of the National Acute Spinal Cord Injury Studies (II and III) of methylprednisolone in acute spinal cord injury. J Spinal Disord 2000;13:185–199

9. Nesathurai S. Steroids and spinal cord injury: revisiting the NASCIS 2 and NASCIS 3 trials. J Trauma 1998;45:1088–1093

10. Bracken MB. The use of methylprednisolone [letter]. J Neurosurg 2000;93(2, Suppl):340–341

11. Short DJ, El Masry WS, Jones PW. High dose methylprednisolone in the management of acute spinal cord injury: a systematic review from a clinical perspective. Spinal Cord 2000;38:273–286

12. Hugenholtz H, Cass DE, Dvorak MF, et al. High-dose methylprednisolone for acute closed spinal cord injury: only a treatment option. Can J Neurol Sci 2002;29:227–235

13. Sayer FT, Kronvall E, Nilsson OG. Methylprednisolone treatment in acute spinal cord injury: the myth challenged through a structured analysis of published literature. Spine J 2006;6:335–343

14. Kiwerski JE. Application of dexamethasone in the treatment of acute spinal cord injury. Injury 1993;24:457–460

15. Aito S, D'Andrea M, Werhagen L. Spinal cord injuries due to diving accidents. Spinal Cord 2005;43:109–116

16. Qian T, Guo X, Levi AD, Vanni S, Shebert RT, Sipski ML. High-dose methylprednisolone may cause myopathy in acute spinal cord injury patients. Spinal Cord 2005;43:199–203

17. Roberts I, Yates D, Sandercock P, et al; CRASH trial collaborators. Effect of intravenous corticosteroids on death within 14 days in 10008 adults with clinically significant head injury (MRC CRASH trial): randomised placebo-controlled trial. Lancet 2004;364:1321–1328

18. Edwards P, Arango M, Balica L, et al; CRASH trial collaborators. Final results of MRC CRASH, a randomised placebo-controlled trial of intravenous corticosteroid in adults with head injury-outcomes at 6 months. Lancet 2005;365:1957–1959

19. Pitts LH, Ross A, Chase GA, Faden AI. Treatment with thyrotropin-releasing hormone (TRH) in patients with traumatic spinal cord injuries. J Neurotrauma 1995;12:235–243

20. Geisler FH, Dorsey FC, Coleman WP. Recovery of motor function after spinal-cord injury: a randomized, placebo-controlled trial with GM-1 ganglioside. N Engl J Med 1991;324:1829–1838

21. Geisler FH, Coleman WP, Grieco G, Poonian D; Sygen Study Group. The Sygen multicenter acute spinal cord injury study. Spine 2001; 26 (24, Suppl):S87–S98

22. George ER, Scholten DJ, Buechler CM, Jordan-Tibbs J, Mattice C, Albrecht RM. Failure of methylprednisolone to improve the outcome of spinal cord injuries. Am Surg 1995;61:659–663, discussion 663–664

23. Gerndt SJ, Rodriguez JL, Pawlik JW, et al. Consequences of high-dose steroid therapy for acute spinal cord injury. J Trauma 1997;42:279–284

24. Otani K, Abe H, Kadoya S, et al. Beneficial effect of methylprednisolone sodium succinate in the treatment of acute spinal cord injury [in Japanese]. Sekitsu Sekizui 1994;7:633–647

25. Pointillart V, Petitjean ME, Wiart L, et al. Pharmacological therapy of spinal cord injury during the acute phase. Spinal Cord 2000;38:71–76

26. Pollard ME, Apple DF. Factors associated with improved neurologic outcomes in patients with incomplete tetraplegia. Spine 2003;28:33–39

27. Poynton AR, O'Farrell DA, Shannon F, Murray P, McManus F, Walsh MG. An evaluation of the factors affecting neurological recovery following spinal cord injury. Injury 1997;28:545–548

28. Prendergast MR, Saxe JM, Ledgerwood AM, Lucas CE, Lucas WF. Massive steroids do not reduce the zone of injury after penetrating spinal cord injury. J Trauma 1994;37:576–579, discussion 579–580

29. Tsutsumi S, Ueta T, Shiba K, Yamamoto S, Takagishi K. Effects of the Second National Acute Spinal Cord Injury Study of high-dose methylprednisolone therapy on acute cervical spinal cord injury-results in spinal injuries center. Spine 2006;31:2992–2996, discussion 2997

III

Imaging

12

Imaging of the Thoracic and Lumbar Spine During the Emergency Department Evaluation

Miguel A. Schmitz, Darren R. Lebl, and Mitchel B. Harris

Advances in imaging that have become available for the evaluation of patients in the emergency setting have been substantial over the course of the last decade. As a result, established clinical and imaging algorithms are being reexamined with the motive of allowing the most thorough and efficient evaluation of such patients to afford the most appropriate and timely care. Despite the advances in trauma care and imaging, thoracic and lumbar spine injuries are missed for a multitude of reasons. In the polytrauma setting, patients may have life-threatening distracting injuries or altered sensorium, which may eliminate any patient complaints regarding thoracic and lumbar sites of pain. The net result of this is missed or delayed diagnosis of thoracolumbar spine injuries.

The incidence of missed or delayed diagnosis has been noted to be as high as 16.5% in a North American trauma center.[1] In the United Kingdom, the incidence of delayed diagnosis of spinal cord injury has been noted to be as high as 9%; and 50% of those were noted to have experienced neurological deterioration.[2] In another study, there was up to a 10.5% incidence of secondary neurological deficit as opposed to 1.4% in those patients with a more timely diagnosis and treatment.[3] Hence the importance of making the diagnosis of spine injuries early cannot be overemphasized. Altered mental status, a patient presenting in extremis, and distracting injuries are common causes of delayed diagnosis. Cooper and colleagues identified a 30% incidence of cognitive deficits among their cohort of 183 patients with thoracolumbar fractures.[4] In the same study, > 50% of the patients with thoracolumbar fractures had other major injuries qualifying as potential distracting injuries. Frankel and colleagues found that only 60% of patients with thoracolumbar spine fractures were symptomatic.[5]

The application of computed tomography (CT) and magnetic resonance imaging (MRI) has substantially improved the ability to identify major and minor spinal injuries. Difficulties

in imaging the upper thoracic spine such as the presence of overlapping ribs on plain lateral radiographs make it intuitive and practical to consider the CT scan to be a useful tool in the emergency setting. As such, the authors sought to identify whether there is sufficient evidence to support this notion. MRI technology has brought revolutionary changes in the ability to directly identify spinal cord and other soft tissue injuries. However, many current trauma resuscitation protocols do not mandate routine utilization of CT and MRI. Outside of utilizing a spine board for the field management of all trauma victims, emergency medical service protocols have principally focused on the management of the cervical spine. It should be recognized that thoracic spine injuries represent 20% of all spine fractures, and that 10% of these patients have associated spinal cord injuries.[6]

Prolonged supine immobilization of trauma patients due to the incompletely evaluated thoracic and lumbar spine can lead to increased risk for pneumonia, aspiration, venous thrombosis, and pressure sores. Historically, when utilizing plain radiographs alone, there have been limitations in the imaging capacities for thoracic and lumbar spine injuries because of the overlying soft tissues and ribs. CT and MRI can predictably and accurately assess the spinal column for bony and soft tissue injuries; however, their routine application in the trauma setting has been brought into question because of the increased costs and time associated with using these tests. In the case of CT, there is an increase in radiation dose when evaluating the thoracic and lumbar spine. Hence, the authors sought to answer two questions using this evidence-based review.

- What is the safest, most reliable and valid imaging modality to screen the thoracic and lumbar spine of trauma patients in the emergency room (ER) setting?
- What is the role of "emergency" MRI for trauma patients identified with a spinal column injury?

◆ Methods

Search Strategy

Three tiers of search criteria were employed in an attempt to answer these questions. OVIDMedline was used as the search engine using multiple search pairs and a search period from 1950 through February 2007. The search pairs are identified in **Table 12.1**. The first tier included articles within the initial search that were categorized by OVIDMedline to be "comparative studies," "controlled clinical trials," "meta-analyses," "multi-center studies," "randomized controlled trials," and "validation studies." The exclusion criteria for the first tier included manuscripts focused on the cervical spine, case reports, nontrauma-related articles, basic reviews, nonspine dedication, and nonemergency issues. The second tier included studies that were relevant to the questions that were identified in the initial search but were not categorized by OVIDMedline to be "comparative studies," "controlled clinical trials," "meta-analyses," "multi-center studies," "randomized controlled trials," and "validation studies." The third tier included studies that were relevant to the questions that were known by the review authors or were identified within the references of the first and second tier search criteria articles.

Appraisal of Included Studies

All articles were graded according to the system of Schünemann et al[7] and Wright et al,[8] as noted in **Table 12.2**. This entailed independent reviews of the articles by the two junior authors (MAS, DL). In the event of disagreements between these two reviewers, the senior author (MBH) independently graded the manuscript. The senior author's grading served as the final grade determination if it was concordant with either of the two gradings by the junior authors. If there was disagreement among all of the three reviewers, then the manuscript was again reviewed by all three authors to derive the final grade that is noted within **Table 12.2**.

This review asks, what is the safest, most reliable and valid imaging modality to screen the thoracic and lumbar spine in trauma patients in the emergency setting? There are many

levels of consideration in answering this question: accuracy, sensitivity, specificity, time of study, cost, and radiation exposure. The correct diagnosis of a spine fracture was considered the "gold standard" by which the terms *accuracy*, *sensitivity*, and *specificity* were defined. *Accuracy* was defined as the closeness of the imaging modality to the true spine diagnosis. *Sensitivity* was defined as the ability of the imaging modality to identify the true presence of a spine injury. *Specificity* was defined as the ability of the imaging modality to identify the true lack of a spine injury. Accuracy, sensitivity, and specificity are all valuable appraisals of imaging studies in the emergency setting. For the purposes of screening patients for injury, specificity is particularly valuable to the clinician, but for the purposes of treating patients with spine injury, sensitivity is most helpful.

◆ Results

There were no "evidence-based reviews" within the searched pairs noted in **Table 12.1** as rated by OVIDMedline. In the broadest search pair, the search for "spine trauma imaging" yielded 109 manuscripts. There was overlap by the other search pairs with this most broad search that brought the initial search to 126 manuscripts. One hundred sixteen articles identified in the primary search were excluded for the reasons noted in **Table 12.3**. The selected first-, second-, and third-tier manuscripts are noted in **Table 12.2**. The first-tier criteria only yielded five manuscripts. The second-tier criteria identified five studies, and the third-tier criteria yielded 30 articles. The review yielded several answers to the primary question noted within the methods.

Indications for Thoracolumbar Imaging

Most clinicians who manage trauma can agree that there are certain traumatic conditions that mandate thoracolumbar imaging. Frankel and colleagues identified the following factors which increase the likelihood that there is a fracture in the thoracolumbar region: pain, cervical spine fracture, fall, neurological deficit, ejection from a moving vehicle, highspeed crash, and Glasgow Coma Score $\leq$ 8.[5] Holmes and colleagues used a panel of "high-risk" criteria to trigger the acquisition of thoracolumbar radiographs in a prospective observational cohort study. This study considered the following to be high-risk criteria: thoracolumbar spine pain, thoracolumbar spine tenderness, diminished level of consciousness, abnormal neurological examination, distracting painful injury, and evidence of intoxication. The presence of any one of these criteria was considered to be a trigger to image the thoracolumbar spine. Among 2404 patients who sustained blunt trauma, one or more "high-risk criteria" were identified in 2158 patients, and thoracolumbar imaging was obtained. Among this group, 152 patients were noted to have acute thoracolumbar spine injuries. Using these criteria, the specificity for thoracolumbar injury was 3.9%, the positive predictive value was 6.6%, and the negative predictive value was 100%.[9] All of the high-risk criteria except for intoxication were important as sole predictors of thoracolumbar spine injury.[9] Durham and associates found three factors in patients with blunt trauma that were associated with the occurrence of thoracolumbar trauma: an Injury Severity Score $\geq$ 15, a positive clinical examination, and a fall of $\geq$ 10 feet. A clinical

Table 12.1 OVIDMedline Search Pairs

Search Criteria	No. of Manuscripts	Evidence-Based Reviews
Spine trauma and imaging	109	0
Spine trauma and CT scan	7	0
Spine trauma and MRI	23	0
Thoracic spine fracture and imaging	3	0
Thoracic spine trauma and imaging	2	0
Lumbar spine fracture and imaging	5	0
Lumbar spine trauma and imaging	4	0
Thoracic spine trauma and CT scan	1	0
Thoracic spine trauma and MRI	1	0
Lumbar spine trauma and CT scan	0	0
Lumbar spine trauma and MRI	0	0

Table 12.2 Level of Evidence Grading and Summary of Reviewed Literature on Spinal Trauma Imaging

Study	Tier	Description	Level of Evidence		History and Physical	X-ray	CT	MRI	(patients)	Accuracy	Sensitivity (%)	Specificity (%)	Positive Predictive Value	Negative Predictive Value	Special Consideration
			Wright	Schünemann											
Adams et al[21]	1	Retrospective	III	Low			x		97		94.0	94.0	75.0	99.0	CT/CAP versus MRI gold standard
Anderson et al[44]	1	Expert opinion	V	Very low											"Appropriateness criteria"
Antevil et al[18]	1	Prospective; nonrandomized	III	Moderate			x		34		100.0				20 patients in x-ray group; 34 patients in CT scan group; mean time in radiology rooms was significantly less in CT group; may not need x-ray with CT scan for spine
						x			20		70.0				20 patients in x-ray group; 34 patients in CT scan group; four-array helical CT scanner with dedicated views of spine
Ballock et al[16]	3	Retrospective	I	Moderate		x			25		80.0	68.0	78.0		No reconstruction of CT; CT gold standard; studied burst fracture discrimination on x-ray; loss of posterior body height, interpedicular widening
Berry et al[13]	3	Retrospective	II	Moderate			x		26		100.0	97.0	93.0	100.0	Helical CT/CAP/pitch 1; 5 mm reconstructions
			II	Moderate		x			26		73.0				
Brandt et al[24]	3	Prospective	II	Low			x		47		100.0	100.0	100.0	92.0	Helical CT scanner with single detector and two-slice acquisition
			II	Low		x			47		72.3				
Brant-Zawadzki et al[14]	2	Retrospective, nonrandomized	IV	Very low			x		15						1981 publication asserts that if the plain radiographs are abnormal, then CT scan is of modest assistance
Brightman et al[38]	3	Prospective	IV	Very Low				x	24				100.0		PPV only noted for surgical confirmation patient (N = 21 of the 24)

(Continued on page 98)

Table 12.2 Level of Evidence Grading and Summary of Reviewed Literature on Spinal Trauma Imaging (*Continued*)

Study	Tier	Description	Level of Evidence		History and Physical	X-ray	CT	MRI	(patients)	Accuracy	Sensitivity (%)	Specificity (%)	Positive Predictive Value	Negative Predictive Value	Special Consideration
			Wright	Schünemann											
Brown et al[17]	3	Retrospective	III	Low			x		236		99.3				One cervical compression fracture missed; one thoracic compression fracture missed; 5 mm slices
Calendine et al[20]	3	Retrospective	III	Low		x	x		235		63.0			100.0	Gold standard is thoracic spine plain radiographs/general clinical condition; study compares CT scan to plain radiographs and CT scan; CT of spine is more sensitive for T-spine fractures
Cooper et al[4]	3	Prospective	III	Low	x (back tender)				110		69.1				Thoracolumbar fracture present, 7/34 required surgical stabilization, GCS = 13–15
					x (back tender)						37.0				Thoracolumbar fracture present, GCS = 13–14
					x (back tender)						78.0				Thoracolumbar fracture present, GCS = 15
Daffner et al[53]	3	Expert opinion	V	Very low											2007 "Appropriateness Criteria"
Durham et al[10]	3		III	Very Low	x										Three factors associated with thoracolumbar spine injury: ISS ≥ 15, positive clinical examination, fall ≥ 10 feet
Emery et al[41]	3		III	Low				x			90.0	100.0			PLC injury in surgery; surgery gold standard
France et al[22]	2	Literature review; expert opinion	IV	Very low			x	x							Anteroposterior/lateral thoracolumbar films are adequate to rule out thoracic and lumbar spine injuries in most cases; CT/CAPs can be very useful (2–3 mm slices recommended); MRI for soft tissue

Table 12.2 Level of Evidence Grading and Summary of Reviewed Literature on Spinal Trauma Imaging (*Continued*)

Study	Tier	Description	Level of Evidence		History and Physical	X-ray	CT	MRI	(patients)	Accuracy	Sensitivity (%)	Specificity (%)	Positive Predictive Value	Negative Predictive Value	Special Consideration
			Wright	Schünemann											
Frankel et al[5]	3	Prospective	II	Moderate		x			15		100.0				Among 167 patients total (with and without fractures); indications for imaging: back pain after accident; fall ≥ 10 feet; ejection from motorcycle or car; GCS ≤ 8, neuro deficit
Gestring et al[54]	3	Prospective	I	Moderate			x		71		100.0	100.0			CT/CAP with 5 mm abdominal slices and 7 mm pelvis slices plus thoracolumbar scanogram (which was helpful to determine alignment)
Grauer et al[49]	1	Expert survey	V	Very low					8						Neurosurgeons tend to obtain more MRIs more often than orthopedists for spine trauma
Haba et al[42]	3	Retrospective	III	Very low				x	35	90.5	89.4	92.3			Supraspinous ligament injury; surgery gold standard
								x	35	94.3	98.5	87.2			Interspinous ligament; surgery gold standard
Hauser et al[23]	3	Prospective	I	Moderate			x		36	99.0	97.0				N = 36 (thoracic and lumbar only); CT/CAP; 5 mm slices; helical scanner with collimation of 5 mm; pitch of 1.6
						x			36	87.0	58.0				N = 36 (thoracic and lumbar only)
Holmes et al[9]	3	Prospective; observational	II	Moderate	x (high-risk criteria)				152			3.9	6.6	100.0	Prospective, observational cohort study; pain/tenderness/altered sensorium/neuro dim/distraction/intoxication
Kulkarni et al[47]	3	Retrospective	III	Very low				x	27		78.0				Intraspinal hemorrhage is poor prognostic sign for SCI recovery; however, cord edema or contusions recover significant neurological function; predict recovery with MRI?

(Continued on page 100)

12 Imaging of the Thoracic and Lumbar Spine During Evaluation

Table 12.2 Level of Evidence Grading and Summary of Reviewed Literature on Spinal Trauma Imaging *(Continued)*

Study	Tier	Description	Wright	Schünemann	History and Physical	X-ray	CT	MRI	(patients)	Accuracy	Sensitivity (%)	Specificity (%)	Positive Predictive Value	Negative Predictive Value	Special Consideration
Lee et al[43]	3	Prospective	II	Moderate				x		90.0	92.9	80.0			Supraspinous ligament injury; surgery gold standard; T1 MRI was more specific than T2
								x			100.0	75.0			Interspinous ligament; surgery gold standard
								x			85.7	88.5			Ligamentum flavum; surgery gold standard
					x					53.6	52.0	66.7			PLC injury; surgery gold standard
						x				66.7	66.7	66.7			PLC injury; surgery gold standard
Lee et al[33]	3	Expert survey	V	Very low	x	x	x	x	33						Since last survey, there have been changes Preferred PLC diagnostic criteria: diastasis of facet joint on CT; MRI posterior edema at PLC on T2STIR or FAT SAT; disrupted PLC on MRI on proton MRI sequence
McAfee et al[15]	3	Retrospective	III	Low			x		100						Consecutive patients underwent thoracolumbar surgery for trauma; CT more sensitive than any other imaging method
Mehta et al[50]	3	Prospective	II	Low		x			28						Supine films to standing: mean Cobb angle increased 11 degrees to 18 degrees; mean anterior vertebral compression increased 34 to 46%; 7/28 (25%) were subjected to surgery because of standing findings
Meldon et al[1]	3	Retrospective	III	Low	x				145		81.0				Of the 27 (19%) that did not have back tenderness with thoracolumbar spine fractures, all (100%) had altered sensorium.
Meyer[6]	2	Review	IV	Very low			x	x							CT is more sensitive in determining canal compromise; MRI can assess the spinal cord well.

Table 12.2 Level of Evidence Grading and Summary of Reviewed Literature on Spinal Trauma Imaging (*Continued*)

Study	Tier	Description	Level of Evidence Wright	Level of Evidence Schünemann	History and Physical	X-ray	CT	MRI	(patients)	Accuracy	Sensitivity (%)	Specificity (%)	Positive Predictive Value	Negative Predictive Value	Special Consideration
Petersilge et al[39]	3	Retrospective	IV	Very low		x	x		21		33.0				Gold standard = MRI (1.0 or 1.4 Tesla); only burst fractures studied
Regnicolo et al[37]	3	Retrospective	IV	Very low				x	50						Suggests that a standardized integrated panel of MRI findings be used to plan improved treatment; selection bias
Rhee et al[19]	3	Retrospective	II	Moderate			x		115		76.8				Single-slice scanner; 5–10 mm slices; 1994–1996; lumbar fracture only; multislice scanner likely better
			II	Moderate		x			115		87.3				Combination of plain radiographs with CT did not miss any fractures; CT of abdomen/pelvis
Roos et al[28]	2	Retrospective	III	Low			x		82		98.0	97.0			N = 50 control group;4-MDCT of chest/abdomen/pelvis; collimation, 4 × 2.5 mm; slice width, 3 mm; reconstruction interval, 1.5 mm
Sampson et al[25]	3	Prospective	II	Low			x		296						16% of multitrauma studies revealed thoracic and lumbar fractures (N = 48)
Samuels et al[11]	3	Retrospective	III	Low	x				24				58.0	100.0	Retrospective; radiographic gold standard; question of physical examination screening validity; N = 24 had positive clinical evidence of thoracolumbar injury
Sheridan et al[55]	3	Prospective	II	Moderate		x			78		62T/86 L				Thoracic N = 35; lumbar N = 43; plain x-ray N = 50; CT N = 74; both N = 46
							x				97T/95L				Thoracic N = 35; lumbar N = 43; plain x-ray N = 50; CT N = 74; both N = 46

(Continued on page 102)

12 Imaging of the Thoracic and Lumbar Spine During Evaluation

TTable 12.2 Level of Evidence Grading and Summary of Reviewed Literature on Spinal Trauma Imaging (Continued)

Study	Level of Evidence			History and Physical	X-ray	CT	MRI	(patients)	Accuracy	Sensitivity (%)	Specificity (%)	Positive Predictive Value	Negative Predictive Value	Special Consideration
	Tier	Wright	Schünemann											
Sledge et al[46]	2	IV	Very low				x	19						MRI is the imaging modality of choice in pediatric population for assessing thoracolumbar injury
Terk et al[40]	3	III	Very low				x	6		100.0				Gold standard of surgery only used in six patients; PLL injury should be appreciated in patients with burst and compression fractures.
Terregino et al[12]	3	IV	Very low	x (overall)				24					95.0	Pain or tenderness of the thoracolumbar spine mandates image evaluation; no radiography if no pain/tenderness, GCS ≥ 14; in patients with no neurological deficits, no distracting injuries
		IV	Very low	x (pain)				24		47.0	89.0	29.0	95.0	
		IV	Very low	x (tenderness)				24		53.0	94.0	45.0	95.0	
Vaccaro et al[32]	1	V	Very low			x	x	28						Top three criteria for diagnosis of PLC injury of thoracolumbar spine include vertebral body translation, increased interspinous spacing, diastasis of facet joint on CT.
Williams et al[36]	3	IV	Very Low				x	22						MRI is helpful to identify acute spinal instability; n = 10 for operative patients; MRI had 100% sensitivity in this group with operative gold standard.

Abbreviations: CT, computed tomography; CT/CAP, Computed Tomography of Chest, Abdomen, and Pelvis; FAT SAT, fat saturated; GCS, Glasgow Coma Score; ISS, Injury Severity Score; MDCT, multidetector computed tomography; MRI, magnetic resonance imaging; NPV, negative predictive value; PLC, posterior ligamentous complex; PPV, positive predictive value; SCI, spinal column injury; T2STIR, T2 short tau inversion recovery.

Table 12.3 Reason for Exclusion of Manuscripts within the Initial OVIDMedline Search

Exclusion Criteria	No. of Manuscripts
Cervical spine focus rather than thoracolumbar spine	74
Case report < 10 cases	5
Not trauma related	8
Review only with no primary research	18
Spine was not central to the manuscript	5
Imaging was not for emergency purposes	6

examination was noted to be positive if there was localized tenderness, bruising, spine deformity, or neurological deficit that was consistent with spinal injury.[10]

On the other hand, Samuels and Kerstein concluded that physical examination is reliable for assessing the thoracolumbar spine, regardless of the other risk factors, except for "equivocal" examinations.[11] Outside of those circumstances in which there is positive clinical evidence for thoracolumbar injury, Samuels and Kerstein concluded that thoracolumbar films are unnecessary.[11] Terregino and coworkers defined the clinical signs with regard to thoracolumbar trauma in greater detail. As noted in **Table 12.2**, the negative predictive value of physical examination in the blunt trauma setting is 95%.[12] With the potential increased morbidity associated with missing spinal injuries, an argument can be made to be aggressive in evaluating the thoracolumbar spine with imaging even though there will likely be more negative studies in patients without significant thoracolumbar injury, particularly in the setting of multiple trauma. The use of the chest/abdomen/pelvis screening trauma CT appears to be an effective option.[13]

Computed Tomographic Scan of the Thoracic and Lumbar Spine

Accuracy, Sensitivity, Specificity, Negative Predictive Value, Positive Predictive Value

The quality, accuracy, and efficiency of the CT scan have evolved substantially since its introduction. In its nascent applications to the spine (a tier 2 study), Brant-Zawadzki and colleagues concluded that computed tomography yields modestly more information than plain radiographs.[14] Since that time, CT has been consistently noted to be more sensitive in identifying fracture and spinal canal compromise than plain radiographs.[6,15] Using the CT scan as the "gold standard," Ballock and colleagues demonstrated that plain radiographs of the thoracic and lumbar spine could identify the presence of a burst component only 80% of the time it was identified on CT scan. The specificity of plain radiographs was 68%, and the positive predictive value was 78%.[16] Hence it was recommended that CT scans be routinely obtained in all patients with acute thoracic and lumbar compression fractures.[16] In a tier 3 study, Brown and colleagues identified a 99.3% sensitivity for all spine fractures among 236 patients who were studied using a four-slice spiral CT with 5-mm collimation and 3-mm reconstructions.[17] The sensitivity for thoracic and lumbar spine fractures was 98.5% and 100%, respectively.[17] In a

tier 1 study, Antevil and colleagues studied two different imaging protocols for the evaluation of the spine. The first group involved patients whose spine image protocol was initiated with plain radiographs. Under certain circumstances, patients in this group underwent CT scans of symptomatic areas. The second group involved patients whose spine image protocol was initiated with CT scan using a four-array CT scanner (Somotom Volume 4-Slice CT Scanner, Siemens Corporation, New York, New York) of symptomatic areas without obtaining plain radiographs. Although both groups in which CT scanning was performed had 100% sensitivity for spinal fractures, the sensitivity for spinal fractures with plain radiographs was 70% in the plain radiograph group and 75% in the plain radiography followed by CT group.[18] The authors found that although CT scans of the spine detected many fractures that were not identified by plain radiographs, the majority of these fractures were of minimal clinical significance. However, one of five patients in this subseries required treatment for potentially unstable spine fractures.[18]

Computed Tomography of Chest, Abdomen, and Pelvis for Assessment of the Thoracic and Lumbar Spine

The use of nonspine-dedicated single-slice CT scanners was initially demonstrated to be problematic. In a study of 115 patients with lumbar fractures, Rhee and associates found a sensitivity of only 76.8% with single-slice CT scans with 5 to 10 mm cuts that were focused on the abdomen and the pelvis as opposed to the spine.[19] Plain radiographs had a sensitivity in this same series of 87.3%. Seven of the 14 missed fractures required surgery or a brace. When single-slice, nonspine-dedicated CT scanning was combined with plain radiographs, the sensitivity increased to 100%.[19] Using plain radiographs of the thoracic spine as the gold standard, Calendine and associates found a 100% negative predictive value for thoracic CT scans that were derived from chest CT scans with 6.5 mm slices every 5 mm.[20] In a tier 1 study, Adams and colleagues identified that chest, abdomen, and pelvis CT scans (CTCAP) among 29 thoracic and lumbar spine trauma patients with neurological complaints was 100% sensitive and specific with 100% positive and negative predictive values. In the obtunded group (*N* = 29) with MRI-confirmed thoracic and lumbar spine injuries, CTCAP had a sensitivity of 83%, specificity of 91%, positive predictive value of 71%, and negative predictive value of 95%.[21] If CT scans of the chest, abdomen, and pelvis are used for screening thoracic and lumbar spine trauma, then 2-to 3-mm slice thickness is recommended.[22] Conversely, Hauser and colleagues demonstrated 99% accuracy and 97% sensitivity with CT scans of the thoracic and lumbar spine derived from CTCAP with 5-mm collimation.[23] In their series of 47 patients with thoracolumbar fractures, Brandt and colleagues found that CT scanning with a single detector and two-slice technology allowed the identification of 33 thoracolumbar spine fractures that were not seen on plain radiographs, even though the CT scans were used primarily for evaluation of the chest, abdomen, and pelvis. Among these latter fractures were three vertebral body fractures, 25 transverse process fractures, and five spinous process fractures.[24] Berry and colleagues found significant improvements in the sensitivity and negative predictive value of CTCAP over plain radiographs with a sensitivity and negative predictive value of 100% for the former and 73% and 92% for the latter.[13] Sampson and colleagues have refined this CTCAP protocol using a 16 section CT machine to identify a 16% thoracolumbar fracture rate in patients undergoing routine "whole body imaging" in multitrauma. This will likely improve resolution and speed of CT scans even further.[25]

Duration of Study

Seventy percent of all deaths from trauma occur within 24 hours of the insult; 1 to 3% of these are preventable.[26] In the radiology department, trauma patients are in a more precarious position because of the lack of trauma resources that are immediately available in the area. Hence it is in the physicians' and patients' best interest to minimize the time spent in the radiology department. With the advent of multidetector CT (MDCT) capacities on newer-generation CT scanners, whole body scanning has shortened scanning times by a factor of 10 compared with single-detector CT when using a four-way MDCT system.[27] Higher-number MDCT systems will be available for clinical purposes in the future, and this is anticipated to further increase the accuracy and speed of CT scans of the thoracic and lumbar spine.[28] Brandt and colleagues previously performed a study that corroborates the findings of Antevil et al.[24] Specifically, spiral CT with single-detector and two-slice acquisition technology of the torso took an average of 55 minutes compared with the 168 minutes associated with obtaining plain radiographs of the torso.[24] Similarly, Hauser et al found that obtaining a single spiral CT of the thoracolumbar spine took 57 minutes on average compared with plain radiographs, which took 295 minutes.[23] Antevil et al identified that the CT group spent 54 minutes fewer in the radiology department ($p < 0.001$) (114 minutes vs 60 minutes) than the plain radiograph group, signifying that using CT as a primary evaluation tool for the spine is more time efficient.[18] The time efficiency of CT/(CAP) (Chest/abdomen/pelvis) has been demonstrated by Berry and colleagues as well.[13]

Radiation Exposure

Antevil and colleagues also identified that there was a similar mean radiation exposure in the plain radiograph group versus that of the CT group, 30 millisieverts versus 39 millisieverts, respectively.[18] When comparing the radiation exposure for evaluating the thoracolumbar spine, plain radiographs exceeded that of spiral CT scan with exposures of 26 millisieverts versus 13 millisieverts, respectively. This was attributed to the multidetector-row spiral CT design of their scanner. At this time, no study has demonstrated an increase in the incidence of malignancy after diagnostic radiography in adults.[29]

Cost

Although spine-dedicated CT scans at Scripps Memorial hospital have patient charges of $1462 for each segment of the spine (cervical, thoracic, and lumbar) as opposed to $157 to $196 for plain radiographs for the respective spine segments, the total cost to the hospital for CT scans for each of these segments is $57 versus $55 for plain radiographs of each part of the spine: cervical, thoracic, or lumbosacral. Although there is an increased charge associated with obtaining CT scans, obtaining plain radiographs as a screening image study does not preclude the eventual need for a CT scan. Obtaining a CT scan initially will allow the physician to forgo obtaining

a plain radiograph. Hence CT scans in the setting of multiple trauma patients are cost-effective. Other authors have identified that performing a CT of the torso without plain radiographs to evaluate the thoracic and lumbar spine is less expensive than obtaining plain radiographs alone: $1487 versus $654.[24] This study did not consider the frequent need to repeat plain radiographs on the grounds that previous studies were inadequate.[24] Indeed, Hauser and colleagues found that 10.5 films were taken on average to obtain an adequate five-view thoracolumbar radiograph series. On the other hand, Hauser emphasized that scrutiny was applied in determining that CT/CAP was necessary for the 222 patients who underwent such screening in that these 222 patients only represented 11% of the trauma activations.[23]

Magnetic Resonance Imaging

The theoretical importance of the integrity of the posterior ligamentous complex (PLC) in the stability of the thoracic and lumbar spine is reflected in the new Thoracolumbar Injury Severity Score (TLISS) system and the Thoracolumbar Injury Classification and Severity Score (TLICS) system, but its clinical relevance or validity has not yet been firmly established.[30,31] In the assessment of the thoracolumbar PLC, most spine surgeons felt that the top three diagnostic criteria suggesting PLC injury in the thoracolumbar spine included vertebral body translation, widened interspinous spacing on anteroposterior spine radiographs, and diastasis of the facet joint on CT, suggesting that plain radiographs still have value in the evaluation of the thoracolumbar spine in trauma.[32] In another survey of Spine Trauma Study Group members, similar findings have been noted. Specifically, the top three predictors of PLC injury in rank order are diastasis of facet joints on CT, posterior edema in the region of the PLC on T2 short tau inversion recovery (T2 STIR) or fat saturation (FAT SAT) sagittal MRI images, and disrupted PLC components on T1 sagittal MRI.[33] The recent emphasis on the PLC does not diminish the relevance of the anterior structures of the thoracolumbar spine in spine stability as emphasized by Denis[34] and by Alanay and associates.[35] One of the significant advantages of MRI is the ability to assess spinal instability as noted in an earlier study by Williams and coworkers[36] and subsequently by Regnicolo and colleagues.[37]

Multiple studies noted within **Table 12.2** have demonstrated the value of MRI in determining the status of the PLC of the thoracic spine, which has been identified as an important stabilizer of the thoracic spine.[32] Brightman and coworkers compared MRI readings to intraoperative findings to demonstrate that MRI was accurate in identifying injury to the posterior longitudinal ligament in 21 of 24.[38] Using MRI as a gold standard, Petersilge and associates found plain radiographic indicators for posterior ligamentous injury in only 33% of the patients who had posterior ligamentous injury, again highlighting the value of MRI over radiographic methods of assessing the posterior ligamentous structures.[39] Terk and colleagues correlated MRI evidence of thoracolumbar PLC injuries with surgical findings in six patients.[40] Among 68 patients with acute thoracolumbar trauma of varying severities who had MRIs in their series, Terk et al found that the incidence of posterior ligamentous injury on MRI was 53%.[40] Emery found that among 37 patients who underwent surgical intervention after the MRI, the sensitivity and specificity of the MRI in predicting PLC injury after thoracolumbar trauma was 90% and 100%, respectively.[41] Haba and colleagues and Lee and colleagues reported similar findings as noted in **Table 12.2**, although these latter two studies stratified the analysis of the PLC to the supraspinous ligament and the interspinous ligaments.[42,43]

Although MRI does not provide optimal definition of spine bone anatomy, it is helpful for identifying neurological and other soft tissue injury, such as herniated disks, disruption of the anterior or posterior longitudinal ligaments, discontinuity of the ligamentum flavum, facet capsule tears, and disruption of the interspinous ligaments. Some suggest that MRI is particularly helpful in the thoracic spine[44] given that there is up to a 50% incidence of neurological injury with thoracic spine trauma.[45] In the pediatric population, MRI was found to be very helpful in identifying thoracolumbar fractures in the young population in which bony structures are not developed.[46] Kulkarni and associates have identified that the pattern of spinal cord edema correlates with neurological recovery.[47] Ishida and Tominaga reaffirmed the value of MRIs in prognosticating neurological recovery in the cervical spine, but this study did not include the thoracic and lumbar spine.[48] Indeed, neurosurgeons are more likely to obtain an MRI than orthopedists who practice spine surgery,[49] perhaps because some locales traditionally have neurosurgeons manage neurologically involved spine trauma.

On the other hand, the limitations of MRI include the duration of the study[22] (which is usually at least 45 minutes), and the inability to scan patients with pacemakers and cardiac defibrillators. In a tier 1 study, Adams and colleagues identified the value of MRI over CT scan in several cases among 97 trauma patients. Within 97 patients with CT criteria suggesting fracture, 12 fractures were reclassified as degenerative changes. Additionally, MRI identified two new injuries. One injury was a stable ligament tear and another was a T7 Chance fracture; the management of both of these patients was significantly altered by virtue of the MRI findings.[21] With the sensitivity of MRI for soft tissue injury associated with spine trauma, the clinician must be aware of the potential of the MRI to identify incidental and inconsequential findings. Hence, MRI findings must be corroborated with the history and clinical examination and other imaging modalities.

With these considerations, the authors suggest reserving MRI for those patients who are hemodynamically stable and who are in question of having a thoracic or lumbar injury that is not completely defined with CT scanning. MRI can be particularly helpful in defining the status of the posterior ligamentous structures and thus potentially determining the surgical approach. MRI along with a proper physical examination can help define and explain the neurological status better than a CT scan.

Figures 12.1 and **12.2** demonstrate a case in which MRI was very helpful in identifying the level of the flexion-distraction injury in a 38-year-old patient who was hit by a snow plow, sustaining a splenic artery injury and a flexion-distraction injury of T12 on L1 associated with T10 level paraplegia. The MRI scans in **Fig. 12.2** served as a useful study in this setting to demonstrate the level of the injury not evident on the CT scans in **Fig. 12.1**.

Plain Radiographs

Although the more recent focus has been on the value of CT scan and MRI in the evaluation of patients with spine injury, the clinician must also remember that plain radiographs are a useful adjunct, particularly when performed in positions of function, such as standing, bending, flexing, and extending. This should be reserved for the alert patient who is medically capable of sitting up. Mehta and colleagues demonstrated the value of weight-bearing radiographs in thoracolumbar fractures in 28 patients with such fractures that had prior CT scans of the thoracolumbar spine. In their series, the mean Cobb angle increased from 11 degrees in a supine position to 18 degrees in the erect position. The mean anterior vertebral compression increased from 34 to 46%.[50] Within this series, 25% of the patients had their treatment course changed from nonoperative to operative because of findings noted on the erect radiographs even though a CT scan of the thoracolumbar spine had already been obtained.[50]

◆ Discussion

In the polytrauma setting, optimal clinical diagnostic conditions do not exist by definition. Two or more traumatic conditions may distract the examiner from a spinal injury in an acute trauma patient. Additionally, patients with polytrauma frequently have altered sensorium, history of loss of consciousness, and exposure to intoxicating substances. Hence, patients with polytrauma frequently do not have clinical examinations that can absolutely rule out thoracolumbar trauma. Furthermore, the physician must also consider that 11% of patients with a cervical spine injury may also have thoracic and/or lumbar injuries that are not contiguous with the cervical spine injury.[51] As such, it is increasingly recognized that the identification of cervical spine injuries begets imaging evaluation of the thoracic and lumbar spine.[52] Therefore the importance of imaging the thoracic and lumbar spine in the polytrauma setting has become an even more important issue than recognized in the past.

As of the year 2000, plain radiographs of the thoracic and lumbar spine were asserted to be the primary imaging modalities for evaluating the thoracic and lumbar spine in the trauma patient, as outlined in "Appropriateness Criteria" by the American College of Radiology. These criteria dictated that plain radiographs are more appropriate than either CT scan or MRI in the evaluation of thoracic and lumbar spine trauma unless there is a neurological injury.[44] With this review, it is evident to the authors that even survey CT scans of the chest, abdomen, and pelvis that are not dedicated to the spine, which are obtained using more advanced CT scanning techniques such as those employing multidetectors with 5 mm or smaller cuts, are of greater value with little downside when compared with plain radiographs. As of 2007, the American College of Radiology Appropriateness Criteria have been updated and they are consistent with the conclusions of this review, although this guideline emphasizes the evaluation of the cervical spine.[53]

With the cost-effectiveness of CT scanning versus that of plain radiographs in the emergency setting for thoracolumbar spine evaluation, the use of CT scanning is further supported. Although MRI requires more time and preparation to carry out versus a CT scan, it can be instrumental in identifying soft tissue trauma in those cases that soft tissue trauma is not evident on CT scan and/or plain radiographs (**Fig. 12.2**). When used to complement radiographic studies under clinical circumstances whereby soft tissue injury is not readily apparent on plain radiographs or CT scan, MRI can also provide a cost-effective imaging option in terms of rendering a timely diagnosis for timely treatment.

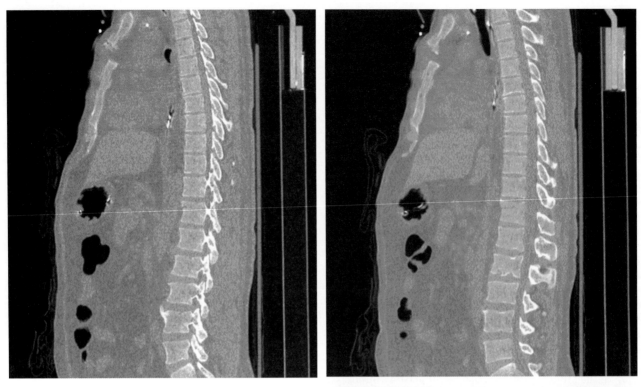

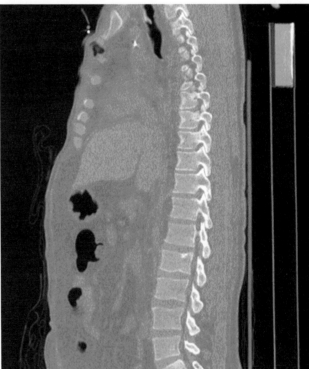

Fig. 12.1 (A–C) Sagittal reconstructions of the spine of a 38-year-old man who was struck from behind by a snow plow, sustaining a splenic artery injury requiring embolization and T10 level paraplegia associated with a flexion-distraction injury of T12. Although the computed tomographic (CT) scan noted in **(A)** suggests possible diastasis at the left T12–L1 facet and a superior end-plate fracture of T12, the remainder of the CT was nondiagnostic (B and C).

◆ Summary and Recommendations

With "high-quality evidence"[7] suggesting that modern CT scan techniques are the most reliable, rapid, and accurate methods for imaging the thoracolumbar spine with an acceptable safety margin, the authors strongly recommend the use of higher-quality CT/CAP scans in the polytrauma setting, while reserving spine-dedicated CT scans for patients that are committed to having spine surgery for the purposes of better osseous definition. The frequent need to repeat plain radiographs and the fact that they often do not preclude the need for an eventual CT scan, makes a CT scan in the primary setting of a polytrauma patient a cost-effective option. The authors do not recommend the use of plain spine radiographs because they have high cost in terms of time and money in a level 2 trauma center prior to transferring the patient to the treating level 1 institution. Also with "strong moderate-quality evidence,"[7] the authors strongly recommend using MRI in the stabilized polytrauma patient to identify the status of the soft tissues of the thoracolumbar spine in cases in which the

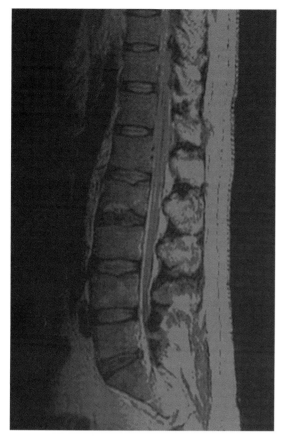 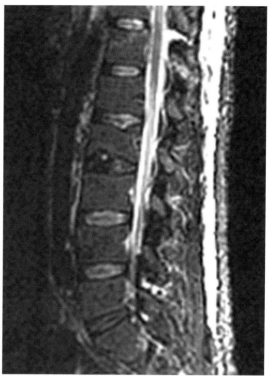

Fig. 12.2 Sagittal views of a magnetic resonance imaging (MRI) scan that was subsequently obtained in the same patient demonstrating **(A)** a T2 image and **(B)** a tear within the ligamentum flavum and associated posterior ligamentous injury. Although the T2 image is not revealing of posterior soft tissue compromise, the inversion recovery image in **(B)** reveals a tear within the ligamentum flavum associated with posterior muscular injury.

integrity of the posterior soft tissues is brought into question and in which there is neurological compromise, after the patient is hemodynamically stabilized.

References

1. Meldon SW, Moettus LN. Thoracolumbar spine fractures: clinical presentation and the effect of altered sensorium and major injury. J Trauma 1995;39:1110–1114
2. Poonnoose PM, Ravichandran G, McClelland MR. Missed and mismanaged injuries of the spinal cord. J Trauma 2002;53:314–320
3. Reid DC, Henderson R, Saboe L, Miller JDR. Etiology and clinical course of missed spine fractures. J Trauma 1987;27:980–986
4. Cooper C, Dunham CM, Rodriguez A. Falls and major injuries are risk factors for thoracolumbar fractures: cognitive impairment and multiple injuries impede the detection of back pain and tenderness. J Trauma 1995;38:692–696
5. Frankel HL, Rozycki GS, Ochsner MG, Harviel JD, Champion HR. Indications for obtaining surveillance thoracic and lumbar spine radiographs. J Trauma 1994;37:673–676
6. Meyer S. Thoracic spine trauma. Semin Roentgenol 1992;27:254–261
7. Schünemann HJ, Jaeschke R, Cook DJ, et al; ATS Documents Development and Implementation Committee. An official ATS statement: grading the quality of evidence and strength of recommendations in ATS guidelines and recommendations. Am J Respir Crit Care Med 2006; 174:605–614
8. Wright JG, Swiontkowski MF, Heckman JD. Introducing levels of evidence to the journal. J Bone Joint Surg Am 2003;85-A:1–3
9. Holmes JF, Panacek EA, Miller PQ, Lapidis AD, Mower WR. Prospective evaluation of criteria for obtaining thoracolumbar radiographs in trauma patients. J Emerg Med 2003;24:1–7
10. Durham RM, Luchtefeld WB, Wibbenmeyer L, Maxwell P, Shapiro MJ, Mazuski JE. Evaluation of the thoracic and lumbar spine after blunt trauma. Am J Surg 1995;170:681–684, discussion 684–685
11. Samuels LE, Kerstein MD. "Routine' radiologic evaluation of the thoracolumbar spine in blunt trauma patients: a reappraisal. J Trauma 1993;34:85–89
12. Terregino CA, Ross SE, Lipinski MF, Foreman J, Hughes R. Selective indications for thoracic and lumbar radiography in blunt trauma. Ann Emerg Med 1995;26:126–129
13. Berry GE, Adams S, Harris MB, et al. Are plain radiographs of the spine necessary during evaluation after blunt trauma? Accuracy of screening torso computed tomography in thoracic/lumbar spine fracture diagnosis. J Trauma 2005;59:1410–1413, discussion 1413
14. Brant-Zawadzki M, Miller EM, Federle MP. CT in the evaluation of spine trauma. AJR Am J Roentgenol 1981;136:369–375
15. McAfee PC, Yuan HA, Fredrickson BE, Lubicky JP. The value of computed tomography in thoracolumbar fractures: an analysis of one hundred consecutive cases and a new classification. J Bone Joint Surg Am 1983;65:461–473
16. Ballock RT, Mackersie R, Abitbol JJ, Cervilla V, Resnick D, Garfin SR. Can burst fractures be predicted from plain radiographs? J Bone Joint Surg Br 1992;74:147–150
17. Brown CVR, Antevil JL, Sise MJ, Sack DI. Spiral computed tomography for the diagnosis of cervical, thoracic, and lumbar spine fractures: its time has come. J Trauma 2005;58:890–895, discussion 895–896
18. Antevil JL, Sise MJ, Sack DI, Kidder B, Hopper A, Brown CVR. Spiral computed tomography for the initial evaluation of spine trauma: a new standard of care? J Trauma 2006;61:382–387
19. Rhee PM, Bridgeman A, Acosta JA, et al. Lumbar fractures in adult blunt trauma: axial and single-slice helical abdominal and pelvic computed tomographic scans versus portable plain films. J Trauma 2002;53:663–667, discussion 667
20. Calendine CL, Fajman WA, Hanna SL, Tigges S. Is there need for thoracic spine radiographs following a negative chest CT in trauma patients? Emerg Radiol 2002;9:254–256
21. Adams JM, Cockburn MI, Difazio LT, Garcia FA, Siegel BK, Bilaniuk JW. Spinal clearance in the difficult trauma patient: a role for screening MRI of the spine. Am Surg 2006;72:101–105
22. France JC, Bono CM, Vaccaro AR. Initial radiographic evaluation of the spine after trauma: when, what, where, and how to image the acutely traumatized spine. J Orthop Trauma 2005;19:640–649

23. Hauser CJ, Visvikis G, Hinrichs C, et al. Prospective validation of computed tomographic screening of the thoracolumbar spine in trauma. J Trauma 2003;55:228–234, discussion 234–235

24. Brandt M-M, Wahl WL, Yeom K, Kazerooni E, Wang SC. Computed tomographic scanning reduces cost and time of complete spine evaluation. J Trauma 2004;56:1022–1026, discussion 1026–1028

25. Sampson MA, Colquhoun KB, Hennessy NLM. Computed tomography whole body imaging in multi-trauma: 7 years experience. Clin Radiol 2006;61:365–369

26. Acosta JA, Yang JC, Winchell RJ, et al. Lethal injuries and time to death in a level I trauma center. J Am Coll Surg 1998;186:528–533

27. Ptak T, Rhea JT, Novelline RA. Experience with a continuous, single-pass whole-body multidetector CT protocol for trauma: the three-minute multiple trauma CT scan. Emerg Radiol 2001;8:250–256

28. Roos JE, Hilfiker P, Platz A, et al. MDCT in emergency radiology: is a standardized chest or abdominal protocol sufficient for evaluation of thoracic and lumbar spine trauma? AJR Am J Roentgenol 2004;183:959–968

29. Kalra MK, Maher MM, Rizzo S, Saini S. Radiation exposure and projected risks with multidetector-row computed tomography scanning: clinical strategies and technologic developments for dose reduction. J Comput Assist Tomogr 2004;28(Suppl 1):S46–S49

30. Vaccaro AR, Lehman RA Jr, Hurlbert RJ, et al. A new classification of thoracolumbar injuries: the importance of injury morphology, the integrity of the posterior ligamentous complex, and neurologic status. Spine 2005;30:2325–2333

31. Vaccaro AR, Zeiller SC, Hulbert RJ, et al. The thoracolumbar injury severity score: a proposed treatment algorithm. J Spinal Disord Tech 2005;18:209–215

32. Vaccaro AR, Lee JY, Schweitzer KM Jr, et al; Spine Trauma Study Group. Assessment of injury to the posterior ligamentous complex in thoracolumbar spine trauma. Spine J 2006;6:524–528

33. Lee JY, Vaccaro AR, Schweitzer KM Jr, et al. Assessment of injury to the thoracolumbar posterior ligamentous complex in the setting of normal-appearing plain radiography. Spine J 2007;7:422–427

34. Denis F. The three column spine and its significance in the classification of acute thoracolumbar spinal injuries. Spine 1983;8:817–831

35. Alanay A, Yazici M, Acaroglu E, Turhan E, Cila A, Surat A. Course of non-surgical management of burst fractures with intact posterior ligamentous complex: an MRI study. Spine 2004;29:2425–2431

36. Williams RL, Hardman JA, Lyons K. MR imaging of suspected acute spinal instability. Injury 1998;29:109–113

37. Regnicolo L, Messori A, Polonara G, Burroni E, Perugini S, Salvolini U. MRI assessment of post-traumatic spinal instability. Eur J Radiol 2002;42:154–159

38. Brightman RP, Miller CA, Rea GL, Chakeres DW, Hunt WE. Magnetic resonance imaging of trauma to the thoracic and lumbar spine: the importance of the posterior longitudinal ligament. Spine 1992;17:541–550

39. Petersilge CA, Pathria MN, Emery SE, Masaryk TJ. Thoracolumbar burst fractures: evaluation with MR imaging. Radiology 1995;194:49–54

40. Terk MR, Hume-Neal M, Fraipont M, Ahmadi J, Colletti PM. Injury of the posterior ligament complex in patients with acute spinal trauma: evaluation by MR imaging. AJR Am J Roentgenol 1997;168:1481–1486

41. Emery SE, Pathria MN, Wilber RG, Masaryk T, Bohlman HH. Magnetic resonance imaging of posttraumatic spinal ligament injury. J Spinal Disord 1989;2:229–233

42. Haba H, Taneichi H, Kotani Y, et al. Diagnostic accuracy of magnetic resonance imaging for detecting posterior ligamentous complex injury associated with thoracic and lumbar fractures. J Neurosurg 2003;99(1, Suppl):20–26

43. Lee HM, Kim HS, Kim DJ, Suk KS, Park JO, Kim NH. Reliability of magnetic resonance imaging in detecting posterior ligament complex injury in thoracolumbar spinal fractures. Spine 2000;25:2079–2084

44. Anderson RE, Drayer BP, Braffman B, et al. Spine trauma. American College of Radiology. ACR Appropriateness Criteria. Radiology 2000;215(Suppl):589–595

45. Brandser EA, el-Khoury GY. Thoracic and lumbar spine trauma. Radiol Clin North Am 1997;35:533–557

46. Sledge JB, Allred D, Hyman J. Use of magnetic resonance imaging in evaluating injuries to the pediatric thoracolumbar spine. J Pediatr Orthop 2001;21:288–293

47. Kulkarni MV, McArdle CB, Kopanicky D, et al. Acute spinal cord injury: MR imaging at 1.5 T. Radiology 1987;164:837–843

48. Ishida Y, Tominaga T. Predictors of neurologic recovery in acute central cervical cord injury with only upper extremity impairment. Spine 2002;27:1652–1658, discussion 1658

49. Grauer JN, Vaccaro AR, Beiner JM, et al. Similarities and differences in the treatment of spine trauma between surgical specialties and location of practice. Spine 2004;29:685–696

50. Mehta JS, Reed MR, McVie JL, Sanderson PL. Weight-bearing radiographs in thoracolumbar fractures: do they influence management? Spine 2004;29:564–567

51. Vaccaro AR, An HS, Lin S, Sun S, Balderston RA, Cotler JM. Noncontiguous injuries of the spine. J Spinal Disord 1992;5:320–329

52. Harris MB, Sethi RK. The initial assessment and management of the multiple-trauma patient with an associated spine injury. Spine 2006;31(11, Suppl):S9–S15, discussion S36

53. Daffner RH, Hackney DB. ACR Appropriateness Criteria on suspected spine trauma. J Am Coll Radiol 2007;4:762–775

54. Gestring ML, Gracias VH, Feliciano MA, et al. Evaluation of the lower spine after blunt trauma using abdominal computed tomographic scanning supplemented with lateral scanograms. J Trauma 2002;53:9–14

55. Sheridan R, Peralta R, Rhea J, Ptak T, Novelline R. Reformatted visceral protocol helical computed tomographic scanning allows conventional radiographs of the thoracic and lumbar spine to be eliminated in the evaluation of blunt trauma patients. J Trauma 2003;55:665–669

13

Clearing the Cervical Spine in the Trauma Patient: A Systematic Review

John C. France

Identifying the existence of or proving the lack of injury to the cervical spine is a high priority in the trauma patient because the potential for devastating spinal cord injury remains a concern until this task is accomplished. Even during the initial evaluation one must be mindful of the possibility of a cervical injury because manipulation of the neck for the purposes of securing an airway could lead to a spinal cord injury in the unstable neck. For some patients cervical clearance can be accomplished before they leave the emergency department; however, the process continues beyond the trauma bay in many patients and can involve a series of imaging and clinical exams. Debate still exists as to the most efficient and reliable means to accomplish the task of cervical clearance. There are essentially two subsets of patients that require different consideration: those patients that are alert and cooperative, and those that are unable to cooperate for a variety of reasons such as being obtunded from closed head injury. This chapter offers some evidence-based guidelines for the purpose of clearing both of these groups.

The following two questions are evaluated:

♦ What is the safest, most reliable, and valid way to clear the cervical spine in an alert cooperative trauma patient?
♦ What is the safest, most reliable, and valid way to clear the cervical spine in the obtunded or uncooperative trauma patient?

◆ Methods

A search of the literature published from 1980 to 2007 was performed using PubMed and EMBASE electronic database search engines. The search was performed using various keyword combinations, including; "cervical spine clearance," "cervical trauma radiographs," and "cervical trauma." The articles were then reviewed by title and abstract to select those pertinent to the questions to be answered. Only those articles published in English in international peer-reviewed journals and those that had abstracts available were considered. To be

selected the focus of the paper had to address the issue of early spine evaluation for the distinct purpose of clearing the cervical spine. Based on this preliminary evaluation the selected articles were obtained in full text form for more extensive and thorough evaluation. These articles were cross-referenced by hand to identify any pertinent articles undetected with the initial search. All articles fulfilling those criteria were reviewed, including case series and case reports so that the entire body of literature was available. The articles were evaluated and the body of literature assessed according to the guidelines outlined by the American Thoracic Society.[1] Using these criteria each study was graded as high quality (I), moderate quality (II), low quality (III), and very low quality (IV), then this grade with potential positive and negative impacts was used to come up with a recommendation for treatment that is simply a strong or weak recommendation. The level of evidence is graded as outlined by Fisher and Wood[2] for diagnostic testing. See **Table 13.1**.

◆ Results

Clearing the Cervical Spine in the Alert and Cooperative Patient

Within the group of patients that are alert and cooperative, there are two subgroups: (1) those that can be cleared without radiographic imaging, and (2) those that require imaging. The literature identified addressed either of these subgroups and will be reviewed separately.

Patients That Do Not Require Imaging

Sixteen studies were identified regarding clinical clearance (without the need for imaging). The most current studies assessed the reliability of either the National Emergency X-ray Utilization Study (NEXUS) criteria or the Canadian C-spine rules to determine which patients require imaging

Table 13.1 Clearing the Cervical Spine in the Alert and Obtunded Patient: An Evidence-Based Analysis

I. The Alert Patient

a. Clinical Exam Only for Clearance

Reference	Description	Level of Evidence	Topic and Conclusion
Stiell et al[4]	Prospective cohort observational	I	8924 blunt trauma patients present to ER, GCS 15. Record 20 clinical findings prior to radiography including three questions of Canadian C-spine rule (energy of trauma important). 100% sensitive for clinically significant injury, 58.2% rate of radiograph ordering.
Hoffman et al[3]	Prospective cohort observational	I	NEXUS multicenter study assess five criteria for clinical only clearance. 34,069 patients. Detect all but two significant injuries. 99.8% negative predictive value. Decrease necessary x-rays by 12.6%
Stiell et al[5]	Prospective cohort observational	I	Multicenter, compare Canadian rule and NEXUS clinical clearance criteria. 8283 patients. Canadian rule 99.4% sensitive versus NEXUS 90.7% ($p < 0.001$)
Kerr et al[12]	Prospective cohort observational, historical control	II	Study x-ray usage before and after implementation of Canadian c-spine rule, 25% relative decrease in imaging in 211 patients studied
Dickinson et al[11]	Prospective cohort observational	I	8924 patients in Canadian ERs as part of Canadian c-spine study, assess NEXUS criteria; only 92.7% sensitive, only 6.1% decrease in radiographs
Panacek et al[9]	Prospective cohort observational	III	Review of NEXUS data to determine if all five criteria necessary, look at 818 patients with injury, even leaving out one criterion can result in missed injury
Duane et al[13]	Prospective cohort observational	III	534 blunt trauma patients evaluated using EAST criteria and clinical exam, compare with CT rather than plain films, 76.9% sensitivity and 95.7% negative predictive value, clinical exam may be unreliable
Heffernan et al[7]	Prospective cohort observational	III	Single center, attempt to define distracting injury, 7/40 patients with fracture but nontender neck had upper torso injury, none with lower torso
Chang et al[8]	Prospective cohort observational	II	336 of 4698 patients had distracting injury as sole reason for x-rays. Eight patients with fracture. Any fracture should be considered distracting injury
Dearden and Hughes[43]	Prospective cohort observational	III	Pre- (252 patients) and post- (268 patients) implementation of NEXUS criteria, no difference in x-rays ordered or missed/identified injuries
Velmahos et al[10]	Prospective cohort observational	III	549 patients, alert, blunt trauma with negative clinical exam. No missed injuries. 2272 x-rays, 78 CT and MRIs. Cost $242,000.
Meldon et al[6]	Prospective cohort observational	III	Compare prehospital personnel to emergency physician's utilization of clinical clearance in 199 prospective cohort observational patients. EMT clear 21% but EP put 61% of these back into collar for radiographs (kappa 0.29), no missed injuries by EMT
Banit et al[44]	Retrospective review, historical control	II	Initiate clearance protocol, 3/2217 patients had missed injury prior and 0/2243 after, included energy of trauma early in decision tree
Barry and McNamara[45]	Case report	IV	Elderly patient, cleared by NEXUS but not by Canadian C-spine rules: odontoid fracture
Maxwell and Jardine[15]	Case report	IV	3-year-old collision, high speed, high energy. Clear by NEXUS, odontoid fracture

b. Plain Radiographs versus Helical CT Imaging

Reference	Description	Level of Evidence	Topic and Conclusion
Mathen et al[17]	Prospective cohort observational	II	667 patients CT and x-rays, 60 injuries, sensitivity CT 100% vs x-ray 45%
McCulloch et al[16]	Prospective cohort observational	I	407 blunt trauma patients had CT and plain films for clearance, films reviewed at later date blinded to each other, only 48% adequate plain films. Plain films 45% sensitve, CT 98% sensitive
Daffner et al[20]	Retrospective cohort review	II	2-year period, 245 patients with cervical fractures, only 44.1% detected by x-ray, 99.2% by CT. Two missed on CT both at C2; one due to dental artifact and other in axial plain

Table 13.1 Clearing the Cervical Spine in the Alert and Obtunded Patient: An Evidence-Based Analysis *(Continued)*

Reference	Description	Level of Evidence	Topic and Conclusion
Griffen et al[22]	Retrospective cohort review	II	All patients receive CT and plain films, 3018 patients, 116 patients with cervical injury, 41 (35.3%) missed on x-ray
Antevil et al[18]	Retrospective review, cohorts	III	Pre- and post- using spiral CT as primary cervical screening tool. Sensitivity improves from 70 to 100%, imaging time decreases 1.9 to 1.0 hours, slight increase in mean overall cost per patient $172 vs $164, increase radiation exposure for cervical but not thoracolumbar
Cohn et al[46]	Retrospective cohort review	III	Study initial lateral c-spine to assess early impact, 60 patients, seven with injury (two missed at C7); maintain collar through emergent imaging, intubation, operations without new deficit; lateral does not appear to alter urgent management but maintain precautions
Gale et al[21]	Retrospective cohort review	III	Review EAST guidelines for head CT to C2 then plain x-rays for remainder of C-spine and return to CT if necessary, plain x-rays inadequate 72.2% of time requiring return to CT, recommend complete cervical CT as initial evaluation
Adams et al[23]	Retrospective cohort review	III	MRI done early on 99 high-risk trauma patients, confirm high sensitivity but less specificity of CT scanning, MRI only necessary to confirm or define cervical trauma

c. The Role of Flexion-Extension Radiographs

Reference	Description	Level of Evidence	Topic and Conclusion
Mauldin et al[24]	Prospective cohort observational	III	159 patients with negative CT but neck persists after blunt trauma, active ROM compared with using a bolster, ROM better actively (51.4 vs 32.0 degrees), positive findings in 3.45 of patients
Wang et al[47]	Retrospective cohort review	III	290 flexion-extension x-rays, one unstable injury identified, 33.5% inadequate excursion
Lewis et al[48]	Retrospective cohort review	III	Four of 141 patients with normal neutral plain films demonstrate instability on flexion-extension, no neuron deficits (three require surgery)

II. The Obtunded Patient

a. MRI

Reference	Description	Level of Evidence	Topic and Conclusion
Diaz et al[42]	Prospective cohort observational	II	85 patients had MRI out of large series of trauma patients (1577 patients), 21 (25%) had ligamentous injury with 7/21 abnormal on helical CT (32% sensitive), only 3/21 abnormal on plain films (16% sensitive), four SCIWORA. MRI clearly more sensitive for ligamentous injury than CT
Stassen et al[35]	Retrospective cohort review	II	52 obtunded patients with x-ray, CT, and MRI. CT day 0.4 but MRI day 4. 44 negative CT of which 13 (30%) had positive MRI for ligamentous injury
Frank et al[36]	Retrospective cohort review	II	Pediatric patients, pre- and post-protocol to utilize MRI within 72 hours if not cleared. ICU stay and hospital stay decreased with savings $7700 per patient
Platzer et al[37]	Retrospective review of prospective database	III	Three (6%) ligamentous injuries missed despite complete x-ray series and CT, these can only be identified with MRI or dynamic imaging
Weinberg et al[38]	Case reports	IV	Two cases of high-energy trauma, obtunded patients with missed ligamentous injury on plain film and CT, later identified on MRI

b. Flexion-Extension

Reference	Description	Level of Evidence	Topic and Conclusion
Bolinger et al[27]	Retrospective cohort review	III	56 consecutive comatose patients, normal CT, flexion-extension at bedside, one occult instability, one missed C6–C7 instability, only 4% visualization of C7 on T1, recommend against its use
Anglen et al[26]	Retrospective radiographic report review	III	837 flexion-extension reports reviewed after normal plain films (mostly obtunded patients), one third of studies inadequate, four positives but not considered significant injury, flexion-extension determined not to be cost-effective and protocol dropped
Freedman et al[29]	Retrospective cohort review	III	123 patients with normal static plain films (initial CT not routine). two true positive and one false positive, four false-negatives (all identified later using CT), no neuron injury, passive flexion-extension inadequate sensitivity to recommend

13 Clearing the Cervical Spine in the Trauma Patient

(Continued on page 112)

Table 13.1 Clearing the Cervical Spine in the Alert and Obtunded Patient: An Evidence-Based Analysis *(Continued)*

Reference	Description	Level of Evidence	Topic and Conclusion
Harris et al[33]	Prospective cohort observational	III	153 patients undergoing anesthesia assessed for instability with initial traction film then flexion-extension, eight inadequate visualization, three positive findings
Brooks and Willett[49]	Prospective cohort observational	III	78 patients cleared using flexion-extension, five injuries identified (three apparent prior to dynamic study), one nondisplaced spinous process fracture would have been seen if CT done, one C1–C2 instability, no false-negative
Cox et al[28]	Prospective cohort observational	IV	110 patients normal plain films (not all had CT), three significant instabilities, no missed injuries identified, no info on % of adequate studies
c. CT scan only			
Sanchez et al[50]	Prospective cohort observational	III	Prospectively collect data based on clearance protocol, in comatose patients who moved all four extremities in the ER only a helical CT was used to clear if negative—no missed pure ligamentous injury and no new deficits (MRI used if not moving extremities)
Padayachee et al[30]	Retrospective review of prospective database	III	276 unconscious patients evaluated with helical CT with three-dimensional reconstructions then flexion-extension, no new injuries identified, only nine inadequate dynamic studies
Widder et al[41]	Prospective cohort observational	III	102 patients with plain films and CT, 100% sensitivity for CT, no late ligamentous injuries identified
Broh et al[40]	Prospective cohort observational	III	437 patients, 61 cervical injuries identified, no missed pure ligamentous injuries
Spiteri et al[31]	Retrospective cohort review	III	839 patients plain films, CT, dynamic imaging. 87 unstable injuries; 85 detected by CT, one required dynamic imaging and the other missed by dynamic imaging at the occipital cervical junction but retrospectively should have been identified on CT, dynamic safe but unnecessary

Abbreviations: CT, computed tomography; EAST, Eastern Association of the Surgery of Trauma; EMT, emergency medical technician; EP, emergency physician; ER, emergency room; GCS, Glasgow Coma Score; ICU, intensive care unit; NEXUS, National Emergency X-ray Utilization Study; ROM, range of motion.

and which can be cleared without further study. The NEXUS criteria include five rules:

1. Absence of midline tenderness
2. Normal level of alertness
3. No evidence of intoxication
4. No neurological findings
5. No painful distracting injuries

The Canadian C-spine rule places emphasis on the energy of the traumatic event and risk factors for a particular patient to have sustained a significant cervical injury given the traumatic event, as well as the ability to actively rotate the neck (**Fig. 13.1**). The initial studies for both of these criteria were multicenter and included a large number of patients and should be considered level I evidence.[3,4] The NEXUS study included 34,069 patients studied prospectively and detected all but two significant injuries for a 99.6% sensitivity, 99.8% negative predictive value, and decreased radiographs by 12.8%. The Canadian C-spine rule study included 8924 blunt trauma patients and had 100% sensitivity for detecting significant injury. A third level I study directly compared the Canadian C-spine rules and the NEXUS low-risk criteria[5] in 8283 patients in nine tertiary emergency rooms. Both criteria were excellent at ruling out injury, with the Canadian C-spine rule performing statistically better. The Canadian rules had a sensitivity of 99.4% and negative predictive value of 100%,

whereas the NEXUS rules had a sensitivity of 90.7% and negative predictive value of 99.4%. Dickinson et al analyzed the dataset from the original Canadian C-spine study looking at the NEXUS rules, which were collected prospectively, and observed a 92.7% sensitivity.[11] Specifically, 11 important cervical injuries were missed in 8924 patients evaluated, five of which required halo or surgical management.

Some studies looked at the details of implementation of clinical criteria. Meldon et al[6] compared the agreement between emergency room physicians and emergency medical technicians implementing clinical criteria for cervical clearance, and disagreement occurred in 23% of the 190 patients assessed. Five injuries were detected, and there was agreement on the need for radiographic imaging in all five, making the actual significance of the disagreement indeterminate. Some of the criteria lacked a specific definition such as a "distracting injury," and two studies were identified looking at what defines a distracting injury. Heffernan et al[7] found that seven of the 40 patients with fractures in their study had nontender, nonpainful necks but did have upper torso injuries as a distraction. There were no lower extremity fractures as a distractor. To the contrary, Chang et al[8] looked at 336 of 4698 patients that had distracting injury given as the sole reason for their radiographs. They identified eight cervical fractures and concluded that any extremity fracture should be considered a distraction and warrants cervical radiographs. The other rules from the NEXUS study were also

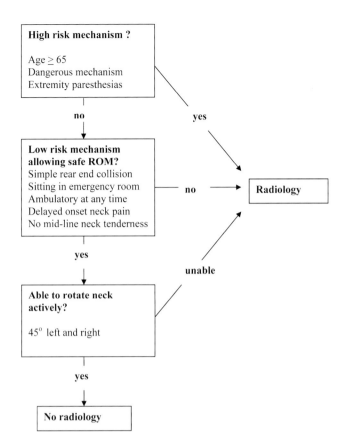

High risk mechanism ?

Age ≥ 65
Dangerous mechanism
Extremity paresthesias

no

Low risk mechanism
allowing safe ROM?
Simple rear end collision
Sitting in emergency room
Ambulatory at any time
Delayed onset neck pain
No mid-line neck tenderness

yes

Able to rotate neck
actively?

45° left and right

yes

No radiology

yes → Radiology

no → Radiology

unable → Radiology

Fig. 13.1 Canadian C-spine rule. To use this rule to determine the need for radiographic imaging the patients must be alert (Glasgow Coma Score 15) and stable. Dangerous mechanism includes fall ≥ 3 feet or five stairs, axial load (i.e., diving), high-speed motor vehicle crash (MVC) ≥ 60 mph or rollover or ejection, involves motorized recreational vehicle, bicycle collision. Simple rear-end collision excludes being pushed into oncoming traffic, being hit by large truck or bus, a rollover, and hit by a high-speed vehicle. (From Stiell IG et al. The Canadian C-spine rule versus the NEXUS low-risk criteria in patients with trauma. N Engl J Med 2003;349(26):2510-2518.)

evaluated individually as to their necessity. Panacek et al[9] found that eliminating any one of the five rules would markedly decrease the sensitivity of the instrument as a whole and make it unacceptable for use.

Prior to the specific guidelines proposed in the NEXUS and Canadian C-spine studies most physicians evaluating blunt trauma patients used their own clinical judgment[10] to determine the need for radiographs. Generally they used criteria similar to that more specifically defined in the referenced studies. Most studies that collected data on radiographic usage before and after implementation of specific rules for clinical clearance were able to show a decrease in the number of images ordered.[11,12] One study prospectively looked at the usage of radiographs 3 months before and after implementation of the NEXUS rules but failed to show a difference in the number of x-rays ordered.

Despite the evidence in support of using guidelines for clinical clearance there are some papers that raise concern, although at a lower level of evidence. One study[13] was done prospectively in which 24 patients with Glasgow Coma Score of 15 out of a total of 534 patients were identified with fractures of the cervical spine. Only 16 of the 24 were identified using the Eastern Association of the Surgery of Trauma (EAST) criteria, identical to the NEXUS rules, resulting in a

sensitivity of only 66.7%. Some case reports[14,15] demonstrate the weaknesses in the elderly and pediatric age groups. The former would only be a weakness using the NEXUS rules because age > 65 is considered high risk, warranting x-rays using the Canadian C-spine rules.

Overall, these studies represent a high level of evidence for using the postulated rules to clear the cervical spine prior to radiographs in a select group of patients and a strong recommendation can be given for using either the NEXUS or the Canadian C-spine rules to clear the cervical spine in blunt trauma patients prior to radiographic imaging.

Patients That Require Imaging

The patients that do not meet criteria for cervical clearance via clinical means alone require radiographic studies. This group generally includes all polytrauma patients because they are typically high-energy injuries with associated, potentially distracting injuries by definition. Traditionally, the radiographic screening in this group begins with plain radiographs; first a cross-table lateral in the trauma bay during the primary survey followed at least by anteroposterior (AP) and odontoid views. Other views such as trauma obliques or pillar views can be used for further evaluation, and CT scanning is done to analyze suspicious areas, define clear injuries, and get a better look at hard-to-visualize areas such as the occipitocervical or cervicothoracic junctions.

As the technology of computed tomographic (CT) scanning has improved there has been a trend toward eliminating plain radiographs and using the cervical CT as the sole means of screening the cervical spine for injury. Over the past several years there have been several studies looking at this issue in attempts to determine the sensitivity and feasibility of using the helical CT as the primary screening tool. Studies by McCulloch et al[16] and Mathen et al[17] show the sensitivity of CT scanning is clearly greater than plain radiographs. In the McCulloch study the sensitivity of plain radiographs overall was only 45%. If only "adequate" plain were considered the sensitivity improved slightly to 52%, whereas the sensitivity of CT was 98% (the only missed injury was definitely apparent on the study and was missed by reader error). Similarly, the Mathen study demonstrated a plain radiograph sensitivity of 45% and CT sensitivity of 100%. Other studies done retrospectively[18-21] also included large numbers of patients, and the sensitivity of plain radiographs ranged 31.6 to 70%, and the sensitivity of CT was 99.2% to 100%. Griffen et al[22] in their review of 3018 blunt trauma patients failed to identify any factors that could predict false-negative plain radiographs and concluded that there did not appear to be a reason to use plain radiographs in the initial screening process. The level of evidence in these studies is high and leaves little doubt that CT imaging is much more likely to detect an existing injury than plain radiographs.

Because the cost and radiographic exposure is greater with CT scanning there has been some hesitancy to adopt a policy that eliminates plain radiographs and uses only CT as the primary screening tool for the polytrauma patient. When the plain radiographs fail to visualize the entire spine due to the complexity of the occipitocervical junction or overlying shadows at the cervicothoracic junction, then a CT becomes necessary. Two studies[16,21] assessed the percentage of films that would be adequate to avoid secondary imaging with a CT scan and found that only 27.8% and 48% of the time were the plain films considered adequate. This means that the remainder of the patients would require a CT even after attempts at plain radiographs. In addition, any patient with neck pain or neurological symptoms would also require further imaging with a CT scan. This leaves a small percentage of patients that could be cleared after plain radiographs. Antevil et al[18] specifically studied the logistics, cost, and radiation exposure of using CT alone versus a protocol that uses plain radiographs supplemented by CT scanning as necessary. Using CT the mean time in the emergency room significantly decreased from 1.9 to 1.0 hours. The radiation exposure for cervical imaging was 26 mSv for CT compared with 4 mSv for plain radiographs, but if one takes into account the fact that ~70% of plain radiographic patients need a supplemental CT the amount of overall radiation between the two groups is more comparable. Although the cost of CT was significantly higher than plain radiographs when the need for CT in addition to plain radiographs is considered the mean costs are similar ($172 vs $164). A cost analysis was also done by McCulloch et al[16] taking the need for CT in those patients with inadequate plain films (the analysis did not take into account the need for even more CT scans in patients with neck pain) and cost was again comparable at $1151 for CT versus $870 for plain films.

One subgroup of alert patients remains and is those patients that after negative CT still complain of neck pain or have neurological complaints and could potentially suffer from a pure soft tissue injury such as a ligamentous disruption in perfect alignment on the CT imaging. The literature was more limited on this topic, with only one paper looking at MRI[23] in 78 patients in this category, and only one patient was identified with ligamentous edema that was treated with collar immobilization. Two studies[23–25] looked at flexion-extension films to finalize the cervical evaluation in these patients. The first study was part of the larger NEXUS study, which identified 818 patients with injuries. Of those 818 injuries, six were identified using flexion-extension films, but it is unclear from this study whether a CT was utilized as part of the initial screening radiographs. The available evidence would have to be considered moderate to low for evaluation of this subgroup.

Overall, the level of evidence is high to support CT as the sole means of screening the polytrauma patient for cervical injury. Given the low risk to the patient, minimal increase in cost, and improved efficiency of the process we can offer a strong recommendation in favor of CT as the primary means of clearance in the alert, cooperative trauma patient that requires imaging.

Clearing the Cervical Spine in the Obtunded Patient

All obtunded patients should have been evaluated with a helical CT based on our foregoing recommendation. The issue becomes the potential for a rare, pure ligamentous injury with possible instability or neurological injury existing in the face of a normal cervical CT. Because the patient is unable to cooperate or communicate the history and physical exam components of the evaluation are lost. The three ways to complete the cervical evaluation to detect or exclude clinically important injury would be (1) use the negative helical CT as the only means, (2) use passive flexion-extension lateral radiographs, or (3) use magnetic resonance imaging (MRI). Attempts to use CT only have been considered in recent years and will be discussed last.

Use of Passive Flexion-Extension Lateral Radiographs

Flexion-extension lateral radiographs are either done at the bedside with a portable fluoroscopy unit or the patient is transported to a fluoroscopy suite in radiology. No studies were identified that directly compared these two methods, no definitive benefit of one or the other could be ascertained, and the method used is institution dependent. The ability to adequately visualize the entire cervical spine is limited. Anglen et al[26] used the radiology suite for 837 patients, both obtunded and alert patients, and 236 (28%) of those inadequately visualized the cervicothoracic junction. Similarly, Bolinger et al[27] looked at 56 consecutive comatose patients with bedside fluoroscopy and were only able to visualize the cervicothoracic junction in 4% of those studied. Some studies[28,29] fail to make observations on the adequacy of the dynamic fluoroscopy to visualize the entire cervical spine, and others have reported 96 to 100% of adequate imaging using a highly sensitive fluoroscopy suite.[30,31] Based on this information it is apparent that the use of dynamic fluoroscopy is technically challenging and frequently fails to visualize the cervicothoracic junction, and additional imaging studies would be required in those patients. The logistical difficulty with transport is discussed by Anglen, but no patient morbidity was tied to the transport. The safety of performing a passive flexion-extension in the potentially unstable spine is an often expressed concern, but in the cumulative 2599 patients of the studies[26–32] reviewed there was only one reported neurological injury,[27] which was a temporary C7 radiculopathy. Harris et al[33] and Bednar et al[32] incorporated a traction test into their dynamic evaluation in an attempt to diminish safety concerns, and again there were no reported patient injuries so the use of dynamic fluoroscopy can be performed with reasonable safety. The remaining issue is the ability of dynamic imaging to detect clinically relevant instability that was not evident on the CT imaging.

Freedman et al[29] used the dynamic fluoroscopy prior to CT or MRI and identified two of 123 (1.6%) abnormal studies suspicious for pure ligamentous injury, but on further study no injury existed, thus they were false-positives. There were also four (3.2%) false-negatives identified at a later date after persistent pain, two of which required surgical intervention. Cox et al[28] also used a plain radiograph series as the initial means of evaluation and followed with dynamic imaging for obtunded patients with negative plain films. They found nine of 110 positive studies, but only three were clinically significant and there were no false-negatives. They failed to reveal any CT results on the three true positives, so it is unclear how many of these would have been detected by CT (as recommended earlier in this chapter), eliminating the need for the dynamic study. Bolinger et al[27] detected one instability due to a fracture in the horizontal plane on CT and missed one C6–C7 subluxation due to poor visualization of the lower cervical spine. Padayachee et al[30] and Spiteri et al[31] included CT in their initial screening protocols. In the latter of these studies 87 unstable cervical spines out of 837 ICU patients were reviewed. Only two were missed by the initial CT, but only one of the two was detected on the subsequent dynamic fluoroscopy, and the other was apparent on the CT in retrospect, so it was considered reader error rather than a failure of the imaging modality to detect the injury. In the former there were no injuries detected by dynamic imaging that were not visible on the CT, and there were six false-positives and one false-negative.

Use of Magnetic Resonance Imaging

The second common means of clearance in the obtunded patient is the MRI. The superior ability of MRI to visualize soft tissue is well established so its seems like the ideal imaging tool to identify pure ligamentous injury or an injury to the spinal cord without apparent structural vertebral injury such as the pediatric spinal cord injury without radiographic abnormality (SCIWORA), elderly central cord, or epidural hematoma. D'Alise et al[34] looked at MRI in 121 comatose patients who were initially evaluated with plain radiographs alone and identified 31 potentially unstable ligamentous injuries with eight requiring surgery, but it is not clear how many of those injuries would have been identified with a helical CT. Stassen et al[35] used helical CT as the initial means of clearance in 52 obtunded patients, followed by an MRI done postinjury day 4 on average. They identified 13 patients of the 44 negative (30%) CT scans who were found on MRI to have a ligamentous injury and who were all managed in a rigid collar for 6 weeks with no additional need for surgical intervention. The true clinical significance of these ligamentous injuries remains unclear. Frank et al[36] used MRI early in obtunded pediatric patients to clear the cervical spine and had clinically significant positive findings in seven of 50 patients. They did not specify how many of these injuries could be detected by CT, but the injuries did include a cord contusion without obvious instability, which is unique to this population. They concluded that an early MRI can improve the efficiency of collar removal. Platzer et al[37] found that plain film and CT failed to detect 6% (three patients) of clinically significant ligamentous injury, but they did not elaborate on the severity or need for treatment in those specific injuries. One case series[38] of two patients who suffered ligamentous injury missed on plain film and CT was identified. One of these patients required surgery, and the other was managed with a rigid collar. None of the foregoing studies reported any patients who had a missed injury with the combination of CT for bony injury and MRI for soft tissue injury.

Use of Computed Tomography Alone

Because the potential for a clinically significant pure ligamentous injury is extremely small and the technology of helical CT has improved substantially there is an increasing interest in using the CT alone to fully evaluate and clear the cervical spine. Schuster et al[39] and Brohi et al[40] both collected prospective data on 1462 and 437 unconscious blunt trauma patients, respectively. MRI was used sparingly in these studies. Neither study identified any unstable, purely ligamentous or disk injuries that were not apparent on the CT imaging and concluded that MRI did not add to the sensitivity of detecting injury beyond the helical CT. Interestingly, Schuster et al reported that there were 15 spinal cord injuries without radiographic abnormality in 15 of the alert patients that were also analyzed in their study. It seems likely that some of these injuries would also exist among the head-injured patients and would be, by definition, missed with CT alone. Similarly, Widder et al[41] prospectively looked at 102 obtunded trauma patients with the purpose of comparing plain radiographs and CT but reported that, with use of CT as the means of clearance, there

were undiagnosed or delayed diagnoses of cervical spine injuries.

To the contrary, Diaz et al[42] studied 1577 consecutive patients with plain films and CT using MRI in those patients that could not be cleared. Their patients had an average Glasgow Coma Score of 13.2, but they did not identify the exact number that would be considered comatose. Eighty-five patients without fracture underwent an MRI, and 21 of these patients were found to have a ligamentous injury. Only seven of the 21 had an injury detected on CT, leaving 14 undetected ligamentous injuries (only two obtunded patients had ligamentous injury, the remainder were alert patients, often with pain). None of the ligamentous injuries detected by MRI only (negative CT) was treated with anything more than a collar. In addition to the ligamentous injuries there were four SCIWORA injuries detected on MRI. Based on this review it is clear that ligamentous injury is more consistently identified with MRI, but it is not clear how clinically significant these injuries are and what the danger of undertreatment may be. Additionally, spinal cord injury without radiographic abnormality in the young or elderly can only be detected using MRI, but true SCIWORA injuries do not represent unstable patterns of injury and the importance of immobilization or early surgery is yet to be determined.

Overall, the level of evidence in support of MRI after CT as a means of detecting clinically important injury in the obtunded patient is moderate, and evidence for dynamic flexion-extension radiographs is weak. The evidence for using only the CT is moderate as well. Given the fact that the danger to the patient of an undetected injury is catastrophic and the rarity of this type of injury requires large numbers of patients to detect even a single significant injury, the recommendation for the use of MRI as an adjuvant to CT to clear the cervical spine in the obtunded patient is strong. As helical CT improves its ability to visualize soft tissue, this could change in favor of CT.

◆ Summary and Recommendations

The level of evidence, risk:benefit ratio, cost, and clinical judgment justify the following recommendations for clearing the cervical spine in the polytrauma patient:

- ◆ Strong in favor of using the NEXUS and/or Canadian C-spine rules to clinically clear a subgroup of patients without the need for radiographs.
- ◆ Strong in favor of using helical CT scanning as the means of initial evaluation in all polytrauma patients requiring imaging eliminating the need for screening plain radiographs. A lateral in the trauma bay should be left to the discretion of the trauma team and can be used in some circumstances. Plain radiographs will still play a role in treatment decisions and follow-up for injured patients but not in screening.
- ◆ Strong in favor of using MRI as an adjuvant to CT for those patients that remain obtunded and no clinical exam is available. A weak recommendation can be made against using dynamic flexion-extension radiographs as a means of detecting clinically important instability in this group of patients. Although if MRI is contraindicated due to metal in sensitive areas, a weak recommendation can be made for either dynamic fluoroscopy or CT alone.

References

1. Schünemann HJ, Jaeschke R, Cook DJ, et al; ATS Documents Development and Implementation Committee. An official ATS statement: grading the quality of evidence and strength of recommendations in ATS guidelines and recommendations. Am J Respir Crit Care Med 2006;174:605–614

2. Fisher CG, Wood KB. Introduction to and techniques of evidence-based medicine. Spine 2007;32(19, Suppl):S66–S72

3. Hoffman JR, Mower WR, Wolfson AB, Todd KH, Zucker MI; National Emergency X-Radiography Utilization Study Group. Validity of a set of clinical criteria to rule out injury to the cervical spine in patients with blunt trauma. N Engl J Med 2000;343:94–99

4. Stiell IG, Wells GA, Vandemheen KL, et al. The Canadian C-spine rule for radiography in alert and stable trauma patients. JAMA 2001;286:1841–1848

5. Stiell IG, Clement CM, McKnight RD, et al. The Canadian C-spine rule versus the NEXUS low-risk criteria in patients with trauma. N Engl J Med 2003;349:2510–2518

6. Meldon SW, Brant TA, Cydulka RK, Collins TE, Shade BR. Out-of-hospital cervical spine clearance: agreement between emergency medical technicians and emergency physicians. J Trauma 1998;45:1058–1061

7. Heffernan DS, Schermer CR, Lu SW. What defines a distracting injury in cervical spine assessment? J Trauma 2005;59:1396–1399

8. Chang CH, Holmes JF, Mower WR, Panacek EA. Distracting injuries in patients with vertebral injuries. J Emerg Med 2005;28:147–152

9. Panacek EA, Mower WR, Holmes JF, Hoffman JR; NEXUS Group. Test performance of the individual NEXUS low-risk clinical screening criteria for cervical spine injury. Ann Emerg Med 2001;38:22–25

10. Velmahos GC, Theodorou D, Tatevossian R, et al. Radiographic cervical spine evaluation in the alert asymptomatic blunt trauma victim: much ado about nothing. J Trauma 1996;40:768–774

11. Dickinson G, Stiell IG, Schull M, et al. Retrospective application of the NEXUS low-risk criteria for cervical spine radiography in Canadian emergency departments. Ann Emerg Med 2004;43:507–514

12. Kerr D, Bradshaw L, Kelly AM. Implementation of the Canadian C-spine rule reduces cervical spine x-ray rate for alert patients with potential neck injury. J Emerg Med 2005;28:127–131

13. Duane TM, Dechert T, Wolfe LG, Aboutanos MB, Malhotra AK, Ivatury RR. Clinical examination and its reliability in identifying cervical spine fractures. J Trauma 2007;62:1405–1408, discussion 1408–1410

14. Hoffman JR, Mower WR. Re: clinical decision rules and cervical spine injury. J Emerg Med 2008;34:99–100, author reply 99–100

15. Maxwell MJ, Jardine AD. Paediatric cervical injury but NEXUS negative. Emerg Med J 2007;24:676

16. McCulloch PT, France J, Jones DL, et al. Helical computed tomography alone compared with plain radiographs with adjunct computed tomography to evaluate the cervical spine after high-energy trauma. J Bone Joint Surg Am 2005;87:2388–2394

17. Mathen R, Inaba K, Munera F, et al. Prospective evaluation of multislice computed tomography versus plain radiographic cervical spine clearance in trauma patients. J Trauma 2007;62:1427–1431

18. Antevil JL, Sise MJ, Sack DI, Kidder B, Hopper A, Brown CV. Spiral computed tomography for the initial evaluation of spine trauma: a new standard of care? J Trauma 2006;61:382–387

19. Barba CA, Taggert J, Morgan AS, et al. A new cervical spine clearance protocol using computed tomography. J Trauma 2001;51:652–656, discussion 656–657

20. Daffner RH, Sciulli RL, Rodriguez A, Protetch J. Imaging for evaluation of suspected cervical spine trauma: a 2-year analysis. Injury 2006;37:652–658

21. Gale SC, Gracias VH, Reilly PM, Schwab CW. The inefficiency of plain radiography to evaluate the cervical spine after blunt trauma. J Trauma 2005;59:1121–1125

22. Griffen MM, Frykberg ER, Kerwin AJ, et al. Radiographic clearance of blunt cervical spine injury: plain radiograph or computed tomography scan? J Trauma 2003;55:222–226, discussion 226–227

23. Adams JM, Cockburn MI, Difazio LT, Garcia FA, Siegel BK, Bilaniuk JW. Spinal clearance in the difficult trauma patient: a role for screening MRI of the spine. Am Surg 2006;72:101–105

24. Mauldin JM, Maxwell RA, King SM, et al. Prospective evaluation of a critical care pathway for clearance of the cervical spine using the bolster and active range-of-motion flexion/extension techniques. J Trauma 2006;61:679–685

25. Pollack CV Jr, Hendey GW, Martin DR, Hoffman JR, Mower WR; NEXUS Group. Use of flexion-extension radiographs of the cervical spine in blunt trauma. Ann Emerg Med 2001;38:8–11

26. Anglen J, Metzler M, Bunn P, Griffiths H. Flexion and extension views are not cost-effective in a cervical spine clearance protocol for obtunded trauma patients. J Trauma 2002;52:54–59

27. Bolinger B, Shartz M, Marion D. Bedside fluoroscopic flexion and extension cervical spine radiographs for clearance of the cervical spine in comatose trauma patients. J Trauma 2004;56:132–136

28. Cox MW, McCarthy M, Lemmon G, Wenker J. Cervical spine instability: clearance using dynamic fluoroscopy. Curr Surg 2001;58:96–100

29. Freedman I, van Gelderen D, Cooper DJ, et al. Cervical spine assessment in the unconscious trauma patient: a major trauma service's experience with passive flexion-extension radiography. J Trauma 2005;58:1183–1188

30. Padayachee L, Cooper DJ, Irons S, et al. Cervical spine clearance in unconscious traumatic brain injury patients: dynamic flexion-extension fluoroscopy versus computed tomography with three-dimensional reconstruction. J Trauma 2006;60:341–345

31. Spiteri V, Kotnis R, Singh P, et al. Cervical dynamic screening in spinal clearance: now redundant. J Trauma 2006;61:1171–1177, discussion 1177

32. Bednar DA, Toorani B, Denkers M, Abdelbary H. Assessment of stability of the cervical spine in blunt trauma patients: review of the literature, with presentation and preliminary results of a modified traction test protocol. Can J Surg 2004;47:338–342

33. Harris MB, Kronlage SC, Carboni PA, et al. Evaluation of the cervical spine in the polytrauma patient. Spine 2000;25:2884–2891, discussion 2892

34. D'Alise MD, Benzel EC, Hart BL. Magnetic resonance imaging evaluation of the cervical spine in the comatose or obtunded trauma patient. J Neurosurg 1999;91(1, Suppl):54–59

35. Stassen NA, Williams VA, Gestring ML, Cheng JD, Bankey PE. Magnetic resonance imaging in combination with helical computed tomography provides a safe and efficient method of cervical spine clearance in the obtunded trauma patient. J Trauma 2006;60:171–177

36. Frank JB, Lim CK, Flynn JM, Dormans JP. The efficacy of magnetic resonance imaging in pediatric cervical spine clearance. Spine 2002;27:1176–1179

37. Platzer P, Jaindl M, Thalhammer G, et al. Clearing the cervical spine in critically injured patients: a comprehensive C-spine protocol to avoid unnecessary delays in diagnosis. Eur Spine J 2006;15:1801–1810

38. Weinberg L, Hiew CY, Brown DJ, Lim EJ, Hart GK. Isolated ligamentous cervical spinal injury in the polytrauma patient with a head injury. Anaesth Intensive Care 2007;35:99–104

39. Schuster R, Waxman K, Sanchez B, et al. Magnetic resonance imaging is not needed to clear cervical spines in blunt trauma patients with normal computed tomographic results and no motor deficits. Arch Surg 2005;140:762–766

40. Brohi K, Healy M, Fotheringham T, et al. Helical computed tomographic scanning for the evaluation of the cervical spine in the unconscious, intubated trauma patient. J Trauma 2005;58:897–901

41. Widder S, Doig C, Burrowes P, Larsen G, Hurlbert RJ, Kortbeek JB. Prospective evaluation of computed tomographic scanning for the spinal clearance of obtunded trauma patients: preliminary results. J Trauma 2004;56:1179–1184

42. Diaz JJ Jr, Aulino JM, Collier B, et al. The early work-up for isolated ligamentous injury of the cervical spine: does computed tomography scan have a role? J Trauma 2005;59:897–903, discussion 903–904

43. Dearden C, Hughes D. Does the National Emergency X-ray Utilization Study make a difference? Eur J Emerg Med 2005;12:278–281

44. Banit DM, Grau G, Fisher JR. Evaluation of the acute cervical spine: a management algorithm. J Trauma 2000;49:450–456

45. Barry T, McNamara R. 2007. Clinical decision rules and cervical spine injury. J Emerg Med 2005;29(4):433–436

46. Cohn SM, Lyle WG, Linden CH, Lancey RA. Exclusion of cervical spine injury: a prospective study. J Trauma 1991;31:570–574

47. Wang JC, Hatch JD, Sandhu HS, Delamarter RB. Cervical flexion and extension radiographs in acutely injured patients. Clin Orthop Relat Res 1999;(365):111–116

48. Lewis LM, Docherty M, Ruoff BE, Fortney JP, Keltner RA Jr, Britton P. Flexion-extension views in the evaluation of cervical-spine injuries. Ann Emerg Med 1991;20:117–121

49. Brooks RA, Willett KM. Evaluation of the Oxford protocol for total spinal clearance in the unconscious trauma patient. J Trauma 2001;50:862–867

50. Sanchez B, Waxman K, Jones T, Conner S, Chung R, Becerra S. Cervical spine clearance in blunt trauma: evaluation of a computed tomography-based protocol. J Trauma 2005;59:179–183

14

Spinal Nomenclature and Image Measurement Techniques for Cervical, Thoracic, Lumbar, and Sacral Injuries

Jared A. Toman and Christopher M. Bono

During the past 3 decades, there have been multiple attempts to formulate a cogent and usable system by which to describe traumatic injuries of the spine. Most simply can be divided into two categories: nomenclature (i.e., the moniker ascribed to a particular injury type) and measurement techniques (i.e., the manner in which various injury characteristics are quantified). Unfortunately, one system has not been adopted by the spine surgical community at large. This has apparently resulted in both a lack of clarity and inconsistency of injury description in the literature. Because treatment decision making and prognosis are influenced by injury type and characteristics, it is important to gain a better understanding of the current literature. To the authors' knowledge, a large-scale systematic review of the literature concerning cervical, thoracolumbar, and sacral spine trauma has not been previously reported.

This chapter presents the results of a systematic review of the literature concerning nomenclature (i.e., descriptions of injury types) and measurement methods for spinal injuries. In addition, it highlights the wide variability with which spinal injuries have been described and measured in peer-reviewed literature.

◆ Methods

Two questions were formulated to perform the systematic review.

- Are there standardized and/or peer-reviewed methods of describing spinal injuries in the cervical, thoracolumbar, and sacral spine?
- Are there standardized and/or peer-reviewed methods of measuring injury characteristics after cervical, thoracolumbar, and sacral spine fractures, and dislocations?

Based on these questions, multiple searches were performed using the following keywords: "cervical," "cervical spine," "trauma," "nomenclature," "injury description,"

"measurement," "measurement technique," "thoracic," "thoracic spine," "lumbar," "lumbar spine," "thoracolumbar spine," "thoracolumbar," "sacrum," "sacral spine." Literature searches were performed using PubMed. The abstracts of all hits were reviewed for eligibility. Full articles were reviewed if they included a system by which to describe traumatic spine injury types or a method of measuring an injury characteristic. Ultimately, articles were included in the evidentiary table (**Table 14.1**) if they detailed a standardized and/or peer-reviewed method of describing injuries or measuring injury characteristics to answer the two systematic review questions. Articles were graded for their levels of evidence as diagnostic studies.

◆ Results

- *Are there standardized and/or peer-reviewed methods of describing spinal injuries in the cervical, thoracolumbar, and sacral spine?* The results of multiple searches were reviewed in detail. Many of the abstracts reviewed included proposals for injury classification, which lies outside the boundaries of the current review. Using the search terms "spine, fracture, nomenclature" or "spine, dislocation, nomenclature," there were no eligible articles for full review. A search with the terms "spine, dislocation, injury description" resulted in one hit.[1]

Using the search terms "spine, fracture, injury description," five abstracts were found eligible for full review. One of the articles[2] was reviewed but subsequently rejected because it was a study of the reproducibility of osteoporotic thoracolumbar fracture detection. The other articles included those by Bono et al,[3,4] Keynan et al,[5] and Kuklo et al,[6] which will be reviewed in detail later in the chapter because they dealt primarily with measurement techniques. There was no article offering a standardized or uniform method of injury description for any

Table 14.1 Evidentiary Table

Reference	Description	Level of Evidence of Primary Question	Topic and Conclusion
Harris et al[7]	Retrospective cohort study	III-diagnostic	The authors tested the accuracy of a new measurement method. They made their newly described measurements on the plain lateral radiographs of 400 normal adults. In 98% and 95% of those cases, respectively, the BAI and BDI were not more than 12 mm.
			In critique of this study, only normal studies were included. Thus conclusions about its utility for traumatic conditions may be limited.
Harris et al[8]	Retrospective cohort study	II-diagnostic	In this retrospective study, the authors compared the BAI and BDI to the Power ratio and the X-line method, which at the time of publication could be considered so-called gold standard measurements. They found that the BAI and BDI method correctly identified the presence and type of occipitocervical dissociation in all cases, whereas the Power ratio and the X-line method could not be even performed in 46% of cases. The authors concluded that the BAI/BDI method was superior.
			In critique of this study, there was no assessment of interobserver or intraobserver variability. Furthermore, these measurements may be limited by relatively common anatomical deficiencies of the posterior arch of C1 and optimal visualization of the required structures on plain radiographs.
Rojas et al[9]	Retrospective case series	III–diagnostic	The paper reports the findings of a study using sagittal CT images to measure the craniocervical relationship as opposed to standard plain films. They found that 95% of normal patients had a BDI less than 8.5 mm on CT but less than 12 mm on plain radiographs.
			In critiquing this study, it is unclear if this was a consecutive series of patients. Moreover, it did not examine the ability of CT to detect an injury as compared with plain radiographs. It did, however, compare a gold standard with a revised measurement protocol. Of note, BAI was poorly reproduced on CT and could not be assessed.
Ahuja et al[10]	Case series	IV–diagnostic	This study reported results of a small case series of survivors following atlanto-occipital dislocation, assessed with plain films and CT. The authors showed that the Power ratio was abnormal in five of six survivors and decreased with operative intervention.
			In critique of this study, there were low patient numbers. In addition, other alternative or complementary measurement strategies were not assessed.
Heller et al[11]	Case series retrospective	IV–diagnostic	Thirty-five consecutive odontoid-view radiographs were analyzed with respect to three radiologists' measurement of C1 on C2 overhand in the setting of Jefferson fractures. A radiographic marker of known length was used as an internal control of true sizing. The authors reported that an average AP magnification of 18% was observed. Therefore, they suggested that to take into account this magnification, contemporary criteria proposed by Spence of 6.9 mm total overhang of C1 on C2 be revised to 8.1 mm as the threshold transverse ligament disruption.
			In critique of this study, the authors made no recommendations based on their findings. Moreover, given the measurements that include fractions of a millimeter, there is no discussion of range of magnification or standard of error.
Westaway et al[13]	Retrospective case series	IV–evaluation of diagnostic evidence	The authors reported results of a retrospective series of patients with suspected craniocervical instability as assessed with the anterior atlantodens interval. Interobserver reliability and measurement error are reported. However, the authors also concluded that the reproducibility of the measure is contingent on head position.
			A critique of the article is that no normal values are presented for comparison, and the clinical application of their finding is unclear, given that both trauma and congenital patients are included.
Bono et al[4]	Literature review	V–expert opinion	This paper presents the results of a literature and expert panel (Spine Trauma Study Group) review of measurement techniques for assessing the radiographic features of the upper cervical spine (C0–C2). The results of previous studies of examining the efficacy of these techniques are reported, pointing out that very few have been objectively evaluated, but no new experimental analysis of reported measurement strategies was undertaken.

Table 14.1 Evidentiary Table *(Continued)*

Reference	Description	Level of Evidence of Primary Question	Topic and Conclusion
			The authors suggested a set of measurement techniques and describe their standardized execution. The study is listed as level V evidence because, although the results of prior studies are referenced, the methods by which those results are derived are not analyzed.
Bono et al[3]	Literature review	V–expert opinion	This paper presents the results of a literature and expert panel (Spine Trauma Study Group) review of measurement techniques for assessing the radiographic features of the subaxial cervical spine (C3–C7). The results of previous studies of examining the efficacy of these techniques are reported, pointing out that very few have been objectively evaluated, but no new evaluation of the reported measurement strategies was undertaken.
			The authors suggested a set of measurement techniques and describe their standardized execution. The study is listed as level V evidence because, although the results of prior studies are referenced, the methods by which those results are derived are sparingly analyzed.
Spector et al[17]	Retrospective consecutive cohort study	III–diagnostic	This retrospective study attempted to define the radiographic features of isolated unilateral facet fractures that would lead to failure of nonoperative management. CT scans of 24 patients with unilateral facet fractures were analyzed, five of which required delayed surgery. The authors identified the percent of the lateral mass involved with the fracture as significantly differing between the two groups. Thus they proposed that facet fractures involving > 40% of the intact lateral mass height or > 1 cm absolute height may benefit from close observation if nonoperative management is pursued.
			The article focused only mechanical (bony) features of injury, and neurological injury was not considered. Moreover, the criteria for a failure of nonop management were not clearly defined in the small patient population. Lastly, although a Power analysis was not performed, the failure group was acknowledged to be very small.
Fehlings et al[18]	Retrospective, comparative cohort study Nonconsecutive	II–diagnostic	This paper reports the results of a multicenter retrospective study using CT and MRI to formulate quantitative radiographic assessment parameters for subaxial cord compression and canal compromise. Seventy-one patients were selected on the basis of completeness of record. The authors found T2-MRI to be the most reliable study for cord compression, and magnitude of compression correlated with recorded degree of neurological deficit at the level of injury. Greater than 25% osseous canal compromise on CT also correlated strongly with cord impingement. However, their results showed that CT alone was not sensitive enough (72%) to quantify cord compression.
			Although, intra- and interobserver values were obtained and used in validating the measurements, the retrospective nature of the study over 16 years, as well as suboptimal precision in correlating the planes of imaging between CT and MRI reconstructions, are potential limitations of the study.
Rao and Fehlings[20]	Literature review	III–systematic review of level II–IV studies	First part of a two-part study surveying the literature for evidence-based analysis of radiographic criteria for evaluating spinal canal compromise. Thirty-seven studies were included. The authors concluded that existing measurement strategies were insufficient to provide the necessary information about the traumatized spinal canal. They found some evidence that AP spinal canal diameter may predispose to cord injury following trauma, but these studies were inconclusive. The authors thus suggested the need for mandatory standards of measurement.
			A potential critique is that the authors included assessment techniques that have been applied to traumatic as well as degenerative canal stenosis. Also, of the considered studies, only 19% and 32% included validity and sensitivity parameters, respectively.
Furlan et al[19]	Observational, blinded survey of experts	III–diagnostic	The authors devised a study to determine if a previously developed measurement technique to assess traumatic spinal cord compromise would prove more accurate and reproducible if digital magnification of the images was used in place of printed films and manual measurement. Five representative images were measured by 13 experienced spine surgeons on 10 occasions.

14 Spinal Nomenclature and Image Measurement Techniques

(Continued on page 120)

Table 14.1 Evidentiary Table *(Continued)*

Reference	Description	Level of Evidence of Primary Question	Topic and Conclusion
			Although the authors showed higher interobserver reliabilities with the digital magnification than did previous studies using the same measurement technique, the results were still well below intrarater scores. Moreover, the same five images were used on all 10 occasions; this may have potentiated results despite ostensibly blinding participants to the clinical findings of the represented patient.
Fehlings et al[21]	Prospective, blinded survey of experts	Level II–diagnostic	Article details a prospective, blinded validation study of a strategy for measuring osseous spinal canal compromise as it relates to cord compression. The method involves expression of sagittal stenosis as a percent of preinjury baseline for both the canal and the cord diameters. Midsagittal MRI and CT cuts were shown to 28 spine surgeons, who were asked to assess the images on two separate occasions. Excellent intraobserver reliability was demonstrated, with canal stenosis proving more accurate in cases of minimal cord compression; measurement of the cord itself via MRI proved more accurate in cases of severe compression.
			A critique of this article is that the interobserver reliability rate was low (below 0.75), which the authors attribute to manual measurement error of the images. However, it may still inhibit the reproducibility of the suggested measurement.
Keynan et al[5]	Literature review	V–expert opinion	The authors surveyed the available literature for studies defining techniques to measure the radiographic features of injury to the thoracolumbar spine. Although a certain methodological quality was sought in the reviewed articles, no new independent analysis of the reported techniques was undertaken. Their conclusions are based on consideration of 18 articles, which themselves vary from level II to V. However, a collection of techniques is recommended, and the authors do critique the practicality and derivation of several reported measurement strategies, albeit not in a systematic fashion.
Kuklo et al[26]	Case series expert survey	Level IV–diagnostic	Five different methods of measuring posttraumatic kyphosis were assessed by way of three experts reviewing films of 50 different fractures. Intra- and interobserver agreement was assessed. The authors concluded that the Cobb angle provided the greatest reliability of measure. However, due to lack of antecedent in the literature, a reference measurement was not employed, and the prognostic importance of these measurements, as well as the comparability of values derived by these measures, has yet to be defined.
Ruan et al[28]	Retrospective consecutive cohort	Level IV–diagnostic	The authors report the use of a measure for assessing thoracolumbar translation in the context of evaluating instrumentation. Ninety-six consecutive thoracolumbar burst fracture patients were treated with Shen instrumentation. The method is detailed as the perpendicular distance between the posterior cortecies of the involved motion segment.
			Although not surprising given the objectives of the articles, there is no discussion of traumatized osseous landmarks or observer reliability analysis; however, there also seems to be no referenced precedent for this measure. Thus practical, prognostic utility of this diagnostic measuring tool is limited at this point.
Vaccaro et al[33]	Prospective, comparative Consecutive	Level II–diagnostic	The paper describes the findings of a prospective observational study of consecutive patients sustaining thoracolumbar burst fracture. Forty-three patients met criteria and were imaged with CT and plain film; postinjury canal dimensions were compared against neurological injury. Their data suggest that a lower AP to transverse diameter ratio correlates with neurological injury. Larger canals were not protective, nor did preinjury geometry impact the potential for neurological injury.
			Measurement acquisition was assessed with interobserver reliability, and results correlate with previous reports in the literature. Although all patients considered were postinjury, neuro-injured were compared against neuro-intact, serving as a loose control.
Hashimoto et al[35]	Consecutive, comparative case series	Level IV–diagnostic	This paper reports the results of digital imaging measurement of 112 consecutive thoracolumbar burst fractures, and percentage canal compromise.
			Posterior element disruption was predictive of neuron deficit, and critical values for imputed stenosis were reported, with the canal being

Table 14.1 Evidentiary Table *(Continued)*

Reference	Description	Level of Evidence of Primary Question	Topic and Conclusion
			increasingly tolerant of encroachment the more distal the injury (ranging from 35 to 55% critical percent stenosis).
			In a critique of the paper, whether the evaluation is prospective or retrospective is not made clear, although they state that conclusions are retrospective. Moreover, although their results are in agreement with other reports in the literature, the clinical application of these findings is not yet clear. A discussion of measurement error is also absent, as is a clearly applied control.
Rasmussen et al[34]	Retrospective case control	Level III–diagnostic	The paper presents the results of a study to determine the efficacy of different measurement strategies for assessing lumbar canal compromise following trauma. Using digital, as compared against manual (control), measurement and area calculations, the authors conclude that transverse area is the more reliable measure. They further report that transverse canal area at L1 has a critical value below which neurological injury was certain; however, no other such conclusions could be reached for other lumbar levels. Lastly, although analysis is limited, they report good agreement between canal area measurements made with computer-aided versus manually calculated means.
Kuklo et al[6]	Literature review	V–expert opinion	Paper presents the results of a literature review of measurement techniques for assessing the radiographic features of the sacral spine fractures. Previously described classification systems and measurement techniques are reported.
			The author suggests a canon of measurement techniques and a standardized methodology for their application. The focus is on diagnosis and defining injury; there is no reference of literature assessing the efficacy of one technique over others, and no attempt is made in the paper to perform such analysis.

Abbreviations: AP, anteroposterior; BAI, basion–posterior axial line interval; BDI, basion–dens interval; CT, computed tomography; MRI, magnetic resonance imaging.

part of the spine. Furthermore, there were no studies that adequately evaluated the reproducibility or reliability of any type of injury description or nomenclature system.

♦ *Are there standardized and/or peer-reviewed methods of measuring injury characteristics after cervical, thoracolumbar, and sacral spine fractures, and dislocations?* Search strings resulted in a substantially greater number of articles for this question. This was likely a result of the search strategy, which targeted any article that proposed a measurement method of any type of spinal injury. The results of this portion of the systematic review will be organized according to injury type. This, of course, has inherent limitations. Based on the paucity of results from the systematic review for Question 1, the injury types included do not have a uniform description between studies. Thus the results presume that injuries with the same moniker (e.g., burst fracture) are truly describing measurement methods for the same type of injury. As an additional disclaimer, the injury list attempts to be comprehensive but could likely exclude some less common injury types.

Upper Cervical Spine

Occipitocervical Dislocation/Dissociation

Harris et al[7,8] described the relationship between the cranium (basion) and C2 as a finite linear measurement to judge the likelihood of an occipitocervical dissociation or dislocation following trauma. It involves two measurements. The first is the basion–dens interval (BDI), which denotes the distance between the tip of the dens (or odontoid process) and the tip of the basion, the most anterior portion of the foramen magnum. The second measurement is the basion–posterior axial line interval (BAI), which denotes the distance from a tangent line drawn along the posterior C2 vertebral body and the basion (**Fig. 14.1**).

Harris et al[7] also tested the accuracy of the measurement method. In one study, they made the measurement on the plain lateral radiographs of 400 normal adults. In 98% and 95% of those cases, respectively, the BAI and BDI were not more than 12 mm. In a second study, the authors compared the BAI and BDI to the Power ratio and the X-line method.[8] They found that the BDI and BAI method correctly identified the presence and type of occipitocervical dissociation in all cases, whereas the Power ratio and the X-line method could not be performed in 46% of cases. The authors concluded that the BAI/BDI method was superior; however, there was no assessment of interobserver or intraobserver variability. Furthermore, these measurements may be limited by relatively common anatomical deficiencies of the posterior arch of C1 and optimal visualization of the required structures on plain radiographs.

The utility of these measurements has recently been performed using computed tomographic (CT) images. Rojas et al[9] studied reconstructed CT images of 200 normal spines. They found that 95% had a BDI less than 8.5 mm on CT but less than 12 mm on plain radiographs, whereas the BAI was reportedly difficult to reproduce on CT and could not be

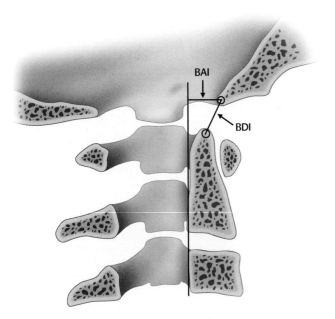

Fig. 14.1 Basion–posterior axial line interval and basion–dens interval according the method of Harris et al.

C1 Bursting (Jefferson) Fractures

A common measurement prescribed to assess a C1 bursting fracture is the degree of lateral displacement of the C1 lateral masses on the C2 lateral masses. Multiple searches using the search terms "Jefferson fracture, C1 bursting fracture, C1 fracture, distance, measurement, displacement" revealed few studies. The only eligible articles were those of Bono et al, Spence et al, and Heller et al.[4,11,12] The original work by Spence et al[12] stated that 6.9 mm of total overhang was suggestive of transverse atlantal ligament (TAL) rupture. However, this was primarily a cadaveric study. Heller et al[11] argued that this number was based on direct measurement and did not take into account radiographic magnification. They found an 18% magnification error and thus concluded that the criterion threshold for lateral displacement should be less than 8.1 mm. Regardless, neither study evaluated the inter- or intraobserver error of these measurements, though both used the same method of measurement, detailed in **Fig. 14.2**. In this systematic review, there were no other studies found regarding the ideal method by which to make these measurements. Therefore, these data offer level IV evidence that the prescribed method of measurement can be considered the standardized mode by which to measure lateral displacement of the C1 and C2 lateral masses after a Jefferson fracture.

Atlantoaxial Instability

A search using the terms "atlantoaxial instability" and "measurement" yielded few abstract hits. In a study of normal volunteers, Westaway et al[13] found extremely high reliability of measurements of the anterior atlantodens interval using plain radiographs. The method by which they made the measurements was identical to that detailed by Bono et al.[4] The review yielded no other articles that denoted a standardized measurement method for the atlantodens interval. These data offer, at best, level IV diagnostic evidence of the manner in which the ADI should be measured.

assessed. In critique of this study, it is unclear if this was a consecutive series of patients. In addition, it did not assess the ability to detect an injury because it was limited to defining the limits of the normal population. It did, however, compare a gold standard (plain radiograph measurement) with a new one (CT measurement). Based on these attributes, the study offers level III evidence that plain radiographs may be more appropriate than CT when making BAI and BDI measurements.

Bono et al[4] performed a systematic review of the literature concerning upper cervical injury measurements. Although not detailed in the published article, a multitude of search strings were employed in an exhaustive attempt to detect eligible articles. In this work, the authors (and members of the Spine Trauma Study Group) felt that the BAI and BDI were the most utilitarian method of occipitocervical dislocation measurement.

The Power ratio has also been advocated. The measurement was assessed by Ahuja et al[10] in six patients. In five of the surviving patients, they found a lower ratio than the one patient who died after an occipitocervical dislocation. Because this was a case series, this study constitutes, at best level IV evidence, that the Power ratio is a useful method to measure an occipitocervical dissociation.

Occipital Condyle Fractures

A search of the terms "occipital condyle, fracture, measurement" yielded only two abstract hits. The only relevant article was that by Bono et al.[4] Though not substantiated by any clinical evidence, the authors introduced a measurement of the size and displacement of the occipital condyle fragment using coronal and sagittal CT images. While potentially useful, these data constitute level V evidence that these measurements are of clinical utility. Notwithstanding articles describing the classification of these injuries, there were no other works found regarding the measurement of occipital condyle fractures.

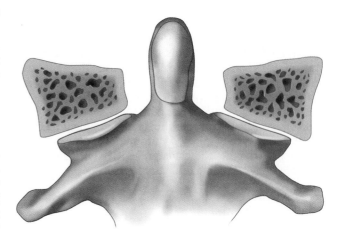

Fig. 14.2 The method of Spence for measuring aggregate overhang of C1 on C2 for transverse atlantal ligament (TAL) disruption. Vertical lines are drawn along the lateral aspect of the bone of the C1 and C2 articular processes. The transverse distance between them is then measured in millimeters on each side and totaled.

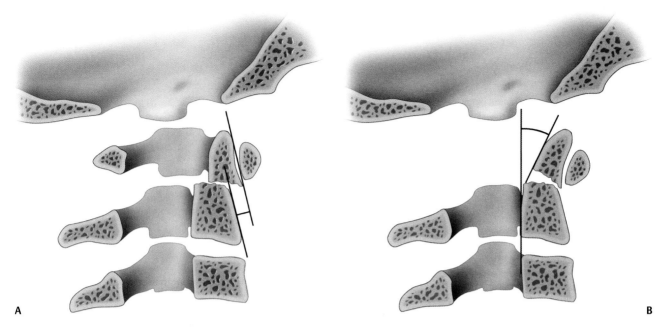

Fig. 14.3 Measurement of type II odontoid fractures. Measurements of translation (A) and measurement of angulation (B).

Odontoid Fractures

Using the search terms "odontoid fracture" and "measurement," few abstract hits were produced. Although some highlighted the importance of measurement of fracture displacement or angulation,[14] only one article detailed a precise measurement method.[4] These limited data offer level V evidence that the most appropriate method of measuring odontoid fracture displacement and angulation is as described in **Fig. 14.3**.

Traumatic Spondylolisthesis (Hangman's Fractures)

Hangman's fractures are classified based on the degree of angulation and displacement of the individual fragments.[15,16] However, in the current systematic review, there was only one article identified that detailed the specific manner in which these injury parameters should be measured.[4] Because it was a compilation of a consensus statement, this work provides only level V evidence that the prescribed measurement methods (**Fig. 14.4**) are the most appropriate for this injury type.

Lower Cervical Spine

In an extensive review of the literature using a multitude of search terms, there was at least some evidence to establish a standardized measurement method to characterize a limited subset of injury characteristics. For other injuries and characteristics, there was insufficient evidence that a single standardized imaging method could be prescribed. In light of these deficiencies, Bono et al[3] have detailed the Spine Trauma Study Group's consensus of the most appropriate measurement methods.

Facet Dislocation and Fracture

With the current search parameters, there were few studies that detailed a measurement method by which to describe the degree of facet fracture or facet subluxation. Bono et al[3] proposed a method to measure articular surface apposition after fracture or subluxation/dislocation. However, this was not based on clinical data. Building upon this concept, Spector et al[17] found, in a retrospective review, that the prescribed measurement of the articular fragment size in relation to the intact articular surface might be predictive of displacement with nonoperative care for unilateral facet fractures. They found that those involving more than 40% of the articular surface are at increased risk for displacement. In critique of this study, there were low patient numbers. However, it does appear to be a consecutive series of patients with a single injury type. These data provide level III prognostic evidence

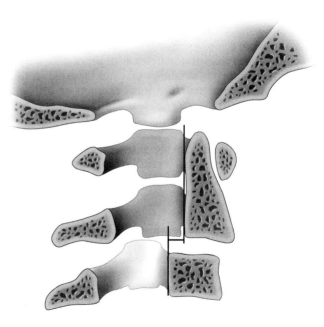

Fig. 14.4 Measurements of translation and angulation in Hangman's fractures: the posterior vertebral body referencing method.

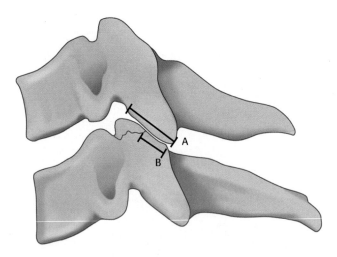

Fig. 14.5 For facet fractures, (A) the length of the inferior articular surface of the superior vertebra measured in millimeters will be used as the denominator, representing normal articular surface. (B) The length of the residual contacting articular surface will be measured and used as the numerator. The percentage of facet apposition is calculated by dividing B/A × 100.

that fracture fragment size measured as detailed in (**Fig. 14.5**) is predictive of late injury displacement.

Canal and Cord Compromise

There have been several studies evaluating a standardized method of measuring spinal cord compression, spinal cord compromise, and its potential influence of neurological deficit.[18–20] In the first of several works, Rao and Fehlings[20] found no precise measurement methods to assess spinal cord compression or canal compromise following trauma in a systematic review. Fehlings et al[18] proposed measurement methods for these injury parameters. Two observers studied and reviewed the images of 71 patients with acute cervical spinal cord injury from subaxial trauma. They found a strong correlation between canal compromise and cord compression measurements. The authors concluded that the midsagittal T1- and T2-weighted MRI is an objective and reliable method of assessing cord compression.

Though various statistical analyses were performed, the inter- and intraobserver variability was not reported in this study. In subsequent investigations, Fehlings et al[21] and Furlan et al[19] found moderate inter- and intraobserver reproducibility of these measurements. These studies provide level II diagnostic and level III prognostic evidence that the prescribed spinal cord and canal measurements are appropriate for the evaluation of subaxial cervical spine trauma.

Kyphosis

The current systematic review identified two techniques of measurement subaxial cervical kyphosis after injury: the Cobb method,[22] and the posterior vertebral body tangent method.[23] However, there have been no studies comparing the reliability or utility of these methods in the setting of spinal trauma. The methods by which these measurements are made have been detailed by Bono et al.[3] Apart from these works, there is no agreement in the literature concerning the most appropriate method by which to make these measurements.

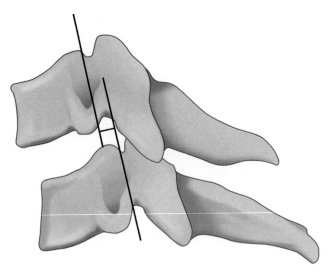

Fig. 14.6 Measurement method for translation.

Translation

White et al detailed a method of measuring translation in the subaxial spine.[24,25] It involves measuring from the posterior portion of the upper (displaced) vertebral body to a perpendicular line drawn along the superior end plate of the lower vertebra. Beyond this description, this measurement method has never been assessed for inter- or intraobserver reproducibility.

In a consensus work by the Spine Trauma Study Group, Bono et al[3] described a measurement method that utilizes posterior vertebral tangent lines of the upper and lower vertebrae (**Fig. 14.6**). Though studies are in progress, the inter- and intraobserver reliability has not been published. These data, therefore, provide level V evidence that the prescribed measurement methods are appropriate for measuring translation.

Vertebral Body Height Loss

In the current systematic review, there was only one report of a method of measuring vertebral body height loss following cervical trauma,[3] which is from the Spine Trauma Study Group. This involves measurement of the height of the vertebral body at, above, and below the level of injury in three locations: anterior, middle, and posterior. Height loss is then calculated by comparing the measurements at the injured segments to the average of the intact uninjured segments above. To date, the inter- and intraobserver reproducibility of this measurement has not been published. These data, therefore, provide level V evidence that the prescribed measurement methods are appropriate for measuring vertebral body height loss.

Thoracolumbar Spine

Keynan et al,[5] in conjunction with the Spine Trauma Study Group, published the results of a systematic review of radiographic measurement parameters for thoracolumbar spine trauma. These authors found various methods of measuring several different injury characteristics, which included sagittal alignment, vertebral body translation, vertebral body compression, and spinal canal compromise.

Sagittal Alignment

Sagittal alignment, a measure of posttraumatic kyphosis, can influence treatment decision making following thoracolumbar fractures. In an assessment of the reliability of five measures for kyphosis after thoracolumbar burst fractures, Kuklo et al[26] found that the Cobb angle was the most reliable and least variable. The authors described the method measurement as the angle subtended between lines drawn along the superior end plate of the supradjacent uninjured vertebra and the lower end plate of the infradjacent uninjured vertebra. This represents a modification of the original intention of the Cobb angle, which was for the measurement of coronal deformity from scoliosis.[22,27]

Kuklo et al[26] also assessed the Gardner segmental deformity method and the sagittal index. The Gardner method is similar to the Cobb method except the lower line is drawn along the inferior end plate of the injured vertebra. The sagittal index relies on lines drawn along the superior and inferior end plates of the injured vertebra only. Beyond the papers in which these measurement methods were initially introduced, the study by Kuklo et al[26] was the only study found that compared the reliability of the measurements.

Because the prognostic importance of these measurements has yet to be clearly determined, these data provide level IV evidence that the Cobb angle is the ideal measurement for assessing sagittal alignment/kyphosis after thoracolumbar trauma.

Vertebral Body Translation

Vertebral body translation is a common radiographic feature following thoracolumbar trauma. It indicates that a substantial amount of force has been delivered to the spine, usually leading to ligamentous disruption. Therefore, it is considered by many to be an indicator of severe mechanical instability.

In the current systematic review, only one study detailed a method of measuring translation of thoracolumbar fractures.[28] In their assessment of 96 consecutive patients with thoracolumbar fractures, Ruan et al[28] measured the perpendicular distance between the posterior vertebral bodies of the involved motion segment, compared as a ratio to the midsagittal diameter of the slipped vertebra. The interobserver or interobserver reliability of this measure was not reported, nor has it been subsequently assessed. Due to a lack of analysis of the prognostic utility of this diagnostic measuring tool, these data provide only level IV evidence that the prescribed measurement method is ideal for quantifying posttraumatic translation.

Spinal Canal Compromise

Spinal canal compromise is a frequent radiographic finding after thoracolumbar trauma. The potential relationship between posttraumatic spinal canal encroachment and the presence or severity of neurological deficit has been studied extensively in terms of both stenosis predisposing to injury and traumatic canal deformation.[29–32] In following, there are a multitude of methods for spinal canal assessment. These include the sagittal canal diameter, the transverse canal diameter, the sagittal:transverse ratio, total canal cross-sectional area, and percentage canal occlusion. Unfortunately, there is no consensus as to which of these measurements are

ideal or should be considered standard. Furthermore, the inter- and intraobserver reliability of these measures has not been assessed.

In a retrospective study, Vaccaro et al[33] found that the propensity for neurological injury correlated more highly with the sagittal:transverse ratio than to the absolute area of the spinal canal. Rasmussen et al[34] compared a computer-digitized method to a manually calculated method of assessing the cross-sectional area of the spinal canal, finding that the former correlated well with the latter. Hashimoto et al[35] calculated the ratio of the canal area at the injured segment in relation to uninjured segments. This group claimed to find critical values above which a neurological deficit was more likely (e.g., greater than 35% occlusion at T11 to T12).

As stated earlier, the wide variation with which previous authors have measured spinal canal compromise suggests that there is currently no standard or one accepted method that can be recommended.

Vertebral Body Compression

Compression of the vertebral body is a common imaging feature following thoracolumbar injury. Surprisingly, however, few methods have been proposed to quantify this injury feature. In a cadaveric study, Isomi et al[36] included measurements of the anterior and posterior vertebral body heights as part of their assessment of experimental thoracolumbar burst fractures. In the current systematic review, a myriad of articles and chapters allege the importance of so-called critical thresholds for vertebral body height loss (e.g., more than 50%). However, none has detailed the method by which this measurement should be made.

In a recent consensus work from the Spine Trauma Study Group, Keynan et al[5] recommended using Isomi et al's formula for measurement of anterior vertebral body height loss. Because reproducibility has yet to be assessed, this work provides only level V evidence that the prescribed measurement method is a reasonable current standard.

Sacrum

The sacrum is the transition zone between the mobile spine and the pelvis, and in most centers, sacral fractures are treated by orthopedic traumatologists. Thus the large majority of the literature and terminology concerning description and measurement of these injuries lies within the orthopedic trauma literature. For the purposes of the current systematic review, the measurement parameters discussed will be those most germane to the spinal surgeon, and will not be, by nature, comprehensive. Data will be derived primarily from the recent review by Kuklo et al,[6] who published recommendations on behalf of the Spine Trauma Study Group.

According to Kuklo et al,[6] anteroposterior displacement is best measured on an axial CT image. However, the authors admittedly recognize the lack of standardization and wide variability by which this measurement is made in the literature. Vertical translation is measured using a coronal CT image, calculated as the linear distance between the most superior portions of the two sacral fragments. Sacral kyphosis is measured using a sagittal CT image by drawing tangent lines along the posterior cortex of the proximal and distal fragments. These data provide only level V evidence that the prescribed measurement methods can be considered standard and accepted.

◆ Summary

Achieving standardization among a diverse population of surgeons and researchers is difficult, especially when considering an entity as protean as spine trauma. Nomenclature and measurement schemata have evolved in parallel, drawing from the insights of a diverse range of experienced observers, and reflect the progress of technology available to diagnose and treat spinal trauma. Fundamental to any clinically relevant classification system, the standardization of terminology as related to the definition of injury characteristics is critical to identifying optimal treatment options.

Ideally a common canon of measurement techniques would be applied to every region of the spinal column, and the lexicon of spinal trauma would be constant regardless of surgical discipline. Although heterogeneity still exists, the Spine Trauma Study Group has been working toward a goal of standardization of these parameters. Only through prospective evaluation and objective validation will the group be able to determine the ultimate utility of these or any other assessment techniques. Toward this end, it is the authors' hope that development of uniform radiographic measurement techniques and nomenclature will facilitate care of the traumatized spine and help codify a common descriptive language.

References

1. Jelsma RK, Kirsch PT, Rice JF, Jelsma LF. The radiographic description of thoracolumbar fractures. Surg Neurol 1982;18:230–236

2. Olmez N, Kaya T, Gunaydin R, Vidinli BD, Erdogan N, Memis A. Intra- and interobserver variability of Kleerekoper's method in vertebral fracture assessment. Clin Rheumatol 2005;24:215–218

3. Bono CM, Vaccaro AR, Fehlings M, et al. Measurement techniques for lower cervical spine injuries: consensus statement of the Spine Trauma Study Group. Spine 2006;31:603–609

4. Bono CM, Vaccaro AR, Fehlings M, et al; Spine Trauma Study Group. Measurement techniques for upper cervical spine injuries: consensus statement of the Spine Trauma Study Group. Spine 2007;32:593–600

5. Keynan O, Fisher CG, Vaccaro A, et al. Radiographic measurement parameters in thoracolumbar fractures: a systematic review and consensus statement of the Spine Trauma Study Group. Spine 2006;31:E156–E165

6. Kuklo TR, Potter BK, Ludwig SC, Anderson PA, Lindsey RW, Vaccaro AR ; Spine Trauma Study Group. Radiographic measurement techniques for sacral fractures consensus statement of the Spine Trauma Study Group. Spine 2006;31:1047–1055

7. Harris JH Jr, Carson GC, Wagner LK. Radiologic diagnosis of traumatic occipitovertebral dissociation, I: Normal occipitovertebral relationships on lateral radiographs of supine subjects. AJR Am J Roentgenol 1994;162:881–886

8. Harris JH Jr, Carson GC, Wagner LK, Kerr N. Radiologic diagnosis of traumatic occipitovertebral dissociation, II: Comparison of three methods of detecting occipitovertebral relationships on lateral radiographs of supine subjects. AJR Am J Roentgenol 1994;162:887–892

9. Rojas CA, Bertozzi JC, Martinez CR, Whitlow J. Reassessment of the craniocervical junction: normal values on CT. AJNR Am J Neuroradiol 2007;28:1819–1823

10. Ahuja A, Glasauer FE, Alker GJ Jr, Klein DM. Radiology in survivors of traumatic atlanto-occipital dislocation. Surg Neurol 1994;41:112–118

11. Heller JG, Viroslav S, Hudson T. Jefferson fractures: the role of magnification artifact in assessing transverse ligament integrity. J Spinal Disord 1993;6:392–396

12. Spence KF Jr, Decker S, Sell KW. Bursting atlantal fracture associated with rupture of the transverse ligament. J Bone Joint Surg Am 1970;52:543–549

13. Westaway MD, Hu WY, Stratford PW, Maitland ME. Intra- and inter-rater reliability of the anterior atlantodental interval measurement from conventional lateral view flexion/extension radiographs. Man Ther 2005;10:219–223

14. Koivikko MP, Kiuru MJ, Koskinen SK, Myllynen P, Santavirta S, Kivisaari L. Factors associated with nonunion in conservatively-treated type-II fractures of the odontoid process. [see comment] J Bone Joint Surg Br 2004;86:1146–1151

15. Effendi B, Roy D, Cornish B, Dussault RG, Laurin CA. Fractures of the ring of the axis: a classification based on the analysis of 131 cases. J Bone Joint Surg Br 1981;63-B:319–327

16. Levine AM, Edwards CC. The management of traumatic spondylolisthesis of the axis. J Bone Joint Surg Am 1985;67:217–226

17. Spector LR, Kim DH, Affonso J, Albert TJ, Hilibrand AS, Vaccaro AR. Use of computed tomography to predict failure of nonoperative treatment of unilateral facet fractures of the cervical spine. Spine 2006;31:2827–2835

18. Fehlings MG, Rao SC, Tator CH, et al. The optimal radiologic method for assessing spinal canal compromise and cord compression in patients with cervical spinal cord injury, II: Results of a multicenter study. Spine 1999;24:605–613

19. Furlan JC, Fehlings MG, Massicotte EM, et al. A quantitative and reproducible method to assess cord compression and canal stenosis after cervical spine trauma: a study of interrater and intrarater reliability. Spine 2007;32:2083–2091

20. Rao SC, Fehlings MG. The optimal radiologic method for assessing spinal canal compromise and cord compression in patients with cervical spinal cord injury, I: An evidence-based analysis of the published literature. Spine 1999;24:598–604

21. Fehlings MG, Furlan JC, Massicotte EM, et al; Spine Trauma Study Group. Interobserver and intraobserver reliability of maximum canal compromise and spinal cord compression for evaluation of acute traumatic cervical spinal cord injury. Spine 2006;31:1719–1725

22. Cobb JR. The American Academy of Orthopedic Surgeons Instructional Course Lectures. Vol 5. Ann Arbor, MI: Edwards; 1948

23. Harrison DE, Harrison DD, Cailliet R, Troyanovich SJ, Janik TJ, Holland B. Cobb method or Harrison posterior tangent method: which to choose for lateral cervical radiographic analysis. Spine 2000;25:2072–2078

24. White AA III, Johnson RM, Panjabi MM, Southwick WO. Biomechanical analysis of clinical stability in the cervical spine. Clin Orthop Relat Res 1975;109:85–96

25. White A, Panjabi M, eds. Clinical Biomechanics of the Spine. 2nd ed. Philadelphia: Lippincott-Raven; 1990

26. Kuklo TR, Polly DW, Owens BD, Zeidman SM, Chang AS, Klemme WR. Measurement of thoracic and lumbar fracture kyphosis: evaluation of intraobserver, interobserver, and technique variability. Spine 2001; 26:61–65, discussion 66

27. Polly DW Jr, Kilkelly FX, McHale KA, Asplund LM, Mulligan M, Chang AS. Measurement of lumbar lordosis: evaluation of intraobserver, interobserver, and technique variability. Spine 1996;21:1530–1535, discussion 1535–1536

28. Ruan DK, Shen GB, Chui HX. Shen instrumentation for the management of unstable thoracolumbar fractures. Spine 1998;23:1324–1332

29. Eismont FJ, Clifford S, Goldberg M, Green B. Cervical sagittal spinal canal size in spine injury. Spine 1984;9:663–666

30. Matsuura P, Waters RL, Adkins RH, Rothman S, Gurbani N, Sie I. Comparison of computerized tomography parameters of the cervical spine in normal control subjects and spinal cord-injured patients. J Bone Joint Surg Am 1989;71:183–188

31. Stagnara P, De Mauroy JC, Dran G, et al. Reciprocal angulation of vertebral bodies in a sagittal plane: approach to references for the evaluation of kyphosis and lordosis. Spine 1982;7:335–342

32. Torg JS, Naranja RJ Jr, Pavlov H, Galinat BJ, Warren R, Stine RA. The relationship of developmental narrowing of the cervical spinal canal to reversible and irreversible injury of the cervical spinal cord in football players. [see comment] J Bone Joint Surg Am 1996;78:1308–1314

33. Vaccaro AR, Nachwalter RS, Klein GR, Sewards JM, Albert TJ, Garfin SR. The significance of thoracolumbar spinal canal size in spinal cord injury patients. Spine 2001;26:371–376

34. Rasmussen PA, Rabin MH, Mann DC, Perl JR II, Lorenz MA, Vrbos LA. Reduced transverse spinal area secondary to burst fractures: is there a relationship to neurologic injury? J Neurotrauma 1994;11:711–720

35. Hashimoto T, Kaneda K, Abumi K. Relationship between traumatic spinal canal stenosis and neurologic deficits in thoracolumbar burst fractures. Spine 1988;13:1268–1272

36. Isomi T, Panjabi MM, Kato Y, Wang JL. Radiographic parameters for evaluating the neurologic spaces in experimental thoracolumbar burst fractures. J Spinal Disord 2000;13:404–411

15

Spinal Stability

Cao Yang, Kirkham B. Wood, and Alexander R. Vaccaro

The determination of spinal stability is one of the most important tasks confronting spinal specialists as its presence significantly affects the treatment strategy of injuries to the spine. This determination, however, remains challenging and continues to evolve, for significant ambiguity exists in its definition despite widespread use of the term.

The concept was first introduced in the Watson-Jones classification of spinal fractures in 1931 and then verified by Nicoll in 1949.[1,2] Since then, numerous classification systems have been proposed. The modern concept of mechanical stability of the spinal column was described by White and Panjabi.[3] They proposed that stability of the spinal column is provided by the interaction of three subsystems: vertebrae providing intrinsic stability, spinal muscles surrounding the spinal column providing dynamic stability, and a neural control system coordinating the muscle response. The authors defined clinical stability as the ability of the spine under physiological loads to maintain relationships between vertebrae in such a way that there is neither damage nor subsequent irritation to the spinal cord or nerve roots, and in addition, there is no development of incapacitating deformity or pain due to structural changes. Denis also concluded that a spine that could withstand normal physiological stresses without progressive deformity or neurological abnormalities, or both, was considered stable.[4]

It is clear in any classification system that some lesions are stable (such as compression fractures), whereas others are clearly unstable (such as fracture–dislocations). The challenge lies in the categories that make up the gray zone such as burst fractures, disk disruptions, and certain flexion–distraction injuries. There is no single system that has been fully validated for assessing spinal stability. This task remains an art form. At present, final determination of spinal stability requires consideration of many different factors taken on a case-by-case basis.

◆ Determining Stability of the Cervical Spine

Upper Cervical Spine

The structures from the occiput to C2 have unique ligamentous and joint configurations and should be considered separately from the lower cervical spine. Making the diagnosis of injury

to the upper cervical ligamentous complex can sometimes be difficult because the radiographic findings can be subtle. Even a hangman's dislocation can be missed if not potentially fatal. By far the most common occipital cervical dislocation is a longitudinal separation, although posterior and anterior dislocations may occur. The relationship of the dens to the basion and the Power ratio are useful for diagnosis of ligamentous disruption and instability. In a normal cervical spine, the distance from the tip of the odontoid to the basion is 4 to 5 mm in adults and up to 10 mm in children.[5,6] The Power ratio uses two distances measured between four points, using a lateral radiograph (**Fig. 15.1**).[7] The distance between the basion and the posterior arch of C1 is measured in relation to the distance between the opisthion and the anterior arch of C1. Because this distance is expressed as a ratio, there is no variability with

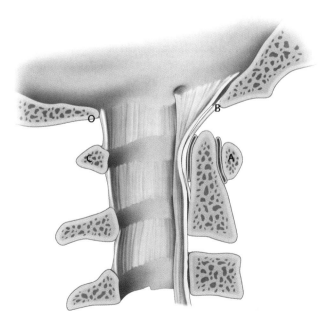

Fig. 15.1 The Power ratio uses four points of reference in the midsagittal section through the craniocervical junction. B, basion; O, opisthion; A, anterior arch of atlas; C, posterior arch of atlas. The ratio BC:OA should always equal 1 or less. If it is greater than 1, the patient most likely has an anterior occipitocervical subluxation dislocation.

head position or magnification. A ratio greater than 1 suggests a radiographic diagnosis of occipitocervical anterior dislocation. Harris et al[8] defined the rostral extension of the posterior cortex of the axis body as the posterior axial line, the distance between the basion (tip of the clivus) and the posterior axial line as the basion–axial interval, and the distance between the basion and the rostral tip of the dens as the basion–dental interval. In adults, the occipitovertebral junction can be considered normal when both the basion–axial interval and the basion–dental interval are 12 mm or less. In children less than 13 years old, the basion–dental interval is not reliable because of the variable age at which complete ossification and fusion of the dens occur. The normal basion–axial interval in children does not exceed 12 mm.

Lee et al[9] developed the X-line method for the diagnosis of traumatic atlantooccipital dislocation. They compared three methods of detecting occipitovertebral relationships on lateral radiographs: the basion–axial interval and basion–dental interval, the Power ratio, and the X-line method. They concluded that direct measurement of occipitovertebral skeletal relationships altered by occipitoatlantal dissociation using the basion–axial and basion–dental intervals provides the most accurate radiological assessment of this injury.[10] Although three-dimensional CT can clearly describe all bony structures, magnetic resonance imaging (MRI) is able to indicate not only the magnitude of displacement but also injuries to neurological and ligamentous structures. Hadley performed a systematic review on diagnosis and management of traumatic atlantooccipital dislocation injuries.[11] The presence of upper cervical prevertebral soft tissue swelling on an otherwise nondiagnostic plain x-ray should prompt additional imaging. If there was clinical suspicion of atlantooccipital dislocation, and plain x-rays were nondiagnostic, computed tomography (CT) or MRI was recommended.

The C1–C2 articulation is principally stabilized by the transverse ligament. Fractures of the atlas may develop C1–C2 instability if the transverse ligament is disrupted.[12] Spence suggested that the transverse ligament should be considered to be ruptured if the total overhang of the lateral masses of C1 in relation to the lateral borders of C2 in the open-mouth-view radiograph is greater than 7 mm.[13] On a lateral radiograph, the atlanto–dens interval should be less than 3 mm in adults and 5 mm in children if the transverse ligament is intact.[14] This parameter, however, is a static one and does not necessarily define instability adequately. Thus dynamic motion analysis should be important for precise assessment of the atlantoaxial instability. Dvorak et al used functional CT scanning to diagnose rotatory instability of the upper cervical spine. They suggested that axial rotation at C0–C1 greater than 8 degrees; at C1–C2 greater than 56 degrees; or a right–left difference C0–C1 greater than 5 degrees and C1–C2 greater than 8 degrees indicates instability.[15]

Lower Cervical Spine

Various anatomical structures have been implicated in maintaining stability within the lower cervical spine. The intervertebral disks. anterior and posterior longitudinal ligaments, paraspinal muscles, interspinous and supraspinous ligaments, and ligamentum nuchae all play an integral role in maintaining stability.[16–18] Using cadaver spines, White and Panjabi analyzed 17 different cervical motion segments and determined that the horizontal and angular displacements between

Table 15.1 Checklist for the Diagnosis of Clinical Instability in the Middle and Lower Cervical Spine

Element	Point Value
Anterior elements destroyed or unable to function	2
Posterior elements destroyed or unable to function	2
Positive stretch test	2
Radiographic criteria	
A. Flexion–extension x-rays	
1. Sagittal plane translation > 3.5 mm or 20%	2
2. Sagittal plane rotation > 20 degrees	2
or	
B. Resting x-rays	
1. Sagittal plane displacement > 3.5 mm or 20%	2
2. Relative sagittal plane angulation > 11 degrees	2
Developmentally narrow spinal canal (sagittal diameter < 13 mm or Pavlov ratio < 0.8)	1
Abnormal disk narrowing	1
Spinal cord damage	2
Nerve root damage	1
Dangerous loading anticipated	1

Note: Score of 5 or more = unstable.

Source: White AA, Panjabi MM. Clinical Biomechanics of the Spine. 2nd ed. Philadelphia: Lippincott; 1990:314.

vertebrae could not exceed 2.67 mm and 10.7 degrees, respectively, without complete failure of the motion segment.[19,20] From these data they proposed a system well suited for the diagnosis of cervical instability using plain radiographic evidence of translation and displacement (**Table 15.1**). Two points are given if the anterior column is destroyed or unable to function, and two points if the posterior column is similarly affected. This list also includes the stretch test.[3] Two points are given if there is a greater than 1.7 mm difference in interspace separation or a greater than 7.5 degree change in angulation between vertebrae when compared with prestretched radiographs after the standard application of incremental cervical traction. Sagittal plane displacement or translation greater than 3.5 mm or 20% respectively on either the resting or flexion–extension films is also considered unstable. This value of 3.5 mm was extrapolated from the 2.67 mm result obtained experimentally and with an assumed radiographic magnification of 30%. Relative sagittal plane angulation of more than 11 degrees on resting radiographs or 20 degrees on flexion–extension views is also considered unstable. Sagittal plane angulation is measured at the inferior end plate (**Fig. 15.2**).

When resting radiographs are used, comparison with the level above or below is necessary because the 11 degree rule is the difference from the expected normal alignment. For instance, if the adjacent normal level has lordosis of −2 degrees, then a measurement of +9 degrees of kyphosis at the affected level represents 11 degrees of relative sagittal plane angulation. Knopp et al[21] performed a prospective, observational study of normal male volunteers between the ages of 18 and 40 years. They obtained radiographs of all participants in neutral, flexion, and extension positions and measured the amount of subluxation and interspinous distance, as well as

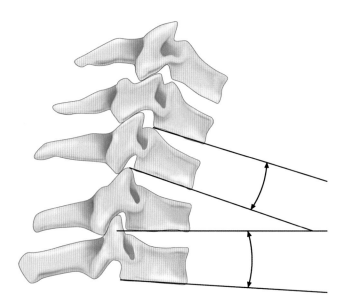

Fig. 15.2 Measurement of regional instability includes angular displacement 11 degrees greater than that at the adjacent vertebral segments and translation greater than 3.5 mm.

the degree of vertebral angulation between C3 and C7. Their study also suggested that subluxation greater than 2 mm in men 18 to 40 years of age may be a useful variable for further study as an indicator of ligamentous injury. Interspinous distance and vertebral angulation appeared less likely to have useful clinical application.

CT is commonly used to fully evaluate the extent of spinal injury and may aid in the analysis of potential instability. The configuration of the facet joints can be evaluated with axial sections, sometimes better appreciated using sagittal reconstructions. Lateral displacement of the facets, fractures into the facets, marked widening of the facet joint, or a "naked facet" will suggest that the joint capsule, which forms part of the posterior column, has been disrupted.[22] These changes can be appreciated even after reduction has been obtained. Perched facets show only minimal continuity between the facet joints on the axial section, whereas overriding facets will have the rounded outer surfaces rather than the flat, articulating surfaces unopposed as seen with a facet dislocation. Unilateral facet fractures are generally stable; however, when there is concomitant disk disruption and anterior longitudinal ligament injury, or significant bone loss, instability may ensue. Lifeso and Colucci reported their series of patients with this injury pattern and noted that patients treated with anterior cervical diskectomy and fusion improved significantly, whereas patients treated nonoperatively fared poorly.[23] In the study of Spector et al they used standard CT evaluation to predict failure of nonoperative treatment in patients with unilateral facet fractures.[24] They suggested that patients with unilateral cervical facet fractures involving >40% of the absolute height of the intact lateral mass or an absolute height >1 cm are at increased risk for failure of nonoperative treatment. Failure of nonoperative treatment was not observed in any patient with a fracture involving less than 40% of the height of the lateral mass or an absolute height < 1 cm.

MRI in recent years has become the standard method for analyzing soft tissue injuries in the spine. Many studies have reported the efficacy of its use for imaging after traumatic lesions to the spinal column because of its ability to detect soft tissue and cord injuries. Unilateral and bilateral facet dislocations of the subaxial spine are associated with damage to numerous soft tissue structures that provide stability to the lower cervical spine.[25] Damage to the posterior longitudinal ligament did not occur consistently in unilateral facet dislocations, whereas bilateral facet dislocations were consistently associated with disruption to both the posterior and the anterior longitudinal ligaments and facet capsule, as compared with unilateral facet dislocations. Horn et al evaluated the utility of using MRI in the acute trauma period to determine cervical spine instability. They found no evidence of spinal instability clinically in patients with normal CT or radiographic studies and signs of instability on MRI. MRI allows visualization of these disruptions as a prediction of cervical spinal stability after trauma.[26]

◆ Determining the Stability of the Thoracic and Lumbar Spine

The thoracic spine is mechanically stiffer and less mobile than the cervical region because it is supported by the rib cage with its costovertebral articulations and ligaments. White and Panjabi's checklist for clinical instability is often used for this region of the spine (**Table 15.2**). Disruption of the costovertebral articulations is given 1 point. Sagittal plane displacement of greater than 2.5 mm or sagittal plane angulation of more than 5 degrees is given 2 points on the checklist. Anterior or posterior disruptions are also given 2 points each. At the lumbar spine, the spinal cord stops at L1–L2, and thus neurological deficits incurred by trauma at this level are less frequent and disabling. There is, however, a high incidence of back pain and deformity from these injuries because higher loads have to be borne by this region of the spine. White and Panjabi's checklist system continues to be useful in this region, as described in **Table 15.3**. Cauda equina damage is given 3 points on the checklist. This higher value is given because the presence of neurological deficit at this region of the spinal column implies significant injury.

Denis's concept of the "three-column" spine, which evolved from a retrospective review of 412 thoracolumbar spine injuries and observations on spinal instability, classified spinal injuries into four different categories, all definable in terms of

Table 15.2 Checklist for the Diagnosis of Clinical Instability in the Thoracic and Thoracolumbar Spine

Element	Point Value
Anterior elements destroyed or unable to function	2
Posterior elements destroyed or unable to function	2
Disruptions of costovertebral articulations	1
Radiographic criteria	
1. Sagittal plane displacement > 2.5 mm	2
2. Relative sagittal plane angulation > 5 degrees	2
Spinal cord or cauda equina damage	2
Dangerous loading anticipated	1

Note: Score of 5 or more = unstable.

Source: White AA, Panjabi MM. Clinical Biomechanics of the Spine. 2nd ed. Philadelphia: Lippincott; 1990:335.

Table 15.3 Checklist for the Diagnosis of Clinical Instability in the Lumbar Spine

Element	Point Value
Anterior elements destroyed or unable to function	2
Posterior elements destroyed or unable to function	2
Radiographic criteria	
A. Flexion–extension x-rays	
1. Sagittal plane translation >4.5 mm or 15%	2
2. Sagittal plane rotation >15 degrees at L1–L2, L2–L3, and L3–L4	2
>20 degrees at L4–L5	2
>25 degrees at L5–S1	2
or	
B. Resting x-rays	
1. Sagittal plane displacement >4.5 mm or 15%	2
2. Relative sagittal plane angulation >22 degrees	2
Cauda equina damage	3
Dangerous loading anticipated	1

Note: Score of 5 or more = unstable.

Source: White AA, Panjabi MM. Clinical Biomechanics of the Spine. 2nd ed. Philadelphia: Lippincott; 1990:352.

the degree of involvement of each of the three columns.[27] The author further incorporated the concept of an unstable spine and classified instability into three degrees: (1) Instability of the first degree is a mechanical instability with risk of chronic kyphosis. An example would be a severe compression fracture with posterior column disruption. (2) Instability of the second degree is neurological instability. The so-called stable burst fracture falls into this category because further vertical collapse of the fractured vertebra may lead to more retropulsion of bone into the canal in the early posttraumatic phase and to higher risks of posttraumatic spinal stenosis after healing of the fracture. Both of these situations may precipitate neurological complications in a previously intact patient. (3) Instability of the third degree represents both mechanical and neurological instability. Fracture-dislocations and unstable burst fractures with or without existing neurological damage are in this category. Panjabi et al used a biomechanical trauma model to test their theory.[28] Burst fractures were produced in cadavers by either simple axial compression or flexion–compression. Multidirectional flexibility was measured before and after the trauma, thus quantifying the instability of the burst fracture. CT scans were taken after the fracture, and an injury scoring scheme quantified the injuries to the anterior, middle, and posterior columns. In the axial compression group, the middle column injury, compared with the other two columns, showed the highest correlations to the flexibility parameters. In the flexion–compression group, again the middle column injury showed the highest correlations to the flexibility parameters. The results allowed the authors to conclude that the concept of a middle column being the primary determinant of mechanical stability of the thoracolumbar spine was valid. James et al, however, used an L1 burst fracture model to evaluate the contribution of the three columns of the spine and came to a different conclusion.[29]

T12–L2 motion measurements after vertebral and ligamentous disruption revealed a statistically significant increase in motion upon anterior and added posterior column compromise, but not for added middle column disruption. This seemed more consistent with the clinical series of burst fractures with anterior and middle column compromise but an intact posterior column that seemed stable and healed satisfactorily. The condition of the posterior column, not the middle column, was thus considered the primary indicator of burst fracture stability.

With this knowledge in hand, Magerl et al described the 3–3–3 scheme of the AO fracture classification, which was really the first system to select a progressive scale of morphological damage by which the degree of instability was determined. The types have a fundamental injury pattern that is determined by the three most important mechanisms acting on the spine: compression, distraction, and axial torque.[30] It is a hierarchical system based on increasing injury severity and increasing instability.

The Spine Trauma Study Group has expanded on this work and developed its own Injury Severity Score as described by Vaccaro et al based on three major variables: the morphology of injury determined by radiographic appearance, the integrity of the posterior ligamentous complex, and the neurological status of the patient, the first classification system to incorporate neurologic stability into a thoracolumbar classification scheme.[31] By systematically assigning specific point values within each category based on the severity of injury, a final severity score may be generated that can be used to help direct treatment. Injuries are generally described or classified morphologically into three major categories: compression injuries (1 point for compression, 1 point for burst injury), translational/rotational injuries (3 points), and distraction injuries (4 points). Within each category as noted, 1 to 4 points are assigned, reflecting the severity of bony and soft tissue disruption. If there are multiple fractures at different spinal levels, the injury level with the most significant morphological descriptor or morphology is given the most points and is the only level that is scored. Multiple morphologies at a single level, such as a distraction translational injury, is only given a single score commensurate with the largest scored morphology (i.e., 4 points for the distraction injury rather than 3 points for the translational component). The neurological status of the patient is divided into four subcategories based on the severity of the deficit as well as the potential for neural recovery with surgical intervention: intact (0 points), nerve root injury (2 points), complete spinal cord injury (motor and sensory, 2 points), and incomplete spinal cord injury (motor or sensory, 3 points) or cauda equina syndrome (3 points).

Finally, the integrity of the posterior ligamentous complex is categorized as intact (0 points), indeterminate disruption (2 points), or definitely disrupted (3 points). The posterior capsular ligamentous complex historically has been assessed by clinical examination (palpable gap between spinous processes), interspinous widening on plain films, or reconstructed CT evaluation. However, diagnostic accuracy of these imaging modality evaluations is low compared with MRI.[31] MRI assessment in the presence of posterior ligamentous disruption may demonstrate hyperintensity in the posterior ligament complex on fat suppression T2-weighted images. Once all major variables have been assigned points, a total score is determined, which is intended to assist the surgeon in selecting the need for nonoperative or operative intervention. Patients with <3 points are considered nonoperative candidates. Patients with > 5 points are considered surgical candidates. Patients with a point total of 4 may be considered for either operative or nonoperative treatment.[32]

Oner et al[33] identified six stages of disk injury following trauma using criteria based on disk morphology and signal intensity of the MRI signal, in the attempt to study the relative stability and instability of the disk adjacent to fractured vertebrae. A type 1 is a normal or near normal disk. There is no significant loss of height or signal abnormality or evidence of herniation. Type 2, a black disk, is morphologically similar to type 1 with diffuse loss of signal on T2 images. Type 3 disk has Schmorl-type changes to the end plates with no significant loss of height or signal. There is a small herniation of the nucleus pulposus into the end plate. Type 4 disk demonstrates anterior disk height collapse. There is disproportional loss of height in the anterior third of the disk, but the middle and posterior sections remain unchanged. Anterior bulging of the disk or herniation of the nucleus pulposus into the end plate is seen in the anterior third. There is no change in the signal intensity of the nucleus pulposus. Type 5 disk describes a central herniation. There is a massive herniation of the nucleus pulposus into the central end plate. As a result of this herniation loss of height in the anterior and posterior disk results in almost complete bony contact between the adjacent end plates. The nucleus pulposus in this type has a normal signal intensity. Type 6 degenerated disk describes loss of disk height and signal intensity in all three sections of the disk (anterior, middle, and posterior).

The identification of different types of disk morphologies using MRI suggests common traumatic patterns that have never been considered previously in contemporary fracture classification systems. In nonoperatively treated patients, changes in disk morphology appeared to influence the progression of kyphosis. Injuries leading to disk types 1, 2, or 3 did not cause progression of the kyphosis, whereas those giving rise to types 4, 5, or 6 were associated with kyphosis progression in some cases. In those managed by surgery, statistical analysis showed no clear relationship between the degree of recurrence of kyphosis and disk type. Recurrent kyphosis after posterior reduction appeared to be a result of creeping of the nucleus pulposus back into the depressed central area.

Understanding spinal stability is a complicated and poorly understood concept. The emergence of new imaging technologies may allow the treating physician to make correlations between anatomical deficiencies and the potential for structural incompetency leading to future loss of alignment and neurological instability. Meticulous registries recording the natural history of fracture healing treated nonoperatively correlating structural deficiencies with symptomatology will be vital in understanding the contributions of invasive interventions on the long-term functional outcome of a spinal trauma patient.

References

1. Nicoll EA. Fractures of the dorso-lumbar spine. J Bone Joint Surg Am 1949;31B:376–394
2. Watson-Jones R. Fracture and Joint Injuries. 3rd ed. Baltimore: Williams & Wilkins; 1943
3. White AP, Panjabi MM, eds. Clinical Biomechanics of the Spine. Philadelphia: Lippincott, Williams & Wilkins; 1990
4. Denis F. Spinal instability as defined by the three-column spine concept in acute spinal trauma. Clin Orthop Relat Res 1984;(189):65–76
5. Wholey MH, Bruwer AJ, Baker HL Jr. The lateral roentgenogram of the neck; with comments on the atlanto-odontoid-basion relationship. Radiology 1958;71:350–356
6. Wiesel SW, Rothman RH. Occipitoatlantal hypermobility. Spine 1979;4:187–191
7. Powers B, Miller MD, Kramer RS, Martinez S, Gehweiler JA Jr. Traumatic anterior atlanto-occipital dislocation. Neurosurgery 1979;4:12–17
8. Harris JH Jr, Carson GC, Wagner LK. Radiologic diagnosis of traumatic occipitovertebral dissociation, I: Normal occipitovertebral relationships on lateral radiographs of supine subjects. AJR Am J Roentgenol 1994;162:881–886
9. Lee C, Woodring JH, Goldstein SJ, Daniel TL, Young AB, Tibbs PA. Evaluation of traumatic atlantooccipital dislocations. AJNR Am J Neuroradiol 1987;8:19–26
10. Harris JH Jr, Carson GC, Wagner LK, Kerr N. Radiologic diagnosis of traumatic occipitovertebral dissociation, II: Comparison of three methods of detecting occipitovertebral relationships on lateral radiographs of supine subjects. AJR Am J Roentgenol 1994;162:887–892
11. Hadley M. Diagnosis and management of traumatic atlanto-occipital dislocation injuries. Neurosurgery 2002;50(3, Suppl):S105–S113
12. Sullivan JD, Farfan HF. The crumpled neural arch. Orthop Clin North Am 1975;6:199–214
13. Spence KF Jr, Decker S, Sell KW. Bursting atlantal fracture associated with rupture of the transverse ligament. J Bone Joint Surg Am 1970;52:543–549
14. Fielding JW, Cochran GB, Lawsing JF III, Hohl M. Tears of the transverse ligament of the atlas: a clinical and biomechanical study. J Bone Joint Surg Am 1974;56:1683–1691
15. Dvorak J, Hayek J, Zehnder R. CT-functional diagnostics of the rotatory instability of the upper cervical spine, II: An evaluation on healthy adults and patients with suspected instability. Spine 1987;12:726–731
16. Bailey R. Observations of cervical intervertebral disc lesion in fracture and dislocations. J Bone Joint Surg Am 1963;45:461–470
17. Holdsworth F. Fractures, dislocations, and fracture-dislocations of the spine. J Bone Joint Surg Am 1970;52:1534–1551
18. Roaf R. Vertebral growth and its mechanical control. J Bone Joint Surg Br 1960;42-B:40–59
19. Panjabi MM, White AA III, Johnson RM. Cervical spine mechanics as a function of transection of components. J Biomech 1975;8:327–336
20. White AA III, Johnson RM, Panjabi MM, Southwick WO. Biomechanical analysis of clinical stability in the cervical spine. Clin Orthop Relat Res 1975;(109):85–96
21. Knopp R, Parker J, Tashjian J, Ganz W. Defining radiographic criteria for flexion-extension studies of the cervical spine. Ann Emerg Med 2001;38:31–35
22. Pech P, Kilgore DP, Pojunas KW, Haughton VM. Cervical spinal fractures: CT detection. Radiology 1985;157:117–120
23. Lifeso RM, Colucci MA. Anterior fusion for rotationally unstable cervical spine fractures. Spine 2000;25:2028–2034
24. Spector LR, Kim DH, Affonso J, Albert TJ, Hilibrand AS, Vaccaro AR. Use of computed tomography to predict failure of nonoperative treatment of unilateral facet fractures of the cervical spine. Spine 2006;31:2827–2835
25. Vaccaro AR, Madigan L, Schweitzer ME, Flanders AE, Hilibrand AS, Albert TJ. Magnetic resonance imaging analysis of soft tissue disruption after flexion-distraction injuries of the subaxial cervical spine. Spine 2001;26:1866–1872
26. Horn EM, Lekovic GP, Feiz-Erfan I, Sonntag VK, Theodore N. Cervical magnetic resonance imaging abnormalities not predictive of cervical spine instability in traumatically injured patients. Invited submission from the Joint Section Meeting on Disorders of the Spine and Peripheral Nerves, March 2004. J Neurosurg Spine 2004;1:39–42
27. Denis F. The three column spine and its significance in the classification of acute thoracolumbar spinal injuries. Spine 1983;8:817–831
28. Panjabi MM, Oxland TR, Kifune M, Arand M, Wen L, Chen A. Validity of the three-column theory of thoracolumbar fractures: a biomechanic investigation. Spine 1995;20:1122–1127
29. James KS, Wenger KH, Schlegel JD, Dunn HK. Biomechanical evaluation of the stability of thoracolumbar burst fractures. Spine 1994;19:1731–1740
30. Magerl F, Aebi M, Gertzbein SD, Harms J, Nazarian S. A comprehensive classification of thoracic and lumbar injuries. Eur Spine J 1994;3:184–201
31. Vaccaro AR, Zeiller SC, Hulbert RJ, et al. The thoracolumbar injury severity score: a proposed treatment algorithm. J Spinal Disord Tech 2005;18:209–215
32. Lee HM, Kim HS, Kim DJ, Suk KS, Park JO, Kim NH. Reliability of magnetic resonance imaging in detecting posterior ligament complex injury in thoracolumbar spinal fractures. Spine 2000;25:2079–2084
33. Oner FC, van Gils AP, Dhert WJ, Verbout AJ. MRI findings of thoracolumbar spine fractures: a categorization based on MRI examinations of 100 fractures. Skeletal Radiol 1999;28:433–443

IV

Problem-Based Approach to the Principles of Spinal Injury Management

16

Treatment and Outcomes of Pediatric Spinal Cord Injury

John R. Dimar and Leah Y. Carreon

Spinal cord injury (SCI) is a devastating event regardless of the age when it occurs. However, when it occurs in the pediatric population it often carries with it dire, lifelong consequences, along with a unique set of complications that significantly differ from those encountered in adults.[1] Unfortunately, due to the rarity of these injuries in the pediatric population, most of the recent published reports are retrospective series or case reports that offer little insight into how to effectively treat these injuries. Outcome measures to assess the patient's long-term neurological and physical function and quality of life after treatment are also unavailable. Anecdotal experience has generally extrapolated the use of adult treatment paradigms to that of children based on the generally accepted opinion that children recover from SCI in a superior fashion to that of adults when treated with similar methods. These commonly accepted adult treatment recommendations include rapid emergent stabilization, traction, rigid orthotic treatment, and, when necessary, rapid surgical decompression and stabilization via internal fixation.

Although certain of these techniques have shown some preclinical and clinical effectiveness in adults there is no definitive evidence proving similar success in the treatment of a pediatric SCI. This lack of level 1 evidence (supporting appropriateness of a specific treatment regimen and the long-term outcomes of such treatment) is rooted in the difficulty of designing a prospective pediatric SCI study with enough power considering that even large centers see so few cases. Therefore, the most appropriate current treatment for a pediatric patient with an acute SCI remains traditional techniques that prevent additional acute injury, reduce secondary posttraumatic inflammatory injury, and stabilize the spine to prevent reinjury.

◆ Preclinical Evidence

There are no preclinical studies that specifically address pediatric SCI and how it compares with adult SCI. However, assuming that the physiology of children does not differ significantly from that of adults, there is encouraging evidence that certain modalities can affect the short- and long-term outcomes of an SCI. There are currently several key preclinical studies that have demonstrated improved neurological outcomes following an SCI. The first series of studies utilized pharmacological agents to modify the secondary injury that occurs after injury. Methylprednisolone, a steroid agent, has been extensively studied to evaluate its effects upon an acute SCI.[2-4] Although some studies have demonstrated the protective effectiveness of steroids, other studies have clearly not supported this contention.[5] Additionally, the dosages suggested for SCI have been found to have significant side effects, including suppression of the immune system, increased infection rates, delayed wound healing, and hyperglycemia.[5-10] Sygen (Fidia Pharmaceuticals, Abano Terme, Italy) (GM-1 ganglioside) also demonstrated enough preclinical protective effect following an SCI to undergo human trials leading to the recent U.S. Food and Drug Administration (FDA) approval for human use.[11]

The second series of studies evaluated the role and effectiveness of surgical intervention with decompression of the injured spinal cord. These studies, which carefully controlled for the severity of the injury, clearly showed that the amount of residual spinal canal narrowing following fracture directly influenced the degree of secondary injury within the spinal cord. Furthermore, the study shows that the longer the duration of the narrowing the less favorable the neurological recovery. The optimum time interval for decompression established in the study was 6 hours or less, whereas persistent spinal canal narrowing longer than 72 hours resulted in no recovery. This was the first study to clearly demonstrate that neurological recovery is directly influenced by both the degree of spinal canal narrowing as well as the duration of the narrowing.[12]

Hypothermia treatment has demonstrated effectiveness in slowing the progression of neurological compromise in animal studies. In a carefully controlled spinal cord contusion model the spinal canal was precisely narrowed with spacers. The control animal group suffered irreversible SCI, whereas the investigational group, in which continuous cooling was applied directly to the area of injury, showed that hypothermia treatment was protective in preventing injury. Other animals within the study that had a contusion combined with persistent narrowing of the spinal canal demonstrated generally poor outcomes.[13] These preclinical studies clearly show that interventional modalities have reasonably strong preclinical evidence of their ability to modify the ultimate degree of permanent SCI. Although these marginal improvements in neurological recovery might not be as dramatic as hoped for, any degree of useful return of function, whether motor or sensory, carries huge ramifications for a patient's ability to successfully carry out activities of daily living. Unfortunately, except in a few rare cases, none of these preclinical studies were specifically performed in immature animals, so their applicability to human pediatric patients cannot be stated with certainty.

◆ Epidemiology

Traumatic SCI in a child or adolescent is devastating, often resulting in quality of life changes that are frequently lifelong. Fortunately, the incidence of such injuries is low in patients younger than 15 years of age, accounting for less than 10% of all patients that suffer an SCI. Sixty to eighty percent of SCIs in children occur in the cervical spine, and 5.4 to 34% occur in the thoracolumbar spine.[14–16] The overall incidence is 1.99 SCI injuries per 100,000 children in the United States; however, there are distinct racial and ethnic differences, with African Americans exhibiting a 1.53 rate, Native Americans a 1.00 rate, Hispanics a 0.87 rate, and Asians a 0.36 rate per 100,000.

Boys were twice as likely to suffer an SCI, whereas motor vehicle accidents are the most common cause, responsible for 50 to 56% of the total injuries.[17] Surprisingly, almost 68% of children suffering an SCI were not wearing seat belts at the time of the accident. Other frequently cited causes of a pediatric SCI are diving injuries, accidental falls, sports injuries, motor vehicle/pedestrian injuries, firearms, and birth injuries.[18–20] SCI resulting from child abuse is rare, constituting less than 1% of the total skeletal injuries suffered, and when seen it frequently involves the upper cervical spine.[21]

Reports in Canada demonstrate similar pediatric SCI rates with an incidence of one per million in young children and a young adult rate of 17 per million.[14] SCI rates reported in Europe are quite variable where Swedish demographic studies from 1985 to 1996 reported SCI rates of 0.46 per 100,000, whereas 41% of the injuries were secondary to sports injuries and 29% followed motor vehicle collisions. This incidence can be contrasted to significantly higher fatal and nonfatal SCI rates of 2.70 per 100,000 in Portugal.[22]

Injuries to the spinal cord in newborns and infants are quite rare, being reported at an incidence of one per 29,000 to 60,000 live births and are believed to be caused by hyperextension of the fetal head during forceps-assisted breech deliveries. Clinical symptomatology includes flaccid quadriplegia, apnea, and death, with 10% of stillborns having injury to the spinal cord upon autopsy. Most of the cases are cervical, but the upper thoracic spine may also be involved. The prognosis for recovery is extremely poor (0%) with a 33% mortality rate before the age of 6.[23] There is frequently no observable fracture necessitating the use of ultrasound or magnetic resonance imaging (MRI) to formulate the diagnosis.[19,24] Unfortunately, the epidemiological outcome information available concerning the long-term recovery of these pediatric SCI patients conveys that they suffer lifelong permanent disabilities requiring tracheostomies, with potential lifelong ventilation for cervical injuries, numerous reconstructive surgeries, assisted ambulation, and the need for long-term-care facilities.[25]

◆ Unique Anatomical Consideration

Children have unique anatomical differences that need to be considered during treatment for spinal trauma along with the need for established protocols to facilitate the clearance of spine following an injury.[26] The infant spinal cord can only stretch $1/_4$ inch during a distraction injury, whereas the spinal column can stretch 2 inches, allowing the spine to distract more than the spinal cord.[27] The mismatch in elasticity results in the classic significant spinal cord injury without radiographic abnormality (SCIWORA) pattern where the spinal cord can sustain a significant traction injury while the spinal vertebrae and ligaments remain uninjured. Additionally, children have an increased head:body ratio shifting the fulcrum of movement to the upper spine (C2–C3). They have less developed musculature, increased elasticity of the ligaments, a flatter slope of the facet joints allowing for more translation, and less developed uncinate processes.[24,28] The general ligamentous laxity of the pediatric spine causes the energy imparted by a traumatic injury to be distributed over multiple levels, frequently resulting in multiple vertebral fractures, particularly in the thoracolumbar spine.[29]

The immature spinal vertebrae contain numerous ossification centers that are often misinterpreted as fractures.[30] These growth centers of the spine differ between the cervical and thoracolumbar spine. The cervical spine is conceptually the most difficult to understand because there are numerous ossification centers within the vertebrae, particularly the C1 and C2 vertebrae. The C1 vertebra develops from three ossification centers consisting of the body and two neural arches. The C2 vertebra has four ossification centers consisting of the body, two neural arches, and the odontoid. The remaining cervical, thoracic, and lumbar vertebrae all have three ossification centers, consisting of two neural arches and one body (**Fig. 16.1**).

There are five secondary ossification centers in the cervical, thoracic, and lumbar spine consisting of one spinous process growth center, two transverse process growth centers, and two ring apophyses on the superior and inferior aspect of the vertebral body. The lumbar spine has two additional mammillary body ossification centers at the dorsal junction of the transverse process and the facet joint.[30] Fractures can occur through any of these growth centers, making the diagnosis difficult if one is not familiar with these anatomical differences. Modern radiographic diagnostic modalities have greatly facilitated the identification of occult ligamentous and bony injuries, even if an occult growth plate injury occurs. Long-term spine abnormalities following spinal trauma can result from damage to the vertebral apophyseal growth plates resulting in the potential for growth arrest and resultant spinal deformity.

Differences in anatomy between adults and children also result in pediatric trauma causing unexpected neurological injuries. For example, in infants the location of the conus is near the sacrum, resulting in SCI occurring at unanticipated levels in the lumbar spine. Young children may experience a SCIWORA, which may occur acutely or in a delayed fashion, thus confounding their ability to be diagnosed. Finally, if a child less than 10 years old suffers paralysis following trauma the resultant loss of thoracolumbar muscle control leads to a 100% chance of developing a significant neuromuscular scoliosis.[14]

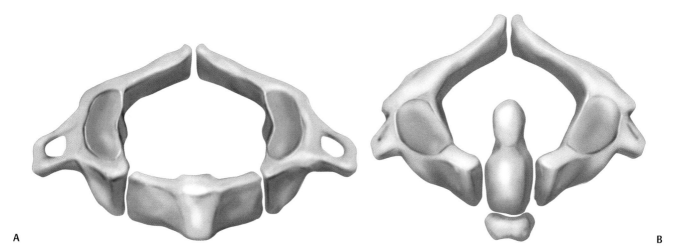

Fig. 16.1 Pediatric growth centers of **(A)** C1 and **(B)** C2 of children 3 to 6 years old.

Spinal Cord Injury without Radiographic Abnormality

SCIWORA occurs in younger children, generally less than 8 years old, and is believed to occur due to the significantly greater elasticity of the stabilizing disk and ligamentous structures of the spinal vertebrae when compared with the spinal cord.[31] The mismatch in elongation capacity between the vertebral column and the spinal cord results in the spinal cord being stretched beyond its elastic capacity, thus resulting in an SCI (**Fig. 16.2**).[24,27]

SCIWORA is responsible for one third of all pediatric SCIs. This cord injury type has the greatest potential recovery among all spinal cord injured children.[14] SCIWORA is more predominant in the cervical spine, with one series reporting

10 injuries between C1 and C5, 33 between C5 and C8, and 12 thoracic injuries. Of these patients 22 had severe SCIs, with all but one occurring before the age of 8, whereas 24 of 33 of the milder injuries occurred in an older pediatric age population. This large series also cautioned about the risk of late-onset SCIWORA, which they believed to be due to undetected instability. Only four of the severely neurologically impaired patients improved enough to walk with prosthetic aids, whereas the 33 incomplete lesion patients all had significant improvement (**Fig. 16.3**).[32] Traditional plain radiographs unfortunately were unable to identify any typical fractures or misalignment of the spinal axis, resulting in coining of the term *SCIWORA*.

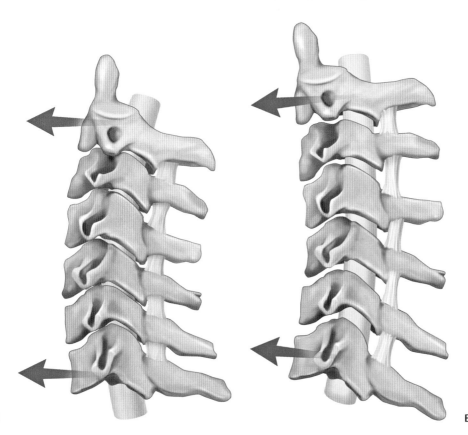

Fig. 16.2 (A–D) Due to the mismatch between the highly elastic vertebral/ligamentous structures of the spinal column and the minimally inflexible spinal cord, acute hyperflexion tears the supporting ligamentous soft tissues, causing a concurrent stretch injury of the spinal cord. *(Continued on page 138)*

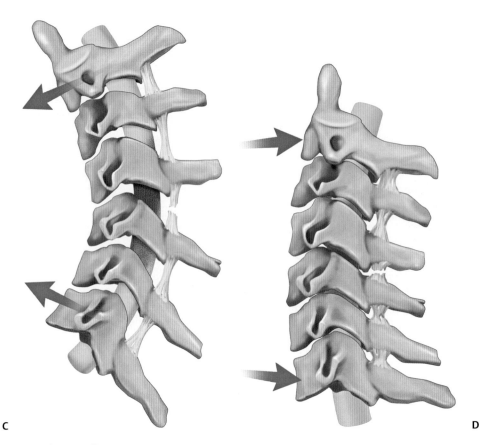

C

D

Fig. 16.2 *(Continued)*

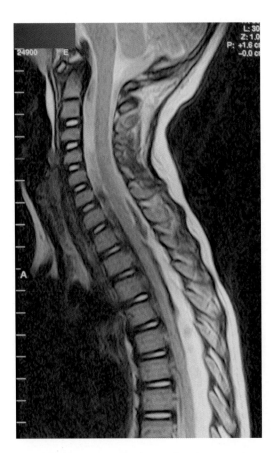

Fig. 16.3 Classic example of a spinal cord injury without radiographic abnormality (SCIWORA) that demonstrates a significant spinal cord injury.

Because many of these patients suffer subtle ligamentous injury, the advent of MRI has allowed for the identification of previously unrecognized pathology.[33] These MRI findings have been useful in predicting the neurological outcome of children suffering an SCI, with complete transection and major hemorrhages having extremely poor recovery, 40% of minor hemorrhage patients improving to a mild level of residual neurological injury, 75% of cord-edema-only patients improving a mild level of neurological injury, along with 25% having complete return of neurological function, whereas patients with a normal MRI all had full neurological recovery.[34]

Several series reporting on SCIWORA provide significant insight into SCI in children because they focus on the recovery from the neurological injury and not vertebral fracture. One meta-analysis showed that, of the 109 pediatric patients whose neurological status was available for review following treatment, complete recovery occurred in only 33% (36 patients), partial recovery in 15% (16 patients), and no recovery in 49% (53 patients), whereas 4% of the patients died. The authors also concluded that the incidence of late or delayed SCIWORA could be diminished by brace treatment along with an improved prognosis for neurological recovery.[35] Another study of 189 pediatric patients suffering a SCIWORA injury demonstrated that the 19 patients presenting with a complete SCI had an ominous prognosis with only one recovering any significant function, confirming the previous literature's dismal report of a 99% chance of having no recovery. The 170 patients that suffered an incomplete injury fared much better, with 95% of the full recovery that the authors contrasted to the currently reported literature rate of 84%. These authors reported that prolonged bracing did little to prevent permanent neurological damage or prevent recurrent SCIWORA once structural instability had been ruled out.[36] Clearly these studies demonstrate that a complete SCI, even in children, carries a grave prognosis with little chance for recovery regardless of the modality of treatment. It would appear that incomplete lesions carry a significantly better prognosis with a high probability of complete recovery, but it is still impossible to quantitate the degree of recovery in children and be able to have any meaningful comparison to that in adults.

Cervical Spinal Cord Injury

Cervical traumatic spinal injuries and fractures, although rare, are the most common cause of SCI in children. These injuries comprise a broad spectrum of injuries, including the classic SCIWORA injury in very young children where the supporting osseous/ligamentous structures remain intact, upper cervical occipital–C1–C4 subluxations or fracture/dislocations in children less than 8 to 9 years old, to adult injury fracture patterns that resemble typical adult injuries in the adolescent population.[24] One large series indicated that up to 32% of pediatric patients present with radiographic evidence of vertebral fracture, with younger children presenting more often with subluxation (39%), whereas the majority of adolescents presented with a fracture (80%).

Patients less than 9 years old tend to suffer more severe neurological injuries than older patients along with a significant rate of concurrent head injuries (40%) that complicate the identification of a concomitant SCI (**Fig. 16.4**). These authors reported 38/46 (86%) patients who suffered incomplete SCIs

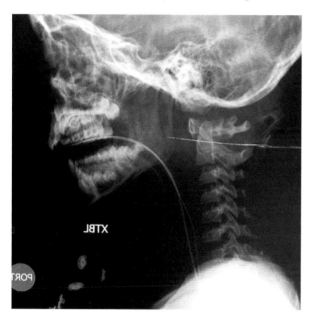

A

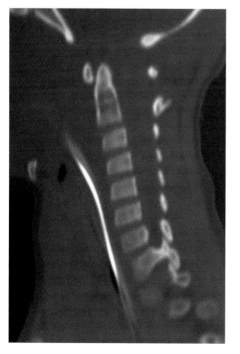

B

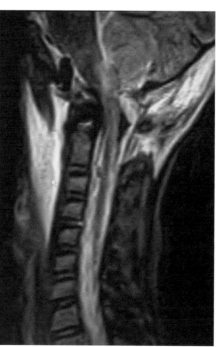

C

Fig. 16.4 An 8-year-old girl involved in a motor vehicle accident found to be unconscious and quadriplegic following a high-speed impact with a wall. Following successful resuscitation and transport **(A)** lateral radiographs and **(B)** computed tomographic scan revealed an occipital, C1, C2 dislocation. **(C)** Magnetic resonance imaging revealed significant spinal cord edema. *(Continued on page 140)*

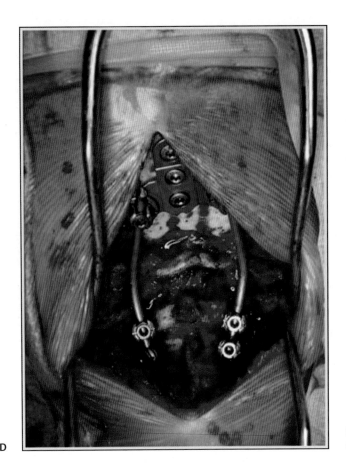

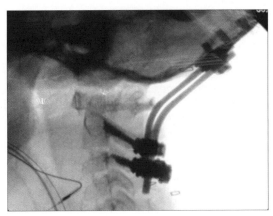

E

D

Fig. 16.4 *(Continued)* **(D,E)** The patient underwent an open reduction, occipital–C3 instrumentation with fusion.

recovered completely, with the remainder improving 1 to 2 Frankel grades. As a result, they concluded that a cervical level incomplete SCI has a good prognosis if the child survives the concomitant injuries.[37] However, other reports looking at younger children involved in higher-energy motor vehicle accidents where they suffered multiple injuries and severe cervical spine injuries reported a permanent SCI rate of 57%.[38]

The direct relationship between the severity of the injury and the presence of an SCI is further illustrated in a series of 56 cervical spine injuries where 66% of the patients had concurrent neurological deficits and the mortality rate was 27%. Of the neurologically injured patients, 25 had complete recovery, three had incomplete recovery, and the eight patients who were graded complete lesions (ASIA A) demonstrated no recovery (14%).[15] It is therefore reasonable to assume that the high-energy injuries associated with motor vehicle accidents appear to result in much more severe SCI when compared with those resulting from falls or sports injuries that impart significantly lower forces to the spine.

Thoracolumbar Spinal Cord Injury

Thoracolumbar spine fractures are more common in older children and adolescents than younger children, with the most common causes being motor vehicle accidents, sports, falls, and pedestrian/motor vehicle accidents (**Fig. 16.5**). They are often associated with lung, liver, spleen, bowel, and kidney injuries, especially seat-belt injuries involving the lumbosacral spine.[39] Thoracolumbar fractures occur mainly in the lumbar spine in older children, followed by the midthoracic spine. In younger children the thoracic region is the more common site of injury (29%), followed by the

lumbar spine (19%), along with a 60% concurrent neurological injury.[1,40] Many reviews of pediatric thoracolumbar fractures devote most of their focus to the bony injuries, with minimal attention to the neurological injuries.[14,16,39]

Surgical stabilization is often required. Nearly one third (23/89) of patients in one large series reported the need for surgical stabilization. The rate of neurological injury following a thoracolumbar fracture has been reported to be 14.6%, with 6/9 complete injuries remaining complete and 2/4 incomplete injuries failing to return to normal. These neurological recovery rates are certainly not encouraging and not significantly different from those in the adult.[16] Another study reported that 27% of pediatric thoracolumbar burst fractures have an SCI and require surgical stabilization with decompression. The authors report that children could have up to 55% narrowing of the spinal canal without affecting neurological recovery. This is an important observation in children, where significant narrowing still showed neurological recovery,[41] highlighting a possible difference between adults and children. Adults, with age-related and degenerative narrowing, are more susceptible to injury.

Seat-Belt Injuries (Flexion-Distraction)

Pediatric lumbar fractures have unique patterns of injury due to the child's smaller pelvis, which allows the lap belt to slide up the abdomen, shifting the axis of rotation superior to the umbilicus. These injuries have a broad spectrum of presentation ranging from simple compression fracture to disruption of the posterior ligamentous complex to fracture/dislocations. Approximately 20 to 30% of children involved in motor vehicle accidents while wearing seat belts present with a neurological deficit.[31,42]

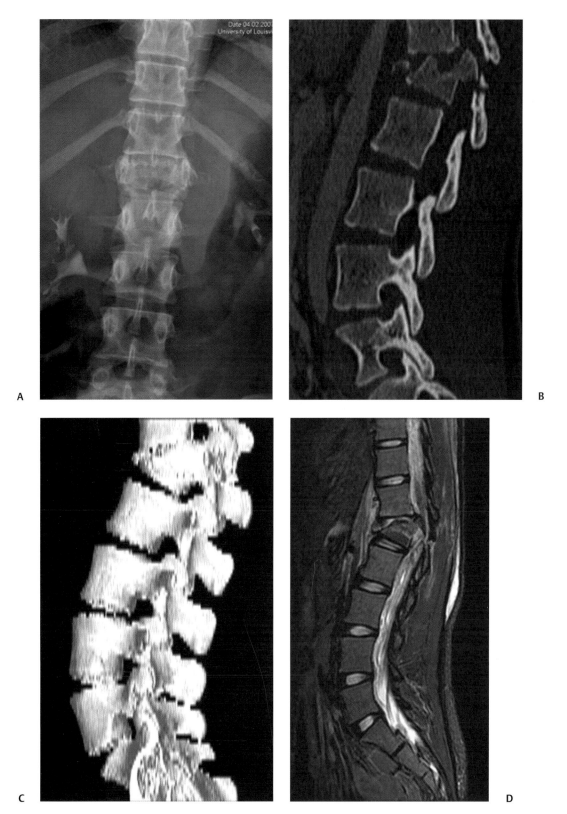

A

B

C

D

Fig. 16.5 A 15-year-old girl involved in a rollover motor vehicle accident who upon arrival to the emergency room was noted to have a flexion-compression burst fracture of L1 on **(A)** plain radiographs and **(B,C)** computed tomographic scans. **(D,E)** Magnetic resonance imaging demonstrated severe canal narrowing at L1. Physical exam demonstrated only mild sacral sparing. *(Continued on page 142)*

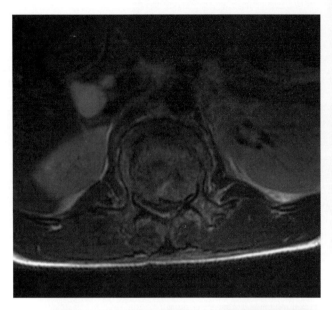

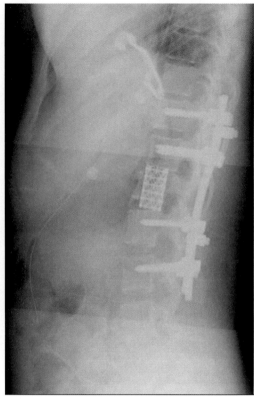

F

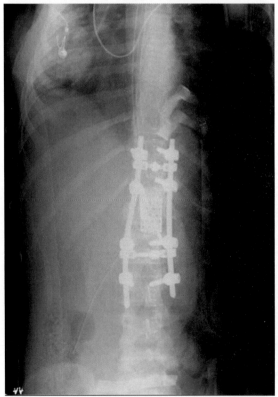

G

Fig. 16.5 *(Continued)* **(F,G)** The patient was taken to surgery where an anterior L1 decompression/vertebrectomy was done followed by a T11–L3 posterior fusion. The patient regained all lower extremity function with the exception of $^3/_5$ dorsiflexion strength 6 months after surgery.

Originally described by Chance in 1948, these fractures are characterized by a horizontal split in the spine and neural arch through the posterior spinous process, pedicles, and vertebral body secondary to a flexion force around an opposing fulcrum.[43] These flexion-distraction injuries were further classified into three types, consisting of type 1: a transverse fracture through bone; type 2: a fracture through the inferior portion of the posterior elements proceeding anteriorly; and type 3: a fracture that is asymmetric, affecting one side or the other.

Seat-belt injuries are more than just the Chance fracture because these higher-energy injuries also have a 31 to 71% incidence of concurrent abdominal injuries and major vessel and lower extremity injuries, which are frequently more life threatening than a simple bony horizontal fracture of the vertebral body.[44,45] When a fracture/dislocation of the spine is combined with a seat-belt sign (severe abdominal ecchymosis across the waist) it is 85% predictive of a significant abdominal injury necessitating an exploratory laparotomy.[46] The most severe of these injuries are typified by the triad of bowel perforation requiring a colostomy, aortic tearing requiring repair and grafting, and a fracture/dislocation of the spine with transection of the spinal cord or cauda equina (**Fig. 16.6**). Although there are no reported outcomes of how

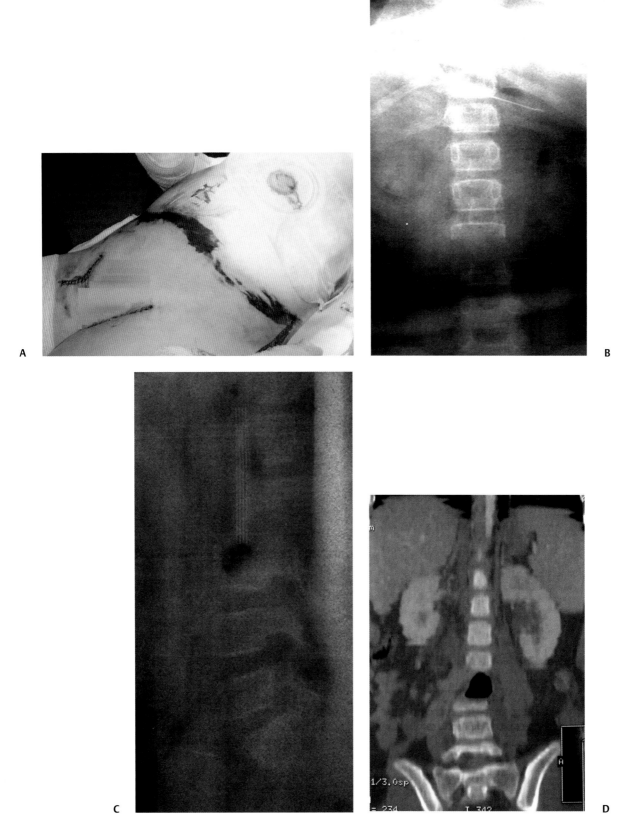

A

B

C

D

Fig. 16.6 A 4-year-old girl was a backseat passenger restrained with a lap belt involved in a motor vehicle accident. In the emergency room she was alert, but unable to move her lower extremities. Upon inspection there was **(A)** a large contusion along the inferior aspect of her abdominal wall, which was consistent with a seat-belt injury. Pulses, motor strength and sensation were absent in both lower extremities. **(B)** Plain anteroposterior and **(C)** lateral radiographs show a fracture dislocation at L2–L3. **(D)** Coronal and *(Continued on page 144)*

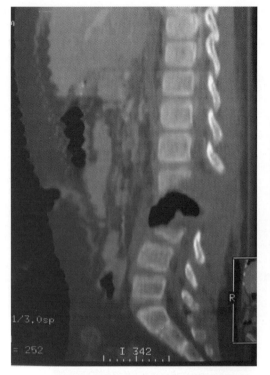

E

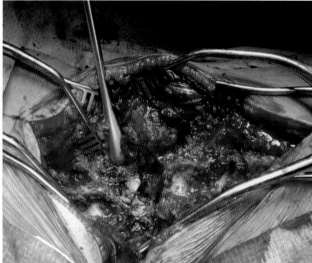

F

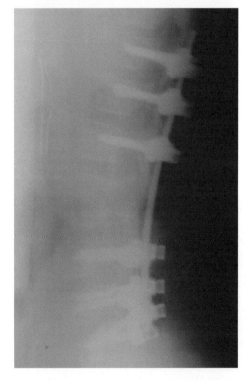

G

Fig. 16.6 *(Continued)* **(E)** sagittal reconstructed computed tomographic scans show disruption of the vertebral column at L3 with interposed bowel. **(F)** Intraoperative photograph shows disrupted vertebral column with avulsed cauda equina. **(G)** Postoperative films show reduction of fracture dislocation. (D, E, and G from Crawford CH, Puno RM, Campbell, MJ, et al. Surgical management of severely displaced pediatric seat-belt fracture-dislocations of the lumbar spine associated with occlusion of the abdominal aorta and avulsion of the cauda equina. SPINE 2008;33(10);E325-E328. Reprinted by permission.)

these severe injuries do long term, it is obvious that they carry an extremely high mortality rate and a minimal chance of neurological recovery.

◆ Summary

Anecdotal experience has generally extrapolated the use of adult treatment paradigms to treatment of children based on the generally accepted opinion that children recover from bony injuries in a superior fashion to that of adults when treated with similar methods. However, there are no conclusive data to support the contention that a pediatric SCI recovers in a similar fashion or has significantly greater chance of recovery than an adult injury. Studies do show that children have unique anatomy that leads to specific injury patterns following trauma. Because the best preclinical evidence supports the prevention of injury and the salvage of remaining function it is prudent to recommend the commonly accepted adult acute spinal cord treatment regimen that includes rapid emergency immobilization, traction, rigid orthotic treatment, and when necessary rapid surgical decompression and stabilization via internal fixation. Perhaps one of the most supportive quoted references of the concept of protection of the spinal cord from secondary injury by the restoration of the spinal canal diameter via decompression and stabilization is the finding that children can have up to 55% static canal narrowing and still have normal neurological function. This fact may be the critical determinant for the hypothesis that children fare better following trauma simply because they are unencumbered by the acquired degenerative changes that cause significant canal narrowing within the adult population increasing the chance of an SCI following a traumatic injury.

References

1. Vialle LR, Vialle E. Pediatric spine injuries. Injury 2005;36(Suppl 2): B104–B112
2. Bracken MB, Collins WF, Freeman DF, et al. Efficacy of methylprednisolone in acute spinal cord injury. JAMA 1984;251:45–52
3. Bracken MB, Shepard MJ, Holford TR, et al. Administration of methylprednisolone for 24 or 48 hours or tirilazad mesylate for 48 hours in the treatment of acute spinal cord injury. Results of the Third National Acute Spinal Cord Injury Randomized Controlled Trial. National Acute Spinal Cord Injury Study. JAMA 1997;277:1597–1604
4. Bracken MB, Shepard MJ, Collins WF, et al. A randomized, controlled trial of methylprednisolone or naloxone in the treatment of acute spinal-cord injury. Results of the Second National Acute Spinal Cord Injury Study. N Engl J Med 1990;322:1405–1411
5. Coleman WP, Benzel D, Cahill DW, et al. A critical appraisal of the reporting of the National Acute Spinal Cord Injury Studies (II and III) of methylprednisolone in acute spinal cord injury. J Spinal Disord 2000;13:185–199
6. Hurlbert RJ. Methylprednisolone for acute spinal cord injury: an inappropriate standard of care. J Neurosurg 2000;93(1, Suppl):1–7
7. Matsumoto T, Tamaki T, Kawakami M, Yoshida M, Ando M, Yamada H. Early complications of high-dose methylprednisolone sodium succinate treatment in the follow-up of acute cervical spinal cord injury. Spine 2001;26:426–430
8. Nesathurai S. Steroids and spinal cord injury: revisiting the NASCIS 2 and NASCIS 3 trials. J Trauma 1998;45:1088–1093
9. Qian T, Guo X, Levi AD, Vanni S, Shebert RT, Sipski ML. High-dose methylprednisolone may cause myopathy in acute spinal cord injury patients. Spinal Cord 2005;43:199–203
10. Sayer FT, Kronvall E, Nilsson OG. Methylprednisolone treatment in acute spinal cord injury: the myth challenged through a structured analysis of published literature. Spine J 2006;6:335–343
11. Geisler FH, Coleman WP, Grieco G, Poonian D ; Sygen Study Group. The Sygen multicenter acute spinal cord injury study. Spine 2001;26(24, Suppl):S87–S98
12. Dimar JR II, Glassman SD, Raque GH, Zhang YP, Shields CB. The influence of spinal canal narrowing and timing of decompression on neurologic recovery after spinal cord contusion in a rat model. Spine 1999;24: 1623–1633
13. Dimar JR II, Shields CB, Zhang YP, Burke DA, Raque GH, Glassman SD. The role of directly applied hypothermia in spinal cord injury. Spine 2000;25:2294–2302
14. Reilly CW. Pediatric spine trauma. J Bone Joint Surg Am 2007;89(Suppl 1):98–107
15. Platzer P, Jaindl M, Thalhammer G, et al. Cervical spine injuries in pediatric patients. J Trauma 2007;62:389–396, discussion 394–396
16. Dogan S, Safavi-Abbasi S, Theodore N, et al. Thoracolumbar and sacral spinal injuries in children and adolescents: a review of 89 cases. J Neurosurg 2007;106(6, Suppl):426–433
17. Brown JK, Jing Y, Wang S, Ehrlich PF. Patterns of severe injury in pediatric car crash victims: Crash Injury Research Engineering Network database. J Pediatr Surg 2006;41:362–367
18. Vitale MG, Goss JM, Matsumoto H, Roye DP Jr. Epidemiology of pediatric spinal cord injury in the United States: years 1997 and 2000. J Pediatr Orthop 2006;26:745–749
19. Caird MS, Reddy S, Ganley TJ, Drummond DS. Cervical spine fracture-dislocation birth injury: prevention, recognition, and implications for the orthopaedic surgeon. J Pediatr Orthop 2005;25:484–486
20. Lallier M, Bouchard S, St-Vil D, Dupont J, Tucci M. Falls from heights among children: a retrospective review. J Pediatr Surg 1999;34:1060–1063
21. Ghatan S, Ellenbogen RG. Pediatric spine and spinal cord injury after inflicted trauma. Neurosurg Clin N Am 2002;13:227–233
22. Augutis M, Levi R. Pediatric spinal cord injury in Sweden: incidence, etiology and outcome. Spinal Cord 2003;41:328–336
23. Vialle R, Piétin-Vialle C, Ilharreborde B, Dauger S, Vinchon M, Glorion C. Spinal cord injuries at birth: a multicenter review of nine cases. J Matern Fetal Neonatal Med 2007;20:435–440
24. McCall T, Fassett D, Brockmeyer D. Cervical spine trauma in children: a review. Neurosurg Focus 2006;20:E5
25. Claret Teruel G, Trenchs Sáinz de la Maza V, Palomeque Rico A. Pediatric acute spinal cord injury [in Spanish]. An Pediatr (Barc) 2006;65:162–165
26. Anderson RC, Scaife ER, Fenton SJ, Kan P, Hansen KW, Brockmeyer DL. Cervical spine clearance after trauma in children. J Neurosurg 2006;105 (5, Suppl):361–364
27. Leventhal HR. Birth injuries of the spinal cord. J Pediatr 1960;56:447–453
28. Pizzutillo PD. Injury of the cervical spine in young children. Instr Course Lect 2006;55:633–639
29. Dogan S, Safavi-Abbasi S, Theodore N, Horn E, Rekate HL, Sonntag VK. Pediatric subaxial cervical spine injuries: origins, management, and outcome in 51 patients. Neurosurg Focus 2006;20:E1
30. Reynolds R. Pediatric spinal injury. Curr Opin Pediatr 2000;12:67–71
31. Akbarnia BA. Pediatric spine fractures. Orthop Clin North Am 1999;30: 521–536, x
32. Pang D, Pollack IF. Spinal cord injury without radiographic abnormality in children—the SCIWORA syndrome. J Trauma 1989;29:654–664
33. Khanna AJ, Wasserman BA, Sponseller PD. Magnetic resonance imaging of the pediatric spine. J Am Acad Orthop Surg 2003;11:248–259
34. Pang D. Spinal cord injury without radiographic abnormality in children, 2 decades later. Neurosurgery 2004;55:1325–1342, discussion 1342–1343
35. Launay F, Leet AI, Sponseller PD. Pediatric spinal cord injury without radiographic abnormality: a meta-analysis. Clin Orthop Relat Res 2005;(433): 166–170
36. Bosch PP, Vogt MT, Ward WT. Pediatric spinal cord injury without radiographic abnormality (SCIWORA): the absence of occult instability and lack of indication for bracing. Spine 2002;27:2788–2800
37. Eleraky MA, Theodore N, Adams M, Rekate HL, Sonntag VK. Pediatric cervical spine injuries: report of 102 cases and review of the literature. J Neurosurg 2000;92(1, Suppl):12–17
38. Zuckerbraun BS, Morrison K, Gaines B, Ford HR, Hackam DJ. Effect of age on cervical spine injuries in children after motor vehicle collisions: effectiveness of restraint devices. J Pediatr Surg 2004;39:483–486
39. Santiago R, Guenther E, Carroll K, Junkins EP Jr. The clinical presentation of pediatric thoracolumbar fractures. J Trauma 2006;60:187–192
40. Reddy SP, Junewick JJ, Backstrom JW. Distribution of spinal fractures in children: does age, mechanism of injury, or gender play a significant role? Pediatr Radiol 2003;33:776–781
41. Lalonde F, Letts M, Yang JP, Thomas K. An analysis of burst fractures of the spine in adolescents. Am J Orthop 2001;30:115–120
42. Sturm PF, Glass RB, Sivit CJ, Eichelberger MR. Lumbar compression fractures secondary to lap-belt use in children. J Pediatr Orthop 1995;15: 521–523
43. Chance GQ. Note on a type of flexion fracture of the spine. Br J Radiol 1948;21:452–453
44. Carreon LY, Glassman SD, Campbell MJ. Pediatric spine fractures: a review of 137 hospital admissions. J Spinal Disord Tech 2004;17:477–482
45. Glassman SD, Johnson JR, Holt RT. Seatbelt injuries in children. J Trauma 1992;33:882–886
46. Tyroch AH, McGuire EL, McLean SF, et al. The association between Chance fractures and intra-abdominal injuries revisited: a multicenter review. Am Surg 2005;71:434–438

17

Principles of Spinal Instrumentation in the Treatment of Pediatric Cervical, Thoracic, and Lumbar Spinal Injuries

Ahmet Alanay and Z. Deniz Olgun

Pediatric spinal injuries, although rare, constitute an important cause of morbidity and mortality, not to mention the economical ramifications of healthy individuals becoming disabled. Mechanisms of injury as well as the treatment methods are unique in the growing spine as opposed to those in adults. This chapter focuses on the most commonly seen pediatric spinal injuries and their management in regard to the specific anatomy and growth potential of the spinal column. The chapter also discusses whether many pediatric fractures should be treated nonoperatively, considering the remodeling capacity of the pediatric spine.

◆ Relevant Developmental Anatomy

Due to the intrinsic properties of the immature spine, injury patterns, especially in the younger child, differ from those encountered in the adult. Some injuries are seen exclusively in children, such as growth-plate-related fractures and SCIWORA.[1] All typical vertebrae, except for the atypical C1 and C2 (atlas and axis, respectively), have three ossification centers: one anterior centrum and two posterior arches.[2] This allows multidimensional growth, especially of the spinal canal. Most of the growth of the diameter of the spinal canal is completed by 6 to 8 years of age.

Longitudinal growth in the human spine occurs not in the primary ossification centers of the vertebral bodies but in the chondroepiphyseal portions of the end plates. These areas are also responsible for circumferential growth. Through a posterior growth plate at the spinous process synchondrosis and at the pedicle/vertebral body junction, the posterior elements also demonstrate circumferential and longitudinal growth. Posterior element growth ceases at 5 to 8 years of age, whereas anterior growth continues until ages 16 to 18. Longitudinal growth is the result of enchondral ossification, whereas circumferential growth is due to perichondral and periosteal apposition.[3] The term *ring apophysis* is a misnomer;

it is the thickened region of the end plates that undergoes shear and compression rather than tension, as a true apophysis. A focus of ossification appears at the ages 12 to 15 around the end plate epiphyses, giving rise to the radiological ring. The ring apophysis has been implicated in fractures, herniating into the spinal canal and mimicking symptoms of a disk protrusion.[4]

The disk in the immature spine is a very firm structure and more resistant to injury than the vertebral bone.[5] When compressive forces act on the immature spinal column, the cartilaginous end plate often fails before the anulus, resulting in Schmorl nodules rather than disk protrusion into the spinal canal as occurs in adults.[1,6,7] Compression forces are also transmitted as a wave to multiple levels by the more elastic disks, resulting in the multiple compression fractures that are seen more commonly in children than in adults.[8,9]

The pediatric spine is in a state of continual change. Leventhal proved that the bony column in the immature spine is far more elastic than the neural elements and can distend up to 2 inches without disruption. The spinal cord, on the other hand, can only tolerate stretching up to 0.25 inch.[10] Children under 8 years of age have increased cervical motion compared with older children and adults. This has been shown to be the result of relative ligamentous laxity, muscle weakness, incomplete ossification, and horizontal orientation of the shallow facet joints found in the developing spine. As the cervical spine approaches adult size, vertebral bodies become more rectangular, facet orientation changes to the configuration seen in the adult, and ligaments and facet capsules increase in tensile strength, resulting in a more adultlike pattern of injury. It is because of these unique anatomical considerations that spinal cord injury without radiological abnormality is more prevalent in the pediatric population. The size of the head relative to the body is larger in children. Added to the inherent hypermobility of the pediatric spine, this results in a higher fulcrum of motion as compared with the adult (C2–C3 in children versus C5–C6 in adults).[11–13]

◆ Injuries of the Cervical Spine

Atlanto-occipital Dislocation

Although injuries to the occipitocervical region are generally fatal and are therefore underreported,[14] with improved immobilization and transportation techniques, more patients are surviving.[15,16] The large head:body ratio of especially younger children and the relative underdevelopment of their neck musculature with ligamentous hyperlaxity make them particularly susceptible to this injury. Anatomically, smaller occipital condyles and a more horizontal plane of the atlanto-occipital joint might explain the predilection of this injury to children.[17,18] Injuries of the occipitocervical junction are usually ligamentous in nature and therefore very unstable. The rupture of the alar ligaments and the tectorial membrane is enough to result in atlanto-occipital dissociation.[19] With the correct immobilization techniques, deformity may reduce, and diagnosis by plain films can be difficult. Despite improvements in transportation, management, and surgical techniques, injuries of the occipitocervical junction still have the poorest prognosis of all spinal injuries.[20]

Traction should never be applied in the patient with possible atlanto-occipital dislocation; focus should be on appropriate immobilization. Surgical treatment is generally an occiput to C2–C4 fusion with or without instrumentation combined with autograft.[15,21,22] Nonoperative treatment consists of Halo-vest immobilization or Minerva casts in selected patients.[15] Recent literature supports the use of occipitocervical plates and contoured titanium rods instead of the more traditional methods of onlay grafting and wiring techniques.[23-25]

Atlantoaxial Subluxation

There are two types of atlantoaxial subluxation: rotatory and translational. Translational atlantoaxial subluxation is a rare injury resulting from high-energy flexion/extension and distraction mechanisms. It occurs when the transverse ligament is torn and the cord is compressed between the odontoid and the posterior arch of the atlas. MRI may show this ligamentous rupture. Treatment is generally surgical, but data regarding this rare injury are scant.

Atlantoaxial rotatory subluxation is thought to result from physiological hypermobility of the atlantoaxial articulation during a sudden and violent turn of the head.[26] It has also been explained as the entrapment of synovial folds between the C1 and C2 joints.[27] The cause can be minor trauma or a nasopharyngeal infection, and patients present with acute acquired torticollis (the so-called cock-robin appearance).[14] Plain x-rays are usually inadequate in diagnosis and dynamic rotation. Computed tomography (CT) performed in neutral, right, and left rotated positions has been suggested as a more accurate modality.[28] However, the interobserver and intraobserver reliability of dynamic CT has been found to be poor, and it has been suggested that dynamic CT should be performed only if acute torticollis caused by a minor trauma fails to respond to a week of soft collar treatment.[29,30] The method of treatment chosen depends on the time that the symptoms have been present. If symptoms have been present less than a week, a course of nonsteroidal antiinflammatory medications with muscle relaxants and a soft collar may be attempted. If symptoms persist for more than a week, halter traction should be attempted. Symptoms lasting for more than a month have been treated with posterior cervical fusion of C1 to C2.[14,31] Crossman et al have reported good functional outcome using open reduction, adjunct fixation, and postoperative halo immobilization in 13 pediatric patients with irreducible atlantoaxial rotatory subluxation.[32]

Odontoid Fractures

Fractures of the odontoid usually occur as a result of motor vehicle accidents or severe falls. In children younger than 5 years of age, the odontoid synchondrosis is still open, predisposing this age group to this injury.[14] Due to the intrinsic anatomical properties of this region, fractures tend to decompress the cord; therefore, neurological injury is rare. Diagnosis is made by lateral cervical x-rays. CT examination and sagittal reconstruction may be needed in questionable cases. Displaced fractures can be reduced safely under sedation, generally in extension. These injuries heal well with adequate immobilization. Nondisplaced fractures can successfully be managed with Minerva style jacket or halo vest application. Anterior fixation may be considered for the treatment of odontoid fractures or nonunions in adolescent patients.[33]

Injuries of the Subaxial Cervical Spine

As the child grows older and the spine becomes more mature, the fulcrum of movement with flexion/extension shifts in a more caudal direction. Therefore, subaxial cervical spine injuries are more common in older children and mimic adult fracture patterns, unlike those that occur in the very young, which are generally above C4.[1] Bony fractures are the most commonly observed among subaxial cervical spine injuries, followed by fractures with dislocation, pure dislocations, and ligamentous injuries.[34] Among fractures, compression fractures with flexion mechanisms predominate.

Literature regarding subaxial cervical injuries is scant, reflecting the rarity of isolated injuries of this region.[34-36] Less severe injuries such as simple compression fractures and burst fractures without neurological injury and posterior ligamentous disruption may be treated by immobilization alone using a collar or Minerva-jacket brace. Unilateral or bilateral facet dislocations should be reduced under conscious sedation and then immobilized with halo vest application for 3 months. Fracture dislocations, compression and burst fractures with ligamentous injuries, and patients with neurological deterioration may warrant surgical treatment as in adults. Dogan et al reported the successful use of instrumentation in the pediatric population, excellent rates of arthrodesis, good clinical outcome, and normal growth of the cervical spine with both anterior and posterior approaches.[34]

◆ Injuries of the Thoracolumbar Spine

Thoracolumbar fractures in children are rare. The pediatric thoracolumbar spine assumes adult characteristics by age 8, after which it shows adult patterns of injury. Thoracolumbar fractures are more common in older children.[37] Thoracolumbar fractures in older children can therefore be classified according to the three-column theory of Denis.[38] Injuries according to this system are grouped into four major types: compression fractures, burst fractures, flexion-distraction or Chance fractures, and fracture-dislocations, which represent the most severe end of the spectrum.

Compression Fractures

Compression fractures of the thoracic spine are relatively common, whereas those involving the lumbar spine are less so. They are incurred oftentimes as the result of falls from a height, and due to the firmness of the immature disk, multiple levels can be fractured. Only the anterior column is involved, rendering these injuries inherently stable and manageable by conservative methods. Vertebral height loss is usually compensated for by residual growth through the vertebral body. There is significant evidence that in compression fractures in children under the age of 10 years, correction of sagittal plane deformity occurs within the remodeling capacity of the pediatric spine.[1,39,40] Frontal plane deformity is not remodeled as effectively.

Treatment is mainly conservative. Mild compression fractures usually respond well to bed rest and immobilization. Those with less than 50% of height loss can be treated nonoperatively but should be followed for a longer time to exclude postinjury deformity (**Fig. 17.1**).[1] Severe compression fractures spanning multiple levels should be treated with a full

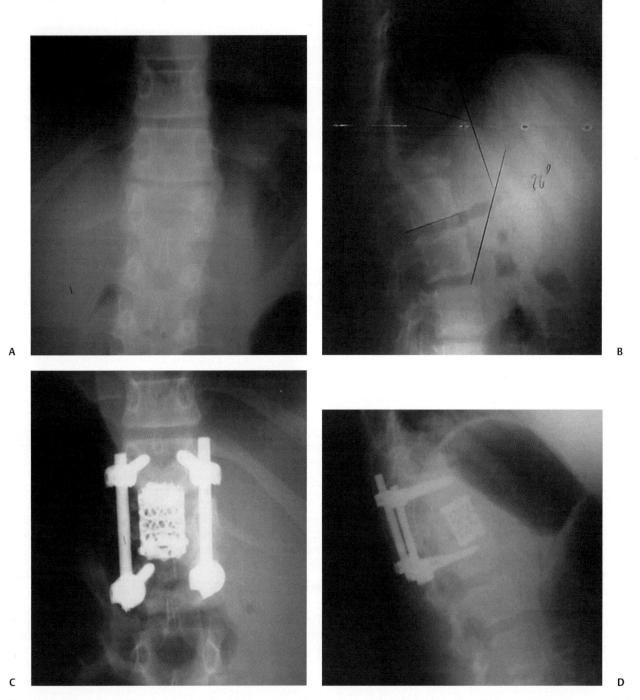

A

B

C

D

Fig. 17.1 **(A)** A 13-year-old female patient. Patient fell from a height 3 years ago but did not seek medical attention until increasingly unremitting back pain developed that failed to respond to conservative measures. **(B)** Lateral radiograph of same patient displaying a T12-compression fracture and segmental kyphosis of 36 degrees as measured by the Cobb method. **(C)** Sequential-simultaneous anterior-posterior surgery was performed on the patient with removal of the T12 vertebral body, cage placement, and posterior instrumentation with pedicle screws, followed by fusion. **(D)** Following surgery sagittal alignment is reestablished. Symptoms resolved completely.

contact thoracolumbosacral orthosis (TLSO) or with posterior compressive instrumentation and fusion if significant instability is present.[41]

Burst Fractures

These generally occur in adolescents and are therefore analogous to their adult counterparts. Anterior and middle columns are involved in this injury, and the mechanism is axial compression as occurs after a high energy fall. By definition, these injuries are unstable, more so in the child with a less effective posterior ligamentous complex as compared with the adult.[1] Burst fractures develop due to end plate fracture by the forceful entrance of the nucleus pulposus into the vertebral body and therefore may lead to growth plate damage. It is for this reason that, depending on the amount of growth remaining, kyphotic deformity may increase with age following burst fractures. Magnetic resonance scanning is essential because

plain radiographs and CT cannot always appreciate an additional injury of the posterior ligamentous complex.

Treatment ranges from hyperextension orthoses to surgical stabilization. Patients without posterior ligamentous complex injury can be managed with hyperextension orthoses, whereas those with ligamentous injury, particularly at the thoracolumbar junction and neurological compromise, should be treated with decompression and stabilization (**Fig. 17.2**). It has been found that residual deformity does not correlate with functional outcome in these patients.[1] Thoracolumbar burst fractures with severe kyphosis may require anterior column reconstruction.[41]

Flexion-Distraction Fractures

First described by Chance in 1948, these injuries have the distinct mechanism of flexion and distraction of the spine as classically occurs during a head-on motor vehicle collision to

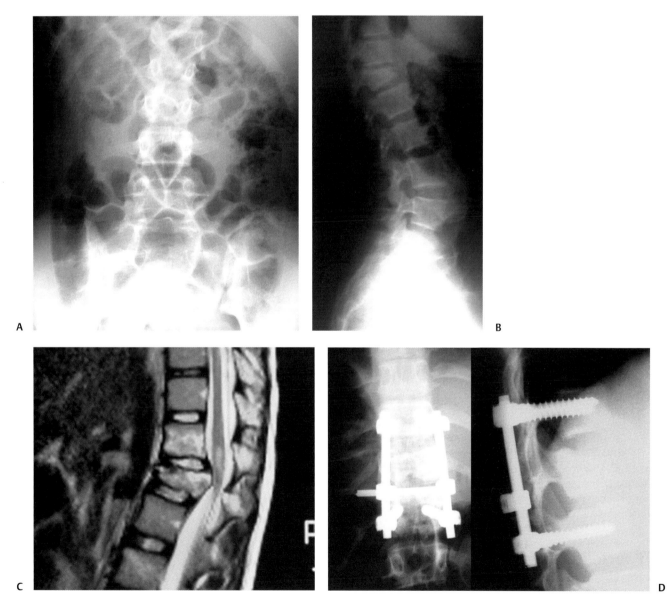

Fig. 17.2 **(A)** A 12-year-old female patient involved in a motor vehicle accident. She presented with an L1 burst fracture and partial neurological deficit. **(B)** Lateral plain x-ray of the same patient. **(C)** Preoperative magnetic resonance imaging of the same patient displaying the fracture and severe compression of the cord. **(D)** Postoperative x-rays displaying posterior distractive instrumentation with pedicle screws and a transverse connector followed by fusion. Sagittal alignment and vertebral height were both restored.

a person restrained by a lap belt. Designed to contact the iliac wings originally, in a small child the lap belt slides up to cross the abdomen and, changing the distribution of forces, causes a hyperflexion moment with the belt as the pivoting point. Although seatbelts have been proven to reduce the risk of injury or death in motor vehicle collisions, they change the axis of rotation of the lumbosacral spine in a child, distributing the hyperflexion forces through the midportion of the spine. This results in a distinct pattern of injuries commonly referred to as seat-belt syndrome.[42–44] Clinical exam often reveals a classic seat-belt sign, a distinct form of abdominal bruising, combined with severe low back pain with palpation and a palpable "gapping of the intraspinous ligaments." Newer designs of lap belts with shoulder harnesses and three-point fixation along with airbags have reduced the prevalence of this mechanism of injury in many regions.

The pathomechanism of these injuries is thought to be the rapid deceleration caused by the seat belt causing compression of the abdominal contents and sudden violent flexion of the upper body.[9,45] Among the injuries included in the seat-belt syndrome are abdominal contusions, intraabdominal injuries (especially hollow viscus perforations), liver and spleen injuries, major vessel injury (aortal and vena cava) and flexion-distraction type lumbar spinal injuries that may result in severe neurological injury.[44] The spinal injuries can be purely osseous, constituting a true Chance fracture, purely ligamentous or combined.[14,46,47] Flexion-distraction injuries are by definition unstable; all three columns are disrupted: posterior and middle columns by distraction and the anterior column by compression.[5,9,48]

Purely osseous injuries generally reduce with hyperextension and heal well with spica cast immobilization, whereas purely ligamentous injuries or those with evidence of severe posterior ligamentous injury should be treated with surgical fusion. Surgical treatment should be considered for patients with neurological deterioration, polytrauma, inadequate reduction, segmental kyphosis of more than 20 degrees, and the inability to tolerate cast treatment.[14,49] Mulpuri et al in a recent study have shown that intervertebral kyphosis remodeling and spontaneous correction are better in surgically treated patients.[49]

Fracture-Dislocations

Fracture-dislocations represent the severest form of injury to the spine. All three columns are disrupted by a high-energy mechanism of injury. In these injuries, a rotational or shear component exists, and these are by definition very unstable injuries. Neurological injury can be encountered. In these rare injuries, treatment should aim to preserve neurological status (**Fig. 17.3**). Due to the inherent instability of these injuries, operative treatment should be considered regardless of neurological injury (**Fig. 17.4**). Periosteal sleeve healing of apparent dislocations can occur in small children (**Fig. 17.5**).

◆ Principles of Instrumentation for the Growing Spine

Children represent a unique challenge for the spinal surgeon. Not only are their mechanisms of injury different, their skeletal immaturity provides controversy as to the prudent course of action. Pediatric vertebral column morphology holds many contrasts to that of the adult spine, the most glaring of which is size and the difficulty it creates for the application of modern spinal instrumentation techniques. Another important issue is the effect of fusion procedures to treat unstable fractures on the growth potential of the spinal column.

Cervical Spine

Pediatric cervical spine instrumentation techniques in the past included interspinous wiring and sublaminar wiring, both of which can be combined with various rod and hook constructs.[23,51,52] Due to the unreliable biomechanical stability of wires and rods, however, there is a requirement for an additional method of external stabilization. Currently there exists a tendency in pediatric spinal surgery to use rigid segmental instrumentation techniques.

Modern segmental instrumentation relies on studies of morphology. To date, there are no studies regarding the morphology of the developing human occiput or cervical spinal lateral masses from the spinal surgery point of view. In a study of human pediatric cadaveric cervical spines by Vara and Thompson, the feasibility of surgical pedicle screw instrumentation of the pediatric cervical spine was evaluated among other objectives.[53] The pedicle axis length, defined as the line parallel to the axis of the pedicle and passing through the center of the same, was found to increase with age. The pedicle diameter, perhaps the most important measurement in the use of pedicle screws, was shown to increase significantly with growth. In the youngest age group (3 to 5 years old), mean pedicle diameter width was 3.0 mm at C3 and 4.2 mm at C7. This shows a dramatic difference in pedicle diameter width when compared with the 18-year group, whose pedicle diameter widths of C3 and C7 were 4.3 and 6.1 mm, respectively. The anteroposterior canal diameter was found to be relatively constant among age groups, and the interpedicular distance reached 80% of adult dimensions by age 3 to 5. The pedicle itself was found to contribute a progressively smaller percentage to overall vertebral growth. Pedicle length was not found to change significantly. The authors concluded that due to small pedicle widths, pedicle screw instrumentation in the cervical spine of children, particularly younger ones, may not be safe.

Despite the lack of detailed morphological studies related to ideal implant shape and size for cervical instrumentation in the pediatric spine, there are a few studies reporting safe and successful application of available adult-size implants for pediatric cervical spine pathologies. C1–C2 transarticular fixation is the most extensively studied technique among other modern instrumentation techniques. Reilly and Choit have reported 12 patients aged 5.8 to 16.9 years who had C1–C2 transarticular fixation for instability with no major complications.[54] Gluf and Brockmeyer have recently reported the results of atlantoaxial transarticular fixation in 67 consecutive pediatric patients with ages ranging from 1.7 to 16 years. One hundred percent of fusion was obtained by successful C1–C2 fixation, and the complication rate was 10.4%, including two vertebral artery injuries that were managed with no long-term problems.[56] Both papers emphasized the importance of preoperative CT evaluation of the anatomy. Rigid plate/rod fixation of the occiput for occipitocervical fusion has also been successfully performed in many case series[54,56,57] with the application of principles available for adult patients.

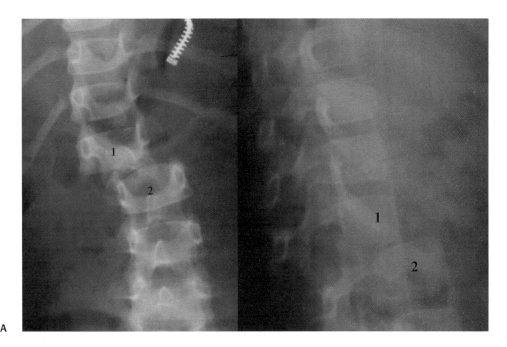

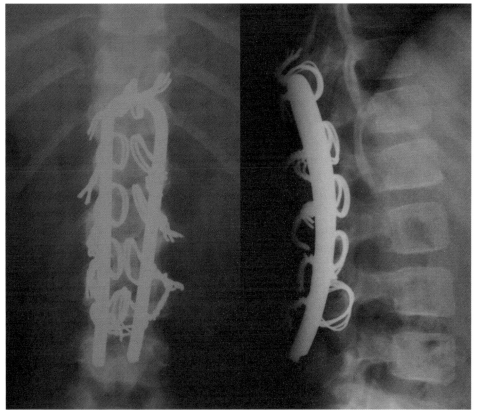

Fig. 17.3 **(A)** A 6-year-old female victim of a farm machine accident. L1–L2 dislocation without fracture is noted on plain x-rays. The patient had incomplete paraplegia on referral. **(B)** Follow-up radiographs after surgical treatment with a modified Luque frame and sublaminar wires. Six months after surgery, patient's neurological deficit recovered completely.

One issue concerning occiput–C1–C2 fusion is the complex anatomical circumstances that make bilateral transarticular fixation difficult. Anderson et al have recently reported alternative fixation techniques in these circumstances and demonstrated that it was also possible to apply other techniques available for adult patients.[25]

Lateral mass fixation of the subaxial spine was described by Hedequist et al. The authors analyzed the safety and efficacy of modern instrumentation techniques in a group of 25 pediatric patients aged 6 to 15 years. Postoperative CT evaluation of 112 implants demonstrated that all were in correct position and fully contained within bone. All the

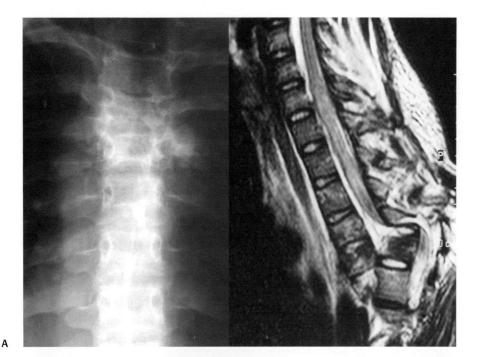

A

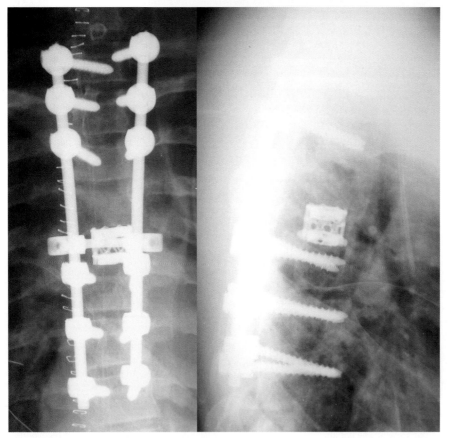

B

Fig. 17.4 (A) A 16-year-old male patient with T4–T5 fracture dislocation after suffering a motor vehicle accident. The patient was kept in the intensive care unit for 3 weeks due to head trauma. His T4–T5 fracture-dislocation was left untreated during this period. The patient had complete neurological deficit below T4. **(B)** After the patient regained consciousness, he was transferred to the authors' institution where removal of the T5 vertebral body was performed along with realignment and cage placement all through a posterior approach. Expectedly, neurological deficit remained unchanged.

patients had successful fusion with no implant-related complications.[55]

There are only few reports in the literature regarding anterior instrumentation techniques.[33,55,58] Two case studies reported successful fixation of odontoid fractures; one in a 15-year-old child[33] and the other[58] in a 2.5-year-old child with no implant-related complications. Hedequist et al performed anterior plate fixation in eight patients, with anterior cages in six of them.

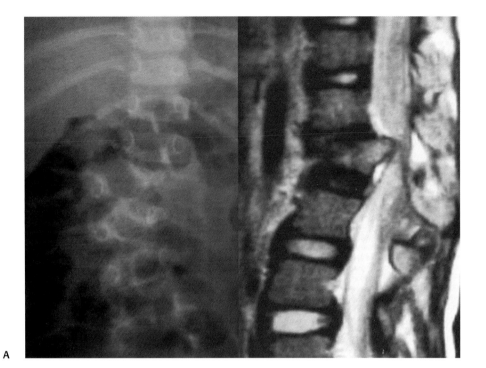

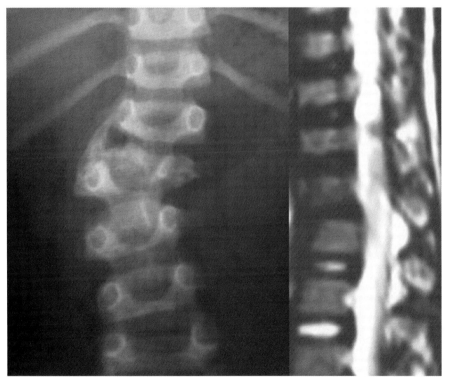

Fig. 17.5 (A) A 3-year-old boy who fell down 5 m feet-first onto concrete. L1–L2 dislocation without fracture was identified in plain x-rays. The patient was neurologically intact. **(B)** X-rays 2 years after the injury. Despite the lack of surgical treatment, coronal realignment was restored. Spinal canal patency was reestablished as demonstrated on sagittal magnetic resonance imaging. (From Guzel A, Belen D, Tatli M, Simsek S, Guzel E. Complete L1–L2 lateral dislocation without fracture and neurologic deficit in a child. Pediatr Neurosurg 2006;42(3): 183–186.[73] Reprinted with permission.)

The ages of these patients requiring anterior surgery ranged from 12 to 16 years. The authors did not encounter any intra-operative or postoperative problems with implant sizes in these adolescent patients, but they caution against potential size mismatches in younger children.[55]

In summary, segmental rigid instrumentation techniques using implants designed for adults may be performed safely in younger children with appropriately downsized systems. Potential benefits may include increasing the rate of fusion and the success of clinical outcomes and obviating the need for additional external immobilization. Meticulous preoperative planning regarding the suitability of morphology and careful patient selection are the key issues leading to safe and successful results.

One of the major concerns following the instrumentation and fusion of the growing spine is the long-term effect of these fusions on the growth and alignment of the cervical spine. There are no reports on the effect of fusion on canal size and the length of the cervical spinal column, which have been major issues following fusion for thoracolumbar spinal problems in growing children. The only well-studied potential complication of fusion is subaxial sagittal alignment after C1–C2 fusion. The few studies that have described the onset of postoperative compensatory subaxial sagittal cervical deformities after the fusion of C1–C2[59–61] demonstrated that any sagittal plane deformity that occurred after C1–C2 fusion corrected gradually with remodeling of the subaxial spine. Later, Anderson et al retrospectively evaluated 17 children under the age of 6 who had posterior C1–C2 fusion performed on them and demonstrated that there were no cases of sagittal malalignment, subaxial instability, or unintended fusion of adjacent levels at final follow-up.[57] There is obviously the need for long-term follow-up studies to determine precisely how children's spines grow and remodel after cervical spinal fusion.

Thoracic and Lumbar Spine

Modern instrumentation techniques for the pediatric thoracolumbar spine have led to the development of special instrumentation sets designed to address the morphology of the pediatric thoracolumbar spine. Pedicle screw instrumentation is the most commonly used instrumentation technique due to its advantage of providing rigid segmental fixation that obviates the need for longer fusions and enables more powerful correction forces to manage posttraumatic deformity. The morphology of thoracic and lumbar pedicles in children has been well studied.[62,63] In a recent clinical study by Senaran et al, the lumbar pedicle morphology of the immature spine was studied using three-dimensional spiral CT. Twenty-one children aged 5 to 10 years were evaluated, and their inner- and outer-pedicle diameters, pedicle angles, and pedicle lengths measured. Lumbar pedicle dimensions were found to decrease progressively from L5 to L1, whereas pedicle angles increased, reflecting the results of previous studies. The authors concluded that, although it is safe to use standard implants in the instrumentation of L4–L5 pedicles in children aged 5 to 8 years and L3–L5 in older children, custom-made implants should be considered for the safe instrumentation of more proximal levels in all age groups.[63] In an effort to develop methods enabling the segmental instrumentation of the pediatric spine with standard implants, Yazici et al studied the possibility of pedicle expansion using immature porcine thoracolumbar spines and stainless steel pedicle dilators.[64] Significant increases in internal and external pedicle width were achieved; however, pullout strengths suffered considerably in return.

The effect of the insertion of pedicle screws on the portion of growth provided by the neurocentral junction is a matter of debate. In an experimental study by Cil et al, newborn pigs were operated on and their pedicles probed, instrumented with screws only or instrumented with screws and washers, exerting compression across the neurocentral cartilage. Pedicle screws passing through the neurocentral cartilage even without compression were found to disturb spinal canal growth significantly, and clinical correlation with young children was questioned.[65] However, a retrospective analysis by Ruf and Harms of 16 1- to 2-year-old children instrumented with pedicle screws showed that in a 6-year-long follow-up period, no adverse effects related to vertebral growth or neurological function could be demonstrated. The authors concluded that pedicle screw fixation could be safely performed in very young children.[66]

Spinal instrumentation and fusion in the thoracic and lumbar spine with the potential for growth remains a controversy. Early fusion may result in shorter trunk height and may interfere with the development of the thoracic cage and subsequently the lungs, resulting in poor pulmonary function.[3,68,69]

The crankshaft phenomenon on the other hand is also a consequence of spinal fusion in children. It occurs when there is solid fusion of the posterior components of the spine, with sufficient anterior growth remaining to produce spinal deformity. This phenomenon occurring after selective posterior fusion was first described by Dubousset et al in a retrospective review of 40 spinal fusions done prior to Risser stage 1 for idiopathic and paralytic scoliosis. Thirty-nine of these patients were shown to have progressive angulation and rotation of the spine, and the more immature the patient, the greater the resultant progression.[70] However, a 1996 experimental study by Kioschos et al comparing fusion without instrumentation and fusion with instrumentation in skeletally immature canines showed that rigid transpedicular constructs overcome the crankshaft phenomenon, resulting in the absence of late deformity.[71] Fortunately, thoracolumbar spine fractures in children may be successfully treated by short segment instrumentation and fusion techniques unless there is a multilevel fracture, rendering these issues of less importance in the management of pediatric spinal fractures.

Anterior procedures in the pediatric trauma patient have been reported in conjunction with severely kyphotic and comminuted burst fractures in adolescents.[72] The question regarding neurocentral growth in the immature spine gave rise to an experimental study in our institute.[68] We evaluated the effect of anterior spinal fusion in the immature porcine spine on the development of the spinal canal. Twelve 8-week-old domestic pigs were used to develop an anterior fusion model. The spines were instrumented and fused from L3 to L5. Spinal canal areas were measured with the help of CT scanning. Anterior arthrodesis was found to result in the iatrogenic retardation of spinal canal growth. Although the clinical impact of this study is unclear, spine surgeons should be aware that every intervention may result in inadvertent deformity due to loss of growth potential.

We performed a systematic review in response to the question that was posed at the outset of this chapter as to whether pediatric fractures should be treated nonoperatively considering the remodeling capacity of the pediatric spine. In this review we searched the National Library of Medicine database of the literature published from 1966 to 2008. The medical subject headings "spine, fracture, child" yielded 1407 citations. Abstracts were reviewed for those that described children who had sustained or were being evaluated for cervical, thoracic, thoracolumbar, and lumbar fractures. Among these, articles describing patients with spinal fractures occurring in childhood (birth to 18 years old) and reevaluated after the growth is completed and specifically focusing on the remodeling capacity of spinal column were used to generate the recommendations. None of the studies on cervical spine fractures fit our criteria. There were only four papers on thoracolumbar fractures fitting the inclusion criteria (**Table 17.1**).

Table 17.1 Literature Review of Treatment of Pediatric Spine Fractures

Investigator	Description	Level of Evidence	Topic and Conclusion
Moller et al[50]	Retrospective case series	Level 4	Investigating the remodeling capacity and outcome of late adolescent thoracolumbar fractures. Conclusions: Thoracolumbar fractures with no neurological compromise in late adolescent children treated nonoperatively have favorable outcome even if a remodeling capacity does not occur. Weaknesses: 40% lost to f/up. No other information on maturity other than age
Pouliquen et al[40]	Retrospective case series	Level 4	Evaluating the natural history of growth of epiphyseal plates and influence of treatment on it after uncomplicated thoracic and lumbar spine fractures. Conclusions: compression fractures in patients with Risser 0–1 and with less than 10 degrees of kyphosis remodels well. Conservative treatment still effective in more than 10 degrees of kyphosis in patients Risser less than 2. Not effective in patients Risser 3 or more. Patients with scoliosis over 15 degrees may not remodel and require surgery. Best results in terms of kyphosis and scoliosis were obtained by surgery with acute correction; however, the vertebral volume did not remodel perhaps due to growth arrest by fusion. Weaknesses: Too many patients dropped out, small sample size.
Magnus et al[67]	Retrospective case series although described as observational cohort study by the authors	Level 4	Aims to determine incidence, localization, and long-term outcome of thoracolumbar fracture under age 16. Conclusion: 30% of patients all under 13 had a remodeling capacity. Long-term clinical outcome is favorable for compression and burst fracture for children under age 16. Weaknesses: retrospective case series with more than 50% dropouts. No comparison group (surgical treatment), no sufficient information about the maturity of patients (menarche, Risser sign, etc.) other than age, small sample size, although the largest in the literature
Parisini et al[61]	Retrospective case series	Level 4	Aims to investigate the long-term outcome of conservatively and surgically treated patients with thoracolumbar and cervical fractures in patients younger than 16 years old. Forty-four patients included, none lost to f/up. Conclusions: conservative treatment is valid for stable fractures, whereas surgery results in a better outcome for the unstable fractures. There is not too much statement on the remodeling capacity; however, according to these results the remodeling capacity is only slightly effective for stable fractures, whereas it does not work for unstable fractures. Of note, only six patients in this series were younger than 12 years, and of six, four had spinal cord injury. Weaknesses: invalid outcome tools, subjective assessments, limited number of patients to conclude on remodeling capacity.

◆ Summary and Recommendations

There is insufficient evidence to support a general conclusion regarding the remodeling capacity of spinal fractures of children. It is difficult to estimate the behavior of the acute deformities in the growing spine relying on the available reports in the literature.

Conservative treatment is recommended in stable thoracic, thoracolumbar, and lumbar compression or burst fractures (strong) due to significant remodeling potential particularly related to the sagittal plane deformity. For unstable fractures or those with coronal plane deformity or neurological impairment surgery is recommended (weak).

References

1. Akbarnia BA. Pediatric spine fractures. Orthop Clin North Am 1999;30: 521–536, x
2. Labrom RD. Growth and maturation of the spine from birth to adolescence. J Bone Joint Surg Am 2007;89(Suppl 1):3–7
3. Dimeglio A. Growth in pediatric orthopaedics. J Pediatr Orthop 2001;21: 549–555
4. Sovio OM, Bell HM, Beauchamp RD, Tredwell SJ. Fracture of the lumbar vertebral apophysis. J Pediatr Orthop 1985;5:550–552
5. Clark P, Letts M. Trauma to the thoracic and lumbar spine in the adolescent. Can J Surg 2001;44:337–345
6. Aufdermaur M. Spinal injuries in juveniles: necropsy findings in twelve cases. J Bone Joint Surg Br 1974;56B:513–519
7. Roaf R. A study of the mechanics of spinal injuries. J Bone Joint Surg Br 1960;42:810–823
8. Hadley MN, Zabramski JM, Browner CM, Rekate H, Sonntag VK. Pediatric spinal trauma: review of 122 cases of spinal cord and vertebral column injuries. J Neurosurg 1988;68:18–24
9. Smith WS, Kaufer H. Patterns and mechanisms of lumbar injuries associated with lap seat belts. J Bone Joint Surg Am 1969;51:239–254
10. Leventhal HR. Birth injuries of the spinal cord. J Pediatr 1960;56:447–453
11. Kokoska ER, Keller MS, Rallo MC, Weber TR. Characteristics of pediatric cervical spine injuries. J Pediatr Surg 2001;36:100–105
12. Roche C, Carty H. Spinal trauma in children. Pediatr Radiol 2001;31: 677–700
13. Lustrin ES, Karakas SP, Ortiz AO, et al. Pediatric cervical spine: normal anatomy, variants, and trauma. Radiographics 2003;23:539–560
14. Hedequist D. Pediatric spine trauma. In: MF Abel, ed. Orthopedic Knowledge Update: Pediatrics 3. Rosemont, IL: AAOS; 2006:323–335
15. Hosalkar HS, Cain EL, Horn D, Chin KR, Dormans JP, Drummond DS. Traumatic atlanto-occipital dislocation in children. J Bone Joint Surg Am 2005;87:2480–2488
16. Bulas DI, Fitz CR, Johnson DL. Traumatic atlanto-occipital dislocation in children. Radiology 1993;188:155–158

17. Saeheng S, Phuenpathom N. Traumatic occipitoatlantal dislocation. Surg Neurol 2001;55:35–40, discussion 40

18. Nischal K, Chumas P, Sparrow O. Prolonged survival after atlanto-occipital dislocation: two case reports and review. Br J Neurosurg 1993;7:677–682

19. Werne S. Studies in spontaneous atlas dislocation. Acta Orthop Scand Suppl 1957;23:1–150

20. Wang MY, Hoh DJ, Leary SP, Griffith P, McComb JG. High rates of neurological improvement following severe traumatic pediatric spinal cord injury. Spine (Phila Pa 1976) 2004;29:1493–1497, discussion E266

21. Cohen MW, Drummond DS, Flynn JM, Pill SG, Dormans JP. A technique of occipitocervical arthrodesis in children using autologous rib grafts. Spine (Phila Pa 1976) 2001;26:825–829

22. Dormans JP, Drummond DS, Sutton LN, Ecker ML, Kopacz KJ. Occipitocervical arthrodesis in children: a new technique and analysis of results. J Bone Joint Surg Am 1995;77:1234–1240

23. Schultz KDJ Jr, Petronio J, Haid RW, et al. Pediatric occipitocervical arthrodesis: a review of current options and early evaluation of rigid internal fixation techniques. Pediatr Neurosurg 2000;33:169–181

24. Nockels RP, Shaffrey CI, Kanter AS, Azeem S, York JE. Occipitocervical fusion with rigid internal fixation: long-term follow-up data in 69 patients. J Neurosurg Spine 2007;7:117–123

25. Anderson RC, Ragel BT, Mocco J, Bohman LE, Brockmeyer DL. Selection of a rigid internal fixation construct for stabilization at the craniovertebral junction in pediatric patients. J Neurosurg 2007;107(1, Suppl):36–42

26. Pang D. Spinal cord injuries. In: D McLone, ed. Pediatric Neurosurgery: Surgery of the Developing Nervous System. Philadephia: WB Saunders; 2001: 660–694

27. Kawabe N, Hirotani H, Tanaka O. Pathomechanism of atlantoaxial rotatory fixation in children. J Pediatr Orthop 1989;9:569–574

28. Rinaldi I, Mullins WJ Jr, Delaney WF, Fitzer PM, Tornberg DN. Computerized tomographic demonstration of rotational atlanto-axial fixation: case report. J Neurosurg 1979;50:115–119

29. Alanay A, Hicazi A, Acaroglu E, et al. Reliability and necessity of dynamic computerized tomography in diagnosis of atlantoaxial rotatory subluxation. J Pediatr Orthop 2002;22:763–765

30. Hicazi A, Acaroglu E, Alanay A, Yazici M, Surat A. Atlantoaxial rotatory fixation-subluxation revisited: a computed tomographic analysis of acute torticollis in pediatric patients. Spine (Phila Pa 1976) 2002;27:2771–2775

31. Pang D, Wilberger JEJ Jr. Spinal cord injury without radiographic abnormalities in children. J Neurosurg 1982;57:114–129

32. Crossman JE, David K, Hayward R, Crockard HA. Open reduction of pediatric atlantoaxial rotatory fixation: long-term outcome study with functional measurements. J Neurosurg 2004;100(3, Suppl Spine):235–240

33. Jones A, Mehta J, Fagan D, Ahuja S, Grant A, Davies P. Anterior screw fixation for a pediatric odontoid nonunion: a case report. Spine (Phila Pa 1976) 2005;30:E28–E30

34. Dogan S, Safavi-Abbasi S, Theodore N, Horn E, Rekate HL, Sonntag VK. Pediatric subaxial cervical spine injuries: origins, management, and outcome in 51 patients. Neurosurg Focus 2006;20:E1

35. Hooley E, Chaput CD, Rahm M. Internal fixation without fusion of a flexion-distraction injury in the lower cervical spine of a three-year-old. Spine J 2006;6:50–54

36. Dickerman RD, Morgan JT, Mittler M. Circumferential cervical spine surgery in an 18-month-old female with traumatic disruption of the odontoid and C3 vertebrae: case report and review of techniques. Pediatr Neurosurg 2005;41:88–92

37. Santiago R, Guenther E, Carroll K, Junkins EP Jr. The clinical presentation of pediatric thoracolumbar fractures. J Trauma 2006;60:187–192

38. Denis F. Spinal instability as defined by the three-column spine concept in acute spinal trauma. Clin Orthop Relat Res 1984;189:65–76

39. Horal J, Nachemson A, Scheller S. Clinical and radiological long term follow-up of vertebral fractures in children. Acta Orthop Scand 1972;43:491–503

40. Pouliquen JC, Kassis B, Glorion C, Langlais J. Vertebral growth after thoracic or lumbar fracture of the spine in children. J Pediatr Orthop 1997;17:115–120

41. Lyon R. Pediatric spine injuries. In: Bridewell KH, et al, eds. The Textbook of Spinal Surgery. Philadelphia, PA: Lippincott Williams & Wilkins; 1997

42. Kulowski J, Rost WB. Intra-abdominal injury from safety belt in auto accident; report of a case. AMA Arch Surg 1956;73:970–971

43. Garrett JW, Braunstein PW. The seat belt syndrome. J Trauma 1962;2:220–238

44. Papavasiliou A, Stanton J, Sinha P, Forder J, Skyrme A. The complexity of seat belt injuries including spinal injury in the pediatric population: a case report of a 6-year-old boy and the literature review. Eur J Emerg Med 2007;14:180–183

45. Prince JS, LoSasso BE, Senac MOJ Jr. Unusual seat-belt injuries in children. J Trauma 2004;56:420–427

46. Chance GQ. Note on a type of flexion fracture of the spine. Br J Radiol 1948;21:452–453

47. Gumley G, Taylor TK, Ryan MD. Distraction fractures of the lumbar spine. J Bone Joint Surg Br 1982;64:520–525

48. Kewalramani LS, Tori JA. Spinal cord trauma in children: neurologic patterns, radiologic features, and pathomechanics of injury. Spine (Phila Pa 1976) 1980;5:11–18

49. Mulpuri K, Jawadi A, Perdios A, Choit RL, Tredwell SJ, Reilly CW. Outcome analysis of chance fractures of the skeletally immature spine. Spine (Phila Pa 1976) 2007;32:E702–E707

50. Moller A, Hasserius R, Besjakev J, et al. Vertebral fractures in late adolescence: a 27 to 47-year follow-up. Eur Spine J 2006;15(8):1247–1254

51. Rodgers WB, Coran DL, Emans JB, Hresko MT, Hall JE. Occipitocervical fusion in children: retrospective analysis and technical considerations. Clin Orthop Relat Res 1999;364:125–133

52. Currier BL, Papagelopoulos PJ, Neale PG, et al. Biomechanical evaluation of new posterior occipitocervical instrumentation system. Clin Orthop Relat Res 2003;411:103–115

53. Vara CS, Thompson GH. A cadaveric examination of pediatric cervical pedicle morphology. Spine (Phila Pa 1976) 2006;31:1107–1112

54. Reilly CW, Choit RL. Transarticular screws in the management of C1–C2 instability in children. J Pediatr Orthop 2006;26:582–588

55. Hedequist D, Hresko T, Proctor M. Modern cervical spine instrumentation in children. Spine (Phila Pa 1976) 2008;33:379–383

56. Gluf WM, Brockmeyer DL. Atlantoaxial transarticular screw fixation: a review of surgical indications, fusion rate, complications, and lessons learned in 67 pediatric patients. J Neurosurg Spine 2005;2:164–169

57. Anderson RC, Kan P, Gluf WM, Brockmeyer DL. Long-term maintenance of cervical alignment after occipitocervical and atlantoaxial screw fixation in young children. J Neurosurg 2006;105(1, Suppl):55–61

58. Godard J, Hadji M, Raul JS. Odontoid fractures in the child with neurological injury: direct anterior osteosynthesis with a cortico-spongious screw and literature review. Childs Nerv Syst 1997;13:105–107

59. Toyama Y, Matsumoto M, Chiba K, et al. Realignment of postoperative cervical kyphosis in children by vertebral remodeling. Spine (Phila Pa 1976) 1994;19:2565–2570

60. Nakagawa T, Yone K, Sakou T, Yanase M. Occipitocervical fusion with C1 laminectomy in children. Spine (Phila Pa 1976) 1997;22:1209–1214

61. Parisini P, Di Silvestre M, Greggi T, Bianchi G. C1–C2 posterior fusion in growing patients: long-term follow-up. Spine (Phila Pa 1976) 2003;28:566–572, discussion 572

62. Zindrick MR, Knight GW, Sartori MJ, Carnevale TJ, Patwardhan AG, Lorenz MA. Pedicle morphology of the immature thoracolumbar spine. Spine (Phila Pa 1976) 2000;25:2726–2735

63. Senaran H, Yazici M, Karcaaltincaba M, et al. Lumbar pedicle morphology in the immature spine: a three-dimensional study using spiral computed tomography. Spine (Phila Pa 1976) 2002;27:2472–2476

64. Yazici M, Pekmezci M, Cil A, Alanay A, Acaroglu E, Oner FC. The effect of pedicle expansion on pedicle morphology and biomechanical stability in the immature porcine spine. Spine (Phila Pa 1976) 2006;31:E826–E829

65. Cil A, Yazici M, Daglioglu K, et al. The effect of pedicle screw placement with or without application of compression across the neurocentral cartilage on the morphology of the spinal canal and pedicle in immature pigs. Spine (Phila Pa 1976) 2005;30:1287–1293

66. Ruf M, Harms J. Pedicle screws in 1- and 2-year-old children: technique, complications, and effect on further growth. Spine (Phila Pa 1976) 2002;27:E460–E466

67. Karlsson MK, Moller A, Hasserius A, et al. A modeling capacity of vertebral fractures exists during growth: an up to 47-year follow-up. Spine 2003;28(18):2087–2092

68. Pekmezci M, Yilmaz G, Daglioglu K, et al. The effect of anterior spinal fusion on spinal canal development in an immature porcine model. Spine (Phila Pa 1976) 2009;34:E501–E506

69. Canavese F, Dimeglio A, Volpatti D, et al. Dorsal arthrodesis of thoracic spine and effects on thorax growth in prepubertal New Zealand white rabbits. Spine (Phila Pa 1976) 2007;32:E443–E450

70. Dubousset J, Herring JA, Shufflebarger HL. The crankshaft phenomenon. J Pediatr Orthop 1989;9:541–550

71. Kioschos HC, Asher MA, Lark RG, Harner EJ. Overpowering the crankshaft mechanism: the effect of posterior spinal fusion with and without stiff transpedicular fixation on anterior spinal column growth in immature canines. Spine (Phila Pa 1976) 1996;21:1168–1173

72. Dogan S, Safavi-Abbasi S, Theodore N, et al. Thoracolumbar and sacral spinal injuries in children and adolescents: a review of 89 cases. J Neurosurg 2007;106(6, Suppl):426–433

73. Guzel A, Belen D, Tatli M, Simsek S, Guzel E. Complete L1–L2 lateral dislocation without fracture and neurologic deficit in a child. Pediatr Neurosurg 2006;42:183–186

18

The Benefits of Early Stabilization of Spinal Fractures in the Trauma Patient

Miguel A. Schmitz, Darren R. Lebl, and Mitchel B. Harris

Although there have been substantial advances in spinal fixation for spinal column injuries, this has not been associated with improvements in neurological recovery. Intuitively, it has been surmised that early surgical decompression of the traumatized spinal cord with associated spinal stabilization would allow better neurological recovery, but this has not been demonstrated with the current definitions of "early" surgery. Early surgical stabilization of the spine after spinal cord injury (SCI) has been demonstrated to improve general medical recovery, particularly in the polytrauma patient. On the other hand, ultra-early surgical intervention has been demonstrated in animal spinal trauma models to improve spinal cord recovery.

There are many complicating treatment issues under consideration in the initial management of the polytrauma patient with an associated spinal injury. Factors favoring subacute surgical intervention include waiting for the best surgical team available that is familiar with spine surgery, having optimal medical resources available for the postoperative period (generally found during daytime hours), and allowing the trauma team to more comprehensively evaluate and thoroughly resuscitate the polytrauma patient prior to additional blood loss from spinal surgery and anesthesia. Factors that support early spinal decompression and stabilization in the patient with SCI include the basic surgical tenet that suggests improved function occurs after restoration of an injury to its premorbid status. Additionally, expedient surgical stabilization of the medically stabilized patient allows more prompt mobilization of the patient that in turn diminishes the risk of pulmonary, gastrointestinal, and skin-related sequelae associated with prolonged immobilization in the polytrauma patient. This review addresses the question, Does the timing of surgical stabilization for spine fractures affect morbidity and mortality in the polytrauma patient?

◆ Methods

Three tiers of search criteria were employed to answer these questions with contemporary studies. OVIDMedline was used as the search engine using multiple search pairs and a search period from 1950 through February 2007. The search pairs are identified in **Table 18.1**. The first tier included articles within the initial search that were categorized by OVIDMedline to be "comparative studies," "controlled clinical trials," "meta-analyses," "multi-center studies," "randomized controlled trials," and "validation studies." The exclusion criteria for the first tier included case reports with fewer than 10 cases, nontrauma-related articles, basic reviews, oncological cases, and cadaver studies. Although some studies were excluded, many of them were utilized as background references, and some are noted in the reference section. The second tier included studies that were relevant to the question that were identified in the initial search but were not categorized by OVIDMedline to be "comparative studies," "controlled clinical trials," "meta-analyses," "multi-center studies," "randomized controlled trials," and "validation studies." The third tier included studies that were relevant to the questions that were known by the review authors or were identified within the references of the first- and second-tier search criteria articles. All articles were graded according to the system of Schünemann et al[8] and Wright et al.[1]

◆ Results

There were no "evidence-based reviews" within any of the search pairs noted in **Table 18.1** as rated by OVIDMedline. In the broadest search pair, the search for "multiple trauma and

Table 18.1 OVIDMedline Search

Screening Criteria	Number of Manuscripts
Polytrauma and spinal stabilization	1
Spine trauma and timing of surgery	3
Multiple trauma and spine fractures	43
Multiple trauma and timing of surgery	11
Spine fracture and surgery	37
Multiple trauma	7314

Table 18.2 Reasons for Exclusion of Manuscripts within the Initial OVIDMedline Search

Exclusion Criteria	Number of Manuscripts
Case reports with less than 10 cases	9
Not trauma related	4
Not focused on spine	37
Not specific to surgery	18
Review only	3
Not specific to the timing of surgery	12
No English translation	1

spine fractures" yielded 43 manuscripts. There was overlap by the other search pairs with this broadest search that brought the initial search to 90 manuscripts. The first-tier criteria only yielded one manuscript. The second-tier criteria identified five studies, and the third tier yielded 14 articles. Eighty-four articles that were identified in the primary search were excluded for the reasons noted in **Table 18.2**. **Table 18.3** describes animal model studies that were used in an attempt to answer the question using third-tier manuscripts. **Table 18.4** shows the first-, second- and third-tier manuscripts that were reviewed to answer the primary question of whether the timing of surgical stabilization for spine fractures affects morbidity and mortality in the polytrauma patient. **Table 18.4** also shows the associated Schünemann and Wright grade as well as whether it is tier 1, 2, or 3.

Animal Models of the Efficacy of Early Surgical Management of Spinal Cord Injury

To answer the question regarding the proper timing of surgical intervention for spine injuries associated with SCI, researchers have turned to animal models given the inherent uncontrolled environment associated with clinical studies on this subject, particularly in those patients with polytrauma. **Table 18.3** summarizes these studies. Guha and associates used a rat spine injury model to identify that spinal decompression at 15 minutes or 60 minutes after spinal cord compression allows

Table 18.3 Animal Studies Relevant to the Timing of Spinal Decompression Surgery for Acute Spinal Cord Injury

Reference	Description	Tier	Level of Evidence of Primary Question	Topic and Conclusion
Carlson et al[4]	Dog study	III	Animal study	In 21 mature beagles, the spinal cord at T13 was loaded until evoked potentials had been reduced by 50%. Spinal cord displacement was maintained for 30 ($n = 7$), 60 ($n = 8$), and 180 ($n = 6$) minutes, and decompression was followed by a 3-hour monitoring period and blood flow was measured. Conclusion: Spinal cord decompression performed within 1 hour of evoked potential loss resulted in significant electrophysiological recovery after 3 hours of monitoring.
Carlson et al[6]	Dog study	III	Animal study	16 dogs underwent spinal cord compression for 30 or 180 minutes by a loading device. SSEPs were monitored during a 60-minute recovery period and after 28 days. Motor recovery was measured after 26 days. Conclusions: The duration of compression of 180 minutes resulted in long-term decreases in SSEPs and greater lesional volumes determined by MRI. Decompression after 30 minutes resulted in early recovery of SSEPs that coincided with histological findings of minimal long-term damage and early functional improvements.
Delamarter et al[3]	Dog study	III	Animal study	Evaluated timing of decompression after compression of 50% of spinal cord diameter in 30 purebred dogs. Dogs that had immediate decompression or decompression after 1 hour recovered the ability to walk as well as control the bowel and bladder; however, when compression lasted 6 hours or more there was no neurological recovery. The percentage of SSEPs by 6 weeks after decompression was significantly related to the duration of the compression ($p < 0.0008$).
Guha A et al[2]	Rat study	III	Animal study	Force of spinal cord injury was studied by different clip strengths (2.3 g, 16.9 g, 53.0 g) under different times of decompression (15, 60, 120, 240 minutes). Conclusions: The time until decompression was a significant determinant of function for the 2.3 gm, 16.9 gm clips ($p < 0.05$). The animals decompressed after 15 or 60 minutes had significantly better function than those decompressed after longer periods.
Dimar JR et al[5]	Rat study	III	Animal study	Evaluated canal narrowing and duration of compression. The canal was precisely narrowed using spacers at 35% or 50% followed by neurological assessment with BBB motor scores and TcMMEPs. The second phase evaluated the effect of time of compression recovery by sequentially removing the spacers from the test groups at 2, 6, 24, and 72 hours. Conclusions: The study demonstrated that the degree of spinal cord injury is directly related to the severity of spinal canal narrowing and the duration of compression.

Abbreviations: BBB, Basso, Beattie, Bresnahan Locomotor Rating Scale; MRI, magnetic resonance imaging; SSEPs, somatosensory evoked potentials; TcMMEPs, transcranial magnetic motor evoked potentials.

Table 18.4 Evidence-Based Review Literature with Study Description and Rating According to Schünemann et al[8] and Wright et al[1]

Investigator	Description	Tier	Level of Evidence of Primary Question	Topic and Conclusion
Aebi et al[17]	Retrospective case series	III	IV (very low)	100 cervical spine injuries that were treated operatively were reviewed. Only 25% had closed manual or open reduction within the first 6 hours. The majority of patients who improved neurologically were reduced within the first 6 hours after the accident. Conclusion: Immediate reduction of the injury is more important for the future neurological outcome than improved surgical techniques.
Chen et al[28]	Retrospective review	III	IV (very low)	114 patients from 1988 to 1994 with acute or chronic traumatic central cord syndrome were reviewed. Conclusions: Better results were achieved in younger patients and in patients with clinically correlated encroaching cord lesions who received early surgical decompression.
Clohisy[22]	Retrospective case series	III	IV (very low)	22 patients with incomplete neurological deficits after thoracolumbar junction fractures were treated by anterior decompression and stabilization. 11 underwent early decompression (< 48 hours) and nine patients underwent late decompression (average 61 days), two were unavailable for follow-up. Patients were followed for an average of 8.5 years. The modified Frankel grade ($p < 0.04$) and ASIA motor point score improvements ($p < 0.01$) were significantly different. Conclusion: In this series, early anterior decompression and stabilization for traumatic injuries at the thoracolumbar spine was associated with improved rates of neurological recovery when compared with late decompression.
Comarr, Kaufman[29]	Retrospective case series	III	IV (very low)	858 patients admitted to the paraplegia service during a 9-year period were studied. Decompressive laminectomy was performed in 579, 279 were not explored. 16% of laminectomized patients were improved, and 8% were ambulatory. In the nonoperative group 29% improved neurologically, and 16% were ambulatory. Among the laminectomized patients, the most favorable interval between injury and operation was 24 hours to 1 month, those operated upon earlier seemed less likely to improve. Lesser rates of improvement were observed in all types of lesion operated on more than 1 month after injury.
Croce et al[16]	Retrospective case series	III	IV (very low)	291 patients had spine fracture fixation, 142 (49%) early and 149 (51%) late, 163 cervical (83 early, 80 late), 79 thoracic (30 early, 49 late), and 49 lumbar (29 early, 20 late). Conclusions: ICU stay was shorter for patients with early fixation, the incidence of pneumonia was lower, fewer ventilator days, and lower charges
Dai et al[14]	Retrospective case series	II	IV (very low)	147 patients w/acute thoracolumbar fractures and multiple trauma from 1988 to 1997 were reviewed retrospectively at a single institution. The incidence of missed injuries and reasons for delay in diagnosis were determined. Conclusions: Delayed diagnosis of thoracolumbar fractures was made in 28 patients (19%). There was an increased incidence of pulmonary complications ($p < 0.01$) and increased hospital LOS ($p < 0.05$) in patients treated nonoperatively. No significant differences in the recovery rate of neurological function ($p > 0.05$), surgical patients had significantly less pain ($p < 0.01$). The relationship between timing of surgery and complications failed to show statistical significance ($p > 0.05$). Neither the severity of injury nor the timing of surgery had any significant effect on recovery rate ($p > 0.05$)
Gaebler et al[21]	Retrospective case series	III	IV (very low)	88 patients were followed up after an average of 5.6 years after short segment pedicle stabilization and fusion in patients with thoracolumbar fractures/dislocations. The highest neurological recovery rates were found in patients operated within 8 hours after initial trauma. High remission rates were still found if the patients had been operated on within 48 hours. After 48 hours there was no significant difference in the neurological outcome compared with the time of operation. Conclusion: Their results suggest that the earlier operative decompression and stabilization take place, the better is the recovery rate in patients with neurological deficits.

(Continued on page 160)

Table 18.4 Evidence-Based Review Literature with Study Description and Rating According to Schünemann et al[8] and Wright et al[1] *(Continued)*

Investigator	Description	Tier	Level of Evidence of Primary Question	Topic and Conclusion
Gertzbein et al[30]	Prospective cohort study, nonrandomized	I	III (low) (not randomized, not consecutive)	$n = 1019$ consecutive cases of thoracolumbar fractures treated nonoperatively and operatively, 64 physicians from 12 countries, followed patients for 2 years. 820 (80.5%) patients were treated operatively, 19.5% (199) were treated conservatively. 67% had posterior surgery, 13.8% had anterior surgery. Conclusions: (1) Surgery led to improved function but rate of improvement was not statistically different; at 1 year the surgical patients showed a significantly greater relative improvement in motor score, only 69.2% compared with 14.0% for the nonsurgical group ($p < 0.00001$). This difference was maintained at the 2-year evaluation point (59% vs 16.0%, $p < 0.0003$). (2) Anterior surgery was not more effective than posterior surgery in improving the neurological function when function was assessed using the Frankel or motor index scales, but it was statistically significant to the Manabe scale. (3) Anterior surgery was more beneficial in improving complete bladder impairment to partial impairment compared to posterior surgery. (4) A kyphotic deformity of > 30 degrees was associated with increased incidence of significant back pain. (5) Patients who had surgery complained less of severe pain. Limitation: Different fracture types and neurological scores in surgical and nonsurgical groups made it difficult to compare effectiveness of treatment.
Kerwin et al[13]	Retrospective case series	III	IV (very low)	Trauma registry review Jan 1988 to Oct 2001 of spinal fractures. 299 required surgical stabilization, 174 (58.2%) had surgical stabilization within 3 days, whereas 125 (41.8%) had surgical stabilization > 3 days. Conclusions: Hospital LOS was significantly shorter (14.3 vs 21.1 days); however, there was no significant difference in ICU LOS, or number of ventilator days.
Krengel et al[20]	Retrospective case series with historical controls	III	IV (very low)	14 patients were identified with incomplete thoracic level paraplegia (T2 to T11): all were treated surgically. 12 patients had surgery within 24 hours, one at 26 hours, and one at 5 days. At an average of 20 months follow-up, average neurological improvement was 2.2 Frankel grades per patient, lower extremity motor index improved from an average of 7 to 44. Conclusions: Early surgical reduction, stabilization, and decompression are safe procedures and improve neurological recovery in comparison with historical controls treated by postural reduction or late surgical intervention.
Hadley et al[24]	Retrospective review	II	IV (very low)	68 patients with acute cervical facet fracture-dislocation injuries were reviewed. 31 patients had unilateral facet injuries and 37 patients had bilateral facet injuries. Neurological morbidity was 90% and was most severe among bilateral face injury patients (84% had complete injuries). 78% of patients improved with closed reduction, 60% improved with ORIF, only 10/68 patients made significant neurological recoveries. Open reduction followed closed reduction in all but two patients. Conclusions: Of the 10 patients who improved neurologically, all were reduced within 8 hours of injury, six patients within 5 hours of injury. Although a small number of patients, it appears that preservation or restoration of neurological function can be improved with early decompression-realignment.
La Rosa et al[26]	Meta-analysis literature review	III	IV (very low)	Medline search from 1966 to 2000 supplemented with manual search. This analysis included 1687 patients. Conclusions: Although statistically the percentage of neurological deficits improving after early decompression appear 89.7% to be better than with other modes of treatment, the authors were unable to determine with any degree of confidence a real neurological advantage to surgery within 24 hours from injury due to heterogeneity of the groups.
Levi et al[10]	Retrospective case series	II	IV (very low)	Retrospective review of 103 patients (50 incomplete deficits, 53 complete deficits) presenting to shock trauma during a 5-year period. Conclusions: No statistically significant difference in outcome between early surgery (< 24 hours) and delayed surgery subgroups. There was no statistically significant difference in hospital LOS in incomplete injuries (20 days early and 22 days delayed). However, in complete SCI hospital LOS was 38.7 early and 45.2 delayed ($p < 0.05$). Authors recommended early surgery because of comparable complication rates, improved ease of patient care, and more rapid discharge to rehab.

Table 18.4 Evidence-Based Review Literature with Study Description and Rating According to Schünemann et al[8] and Wright et al[1] *(Continued)*

Investigator	Description	Tier	Level of Evidence of Primary Question	Topic and Conclusion
McKinley et al[15]	Retrospective case series	III	III (low)	Compared outcomes between surgical and nonsurgical groups during acute care, rehabilitation, and at 1-year follow-up. Motor and sensory levels, motor index score, ASIA impairment scale, medical complications, and functional outcomes (acute and rehabilitation LOS, hospital charges, were analyzed. Conclusions: Those with late surgery (> 72 hours) had significantly ($p < 0.05$) increased acute care, total LOS, and hospital charges, along with higher incidence of pneumonia and atelectasis. No differences between groups were found for changes in neurological levels, AIS grade, or FIM motor efficiency.
McLain et al[25]	Prospective, nonrandomized longitudinal study of fractures treated with segmental instrumentation with historical control	II	III (low)	75 patients met inclusion criteria, minimum 2-year follow-up to assess outcome. Urgent treatment (< 24 hours) $n = 14$, early treatment (24 to 72 hours) $n = 13$, delayed treatment (> 72 hours) $n = 0$. Conclusions: EBL for urgent stabilization was significantly higher for anterior procedures, but EBL for posterior procedures was similar in both groups. Urgent surgical intervention is not more dangerous than surgery performed 24 to 72 hours after injury. Neurological improvement was better in the urgently treated group than in the early group (all three patients with complete neurological recovery were in the urgent group; both patients with > 2 Frankel grades of recovery were treated urgently), but the numbers were too small for statistical significance.
Mirza et al[18]	Retrospective cohort study	III	III (low)	Patients undergoing surgical treatment for acute cervical SCI at two institutions between 1989 and 1991 were reviewed. 15 patients underwent early surgery (< 72 hours) mean 1.8 days, and 15 patients underwent late surgery (> 72 hours) mean 14.1 days. There was no significant difference in number of ventilator days of ICU LOS. The change in motor index score from preop to postop was statistically significant in the group of patients who underwent early surgery ($p = 0.0063$), but not in the group of patients who had late surgery ($p = 0.14$). The change in Frankel grade from preop to postop was statistically significant in the patients who underwent early surgery ($p = 0.0026$) but not in the late surgery group ($p = 0.30$). There was no difference in the number of complications. Conclusion: Patients may benefit from early surgery. Early surgery is not associated with more complications and may improve neurological recovery and decrease hospitalization time.
Papadopoulos et al[19]	Prospective, nonrandomized cohort study	III	II (moderate)	91 consecutive patients with acute, traumatic cervical SCI were enrolled in a protocol group (emergent MRI to determine cord compression and surgery if indicated or a reference group—no MRI/surgery. 50% of protocol patients compared with 24% reference patients improved their Frankel grade. 32 patients (46%) in the protocol group were treated with skeletal traction and 24 patients (54%) were decompressed. Eight protocol patients, but no reference patients, improved from complete motor quadriplegia to independent ambulation. Conclusions: Immediate spinal column stabilization and spinal cord decompression, based on MRI, may significantly improve neurological outcome.
Randle et al[9]	Retrospective case series	II	IV (very low)	54 patients underwent anterior stabilization and Caspar plating for acute cervical spine injury. 32 patients had complete neurological deficit at presentation, 14 had partial SCI, and 8 were neurologically intact. Conclusions: Early intervention (< 24 hours) ($n = 22$) was frequently performed in the neurologically compromised patients. 12/22 regained significant neurological function, 13/22 had postoperative complications. In the delayed group (> 24 hours, mean 14.3 days), 14 patients had postop complications, 15/24 had neurological improvement. Hospital LOS was lower in the early surgery group with complete injuries 39.8 ± 27.7 versus 53.3 ± 24.1 days, but not statistically significant $p = 0.18$.
Schlegel et al[11]	Retrospective case series	III	IV (very low)	138 patients requiring operative decompression between Jan 1986 and April 1989 were reviewed. Patients had fewer complications if they underwent surgery within 72 hours. Morbidity was higher in patients with a neurological deficit compared with neurologically intact patients. Conclusion: Surgical decompression within the first 72 hours is indicated in patients with polytrauma (ISS ≥ 18) and cervical injuries with neurological deficit.

(Continued on page 162)

Table 18.4 Evidence-Based Review Literature with Study Description and Rating According to Schünemann et al[8] and Wright et al[1] *(Continued)*

Investigator	Description	Tier	Level of Evidence of Primary Question	Topic and Conclusion
Vaccaro et al[12]	Prospective, randomized, nonblinded	III	II (moderate)	64 patients with traumatic cervical SCI (C3–T1) met inclusion criteria and were randomized to early (< 72 hours) and late (> 5 days) surgical treatment protocols. 34 patients in the early group had surgery at an average of 1.8 days. 28 patients in the late group had surgery at an average of 16.8 days. Conclusions: No significant neurological benefit with early surgery

Abbreviations: AIS, Abbreviated Injury Scale; ASIA, American Spinal Injury Association; EBL, estimated blood loss; FIM, functional independence motor; ICU, intensive care unit; ISS, injury severity score; LOS, length of stay; SCI, spinal cord injury; ORIF, Open Reduction and Internal Fixation.

better function than those that are decompressed after a longer period of time of cord compression.[2] Delamarter and colleagues used a dog spinal injury model to study the influence of early versus late spinal cord decompression.[3] The investigators compressed the cord 50% of the normal spinal cord diameter in 30 dogs. Dogs that had immediate decompression or decompression within 1 hour recovered the ability to walk as well as control of bowel and bladder. When compression lasted 6 hours or more, there was no neurological recovery. The percentage of somatosensory evoked potentials (SSEPs) recovery at 6 weeks postdecompression was inversely related to the duration of compression.[3] Carlson and colleagues studied beagles after a T13 SCI that was produced in a controlled fashion. SSEPs and regional blood flow were monitored in 21 of these dogs that were decompressed for 30 minutes, 60 minutes, or 180 minutes after the experimental SCI. This study revealed that the degree of early reperfusion after decompression was inversely proportional to the duration of spinal cord compression and proportionate to the electrophysiological recovery. These authors concluded that in beagles, there is a critical time period between 1 and 3 hours after the injury in which neurological recovery can be rendered.[4] Dimar et al evaluated the effects of canal narrowing and the duration of narrowing in the rat model where the New York weight drop technique was used to create mild, moderate, and severe SCIs.[5] Following injury the canal was precisely narrowed using spacers that narrowed the canal 35% or 50% followed by neurological assessment with Basso, Beattie, Bresnahan (BBB) motor scores and transcranial magnetic motor evoked potentials (TcMMEPs) monitoring.

The second phase of the study evaluated the effect of time of compression on spinal cord recovery by evaluating sequentially removing the spacers from the test groups at 2, 6, 24, and 72 hours. The study demonstrated that the degree of SCI is directly related to the severity of spinal canal narrowing and the duration of compression.[5] Subsequent to this, Carlson et al conducted a study on 16 dogs that underwent spinal cord compression for either 30 minutes or 180 minutes by a loading device. SSEPs were monitored 60 minutes after decompression and 28 days after decompression. Motor recovery was monitored 26 days after decompression.[6] It was identified that a compression duration of 180 minutes resulted in long-term decreases in SSEP and greater lesional volumes determined by magnetic resonance imaging (MRI).[6] Decompression after 30 minutes resulted in early recovery of SSEPs that coincided with histological findings and early functional recovery.[6]

Part of the problem with spinal injuries associated with SCI is that there is a secondary injury response, which has been discussed in detail as reviewed and investigated by Kwon and others and is outside the scope of this review.[7] Nevertheless, this is an important consideration, and it can most briefly

be described as an interaction at the cord level that occurs between the immediate trauma and acute vascular disruptions, secondary vascular disruption from clotting, ischemia, inflammation, excitotoxicity, electrolyte imbalance, free radical generation, and lipid peroxidation. The net effect is secondary injury to the cord that is often greater than that of the primary injury.[7]

Does Early Surgical Management of Spinal Cord Injuries Result in Better Outcomes?

Table 18.4 summarizes the studies that were found to be germane to this question. This review found that there were two main conclusions from these studies. Some studies found that "early" surgical intervention does not result in neurological improvement more so than "delayed" surgical intervention, but that there was a trend toward decreased medical complications and decreased hospital length of stay and intensive care unit stay. Another set of studies found that "early" surgical intervention resulted in better neurological outcome as well as better medical outcomes. There were no high-quality studies in this regard as rated using the Schünemann scale,[8] and there were no level I studies as rated using the Wright scale.[1]

Early Surgery Yields Decreased Length of Stay but No Significant Neurological Recovery

Cervical Spine   Although there are few dissentions regarding indications for surgery, there is considerable controversy regarding the timing of surgical intervention. In a retrospective series of 54 patients, Randle and coworkers did not find that there was a difference between early (< 24 hours postinjury) and late (> 24 hours postinjury) intervention for cervical spine injuries treated with reduction and anterior stabilization in terms of neurological improvement. However, the length of hospitalization was lesser in the early group. This was not statistically significant.[9] Similar findings were noted in a retrospective review by Levi and colleagues; however, there was a statistically significant shorter length of stay with early surgical intervention.[10] Schlegel and colleagues in a retrospective case series identified 138 patients who underwent surgical decompression for cervical injuries. They found that patients who underwent surgery within 72 hours had fewer complications than those patients who had surgery after 72 hours.[11] In the only prospective, randomized, nonblinded study in this literature review, Vaccaro and colleagues studied 62 patients with cervical (C3–T1) SCIs who were randomized to early (< 72 hours) or late (> 5 days) surgical treatment protocols.[12] The 34 patients in the early group had surgery an average of 1.8 days postinjury, and the 28 patients in the late group had surgery an average of 16.8 days after the injury. There was no difference in the neurological recovery between the early and the late group, and there was no difference in the length of stay, although it is important to note that 20 of the 62 patients were lost to follow-up.[12]

Although most studies indicate that early surgical intervention for SCI at least yields better medical outcomes and shorter hospital stays, Kerwin and associates did not find this to be the case entirely.[13] In a retrospective case review of 299 patients that had surgical stabilization for spine fractures associated with SCI, 174 had surgical stabilization within 3 days, whereas 125 patients had surgical stabilization beyond 3 days. These investigators found that the hospital length of stay was significantly shorter (14.3 days vs 21.1 days); however, there was no significant difference in intensive care unit (ICU) length of stay or the number of ventilator days, and the mortality was higher in the early surgical group.[13]

Thoracolumbar Spine   In a retrospectively study group of 147 patients with thoracolumbar fractures and polytrauma, Dai and colleagues identified that surgical stabilization diminished the length of stay, but there was no difference in the neurological recovery nor was there a difference in the rate of pulmonary complications when 72 hours postinjury is used as the early threshold.[14] This study did not identify that early surgery allowed better neurological recovery than delayed surgery.[14] In a retrospective study by McKinley and colleagues, similar findings were noted with the threshold of early surgery being defined as 3 days, though they specifically noted a higher incidence of pneumonia and atelectasis in the delayed surgery group.[15]

Any Spine Level   Croce and coworkers identified in a retrospective review that patients with spine fractures at any level in which operative procedures were indicated, had better outcomes in terms of shorter intensive care unit stays, lower incidence of pneumonia, fewer ventilator days, and fewer hospital charges when spine operative intervention was performed earlier rather than later.[16]

Early Surgery Yields Improved Neurological Recovery over Delayed Surgery

Cervical Spine   There are many studies that have demonstrated that early surgical intervention improves neurological recovery over delayed surgery. In a retrospective case series, Aebi and associates studied 100 cervical spine injuries associated with SCI. They found that the 25% who underwent closed manual or open reduction within the first 6 hours represented the majority of patients with improved neurological outcome.[17]

In a retrospective cohort study, Mirza and coworkers found that, among the 15 patients with cervical SCI who underwent early intervention (< 72 hours; mean 1.8 days) after injury, there was no significant difference in the number of ventilator days and the length of stay in the intensive care unit compared with the 15 patients that underwent late surgery (< 72 hours; mean 14.1 days). However, the improvement in the motor index score from preop to postop was statistically significant in the group of patients who underwent early surgery ($p = 0.0063$) compared with the patients who had late surgery ($p = 0.14$).[18] Likewise, there was an improvement in

the Frankel grade from preop to postop in the early group ($p = 0.0026$) as opposed to the delayed group ($p = 0.30$). There was no difference between the two groups in terms of complications.

Papadopoulos and colleagues performed a prospective, nonrandomized cohort study of 91 consecutive patients with acute, traumatic cervical SCI. One group received immediate MRI and surgery or traction as indicated, and the other group did not receive immediate MRI and surgery/traction. Fifty percent of the immediate MRI/surgery or traction patients had improvement in their Frankel grade compared with 24% of the patients who did not receive immediate MRI and surgery or traction.[19] Eight patients in the immediate MRI and surgery or traction group improved from complete motor quadriplegia to independent ambulation, whereas none of the patients that received delayed intervention improved.[19]

Thoracolumbar Spine   In a retrospective case series with historical controls, Krengel and colleagues studied 14 patients with acute SCIs with levels from T2 to T11 who were treated with early surgical intervention, 12 patients within 24 hours of injury, one patient at 26 hours of injury, and one patient at 5 days from the injury.[20] The average neurological improvement in the Frankel score was 2.2 units. The lower extremity motor index improved from an average of 7 to 44. In comparison with historical controls, the authors found that early surgery was safe while providing for better neurological recovery.[20]

In a retrospective study of 88 patients that underwent surgical treatment for thoracolumbar fracture/dislocations, 26 patients received operative intervention within 8 hours of injury, and 50 had operative intervention longer than 8 hours after the injury.[21] The remaining 12 patients were operated on after 10 days in this series. These authors found the greatest neurological recovery in the patients that were operated on within 8 hours after the initial trauma.[21]

In another retrospective analysis of 22 patients with incomplete neurological deficits after thoracolumbar (T12–L1) fractures, Clohisy and colleagues compared the results of 11 patients who underwent anterior decompression within 48 hours to nine patients who underwent decompression after 48 hours (mean 6.1 days). The anterior approach was selected due to significant (> 40%) impingement on the cord. Nine of the 11 patients who underwent surgical intervention prior to 48 hours had at least one Frankel grade of improvement compared with five of nine in the delayed group. Two of the 11 patients who had early surgical intervention had the same Frankel grade as prior to the operation.[22] The mean American Spinal Injury Association (ASIA) motor score improvement in the early group was 21.1 ± 4.1, and in the delayed group, it was 7.6 ± 1.7.[22]

Some spinal injuries associated with neurological injury do not engender much controversy, and there is significant support for early surgical intervention in these cases.[23] Cervical facet dislocations, for instance, are typically treated with immediate reduction in either an open or a closed fashion. Hadley and associates, for instance, retrospectively reviewed 68 patients with either bilateral or unilateral facet dislocations to identify that the neurological morbidity was 90% and that it was most severe in the patients with bilateral facet injuries. Of their bilateral group, 84% experienced complete SCIs.[24] These authors found that 78% of these patients improved with closed reduction, and 60% improved with open reduction internal fixation. Open reduction followed attempted closed reduction in all but two patients, but only 10 of 68 patients had substantial neurological recoveries.[24]

Any Spine Level McLain and colleagues presented 14 patients who had early (< 24 hours) surgical spine stabilization and 13 patients that had delayed (24 to 72 hours) surgical stabilization who were followed prospectively. Although early surgical stabilization had greater blood loss, it was not found to be associated with higher morbidity. Additionally, there was a trend for greater neurological improvement in the early (< 24 hour) group compared with the delayed (24 to 72 hour) group, but this was not statistically significant. Of note, all three patients that had complete neurological recovery and the two patients with > 2 Frankel grade neurological improvements were in the early surgical intervention group.[25]

La Rosa and colleagues performed a meta-analysis of studies that were identified via a Medline search from 1966 to 2000 that were relevant to the appropriate timing of surgery after spine injury.[26] This analysis yielded 1687 patients. The authors found a 90% incidence of neurological improvement after early decompression performed within 24 hours of the injury; however, the heterogeneity of the groups was not conducive to making the definitive conclusion that early surgery after spinal injury associated with neurological injury yields better outcomes.[26]

◆ Discussion

This review echoes the assertions put forth by Albert, in that it recognizes that pulmonary complications and pneumonia are the leading cause of death in SCI patients, and that early stabilization and mobilization tend to reduce the risk of these complications.[27] Our exhaustive review draws similar conclusions to those found by Fehlings and Perrin[23] in their literature review on this topic: there are no evidence-based recommendations on the timing of surgical intervention for SCI or for spine trauma without SCI with surgical indications. The most significant controversy in ascertaining the most appropriate time interval for surgical management of the acute spinal cord injury is the definition of an early versus a late injury. Early has been defined as less than 24 hours, 72 hours, and 5 days. At those time thresholds, it may be that there is already permanent damage to the cord as is suggested by the animal models, which have demonstrated variability in the optimal time threshold for surgical decompression of the cord, including 1 hour,[2] 3 hours,[4,6] or 6 hours.[3] Nevertheless, these animal models take place in a laboratory environment where various injury parameters can be precisely controlled and immediate surgical intervention is technically feasible and concurrent polytrauma is not a concern. Additionally, study animals are generally juveniles, which is not the case in a typical human polytrauma population. The timing of surgery within the emergency patient population is exceedingly variable because numerous technical hurdles have to be overcome to present a patient to the operating room within a 6-hour or less time window. Nevertheless, urgent surgical decompression has been demonstrated to be safe, and there is evidence to suggest that early surgical intervention for patients with SCI have decreased length of stays within the hospital and the intensive care unit as well as diminished medical complications. The question of timing for surgical intervention becomes less of an issue with unstable fractures that have no concurrent neurological injury, although it is logical that there is a similar impact of timing on medical complications in these circumstances as well.

The authors of this review concur with other authors that there is a need for a well-controlled randomized prospective study on this subject that studies time thresholds more in line with what has been identified in animal models. This would imply that the definition of early in terms of surgical decompression and spine stabilization may be as soon as 3 hours after an SCI. If this were to become the new threshold for early surgical intervention, then this will have to be balanced against the realities of the circumstances that surround SCI. First, there may be significant delays in transporting the patient from the site of injury to the emergency room of a hospital that is capable of managing SCI. Second, upon arrival the emergency treatment of the concurrent polytrauma whereby vital organs have to be managed may also significantly delay the treatment of the SCI. These compounding issues all serve to variably delay the emergent decompression of the spinal cord following injury.

◆ Summary and Recommendations

The available evidence strongly supports that surgical stabilization for unstable spine fractures be performed as quickly as possible, generally within 24 hours in the physiologically stable polytrauma patient. The authors highlight the fact that the evidence is weak for supporting the benefit of surgical stabilization for unstable spine fractures performed within 48 hours being more conducive to improved neurological recovery compared with the same surgery performed after 48 hours. The authors are not able to draw any conclusions regarding the effect of surgical timing on mortality associated with spinal injuries. Clearly, additional clinical studies are necessary to identify whether surgical spine stabilization of unstable spine injuries with concurrent neurological injury within earlier time periods is either feasible or conducive to improved neurological outcome.

References

1. Wright JG, Swiontkowski MF, Heckman JD. Introducing levels of evidence to the journal. J Bone Joint Surg Am 2003;85-A:1–3

2. Guha A, Tator CH, Endrenyi L, Piper I. Decompression of the spinal cord improves recovery after acute experimental spinal cord compression injury. Paraplegia 1987;25:324–339

3. Delamarter RB, Sherman J, Carr JB. Pathophysiology of spinal cord injury: recovery after immediate and delayed decompression. J Bone Joint Surg Am 1995;77:1042–1049

4. Carlson GD, Minato Y, Okada A, et al. Early time-dependent decompression for spinal cord injury: vascular mechanisms of recovery. J Neurotrauma 1997;14:951–962

5. Dimar JR II, Glassman SD, Raque GH, Zhang YP, Shields CB. The influence of spinal canal narrowing and timing of decompression on neurologic recovery after spinal cord contusion in a rat model. Spine 1999;24:1623–1633

6. Carlson GD, Gorden CDMA, Oliff HS, Pillai JJ, LaManna JC. Sustained spinal cord compression, I: Time-dependent effect on long-term pathophysiology. J Bone Joint Surg Am 2003;85-A:86–94

7. Kwon BK, Tetzlaff W, Grauer JN, Beiner J, Vaccaro AR. Pathophysiology and pharmacologic treatment of acute spinal cord injury. Spine J 2004;4:451–464

8. Schünemann HJ, Jaeschke R, Cook DJ, et al; ATS Documents Development and Implementation Committee. An official ATS statement: grading the quality of evidence and strength of recommendations in ATS guidelines and recommendations. Am J Respir Crit Care Med 2006;174:605–614

9. Randle MJ, Wolf A, Levi L, et al. The use of anterior Caspar plate fixation in acute cervical spine injury. Surg Neurol 1991;36:181–189

10. Levi L, Wolf A, Rigamonti D, Ragheb J, Mirvis S, Robinson WL. Anterior decompression in cervical spine trauma: does the timing of surgery affect the outcome? Neurosurgery 1991;29:216–222

11. Schlegel J, Bayley J, Yuan H, Fredricksen B. Timing of surgical decompression and fixation of acute spinal fractures. J Orthop Trauma 1996;10: 323–330

12. Vaccaro AR, Daugherty RJ, Sheehan TP, et al. Neurologic outcome of early versus late surgery for cervical spinal cord injury. Spine 1997;22: 2609–2613

13. Kerwin AJ, Frykberg ER, Schinco MA, Griffen MM, Murphy T, Tepas JJ. The effect of early spine fixation on non-neurologic outcome. J Trauma 2005;58:15–21

14. Dai LY, Yao WF, Cui YM, Zhou Q. Thoracolumbar fractures in patients with multiple injuries: diagnosis and treatment-a review of 147 cases. J Trauma 2004;56:348–355

15. McKinley W, Meade MA, Kirshblum S, Barnard B. Outcomes of early surgical management versus late or no surgical intervention after acute spinal cord injury. Arch Phys Med Rehabil 2004;85:1818–1825

16. Croce MA, Bee TK, Pritchard E, Miller PR, Fabian TC. Does optimal timing for spine fracture fixation exist? Ann Surg 2001;233:851–858

17. Aebi M, Mohler J, Zäch GA, Morscher E. Indication, surgical technique, and results of 100 surgically-treated fractures and fracture-dislocations of the cervical spine. Clin Orthop Relat Res 1986;203:244–257

18. Mirza SK, Krengel WF III, Chapman JR, et al. Early versus delayed surgery for acute cervical spinal cord injury. Clin Orthop Relat Res 1999;359: 104–114

19. Papadopoulos SM, Selden NR, Quint DJ, Patel N, Gillespie B, Grube S. Immediate spinal cord decompression for cervical spinal cord injury: feasibility and outcome. J Trauma 2002;52:323–332

20. Krengel WF III, Anderson PA, Henley MB. Early stabilization and decompression for incomplete paraplegia due to a thoracic-level spinal cord injury. Spine 1993;18:2080–2087

21. Gaebler C, Maier R, Kutscha-Lissberg F, Mrkonjic L, Vècsei V. Results of spinal cord decompression and thoracolumbar pedicle stabilisation in relation to the time of operation. Spinal Cord 1999;37:33–39

22. Clohisy JC, Akbarnia BA, Bucholz RD, Burkus JK, Backer RJ. Neurologic recovery associated with anterior decompression of spine fractures at the thoracolumbar junction (T12-L1). Spine 1992;17(8, Suppl):S325–S330

23. Fehlings MG, Perrin RG. The timing of surgical intervention in the treatment of spinal cord injury: a systematic review of recent clinical evidence. Spine 2006;31(11, Suppl):S28–S35, discussion S36

24. Hadley MN, Fitzpatrick BC, Sonntag VK, Browner CM. Facet fracture-dislocation injuries of the cervical spine. Neurosurgery 1992;30:661–666

25. McLain RF, Benson DR. Urgent surgical stabilization of spinal fractures in polytrauma patients. Spine 1999;24:1646–1654

26. La Rosa G, Conti A, Cardali S, Cacciola F, Tomasello F. Does early decompression improve neurological outcome of spinal cord injured patients? Appraisal of the literature using a meta-analytical approach. Spinal Cord 2004;42:503–512

27. Albert TJ, Kim DH, David H. Timing of surgical stabilization after cervical and thoracic trauma. Invited submission from the Joint Section Meeting on Disorders of the Spine and Peripheral Nerves, March 2004. J Neurosurg Spine 2005;3:182–190

28. Chen TY, Lee ST, Lui TN, et al. Efficacy of surgical treatment in traumatic central cord syndrome. Surg Neurol 1997;48:435–440, discussion 441

29. Comarr AE, Kaufman AA. A survey of the neurological results of 858 spinal cord injuries; a comparison of patients treated with and without laminectomy. J Neurosurg 1956;13:95–106

30. Gertzbein SD. Scoliosis Research Society. Multicenter spine fracture study. Spine 1992;17:528–540

19

Principles of Cervical Whiplash Management

Paul M. Arnold, Karen K. Anderson, and Neal G. Haynes

Few topics in medicine are as controversial as cervical whiplash injury. The very name of the syndrome is vociferously debated. Chronic debilitating pain attributed to whiplash injury has been linked to anatomical or psychosocial causes, but in general, whiplash injury has failed to gain universal acceptance as a pathological entity.[1] The term *whiplash* was introduced in 1928 by Crowe[2] to describe the manner in which the cervical spine is injured when the head moves forward and backward in relation to the cervical spine in a "lash-like effect."[3-5] The term was intended to be a description of motion, not the name of a disease. The term *whiplash* has been misused and misunderstood, particularly because it has become widely accepted by the popular press. In 1963, Crowe himself expressed regret for his use of the term and the ensuing confusion it caused.

In 1995, the Quebec Task Force on Whiplash Associated Disorders defined whiplash as an acceleration–deceleration mechanism of energy transfer to the neck, which may result from rear-end or side-impact motor vehicle collisions, but may also result from diving or other mishaps.[6] The Quebec Task Force introduced the term *whiplash-associated disorders* (*WADs*) to distinguish between the bony or soft tissue injuries that may result from the impact and the mechanism of injury.

Whiplash injuries can be severe enough to cause at least transient pain in the majority of patients and permanent disability in some, and they can lead patients to seek medical attention for a broad array of medical complaints that are not easily classified. Whiplash-associated disorder ranges from mild to severe and can be acute, subacute, or chronic. This disorder has become a huge societal problem involving millions of dollars in lost wages, medical bills, legal fees, insurance compensation, and public and private payment of disability and compensation claims. Cervical whiplash injury is the single major cause of compensated claims following traffic accidents[7] and is one of the most common reasons for emergency room visits following automobile accidents.[8]

◆ Cervical Whiplash

Epidemiology

The incidence of whiplash injuries has increased dramatically in Western countries during the last several decades.[1,9] The reasons for this observed increase are not clear; it may reflect a change in care-seeking behavior for suspected neck injuries after traffic collisions, or reflect changes in how such injuries are recorded in health records.[9] Several causative factors associated with the increased incidence of whiplash injury that have been suggested in the literature include use of seat belts, changes in vehicle design, changed traffic patterns, poor driving habits, social copying, psychosocial factors, and increased litigation.[1,10] The current incidence in the United States is estimated to be as high as 1 million new cases annually.[1] In the Western world, the annual incidence of reported WAD is at least 300 per 100,000 inhabitants.[9]

Neck pain following a motor vehicle accident (MVA) begins the day of the collision in ~80% of patients; in 20% of those who develop chronic pain, there is a delay between the time of the MVA and the onset of pain.[11] Between 60 and 85% of those who suffer acute neck pain after whiplash injury go on to recover completely.[11-15] Up to 40% of patients who suffer whiplash injury develop chronic pain (usually mild), but 5 to 12% experience chronic moderate to severe pain. Approximately 5 to 10% of patients have permanent partial or total disability.[11-13,16,17] Chronic whiplash injury appears to affect older people more than younger people, and women more often than men, though acute whiplash appears to more frequently affect the opposite groups, young male drivers between the ages of 20 and 24, and male passengers between the ages of 15 and 19.[18]

Unique Clinical and Diagnostic Features

Whiplash injury was traditionally associated with rear-end vehicle impacts resulting in flexion-extension injury to the neck. Recently, however, this simplistic biomechanical explanation has been largely replaced by an understanding of more complex neck kinetics involving axial compression and biphasic cervical configuration. These kinetics contribute to potential damage to distinct anatomical components of the cervical spine in response to inertia loading.[1]

The normal cervical spine can allow ~60 degrees of flexion, 60 degrees of extension, 90 degrees of side-to-side rotation, and 30 degrees of lateral bending to either side.[19] Anatomical concerns involving injury occur when any of these natural motions are exceeded. The exact pathophysiology of WADs is not known, but it is likely that WADs result from cervical myofacial sprain or strain.[9] There may or may not be damage to soft tissue, including the joints, ligaments, and muscles in the neck, posterior shoulder, and upper thoracic regions.[9] Even though cervical fractures may occur as a result of a whiplash mechanism, they are generally excluded from WADs.[9] It has not been possible to ascertain a definite etiopathological pathway in the causation of whiplash injury. This is largely because whiplash injury is determined by several factors, namely, energy of the trauma, direction of force, biomechanics, preparedness for the injury, social awareness, psychosocial attributes, and medicolegal aspects.[1]

The most frequent complaints of WADs are neck pain and headache, which may begin immediately or 24 to 48 hours after the trauma. Up to 10% of patients reported a brief loss of consciousness after the accident in one series.[20] Confusion, amnesia, mental dullness, soreness, and stiffness in the neck and upper shoulders are also common. Radiculopathy can be a sign of brachial plexus involvement, whereas radiating headache can indicate injury to the occipital nerve. Nondermatomal radiation of pain may indicate damage to the disk end plates or damage to the cervical muscles themselves. Dizziness, tinnitus, Horner syndrome, and disturbance of circadian rhythms may be signs of sympathetic disruption, damage to the great vessels of the neck, or disruption of the spinal trigeminal tract.[21] Unusual presentations may include hoarseness or dysphagia from retropharyngeal hematoma, esophageal and larynx tears, or stretching of the recurrent laryngeal nerve. Damage to the long thoracic and spinal accessory nerves has also been reported.[22] As time passes patients may also complain of psychological symptoms, including anxiety, depression, nervousness, chronic daily headache, whole body ache or pain, weakness or numbness, difficulty coping, difficulty with activities of daily living, difficulty concentrating or working, and fatigue.[20] Although pending litigation and hope for secondary gain may influence some of these complaints, they should all be recorded and treated seriously.

The grading system most often used for WADs is that of Gargan and Bannister, published in 1990.[23] The system has been frequently used because it is simple, reproducible, and validated and is based on the severity of symptoms. Present in all grades can be other symptoms such as dizziness, tinnitus, headache, memory loss, dysphagia, and temporomandibular joint pain. The grading system is summarized as follows:

- *Grade 0.* No neck complaints and no physical sign of injury
- *Grade 1.* Complaints of neck pain, stiffness, or tenderness but no physical signs of injury
- *Grade 2.* Complaints of neck pain, stiffness, or tenderness accompanied by decreased range of motion and point tenderness

- *Grade 3.* Neck complaints accompanied by neurological signs such as decreased or absent deep tendon reflexes, weakness, and/or sensory deficits
- *Grade 4.* Injuries in which neck complaints are accompanied by fracture or dislocation and thus no longer considered whiplash-type injuries.

An update of this system was proposed in 2008 by the Bone and Joint Decade 2000–2010 Task Force on Neck Pain and Its Associated Disorders (the Neck Pain Task Force). The Task Force recommends that in the initial clinical assessment of patients with neck pain, clinicians should triage patients into four simple descriptive categories rather than establish a specific structural diagnosis as the origin of the pain.[24] Different investigations and management are required by each grade, and different assessment and management strategies are required in different clinical settings.[24] The classification is based on five axes, including the source of subjects, the setting and sampling of subjects, and the severity, duration, and pattern of neck pain.[24,25] Briefly, these categories are as follows:

- *Grade I* (common). Neck pain with no signs of serious pathology and no or little interference with daily activities
- *Grade II.* Neck pain with no signs of serious pathology but with interference with daily activities
- *Grade III* (uncommon). Neck pain with neurological signs of nerve compression
- *Grade IV* (rare). Neck pain with signs of major structural pathology

There are several significant differences between the Neck Pain Task Force system and that of Gargan and Bannister: (1) there is no grade 0; (2) grade II is distinguished from grade I by the presence of major interference with activities of daily living, rather than localized tenderness or restricted range of motion; interference with daily living has larger prognostic and management implications than those relatively unreliable physical signs[24]; (3) grade IV includes all major structural pathology, not just fractures; and (4) this new classification system is applicable to all neck pain and associated disorders, not just WADs.[24]

Nonoperative Initial Management

Multiple treatment modalities for cervical neck pain exist, but there is little scientific evidence for their use or efficacy. There are remarkably few evidence-based treatments for whiplash-associated disorder, although several systematic reviews and clinical practice guidelines do exist. **Table 19.1**, based on results of the Neck Pain Task Force[24] and endorsed by the authors, is a summary of nonoperative interventions for patients with neck pain.

Surgical Management

For the patient with cervical neck pain, the role of surgery is controversial. In 2002, Garvey et al[26] reported on 87 patients, including 25 with chronic whiplash-associated injury, who underwent ACDF for axial neck pain with good to excellent results at 4 years.[26] In 1999, Palit et al[27] reported on 38 patients who underwent anterior cervical discectomy and fusion (ACDF) for chronic axial neck pain, with 79% of patients satisfied with

Table 19.1 Summary of Nonoperative Interventions for Patients with Neck Pain

Situation	Moderate Level of Evidence	Low Level of Evidence	Very Low Level of Evidence	Not Enough Evidence
Acute: Post MVA, neck pain grade I and II	Mobilization, exercises, mobilization plus exercises, educational video	Pulsed electromagnetic therapy	Neck pamphlet alone, methylprednisolone, collars, passive modalities (heat, cold, diathermy, hydrotherapy), referral to fitness or rehab program, frequent early health-care use	NSAIDs, other drugs, manipulation, traction
Nonacute: post-MVA, neck pain grade I and II		Coordinated multidisciplinary care, supervised exercises	Corticosteroid injections, passive modalities (TENS, ultrasound)	NSAIDS, other drugs, manipulation, traction
Nontraumatic neck pain, neck pain grade I and II	Analgesics, acupuncture, low-level laser therapy, manipulation, mobilization, supervised exercises, manual therapy (manipulation, mobilization, massage) plus exercises	Brief intervention using cognitive behavioral principles, percutaneous neuromuscular therapy	Exercise instruction, botulinum toxin A, advice alone, collars, passive modalities (TENS, electrical muscle stimulation, heat therapy, ultrasound)	NSAIDs, other drugs, magnetic stimulation, massage alone, traction
Suspected cervical radiculopathy: neck pain grade III	Not enough evidence	Not enough evidence	Not enough evidence	Not enough evidence

Abbreviations: MVA, motor vehicle accident; NSAIDs, nonsteroidal antiinflammatory drugs; TENS, transcutaneous electrical nerve stimulation.

their outcome. These results are little better than those expected with most other nonoperative treatment modalities.[27] However, although neither of these studies were randomized, controlled trials (RCTs), they do stand out in the literature compared with studies of conservative treatments because of the high number of responders and the definitive nature of the treatment. **Table 19.2**, based on results of the Neck Pain Task Force[24] and endorsed by the authors, is a summary of invasive (surgical) interventions for patients with neck pain.

Potential Complications and Their Avoidance

Although rare, there are possible complications of common treatments for neck pain. **Table 19.3**, based on research by

the Neck Pain Task Force[24] and endorsed by the authors, summarizes these possible complications.

Rehabilitation and Prognosis

Determining the prognostic factors involved in recovery from WAD is important in planning effective health care interventions, health policies, and lifestyle changes.[28] Numerous studies have documented the natural history of whiplash-associated disorder.[6,14,29–36] After an MVA, pain begins the day of the collision in ~80% of patients, and in 20% of those who develop chronic pain, there is a delay between the time of the MVA and the onset of pain.[11] Most people involved in MVAs do not develop neck pain. Of those who do suffer acute neck

Table 19.2 Summary of Invasive (Surgical) Interventions for Patients with Neck Pain

Situation	Moderate Level of Evidence	Low Level of Evidence	Very Low Level of Evidence	Not Enough Evidence
Neck pain grade III	Diskectomy or diskectomy with fusion	Diskectomy with fusion and instrumentation; trial of corticosteroid injections (< 4) for short-term relief; cervical disk replacement	Heating of the dorsal root ganglion	Nothing in this category
Neck pain grade I or II	Nothing in this category	Nothing in this category	Corticosteroid injections to cervical facets	RF neurotomy to cervical facet nerves; anterior cervical fusion (any method); cervical decompression; cervical disk replacement
Neck pain grade I or II after MVA	Nothing in this category	Nothing in this category	Corticosteroid injections to cervical facets	RF neurotomy to cervical facet nerves; anterior cervical fusion (any method); cervical decompression; cervical disk replacement

Table 19.3 Possible Complications of Common Treatments for Neck Pain

Intervention	> 10% Incidence (common)	1–10% Incidence (occasional)	0.001–1% Incidence (rare)	< 0.001% Incidence (remote)	Not Enough Evidence
NSAIDs	Dyspepsia	GI bleeding	Heart attacks	–	–
Muscle relaxants	Drowsiness	–	–	–	–
Exercise	Transient discomfort, dizziness	–	–	–	–
Mobilization	–	Minor, transient discomfort	–	–	–
Manipulation	Minor, transient discomfort	–	–	VBA stroke	–
Epidural injections	–	Headache, increased pain	Dural puncture	–	Infection; major neurologic injury
Cervical root injections	Lightheadedness; pain at injection; increased radicular pain	Headache; nausea; increased neck pain	Transient weakness	–	Infection; major neurologic injury
RF facet ablation	Permanent numb patch to neck; transient increased pain	–	–	–	–
Surgery: diskectomy with or without fusion	Nonunion; dysphagia; hoarseness; serious early complication with use of BMP; any serious complications in > 75 years old	Donor site pain (persistent); vocal cord paralysis (symptomatic)	Root or cord injury; vertebral artery injury; permanent symptomatic vocal cord dysfunction	As for any surgery, other medical, anesthetic and surgical complications	Infection; major neurologic injury

Abbreviations: BMP, bone morphogenetic protein; GI, gastrointestinal; VBA, vertebrobasilar artery.

pain after whiplash injury, between 60 and 85% go on to recover completely.[11–15] In adults, strong evidence indicates that recovery from WADs is prolonged, with approximately half of those affected reporting persistent WAD symptoms 1 year after the injury.[28] In the context of the high prevalence of neck pain in the general population, only 12% of those with WADs reported daily pain at 1 year, and fewer than 12% reported symptoms that had a significant impact on their health.[24] Up to 40% of patients who suffer whiplash injury develop chronic mild pain, but 5 to 12% experience chronic moderate to severe pain and ~5 to 10% have permanent partial or total disability.[11–13,16,17]

◆ Two Key Questions about Cervical Whiplash Management and Evidence-based Answers

During our comprehensive medical literature review, we searched the bibliographic databases of the Cochrane Library, PubMed, and the Cumulative Index to Nursing and Allied Health Literature (CINAHL), limiting our findings to those studies of adults (18 years or older), published in English in peer-reviewed journals, and including neck disorders that are acute (less than 30 days), subacute (30 days to 90 days), or chronic (longer than 90 days). We evaluated several clinical practice guidelines from leading specialty societies as well as several Cochrane reviews. We looked for any supplementary information in the citations from the reference lists of those guidelines and reviews. In addition,

we included the results of the Bone and Joint Decade 2000–2010 Task Force on Neck Pain and Its Associated Disorders, which were released in February 2008. This Neck Pain Task Force conducted a systematic search and critical review of studies on neck pain and its associated disorders and from that data produced a Best Evidence Synthesis of the 552 studies accepted as scientifically admissible. For this chapter, evidence was graded on a four-point scale[37,38] as follows:

- ◆ *High.* It is very unlikely that further research will change our confidence in the estimation of effect.
- ◆ *Moderate.* It is likely that further research will change our confidence in the estimation of effect, and it may even change our estimate.
- ◆ *Low.* It is very likely that further research will change our confidence in the estimation of effect, and is likely to change our estimate.
- ◆ *Very low.* Any estimate of effect is very uncertain.

What Is the Optimal Management of the Patient with Acute Whiplash?

Assessment

To make a diagnosis of cervical whiplash injury there must be a history of trauma, though even a seemingly minor injury can be a causative factor. It is important for the clinician to exclude more severe pathology such as subluxation, fracture-dislocation, disk herniation, spinal cord contusion, and vascular injury.

Other diagnoses to consider include myofascial neck pain, mechanical neck disorder, and occipital neuralgia. A presumptive diagnosis of a whiplash injury should be considered when a computed tomographic (CT) scan is negative for fractures or subluxation; when a magnetic resonance imaging (MRI) scan is negative for soft tissue injuries such as disk herniation, end plate separation, or ligamentous disruption; and when serial flexion-extension films are negative for movement. There is no evidence that the degree of cervical lordosis or kyphosis can distinguish patients with WADs from those without WADs or accurately identify "cervical muscle spasm." In identifying acute whiplash injury in the upper cervical spine ligaments, the validity of high-intensity-signal MRI findings has not been demonstrated.

A gold standard diagnostic test for WADs does not exist.[9] Neither history nor physical examination can elicit specific findings that point to any one structural cause of chronic axial neck pain.[11] Data from the history and physical examination are very important, however, to exclude serious medical problems or causes of pain other than neck pain.[11] Whiplash injuries are usually not apparent on radiographic imaging except for flattening of the cervical lordosis, presumed to be secondary to myofascial spasm. Therefore, the diagnosis is based on clinical findings and is derived by exclusion of more severe pathologies.

In patients seeking care for neck pain who have no exposure to blunt trauma, the Neck Pain Task Force recommends a system of "red flags" to enable clinicians to rule out serious pathology. These conditions include trauma (minor, or no trauma with osteoporosis or corticosteroid treatment); pathological fractures (spontaneous or following minor trauma); tumor/cancer/malignancy; systemic inflammatory diseases (e.g., ankylosing spondylitis, inflammatory arthritis), infections (e.g., urinary tract infection, skin infection, IV drug abuse); spinal cord compromise (cervical myelopathy); and previous cervical spine surgery, neck surgery, or open injury.[25]

Regarding assessment in the emergency setting, the Neck Pain Task Force reports strong consistent evidence[25] for the use of screening protocols [e.g., Canadian C-Spine Rule (CCR), Nexus Low Risk Criteria (NLC)] for low-risk adult patients with blunt trauma to the neck and the use of CT scan for high-risk adults with blunt trauma to the neck; there is strong consistent evidence against the use of flexion-extension or five-view x-ray. There is consistent evidence that a CT scan is more sensitive for finding significant cervical spine injury than a plain three-view x-ray in high-risk or multiinjured blunt trauma neck patients.

Regarding assessment in the primary care setting, the Neck Pain Task Force reports evidence[25] supporting the use of manual provocation tests of the neck and upper extremity for suspected radiculopathy; the combined use of history, physical examination, needle electromyography (EMG), and modern imaging techniques to diagnose the cause and site of cervical radiculopathy; and the use of patient self-reported assessments to evaluate function, disability, perceived pain, and psychosocial status.

According to the Neck Pain Task Force and endorsed by the authors, the Canadian C-spine and NEXUS criteria are likely helpful during the initial assessment in the emergency room after blunt trauma to the neck. For those patients at high risk of fracture, a CT scan and standard three-view x-rays are also likely helpful; those tests likely not helpful include flexion-extension x-rays, five-view x-rays, and blood work. At the initial assessment in the primary care of patients without trauma to the neck, those tests likely helpful include self-assessment questionnaires and clinical examination. For those patients in primary care who present with grade I or II neck pain, those tests likely not helpful include x-ray, CT scan, MRI, and discography.[24]

Nonoperative Management

Table 19.4, based on results of the Neck Pain Task Force[39] and endorsed by the authors, summarizes noninvasive interventions for WADs and other neck disorders. A systematic review of the literature in 2007 by Gross et al[8] evaluated conservative treatments of mechanical neck disorders, including whiplash-associated disorder. They found that for acute WADs, studies of IV glucocorticoid showed reduction of work disability at 1 year, whereas stretching exercises and low-frequency pulse electromagnetic field reduced pain. For chronic neck disorder with radicular findings (NDR), they determined that epidural methylprednisolone and lidocaine improved function and pain in the short and long term, whereas intermittent traction improved pain in the short term. Additionally, for treatment of subacute and chronic mechanical neck disorder (MND) or neck disorder with headache (NDH), their review revealed evidence favoring a multimodal strategy (exercise and mobilization/manipulation); exercise alone; intramuscular (IM) lidocaine injection; and low-level laser therapy [for osteoarthritis (OA)] for pain, function, and global perceived effect in the short and long term. Acupuncture, low-frequency pulsed electromagnetic field, repetitive magnetic stimulation, cervical orthopedic

Table 19.4 Summary of Noninvasive Interventions for WAD and Other Neck Disorders

Situation	Moderate Level of Evidence	Low Level of Evidence	Very Low Level of Evidence	Not Enough Evidence
Acute WAD (neck pain grade I or II)	Mobilization, educational video, exercises, mobilization and exercises	Pulsed electromagnetic therapy	Collars, pamphlet/booklet alone, passive modalities, referral to fitness or rehab program, methylprednisolone, frequent early health-care use	NSAIDs, other drugs, manipulation, traction
Nonacute WAD (neck pain grade I or II)	–	Coordinated multidisciplinary care, supervised exercises	Corticosteroid injections, passive modalities	NSAIDs, other drugs, manipulation, traction

Abbreviations: NSAIDs, nonsteroidal antiinflammatory drugs; WAD, whiplash-associated disorder.

pillow, and traditional Chinese massage were favored for either immediate or short-term pain management.

A Cochrane review of the literature in 2007 by Verhagen et al[40] concluded that because the overall quality of the included studies was poor, there is still conflicting evidence about whether active or passive treatments are more effective for treating acute, subacute, or chronic grade I or II WADs. Although no clear conclusions could be drawn, the authors described a trend that active interventions are probably more effective than passive interventions.

A Cochrane systematic review of the literature in 2006 by Peloso et al evaluated 32 medication trials for mechanical neck disorders, including WADs.[41,42] They reported that the most promising therapies appear to be intravenous (IV) methylprednisolone for acute whiplash and IM lidocaine for chronic WADs. For acute WADs, a single trial of IV methylprednisolone given within 8 hours of injury was superior to placebo, with short-term improvement in pain and reduced long-term sick leave. For chronic MND or neck disorder with radicular findings (NDR), oral psychotropics gave mixed results. For chronic neck pain, nonsteroidal antiinflammatory drugs (NSAIDs) were not effective, and for chronic neck pain with radiation, a single study showed that epidural methylprednisolone and lidocaine improved pain and function at 1 year. For chronic WADs, two trials showed that IM injection of lidocaine provided short-term benefit. For chronic neck disorders with or without radicular findings or headache, Botox-A (Allergan, Inc., Irvine, CA) had no advantage over saline injection, based on five trials and one meta-analysis.

Surgical Management

In treating more common kinds of neck pain, with or without radiculopathy, the role of invasive interventions is less clear than in the treatment of neck pain associated with serious structural disease. There is little evidence that surgery for WAD-associated neck pain alone is efficacious. **Table 19.5**, based on results of the Neck Pain Task Force[43] and endorsed by the authors, summarizes invasive (surgical) interventions for WADs and other neck disorders.

What Are the Prognostic Variables with Respect to Health-Related Quality of Life, Chronic Pain, and Return to Work in the Patient with Acute Whiplash?

Identifying and understanding prognostic factors have implications for patient management. The factors that *increase* the chances of recovery from an episode of neck pain, summarized

Table 19.5 Summary of Invasive (Surgical) Interventions for WAD and Other Neck Disorders

Situation	Moderate Level of Evidence	Low Level of Evidence	Very Low Level of Evidence	Not Enough Evidence
Neck pain grade III (with cervical radiculopathy)	ACD (benefit over nonsurgical treatment most clearly seen in 1st yr post-surgery = "short-term"); ACDF ("short-term")	Limited (< 4 injections) epidural or root corticosteroid injections ("short-term"); ACDF + instrumentation/cages ("short-term"); Single-level cervical disk replacement ("short-term")	Thermal heating of the dorsal root ganglion	Multilevel cervical disk replacement; spinal cord stimulator implantation or implantable intrathecal narcotic pump; disk nucleoplasty or annuloplasty
Neck pain grade I or II; axial neck pain without radiculopathy	None in this category	None in this category	Corticosteroid injections to cervical facets; RF neurotomy to cervical facet nerves w/o confirmed zygapophyseal pain; cervical decompression; cervical fusion or disk replacement (with comorbidities)	RF neurotomy to cervical facet nerves with confirmed zygapophyseal pain; cervical fusion (no comorbidities); cervical disk replacement; spinal cord stimulator implantation or implantable intrathecal narcotic pump; disk nucleoplasty or anuloplasty
WAD-related axial neck pain without fracture, dislocation, or instability	None in this category	None in this category	Corticosteroid injections to cervical facets; RF neurotomy to cervical facet nerves w/o confirmed zygapophyseal pain; cervical decompression; cervical fusion or disk replacement (with comorbidities)	RF neurotomy to cervical facets nerves with confirmed zygapophyseal pain; craniocervical or upper cervical fusion; cervical fusion (w/o comorbidities); cervical disk replacement; spinal cord stimulator implantation or implantable intrathecal narcotic pump; disk nucleoplasty or anuloplasty

Abbreviations: ACD, anterior cervical discectomy; ACDF, anterior cervical discectomy and fusion; RF, radio frequency.

Table 19.6 Factors That Increase the Chances of Recovery from an Episode of Neck Pain

Group	Likely to Increase Chances of Recovery	Might Increase Chances of Recovery	No Effect on Recovery	Not Enough Evidence
General population	Younger age, good physical and psychological health, no previous neck pain, good coping, good social support	Being employed	–	Cervical disk changes, gender, general exercise or fitness prior to pain episode
After a traffic collision	Fewer initial symptoms, no prior pain or sick leave, no early "overtreatment," less symptom severity, grade I WAD, good psychological health (e.g., no fear of movement)	Good prior health, no prior pain problems, non–tort insurance, no lawyer involvement, lower collision speed	Collision-specific factors (e.g., position of vehicle, head position when struck, direction of collision)	Cervical disk changes, gender, age, prior physical fitness, culture

Abbreviations: WAD, whiplash-associated disability.

by the Neck Pain Task Force[28] and endorsed by the authors, are noted in **Table 19.6**. The factors that *decrease* the chances of recovery from an episode of neck pain, summarized by the Neck Pain Task Force[28] and endorsed by the authors, are noted in **Table 19.7**.

In 2003, Scholten-Peeters et al[44] conducted a systematic review of the prognostic factors of WADs that are associated with functional recovery in terms of symptoms or disability. The authors used overall analysis on which to base their final conclusions because the methodological quality of the cohort studies was highly variable. The authors' findings are noted in **Table 19.8**.

In 2007, an updated systematic review was conducted by Williamson et al[45] because of new articles published since 2003, and because of the diversified range of psychological factors now being studied. It was not possible for a meta-analysis to be conducted because of the use of different prognostic factors and outcome measures. Williamson et al reported that the majority of their findings were inconclusive or based on limited evidence (**Table 19.9**).

Table 19.7 Factors That Decrease the Chances of Recovery From an Episode of Neck Pain

Substantial Predictors of Poorer Recovery	Initial postinjury pain intensity; number and severity of injury-related symptoms; WAD grade III versus WAD grade I
Consistent Evidence of Slower Recovery and Poorer Outcome	Increased initial symptom severity (such as greater initial pain, greater number of symptoms, more parts of the body in pain, and pain-related limitations); (on average) frequent, early health care use
Evidence for Slower Recovery and Poorer Outcome	Postinjury psychological distress; later passive types of coping; helplessness; depression; fear of movement; catastrophizing; and anxiety
Some Evidence for Slower Recovery	Greater health care utilization in the first month after a whiplash injury
Varied Evidence of Effect on Recovery	Age, gender, and preinjury neck pain
Preliminary Evidence for Slower Recovery	Compensation and litigation
Evidence of No Prognostic Association	Most collision factors (studies were adjusted for initial pain and symptom severity); coping behaviors used within the first few days of injury

Table 19.8 Scholten-Peeters et al Review

Strong Evidence	High initial pain intensity is associated with persisting symptoms
Moderate Evidence	No prognostic factors found for this level
Limited Evidence	The association of the following prognostic factors with persisting symptoms and continuing disability: nervousness, accidents happening on the highway, stationary cars, need to resume physiotherapy, a driving occupation, high initial pain intensity, restricted cervical range of motion, low muscle workload, high number of complaints, and previous psychological problems
Inconclusive Evidence	Radicular symptoms, sleep disturbances, cognitive impairments, unpreparedness for collision, turned head positions, previous headache, cervical degenerative changes, and bulging disks
Did Not Find Any Evidence	The influence of coping, anxiety, cognition, education level, head restraint, or seat belt
Strong Evidence	Older age, female gender, high acute psychological response, rear-end collision, angular deformity of the neck, and compensation have no prognostic value for delayed functional recovery. (In contrast, in 2001 Côté et al[14] found evidence that gender and age do have an influence on recovery after a whiplash injury.)

Table 19.9 Williamson et al Review

No Strong Evidence	Any psychological factors supporting a positive or negative association with the development of LWS
Limited Evidence	Supporting an association with the development of LWS for lower levels of self-efficacy and greater posttraumatic stress (a stress reaction, not a true diagnosis of posttraumatic stress disorder
Moderate Evidence	No association between personality traits (which Scholten-Peeters et al[44] deemed inconclusive), or general psychological distress (in agreement with Scholten-Peeters) and the development of LWS
Limited Evidence	No association found between well-being, social support, life control, or psychosocial work factors
Inconclusive	The following prognostic factors: psychosocial stress not associated with the accident, previous psychological problems (which Scholten-Peeters et al[43] found to be associated with poor outcome), blame and anger, perceived threat at the time of the accident, cognitive function, anxiety, depression, somatization, irritability, familiarity with whiplash symptoms, fear avoidance beliefs, catastrophizing, and coping strategies

Abbreviation: LWS, late whiplash syndrome.

◆ Summary

In summary, there are no definitive nonsurgical treatments that will "cure" WADs. Multimodal strategies are probably better than single treatments, but therapy must be individualized. Appropriate x-ray workup should be performed to rule out serious bony or spinal cord injury. As with most diseases, treatment should be tailored to the particular situation. Patients who are younger, in good physical health, with good social support, and harbor fewer initial symptoms tend to achieve a better recovery than those who do not have these advantages.

References

1. Giannoudis PV, Mehta SS, Tsiridis E. Incidence and outcome of whiplash injury after multiple trauma. Spine 2007;32:776–781
2. Crowe HE. Injuries to the cervical spine. Presented at the Annual Meeting of the Western Orthopedic Association, San Francisco, CA, 1928
3. Wallace DJ. Whiplash: a case of regretting being responsible for naming a condition. J Clin Rheumatol 2005;11:61
4. Evans RW. Whiplash around the world. Headache 1995;35:262–263
5. Bonuccelli U, Pavese N, Lucetti C, et al. Late whiplash syndrome: a clinical and magnetic resonance imaging study. Funct Neurol 1999;14:219–225
6. Spitzer WO, Skovron ML, Salmi LR, et al. Scientific monograph of the Quebec Task Force on Whiplash-Associated Disorders: redefining "whiplash" and its management. Spine 1995;20(8, Suppl):1S–73S
7. Smed A. Cognitive function and distress after common whiplash injury. Acta Neurol Scand 1997;95:73–80
8. Gross AR, Goldsmith C, Hoving JL, et al; Cervical Overview Group. Conservative management of mechanical neck disorders: a systematic review. J Rheumatol 2007;34:1083–1102
9. Holm LW, Carroll LJ, Cassidy JD, et al; Bone and Joint Decade 2000-2010 Task Force on Neck Pain and Its Associated Disorders. The burden and determinants of neck pain in whiplash-associated disorders after traffic collisions: results of the Bone and Joint Decade 2000-2010 Task Force on Neck Pain and Its Associated Disorders. Spine 2008;33(4, Suppl):S52–S59
10. Kroeling P, Gross AR, Goldsmith CH; Cervical Overview Group. A Cochrane review of electrotherapy for mechanical neck disorders. Spine 2005;30:E641–E648
11. Schofferman J, Bogduk N, Slosar P. Chronic whiplash and whiplash-associated disorders: an evidence-based approach. J Am Acad Orthop Surg 2007;15:596–606
12. Radanov BP, Sturzenegger M, Di Stefano G. Long-term outcome after whiplash injury: a 2-year follow-up considering features of injury mechanism and somatic, radiologic, and psychosocial findings. Medicine (Baltimore) 1995;74:281–297
13. Berglund A, Alfredsson L, Cassidy JD, Jensen I, Nygren A. The association between exposure to a rear-end collision and future neck or shoulder pain: a cohort study. J Clin Epidemiol 2000;53:1089–1094
14. Côté P, Cassidy JD, Carroll L, Frank JW, Bombardier C. A systematic review of the prognosis of acute whiplash and a new conceptual framework to synthesize the literature. Spine 2001;26:E445–E458
15. Scholten-Peeters GG, Bekkering GE, Verhagen AP, et al. Clinical practice guideline for the physiotherapy of patients with whiplash-associated disorders. Spine 2002;27:412–422
16. Gozzard C, Bannister G, Langkamer G, Khan S, Gargan M, Foy C. Factors affecting employment after whiplash injury. J Bone Joint Surg Br 2001; 83:506–509
17. Hendriks EJ, Scholten-Peeters GG, van der Windt DA, Neeleman-van der Steen CW, Oostendorp RA, Verhagen AP. Prognostic factors for poor recovery in acute whiplash patients. Pain 2005;114:408–416
18. Sizer PS Jr, Poorbaugh K, Phelps V. Whiplash associated disorders: pathomechanics, diagnosis, and management. Pain Pract 2004;4:249–266
19. Gibson JW. Cervical syndromes: use of a comfortable cervical collar as an adjunct in their management. South Med J 1974;67:205–208
20. Hohl M. Soft tissue injuries of the neck. Clin Orthop Relat Res 1975; 109:42–49
21. Levine RA. Somatic (craniocervical) tinnitus and the dorsal cochlear nucleus hypothesis. Am J Otolaryngol 1999;20:351–362
22. Omar N, Alvi F, Srinivasan MS. An unusual presentation of whiplash injury: long thoracic and spinal accessory nerve injury. Eur Spine J 2007; 16(Suppl 3):275–277
23. Gargan MF, Bannister GC. Long-term prognosis of soft-tissue injuries of the neck. J Bone Joint Surg Br 1990;72:901–903
24. Guzman J, Haldeman S, Carroll LJ, et al; Bone and Joint Decade 2000-2010 Task Force on Neck Pain and Its Associated Disorders. Clinical practice implications of the Bone and Joint Decade 2000-2010 Task Force on Neck Pain and Its Associated Disorders: from concepts and findings to recommendations. Spine 2008;33(4, Suppl):S199–S213
25. Nordin M, Carragee EJ, Hogg-Johnson S, et al; Bone and Joint Decade 2000-2010 Task Force on Neck Pain and Its Associated Disorders. Assessment of neck pain and its associated disorders: results of the Bone and Joint Decade 2000-2010 Task Force on Neck Pain and Its Associated Disorders. Spine 2008;33(4, Suppl):S101–S122
26. Garvey TA, Transfeldt EE, Malcolm JR, Kos P. Outcome of anterior cervical discectomy and fusion as perceived by patients treated for dominant axial-mechanical cervical spine pain. Spine 2002;27:1887–1895, discussion 1895
27. Palit M, Schofferman J, Goldthwaite N, et al. Anterior discectomy and fusion for the management of neck pain. Spine 1999;24:2224–2228
28. Carroll LJ, Holm LW, Hogg-Johnson S, et al; Bone and Joint Decade 2000-2010 Task Force on Neck Pain and Its Associated Disorders. Course and prognostic factors for neck pain in whiplash-associated disorders (WAD): results of the Bone and Joint Decade 2000-2010 Task Force on Neck Pain and Its Associated Disorders. Spine 2008;33(4, Suppl): S83–S92
29. Bogduk N, Yoganandan N. Biomechanics of the cervical spine, III: Minor injuries. Clin Biomech (Bristol, Avon) 2001;16:267–275
30. Radanov BP, di Stefano G, Schnidrig A, Ballinari P. Role of psychosocial stress in recovery from common whiplash [see comment]. Lancet 1991;338:712–715
31. Radanov BP, Sturzenegger M, Di Stefano G, Schnidrig A, Aljinovic M. Factors influencing recovery from headache after common whiplash. BMJ 1993;307:652–655
32. Radanov BP, Di Stefano G, Schnidrig A, Sturzenegger M, Augustiny KF. Cognitive functioning after common whiplash: a controlled follow-up study. Arch Neurol 1993;50:87–91
33. Radanov BP, Di Stefano G, Schnidrig A, Sturzenegger M. Common whiplash: psychosomatic or somatopsychic? J Neurol Neurosurg Psychiatry 1994;57:486–490
34. Radanov BP, Sturzenegger M, De Stefano G, Schnidrig A. Relationship between early somatic, radiological, cognitive and psychosocial findings and outcome during a one-year follow-up in 117 patients suffering from common whiplash. Br J Rheumatol 1994;33:442–448

35. Radanov BP, Begré S, Sturzenegger M, Augustiny KF. Course of psychological variables in whiplash injury: a 2-year follow-up with age, gender and education pair-matched patients. Pain 1996;64:429–434

36. Radanov BP, Sturzenegger M. Predicting recovery from common whiplash. Eur Neurol 1996;36:48–51

37. Schünemann HJ, Jaeschke R, Cook DJ, et al; ATS Documents Development and Implementation Committee. An official ATS statement: grading the quality of evidence and strength of recommendations in ATS guidelines and recommendations. Am J Respir Crit Care Med 2006;174:605–614

38. Fisher CG, Wood KB. Introduction to and techniques of evidence-based medicine. Spine 2007;32(19, Suppl):S66–S72

39. Hurwitz EL, Carragee EJ, van der Velde G, et al; Bone and Joint Decade 2000-2010 Task Force on Neck Pain and Its Associated Disorders. Treatment of neck pain: noninvasive interventions: results of the Bone and Joint Decade 2000–2010 Task Force on neck pain and its associated disorders. Spine 2008;33(4, Suppl):S123–S152

40. Verhagen AP, Scholten-Peeters GGGM, van Wijngaarden S, de Bie RA, Bierma-Zeinstra SM. Conservative treatments for whiplash. Cochrane Database Syst Rev 2007;(2):CD003338

41. Peloso P, Gross A, Haines T, Trinh K, Goldsmith CH, Burnie S ; Cervical Overview Group. Medicinal and injection therapies for mechanical neck disorders. Cochrane Database Syst Rev 2007;(3, Issue 3)CD000319

42. Peloso PM, Gross AR, Haines TA, Trinh K, Goldsmith CH, Aker P. Medicinal and injection therapies for mechanical neck disorders: a Cochrane systematic review. J Rheumatol 2006;33:957–967

43. Carragee EJ, Hurwitz EL, Cheng I, et al; Bone and Joint Decade 2000-2010 Task Force on Neck Pain and Its Associated Disorders. Treatment of neck pain: injections and surgical interventions: results of the Bone and Joint Decade 2000–2010 Task Force on neck pain and its associated disorders. Spine 2008;33(4, Suppl):S153–S169

44. Scholten-Peeters GGM, Verhagen AP, Bekkering GE, et al. Prognostic factors of whiplash-associated disorders: a systematic review of prospective cohort studies. Pain 2003;104:303–322

45. Williamson E, Williams M, Gates S, Lamb SE. A systematic literature review of psychological factors and the development of late whiplash syndrome. Pain 2008;135:20–30

46. Graham N, Gross AR, Goldsmith C; the Cervical Overview Group. Mechanical traction for mechanical neck disorders: a systematic review. J Rehabil Med 2006;38:145–152

47. Vernon H, Humphreys BK. Manual therapy for neck pain: an overview of randomized clinical trials and systematic reviews. Eura Medicophys 2007;43:91–118

48. Mealy K, Brennan H, Fenelon GC. Early mobilization of acute whiplash injuries. Br Med J (Clin Res Ed) 1986;292:656–657

49. McKinney LA. Early mobilisation and outcome in acute sprains of the neck. BMJ 1989;299:1006–1008

50. Provinciali L, Baroni M, Illuminati L, Ceravolo MG. Multimodal treatment to prevent the late whiplash syndrome. Scand J Rehabil Med 1996;28:105–111

51. Bonk A, Ferrari R, Giebel GD, et al. Prospective, randomized controlled study of activity versus collar, and the natural history for whiplash injury in Germany. J Musculoskeletal Pain 2000;8:123–132

52. Schnabel M, Ferrari R, Vassiliou T, Kaluza G. Randomised, controlled outcome study of active mobilisation compared with collar therapy for whiplash injury. Emerg Med J 2004;21:306–310

53. Fernandez-de-las-Penas C, Fernandez-Carnero J, Palomeque del Cerro L, Miangolarra-Page JC. Manipulative treatment vs conventional physiotherapy treatment in whiplash injury: a randomized controlled trial. J Whip Rel Dis 2004;3:73–90

54. Peeters GG, Verhagen AP, de Bie RA, Oostendorp RA. The efficacy of conservative treatment in patients with whiplash injury: a systematic review of clinical trials. Spine 2001;26:E64–E73

55. Foley-Nolan D, Moore K, Codd M, Barry C, O'Connor P, Coughlan RJ. Low energy high frequency pulsed electromagnetic therapy for acute whiplash injuries: a double blind randomized controlled study. Scand J Rehabil Med 1992;24:51–59

56. Borchgrevink GE, Kaasa A, McDonagh D, Stiles TC, Haraldseth O, Lereim I. Acute treatment of whiplash neck sprain injuries: a randomized trial of treatment during the first 14 days after a car accident. Spine 1998;23:25–31

57. Morley S, Eccleston C, Williams A. Systematic review and meta-analysis of randomized controlled trials of cognitive behaviour therapy and behaviour therapy for chronic pain in adults, excluding headache. Pain 1999;80:1–13

58. Barnsley L, Lord SM, Wallis BJ, Bogduk N. Lack of effect of intraarticular corticosteroids for chronic pain in the cervical zygapophyseal joints. N Engl J Med 1994;330:1047–1050

59. Brison RJ, Hartling L, Dostaler S, et al. A randomized controlled trial of an educational intervention to prevent the chronic pain of whiplash associated disorders following rear-end motor vehicle collisions. Spine 2005;30:1799–1807

60. Bunketorp L, Lindh M, Carlsson J, Stener-Victorin E. The effectiveness of a supervised physical training model tailored to the individual needs of patients with whiplash-associated disorders: a randomized controlled trial. Clin Rehabil 2006;20:201–217

61. Cassidy JD, Carroll LJ, Côté P, Frank J. Does multidisciplinary rehabilitation benefit whiplash recovery?: results of a population-based incidence cohort study. Spine 2007;32:126–131

62. Ferrari R, Rowe BH, Majumdar SR, et al. Simple educational intervention to improve the recovery from acute whiplash: results of a randomized, controlled trial. Acad Emerg Med 2005;12:699–706

63. Gennis P, Miller L, Gallagher EJ, Giglio J, Carter W, Nathanson N. The effect of soft cervical collars on persistent neck pain in patients with whiplash injury. Acad Emerg Med 1996;3:568–573

64. Kongsted A, Qerama E, Kasch H, et al. Neck collar, "act-as-usual" or active mobilization for whiplash injury? A randomized parallel-group trial. Spine 2007;32:618–626

65. Oliveira A, Gevirtz R, Hubbard D. A psycho-educational video used in the emergency department provides effective treatment for whiplash injuries. Spine 2006;31:1652–1657

66. Pettersson K, Toolanen G. High-dose methylprednisolone prevents extensive sick leave after whiplash injury: a prospective, randomized, double-blind study. Spine 1998;23:984–989

67. Rosenfeld M, Gunnarsson R, Borenstein P. Early intervention in whiplash-associated disorders: a comparison of two treatment protocols. Spine 2000;25:1782–1787

68. Rosenfeld M, Seferiadis A, Carlsson J, Gunnarsson R. Active intervention in patients with whiplash-associated disorders improves long-term prognosis: a randomized controlled clinical trial. Spine 2003;28: 2491–2498

69. Rosenfeld M, Seferiadis A, Gunnarsson R. Active involvement and intervention in patients exposed to whiplash trauma in automobile crashes reduces costs: a randomized, controlled clinical trial and health economic evaluation. Spine 2006;31:1799–1804

70. Scholten-Peeters GG, Neeleman-van der Steen CW, van der Windt DA, Hendriks EJ, Verhagen AP, Oostendorp RA. Education by general practitioners or education and exercises by physiotherapists for patients with whiplash-associated disorders? A randomized clinical trial. Spine 2006;31:723–731

71. Stewart MJ, Maher CG, Refshauge KM, Herbert RD, Bogduk N, Nicholas M. Randomized controlled trial of exercise for chronic whiplash-associated disorders. Pain 2007;128:59–68

72. Suissa S, Giroux M, Gervais M, et al. Assessing a whiplash management model: a population-based non-randomized intervention study. J Rheumatol 2006;33:581–587

20

Timing of Surgical Intervention in the Setting of Acute Spinal Cord Injury

Michael G. Fehlings and Marcus M. Timlin

The role of timing of surgical decompression after an acute spinal cord injury (SCI) remains an area of great debate. Despite a wealth of preclinical animal literature and many case series, the question of whether early decompression following SCI should be the recommended course of action remains controversial because of concerns regarding safety and skepticism as to whether neurological outcomes can be influenced. In this context, this chapter uses the techniques of systematic review to address the following two questions, which are of key clinical relevance when considering the option of whether to consider early decompression in the setting of acute SCI:

- Is there a compelling biological rationale to consider early decompression as a therapeutic principle in the management of patients with traumatic SCI based on relevant preclinical animal models of SCI?
- Is there clinical evidence to support the safety and possible efficacy of early decompression in patients with traumatic SCI?

This chapter presents evidence that acute SCI involves both primary and secondary mechanisms of injury.[1] Moreover, there is compelling evidence from laboratory studies in animal models that persistent compression of the spinal cord is a potentially reversible form of secondary injury. Furthermore, there is emerging evidence suggesting that early surgical intervention is safe and effective, and even delayed decompression may convey a neurological benefit.[2]

◆ Primary and Secondary Injury to the Spinal Cord

It is now well recognized that acute SCI involves both primary and secondary injury mechanisms.[1,3] The primary mechanism involves the initial mechanical injury due to local deformation and energy transformation that occurs within the spinal cord at the moment of injury, which is irreversible.

In the majority of cases, primary SCI is caused by rapid spinal cord compression due to bone displacement from a fracture-dislocation or burst fracture.[4–6] Other potential mechanisms include acute spinal cord distraction, acceleration-deceleration with shearing, gunshot wounds, and laceration from penetrating injuries.[7,8]

The concept of secondary mechanisms of injury following primary SCI was first postulated by Allen in 1911.[20] There is now considerable evidence that the primary mechanical injury initiates a cascade of secondary injury mechanisms such as vascular changes, including ischemia, loss of autoregulation, neurogenic shock, hemorrhage, loss of microcirculation, vasospasm, and thrombosis[1,21]; electrolyte derangements, including increased intracellular calcium, increased extracellular potassium, and accumulation of intracellular sodium[22,23]; accumulation of neurotransmitters, including serotonin, catecholamines, and extracellular glutamate[24,25]; excitotoxicity,[26] arachidonic acid release, production of eicosanoids and free radicals, and lipid peroxidation[2,27–29]; endogenous opioids,[30,31] edema,[32] inflammation,[32] loss of energy metabolism, including adenosine triphosphate-dependent cellular processes[27]; and apoptosis.[34–37] Most important is the fact that secondary injury is preventable and may be reversible. The increased understanding of the pathophysiology of acute SCI has led to clinically relevant neuroprotective therapies to attenuate the effects of the secondary injury. The National Acute Spinal Cord Injury Studies (NASCIS II and NASCIS III) have reported a modest beneficial effect of high-dose methylprednisolone if given within 8 hours of injury in patients with SCI,[38,39] and suggest that treatment within 3 hours may be better than treatment initiated 3 to 8 hours after trauma.[40] These studies support the concept of targeting secondary mechanisms in acute SCI and also emphasize the importance of the timing of intervention. The development of these secondary injury events, which lead to tissue destruction during the first few hours after injury, is relevant to the surgical treatment of SCI as well. There is experimental evidence that persistent compression of the spinal cord is a potentially reversible form of secondary injury.[21,41–56] However, despite its widespread use in patients

Table 20.1 Experimental Studies Assessing the Role of Decompression in Animal Models of Acute Spinal Cord Injury

Study	Species	Injury Model	Timing of Decompression	Effective Time Window	Conclusion
Carlson et al (2003)[43]	Dogs	Piston	30 min, 3 h	30 min	Early decompression promotes neurological injury
Dimar et al (1999)[47]	Rats	Extradural pacer and impactor	0–72 h		Early decompression with minimal canal compromise promotes NR
Carlson et al (1997)[44]	Dogs	Piston	5 min, 1 h, 3 h	5 min, 1 h	Recovery of evoked potentials in 5 min and 1 h groups
Delamarter et al (1995)[46]	Dogs	Circumferential cable	1 h–1 wk	1 h	Decompression at 1 hour improves NR
Zhang et al (1993)[59]	Rats	Static load	5 min		Increased levels of lactate, inosine, hypoxanthine with SCI; reversal of metabolic changes with decompression
Nyström and Berglund (1988)[51]	Rats	Static load	1 min, 5 min, 10 min		Neurological impairment increased with greater severities of injury
Guha et al (1987)[48]	Rats	Clip compression	15 min, 1 h, 2 h, 4 h	15 min, 1 h	Early decompression at milder severities of injury promotes NR
Aki and Toya (1984)[21]	Dogs	Static load 30–60 g	30, 60 min		Vascular changes more severe with greater degrees of compression
Dolan et al (1980)[19]	Rats	Clip compression			Neurological impairment increased with greater severities of injury
Bohlman et al (1979)[41]	Dogs	Anterior piston	3–8 wk		Decompression promotes NR
Kobrine et al (1978),[49] (1979)[50]	Primates	Extradural balloon	1–15 min	1–15 min	Early decompression promotes NR
Thienprasit et al (1975)[55]	Cats	Extradural balloon	6 h		Laminectomy ineffective in promoting NR
Brodkey et al (1972)[42]	Cats	Static weight	Min	min	Early removal of weight restores axonal conduction
Croft et al (1972)[45]	Cats	Static weight	5–20 min	20 min	Early decompression at milder severities promotes NR

Abbreviations: NR, neurological recovery; SCI, spinal cord injury.

with acute SCI in North America, the role of surgery in improving neurological recovery remains controversial because of the absence of well-designed and well-executed prospective, randomized, controlled trials. The presence and duration of a therapeutic window, during which surgical decompression could mitigate the secondary mechanisms of SCI, remains unclear.

◆ Preclinical Evidence from Animal Models of Acute Spinal Cord Injury

There is convincing evidence from laboratory studies in various animal models that persistent compression of the spinal cord is a potentially reversible form of secondary injury.[21,41–52,54,56–60] These studies have consistently shown that neurological recovery is enhanced by early decompression. In 1999, Dimar et al[47] provided the most compelling experimental evidence that spinal cord decompression after SCI is beneficial. Using a weight drop model followed by placement of an epidural spacer to simulate persistent compression, a thoracic SCI was performed in rats. Quantitative analysis of locomotor recovery, lesion volume, and electrophysiology was then used to assess the effect of decompression at 0, 2, 6, 24, and 72 hours after SCI. Neurological recovery was inversely related to the duration of compression, with statistically significant differences seen in all

experimental groups. Carlson et al[43] also reported similar results in dogs. Animals undergoing early decompression showed significantly better functional recovery and significantly smaller lesion volumes (**Table 20.1**).

◆ Safety of Early Decompression for Spinal Cord Injury

The issue of whether surgery, especially early surgery, increases the rate of complications in patients with SCI has been one that has generated considerable controversy and debate. Many patients with SCI with high tetraplegia or significant associated systemic injuries are critically ill because of cardiorespiratory compromise. Many investigators have argued against surgery, especially early intervention in these critically ill patients.[61–65] However, modern techniques of spine surgery as well as advances in critical care and neuroanesthesia have allowed these patients to undergo surgery with minimal differences in complication rates between operative and nonoperative cases.[66–75] Indeed, Duh et al[76] showed that those patients operated on in the first 24 hours had a lower rate of complications than those undergoing operative intervention at later times. In a prospective study of 2204 cases, Waters et al[77,78] found that there was no difference in the complication rates of cases treated by nonoperative or surgical techniques. McLain and Benson prospectively looked at the safety of urgent spinal stabilization ($<$24 hours) as compared with those that had early spinal stabilization (between 24 and 72 hours) in patients with severe injury [Injury Severity Score (ISS) > 26].[79] There were no differences in the perioperative complications between the two groups. Unexpectedly, they noted a trend toward better neurological outcome in patients undergoing urgent stabilization. In a study from our unit, the only difference in morbidity between the surgical and nonsurgical cases was a slight increase in the incidence of deep venous thrombosis in the operated group.[69] Furthermore, the length of stay in the two groups did not differ. Despite the concept of damage control orthopedics[80] in the severely injured patient, many authors have found improved nonneurological outcomes with early spine fixation.[81-83] Early fixation was associated with a lower incidence of pneumonia, a shorter intensive care unit stay, and fewer ventilator days.

In the prospective, randomized trial by Vaccaro et al,[84] there was no significant difference in length of acute postoperative intensive care stay or length of inpatient rehabilitation between the early and late groups, which has been reiterated by others as well.[85,86] McKinley et al[87] have reported that early surgery is associated with shorter hospitalization, reduced pulmonary complications, and equivalent neurological outcomes as delayed surgery. Accordingly, there is class II evidence to support the safety of operative treatment within the first 72 hours, and whenever possible, we recommend decompression within 24 hours of injury.

Role of Conservative Treatment in Acute Spinal Cord Injury

To evaluate the possible role of surgery in the treatment of SCI in the appropriate context, it is essential to examine the outcomes of conservative, nonoperative treatment.[86,88-94] Guttman[61,62] advocated the use of postural techniques combined with bed rest to achieve reduction and spontaneous fusion of the spine. Operative treatment was avoided because laminectomy was associated with a higher incidence of neurological complications and worse clinical outcomes.[62,63,89,95,96] Frankel et al,[97] who adhered to these principles, reported on a cohort of 612 patients with closed spinal injuries. Delayed instability developed in only four patients. Importantly, 29% of patients with Frankel A (i.e., complete motor and sensory paralysis below the level of the injury) had improvement of at least 1 Frankel grade during their hospital stay. This high rate of apparent conversion from complete to incomplete status may reflect some of the recognized challenges in obtaining an accurate neurological examination in the first 24 hours. Nonetheless, these data illustrate the importance of controls in assessing any intervention for SCI.

Other investigators[62,63,84,89,95,98-101] have also reported spontaneous neurological improvement with nonoperative treatment. Some investigators have indicated that neither spinal surgery nor anatomical realignment of the spinal column improved neurological outcome in patients with acute SCI, with the possible exception of bilateral locked facets.[62,101,102] However, to our knowledge, all nonoperative treatment studies to date have been limited to noncontrolled, retrospective analyses of clinical databases (class III evidence). Furthermore, surgeons are now aware that laminectomy without fusion is contraindicated in most cases of acute SCI because it usually

provides inadequate decompression of the spinal cord and may exacerbate the underlying spinal instability, potentially leading to worsening of the neurological injury.[103,104] Although meticulous nonoperative treatment remains an essential component to the care of patients with SCI, modern spine surgery has advanced significantly over the past 2 decades. Furthermore, nonoperative treatment is not without its attendant risks; up to 10% of patients with incomplete cervical SCI have neurological deterioration while being treated in an exclusively nonoperative manner.[93]

Possible Efficacy of Decompression in the Treatment of Acute Spinal Cord Injury

Our review of the literature identified 10 prospective, controlled studies of surgical decompression in acute SCI.[65,68,75-77,84,86,106-108] Recently, Papadopoulos et al[106] evaluated 91 patients with acute cervical SCI to assess the feasibility and outcome of an immediate decompression treatment protocol. All patients except one were admitted within 9 hours of their injury. The investigators reported that 39/66 patients in the protocol group had improvement, including some presenting with a complete SCI, compared with 6/25 in the control group. This study was classified as class II evidence because of the lack of randomization. La Rosa et al[109] performed a systematic review of all available studies published between 1966 and 2000. They concluded that early ($\leq$24 hours) surgical decompression in patients with incomplete injuries resulted in better neurological outcomes than patients treated with either delayed decompression ($>$24 hours) or nonoperative treatment. This study is considered class II evidence because of the lack of randomized, controlled trials available for inclusion in the systematic review.

In contrast, several prospective studies[65,76,84,87,107] have failed to document a beneficial effect of surgical decompression. However, to our knowledge, no study to date has truly examined in a systematic way a large cohort of patients who underwent decompression earlier than 24 hours. For example, all patients underwent delayed operative treatment in the study by Waters et al.[77] Moreover, although the study by Vaccaro et al[84] was a prospective, randomized trial, 20 of the 62 patients were lost to follow-up, and "early" surgery was defined as being within 72 hours after SCI. In view of the large number of patients lost to follow-up, we have considered this study to provide class II evidence. In addition, Pollard and Apple[110] undertook a retrospective analysis of 412 patients with incomplete cervical SCI. Unfortunately, only 49% of patients (n = 202) had baseline neurological assessments, and 168 were lost to follow-up. Although the investigators concluded that early surgery ($\leq$24 hours) was not associated with improved neurological outcome, these conclusions must be interpreted very cautiously, given the major concerns regarding incompleteness of the dataset. **Table 20.2** summarizes the data from studies published in the last 5 years, whereas **Table 20.3** shows data from studies published in the last 6 to 10 years. Several investigators have advocated early reduction (4 to 10 hours) and operative fixation of spinal fractures in patients with acute SCI.[111-114] These studies suggest that early decompression may enhance neurological recovery in select patients with SCI. However, most of these studies lack randomization or appropriate controls and, thus, represent class III evidence only. The

Table 20.2 Evidentiary Table of Clinical Studies of Surgical Decompression in Acute Spinal Cord Injury

Study	No. Patients (Level)	Timing of Intervention	Study Design (Class of Evidence)	Conclusions
La Rosa et al (2004)[109]	1683 (all):793 decompressed, 890 nonoperative	226 underwent surgical decompression <24 h	Systematic review of literature up to 2000 (III)	Early decompression improves NR in patients with incomplete neurological deficits
McKinley et al (2004)[87]	779 (all): 603 compressed, 176 nonoperative	73 underwent surgical decompression <24 h	Retrospective case series (III)	Early (<72 h) decompression did not improve NR but was associated with shorter hospital stay and fewer complications
Pollard and Apple (2003)[110]	412 (cervical) incomplete injuries		Retrospective case series; baseline neurological assessment not available in 51% of cases (III)	Baseline neurological assessment only available in 202 cases; 169 patients not available for follow-up. Early surgery (<24 h) not associated with improved neurological recovery
Papadopoulos et al (2002)[106]	91 (cervical): 66 decompressed, 25 nonoperative	34 underwent surgical decompression <10 h	Prospective, nonrandomized (II)	Early surgical decompression is feasible, may improve NR and reduces hospital stay
Pointillart et al (2000)[107]	106 (all levels): 58 (cervical)	49 underwent surgical decompression <8 h	Prospective, nonrandomized (II)	Early surgery did not improve NR
Waters et al (1999)[78]	2204 (all)	88% admitted <72 h	Prospective, nonrandomized (II)	Surgery does not increase complication rates of SCI patients
Tator et al (1999)[124]	585 (all)	23.5% underwent surgery <24 h	Retrospective case series (III)	65% of patients in North America with SCI undergo surgery; no consensus on timing of intervention
Mirza et al (1999)[85]	30 (cervical)	15 <72 h, 15 >72 h	Retrospective case series (III)	Early (<72 h) decompression improves NR and does not increase complication rates
Ng et al (1999)[108]	26 (cervical)	7 underwent surgical decompression <12 h	Prospective, nonrandomized (II)	Surgical decompression within 8 h of injury was feasible in 8% and not associated with increased complication rates
Chen et al (1998)[86]	37 (cervical): 16 decompressed, 21 nonoperative	<2 wk	Prospective, nonrandomized (II)	Surgery associated with improved NR, shorter hospital stay, and fewer complications.
Vaccaro et al (1997)[84]	62 (cervical): early 34, late 38	Early <72 h, late <5 d	Prospective, randomized (II; 20 lost to follow-up)	No difference in NR or length of hospital stay between early and late surgical groups
Vale et al (1997)[66]	77 (all): 58 operated	11 <24 h, 13 24–72 h, 34 <72 h	Prospective nonrandomized (II)	No clear relationship between NR and timing of surgery, but aggressive medical treatment enhanced any potential benefit provided with surgery
Bötel et al (1997)[104]	255 (all): 178 decompressed 51.4% early, 10.5% late	Early <24 h, late >2 wk	Retrospective case series (III)	No NR in complete SCI; no association of NR to timing of decompression
Waters et al (1996)[77]	269 (all): 127 decompressed, 142 nonoperative	Average > 14 d	Prospective nonrandomized (II)	Surgery of no benefit; however, all patients underwent delayed surgery
Petitjean et al (1995)[88]	49 (thoracic)	Early average 12 h, late average 9 d	Retrospective case series (III)	Decompression of no benefit in complete thoracic paraplegia

Abbreviation: NR, neurological recovery.

clinical benefits of early reduction of fracture dislocations of the spine by closed techniques or open surgery are difficult to assess in the absence of class I data.[69,85,107,111,114–117] Although reports of significant neurological improvement in some cervical cases decompressed by early traction are encouraging, they do not provide sufficient evidence to support standards or guidelines.[106,113,115,118,119] Moreover, several studies did not find any neurological benefit with reduction,[76,101,120] with the possible exception of patients with bilateral facet dislocation.[121] Cotler et al[70] examined the safety and efficacy of early reduction and

Table 20.3 Evidentiary Table of Clinical Studies Suggesting Safety of Early Decompression for Spinal Cord Injury

Study	No. of Patients	Timing of Intervention	Study Design (level of evidence)	Conclusions
Schinkel et al (2006)[83]	205 (thoracic) ISS > 15 (all)	156 < 72 h, 49 > 72 h	Retrospective case series (III)	Early group had reduced ICULOS, LOS, and Lung failure
Kerwin et al (2005)[82]	86 (cervical)	59 < 72 h, 27 > 72 h	Retrospective case series (III)	Early group; some improvement in NR, earlier discharge, reduced morbidity
McKinley et al (2004)[87]	605 (all)	307 < 24 h, 296 > 24 h	Retrospective case series (III)	Early group had reduced LOS, pneumonia, and atelectasis
Croce et al (2001)[81]	291 (all)	142 < 72 h, 149 > 72 h	Retrospective case series (III)	Early group had reduced ICULOS, LOS, pneumonia, and hospital charges
Mirza et al (1999)[85]	30 (cervical) ISS < 30	15 < 72 h, 15 < 72 h	Retrospective case series (III)	Reduced LOS, no increase in complication rate
Waters et al (1999)[78]	3756 (all), 1747 (surgery)	Admitted within 24 h (timing of surgery not discussed)	Retrospective case series (III)	No increased complications in surgical group
McLain and Benson (1999)[79]	27 (ISS > 25)	14 < 24 h, 13 > 48 h	Prospective non randomized (III)	No difference in pre- or postop complications
Vaccaro et al (1997)[84]	62 (cervical): early 34, late 38	Early < 72 h, late < 5 d	Prospective, randomized (II; 20 lost to follow up)	No difference in NR or LOS between early and late surgical groups
Duh et al (1994)[76]	298 (all)	38 < 24 h, 260 > 24 h	Review of data from a prospective randomized study (II)	No difference in NR, lower complication rate with early group

Abbreviations: NR, neurologic recovery; ISS, Injury Severity Score; LOS, length of stay; ICULOS, intensive care unit length of stay.

undertook a prospective study of early reduction by traction in 24 patients (class II evidence). They found no neurological deterioration in any of the patients, most of whom had successful reduction with closed techniques within 24 hours of injury. Papadopoulos et al[106] prospectively examined 91 patients with cervical SCI, 32 of whom had immediate spinal cord decompression by traction alone. They suggested that patients who had decompression with closed reduction alone (mean time to decompression 6.0 hours) had better neurological outcomes than those requiring surgical decompression (mean time to decompression 12.6 hours). Moreover, in a retrospective case series that included 46 patients with SCI, Grant et al[123] concluded that cervical traction was safe (one patient, 2.2% deteriorated neurologically) and was associated with improved neurological recovery.

Based on these data and several other class II studies,[102,103,106,108,111,114,116,117,124–126] we can support a recommendation for urgent reduction of bilateral locked facets in a patient with incomplete tetraplegia or in a patient with neurological deterioration. Despite the potential appeal of aggressive, closed reduction of locked cervical facets, Tator et al[124] documented an 8.1% rate of neurological deterioration with attempts at closed reduction in 585 cases. However, it should be emphasized that the majority of the neurological changes related to transient radicular deficits cleared with reduction in weight. Moreover, the retrospective nature of the study design did not allow for precise control of critical variables, such as presence or absence of sedation, fluoroscopic control versus general radiographic imaging, and the method of applying traction. It is recognized that, in experienced hands with control of the aforementioned variables, the rate of serious permanent neurological deterioration with traction is low.[123]

Nonetheless, these sobering data emphasize the difficulty in interpreting accounts of the beneficial effects of rapid closed reduction by traction in the absence of class I data.

In contrast to the aforementioned studies of early decompression, Larson et al[127] advocated operating a week or more after SCI to allow medical and neurological stabilization of the injured patient. This remains the practice in many institutions, particularly in light of early reports suggesting an increased rate of medical complications with early surgery (≤5 days after SCI).[65] Interestingly, several investigators have documented recovery of neurological function after delayed decompression of the spinal cord (months to years) after the injury.[111,127–131] Although these studies are retrospective in design (class III evidence), the improvement in neurological function with delayed decompression in patients with cervical or thoracolumbar SCI who have had a plateau in their recovery is noteworthy and suggests that compression of the cord is an important contributing cause of neurological dysfunction.

La Rosa et al[109] recently published a systematic review of the literature addressing the issue of early decompression and its role in acute SCI. They reviewed all the published clinical studies up to the year 2000 and were able to extract data on 1687 patients. Patients were divided into three treatment groups: early decompression (≤24 hours), delayed decompression (>24 hours), and conservative treatment. Statistically, early decompression resulted in better outcomes compared with both delayed decompression and conservative treatment. However, the investigators performed an analysis of homogeneity, and only data regarding patients with incomplete SCI who underwent early decompression were reliable. They concluded that early decompression can only be considered as a practice option.[109]

◆ Current Studies of the Role of Decompression in Acute Spinal Cord Injury

The Spine Trauma Study Group (STSG) is currently conducting a multicenter, prospective observational study to evaluate the effect of early (≤24 hours after injury) versus late (>24 hours)

decompressive surgery for cervical SCI, the Surgical Timing in Acute Spinal Cord Injury Study (STASCIS) (**Fig. 20.1**).

Although such aggressive treatment protocols demand expedient care and cooperation between spine surgeons and radiologists, they are feasible.[106] The study is not randomized because of ethical concerns about allocating a deteriorating patient to delayed decompression. In addition, logistical and

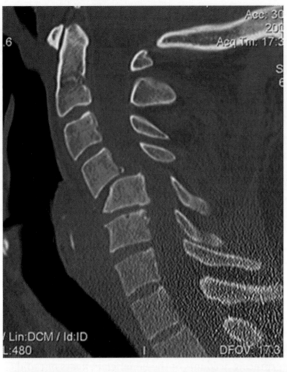

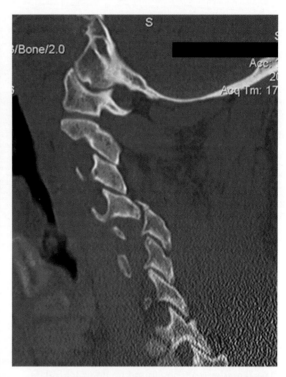

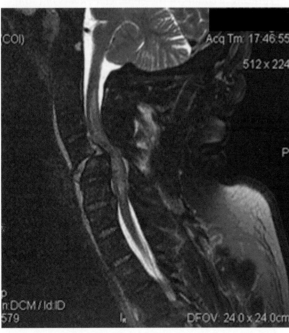

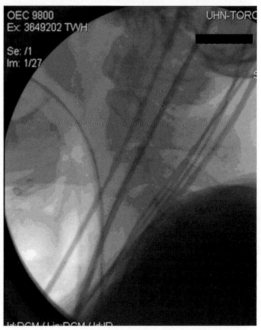

Fig. 20.1 (A–H) Example of a Surgical Timing in Acute Spinal Cord Injury Study (STASCIS) case. A 39-year-old dove into shallow water and suffered a C4/5 bifacetal fracture dislocation with complete paralysis (American Spinal Injury Association grade A)–isolated injury. Admitted to our unit within 8 hours of injury. Appropriate radiology obtained pre-reduction and surgery. Reduction performed in operating room (OR) under fluoroscopic guidance and surgery anterior and posterior performed immediately following reduction. **(A)** Midsagittal right and **(B)** left preoperative computed tomographic (CT) scans show fracture

dislocation > 50% subluxation C4 on C5 with bifacetal dislocation. **(C)** Midsagittal T2-weighted magnetic resonance imaging (MRI) showing fracture subluxation with disruption of anterior longitudinal ligament (ALL), posterior ligamentous complex (PLC) and signal change in spinal cord extending up to C2. Patient was self-ventilating and awake for reduction following this. **(D)** Screening film post-awake reduction in OR. Traction applied in OR, patient awake and C-arm available for screening throughout procedure. Once-reduced surgical decompression performed expeditiously.

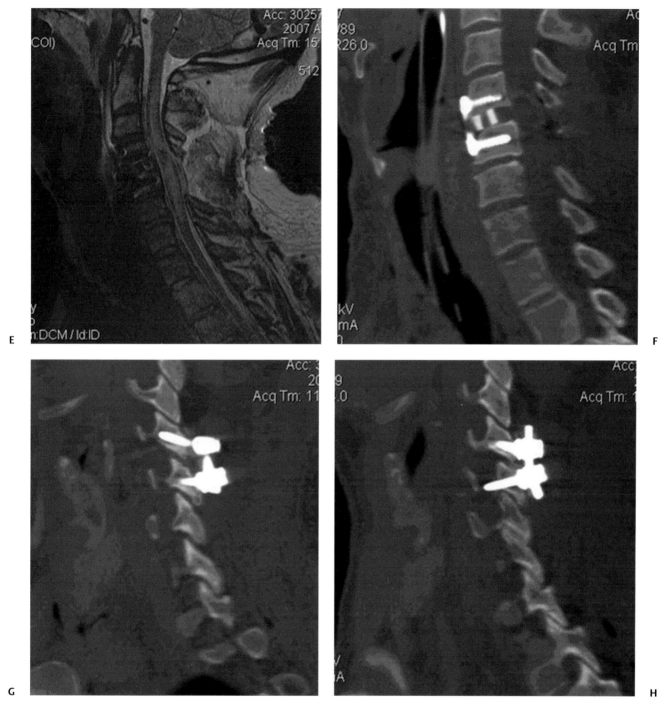

Fig. 20.1 (*Continued*) **(E)** Postoperative midsagittal MRI shows wide decompression of spinal cord. This was achieved by an anterior cervical decompression and fusion (ACDF) of C4/5 followed by posterior lateral mass fixation and laminectomy and decompression. **(F)** Postoperative CT scans with sagittal reconstruction showing full reduction adequate bony decompression and **(G)** and **(H)** showing bilateral posterior lateral mass screw and rod fixation.

Table 20.4 Summary Table of Evidence and Expert Opinion Regarding Early Decompression for Acute Spinal Cord Injury

Question	Level of Recommendation	Expert Recommendation
Biological rationale to support early decompression	Strong–strong evidence	Yes
Safety of early decompression	Strong–moderate evidence	Yes
Possible efficacy of early decompression	Strong–weak evidence	Yes

technical factors limit the number of patients who arrive at a spinal cord center for definitive treatment within 24 hours of injury, thus limiting the number of patients eligible for randomization. This promising study may more clearly delineate whether early intervention and decompression is key to improved neurological outcomes (**Table 20.4**).

References

1. Tator CH, Fehlings MG. Review of the secondary injury theory of acute spinal cord trauma with emphasis on vascular mechanisms. J Neurosurg 1991;75:15–26

2. Hung TK, Albin MS, Brown TD, Bunegin L, Albin R, Jannetta PJ. Biomechanical responses to open experimental spinal cord injury. Surg Neurol 1975;4:271–276

3. Tator CH. Update on the pathophysiology and pathology of acute spinal cord injury. Brain Pathol 1995;5:407–413

4. Sekhon LH, Fehlings MG. Epidemiology, demographics, and pathophysiology of acute spinal cord injury. Spine 2001;26(24, Suppl):S2–S12

5. DeVivo MJ. Causes and costs of spinal cord injury in the United States. Spinal Cord 1997;35:809–813

6. Kraus JF, Franti CE, Riggins RS, Richards D, Borhani NO. Incidence of traumatic spinal cord lesions. J Chronic Dis 1975;28:471–492

7. Cardenas DD, Hoffman JM, Kirshblum S, McKinley W. Etiology and incidence of rehospitalization after traumatic spinal cord injury: a multicenter analysis. Arch Phys Med Rehabil 2004;85:1757–1763

8. Carter RE Jr. Etiology of traumatic spinal cord injury: statistics of more than 1,100 cases. Tex Med 1977;73:61–65

9. Kraus JF. Epidemiologic features of head and spinal cord injury. Adv Neurol 1978;19:261–279

10. Claxton AR, Wong DT, Chung F, Fehlings MG. Predictors of hospital mortality and mechanical ventilation in patients with cervical spinal cord injury. Can J Anaesth 1998;45:144–149

11. Kraus JF. Injury to the head and spinal cord: the epidemiological relevance of the medical literature published from 1960 to 1978. J Neurosurg 1980;Suppl:S3–S10

12. Heinemann AW, Yarkony GM, Roth EJ, et al. Functional outcome following spinal cord injury: a comparison of specialized spinal cord injury center vs general hospital short-term care. Arch Neurol 1989;46:1098–1102

13. DeVivo MJ, Kartus PL, Stover SL, Rutt RD, Fine PR. Cause of death for patients with spinal cord injuries. Arch Intern Med 1989;149:1761–1766

14. Griffin MR, Opitz JL, Kurland LT, Ebersold MJ, O'Fallon WM. Traumatic spinal cord injury in Olmsted County, Minnesota, 1935-1981. Am J Epidemiol 1985;121:884–895

15. Amar AP, Levy ML. Pathogenesis and pharmacological strategies for mitigating secondary damage in acute spinal cord injury. Neurosurgery 1999;44:1027–1039, discussion 1039–1040

16. Tator CH. Spine-spinal cord relationships in spinal cord trauma. Clin Neurosurg 1983;30:479–494

17. Kakulas BA. Pathology of spinal injuries. Cent Nerv Syst Trauma 1984;1:117–129

18. Bunge RP, Puckett WR, Becerra JL, Marcillo A, Quencer RM. Observations on the pathology of human spinal cord injury: a review and classification of 22 new cases with details from a case of chronic cord compression with extensive focal demyelination. Adv Neurol 1993;59:75–89

19. Dolan EJ, Tator CH, Endrenyi L. The value of decompression for acute experimental spinal cord compression injury. J Neurosurg 1980;53:749–755

20. Allen A. Surgery for experimental lesions of spinal cord equivalent to crush injury of fracture dislocation of spinal column: a preliminary report. JAMA 1911;57:878–880

21. Aki T, Toya S. Experimental study on changes of the spinal-evoked potential and circulatory dynamics following spinal cord compression and decompression. Spine 1984;9:800–809

22. Agrawal SK, Fehlings MG. Mechanisms of secondary injury to spinal cord axons in vitro: role of Na+, Na(+)-K(+)-ATPase, the Na(+)-H+ exchanger, and the Na(+)-Ca2+ exchanger. J Neurosci 1996;16:545–552

23. Young W, Koreh I. Potassium and calcium changes in injured spinal cords. Brain Res 1986;365:42–53

24. Agrawal SK, Fehlings MG. Role of NMDA and non-NMDA ionotropic glutamate receptors in traumatic spinal cord axonal injury. J Neurosci 1997;17:1055–1063

25. Osterholm JL, Mathews GJ. Altered norepinephrine metabolism, following experimental spinal cord injury, II: Protection against traumatic spinal cord hemorrhagic necrosis by norepinephrine synthesis blockade with alpha methyl tyrosine. J Neurosurg 1972;36:395–401

26. Faden AI, Simon RP. A potential role for excitotoxins in the pathophysiology of spinal cord injury. Ann Neurol 1988;23:623–626

27. Anderson DK, Hall ED. Pathophysiology of spinal cord trauma. Ann Emerg Med 1993;22:987–992

28. Anderson DK, Means ED, Waters TR, Spears CJ. Spinal cord energy metabolism following compression trauma to the feline spinal cord. J Neurosurg 1980;53:375–380

29. Demopoulos HB, Flamm ES, Pietronigro DD, Seligman ML. The free radical pathology and the microcirculation in the major central nervous system disorders. Acta Physiol Scand Suppl 1980;492:91–119

30. Faden AI, Jacobs TP, Holaday JW. Comparison of early and late naloxone treatment in experimental spinal injury. Neurology 1982;32:677–681

31. Faden AI, Jacobs TP, Holaday JW. Neuropeptides and spinal cord injury. Adv Biochem Psychopharmacol 1982;33:131–138

32. Wagner FC Jr, Stewart WB. Effect of trauma dose on spinal cord edema. J Neurosurg 1981;54:802–806

33. Dietrich WD, Chatzipanteli K, Vitarbo E, Wada K, Kinoshita K. The role of inflammatory processes in the pathophysiology and treatment of brain and spinal cord trauma. Acta Neurochir Suppl (Wien) 2004;89:69–74

34. Casha S, Yu WR, Fehlings MG. Oligodendroglial apoptosis occurs along degenerating axons and is associated with FAS and p75 expression following spinal cord injury in the rat. Neuroscience 2001;103:203–218

35. Crowe MJ, Bresnahan JC, Shuman SL, Masters JN, Beattie MS. Apoptosis and delayed degeneration after spinal cord injury in rats and monkeys. Nat Med 1997;3:73–76

36. Emery E, Aldana P, Bunge MB, et al. Apoptosis after traumatic human spinal cord injury. J Neurosurg 1998;89:911–920

37. Lou J, Lenke LG, Ludwig FJ, O'Brien MF. Apoptosis as a mechanism of neuronal cell death following acute experimental spinal cord injury. Spinal Cord 1998;36:683–690

38. Bracken MB, Shepard MJ, Collins WF, et al. A randomized, controlled trial of methylprednisolone or naloxone in the treatment of acute spinal-cord injury: results of the Second National Acute Spinal Cord Injury Study. N Engl J Med 1990;322:1405–1411

39. Bracken MB, Holford TR. Effects of timing of methylprednisolone or naloxone administration on recovery of segmental and long-tract neurological function in NASCIS 2. J Neurosurg 1993;79:500–507

40. Bracken MB, Shepard MJ, Holford TR, et al. Administration of methylprednisolone for 24 or 48 hours or tirilazad mesylate for 48 hours in the treatment of acute spinal cord injury: results of the Third National Acute Spinal Cord Injury Randomized Controlled Trial. National Acute Spinal Cord Injury Study. JAMA 1997;277:1597–1604

41. Bohlman HH, Bahniuk E, Raskulinecz G, Field G. Mechanical factors affecting recovery from incomplete cervical spinal cord injury: a preliminary report. Johns Hopkins Med J 1979;145:115–125

42. Brodkey JS, Richards DE, Blasingame JP, Nulsen FE. Reversible spinal cord trauma in cats: additive effects of direct pressure and ischemia. J Neurosurg 1972;37:591–593

43. Carlson GD, Gorden CD, Oliff HS, Pillai JJ, LaManna JC. Sustained spinal cord compression, I: Time-dependent effect on long-term pathophysiology. J Bone Joint Surg Am 2003;85-A:86–94

44. Carlson GD, Minato Y, Okada A, et al. Early time-dependent decompression for spinal cord injury: vascular mechanisms of recovery. J Neurotrauma 1997;14:951–962

45. Croft TJ, Brodkey JS, Nulsen FE. Reversible spinal cord trauma: a model for electrical monitoring of spinal cord function. J Neurosurg 1972;36:402–406

46. Delamarter RB, Sherman J, Carr JB. Pathophysiology of spinal cord injury. Recovery after immediate and delayed decompression. J Bone Joint Surg Am 1995;77:1042–1049

47. Dimar JR II, Glassman SD, Raque GH, Zhang YP, Shields CB. The influence of spinal canal narrowing and timing of decompression on neurologic recovery after spinal cord contusion in a rat model. Spine 1999;24:1623–1633

48. Guha A, Tator CH, Endrenyi L, Piper I. Decompression of the spinal cord improves recovery after acute experimental spinal cord compression injury. Paraplegia 1987;25:324–339

49. Kobrine AI, Evans DE, Rizzoli H. Correlation of spinal cord blood flow and function in experimental compression. Surg Neurol 1978;10:54–59

50. Kobrine AI, Evans DE, Rizzoli HV. Experimental acute balloon compression of the spinal cord: factors affecting disappearance and return of the spinal evoked response. J Neurosurg 1979;51:841–845

51. Nyström B, Berglund JE. Spinal cord restitution following compression injuries in rats. Acta Neurol Scand 1988;78:467–472

52. Tarlov IM. Spinal cord compression studies, III: Time limits for recovery after gradual compression in dogs. AMA Arch Neurol Psychiatry 1954;71:588–597

53. Tarlov IM. Spinal cord injuries: early treatment. Surg Clin North Am 1955;35:591–607

54. Tarlov IM, Klinger H. Spinal cord compression studies, II: Time limits for recovery after acute compression in dogs. AMA Arch Neurol Psychiatry 1954;71:271–290

55. Thienprasit P, Bantli H, Bloedel JR, Chou SN. Effect of delayed local cooling on experimental spinal cord injury. J Neurosurg 1975;42:150–154

56. Yoshida H, Okada Y, Maruiwa H, et al. Synaptic blockade plays a major role in the neural disturbance of experimental spinal cord compression. J Neurotrauma 2003;20:1365–1376

57. Dolan EJ, Transfeldt EE, Tator CH, Simmons EH, Hughes KF. The effect of spinal distraction on regional spinal cord blood flow in cats. J Neurosurg 1980;53:756–764

58. Carlson GD, Gorden CD, Nakazawa S, Wada E, Smith JS, LaManna JC. Sustained spinal cord compression, II: Effect of methylprednisolone on regional blood flow and recovery of somatosensory evoked potentials. J Bone Joint Surg Am 2003;85-A:95–101

59. Zhang Y, Hillered L, Olsson Y, Holtz A. Time course of energy perturbation after compression injury of the spinal cord: an experimental study in the rat using microdialysis. Surg Neurol 1993;39:297–304

60. Shields CB, Zhang YP, Shields LB, Han Y, Burke DA, Mayer NW. The therapeutic window for spinal cord decompression in a rat spinal cord injury model. J Neurosurg Spine 2005;3:302–307

61. Guttmann L. Initial treatment of traumatic paraplegia and tetraplegia. In: Harri P, ed. Spinal Injuries Symposium. Edinburgh, UK: Royal College of Surgeons; 1963:80–92

62. Guttmann L. Spinal Cord Injuries: Comprehensive Management and Research. 2nd ed. Oxford: Blackwell; 1976

63. Bedbrook GM, Sakae T. A review of cervical spine injuries with neurological dysfunction. Paraplegia 1982;20:321–333

64. Wilmot CB, Hall KM. Evaluation of the acute management of tetraplegia: conservative versus surgical treatment. Paraplegia 1986;24:148–153

65. Marshall LF, Knowlton S, Garfin SR, et al. Deterioration following spinal cord injury. A multicenter study. J Neurosurg 1987;66:400–404

66. Vale FL, Burns J, Jackson AB, Hadley MN. Combined medical and surgical treatment after acute spinal cord injury: results of a prospective pilot study to assess the merits of aggressive medical resuscitation and blood pressure management. J Neurosurg 1997;87:239–246

67. Benzel EC, Larson SJ. Recovery of nerve root function after complete quadriplegia from cervical spine fractures. Neurosurgery 1986;19:809–812

68. Benzel EC, Larson SJ. Functional recovery after decompressive operation for thoracic and lumbar spine fractures. Neurosurgery 1986;19:772–778

69. Tator CH, Duncan EG, Edmonds VE, Lapczak LI, Andrews DF. Comparison of surgical and conservative management in 208 patients with acute spinal cord injury. Can J Neurol Sci 1987;14:60–69

70. Cotler JM, Herbison GJ, Nasuti JF, Ditunno JF Jr, An H, Wolff BE. Closed reduction of traumatic cervical spine dislocation using traction weights up to 140 pounds. Spine 1993;18:386–390

71. Ahn JH, Ragnarsson KT, Gordon WA, Goldfinger G, Lewin HM. Current trends in stabilizing high thoracic and thoracolumbar spinal fractures. Arch Phys Med Rehabil 1984;65:366–369

72. Wilberger JE Diagnosis and management of spinal cord trauma. J Neurotrauma 1991;8(Suppl 1):S21–S28,discussion S29–S30

73. Rosner MJ, Elias Z, Coley I. New principles of resuscitation for brain and spinal injury. N C Med J 1984;45:701–708

74. Levi L, Wolf A, Belzberg H. Hemodynamic parameters in patients with acute cervical cord trauma: description, intervention, and prediction of outcome. Neurosurgery 1993;33:1007–1016, discussion 1016–1017

75. Rizzolo SJ, Vaccaro AR, Cotler JM. Cervical spine trauma. Spine 1994;19:2288–2298

76. Duh MS, Shepard MJ, Wilberger JE, Bracken MB. The effectiveness of surgery on the treatment of acute spinal cord injury and its relation to pharmacological treatment. Neurosurgery 1994;35:240–248, discussion 248–249

77. Waters RL, Adkins RH, Yakura JS, Sie I. Effect of surgery on motor recovery following traumatic spinal cord injury. Spinal Cord 1996;34:188–192

78. Waters RL, Meyer PR Jr, Adkins RH, Felton D. Emergency, acute, and surgical management of spine trauma. Arch Phys Med Rehabil 1999;80:1383–1390

79. McLain RF, Benson DR. Urgent surgical stabilization of spinal fractures in polytrauma patients. Spine 1999;24:1646–1654

80. Pape HC, Giannoudis P, Krettek C. The timing of fracture treatment in polytrauma patients: relevance of damage control orthopedic surgery. Am J Surg 2002;183:622–629

81. Croce MA, Bee TK, Pritchard E, Miller PR, Fabian TC. Does optimal timing for spine fracture fixation exist? Ann Surg 2001;233:851–858

82. Kerwin AJ, Frykberg ER, Schinco MA, Griffen MM, Murphy T, Tepas JJ. The effect of early spine fixation on non-neurologic outcome. J Trauma 2005;58:15–21

83. Schinkel C, Frangen TM, Kmetic A, Andress HJ, Muhr G; German Trauma Registry. Timing of thoracic spine stabilization in trauma patients: impact on clinical course and outcome. J Trauma 2006;61: 156–160, discussion 160

84. Vaccaro AR, Daugherty RJ, Sheehan TP, et al. Neurologic outcome of early versus late surgery for cervical spinal cord injury. Spine 1997;22:2609–2613

85. Mirza SK, Krengel WF III, Chapman JR, et al. Early versus delayed surgery for acute cervical spinal cord injury. Clin Orthop Relat Res 1999;(359):104–114

86. Chen TY, Dickman CA, Eleraky M, Sonntag VK. The role of decompression for acute incomplete cervical spinal cord injury in cervical spondylosis. Spine 1998;23:2398–2403

87. McKinley W, Meade MA, Kirshblum S, Barnard B. Outcomes of early surgical management versus late or no surgical intervention after acute spinal cord injury. Arch Phys Med Rehabil 2004;85:1818–1825

88. Petitjean ME, Mousselard H, Pointillart V, Lassie P, Senegas J, Dabadie P. Thoracic spinal trauma and associated injuries: should early spinal decompression be considered? J Trauma 1995;39:368–372

89. Bedbrook GM. Spinal injuries with tetraplegia and paraplegia. J Bone Joint Surg Br 1979;61-B:267–284

90. Bohlman HH, Freehafer A, Dejak J. The results of treatment of acute injuries of the upper thoracic spine with paralysis. J Bone Joint Surg Am 1985;67:360–369

91. McEvoy RD, Bradford DS. The management of burst fractures of the thoracic and lumbar spine. Experience in 53 patients. Spine 1985;10:631–637

92. Donovan WH, Cifu DX, Schotte DE. Neurological and skeletal outcomes in 113 patients with closed injuries to the cervical spinal cord. Paraplegia 1992;30:533–542

93. Katoh S, el Masry WS, Jaffray D, et al. Neurologic outcome in conservatively treated patients with incomplete closed traumatic cervical spinal cord injuries. Spine 1996;21:2345–2351

94. Kinoshita H, Nagata Y, Ueda H, Kishi K. Conservative treatment of burst fractures of the thoracolumbar and lumbar spine. Paraplegia 1993;31:58–67

95. Bedbrook GM, Sedgley GI. The management of spinal injuries: past and present. Int Rehabil Med 1980;2:45–61

96. Collins WF. A review and update of experiment and clinical studies of spinal cord injury. Paraplegia 1983;21:204–219

97. Frankel HL, Hancock DO, Hyslop G, et al. The value of postural reduction in the initial management of closed injuries of the spine with paraplegia and tetraplegia, I. Paraplegia 1969;7:179–192

98. Comarr AE, Kaufman AA. A survey of the neurological results of 858 spinal cord injuries; a comparison of patients treated with and without laminectomy. J Neurosurg 1956;13:95–106

99. Ditunno JF Jr, Sipski ML, Posuniak EA, Chen YT, Staas WE Jr, Herbison GJ. Wrist extensor recovery in traumatic quadriplegia. Arch Phys Med Rehabil 1987;68(5 Pt 1):287–290

100. Tator CH, Duncan EG, Edmonds VE, Lapczak LI, Andrews DF. Neurological recovery, mortality and length of stay after acute spinal cord injury associated with changes in management. Paraplegia 1995;33:254–262

101. Wu L, Marino RJ, Herbison GJ, Ditunno JF Jr. Recovery of zero-grade muscles in the zone of partial preservation in motor complete quadriplegia. Arch Phys Med Rehabil 1992;73:40–43

102. Dall DM. Injuries of the cervical spine, II: Does anatomical reduction of the bony injuries improve the prognosis for spinal cord recovery? S Afr Med J 1972;46:1083–1090

103. Harris P, Karmi MZ, McClemont E, Matlhoko D, Paul KS. The prognosis of patients sustaining severe cervical spine injury (C2–C7 inclusive). Paraplegia 1980;18:324–330

104. Bötel U, Gläser E, Niedeggen A. The surgical treatment of acute spinal paralysed patients. Spinal Cord 1997;35:420–428

105. Fehlings MG, Cooper PR, Errico TJ. Posterior plates in the management of cervical instability: long-term results in 44 patients. J Neurosurg 1994;81:341–349

106. Papadopoulos SM, Selden NR, Quint DJ, Patel N, Gillespie B, Grube S. Immediate spinal cord decompression for cervical spinal cord injury: feasibility and outcome. J Trauma 2002;52:323–332

107. Pointillart V, Petitjean ME, Wiart L, et al. Pharmacological therapy of spinal cord injury during the acute phase. Spinal Cord 2000;38:71–76

108. Ng WP, Fehlings MG, Cuddy B, et al. Surgical treatment for acute spinal cord injury study pilot study #2: evaluation of protocol for decompressive surgery within 8 hours of injury. Neurosurg Focus 1999;6:e3

109. La Rosa G, Conti A, Cardali S, Cacciola F, Tomasello F. Does early decompression improve neurological outcome of spinal cord injured patients? Appraisal of the literature using a meta-analytical approach. Spinal Cord 2004;42:503–512

110. Pollard ME, Apple DF. Factors associated with improved neurologic outcomes in patients with incomplete tetraplegia. Spine 2003;28:33–39

111. Aebi M, Mohler J, Zäch GA, Morscher E. Indication, surgical technique, and results of 100 surgically-treated fractures and fracture-dislocations of the cervical spine. Clin Orthop Relat Res 1986;(203):244–257

112. Wiberg J, Hauge HN. Neurological outcome after surgery for thoracic and lumbar spine injuries. Acta Neurochir (Wien) 1988;91:106–112

113. Levi L, Wolf A, Rigamonti D, Ragheb J, Mirvis S, Robinson WL. Anterior decompression in cervical spine trauma: does the timing of surgery affect the outcome? Neurosurgery 1991;29:216–222

114. Hadley MN, Fitzpatrick BC, Sonntag VK, Browner CM. Facet fracture-dislocation injuries of the cervical spine. Neurosurgery 1992;30:661–666

115. Weinshel SS, Maiman DJ, Baek P, Scales L. Neurologic recovery in quadriplegia following operative treatment. J Spinal Disord 1990;3:244–249

116. Brunette DD, Rockswold GL. Neurologic recovery following rapid spinal realignment for complete cervical spinal cord injury. J Trauma 1987; 27:445–447

117. Star AM, Jones AA, Cotler JM, Balderston RA, Sinha R. Immediate closed reduction of cervical spine dislocations using traction. Spine 1990; 15:1068–1072

118. Sussman BJ. Letter: Early management of spinal cord trauma. J Neurosurg 1976;44:766–767

119. Wolf A, Levi L, Mirvis S, et al. Operative management of bilateral facet dislocation. J Neurosurg 1991;75:883–890

120. Burke DC, Berryman D. The place of closed manipulation in the management of flexion-rotation dislocations of the cervical spine. J Bone Joint Surg Br 1971;53:165–182

121. Harvey C, Rothschild BB, Asmann AJ, Stripling T. New estimates of traumatic SCI prevalence: a survey-based approach. Paraplegia 1990; 28:537–544

122. Anderson PA, Bohlman HH. Anterior decompression and arthrodesis of the cervical spine: long-term motor improvement, II: Improvement in complete traumatic quadriplegia. J Bone Joint Surg Am 1992;74: 683–692

123. Grant GA, Mirza SK, Chapman JR, et al. Risk of early closed reduction in cervical spine subluxation injuries. J Neurosurg 1999;90(1, Suppl): 13–18

124. Tator CH, Fehlings MG, Thorpe K, Taylor W. Current use and timing of spinal surgery for management of acute spinal surgery for management of acute spinal cord injury in North America: results of a retrospective multicenter study. J Neurosurg 1999;91(1, Suppl):12–18

125. Sonntag VK. Management of bilateral locked facets of the cervical spine. Neurosurgery 1981;8:150–152

126. Lee AS, MacLean JC, Newton DA. Rapid traction for reduction of cervical spine dislocations. J Bone Joint Surg Br 1994;76:352–356

127. Larson SJ, Holst RA, Hemmy DC, Sances A Jr. Lateral extracavitary approach to traumatic lesions of the thoracic and lumbar spine. J Neurosurg 1976;45:628–637

128. Transfeldt EE, White D, Bradford DS, Roche B. Delayed anterior decompression in patients with spinal cord and cauda equina injuries of the thoracolumbar spine. Spine 1990;15:953–957

129. Bohlman HH, Anderson PA. Anterior decompression and arthrodesis of the cervical spine: long-term motor improvement, I: Improvement in incomplete traumatic quadriparesis. J Bone Joint Surg Am 1992;74: 671–682

130. Bohlman HH, Kirkpatrick JS, Delamarter RB, Leventhal M. Anterior decompression for late pain and paralysis after fractures of the thoracolumbar spine. Clin Orthop Relat Res 1994;(300):24–29

131. Brodkey JS, Miller CF Jr, Harmody RM. The syndrome of acute central cervical spinal cord injury revisited. Surg Neurol 1980;14:251–257

21

Management of Spinal Cord Injury in the Setting of a Closed Head Injury

Peter G. Campbell, Bizhan Aarabi, and James S. Harrop

The treatment, diagnosis, and management of the spine and spinal cord injured patients can be difficult due to polytrauma, inconsistent examinations, and concurrent neurological injuries. Physical examination in the closed head injury population is often limited. Therefore, patients with concurrent neurological injuries, whether peripheral or central, can be particularly difficult to diagnose and manage. There is a need to identify and manage concurrent injuries, particularly closed head injuries. The Advanced Trauma Life Support (ATLS) program manual states, "Any patient sustaining an injury above the clavicle or a head injury resulting in an unconscious state should be suspected of having an associated cervical spinal column injury," and obligates the care provider to immobilize the patient until cervical spine injury can be excluded (ATLS guidelines).

In the United States, traumatic brain injury (TBI) can cause significant mortality of the neurotrauma population and accounts for nearly 40% of deaths from acute injuries. In 2001, 157,078 people died from acute traumatic injury according to the Centers for Disease Control and Prevention 2002 statistics. It is reported that roughly 52,000 were a direct result of brain injury.[1] In the closed head injury, there is a limited ability to obtain a detailed examination. Therefore, if a patient is unable to provide an accurate history or reliably report symptoms, assume an associated spinal cord injury until proven otherwise.

Specifically, the evaluation of the patient with a concurrent TBI is particularly challenging because these patients are unable to report neck pain or cooperate for a detailed neurological examination. Patients unable to cooperate with an exam may have an associated spinal cord injury in 2 to 8% of cases[2–6]. Chiu et al evaluated 2615 blunt trauma victims with a Glasgow Coma Scale (GCS) score of less than 15. Among this group there were 143 (5.5%) cervical spine injuries.[7] Another analysis by Piatt found that, among 41,142 cases of severe TBI (GCS 3 to 8) there was an 8% risk of cervical spine injury.[5] Michael et al evaluated 359 head injuries and 92 cervical spine injuries. Of the 92 patients with "primary" cervical spine injury a coincident head injury was noted in 22 (24%).

In the patients being treated for a "primary" brain injury, the incidence of a cervical spine injury was 6% (22). However, the head injury most commonly described in the patients with cervical spine fracture was mild to moderate in nature.[3] In an analysis of injuries distal to the cervical spine, the incidence of thoracic, lumbar, and sacral injury for 4142 patients arriving at a level I trauma center was 4.4%. However, patients with GCS scores of 13 to 14 had significantly less likelihood of complaining of back pain or tenderness as compared with neurologically intact patients, whereas the incidence of fractures remained evenly divided among the two groups.[8]

The detection of concomitant injuries in the neurotrauma patient requires diligence during physical examination as well as assiduous attention to diagnostic imaging studies, particularly since the prognosis for neurological recovery may be worse in patients with TBI and SCI.[9]

◆ Mechanism and Types of Traumatic Brain Injuries

Given the broad spectrum of the degree and extent of injury, few studies have been able to accurately determine the prevalence of TBI. In fact, the majority of cases are not fatal and do not result in significant focal morbidity. Therefore, many patients do not initially seek professional medical attention until a specific and focused neurological deficit is noted, often difficulty with concentration and memory. Patients with mild and moderate TBI are often not admitted to the hospital or referred for medical evaluation. Mild TBI is defined as GCS scores between 13 and 15, moderate closed head injury (CHI) as a GCS score of 9 to 12, and severe TBI as a GCS score of 8 or lower.

The majority of TBIs are a result of transportation-related injuries (72.5%).[10] Although a variety of mechanisms may create a TBI, there is also great variety in the neuroanatomical pathology of the injury. The cranium provides an osseous vault that protects the neural elements; therefore skull fractures, the result of focal injury to the skull, may be associated with injuries to the cranial nerves, blood vessels at the skull base, and dural lacerations. An epidural hematoma is formed from local impact with a rupture of underlying dural arteries or veins, most frequently caused by a fractured bone edge. Epidural hematomas frequently form over lateral surfaces of the cerebral hemispheres and are at high risk of rapid expansion if arterial in origin, but fortunately are not typically related to an underlying brain injury.

Another source of intraparenchymal injury is a cerebral contusion. It may be the result of contact forces (coup) and/or inertial forces (countercoup) on the neural tissue. Traumatic contusions typically extend from the cortex into the white matter and are differentiated from an intracerebral hematoma (which is rare in trauma) because they are typically caused by damage to smaller cortical vessels, and blood makes up less than two thirds of the volume of the traumatized area in question.[10] Subdural hematomas are located over the cerebral convexities and typically result from injury of the veins that bridge from the cortex to the venous system throughout the subarachnoid space. These veins are susceptible to rupture from brief, high-velocity injury to the head such as a fall. Gennarelli and Thibault reported that 72% of acute subdural hematomas resulted from a fall or an assault, and only 24% were from a transportation-related injury.[11]

Traumatic subarachnoid hemorrhage results when angular acceleration produces forces sufficient to damage the superficial vessels traversing the subarachnoid space. These are common injuries seen in the trauma population. It can be difficult to predict the degree or severity of underlying parenchymal injury. Similarly, traumatic intraventricular hemorrhage is caused by strain to the subependymal veins. However, this type of hemorrhage requires severe force and energy; therefore the resulting concurrent neurological injury carries a poor prognosis.

Concussion, defined as a temporary alteration of sensorium as the result of a traumatic injury, is believed by some to be a mild form of diffuse axonal injury (DAI) caused by angular acceleration.[9] In milder forms, the strain produced is insufficient to cause structural damage but may lead to permanent neurological impairment. Unlike brain trauma that occurs due to direct impact and deformation of the brain, DAI is the result of traumatic shearing forces that occur when the head is rapidly accelerated or decelerated. DAI is caused primarily by angular forces induced by the falx and tentorium.[11,12] Small tissue-tear lesions (Strich hemorrhages) are often noted parasagittally in the white matter as well as in the corpus callosum and cerebral peduncles, which are regions where the nervous tissue is tethered and unable to accommodate external forces.

The brain is contained in the osseous confines of the cranium. Therefore, with an increase in volume either through swelling from trauma or mass effect from hemorrhage there is limited ability to accommodate the increased volume. The resulting expansion forces the brain tissue into nonanatomical regions and can result in the "herniation" of the tissue. Supratentorial brain herniation typically occurs in three patterns: subfalcine, central transtentorial, and uncal. Subfalcine herniation, the most common type, is caused by a mass effect on the cingulate gyrus beneath the falx. This lesion has the ability to compress the ipsilateral anterior cerebral artery, but it typically does not cause tissue infarction. Transtentorial herniation is caused by lesions in the parietal, frontal, or occipital lobes and effectively displaces the midbrain downward through the tentorial notch at the base of the skull. Uncal herniation is caused by a mass lesion in the temporal lobes or middle fossa and results in compression of the oculomotor nerve, ipsilateral cerebral peduncle, and then the brainstem, which can result in rapid progression to coma and death.

◆ Nature of Head and Spinal Cord Injuries

The incidence of concomitant head and spinal cord injuries is quite high. Roughly 2 to 8% of head-injured patients have an associated spine injury; conversely, 25 to 50% of spinal injury patients were noted to sustain a closed head injury as defined by evidence of loss of consciousness or posttraumatic amnesic episode.[13] Bucholz et al performed postmortem radiography and autopsy inspections in 100 consecutive victims of traffic fatalities; they reported a cervical spine injury rate of 24%. Half of these victims were not suspected of having spine injury before detailed postmortem examination.[14] Iida et al examined 188 patients with upper and lower cervical spine injuries and found that 35% had associated moderate to severe head injuries. Of the two groups reviewed, the patients with upper cervical spine injuries had an increased risk of suffering from basilar skull fractures, traumatic subarachnoid hemorrhage, and contusions.[15] Shrago also compared head trauma and the location of spinal cord injury. In this study, of the head trauma victims with spine injuries, 56% had upper cervical injury, 34% had midcervical injury, and 10% had lower cervical injury. However, the types of head trauma were not analyzed.[16] Holly et al reviewed 447 moderate to severely head injured patients and 24 (5.4%) suffered a cervical spine injury. Of these 24 patients, 14 sustained injuries in the occiput to C3 region. As such, they concluded that a disproportionate number of these patients sustain high cervical injuries, the majority of which are mechanically unstable and involve an SCI.[17] Pagni and Massaro reviewed 2304 blunt trauma patients and found 121 with concomitant head and spine fractures. They reported 59 cervical fractures, 27 thoracic lesions (T2–T9), 30 thoracolumbar lesions (T10–L2), and five lumbosacral injuries.[4] A series of 8285 blunt trauma victims showed that patients with clinically significant head injuries were at greater risk of cervical spine injuries than those without head trauma (4.5% vs 1.1%). Analysis with lower GCS scores yielded an even more significant link.[18]

It would seem that, given the concomitance of head and cervical spine injuries, similar mechanisms would be responsible. However, it is likely the biomechanical forces which produce head injuries differ from those that produce the spine injury. In their review Gennarelli and Thibault surmised that mechanisms which produce concussions and DAI are quite different from those that are necessary to produce cervical spine injury (G & T, biological models of head injury, CNS trauma status report—1985, NIH 391–404)[19]. In the series by Michael et al it was noted that only one case out of 22 with concomitant head and cervical spine injury could have theoretically been caused by just a single blow.[3] In patients with singular trauma to the head, such as gunshot wounds localized to the brain, clinical evidence showing concomitant spinal injury is lagging, leading one author to recommend against cervical stabilization in these patients.[20]

Initial Evaluation and Management of the Brain and Spinal Cord Injured Patient

The management principles that govern initial injury management are identical regardless of patient specifics. These principles have been described in the American College of

Surgeons ATLS course (ATLS guidelines). In the primary survey, life-threatening injuries are identified and treated. Patients with neurological injury, be it TBI or SCI, may present some special challenges. Patients with TBI often have a depressed level of consciousness; therefore, a history is unobtainable. More importantly, patients with moderate to severe brain injury are unable to voice specific complaints. Patients with spinal cord injuries, particularly if located in the cervical spine, may also be unable to fully describe their complaints if injuries are located below the level of their spinal injury.

Airway control is the highest priority following injury. Patients who present with any signs or symptoms of airway compromise should be promptly intubated. Patients with TBI are at great risk for developing either or both hypoxia and hypercarbia from their depressed mental status, thus exacerbating their underlying condition.[21,22] Patients with TBI are also at high risk for aspiration. Ninety-five percent of high cervical spinal cord injuries require intubation within 24 hours of admission. Therefore, this patient population should be evaluated for early intubation with a low threshold for securing the airway as a tenet of initial management.

Breathing, the second-highest priority, refers to identification of immediately life-threatening thoracic injuries. Patients with TBI or SCI are certainly at risk for developing any life-threatening thoracic injuries such as tension pneumothorax, massive hemothorax, cardiac tamponade, open pneumothorax, or a flail chest. Following airway control and initiation of mechanical ventilation if necessary, a rapid search should be made for these conditions and they should be treated if present.

Assessing the adequacy of circulation and treating hemorrhage are evaluated next in the ATLS algorithm. A rapid search of hemorrhage should identify the location of bleeding. There are five body cavities into which a patient can lose significant amounts of blood: the abdomen, thorax, muscle compartments, and pelvis and outside the torso. Patients with cervical spinal cord injury may be hypotensive from neurogenic shock, hemorrhagic shock, or a combination of both. Hemorrhage control and rapid resuscitation are particularly important in patients with TBI because hypotension has been shown to markedly worsen outcome by producing secondary brain injury.[21,22]

Patients with neurological injury are often multiply injured. Evaluation and treatment must proceed simultaneously. A full evaluation may not be possible until the patient is stabilized. Even urgent studies such as computed tomographic (CT) scans of the head and cervical spine may have to be deferred until after a laparotomy or thoracotomy is performed for hemorrhage control. Decision making must be fluid and will often require input from various services to obtain optimal patient care.

Clinical Examination of a Traumatic Brain Injury Patient to Evaluate an Associated Spinal Injury

As previously mentioned, it is appropriate to assume that a spinal injury exists in every head-injured or obtunded patient. Several clinical clues that alert the examiner to an underlying spinal injury may exist in the obtunded patient (**Table 21.1**). Inspection of the spine to visualize ecchymosis should initially be undertaken. Respiratory movements should also be visualized at this juncture to assess for the presence of paradoxical respiration, which generally implicates a severe spinal cord injury at C5 or below. Palpation of the entire spine, with caution not to cause movement thereof, should be performed to assess for deformity or tenderness. Priapism is occasionally observed in patients with a spinal cord injury, but never in patients with an isolated head injury. The presence of bilateral flaccid paralysis is common in spinal shock, whereas most severe brain injuries cause hypertonicity. Bilateral weakness or paralysis in the arm greater than in the legs is more suggestive of a central cord type injury, although lesions in the cervicomedullary junction can have a similar presentation.[9] In obtunded patients with a GCS score of 4 or greater response to noxious stimuli may be tested. The presence of a sensory level below which there is no response to pain is an indication of spinal cord damage. Additionally, if there is facial grimacing to noxious stimuli this supports an incomplete injury with motor paralysis but preserved sensory tracts. There are also several clues provided by disturbance to the sympathetic nervous system. The loss of sweat below a certain level denotes the sympathectomy effect of a spinal cord injury. Also, Horner syndrome is typically only present in patients with major cervical spine injury and seldom present in TBI alone. Of the classical triad, anhydrosis and miosis are typically discernable, whereas ptosis is exceedingly difficult to appreciate in the comatose or obtunded patient. Although not as sensitive as imaging studies, any of the previous clinical findings in a trauma victim with depressed level of consciousness should raise one's index of suspicion for the presence of spinal cord injury.[9]

Table 21.1 Clinical Clues to Underlying Spine Injury in a Comatose Patient

1. Vital signs suggestive of neurogenic shock (bradycardia and hypotension)

2. Paradoxical breathing; pronounced contraction of diaphragm without proportional movement of chest wall

3. Priapism

4. Flaccid paralysis of arms and legs, in the absence of paralytics, is usually not expected in severe head injury

5. Paralysis of arms more than legs, reminiscent of central cord syndrome

6. Brown-Séquard syndrome; when weakness and sensory loss are on opposite sides

7. No motor response to painful stimuli, or only by facial grimacing

8. Presence of a level of response to painful stimuli

9. Horner syndrome (ptosis, miosis, anhydrosis of affected side)

10. Presence of a sweating level

11. Dissociation of core and surface body temperatures (suggesting sympathectomy)

Radiological Examination of the Spine in a Traumatic Brain Injury Patient

In a patient with moderate to severe head injury, the single most common cause of missed cervical spine injury seems to be failure to adequately visualize the region of injury. This can be caused by failure to obtain radiographs, or by making judgments on technically suboptimal films. For patients who are unable to reliably describe the presence or absence of neck pain there is persistent debate about the most appropriate studies for clearance of the cervical spine. There are no class I data on which to base a standard imaging protocol. Additionally, patients with closed head injury are frequently uncooperative, young males with well-developed musculature, thus further complicating complete evaluation of the cervical and upper thoracic spine. The Eastern Association for the Surgery of Trauma (EAST) guidelines committee formulated an algorithm based on an extensive literature review for radiographic evaluation of the cervical[23] spine in the trauma population. The standard presented in their guideline as well as other current literature reviews[24] state that a three-view cervical spine series [anteroposterior (AP), lateral, and odontoid views] is recommended for initial radiographic evaluation of the cervical spine in patients who are symptomatic or suffer from altered mental status after traumatic injury. This should be supplemented with axial CT images at 3 mm intervals obtained through suspicious or poorly visualized areas identified on three-view cervical spine x-rays. If the initial evaluation is without evidence of abnormality, cervical spine immobilization may be discontinued after flexion/extension lateral cervical spine fluoroscopy is obtained with static imaging at extremes of flexion and extension[23,25,26] or a magnetic resonance imaging (MRI) scan within 48 hours of injury.[24]

Evaluation of the thoracolumbar spine is also difficult in the head-injured patient. Although there are numerous clinical studies addressing screening of the thoracolumbar spine, to date there are no randomized studies and only a few prospective studies specifically addressing the subject. Unfortunately, delay in diagnosis of thoracolumbar fractures is not uncommon. In a retrospective review, Dai et al identified 147 patients with acute thoracolumbar injuries. In this population, 28 patients (19%) had a thoracolumbar fracture that was not diagnosed at the time of admission, with an average diagnosis made by 47.8 hours (12 to 240 hours) after presentation.[27] A study by Reid et al showed fractures of the thoracolumbar spine that were diagnosed in a delayed fashion had a higher incidence of a new neurological deficit compared with those diagnosed at the time of admission (10.5% vs 1.4%).[28] The EAST practice management guideline committee released recommendations based on an English language literature review and determined due to a lack of appropriate studies that there can be no "standard" practice guideline (EAST thoracolumbar spine). In a blunt trauma patient with altered mental status the EAST group has a level II recommendation that radiological workup is indicated, and multidetector CT scan with reformatted axial collimation is superior to plain films in the screening of the thoracolumbar spine for bony injury. By using a single imaging modality that can increase the efficiency and decrease the delay in diagnosis of an unstable injury, the provider can initiate treatment sooner and decrease any potential loss of neurological function. Although ligamentous injury without bony injury of the thoracolumbar spine is extremely rare, MRI is likely indicated for patients with neurological deficits, abnormal CT scans, or clinical suspicion despite normal radiographic evaluation suggesting an unstable injury.[29]

◆ Treatment of Concomitant Head and Spinal Cord Injuries

In polytrauma, the brain is the most commonly injured organ system.[30] First-responders should begin the assessment, stabilization, and resuscitation. The priorities of trauma management (airway, breathing, and circulation) are especially important given the potential for secondary injury to the brain and spinal cord after a traumatic insult. The acutely injured brain maintains a strong sensitivity to hypotension, hypercarbia, hypoxemia, elevated intracranial pressures (ICPs), and hypoperfusion.[10] Hypotension (systolic blood pressure <90 mm Hg) or hypoxia [apnea, cyanosis, or an oxygen (O_2) saturation <90% in the field or a PaO_2 <60 mm Hg] must be monitored and avoided or immediately corrected.

The damage to the brain after TBI is incomplete at the time of admission and typically evolves over the course of the first several days postinjury. The acutely injured brain is exquisitely sensitive to secondary insults likely as a result of damage to the autoregulatory process that normally maintains proper cerebral blood flow over a wide range of metabolic variables. Disruption of autoregulation caused by TBI is believed to impair cerebral oxygenation resulting in global or regional secondary brain insults.[10] Many medical and critical care initial management goals exist to avoid or lessen the impact of secondary injury. In the absence of any reliable noninvasive indicators of ICP, patients with a GCS score of 8 or less after resuscitation combined with any of the following: CT findings suggestive of elevated ICP, systolic blood pressure less than 90 mm Hg, age greater than 40 years, and evidence of posturing should undergo ICP monitoring, with placement of a ventriculostomy being the gold standard device (brain trauma foundation). If an ICP upper threshold of 20 to 25 mm Hg is reached, treatment should be initiated. Cerebral perfusion pressure (CPP) should be maintained at a minimum of 60 mm Hg. An established standard in TBI is a recommendation against the use of steroids in improving outcome. The final tenet of head injury management is the use of high-dose barbiturate therapy in hemodynamically stable salvageable patients with intracranial hypertension refractory to maximal medical and surgical ICP therapy.

In TBI patients with suspected SCI, high-dose steroid protocols should be initiated early. Immobilization of the spine may then be established with rigid cervical collars, halo vest orthosis, and cervical traction. Patients with depressed skull fractures or who may require extensive craniotomies are typically not candidates for ring or Gardner-Wells tong placement. In concomitantly injured patients, the jugular venous outflow restriction caused by placement in a rigid collar may exacerbate ICP in severe head injury. There is evidence describing a statistically significant increase in ICP with placement in a rigid cervical collar.[31–33] Although the clinical significance of this phenomenon has not been fully demonstrated, the effects of increased ICP in head-injured patients are well documented.[34] In patients with clear evidence of increased ICP, collar repositioning should first be attempted with the goal of cervical spine clearance in an expeditious fashion.

The first operative priority for patients with concomitant injuries is an intracranial mass lesion. Patients with an acute subdural hematoma causing significant midline shift 5 mm or more and demonstrating a poor neurological exam are typically evacuated. Acute epidural hematomas are resected more aggressively secondary to their "classic" presentation of a lucid interval followed by a lapse into a coma. Nonoperative management of these lesions mandates careful ICU observation and immediate neurosurgical availability.[10] Posttraumatic contusions and intracerebral hematomas are evacuated when causing significant mass effect or clinical neurological deterioration. These lesions tend to evolve over time and may cause delayed intracranial hypertension up to 7 to 10 days postinjury.[35] Prompt surgical resection of mass lesions and close postoperative intensive care management are central to reducing elevated ICP, mitigating secondary brain injury, and improving final outcomes in the head-injured patient.

Cervical dislocations should, secondarily, be addressed by traction and immobilization in a halo. Unfortunately, patients requiring operative treatment of an intracranial lesion through a large craniotomy are not candidates for cervical traction. Patients with poor GCS scores, various types of skull fractures, and severe distracting injuries are not candidates for spinal traction. Spinal lesions requiring surgical decompression would typically be addressed within several days of the craniotomy at the discretion of the treating neurosurgeon. Surgical treatment for spinal stability alone is typically assigned a lower priority and may be delayed.[9] The optimal timing of surgical intervention of the spine-injured patient with head injury is controversial and widely debated. Treatment of patients with both a head injury as well as spine injuries poses many challenges and mandates a multidisciplinary solution.

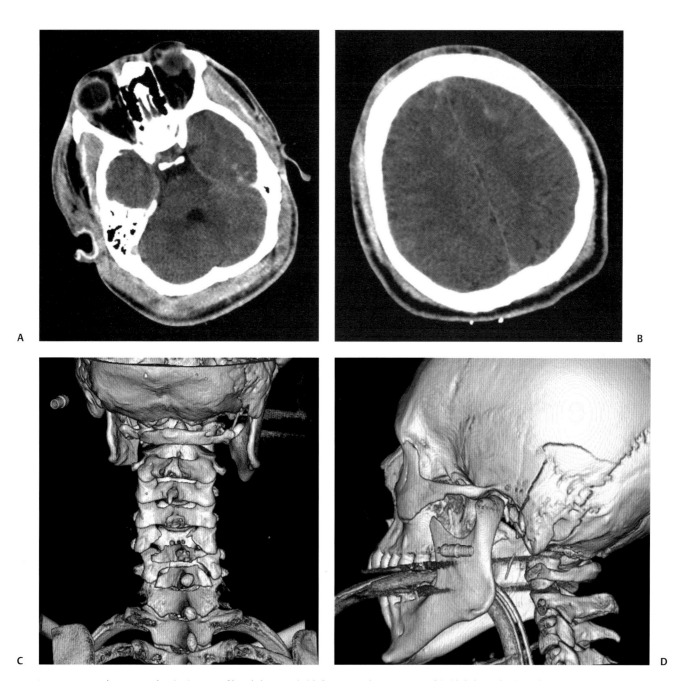

Fig. 21.1 Computed tomographic (CT) scans of head showing **(A)** left temporal contusion and **(B)** left frontal subarachnoid hemorrhage. **(C)** Reconstructed CT revealing extent of C5–C6 posterior laminar fractures. **(D)** CT reconstruction of left temporal bone fracture.

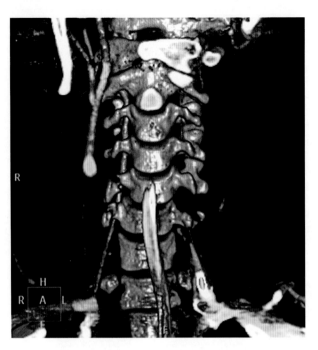

Fig. 21.2 Computed tomographic angiography demonstrating the absence of the left vertebral artery superior to the cervical fracture.

left temporal bone fracture extending into the sphenoid sinus, left vertebral artery injury, multiple lamina fractures of C4 through C6, bilateral pulmonary contusions with a right pneumothorax, and a small splenic laceration (**Fig. 21.1A–D**). The patient was stabilized hemodynamically and a right-sided chest tube was placed on initial resuscitation. High-dose steroid protocol was initiated on arrival. An ICP monitor was placed within 4 hours of arrival. MRI brain and cervical spine with CT angiography were performed to evaluate the severity of his TBI and concomitant spinal column fractures (**Fig. 21.2**). Given the patient's neurological exam, spinal fixation was delayed. Given the severity of his cervical spine injury, a halo vest was placed to immobilize his cervical spine to allow for proper nursing care. Over the course of 5 days, his neurological exam improved to eye opening to pain and left upper extremity localization (GCS 8T). Subsequently, an anterior-posterior spinal fusion was performed with the benefit of intraoperative ICP monitoring on hospital day 6 as definitive management of the unstable cervical spine fractures (**Fig. 21.3A,B**). Throughout his hospital course, he improved neurologically to spontaneous eye opening and continued left upper extremity localization. He remained nonverbal on discharge to a brain injury rehabilitation unit (GCS 10).

◆ Case Report

A 27-year-old male was ejected from a vehicle in a high-speed motor vehicle accident. On initial exam he would withdraw his right upper extremity, was intubated, and did not open his eyes (GCS 6T). After a full radiographic evaluation, the patient was determined to have bilateral cortical subarachnoid hemorrhages, a small left temporal contusion, a

◆ Summary

The trauma patient with a head injury requires a high degree of suspicion for an underlying cervical or thoracolumbar spine injury. The potential for a new or worsening neurological injury from an undiagnosed fracture strongly supports radiographic screening of the spine in these patients. Cervical spine screening has been well documented, and clinical guidelines exist for initial evaluation. CT has been shown in the literature to be superior to plain radiographs in the acute

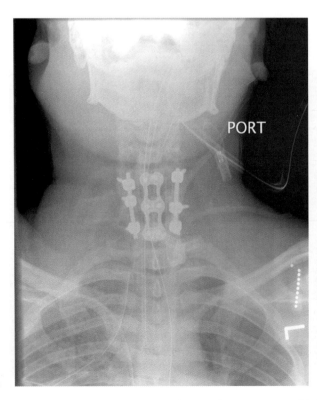

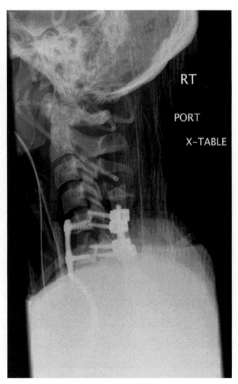

Fig. 21.3 Postoperative x-rays showing **(A)** anterior/posterior view and **(B)** lateral view of anterior/posterior cervical fusion.

evaluation of the thoracolumbar spine. The treatment of an associated spine fracture in the setting of TBI requires a multidisciplinary team of experts to determine the proper course and timing of treatment. After achievement of hemodynamic stability and repair of life-threatening injuries, a delay in treatment of associated injuries is generally recommended to avoid a secondary injury and exacerbate the severity of a brain injury.

References

1. Silver JM, McAllister TW, Yudofsky SC. Textbook of Traumatic Brain Injury. 1st ed. Washington, DC: American Psychiatric Publishing; 2005
2. Bayless P, Ray VG. Incidence of cervical spine injuries in association with blunt head trauma. Am J Emerg Med 1989;7:139–142
3. Michael DB, Guyot DR, Darmody WR. Coincidence of head and cervical spine injury. J Neurotrauma 1989;6:177–189
4. Pagni CA, Massaro F. Concomitant cranio-cerebral and vertebro-medullary injuries: analysis of 121 cases. Acta Neurochir (Wien) 1991;111:1–10
5. Piatt JH Jr. Detected and overlooked cervical spine injury in comatose victims of trauma: report from the Pennsylvania Trauma Outcomes Study. J Neurosurg Spine 2006;5:210–216
6. Ross SE, O'Malley KF, DeLong WG, Born CT, Schwab CW. Clinical predictors of unstable cervical spinal injury in multiply injured patients. Injury 1992;23:317–319
7. Chiu WC, Haan JM, Cushing BM, Kramer ME, Scalea TM. Ligamentous injuries of the cervical spine in unreliable blunt trauma patients: incidence, evaluation, and outcome. J Trauma 2001;50:457–463, discussion 464
8. Cooper C, Dunham CM, Rodriguez A. Falls and major injuries are risk factors for thoracolumbar fractures: cognitive impairment and multiple injuries impede the detection of back pain and tenderness. J Trauma 1995;38:692–696
9. Tator CH. Management of associated spine injuries in head injured patients. In: Narayan RK, Wilberger JE, Povlishock JT, eds. Neurotrauma. New York: McGraw-Hill, Health Professions Division; 1996
10. Halliday AL. Pathophysiology. In: Marion DW, ed. Traumatic Brain Injury. New York: Thieme Medical; 1999
11. Gennarelli TA, Thibault LE. Biomechanics of acute subdural hematoma. J Trauma 1982;22:680–686
12. Wilkins RH, Rengachary SS. Neurosurgery. 2nd ed. New York: McGraw-Hill, Health Professions Division; 1996
13. Chestnut RM. Emergency management of spinal cord injury. In: Narayan RK, Wilberger JE, Povlishock JT. Neurotrauma. New York: McGraw Hill, Health Professions Disivion, 1995.
14. Bucholz RW, Burkhead WZ, Graham W, Petty C. Occult cervical spine injuries in fatal traffic accidents. J Trauma 1979;19:768–771
15. Iida H, Tachibana S, Kitahara T, Horiike S, Ohwada T, Fujii K. Association of head trauma with cervical spine injury, spinal cord injury, or both. J Trauma 1999;46:450–452
16. Shrago GG. Cervical spine injuries: association with head trauma: a review of 50 patients. Am J Roentgenol Radium Ther Nucl Med 1973;118:670–673
17. Holly LT, Kelly DF, Counelis GJ, Blinman T, McArthur DL, Cryer HG. Cervical spine trauma associated with moderate and severe head injury: incidence, risk factors, and injury characteristics. J Neurosurg 2002;96(3, Suppl): 285–291
18. Hills MW, Deane SA. Head injury and facial injury: is there an increased risk of cervical spine injury? J Trauma 1993;34:549–553, discussion 553–554
19. Genarelli TA, Thibault LE. Biological models of head injury. In: Povlishock JT, Becker T, eds. Central nervous system trauma status report. Bethesda, MD: National Institute of Neurological and Communicative Disorders and Strokes; 1985
20. Kaups KL, Davis JW. Patients with gunshot wounds to the head do not require cervical spine immobilization and evaluation. J Trauma 1998; 44:865–867
21. Chesnut RM. The management of severe traumatic brain injury. Emerg Med Clin North Am 1997;15:581–604
22. Chesnut RM, Marshall SB, Piek J, Blunt BA, Klauber MR, Marshall LF. Early and late systemic hypotension as a frequent and fundamental source of cerebral ischemia following severe brain injury in the Traumatic Coma Data Bank. Acta Neurochir Suppl (Wien) 1993;59:121–125
23. Pasquale M, Fabian TC. Practice management guidelines for trauma from the Eastern Association for the Surgery of Trauma. J Trauma 1998;44: 941–956, discussion 956–957
24. Hadley MN, Walters BC, Grabb PA, et al. Guidelines for the management of acute cervical spine and spinal cord injuries. Clin Neurosurg 2002; 49:407–498
25. Davis JW, Parks SN, Detlefs CL, Williams GG, Williams JL, Smith RW. Clearing the cervical spine in obtunded patients: the use of dynamic fluoroscopy. J Trauma 1995;39:435–438
26. Sees DW, Rodriguez Cruz LR, Flaherty SF, Ciceri DP. The use of bedside fluoroscopy to evaluate the cervical spine in obtunded trauma patients. J Trauma 1998;45:768–771
27. Dai LY, Yao WF, Cui YM, Zhou Q. Thoracolumbar fractures in patients with multiple injuries: diagnosis and treatment-a review of 147 cases. J Trauma 2004;56:348–355
28. Reid DC, Henderson R, Saboe L, Miller JD. Etiology and clinical course of missed spine fractures. J Trauma 1987;27:980–986
29. Diaz JJ Jr, Cullinane DC, Altman DT, et al; EAST Practice Management Guideline Committee. Practice management guidelines for the screening of thoracolumbar spine fracture. J Trauma 2007;63:709–718
30. Kraus MF. The neuropsychiatry of TBI: an overview of assessment and pharmacologic interventions. In: Marion D, ed. Traumatic brain injury. New York: Thieme; 1999:175–185
31. Davies G, Deakin C, Wilson A. The effect of a rigid collar on intracranial pressure. Injury 1996;27:647–649
32. Kolb JC, Summers RL, Galli RL. Cervical collar-induced changes in intracranial pressure. Am J Emerg Med 1999;17:135–137
33. Raphael JH, Chotai R. Effects of the cervical collar on cerebrospinal fluid pressure. Anaesthesia 1994;49:437–439
34. Ho AM, Fung KY, Joynt GM, Karmakar MK, Peng Z. Rigid cervical collar and intracranial pressure of patients with severe head injury. J Trauma 2002;53:1185–1188
35. Unterberg A, Kiening K, Schmiedek P, Lanksch W. Long-term observations of intracranial pressure after severe head injury: the phenomenon of secondary rise of intracranial pressure. Neurosurgery 1993;32:17–23, discussion 23–24

22

Closed Skeletal Reduction and Bracing of Cervical, Thoracic, and Lumbar Spinal Injuries

Nestor D. Tomycz, David O. Okonkwo, and Paul A. Anderson

Nonoperative management of spinal column injuries is a critical component of the treatment of spinal trauma. This chapter discusses closed skeletal reduction of traumatic cervical misalignment and bracing of cervical, thoracic, and lumbar injuries. Closed skeletal reduction is a nonoperative means of decompressing the spinal cord and nerve roots that is often performed on an urgent basis for traumatic injuries of the cervical spine. Thus, closed skeletal reduction must be treated with the same deference shown to spinal surgical interventions and should be performed only by trained spine surgeons. Bracing encompasses an array of means to nonoperatively immobilize spinal segments and is important in the prehospital care of the trauma patient and the conservative management of spinal injuries. There is a dearth of studies that address the indications, contraindications, safety, and efficacy of bracing and closed skeletal reduction. As an amalgam of best available literature and expert opinion, this chapter aims to provide concise, evidence-based recommendations on the use of closed skeletal reduction and bracing of cervical, thoracic, and lumbar spine injuries.

◆ Closed Skeletal Reduction

Skull traction to reduce a cervical spine fracture was first described by Crutchfield in 1933.[1] Since that time, closed reduction via skull traction has been routinely employed for five types of traumatic cervical spine injury: subaxial facet fracture/dislocations, atlantoaxial rotatory subluxation, burst fractures, flexion teardrop fractures, and subaxial traumatic spondylolisthesis.[2–4] Failed closed reduction has traditionally prompted urgent surgery for open reduction and stabilization.

◆ Subaxial Cervical Facet Dislocation

Acute cervical facet dislocation is commonly accompanied by devastating neurological deficits from spinal cord injury.[5] The clinically manifested spinal cord injury is likely a combination of both a direct primary injury (e.g., spinal cord contusion) and persistent neural element compression caused by bony malalignment and resultant spinal canal narrowing. Soft tissue elements such as blood, bone fragments, and herniated disk material may also contribute to spinal cord compression in this setting.[6] This ongoing neural compression may be interpreted as a form of reversible secondary injury that avails itself to a therapeutic intervention. The sense of urgency often surrounding attempts at closed reduction is derived from experimental studies, which have shown that neurological recovery after spinal cord injury is directly correlated with the duration of external spinal cord compression.[7] Moreover, the theoretical benefit of rapidly restoring bony alignment in the cervical spine is supported by clinical reports of neurological improvement—as dramatic as reversal of quadriplegia—soon after closed reduction in patients with various cervical fracture-dislocations.[8–10]

Hyperflexion is the mechanism most commonly attributed to facet fracture/dislocations of the cervical spine.[5] A locked or jumped facet, which may occur unilaterally or bilaterally, results when the inferior facet of the upper vertebrae becomes trapped anterior to the superior facet of the lower vertebrae (**Fig. 22.1B**); a "perched' facet is a milder degree of facet dislocation in which the inferior facet of the upper vertebrae has not completely crossed over the superior facet below but instead has become suspended above it in piggyback fashion (**Fig. 22.1A**). Magnetic resonance imaging (MRI) has demonstrated that both unilateral and bilateral subaxial cervical facet dislocations are frequently associated with severe disruption of soft tissue structures such as the anterior and posterior longitudinal ligaments.[11] Even when facet dislocations are diagnosed in the absence of a neurological deficit, closed reduction is still commonly attempted to temporize the instability of the injury and protect the patient from neurological deterioration before definitive surgical instrumentation and fusion. To achieve closed reduction, cervical traction is usually applied with Gardner-Wells skull tongs or a halo (**Fig. 22.2**), and the basic techniques have been well

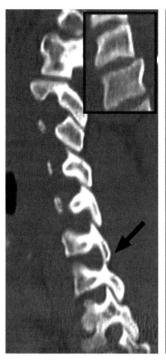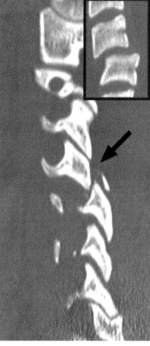

A,B

Fig. 22.1 **(A)** Sagittal reconstruction of a cervical spine computed tomographic (CT) scan demonstrating a C6–C7 perched facet with slight anterolisthesis of the C6 on C7 vertebral body (inset). **(B)** Sagittal CT reconstruction of a C4–C5 jumped or locked facet with an associated fracture fragment. Note the more marked anterolisthesis (inset) in this example of facet fracture-dislocation compared with the example in **(A)**.

described.[8,12–15] Closed reduction should take place in a monitored setting where close supervision may quickly detect changes in the neurological examination.

The hypothesis that early closed reduction of cervical spine fracture-dislocations with craniocervical traction will improve neurological outcome is buttressed by both laboratory experiments and class III clinical evidence. In a retrospective series of 82 patients with either unilateral or bilateral locked cervical facets, Grant et al reported that 97.6% of patients were successfully reduced. Neurological improvement of the American Spinal Injury Association (ASIA) motor scores were 9 and 12 points for complete and incomplete patients, respectively,

at 24 hours after reduction.[16] In another retrospective review of 68 patients with facet fracture dislocations or locked facets, Hadley et al achieved successful closed reduction in only 58% of the patients, whereas 78% exhibited neurological improvement.[17] Combining studies on closed reduction of cervical spine fracture-dislocation injuries yields a success rate of ~80%; however, from a guidelines perspective, closed reduction currently lacks the prospective studies needed to achieve more than an "option" recommendation.[16–20] The largest clinical series ($n \geq 50$) on closed reduction for cervical injuries is summarized in **Table 22.1**.

Craniocervical traction is not without risks, yet the general safety of closed reduction has been supported by several reports. Gardner-Wells tongs have very rarely caused serious morbidities (such as skull perforation and brain abscess) and are contraindicated in a patient with comminuted skull fractures.[21,22] Early neurological deterioration (<24 hours) in cervical spinal cord injury has been mainly attributed to inadequate immobilization and cervical traction.[23] The risk of sustaining a permanent neurological deficit from closed reduction is less that 1.0%.[19,24–27] Transient neurological deficits have been reported with higher frequency (2 to 4%) and tend to resolve or improve after reduction of the traction weight or after open reduction.[18,28] The potential to engender new neurological deficits (as severe as acute quadriplegia) has led most to advocate for closed reduction only in awake and cooperative patients. The manipulation of a cervical fracture dislocation under anesthesia must be done with extreme caution because a comparison study found a lower success rate and higher incidence of complications as compared with skull traction in the oriented patient.[29] Nevertheless, closed manipulation under anesthesia has been utilized safely within the context of a protocol where patients who failed awake craniocervical traction were next treated with manipulation under anesthesia and surgery as a last resort.[27,30]

Neurological worsening after closed reduction with craniocervical traction has been attributed to several factors: overdistraction; failure to recognize a different more rostral, noncontiguous lesion; disk herniation; epidural hematoma; fractures in patients with ankylosing spondylitis; and spinal cord edema.[31–35] A large percentage of overdistraction cases in the literature has been associated with missed atlanto-occipital and atlantoaxial dislocations.[36] In particular, a synchronous longitudinal atlanto-occipital dislocation is difficult

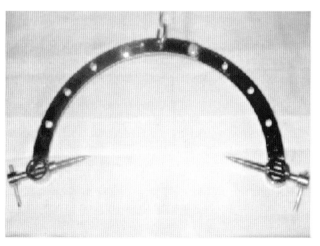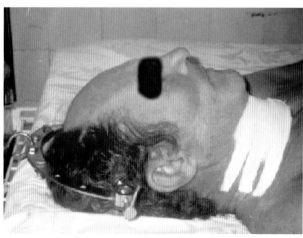

A

B

Fig. 22.2 **(A)** Gardner-Wells tongs applied to **(B)** a patient undergoing cervical spine traction for a traumatic C5–C6 fracture-dislocation.

Table 22.1 Evidentiary Table of Closed Reduction for Subaxial Cervical Spine Trauma

Study Study Type	No. of Patients	Injury Type	Complications	Neurological Change Success rate (%)	Conclusion
Grant et al (1999)[16] Retrospective	82	Facet dislocations Burst Fx Extension injury Pedicle Fx	1 patient (1.3%) Lost ASIA motor points > 6 h postreduction	Average ASIA motor score: Prereduction 54.6 24 h Postreduction 59.3 **97.6%**	Safe and effective
Vital et al (1998)[27] Retrospective	168	Facet dislocations	None	Bilateral dislocation **43%** with traction **27%** with MUA Unilateral dislocation **23%** with traction **36%** with MUA	Safe and effective
Lee et al (1994)[29] Retrospective	210	Facet dislocations	6 MUA lost ASIA motor 1 traction lost ASIA motor	**88%** with traction **73%** with MUA	Traction more effective and safer than MUA
Mahale et al (1993)[19] Retrospective	341	Facet dislocations Different reduction methods including surgery	16 patients worse postreduction 4 reduced with traction 4 reduced with manipulation 8 reduced with surgery	Cannot be determined	Neurological worsening possible
Hadley et al (1992)[17] Retrospective	68	Facet dislocations	7 patients worse with traction	**58%**	Early reduction improves outcome
Star et al (1990)[20] Retrospective	57	Facet dislocations	2 patients lost root function No patient lost Frankel grade	**93%**	Safe and effective
Kleyn (1984)[102] Retrospective	101	Facet dislocations MUA initially MUA if traction failed	None	**81%** with traction/MUA	Safe, effective, and may improve neurological function
Shrosbree (1979)[30] Retrospective	216	Facet dislocations Traction + MUA	None	Cannot be determined	Safe and effective Reduction may improve outcome

Abbreviations: ASIA, American Spinal Injury Association; FX, fracture; MUA, manipulation under anesthesia.

to diagnose and may be one of the most serious contraindications to craniocervical traction.[37,38]

A major controversy surrounding closed reduction of cervical injuries has been the suspicion that neurological deterioration may be caused by disk herniations, urging some to recommend prereduction MRI.[17,39–42] However, only two cases in the literature have associated new neurological deficit after closed reduction with cervical disk herniation.[24,43] Vaccaro et al published the only prospective study designed to investigate disk herniations in this setting and found that, although closed reduction increases the incidence of cervical disk herniations, there was no apparent neurological consequence of disk herniations on closed reduction.[44] In fact, a recent prospective study involving the use of an MRI-guided craniocervical traction system in 17 patients with cervical spine fracture-dislocations has

helped clarify the neuroanatomical consequences of closed reduction; in all cases, traction pulled the herniated disk back toward the disk space, and the cervical canal diameter improved in 11 of 17 patients.[45]

Thus prereduction MRI is not currently recommended for most patients and may even be harmful by delaying the decompressive benefit of closed reduction. Obtaining an MRI is a reasonable option when the patient is obtunded and cannot provide feedback during closed reduction. Even though the clinical significance of prereduction disk herniations remains uncertain, the presence of a large disk herniation in an unreliable patient may encourage a spine surgeon to perform a ventral decompression prior to attempting reduction.[18] MRI might also be valuable for surgical planning after a failed closed reduction. Future studies may help elucidate whether the risks of closed reduction are significantly higher in patients with certain spinal comorbidities such as ossification of the posterior longitudinal ligament and ankylosing spondylitis.

◆ Atlantoaxial Rotatory Subluxation

Closed reduction via tongs or halter traction has also become a standard practice for atlantoaxial rotatory subluxation (AARS). Posttraumatic AARS is primarily seen in the pediatric population; however, adults are also affected.[46] MRI studies suggest that the formation of a fixed atlantoaxial joint subluxation requires disruption of the alar ligaments that tether the odontoid apex to the lateral occipital processes.[47] Patients present with neck discomfort, decreased cervical range of motion, and torticollis, which may manifest as the classic "cock-robin" head appearance. Neurological deficit is rare, but a delay in diagnosis remains common despite the advent of dynamic computed tomographic (CT) and three-dimensional CT reconstructions. In a retrospective study of 20 children, Subach et al successfully restored normal atlantoaxial alignment in 94% of patients using cervical halter traction; reduction was obtained more rapidly and more effectively with the use of traction versus a cervical collar alone.[48] Although CT is the best diagnostic modality, MRI is recommended to assess the integrity of the transverse ligament. If the transverse ligament is intact, successful closed reduction via traction is usually a sufficient cure.[49] Early recognition and treatment are crucial given that the major factor predicting failure of conservative management is the duration of subluxation prior to reduction.[48,50] Associated fractures of the odontoid or facets may lower the success rate of traction for

AARS and encourage one to proceed with open surgical reduction and fixation.[51]

◆ Cervical Burst Fractures, Flexion Teardrop Fractures, and Subaxial Spondylolisthesis

Cervical burst fractures, flexion teardrop fractures, and subaxial cervical spondylolisthesis (**Fig. 22.3**) are additional traumatic cervical injuries that have been treated with initial closed reduction via skull traction or a halo vest. Although the role of conservative management for such injuries has decreased in recent years, there are reports of successful nonoperative management with closed reduction and immobilization alone.[2,52,53] There is a paucity of studies comparing conservative and operative treatments for cervical burst fractures, flexion teardrop fractures, and traumatic cervical spondylolisthesis, and definitive recommendations cannot be made. However, closed reduction should be viewed as a complementary or adjunctive treatment rather than an alternative to surgery.[54] Even if closed reduction does not obviate the need for surgery, arriving in the operating room with restored anatomical alignment likely simplifies and expedites the required surgical intervention. Furthermore, biomechanical studies have shown that traction may reduce spinal cord compression from retropulsed bone fragments in a cervical burst fracture.[55]

In conclusion, closed reduction via skull traction is currently recommended as an effective and safe primary intervention

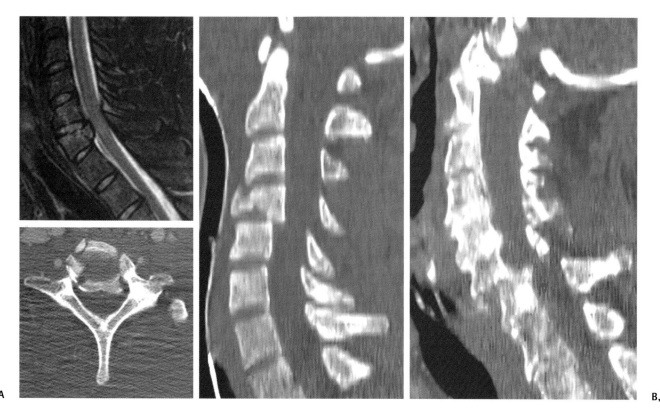

A
B,C

Fig. 22.3 **(A)** Sagittal magnetic resonance imaging (MRI) T2-weighted sequence (*top*) and axial computed tomography (CT) of the cervical spine (*bottom*) of a C6 burst fracture with bony retropulsion into the spinal canal and resultant spinal cord compression. **(B)** Sagittal reconstruction of a cervical spine CT scan showing a C4 flexion teardrop fracture. Note the retrolisthesis at C4–C5, indicative of posterior column incompetence and an unstable injury. **(C)** Sagittal reconstruction of a cervical spine CT scan showing an anterolisthesis of C6 on C7 secondary to bilateral facet fracture-dislocations.

IV Problem-Based Approach to the Principles of Spinal Injury Management

for cervical facet fracture-dislocations and atlantoaxial rotatory subluxation. The role of closed reduction in other unstable cervical injuries such as burst fracture, teardrop fractures, and spondylolisthesis is less defined. However, the principle of indirect neural decompression in patients with spinal cord injury should still apply for these injury types. For all these cervical injuries, closed reduction may strongly influence both the timing and the type of subsequent operative management and may obviate the need to perform longer and more complex fixation operations. Unfortunately, there is currently no class I or even class II evidence that can help guide management decisions regarding closed reduction. Moreover, whereas the basic goals and techniques of traction-mediated closed reduction have not changed for many decades, new operative fixation strategies (many of which are increasingly less invasive) have emerged and must be considered as a first-line reduction and stabilization strategy for complex cervical injuries. Nevertheless, it is likely that comorbid traumatic injuries or hemodynamic instability will continue to preclude emergent surgery for some patients with spinal cord damage and an unstable cervical injury.

◆ Spinal Bracing

Various means for externally immobilizing or bracing injuries along the entire spinal axis have been devised. Similar to closed reduction, bracing has a fundamental role in both the nonoperative and the operative management of traumatic spinal injuries.

◆ Cervical Collar and Halo Vest Immobilization

Although spinal immobilization has become a cornerstone of the emergency medical service response to trauma victims, there is unfortunately no class I or class II evidence to support this practice. However, multiple class III evidence reports have ascribed neurological worsening among trauma patients to a lack of proper immobilization.[56-58] The combination of a hard cervical collar flanked by supportive head blocks on a backboard with straps remains one of the most effective ways to ensure spinal immobilization in a trauma patient prior to transport.[59]

As monotherapy, cervical collars (**Fig. 22.4A**) have proven efficacy and are recommended for the treatment of various isolated cervical spine fractures. Multiple class III reports support the cervical collar as the primary treatment for traumatic occipital condyle fractures, particularly the potentially unstable Anderson-Montesano type III variant, which involves an avulsion of part of the occipital condyle.[60-64] Moreover, isolated fractures of the atlas with an intact transverse ligament have been successfully treated solely with a cervical collar.[65-68] Transverse ligament disruption inferred from MRI signal change, a predental space > 3.0 mm in adults, or by the sum displacement of the lateral masses of C1 on C2 of more than 8.1 mm (adjusted rule of Spence) should prompt one to treat an isolated atlas fracture with either rigid halo-vest immobilization or a C1–C2 operative fixation (**Figs. 22.4B, 22.5**).[65] Type I odontoid fractures have a very high union rate with rigid collar immobilization and type III odontoid fractures have fairly good union rates with a collar alone (50 to 65%).[69-73] Based on a landmark analysis of the literature, Julien et al found no difference in outcomes among patients with type III odontoid fractures treated by halo versus cervical collar immobilization.[74] The type II odontoid fracture has a fairly poor healing rate with a cervical collar alone. Halo vest immobilization alone increases healing to between 43 and 88%.[74,75] Combined C1–C2 fractures have been traditionally managed by focusing on the type of C2 injury. There are several reports of successful union for combined C1–C2 fractures with a collar alone, but patient numbers are very small and most treatment stratagems for such combination fractures have utilized either a more rigid external immobilization (halo or sternal occipital mandibular immobilizer (SOMI) device) or surgery.[76-78] Cervical collars are not

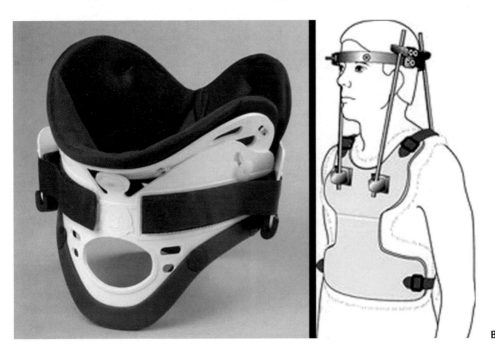

Fig. 22.4 **(A)** The Miami-J collar, one of several commercially available rigid cervical collars, is available in six adult and four pediatric sizes and should be appropriately sized. **(B)** A schematic diagram demonstrating a patient wearing a halo ring-vest orthosis.

196

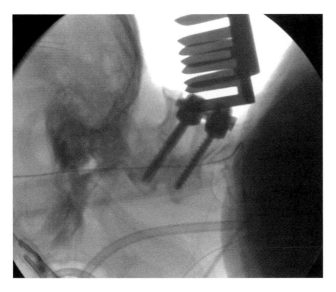

Fig. 22.5 An intraoperative fluoroscopic view of a C1–C2 posterior fixation for traumatic atlantoaxial instability via Harms or Goyel technique. Bilateral polyaxial screws have been placed into the C1 lateral masses and are connected by rods to bilateral C2 pedicle screws.

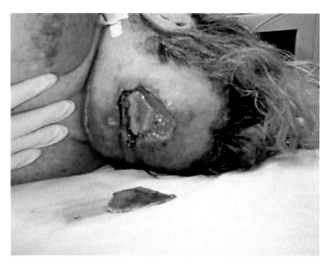

Fig. 22.6 A rigid cervical collar has produced a grade IV (extending down to bone) decubitus skin ulceration on the occipital scalp of an obtunded patient in the intensive care unit.

completely benign and have been associated with patient discomfort, pressure sores (**Fig. 22.6**), increasing intracranial pressure, greater aspiration, and worsened pulmonary function.[79–82]

The halo vest is an important tool in the management of occipitoatlantoaxial trauma. In addition to providing immobilization, the halo vest can also function as a cervical traction apparatus.[83] However, it is associated with intersegmental motion due to snaking of the spinal column, especially at the fracture site. Anderson et al demonstrated that 1.7 mm of translation and 7 degrees of angulation occur at the injury level when patients move from a supine to an upright position (**Table 22.2**).[84] In 2001, Vieweg and Schultheis reported on the outcome analysis of 682 patients from the literature who were treated with conservative therapy consisting of a halo vest for 709 different injuries.[85] **Table 22.3** summarizes the outcomes for halo vest treatment of different upper cervical fractures. The best union results have been seen with isolated Jefferson fractures, stable hangman's fractures, and type I and type II odontoid fractures with minimal dislocation. Despite its efficacy when applied correctly, the halo vest is often criticized for its

multiple complications and impact on quality of life. In particular, halo vest treatment in elderly patients has been linked to significant increases in both early morbidity and mortality.[86–88] Halo complications are not rare and include pin loosening, pin site infection, periorbital edema, superior pressure sores, pin penetration, osteomyelitis, subdural abscess, nerve palsies, and fracture overdistraction.[89] Many halo-related complications can be avoided with meticulous attention to pin care.

◆ Thoracic, Lumbar, and Sacral Orthoses

Fractures of the thoracolumbosacral spine occur in as many as 4% of trauma patients arriving at a level I trauma center.[90] Multidetector spiral CT with reconstructions has become a formidable tool in the diagnosis of acute thoracolumbar spine fractures.[91] Bracing has been a fundamental part of the conservative management of traumatic thoracolumbar compression and burst fractures since the time of Hippocrates. Braces stabilize the spine by limiting overall trunk motion, decreasing isotonic back and abdominal muscular activity, and increasing intraabdominal pressure.[92] Today many companies will provide

Table 22.2 Motion at Fracture Site in Patients Treated with Halo Orthosis

	No. of Cases	Translation (mm)	Angulation (degrees)
Occipital condyle fracture	1	0	16
Jefferson fracture	2	2.0	3.0
Odontoid fracture			
Type I	10	1.85	9.0
Type II	9	1.6	6.3
Hangman's fracture	13	2.0	8.4
Facet fracture dislocation	9	1.6	3.3
Total	44	1.7 ± 1.4*	7.0 ± 6.4*

*Mean ± standard deviation.[84]

Table 22.3 Halo Vest Outcomes for High Cervical Fractures

Injury	Success Rate (%)
Atlas ring fractures	100
Combined atlas ring and odontoid fractures	20
Type II odontoid fractures	85
Combined type II odontoid and other C1 or C2 fractures	67
Type III odontoid fractures	97
Combined type III odontoid and C1 fractures	80
Hangman's fractures	99
Combined hangman's and C1 fractures	100

Source: Vieweg U, Schultheis R. A review of halo vest treatment of upper cervical spine injuries. Arch Orthop Trauma Surg 2001;121:50–55. Adapted with permission.

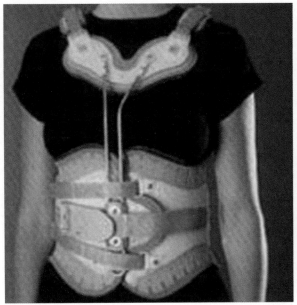
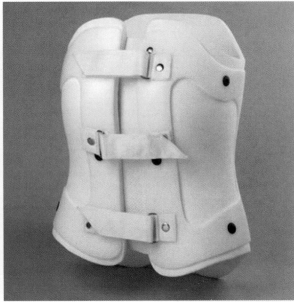

A   B

Fig. 22.7 Several different types of thoracolumbosacral orthoses (TLSOs) are available. Two commonly used varieties are **(A)** the adjustable Aspen TLSO (Aspen Medical Products, Irvine, CA) and **(B)** the custom-fitted "tortoise shell" TLSO.

custom-fitted orthoses on an urgent basis to inpatients with spinal fractures. The ability of thoracolumbosacral orthoses (TLSOs) to significantly reduce both total vertebral motion and intervertebral motion in the lumbar spine has been confirmed by in vivo fluoroscopic studies.[93] There is a wide variety of external bracing options that range from the simple one-size-fits-all lumbosacral corset to the plastic molded TLSO (**Fig. 22.7**). Both retrospective and prospective studies have supported the use of spinal bracing for stable traumatic thoracolumbar burst fractures in the absence of neurological deficit.[94–99] Vertebral compression fractures tend to be stable fractures, and conservative management with bracing is usually successful; surgery is generally advocated when there is a failure of conservative care, kyphosis angle >30 degrees, or anterior height loss > 40%.[100] However, others have argued through retrospective analysis that bracing for lumbar compression fractures (with up to 30% loss of height) may not improve radiographic healing.[92,101] Thus one must recognize that currently there is insufficient evidence to make definitive statements regarding the use of bracing for thoracolumbar spine injuries. Moreover, there are no good comparison studies to prove that the more expensive plastic external braces are superior to over-the-counter cloth braces in facilitating patient recovery. Future studies may help to investigate the influence of bracing on patient comfort and quality of life. Although difficult to measure, braces, as the conspicuous garb of spinal trauma, likely exert a behavioral influence on patients by continually reminding the patient and those around them that a serious injury has been sustained.

References

1. Crutchfield WG. Skeletal traction for dislocations of the cervical spine. Report of a case. South Surg 1933;2:156–159
2. Koivikko MP, Myllynen P, Karjalainen M, Vornanen M, Santavirta S. Conservative and operative treatment in cervical burst fractures. Arch Orthop Trauma Surg 2000;120:448–451
3. Subach BR, McLaughlin MR, Albright AL, Pollack IF. Current management of pediatric atlantoaxial rotatory subluxation. Spine 1998;23:2174–2179
4. Yashon D, Tyson G, Vise WM. Rapid closed reduction of cervical fracture dislocations. Surg Neurol 1975;4:513–514
5. Sonntag VKH. Management of bilateral locked facets of the cervical spine. Neurosurgery 1981;8:150–152
6. Vaccaro AR, Falatyn SP, Flanders AE, Balderston RA, Northrup BE, Cotler JM. Magnetic resonance evaluation of the intervertebral disc, spinal ligaments, and spinal cord before and after closed traction reduction of cervical spine dislocations. Spine 1999;24:1210–1217
7. Delamarter RB, Sherman J, Carr JB. Pathophysiology of spinal cord injury: recovery after immediate and delayed decompression. J Bone Joint Surg Am 1995;77:1042–1049
8. Cotler HB, Miller LS, DeLucia FA, Cotler JM, Davne SH. Closed reduction of cervical spine dislocations. Clin Orthop Relat Res 1987;214:185–199
9. Star AM, Jones AA, Cotler JM, Balderston RA, Sinha R. Immediate closed reduction of cervical spine dislocations using traction. Spine 1990;15:1068–1072
10. Brunette DD, Rockswold GL. Neurologic recovery following rapid spinal realignment for complete cervical spinal cord injury. J Trauma 1987;27:445–447
11. Vaccaro AR, Madigan L, Schweitzer ME, Flanders AE, Hilibrand AS, Albert TJ. Magnetic resonance imaging analysis of soft tissue disruption after flexion-distraction injuries of the subaxial cervical spine. Spine 2001;26:1866–1872
12. Kilburn MP, Smith DP, Hadley MN. The initial evaluation and treatment of the patient with spinal trauma. In: Batjer HH, Loftus CM, eds. Textbook of Neurological Surgery: Principles and Practice. Philadelphia: Lippincott Williams & Wilkins; 2002
13. Wilberger JE. Immobilization and traction. In: Tator CH, Benzel EC, eds. Contemporary Management of Spinal Cord Injury: From Impact to Rehabilitation. Park Ridge: AANS; 2000:91–98
14. Cotler JM, Herbison GJ, Nasuti JF, Ditunno JF Jr, An H, Wolff BE. Closed reduction of traumatic cervical spine dislocation using traction weights up to 140 pounds. Spine 1993;18:386–390
15. Sabiston CP, Wing PC, Schweigel JF, Van Peteghem PK, Yu W. Closed reduction of dislocations of the lower cervical spine. J Trauma 1988;28:832–835
16. Grant GA, Mirza SK, Chapman JR, et al. Risk of early closed reduction in cervical spine subluxation injuries. J Neurosurg 1999;90(1, Suppl):13–18
17. Hadley MN, Fitzpatrick BC, Sonntag VKH, Browner CM. Facet fracture-dislocation injuries of the cervical spine. Neurosurgery 1992;30:661–666
18. [no author listed]. Initial closed reduction of cervical spine fracture-dislocation injuries. Neurosurgery 2002;50(3, Suppl):S44–S50
19. Mahale YJ, Silver JR, Henderson NJ. Neurological complications of the reduction of cervical spine dislocations. J Bone Joint Surg Br 1993;75:403–409
20. Star AM, Jones AA, Cotler JM, Balderston RA, Sinha R. Immediate closed reduction of cervical spine dislocations using traction. Spine 1990;15:1068–1072
21. Feldman RA, Khayyat GF. Perforation of the skull by a Gardner-Wells tong. Case report. J Neurosurg 1976;44:119–120

22. Soyer J, Iborra JP, Fargues P, Pries P, Clarac JP. Brain abscess following the use of skull traction with Gardner-Wells tongs [in French]. Chirurgie 1999;124:432–434

23. Harrop JS, Sharan AD, Vaccaro AR, Przybylski GJ. The cause of neurologic deterioration after acute cervical spinal cord injury. Spine 2001;26:340–346

24. Farmer J, Vaccaro A, Albert TJ, Malone S, Balderston RA, Cotler JM. Neurologic deterioration after cervical spinal cord injury. J Spinal Disord 1998;11:192–196

25. Fehlings MG, Tator CH. An evidence-based review of decompressive surgery in acute spinal cord injury: rationale, indications, and timing based on experimental and clinical studies. J Neurosurg 1999;91(1, Suppl):1–11

26. Mahale YJ, Silver JR. Progressive paralysis after bilateral facet dislocation of the cervical spine. J Bone Joint Surg Br 1992;74:219–223

27. Vital JM, Gille O, Sénégas J, Pointillart V. Reduction technique for uni- and biarticular dislocations of the lower cervical spine. Spine 1998;23:949–954, discussion 955

28. Wimberley DW, Vaccaro AR, Goyal N, et al. Acute quadriplegia following closed traction reduction of a cervical facet dislocation in the setting of ossification of the posterior longitudinal ligament: case report. Spine 2005;30:E433–E438

29. Lee AS, MacLean JC, Newton DA. Rapid traction for reduction of cervical spine dislocations. J Bone Joint Surg Br 1994;76:352–356

30. Shrosbree RD. Neurological sequelae of reduction of fracture dislocations of the cervical spine. Paraplegia 1979;17:212–221

31. Scher AT. Overdistraction of cervical spinal injuries? S Afr Med J 1981;59:639–641

32. Gruenberg MF, Rechtine GR, Chrin AM, Solá CA, Ortolán EG. Overdistraction of cervical spine injuries with the use of skull traction: a report of two cases. J Trauma 1997;42:1152–1156

33. Key A. Cervical spine dislocations with unilateral facet interlocking. Paraplegia 1975;13:208–215

34. Schaefer DM, Flanders A, Northrup BE, Doan HT, Osterholm JL. Magnetic resonance imaging of acute cervical spine trauma: correlation with severity of neurologic injury. Spine 1989;14:1090–1095

35. Fried LC. Cervical spinal cord injury during skeletal traction. JAMA 1974;229:181–183

36. Bohlman HH. Acute fractures and dislocations of the cervical spine: an analysis of three hundred hospitalized patients and review of the literature. J Bone Joint Surg Am 1979;61:1119–1142

37. Guigui P, Milaire M, Morvan G, Lassale B, Deburge A. Traumatic atlantooccipital dislocation with survival: case report and review of the literature. Eur Spine J 1995;4:242–247

38. Steinmetz MP, Lechner RM, Anderson JS. Atlantooccipital dislocation in children: presentation, diagnosis, and management. Neurosurg Focus 2003;14:ecp1

39. Berrington NR, van Staden JF, Willers JG, van der Westhuizen J. Cervical intervertebral disc prolapse associated with traumatic facet dislocations. Surg Neurol 1993;40:395–399

40. Doran SE, Papadopoulos SM, Ducker TB, Lillehei KO. Magnetic resonance imaging documentation of coexistent traumatic locked facets of the cervical spine and disc herniation. J Neurosurg 1993;79:341–345

41. Eismont FJ, Arena MJ, Green BA. Extrusion of an intervertebral disc associated with traumatic subluxation or dislocation of cervical facets: case report. J Bone Joint Surg Am 1991;73:1555–1560

42. Hart RA, Vaccaro AR, Nachwalter RS. Cervical facet dislocation: when is magnetic resonance imaging indicated? Spine 2002;27:116–117

43. Maiman DJ, Barolat G, Larson SJ. Management of bilateral locked facets of the cervical spine. Neurosurgery 1986;18:542–547

44. Vaccaro AR, Falatyn SP, Flanders AE, Balderston RA, Northrup BE, Cotler JM. Magnetic resonance evaluation of the intervertebral disc, spinal ligaments, and spinal cord before and after closed traction reduction of cervical spine dislocations. Spine 1999;24:1210–1217

45. Darsaut TE, Ashforth R, Bhargava R, et al. A pilot study of magnetic resonance imaging-guided closed reduction of cervical spine fractures. Spine 2006;31:2085–2090

46. Crook TB, Eynon CA. Traumatic atlantoaxial rotatory subluxation. Emerg Med J 2005;22:671–672

47. Willauschus WG, Kladny B, Beyer WF, Glückert K, Arnold H, Scheithauer R. Lesions of the alar ligaments. In vivo and in vitro studies with magnetic resonance imaging. Spine 1995;20:2493–2498

48. Subach BR, McLaughlin MR, Albright AL, Pollack IF. Current management of pediatric atlantoaxial rotatory subluxation. Spine 1998;23:2174–2179

49. Weisskopf M, Naeve D, Ruf M, Harms J, Jeszenszky D. Therapeutic options and results following fixed atlantoaxial rotatory dislocations. Eur Spine J 2005;14:61–68

50. Maile S, Slongo T. Atlantoaxial rotatory subluxation: realignment and discharge within 48 h. Eur J Emerg Med 2007;14:167–169

51. Kim YS, Lee JK, Moon SJ, Kim SH. Post-traumatic atlantoaxial rotatory fixation in an adult: a case report. Spine 2007;32:E682–E687

52. Lind B, Sihlbom H, Nordwall A. Halo-vest treatment of unstable traumatic cervical spine injuries. Spine 1988;13:425–432

53. Johnson JL, Cannon D. Nonoperative treatment of the acute tear-drop fracture of the cervical spine. Clin Orthop Relat Res 1982;168:108–112

54. Ido K, Murakami H, Kawaguchi H, Urushidani H. An unusual reduction technique prior to surgical treatment for traumatic spondylolisthesis in the lower cervical spine. J Clin Neurosci 2002;9:664–666, discussion 667

55. Ching RP, Watson NA, Carter JW, Tencer AF. The effect of post-injury spinal position on canal occlusion in a cervical spine burst fracture model. Spine 1997;22:1710–1715

56. Bohlman HH. Acute fractures and dislocations of the cervical spine: an analysis of three hundred hospitalized patients and review of the literature. J Bone Joint Surg Am 1979;61:1119–1142

57. Jeanneret B, Magerl F, Ward JC. Overdistraction: a hazard of skull traction in the management of acute injuries of the cervical spine. Arch Orthop Trauma Surg 1991;110:242–245

58. Garfin SR, Shackford SR, Marshall LF, Drummond JC. Care of the multiply injured patient with cervical spine injury. Clin Orthop Relat Res 1989;239:19–29

59. [no author listed]. Cervical spine immobilization before admission to the hospital. Neurosurgery 2002;50(3, Suppl):S7–S17

60. Anderson PA, Montesano PX. Morphology and treatment of occipital condyle fractures. Spine 1988;13:731–736

61. Desai SS, Coumas JM, Danylevich A, Hayes E, Dunn EJ. Fracture of the occipital condyle: case report and review of the literature. J Trauma 1990;30:240–241

62. Emery E, Saillant G, Ismail M, Fohanno D, Roy-Camille R. Fracture of the occipital condyle: case report and review of the literature. Eur Spine J 1995;4:191–193

63. Goldstein SJ, Woodring JH, Young AB. Occipital condyle fracture associated with cervical spine injury. Surg Neurol 1982;17:350–352

64. Harding-Smith J, MacIntosh PK, Sherbon KJ. Fracture of the occipital condyle: a case report and review of the literature. J Bone Joint Surg Am 1981;63:1170–1171

65. [no author listed]. Isolated fractures of the atlas in adults. Neurosurgery 2002;50(3, Suppl):S120–S124

66. Fowler JL, Sandhu A, Fraser RD. A review of fractures of the atlas vertebra. J Spinal Disord 1990;3:19–24

67. Hadley MN, Dickman CA, Browner CM, Sonntag VKH. Acute traumatic atlas fractures: management and long term outcome. Neurosurgery 1988;23:31–35

68. Kesterson L, Benzel EC, Orrison W, Coleman J. Evaluation and treatment of atlas burst fractures (Jefferson fractures). J Neurosurg 1991;75:213–220

69. Anderson LD, D'Alonzo RT. Fractures of the odontoid process of the axis. J Bone Joint Surg Am 1974;56:1663–1674

70. Chiba K, Fujimura Y, Toyama Y, Fujii E, Nakanishi T, Hirabayashi K. Treatment protocol for fractures of the odontoid process. J Spinal Disord 1996;9:267–276

71. Clark CR, White AA III. Fractures of the dens: a multicenter study. J Bone Joint Surg Am 1985;67:1340–1348

72. Wang GJ, Mabie KN, Whitehill R, Stamp WG. The nonsurgical management of odontoid fractures in adults. Spine 1984;9:229–230

73. [no author listed]. Isolated fractures of the axis in adults. Neurosurgery 2002;50(3, Suppl):S125–S139

74. Julien TD, Frankel B, Traynelis VC, Ryken TC. Evidence-based analysis of odontoid fracture management. Neurosurg Focus 2000;8:e1

75. Polin RS, Szabo T, Bogaev CA, Replogle RE, Jane JA. Nonoperative management of types II and III odontoid fractures: the Philadelphia collar versus the halo vest. Neurosurgery 1996;38:450–456, discussion 456–457

76. Coric D, Wilson JA, Kelly DL Jr. Treatment of traumatic spondylolisthesis of the axis with nonrigid immobilization: a review of 64 cases. J Neurosurg 1996;85:550–554

77. Esses SI, Bednar DA. Screw fixation of odontoid fractures and nonunions. Spine 1991;16(10, Suppl):S483–S485

78. Lee TT, Green BA, Petrin DR. Treatment of stable burst fracture of the atlas (Jefferson fracture) with rigid cervical collar. Spine 1998;23:1963–1967

79. Bauer D, Kowalski R. Effect of spinal immobilization devices on pulmonary function in the healthy, nonsmoking man. Ann Emerg Med 1988;17:915–918

80. Chan D, Goldberg R, Tascone A, Harmon S, Chan L. The effect of spinal immobilization on healthy volunteers. Ann Emerg Med 1994;23:48–51

81. Davies G, Deakin C, Wilson A. The effect of a rigid collar on intracranial pressure. Injury 1996;27:647–649

82. Linares HA, Mawson AR, Suarez E, Biundo JJ. Association between pressure sores and immobilization in the immediate post-injury period. Orthopedics 1987;10:571–573

83. Kyoshima K, Kakizawa Y, Tokushige K. Simple cervical spine traction using a halo vest apparatus: technical note. Surg Neurol 2003;59:518–521, discussion 521

84. Anderson PA, Budorick TE, Easton KB, Henley MB, Salciccioli GG. Failure of halo vest to prevent in vivo motion in patients with injured cervical spines. Spine 1991;16(10, Suppl):S501–S505

85. Vieweg U, Schultheiss R. A review of halo vest treatment of upper cervical spine injuries. Arch Orthop Trauma Surg 2001;121:50–55

86. Tashjian RZ, Majercik S, Biffl WL, Palumbo MA, Cioffi WG. Halo-vest immobilization increases early morbidity and mortality in elderly odontoid fractures. J Trauma 2006;60:199–203

87. Lögters T, Hoppe S, Linhart W, et al. On the problem of halo vest treatment in the elderly. Results of a retrospective analysis [in German]. Unfallchirurg 2006;109:306–312

88. Majercik S, Tashjian RZ, Biffl WL, Harrington DT, Cioffi WG. Halo vest immobilization in the elderly: a death sentence? J Trauma 2005;59: 350–356, discussion 356–358

89. Hayes VM, Silber JS, Siddiqi FN, Kondrachov D, Lipetz JS, Lonner B. Complications of halo fixation of the cervical spine. Am J Orthop 2005; 34:271–276

90. Diaz JJ Jr, Cullinane DC, Altman DT, et al; EAST Practice Management Guideline Committee. Practice management guidelines for the screening of thoracolumbar spine fracture. J Trauma 2007;63:709–718

91. Gong JS, Xu JM. Value of multidetector spiral CT in diagnosis of acute thoracolumbar spinal fracture and fracture-dislocation. Chin J Traumatol 2004;7:289–293

92. Ohana N, Sheinis D, Rath E, Sasson A, Atar D. Is there a need for lumbar orthosis in mild compression fractures of the thoracolumbar spine? A retrospective study comparing the radiographic results between early ambulation with and without lumbar orthosis. J Spinal Disord 2000; 13:305–308

93. Vander Kooi D, Abad G, Basford JR, Maus TP, Yaszemski MJ, Kaufman KR. Lumbar spine stabilization with a thoracolumbosacral orthosis: evaluation with video fluoroscopy. Spine 2004;29:100–104

94. Dai LY, Jiang SD, Wang XY, Jiang LS. A review of the management of thoracolumbar burst fractures. Surg Neurol 2007;67:221–231, discussion 231

95. Dai LY. Remodeling of the spinal canal after thoracolumbar burst fractures. Clin Orthop Relat Res 2001;382:119–123

96. Denis F, Armstrong GW, Searls K, Matta L. Acute thoracolumbar burst fractures in the absence of neurologic deficit: a comparison between operative and nonoperative treatment. Clin Orthop Relat Res 1984;189: 142–149

97. Hitchon PW, Torner JC, Haddad SF, Follett KA. Management options in thoracolumbar burst fractures. Surg Neurol 1998;49:619–626, discussion 626–627

98. Shen WJ, Liu TJ, Shen YS. Nonoperative treatment versus posterior fixation for thoracolumbar junction burst fractures without neurologic deficit. Spine 2001;26:1038–1045

99. Yazici M, Atilla B, Tepe S, Calisir A. Spinal canal remodeling in burst fractures of the thoracolumbar spine: a computerized tomographic comparison between operative and nonoperative treatment. J Spinal Disord 1996;9:409–413

100. Tezer M, Erturer RE, Ozturk C, Ozturk I, Kuzgun U. Conservative treatment of fractures of the thoracolumbar spine. Int Orthop 2005;29:78–82

101. Weitzman G. Treatment of stable thoracolumbar spine compression fractures by early ambulation. Clin Orthop Relat Res 1971;76:116–122

102. Kleyn PJ. Dislocations of the cervical spine: closed reduction under anaesthesia. Paraplegia 1984;22:271–281

23

Management of Cervical Spine Injuries in the Athlete: Return-to-Play Criteria

Ahmad Khaldi and Russ P. Nockels

Returning players to a competitive contest after a cervical spine injury is a task fraught with opinion and bias and without clear consensus.[1] For example, a questionnaire of physicians' responses to different sports-related cervical spine injuries revealed a statistical deviation from reported guidelines.[1] In addition, experts disagree on whether cervical stenosis in asymptomatic athletes is an absolute contraindication,[2] or indeed whether an absolute contraindication exists to returning a player to contact sports[3] (**Table 23.1**).

◆ Cervical Spine Injuries in the Athlete

Epidemiology

Spinal cord injury is estimated to occur ~11,000 times annually in North America, with sports injury contributing between 2 and 10% of the total.[4–9] Approximately 1000 sports-related spinal cord injuries occur in the United States annually.[10,11] Most of those injuries occur during unsupervised sports-related activities such as diving, surfing, or skiing. However, competitive activities such as football, wrestling, ice hockey, and gymnastics all pose a significant risk.[8,10] Diving accidents constitute ~7 to 10% of all spinal injuries,[8] although it is thought that many recreational diving injuries go unreported.[9]

Of the 3200 spine injuries that were seen at Northwestern University Midwest Regional Spinal Cord Unit over a 12-year period (1975 to 1987), 63 (2%) were sports related. Football injuries constituted the majority of cases with 37, whereas wrestling,[12] skiing,[5] and gymnastics[5] were also represented. Of those 63 patients, 45 had sustained permanent damage, and 18 had transient spinal cord symptoms. The 45 patients with permanent injury included 12 with complete spinal cord injury, 14 with incomplete spinal cord injury, and 19 with vertebral column injury. Treatment included 25 surgeries and 20 orthotics.[5]

Football has the largest number of spinal injuries per year involving contact sports.[13] Although the rate per number of players of catastrophic injuries is lower in football than in other sports, the large number of participants makes football the highest-ranking sport with severe neck injures per year in the United States.[9] Although improved protective capabilities of modern helmets have resulted in a decline in head injuries, an increase in neck injuries occurred, possibly due to players using the crown of the helmet as the initial point of contact during the period 1971 to 1975.[12] In 1976, the National Collegiate Athletic Association banned "spear" tackling as well as techniques using the helmet as the initial point of contact. As a result, there has been a decrease in the incidence of permanent spinal cord injury from 20 per year (1971 to 1975) to 7.2 per year (1991 to 2001) in football. This decline in annual injuries probably resulted from the implementation of rule changes (1976) and improved education of better tackling techniques, as well as better treatment of spinal cord injury.[14] The incidence rate for catastrophic spine injury per 100,000 athletes is 0.52 in high school, 1.55 in college, and 14 in professional football.[15]

Spinal injury is also associated with numerous other sports activities. There was one catastrophic spinal cord injury per 100,000 participants in wrestling between the years 1981 and 1999, with cervical fracture or major cervical ligament injuries constituting the majority of the traumatic pathology.[15] The wrestling position most frequently associated with spinal injury is the takedown maneuver.[15] There are also isolated case reports of severe neck injuries in soccer.[16] The incidence of catastrophic injury in ice hockey is high and is mostly associated with checking from behind and being hurled horizontally into the boards.[9,17] There was an increase in hockey injuries after 1976 with the advent of better protective head gear that allowed more aggressive play, with a peak in the late 1980s and a subsequent decline with changes in rules.[18] This has not been substantiated because there was no increase in neck injuries with wearing full protection.[19] Water-related cervical spine injuries are most commonly a result of shallow water dives.[9,20] The injury occurs when a swimmer dives head first into shallow water.[21] The incidence of spinal injury among skiers is around one in 100,000 skier-days and four in

Table 23.1 Summary of Sports-related Cervical Injuries and their Relative Indications Regarding Return-to-play

Pathology	Torg	Bailes	Vaccaro
Cervical stenosis < 0.8	No contraindication	Relative contraindication	No contraindication
Cervical stenosis with neurapraxia	Relative contraindication	No contraindication (first time) Relative contraindication (repeat offender)	Relative contraindication (MRI is negative for cord abnormality)
Odontoid abnormalities, i.e., os odontoideum (C1/C2 instability), odontoid agenesis, odontoid hypoplasia	Absolute contraindication	n/a	Absolute contraindication
Atlanto-occipital fusion	Absolute contraindication	n/a	Relative contraindication
Klippel-Feil, above C3	Absolute contraindication	n/a	Absolute contraindication
Klippel-Feil fusion below C3	No contraindication	n/a	No contraindication
Ligamentous injury (3 mm or 11 degrees)	Absolute contraindication	Absolute contraindication	Absolute contraindication
Healed Jefferson fracture, healed odontoid fracture (I or II), healed lateral mass of C2 (no pain and full range of motion)	Relative contraindication	Relative contraindication	No contraindication
Healed compression fracture	No contraindication	Relative contraindication	No contraindication
Healed end plate fracture	No contraindication	Relative contraindication	No contraindication
Healed spinous process fracture	No contraindication	Relative contraindication	No contraindication
Spear tackler spine	Absolute contraindication	Absolute contraindication	Absolute contraindication
Acute fracture with instability (including fracture with displacement into the spinal canal and fracture with facet incongruity)	Absolute contraindication	Absolute contraindication	Absolute contraindication
Stinger	n/a	Relative contraindication	3 or more stinger (relative contraindication)
Herniated disk with neurapraxia	Relative contraindication	Relative contraindication	No contraindication (treated conservatively)
Acute herniated disk	Absolute contraindication	n/a	Absolute contraindication (symptomatic)
1 level fusion	No contraindication	In 6–12 months	No contraindication
2–3 levels fusion	Relative contraindication	Relative contraindication	Relative contraindication
> 3 levels fusion	Absolute contraindication	n/a	Absolute contraindication

Abbreviations: MRI, magnetic resonance imaging; n/a, not applicable.

100,000 snowboarder-days.[22,23] The risk of spinal cord injury in skiing is highest when intentional jumps are over 2 m.[22] The incidence of cervical spinal injury from rugby in the United States is approximately two per year with more than 50% of the injuries caused during scrum.[24] Cheerleading constitutes the highest percentage of catastrophic neck injuries in female athletes. Between 1982 and 2002, there were eight cervical fractures, three spinal cord contusions, and one cervical fracture associated with a head injury.[25]

Clinical and Diagnostic Features of Catastrophic Cervical Spinal Injury

Structural distortion of the cervical spinal column producing either actual damage or potential damage to the spinal cord is considered a catastrophic injury.[7] Conceptually, the cervical spinal column anatomy can be divided into upper region and lower region. The upper region consists of the occiput

and the first two vertebrae, and the lower region consists of the C3–C7 vertebrae. The spinal canal is comparatively larger in the upper cervical than the lower cervical spine. The catastrophic cervical trauma spectrum includes unstable fractures and dislocations, cervical cord neurapraxia, and intervertebral disk herniation.[7] The mechanism associated with most catastrophic cervical injuries is an axial load with the head and neck slightly flexed.[12] Sports-related cervical spine injuries include, but are not limited to, the following (see **Table 23.2** for different classification schemes).[26]

- Ligamentous injury, sprain/strain
- Spear tackler spine
- Cervical fracture
- Spinous process or laminar fracture
- Bilateral pars fracture
- Cervical 2 (hangman's) fracture
- Comminuted body fracture
- Odontoid fracture

Table 23.2 Three Different Classifications of Spinal Cord Injuries in Sports

Eddy's Classification[4]

1—Cervical spinal stenosis

2—Cervical cord neurapraxia

3—Odontoid abnormalities

4—Atlanto-occipital fusion

5—Klippel-Feil fusion above C3

6—Compression fracture

7—End plate fracture

8—Spinous process fracture

9—Spear tackler spine

10—Acute fracture with instability

11—Stinger

12—Herniated nucleus pulposus

13—Spondylosis

14—Spondylolisthesis

Torg Classification[3,12,27,36,54]

1—Congenital conditions: odontoid anomalies, spina bifida occulta, atlanto-occipital fusion, Klippel-Feil anomaly

2—Developmental conditions: cervical spinal canal stenosis, spear tackler spine

3—Traumatic condition of the upper spine (C1–C2): Jefferson fracture and odontoid fractures

4—Traumatic condition of the middle and lower spine: ligamentous injury, acute fracture of either body or posterior elements

5—Disk injury

Bailes Classification[2,5,8,10,13,28]

1—Type I. Permanent spinal cord injury: complete, anterior cord, central cord, Brown-Séquard, mixed

2—Type II. Transient: concussion, burning hand, neurapraxia

3—Type III. No neurological deficit, radiological abnormality: spinal stenosis, (congenital or acquired), herniated disk, unstable fracture, stable fracture (lamina, spinous process, minor body), ligamentous (unstable), spear tackle

These bony injuries are often associated with concurrent neurological injuries, including spinal cord injury without radiographic abnormality (SCIWORA), spinal cord injury, (complete or incomplete) or peripheral nerve injuries such as burners, transient neurapraxia, or brachial plexus injuries. Underlying congenital conditions, such as congenital cervical stenosis or Klippel-Feil anomaly may worsen the chance of injury.

Neurapraxia/Spinal Cord Concussion

Acute, transient neurological sequela with initial neck pain that is associated with sensory changes of burning pain, numbness, tingling, or loss of sensation with or without motor changes is termed neurapraxia or spinal cord concussion.[12] The prevalence of this injury is estimated to be seven per 10,000 in football participants.[12] Recovery usually occurs within 10 to 15 minutes, although occasionally symptoms may last 24 to 36 hours.[27] The risk of recurrence is ~50% and is related to canal diameter.[27]

There appear to be two groups of patients with spinal cord concussion; one group with normal radiographs and the other group with cervical stenosis.[28] Cervical spinal stenosis can be assessed using the vertebral body ratio method on plain radiographs.[29] Others have suggested using space available for the cord as an indication of spinal stenosis.[30] Meanwhile,

some have proposed magnetic resonance imaging (MRI) as the preferred method of assessing relative anatomy of stenosis as well as evaluating the spinal cord, cerebrospinal fluid (CSF), and spinal canal.[28]

In an epidemiological study, Torg et al evaluated five different groups of football players to assess the importance of transient neurapraxia (TN).[27] Cohort I included 227 college football players with no previous TN, cohort II included 97 professional football players with no previous TN, cohort III included 45 football players (high-school, college, and professional) with previous TN, cohort IV included 77 quadriplegic players who were injured while playing, and cohort V included 105 control subjects. In cohort III, seven athletes were found to have a bulging disk, five had evidence of instability, five had spondylosis, and five had congenital fusion. With regard to harboring a spinal diameter:vertebral body ratio of < 0.8 (**Fig. 23.1**), cohort I was found to have a 41% (93/227) and cohort II a 42% (41/97) incidence. In comparison, players in cohort III were found to have a 93% (42/45) incidence. Cohort V (control) had a significant difference in the ratio of the spinal canal diameter to the vertebral body when compared with athletes (cohorts I, II, and IV), which is consistent with the large vertebral body size in athletes. On the other hand, the positive predictive value of utilizing these findings to assess neurological risk was 0.2%, which is very low to be used as a screening mechanism.[27] Conversely, others have not found that vertebral body to canal ratio is related to spinal cord

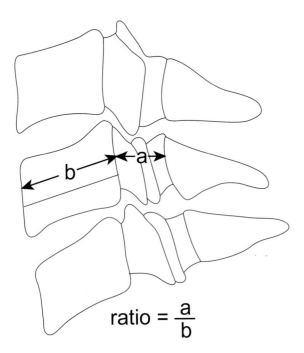

$$ratio = \frac{a}{b}$$

Fig. 23.1 Representation of the Pavlov ratio, the vertebral canal:vertebral body ratio on plain radiograph.

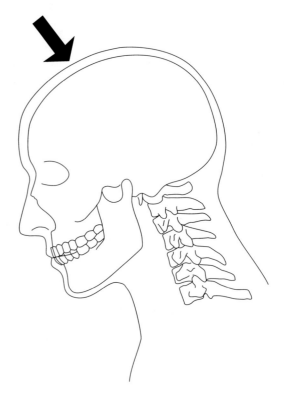

Fig. 23.2 Axial load with the neck slightly flexed, which leads to loss of lordosis and thus the transmitted force is directed along the spine causing a large amount of energy to be transferred directly to the vertebrae as opposed to the soft tissue.

concussion.[31] Of the 19 (16 cervical) patients in this study who had spinal cord concussion, only one had cervical stenosis.[31]

The largest series of cervical cord concussion included 110 athletes followed prospectively after a symptomatic episode.[3] Most of these athletes played football (96; 87%), where 28 (25%) were professional players, 49 (45%) were collegiate players, 29 (26%) were high school athletes, and 4 were recreational players. Of these 110 athletes, 104 had plain radiographs taken and 53 had cervical MRI scans. On plain radiographs, 89 (86%) had a ratio < 0.8 of vertebral canal to vertebral body and 43 (81%) had a degenerative disk on MRI. Of the 63 (57%) athletes who returned to play, 35 (56%) suffered recurrent episodes of transient neuritis, and none suffered permanent neurological deficit.[3] Therefore, there was no increased risk of permanent neurological injury after cervical cord neurapraxia. In addition, there was an increased risk of recurrence of transient neuritis that was inversely correlated to the space available for the spinal cord.[3]

In a smaller series, 10 athletes with transient spinal cord injury were evaluated with MRI in addition to CT scan and plain radiographs.[28] MRI was preferred to plain radiograph in assessing the relative anatomy of the spinal cord canal. Of these 10 athletes, three had no CSF reserve (< 1 mm CSF signal), and all players had spinal stenosis (< 13 mm) on cervical MRI. Six players had recurrence of symptoms within 1 month to 3 years of initial injury.[28]

More recently, five elite athletes were treated with anterior cervical diskectomy and fusion following neurapraxia.[32] All five athletes had either a herniated disk or a focal cord compression, but no parenchymal changes on MRI of the cervical spine. All five returned to play after rehabilitation, and two suffered recurrent disk herniation at adjacent levels.[32]

Burners or Stingers

A burner is characterized as a painful sensation that radiates from the neck to the finger tips that involves deltoid, biceps, and spinatus muscles and lasts 10 to 15 minutes.[6,33] Temporary weakness of the arm might also occur.[34] The incidence of burners has been reported as high as 65% of college football players.[34] A burner is associated with head and shoulder contact in which the head is laterally flexed to the opposite side with downward traction to the ipsilateral shoulder causing traction on the upper trunk of the brachial plexus, or by axial loads to the head or shoulders causing injury to the cervical root within the foramen[13] (**Fig. 23.2**). The mechanism of the injury is not well understood but is proposed to include either a stretch injury to the brachial plexus, extension of the spine with nerve root compression in the foramina, or a direct blow to the brachial plexus.[6,33,34]

A stinger is defined as a temporary episode of upper extremity unilateral burning dysesthesia with motor weakness. It is estimated to occur in 50% of athletes involved in contact/collision sports such as rugby or football.[6] It is conjectured that stingers are caused by an extension-compression mechanism and not due to brachial plexus traction.[33] The risk of stingers is increased in cervical spinal stenosis. A narrow cervical foraminal dimension increases the likelihood of cervical root pinch as described by the Pavlov ratio (foramen:intervertebral body ratio).[34]

Either phenomenon should be investigated with an MRI scan of the cervical spine to rule out a significant disk herniation, congenital spinal stenosis, or other structural abnormality.[6] Athletes with burners may be considered healed when their symptoms resolve and exam shows no abnormal results.[10] The necessity of imaging or electrodiagnostics depends on the persistence of symptoms and signs as well as the number of stingers the athlete has sustained.[35] Electromyography (EMG) is reasonable to perform 2 weeks following injury if persistent weakness is present to confirm cervical nerve root injury versus brachial plexus injury.[35]

Spear Tackler Spine

This is an absolute contraindication to participation in contact sports.[12] Spear tackler spine is found in a subset of football players who have used spear tackling techniques and who have a narrow cervical canal (canal:vertebral body ratio < 0.8), straightening or reversal of normal cervical lordosis, and post-traumatic radiographic abnormality such as spondylosis.[12,36] Between 1987 and 1990, four out of 15 patients who met the foregoing criteria had permanent neurological damage.[37]

Initial Management: Emergency Stabilization and Transport

With a conscious player, any radiating pain, loss of function, or loss of cervical range motion prompts removing the player from the game.[38] After physical exam, criteria for removing a player from the game include any new neurological deficit or any loss of cervical range of motion.[38] A limited examination to identify neurological deficits such as weakness, numbness, or significant pain from palpation of the cervical spine is essential.[12] With a suspicion of vertebral column or neurological injury, the player should be promptly transferred to an adequate facility for treatment in a neutral and immobilized position.[5] A rigid cervical collar (or a helmet and pads) with supportive blocks in combination with a rigid backboard with straps is effective in immobilizing the spine for transport.[39]

An unconscious player should be treated as harboring an unstable cervical spine until proven otherwise.[38] The initial evaluation follows the ABCDE guidelines (airway-while maintaining cervical alignment, breathing, circulation, disability-neurological, exposure of the athlete).[40] It is important to obtain a proper airway without moving the player inappropriately. The evaluation should also include an examination to determine motor or sensory loss, spinal pain, neck pain, and arm pain.[38] Cervical spine precautions should be maintained at all times, especially while removing the helmet. This may require special instruments such as a large bolt cutter.[8] Flexing or extending the neck should be avoided.[8] In the majority of cases of potential cervical spinal cord injury, the athlete is best immobilized and transported with the helmet and shoulder pads in place.[40] The exception to the rule is access to the airway, where the face mask can be removed or if the helmet prevents immobilization for transport.[13,40]

When presenting for definitive medical care, the shoulder pads and helmet should either be left in place or removed at the same time.[41] Multiple studies have shown that the athlete[42] and cadaveric heads/shoulders[41] are more aligned with either no protective equipment at all or with both the helmet and shoulder pads left in place. On the other hand, there was a significant difference in angulations in the intact specimen as well as with the injured specimen when either the helmet or the shoulder pads were left in place.[41] The same principle applied to hockey players, where players revealed changes in lordosis of the computerized lateral scout scan after the helmet was removed while shoulder pads were left in place.[42] The best plan is to leave the player's shoulder pads and helmet in place, which is consistent with the recommendation of the Inter-Association Task Force for the Appropriate Care of the Spine-Injured Athlete.[13] Turning the patient should involve 5 or 6 people, with one person stabilizing the cervical spine while controlling the head and shoulders, and others on each side of the shoulders and waist. An additional person can

be present at the feet.[38] To remove the helmet, the face mask must be cut off. One person should maintain cervical alignment while two assistants pull the sides of the helmet and remove it in a cephalad direction.[38]

Plain radiographs of the cervical spine are a good initial means of evaluating the integrity of bone structures. This includes anterior-posterior, lateral, and odontoid views. There should be no translation greater than or equal to 3.5 mm or angulation greater than or equal to 11 degrees at adjacent vertebrae on lateral radiographs and later on flexion/extension views.[43] If there is historical or objective evidence of spinal column or spinal cord involvement, further evaluation is needed. Computed tomography (CT) of the cervical spine provides the ability to view fractures that were not fully appreciated on plain radiographs.[8,44,45] A CT scan of the occiput to the third cervical vertebra was superior to five views using plain radiography in early identification of upper cervical spine injury. In one series, plain radiographs failed to identify 45% of upper cervical spine injuries.[46] In addition, the updated Eastern Association for the Surgery of Trauma (EAST) cervical spine clearance protocol recommends MRI of the cervical spine in the presence of a neurological deficit.[47]

MRI provides an unparalleled visualization of the nonbony structures of the cervical spine. As a result, MRI is superior in identifying soft tissue injuries such as ligamentous injury (100%) and spinal cord injury (100%) compared with CT scanning. However, CT scan performs better in identifying bony injuries such as an osseous fracture (97%), subluxation/dislocation (86%), and bilateral facet dislocations (97%).[48] In addition, complete spinal cord injured patients had a more substantial maximum spinal cord compression and maximum canal compromise with greater lesion length when compared with incomplete spinal cord injured patients.[49] Extent of the maximum spinal cord compression is more reliable than the presence of canal stenosis in predicting neurological outcome after spinal cord injury.[49] In addition, cord swelling, substantial maximum spinal cord compression, and maximum canal compromise correlated with worsening exam.[49,50]

Initial cervical traction using Gardner-Wells tongs or halo ring should be applied to reduce fracture and achieve anatomical alignment followed by a method of spinal stabilization.[5,8,13] There is a need for repeated exam and constant radiographic assessment.[13] Patients with minor fractures such as laminar fracture or spinous process fracture require flexion-extension films to document ligamentous status.[13,38,47]

The use of methylprednisolone within 8 hours in the treatment of acute spinal cord injury can be considered a treatment option.[51]

Surgical Management

Surgical treatment is usually required for comminuted fractures of the vertebral body, fracture of the posterior elements with extreme instability, or acute herniated disks (see earlier discussion), type II odontoid fractures, and spinal cord injuries with canal or cord compromise.[5,8,13]

Prevention

The majority of cervical spine injuries in football are the result of an axial load applied with the cervical spine in flexion.[12] The primary prevention of burners in football is

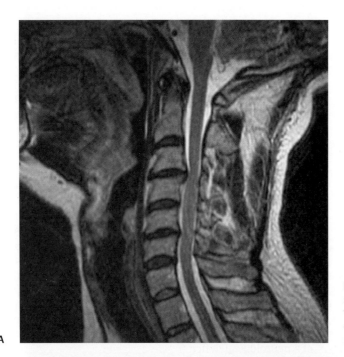

A

Fig. 23.3 (A–C) Sagittal and axial magnetic resonance imaging scans demonstrating severe congenital stenosis. Patient had transient spinal cord injury during a hockey game. The patient elected to have surgery to decompress his spine, and he decided not to return to contact sports.

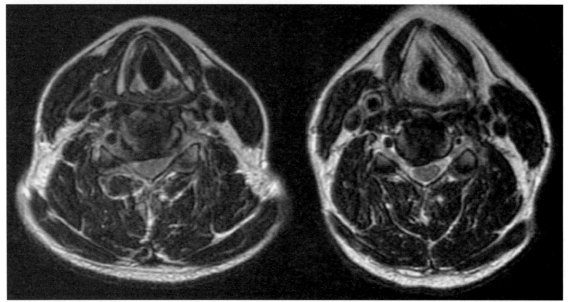

B   C

wearing properly fitting shoulder pads with lifters and shock absorbing capability.[38] The best preventive measures toward avoiding a spinal cord injury are coaches teaching proper tackling techniques and players building their neck muscles through weight lifting, which increases their chances of weathering a potentially dangerous blow. The major factor in the occurrence of cervical quadriplegia in football players is a playing technique in which the head is used as the primary point of contact, resulting in subsequent failure of the cervical spine.[13] In ice hockey, checking from behind has been implicated as a potential cause of cervical injury; thus education regarding rules of cross checking should reduce the incidence of neck injury in hockey.[40] Neck strengthening is critical in protecting the spine and allowing for full range of motion.[8,38]

Catastrophic spinal cord injury is not usually associated with recurrent symptoms for obvious reasons. Spinal stenosis alone does not result in a high risk of future catastrophic spinal cord injury.[13]

Rehabilitation

There are different types of intensive rehabilitation recommended for an injured athlete. Polymetric exercise is the lengthening of the muscle tendon unit followed directly by shortening. This stretch–shortening cycle has been shown to promote quick and safe return to sport after injury.[52] Polymetric exercise should be implemented after the patient is first able to tolerate the activity of daily living without pain or swelling.[52]

Table 23.3 Evidence Table for Return-to-play Criteria Following Transient Spinal Cord Injury

Study	No Cervical Stenosis	Cervical Stenosis	Strength of the Study
Zwimpfer and Bernstein (1990)[31]	No contraindication	No contraindication	Level IV
Torg et al (1996)[27]	No contraindication	Relative contraindication	Level II
Torg et al (1997)[3]	No contraindication	Relative contraindication	Level II
Brigham and Adamson (2003)[53]	Not applicable	Relative contraindication	Level IV
Bailes (2005)[28]	No contraindication	Relative contraindication	Level III
Maroon (2007)[32]	No contraindication	Relative contraindication	Level III

◆ Two Key Questions about Cervical Spine Injury in the Athlete and Evidence-Based-Medicine Answers

Can an athlete with a transient spinal cord "concussion" in the setting of normal cervical spine anatomy safely return to an athletic contest following full recovery?

There are two groups of patients with spinal cord "concussion": one with normal cervical spine anatomy and the other with cervical stenosis (**Fig 23.3**).[28] Torg and colleagues studied 110 athletes with cervical neurapraxia. Of the 63 who returned to contact sports, 35 (56%) experienced recurrent episodes of neurapraxia, but none suffered permanent neurological injury. Therefore, although the risk of neurapraxia is inversely correlated with spinal canal diameter, there is no increased risk of producing permanent damage with a narrow canal. Furthermore, there was no correlation between permanent neurological injury and a narrow spinal cord.[27] Therefore, there is no contraindication for athletes with a narrow cervical canal to participate in contact sports.[27] There are reports of case studies that have evaluated the relationship between cervical stenosis and neurapraxia as well as with permanent neurological damage in athletes. This includes a single case report of an athlete with congenital stenosis who had experienced previous transient spinal cord concussion and an injury that caused permanent neurological deficit.[53] An additional 10 patients were evaluated for cervical concussion

where all were found to have cervical stenosis on MRI. None of the four athletes who returned to play had a recurrent episode of concussion.[28] On the other hand, cervical stenosis due to a herniated disc or focal cord compression was treated with anterior cervical discectomy and fusion in five cases. All five returned to play, with two, however, suffering recurrent disc at an adjacent disc space, with one requiring additional surgery (**Table 23.3**)

Although the studies in **Table 23.3** are mainly classified as level II and level III, it should be noted that a lack of uniformity exists in these studies regarding the type of imaging used to quantify canal size. While MRI is preferred to plain radiology to assess spinal cord and spinal canal anatomy, it was used sporadically in these studies. There is, however, no large study examining the risk of athletes returning to sports in lieu of spinal stenosis as assessed by MRI. Thus the Spine Trauma Study Group gives only a weak recommendation for an athlete to return to sports with a transient spinal cord concussion in the setting of cervical spine stenosis.

Can an athlete with a transient spinal cord concussion in a setting of an abnormal cervical spine anatomy safely return to an athletic contest following full recovery?

Table 23.4 demonstrates the literature consensus regarding return-to-play following recognition of abnormal cervical spine and following anterior cervical discectomy and fusion (ACDF).

Table 23.4 Evidence Table for Return-to-play Criteria Following Transient Spinal Cord Injury in the Setting of Abnormal Cervical Spine Anatomy

Study	Disk Herniation	Single Level ACDF	Single ACDF Associated with Narrow Canal	Strength of the Study
Bailes (2005)[28]	Absolute contraindication	No contraindication	Absolute contraindication	Level V
Torg and Glasgow (1991)[54]	Absolute contraindication	No contraindication	Absolute contraindication	Level V
Cantu et al (1998)[2]	Absolute contraindication	No contraindication	Absolute contraindication	Level V
Vaccaro et al (2002)[6]	Absolute contraindication	No contraindication	Absolute contraindication	Level V
Maroon (2007)[32]	Absolute contraindication	No contraindication	Not applicable	Level III

References

1. Morganti C. Recommendations for return to sports following cervical spine injuries. Sports Med 2003;33:563–573
2. Cantu RC, Bailes JE, Wilberger JE Jr. Guidelines for return to contact or collision sport after a cervical spine injury. Clin Sports Med 1998;17:137–146
3. Torg JS, Corcoran TA, Thibault LE, et al. Cervical cord neurapraxia: classification, pathomechanics, morbidity, and management guidelines. J Neurosurg 1997;87:843–850
4. Eddy D, Congeni J, Loud K. A review of spine injuries and return to play. Clin J Sport Med 2005;15:453–458
5. Bailes JE, Hadley MN, Quigley MR, Sonntag VK, Cerullo LJ. Management of athletic injuries of the cervical spine and spinal cord. Neurosurgery 1991;29:491–497

6. Vaccaro AR, Klein GR, Ciccoti M, et al. Return to play criteria for the athlete with cervical spine injuries resulting in stinger and transient quadriplegia/paresis. Spine J 2002;2:351–356

7. Banerjee R, Palumbo MA, Fadale PD. Catastrophic cervical spine injuries in the collision sport athlete, I: Epidemiology, functional anatomy, and diagnosis. Am J Sports Med 2004;32:1077–1087

8. Bailes JE, Maroon JC. Management of cervical spine injuries in athletes. Clin Sports Med 1989;8:43–58

9. Boden BP, Prior C. Catastrophic spine injuries in sports. Curr Sports Med Rep 2005;4:45–49

10. Maroon JC, Bailes JE. Athletes with cervical spine injury. Spine 1996;21:2294–2299

11. Ghiselli G, Schaadt G, McAllister DR. On-the-field evaluation of an athlete with a head or neck injury. Clin Sports Med 2003;22:445–465

12. Torg JS, Guille JT, Jaffe S. Injuries to the cervical spine in American football players. J Bone Joint Surg Am 2002;84-A:112–122

13. Bailes JE, Petschauer M, Guskiewicz KM, Marano G. Management of cervical spine injuries in athletes. J Athl Train 2007;42:126–134

14. Cantu RC, Mueller FO. Catastrophic spine injuries in American football, 1977-2001. Neurosurgery 2003;53:358–362, discussion 362–363

15. Boden BP, Lin W, Young M, Mueller FO. Catastrophic injuries in wrestlers. Am J Sports Med 2002;30:791–795

16. Silva P, Vaidyanathan S, Kumar BN, Soni BM, Sett P. Two case reports of cervical spinal cord injury in football (soccer) players. Spinal Cord 2006;44:383–385

17. Tator CH, Carson JD, Edmonds VE. Spinal injuries in ice hockey. Clin Sports Med 1998;17:183–194

18. Tator CH, Carson JD, Cushman R. Hockey injuries of the spine in Canada, 1966–1996. CMAJ 2000;162:787–788

19. Stuart MJ, Smith AM, Malo-Ortiguera SA, Fischer TL, Larson DR. A comparison of facial protection and the incidence of head, neck, and facial injuries in Junior A hockey players: a function of individual playing time. Am J Sports Med 2002;30:39–44

20. Chang SK, Tominaga GT, Wong JH, Weldon EJ, Kaan KT. Risk factors for water sports-related cervical spine injuries. J Trauma 2006;60: 1041–1046

21. Aito S, D'Andrea M, Werhagen L. Spinal cord injuries due to diving accidents. Spinal Cord 2005;43:109–116

22. Tarazi F, Dvorak MF, Wing PC. Spinal injuries in skiers and snowboarders. Am J Sports Med 1999;27:177–180

23. Meyers MC, Laurent CM Jr, Higgins RW, Skelly WA. Downhill ski injuries in children and adolescents. Sports Med 2007;37:485–499

24. Wetzler MJ, Akpata T, Laughlin W, Levy AS. Occurrence of cervical spine injuries during the rugby scrum. Am J Sports Med 1998;26:177–180

25. Boden BP, Tacchetti R, Mueller FO. Catastrophic cheerleading injuries. Am J Sports Med 2003;31:881–888

26. Morganti C, Sweeney CA, Albanese SA, Burak C, Hosea T, Connolly PJ. Return to play after cervical spine injury. Spine 2001;26:1131–1136

27. Torg JS, Naranja RJ Jr, Pavlov H, Galinat BJ, Warren R, Stine RA. The relationship of developmental narrowing of the cervical spinal canal to reversible and irreversible injury of the cervical spinal cord in football players. J Bone Joint Surg Am 1996;78:1308–1314

28. Bailes JE. Experience with cervical stenosis and temporary paralysis in athletes. J Neurosurg Spine 2005;2:11–16

29. Pavlov H, Torg JS, Robie B, Jahre C. Cervical spinal stenosis: determination with vertebral body ratio method. Radiology 1987;164:771–775

30. Kang JD, Figgie MP, Bohlman HH. Sagittal measurements of the cervical spine in subaxial fractures and dislocations: an analysis of two hundred and eighty-eight patients with and without neurological deficits. J Bone Joint Surg Am 1994;76:1617–1628

31. Zwimpfer TJ, Bernstein M. Spinal cord concussion. J Neurosurg 1990; 72:894–900

32. Maroon JC, El-Kadi H, Abla AA, et al. Cervical neurapraxia in elite athletes: evaluation and surgical treatment: report of five cases. J Neurosurg Spine 2007;6:356–363

33. Meyer SA, Schulte KR, Callaghan JJ, et al. Cervical spinal stenosis and stingers in collegiate football players. Am J Sports Med 1994;22: 158–166

34. Kelly JD IV, Aliquo D, Sitler MR, Odgers C, Moyer RA. Association of burners with cervical canal and foraminal stenosis. Am J Sports Med 2000;28:214–217

35. Chang D, Bosco JA. Cervical spine injuries in the athlete. Bull NYU Hosp Jt Dis 2006;64:119–129

36. Torg JS, Ramsey-Emrhein JA. Suggested management guidelines for participation in collision activities with congenital, developmental, or postinjury lesions involving the cervical spine. Med Sci Sports Exerc 1997;29(7, Suppl):S256–S272

37. Torg JS, Sennett B, Pavlov H, Leventhal MR, Glasgow SG. Spear tackler's spine. An entity precluding participation in tackle football and collision activities that expose the cervical spine to axial energy inputs. Am J Sports Med 1993;21:640–649

38. Watkins RG. Neck injuries in football players. Clin Sports Med 1986; 5:215–246

39. Cervical spine immobilization before admission to the hospital. Neurosurgery 2002;50(3, Suppl):S7–S17

40. Banerjee R, Palumbo MA, Fadale PD. Catastrophic cervical spine injuries in the collision sport athlete, II: Principles of emergency care. Am J Sports Med 2004;32:1760–1764

41. Palumbo MA, Hulstyn MJ, Fadale PD, O'Brien T, Shall L. The effect of protective football equipment on alignment of the injured cervical spine: radiographic analysis in a cadaveric model. Am J Sports Med 1996; 24:446–453

42. Laprade RF, Schnetzler KA, Broxterman RJ, Wentorf F, Gilbert TJ. Cervical spine alignment in the immobilized ice hockey player: a computed tomographic analysis of the effects of helmet removal. Am J Sports Med 2000;28:800–803

43. White AA III, Panjabi MM. Clinical Biomechanics of the Spine. 2nd ed. Philadelphia: JB Lippincott; 1990

44. Hoffman JR, Mower WR, Wolfson AB, Todd KH, Zucker MI; National Emergency X-Radiography Utilization Study Group. Validity of a set of clinical criteria to rule out injury to the cervical spine in patients with blunt trauma. N Engl J Med 2000;343:94–99

45. Holmes JF, Akkinepalli R. Computed tomography versus plain radiography to screen for cervical spine injury: a meta-analysis. J Trauma 2005;58:902–905

46. Schenarts PJ, Diaz J, Kaiser C, Carrillo Y, Eddy V, Morris JA Jr. Prospective comparison of admission computed tomographic scan and plain films of the upper cervical spine in trauma patients with altered mental status. J Trauma 2001;51:663–668, discussion 668–669

47. Pasquale M, Fabian TC. Practice management guidelines for trauma from the Eastern Association for the Surgery of Trauma. J Trauma 1998;44:941–956, discussion 956–957

48. Holmes JF, Mirvis SE, Panacek EA, Hoffman JR, Mower WR, Velmahos GC; For the NEXUS Group. Variability in computed tomography and magnetic resonance imaging in patients with cervical spine injuries. J Trauma 2002;53:524–529, discussion 530

49. Miyanji F, Furlan JC, Aarabi B, Arnold PM, Fehlings MG. Acute cervical traumatic spinal cord injury: MR imaging findings correlated with neurologic outcome: prospective study with 100 consecutive patients. Radiology 2007;243:820–827

50. Fehlings MG, Furlan JC, Massicotte EM, et al; Spine Trauma Study Group. Interobserver and intraobserver reliability of maximum canal compromise and spinal cord compression for evaluation of acute traumatic cervical spinal cord injury. Spine 2006;31:1719–1725

51. Bracken MB, Shepard MJ, Collins WF, et al. A randomized, controlled trial of methylprednisolone or naloxone in the treatment of acute spinal-cord injury: results of the Second National Acute Spinal Cord Injury Study. N Engl J Med 1990;322:1405–1411

52. Chmielewski TL, Myer GD, Kauffman D, Tillman SM. Plyometric exercise in the rehabilitation of athletes: physiological responses and clinical application. J Orthop Sports Phys Ther 2006;36:308–319

53. Brigham CD, Adamson TE. Permanent partial cervical spinal cord injury in a professional football player who had only congenital stenosis: a case report. J Bone Joint Surg Am 2003;85-A:1553–1556

54. Torg JS, Glasgow SG. Criteria for return to contact activities following cervical spine injury. Clin J Sport Med 1991;1:12–26

V

Upper Cervical Injuries and Their Management

24

Craniocervical Disruption: Injuries of the Occiput–C1–C2 Region

Ignacio Madrazo, Carlos Zamorano, Richard J. Bransford, and Jens R. Chapman

We performed a systematic review and analysis of the English language literature regarding traumatic disruption of the craniocervical junction extending from the occiput through the axis. Standard databases were queried using the keywords "spinal injury," "medulla and C1–C2 spinal cord injury," "CO–C1–C2 spinal injuries," "traumatic CO–C1–C2 instability," and "traumatic CO–C1–C2 dissociation/dislocation." We collected and then stratified the data in regard to epidemiology, diagnosis, treatment, and outcome on this set of injuries. We reviewed the references of known key articles and reviewed the bibliography of all major textbooks on spine surgery for any omissions and included such studies in our database. Our search yielded 132 articles. We finally removed all such studies that did not meet our predetermined set of inclusion and exclusion criteria. The essence and spirit of the included studies set the general tone and direction of our chapter, and we used specific data points to answer two basic questions directed at optimizing treatment. We found no class I articles, one class II, four class III studies, and 25 class IV reports. Due to the relatively low incidence of these injuries, we chose to include case reports as long as they fulfilled our inclusion criteria. We found 191 patients with craniocervical disruption. **Table 24.1** lists the peer-reviewed publications from 1994 to 2007.

Table 24.1 Evidentiary Table of the Peer-Reviewed Publications from 1994 to 2007

Study	Description	Level of Evidence of Primary Question	Topic and Conclusion
Elaraky (2000)[142]	Retrospective pediatric cohort study	II	24 cases that satisfied our inclusion criteria. 7 unreduced dislocations treated with (OC) fusion and 1 with lateral mass plate system; 16 treated with halo or hard collars. No incidence of complications or related death in both groups. CONCLUSION: Pediatric population should be clearly separated in those surgical and nonsurgical cases because both techniques will give good results.
Bellabarba (2006)[45]	Retrospective cohort study	III	18 patients. All diagnosed by plain x-rays as craniocervical dislocation. Treatment was OC fusion in all cases. Outcomes not mentioned. CONCLUSION: Surgical treatment produced good results in all cases. No control group.
Sai-cheung Lee (2006)[143]	Retrospective case series	III	16 patients. Surgical treatment in all cases was OC fusion with plate screw (titanium construct). 1 patient died. All others uncomplicated. CONCLUSION: Surgical treatment was successful in most cases. No control group.
Stulik (2005)[144]	Retrospective case series	III	10 cases satisfied our inclusion criteria. Treatment was Harms technique. Only 1 patient Frankel C neurological deficit on admission. Solid bony fusion in all patients. CONCLUSION: Harms fixation enables to provide temporary fixation without damage to the AA joint after the screws and rods had been inserted. Operative technique done in 45 min. No clinical consequences. Control with 2 patients treated nonoperatively.
Harms & Melcher (2001)[145]	Retrospective cohort study	III	37 cases. OC dislocation. Minimal clinical information. Treatment in all cases with posterior C1–C2 fusion with polyaxial screw and rod fixation. Outcome not mentioned. CONCLUSION: Posterior C1–C2 fusion with polyaxial screw and rod fixation technique is an easy and effective procedure in trained hands.

(Continued on page 212)

Study	Description	Level of Evidence of Primary Question	Topic and Conclusion
Gautschi (2007)[146]	Case report	IV	1 patient. Complete medulla/cervical spine transection. Injury severity score 7.5. Survive long term with neurological damage. Treated surgically (OC stabilization). CONCLUSION: Even very severe cases should be treated because they can survive, but is it worth it to treat these patients surgically?
Behari (2006)[147]	Retrospective case series	IV	4 patients. CT done to delineate osseous anatomy and course of vertebral arteries. Outcomes not mentioned. Treatment was in all cases posterior cervical polyaxial screws and rod system. CONCLUSION: Surgical treatment was successful in all cases. No control group.
Anderson (2006)[148]	Case report	IV	1 case. OC disruption. Treatment was AO fusion with cancellous bone autografting, supported by an occipital plate linked by rods to lateral mass screws in the atlas. No neurological deficit. Successful radiological fusion at 1 year. AA rotation preserved. CONCLUSION: Surgical treatment. Good fusion after 1 year. Good results with preservation of AA rotation.
Violas (2006)[149]	Case report	IV	1 case. AO and AA traumatic dislocation. Paraplegia from thoracic spine lesion. Decision was to treat nonoperatively. Outcome without cervical damage. CONCLUSION: The double neurological lesion took to the decision of treating this patient nonoperatively, with good results related to the cervical problem.
Hamai (2006)[105]	Case report	IV	1 case. AO dislocation with AA subluxation. First report of survival. Plain x-rays with widening of distance between basion and tip of dens, and separation of spinous processes of C1 and C2. CT with anterior dislocation of bilateral occipital condyles from superior articular facets of C1+ AA subluxation. MRI (T2) with disruption of both tectorial membranes and alar ligaments, prevertebral soft tissue swelling, contusion of medulla and intact spinal cord. GCS score: 6, disturbed consciousness, no response to pain, hyperreflexia of extremities, and bilateral Babinski. Treatment was cervical traction-realignment under fluoroscopy–halo vest–surgical reduction and posterior spinal fusion of occiput to C3 with iliac crest graft. Outcome: 2 years after surgery, able to stand on her own, get up from wheelchair and go to bed, eat with a spoon. CONCLUSION: Good example of a case that requires the intelligent combination of all treatment options, finally obtaining good results.
QingShui Yin (2005)[150]	Retrospective case series	IV	5 cases with irreducible anterior AA dislocation. All with ventral spinal cord compression. Treatment was transoral AA fixation and fusion. All cases with stable AA segment after surgery, and important clinical benefit. CONCLUSION: Transoral surgery of the spinal cord is helpful when ventral compression is present.
Seibert (2005)[151]	Case report	IV	1 case. AO dislocation. No neurological deficit. Treatment was craniocervical stabilization from occiput to C3 with lateral mass screws (C1–C3) and transarticular screws (C2–C3) and occipital bone screws. Good outcome. CONCLUSION: Surgical treatment as first and unique option.
Ames (2005)[152]	Case report	IV	1 case. C1 fracture with transverse ligament avulsion. Clinical data was flexion-extension pain. CT with C1 ring fracture, basilar invagination, and severe lateral splaying of C1 lateral masses. Treatment was horizontal reduction of C1 lateral masses with direct C1 lateral mass screws, a rod compressor and a cross-link. Outcome without neurological deficit, and disappearance of pain. CONCLUSION: Minimal clinical data after a neck lesion should be radiologically revised.
Ramaré (1999)[153]	Case report	IV	1 case. AA dislocation. Treatment was OA stabilization. Outcome: excellent in mobility and pain. CONCLUSION: Surgical treatment as the first and unique option.
Govender (2003)[154]	Retrospective case series	IV	4 cases. AO dislocation. 1 neurologically intact. 3 with neurological deficit. Treatment in 3 cases was OC fusion. 1 case (the neurologically intact) nonsurgical. All cases had a complete neurological recovery. CONCLUSION: When indicated patients may have a good outcome with nonsurgical treatment.
Horn (2003)[155]	Retrospective case series	IV	5 cases. As very rare cases, the treatment was selected according each case: Case 1: Steinman pin, Songer cables, and autograft. Case 2: Screws and titanium rods from CO to C2. Case 3: Transarticular screws CO-C2. Case 4: Polyaxial titanium screws bilaterally into lateral masses of C1 and C2. Case 5: Atlantoaxial transarticular screws. Outcome not mentioned. CONCLUSION: Relevant information in surgical techniques. No control group.

Study	Description	Level of Evidence of Primary Question	Topic and Conclusion
Rahimi (2003)[156]	Retrospective pediatric cohort study	IV	23 cases: 6 with AA rotatory subluxation; 10 with anterior posterior AA instability; 5 with AA fracture with or without dislocation, and 2 with AO dislocation. All cases had marked neurological improvement. No data on treatments. CONCLUSION: Surviving pediatric population seems to have better evolution than adults.
Fiore (2002)[157]	Two cases report	IV	2 cases. AA subluxation. Treatment was performing rigid fixations. No outcome mentioned.
Lo (2002)[158]	Retrospective case series	IV	3 pediatric cases. Avulsion of transverse ligament, with instability of AA complex. All patients with neck pain, without neurological deficit. Treatment was halo vest for 6 to 12 weeks. Outcome with disappearance of pain. CONCLUSION: In pediatric ligament instability, the treatment of choice is nonsurgical.
Razif (2001)[159]	Case report	IV	1 pediatric case. Chronic C1–C2 subluxation. Tetraplegia for 18 months presurgical. Treatment was cervical cord decompression and OC fusion. Satisfactory outcome with neurological improvement sufficient to allow self-care for personal hygiene. CONCLUSION: Even delayed surgery can be useful.
Heidecke (1998)[160]	Retrospective case series.	IV	14 cases. (Not clear if all were trauma cases.) No clinical data. In all cases treatment was OC fusion with Cotrel-Dubousset rod system + bone or hydroxyapatite. Outcome: No morbidity or mortality. No neurological deterioration. No halo after surgery. CONCLUSION: In trained hands this is a good surgical procedure.
Dickman (1998)[161]	Retrospective case series	IV	11 cases who satisfied our inclusion criteria. Transverse ligament disruption. In all cases treatment was posterior C1–C2 transarticular screw fixation. Outcome with 98% fusion rate. CONCLUSION: Surgical technique article, depicting a good procedure.
Faure (1998)[162]	Case report	IV	1 case. OC dislocation. Treated by OC fixation with a single occipital clamp using inverted hooks. Obtained immediate stability. CONCLUSION: Surgical technique article.
Rainov (1998)[163]	Case report	IV	1 case. Vertebral fracture of the axis body. Dislocation of the anterior part of the axis. Treatment was one time combined ventrodorsal approach using anterior C2–C3 locking plate fusion and C2 bilateral dorsal transpedicular screw fixation. Outcome: stable bony fusion, with minimal restriction of head mobility. CONCLUSION: These lesions require combined treatment.
Schultz (1997)[164]	Retrospective case series	IV	8 cases. Craniocervical dislocation. No clinical data. Treatment was occipitocervical fusion with rectangular rod. No outcome mentioned. CONCLUSION: Surgical technique article.
Song (1997)[165]	Retrospective case series	IV	1 case. AA instability and unilateral anomalies. No clinical data. Treatment was single contralateral transarticular screw across C1–C2 facet + interspinous bone grafting wiring. Outcome: Philadelphia collar (6 to 12 weeks). CONCLUSION: As in most of these initial articles, the emphasis is clearly on surgical technical aspects.
Malcom (1994)[166]	Retrospective case series	IV	3 cases. OC instability. Plain x-rays with occipito–C1–C2 hypermobility. Treatment was posterior fixation with Hartshill-Ransford contours loop. Outcome: No neurological deterioration. Neck stiffness. CONCLUSION: Surgical technique article.
Zigler (1986)[112]	Case report	IV	1 case. OC dislocation. CT with ligamentous instability between the occiput and the cervical spine. Quadriplegic C1 level. Breathing support. Treatment was fusion of the occiput to cervical spine and cervical spine to thoracic spine. Outcome: No need for external neck support. No change in neurological status. CONCLUSION: Initial work looking for treatment of these severe cases.
Gerrit van de Pol (2005)[93]	Case report	IV	1 case. Pediatric redislocation in a halo of an AOD. GCS score: 3. Treatment was halo vest reduction under image intensification occiput–C1–C2 fusion using internal fixation and allograft bone. Wheelchair dependent at 7 months as a result of spasticity of legs. CONCLUSION: Another case of intelligent use of all treatment resources in a very ill patient, with good results. These types of approaches are mostly seen in pediatric patients. This patient had a redislocation with the halo vest.

(Continued on page 214)

24 Craniocervical Disruption: Injuries of the Occiput–C1–C2 Region

Study	Description	Level of Evidence of Primary Question	Topic and Conclusion
Labler (2004)[32]	Retrospective case series	IV	4 cases. AO dislocation. 2 died in hospital. Case 3 survived: GCS score: 3, tetraplegia, "locked in" syndrome, bilateral VI nerve palsy. Case 4: GCS score: 15, shortness of breath, bilateral sensorimotor deficiency on C4–C6. Treatment was in case 3 dorsal fusion between occiput and C5 (CerviFix, Synthes, Inc., West Chester, PA); and in case 4 dorsal fusion of CO–C5 with CerviFix. Outcome of case 3: 16 months after surgery fully ambulatory. Incomplete paraplegia, persistent hoarseness, and bilateral VI nerve palsy. Outcome of case 4: 3 months after surgery fully ambulatory. Sensorimotor shortage of right arm at C4–C5. CONCLUSION: AO dislocations are frequently lethal. Those patients arriving at the hospital should be actively treated. Alignment, decompression, and stabilization are the priorities.

Abbreviations: AA, atlantoaxial; AO, atlanto-occipital; AOD, atlanto-occipital dissociation; CT, computed tomography; GCS, Glasgow Coma Scale; OC, occipitocervical.

◆ **Topic Overview**

Serious occipital-cervical trauma, usually considered fatal in the past, has become increasingly better recognized in trauma patients who survive beyond the initial retrieval and resuscitation efforts.[1–3] We found an increasing number of reports on traumatic atlanto-occipital dissociation (AOD) and atlantoaxial disruption (AAD) perhaps reflective of this trend. This injury entity, with dislodgment of the head relative to its cervical spine anchor, frequently results in almost immediate death and, therefore, has remained a rather infrequent occurrence in general practices. The implementation of more systematic injury retrieval and resuscitation algorithms from the point of first encounter to the emergency room along with improved diagnostic possibilities has likely played a major role in the earlier detection of these injuries.

The functional anatomy of the craniocervical junction is complex and lends itself to a wide range of injuries relative to injury mechanisms. Between the three major bony components that form the craniocervical junction—the occiput (Oc), the atlas (C1), and the axis (C2), an intricate arrangement of ligaments provides inherent stability. In a traumatic situation virtually every injury combination among the osteoligamentous structures of this region is imaginable. There are, however, some typical injuries that have been described with some regularity, including occipital condyle fractures, occipitoatlantal dislocations, subluxations and dislocations of the atlantoaxial articulation, atlas fractures, odontoid fractures, and fractures of the neural arch of the axis. Injuries to this region are rather common and can be easily unnoticed because these patients may have an associated head injury, which can alter their level of consciousness and make it difficult obtaining a precise history and physical examination.

◆ **Anatomy**

In view of the structural complexity and functional demands placed upon the upper cervical spine we will discuss the anatomy sequentially. Study of the functional bony anatomy of this region reflects an arrangement that facilitates an extensive range of motion while offering only a modicum of protection for the neurovascular structures it contains. The atlas, which largely consists of a relatively fragile bony ring structure, mainly assumes a washer function and serves as a motion modulator between the skull base and the C2 segment. Its integrity is important to maintain a physiological spacing between the skull base and the odontoid to prevent impingement of the spinal cord and medulla oblongata.

The bony foundation of the upper cervical spine includes the paired semiconstrained ball and open socket articulations formed by the occiput with the atlas and the three joints that link the atlas with the axis. The atlantoaxial facet joints connect the lateral masses of these two vertebrae, and the atlantodental articulation allows a pivot point of contact for the odontoid tip. The facet joints of the atlantoaxial junction allow for some translational displacement thus facilitating the extraordinary coronal plane rotation seen at this motion segment.[4,5] The atlantodental articulation provides the center of rotation anchor for this particular motion. It is apparent that this craniocervical bony setup offers little to no inherent bony stability and largely relies on ligamentous integrity for smooth function.[6]

The ligaments that protect the craniocervical junction consist of the tectorial membrane, the paired alar ligaments, the single midline apical ligament of the dens, the anterior and posterior atlanto-occipital and atlantoaxial membranes, and the respective joint capsules (**Fig. 24.1**). The alar ligaments prevent excessive rotation, abnormal extension is limited by the tectorial membrane, and flexion is checked by the anterior atlas ring abutting the basion.[6–8] The atlantoaxial stability is predominantly provided by the transverse atlantal ligament (TAL), which provides the foundation for the cruciate ligaments, which lock the odontoid to the atlas in a criss-cross fashion. Any injury to any component of the bony or ligament structures of the craniocervical junction may impair stability of this area in general.[4] Disruption of the major ligamentous check reins in this area will leave this transition zone unstable and defenseless to further manipulation. Catastrophic secondary neurological deterioration may be expected if there is a delay in diagnosis of an unstable craniocervical junction.[9]

In general, the pediatric age group appears to be at a 2.5-fold higher risk of incurring craniocervical dissociation resulting

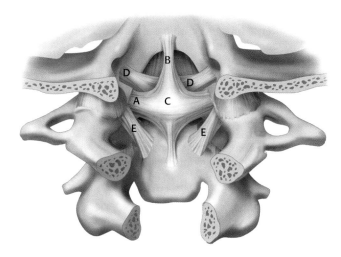

Fig. 24.1 Ligaments anatomy: **(A)** Cruciform ligament, **(B)** upper vertical limb of cruciform ligament, **(C)** transverse ligament of atlas (horizontal portion of cruciform ligament), **(D)** lateral alar odontoid ligament, **(E)** accessory portion of tectorial membrane.

from deceleration trauma than adults.[10–12] The reasons for this lie in higher ligamentous laxity, proportionally larger head size and weight, and less inclined lateral masses.

◆ Classification

For the sake of consistent nomenclature we suggest using *craniocervical dissociation (CCD)* as an overarching term for any and all stages and levels of distractive injuries between the occiput and its C2 base. In contrast, *AOD* describes the more specific injury location between the skull base and atlas and AAD, a dissociative injury to the C1–C2 motion segment.

In the English-speaking world occipital condyle fractures are most commonly classified according to the description offered by Anderson and Montesano.[13] Type I injuries demonstrate comminution of the condyle and are usually stable. Type II injuries consist of a skull-base fracture extending through one of the condyles. Although it is believed that these are shear injuries they are generally considered stable. In contrast, type III injuries consist of a bony avulsion of the occipital condyle through its alar ligament attachment. These latter injuries can be reflective of a CCD and therefore should be viewed with suspicion.[14] Any patient with bilateral occipital condyle fractures should be assumed to have an unstable CCD unless proven otherwise.

AADs have received only sparse attention as to injury classification. Traynelis et al[15] described three different types of AOD dislocation: type I is an anterior dislocation with the occiput displaced anteriorly to the atlas. Type II consists of a vertical dislocation, and type III is posteriorly displaced. The author found type I and II dislocations to be most common, each accounting for ~40% of cases. A type III dislocation was found in only 5% of cases. The remaining 15% of cases consisted of other unclassifiable dislocations. This classification has been criticized for being too focused on the direction of injury displacement and not accounting for injury severity or neurological status of an affected patient. Moreover, the nature of the injury is such that the head can be displaced arbitrarily relative to the C-spine, thus rendering the observation regarding direction of displacement to be of secondary

relevance. This statement is supported by the author's finding that type II injuries were the most unstable subtype because they usually progressed to a type I dislocation.

The Harborview AOD classification (HMC) has been introduced with an emphasis on craniocervical injury severity.[16] In this system type I injuries consist of incomplete ligament injuries, such as unilateral alar ligament tears. Type II injuries consist of complete CCDs with initial lateral radiographs showing borderline screening measurement values. These injuries, however, feature a complete disruption of key ligaments of the craniocervical junction and are unstable. A spontaneous partial reduction of the cranium to its cervical attachments through some remaining residual ligamentous attachments may provide false reassurance to a reviewer. Type IIIa injuries demonstrate obvious major craniocervical displacement on plain radiographs, whereas type IIIb injuries identify death from CCD in the first 24 hours following injury. Neither the Traynelis nor the HMC classification systems have been validated in terms of their observer reliability. Injury severity is not addressed in the Traynelis system. Although the HMC classification is founded on the principle of a severity scale, its subcategories may lack distinctiveness between types II and IIIa to make it clinically meaningful.

Traumatic AAD has not been formally classified outside of basic injury categories. These differentiations may be of partial (subluxation) or complete (dislocation) severity and can be considered a variant of AOD. This injury can also be differentiated by the type of displacement with vertical, translational, or rotatory displacement and may also include fractures of the upper C-spine segments.

◆ Epidemiology

Grossman et al[17] reported the overall incidence of cervical spine injuries to be 4.3%. The incidence of cervical spine injuries following blunt trauma in children was estimated to be 1.3 to 1.5%.[11,12,18–22] The upper C-spine accounted for 10% of C-spine injuries due to blunt trauma in a series of 300 patients.[23] However, in a study on cause of death of 312 traffic victims, radiological findings of major upper C-spine injuries were elicited in 93% of cases.[11,24] Pure ligamentous injuries to the C-spine were found in only 14 patients of 14,577 with blunt trauma.[25] Injuries to the upper cervical spine are frequent in traffic accidents, with the highest prevalence for pedestrians and motorcyclists.[26–28] The incidence of cervical spine injuries in children following blunt trauma was ~1.5%.[12,18,22,29] There is a strong correlation between age of patient and location of cervical spine injury, with patients below age 9 predominantly having upper C-spine injuries.[30] AOD was found in 10% of traumatic cervical spine injuries in skeletally immature patients.[11,29]

To date, AOD remains an uncommon injury after having initially been described in 1908.[1] Among 155 traffic victims, 12 patients with AOD were found with additional various fractures in the OCJ.[8] Other authors report an incidence of AOD of 8 to 31% in fatal traffic accidents[28] and of nearly 10% in fatal cervical spine injuries.[11,15] Autopsy information in pediatric multitrauma cases associated with cervical spine injuries showed AOD to be present in 8 to 27%.[8,11,31]

A meta-analysis of the literature published by Labler et al[32] covering the years of 1948 to 2004 showed 211 patients surviving AOD initially and 108 cases (57%), mainly children and young adults, with long term survival. Our systematic review

(1994 to 2007) of OC dissociations/dislocations, showed 197 cases with 118 survivals, potentially demonstrating a better outcome of patients in recent years. Less prominent dislocations or spontaneously reduced AOD is easily overlooked despite the comprehensive radiological workup.[9,32–36] An analysis of 79 patients with known AOD found that the diagnosis was missed in 19 of 50 (38%) children and in 17 of 29 (59%) adults.[37]

◆ Mechanism of Injury

CCD is typically associated with blunt injury mechanisms such as motor vehicle crashes, falls, and collisions. For very young patients child restraint mechanisms leave the head exposed to whiplash during major deceleration trauma.[38] In a retrospective study on 149 forensic autopsy cases, Ohshima and Kondo studied brain stem and/or upper cervical spinal cord (UCSC) injuries as a result of traffic accidents.[39] Pedestrians were the most common victims, followed by drivers. In another series 11 of the 12 victims were pedestrians. The total ratio of pedestrian victims gradually increased with age. The pontomedullary junction was the most frequent injured site. A total of 146 cases demonstrated basal skull fractures and/or dislocation of the upper cervical joints: atlanto-occipital joint, or the C2–C3 motion segment. However, in three cases,

hyperextension of the neck unexpectedly caused brain stem injury neither associated with basal skull fracture nor with cervical dislocation. Intraventricular hemorrhage was found in 96 cases, suggesting a common feature associated with brain stem or UCSC injury. A tear of the basilar artery and that of the carotid artery was found in 17 and 20 cases, respectively. A total of 39 victims demonstrated a blood alcohol concentration of over 0.5 mg/mL, and hyperextension of the neck occurred more frequently in these cases. In spite of the marked predominance of immediate death (138 cases), 11 cases (nine of brainstem injury and two of UCSC injury) had unexpected survival times of from 45 minutes to 12 hours.[39]

The tensile load capacity to failure of each alar ligament has been described as being half of an anterior cruciate ligament. Although individual ligaments of the craniocervical junction are relatively frail, the overall combination and arrangement of these structures offers reasonable protection against trivial trauma to this area.[4,7] For CCD to occur a combination of major forces needs to occur virtually simultaneously, leading to a catastrophic failure of the craniocervical ligaments. Such a scenario would likely entail hyperextension with disruption of the tectorial membrane, and lateral or hyperflexion with disruption of the alar ligaments and posterior atlanto-occipital ligament. A single ligament rupture, such as an isolated alar ligament injury, is unlikely to give atlanto-occipital instability (**Fig. 24.2**).[4,5]

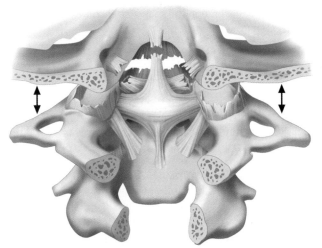

A

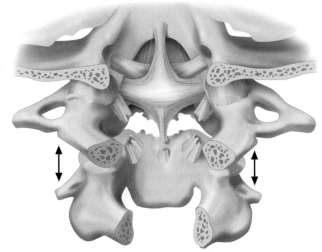

B

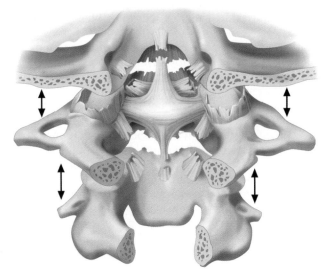

C

Fig. 24.2 Mechanisms of dissociation/dislocation of the upper cervical joints. **(A)** Atlanto-occipital joint: produced by the rupture of the lateral alar and upper vertical limb of cruciform ligament. **(B)** The joint between the second and third cervical vertebrae: produced by the rupture of the accessory portion of tectorial membrane. **(C)** Occipital-atlantoaxial dislocation: a combination of **(A)** and **(B)**.

Judicial hanging has been falsely associated with the "hangman's fracture." In fact it appears that judicial hanging appears to more commonly result in a vertical type of AAD, with the other variants of this injury occurring with associated rotatory head displacements.[40–42] As the various injury patterns seen in AAD and AOD reaffirm, any injury to any component of the craniocervical junction may adversely affect the overall structural integrity of this functional unit

◆ Diagnosis

Clinical Findings

Timely diagnosis of CCD has historically been elusive due to several factors. For many years the low incidence of this injury and its low chances for survival may have lessened physicians' awareness. Moreover this injury was felt to be simply nonsurvivable, thus lessening the sense of urgency to detect and treat this injury entity. Plain radiographs alone can require a fair bit of experience in details of craniocervical anatomy for patients who have sustained less displaced injuries.[43–45] Frequently, an established trauma care algorithm can be derailed through primary attention directed at ostensibly life-saving intervention, thus missing the initial window for rapid CCD diagnosis and implementation of countermeasures.[46,47] Often a closed head injury is the main focus, making it very difficult to recognize cervical spine injury.[48] Finally, there are few, if any, concrete clinical signs hinting at the presence of CCD. There can be massive swelling of the head and neck, and in a nonobtunded patient an astute observer may detect focal suboccipital or severe neck tenderness. Airway disruption, or sequelae of neck and skull base vascular injuries may be indirect indicators of serious craniocervical injury as well.[49–52] Neurological injuries are commonly associated with CCD but can vary widely and can range from tetraplegia with lack of respiratory drive ("pentaplegia") to a perplexing variety of incomplete cervicomedullary injury syndromes and isolated cranial nerve injuries, such as the cruciate paralysis of Bell and the Wallenberg syndrome.[53–56]

In addition to neurological damage, pulmonary problems are commonly found in CCD patients. Respiratory distress can be caused by a variety of reasons. A retropharyngeal hematoma or pseudomeningocele as a result of ligamentous disruption of the atlanto-occipital joint or due to vertebral artery injury can result in dyspnea. Direct brain stem damage, diaphragmatic paralysis, or pulmonary contusions can also result in respiratory distress. In the presence of a combination of respiratory insufficiency, irregular cardiac activity up to cardiac arrest, or hypotension caused by traumatic lesions of the brain stem, AOD should be suspected.[57–60]

Radiographic Findings

Historically, the diagnosis of AOD has been made on a lateral cervical spine radiograph. Because this was the screening tool of choice in the Advanced Trauma Life Support (ATLS) protocols a high degree of emphasis has been placed on interpretation of screening lines to warn of the possibility of CCD.[41,61,62] Presence of prevertebral soft tissue swelling on the lateral cervical radiograph may be the first clue for presence of an unstable cervical spine lesion.[62] Of many screening measurements Powers' BC:AO ratio, which relates the distance between the basion and the posterior arch of the atlas (BC) and the distance between the anterior arch of the atlas and the opisthion (AO), had been considered a standard for many years.[63] The BC:AO ratio, in normal cases, should be less than 1. This tool, however, is limited by being valid only for anterior AOD cases. In the case of a longitudinal distraction or when the head is displaced dorsally, this screening tool inherently bears no relevance. The atlanto–odontoid–basion distance, initially described by Wholey et al,[64] is in principle applicable at all times but may show more variability due to parallaxis. In a normal child, the distance should be less than 10 mm. The problem with the dens:basion ratio is that the not yet ossified bones in children can make them difficult to identify. Harris later refined the dens–basion interval (DBI) and added the axis–basion interval (ABI).[65,66] Both, the ABI and the BDI should remain less than 12 mm in 95% of adults ("rule of twelves"). He demonstrated a higher degree of specificity and sensitivity in detecting AOD with this method compared with Power's ratio and Lee's x-lines.[63,67]

As already implied, radiographic representation of the craniocervical distance also varies with age. Kaufman et al[41] proposed to measure the actual distance between the articular surfaces of the occiput and the superior facet of the atlas on a lateral cervical spine radiograph. These authors held 5 mm as the maximum distance. However, obliquity and rotatory malposition of the head by even a few degrees as well as superimposition of the mastoid process over the occipital condyles can make this measurement attempt nearly impossible. More recently Pang et al have used high-resolution CT scans with reformatted views to obtain measurements of the cranial–C1 interval (CCI). They identified an average CCI of 1.28 mm in children 0 to 18 years of age with a high degree of conformity from left- to right-sided measurements. None of the CCIs exceeded 1.95 mm.[68] Using a cohort of 16 pediatric patients with AOD and a comparison group of 138 intact patients the authors identified significant false-positive rates for other screening tests, such as Sun's, Harris, Wholey's and Powers[29,69–71]

Functional examination can be performed under an image intensifier. Axial traction can readily demonstrate instability of the craniocervical junction. This can be performed with head tongs and weighted traction or manual in-line traction by an experienced surgeon who monitors AOJ alignment under image intensification.[9,16,45,72,73] Opinions vary on how much traction should be applied; however, any displacement of more than 1 mm distraction beyond baseline joint alignment can be considered unstable. In an awake patient, feedback is helpful to avoid overdistraction leading to neurological impairment. In obtunded patients application of somatosensory evoked potentials has been described as a safeguard against neurological injury from manipulation (**Fig. 24.3**).[74,75]

In summary, the diagnosis of AOD is often missed on plain radiographs (sensitivity 0.57). Using a combination of measuring techniques, the sensitivity of radiographs can be increased to 0.76.[21] The use of plain radiographs in the assessment of trauma patients is waning in light of increasing availability of helical screening CTs in the management of trauma patients.[76] Inclusion of the upper C-spine in routine head CTs obtained for the assessment of patients with altered mental status on arrival can reveal the presence of a suboccipital hematoma, which may be indicative of CCD.[37] The inclusion of the foramen magnum in routine cranial CT scans has also increased the rate of detection of occipital condyle and type I odontoid fractures, which may be indicators for a

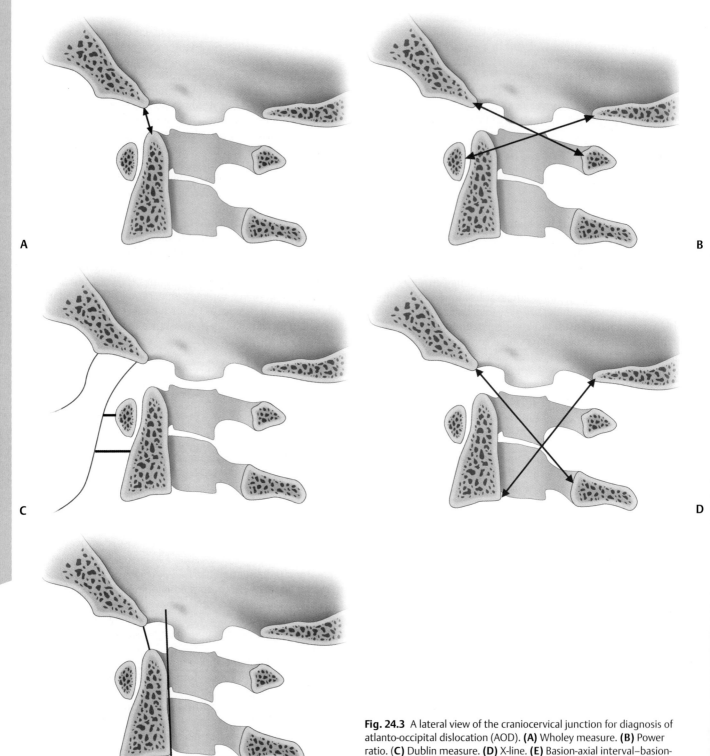

A

B

C

D

E

Fig. 24.3 A lateral view of the craniocervical junction for diagnosis of atlanto-occipital dislocation (AOD). **(A)** Wholey measure. **(B)** Power ratio. **(C)** Dublin measure. **(D)** X-line. **(E)** Basion-axial interval–basion-dens interval (BAI-BDI) method.

CCD as well.[77,78] Definitive CT scan of the cervical spine should include reformatted views, including sagittal and coronal views, especially of the transition zones. These images can provide crucial indicators for the presence of CCD and delineate commonly present accompanying fractures.[40,79,80] Upon arriving at the suspicion of CCD it is preferable to obtain an MRI expediently, if clinical circumstances permit.[81–83] Any patient transfer needs to be contemplated with care because there is no reliable way to externally brace the craniocervical junction. The prospect of concurrent vascular damage commonly prompts CT- or MRI-based angiography. MRI can aid in identifying ligament injuries, intramedullary changes, and hematoma formation in the epidural or paravertebral spaces.[84–86] In the rare cases of demonstrated cord disruption it may play an important role in the discussion of life-prolonging interventions.[87] Despite the availability of definitive diagnostics patients with CCD appear to continue to be subject to critical delays in timely diagnosis. Diagnostic delays of 2 years have been reported (**Fig. 24.4**).[88]

The prognosis of patients with AOD appears to be related to the severity of the initial neurological findings. If patients survive AOD, there appears to be a trend to improve neurologically, with some patients returning to normal but most being left with some residual deficit.[45]

Treatment

Initial Management and Nonoperative Treatment

The emphasis on initial management is clearly focused on assuring best possible chances for patient survival. Despite not having been updated for more recent advances in diagnostic modalities, the ATLS principles remain unchallenged in their organized role of following a principled resuscitation and diagnostic pathway.[61] After establishing vital functions and securing airway control, efforts are directed at providing protection to the disrupted spinal column and if possible effecting reduction of the injury deformity with closed

means. For a patient with true CCD, nonoperative care is largely limited to the role of temporary stabilization as a bridging measure until definitive surgical care can be rendered. Immobilization with a neck collar and skeletal traction, for instance with Gardner-Wells tongs, have to be performed judiciously due to their inherent propensity toward distraction of the cervical spine.[89] Some studies recommend minimal traction (1 to 2 kg) as a temporary stabilization measure.[33,90–92] Others doubt the necessity and point out the danger of a worsening neurological status, especially if a longitudinal dislocation is present.[41] Donahue et al described a case in which traction applied on a ventrally displaced occiput caused a neurological deterioration.[31] On the other hand, Evarts reported a sudden improvement after reduction with traction.[2] Overall, there are ~20 cases presented in the literature in which traction was applied. In two (10%) of these cases, a neurological worsening was noted. Realignment with a halo vest assembly has been suggested as a preferable acute temporary stabilization option but has also been identified as offering inadequate immobilization of the craniocervical

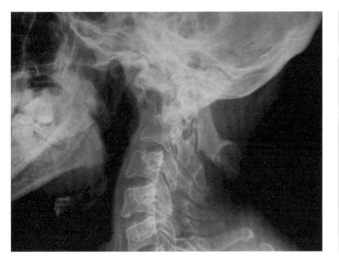

A

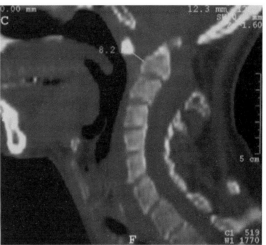

B

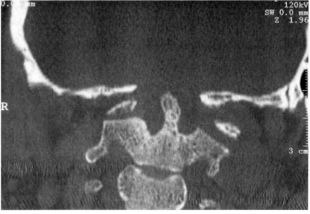

C

D

Fig. 24.4 A case from our department. **(A)** Lateral plain x-ray depicting atlanto-occipital dislocation. **(B)** Sagittal computed tomographic (CT) scan showing a displacement of 8.2 mm from the anterior arch of the atlas to the ventral part of the axis. **(C)** Sagittal T2-weighted magnetic resonance imaging (MRI) demonstrating a severe compression of the medulla and upper spinal cord due to the dislocation of C2. **(D,E)** CT and CT three-dimensional (3-D) reconstruction showing the atlanto-occipital dislocation, with integrity of the odontoid process. (Continued on page 220)

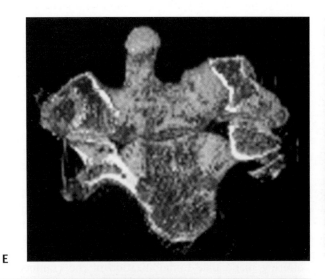

E

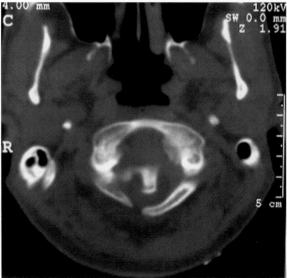

F

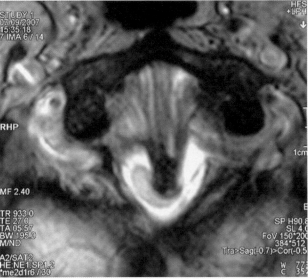

G

Fig. 24.4 *(Continued)* **(F)** Axial CT scan depicting the severe rostral displacement of the odontoid. **(G)** Axial T2-weighted MRI showing the severe displacement of the odontoid process and the extreme elongation of the ligaments.

junction in cases of serious traumatic instability.[92–95] Conservative treatment with extension or halo vest as further management is usually recommended in children and in the case of little instability of AOD[72,92]; however, from the aforementioned literature it is not clear how much instability may be tolerated. Complete closed reduction of a CCD more often than not will leave an unsatisfactory closed reduction result due to interposition of osseous/ligamentous fragments or the presence of deforming muscle forces.

In children, there remains continued controversy as to the historically preferred role of nonoperative care with CCD trauma. There seems to be a greater inherent capacity for the very young to achieve a stable atlanto-occipital segment through a fibrous ankylosis with nonoperative care than comparatively at the atlantoaxial motion segment, where persistent instability has been found in children treated with a halo ring/vest and bed rest over several weeks.[72,96–98] Nonsurgical management in children also holds a fair bit of appeal for fear of disrupting normal craniocervical junction development by surgically interfering with growth centers in that area. More recent studies suggest early surgery due to concern for the failure of any nonsurgical measures to provide sufficient stability to this inherently unstable

region.[99–103] Van de Pol reported on a patient with AOD who sustained a repeat dislocation while in a halo vest assembly.[93] Respiratory problems can be further enhanced with halo vest wear in a predispositioned patient.[94,95] In conclusion, nonoperative care of CCD largely has a temporizing holding function until the patient can be surgically reduced and stabilized. There appears to be a limited role for nonsurgical management in patients with isolated trauma, such as patients with isolated unilateral alar ligament injuries, and in the very young who have an intact TAL. In most other patients with CCD the most desirable care consists of expedient surgical reposition and fixation.

Surgical Options

If the increasing number of case reports and series published on CCD is any measure of real life, there appears to have been a shift toward an increased number of patients surviving these devastating injuries.[20,104–107] Aside from improved resuscitation techniques and diagnostic modalities, urgently performed rigid posterior fixation of the occiput to the cervical spine may play a role in this trend.

Surgical management with arthrodesis of the injured motion segments is usually indicated for patients who have an unstable craniocervical junction or have sustained a spinal cord injury in this region.[20,105,106,108] This simple-sounding premise is, however, somewhat complicated by the ethical questions that can be raised on the question of prolonging survival of patients with severe high-level cord or anoxic brain stem or brain injuries.[87] Spine surgeons may find themselves thrust into a key role of deciding further resuscitation of such unfortunate patients early on or being instrumental in withdrawing life support. On the other hand there are some borderline cases with partial craniocervical ligament disruptions such as unilateral alar ligament tears, which require judicious assessment of residual stability and nonoperative healing potential prior to deciding on surgery. Based on case reports, isolated ligament injuries, such as unilateral alar ligament tears, can usually be treated nonoperatively, whereas certain ligamentous injuries, such as TAL tears, have been reported to have an invariably poor healing rate without surgical stabilization.[16,72,106] Instability of the craniocervical junction was defined by Dickman et al and Dvorak et al as clear evidence of mobile subluxation of more than 1 mm in any direction of its osseous components under fluoroscopic manipulation.[4,5,73]

Achieving stable fixation at the craniocervical junction is technically demanding because of the unique musculoskeletal, neurological, and vascular anatomy of this region. Furthermore, the significant physiological three-plane motion that normally occurs between the occiput and axis places a high biomechanical demand on any fixation device placed into this region until bony healing of the injury region has occurred. The basic surgical concepts of treatment are relatively straightforward and consist of decompression of compromised neural elements and rigid posterior stabilization of the destabilization motion segments, preferably with segmental fixation and suitable bone graft after anatomical reduction of the craniocervical junction. Actual surgical care can be a daunting task and requires experience and resources usually limited to larger trauma centers. It usually requires neurotrauma intensive care, intraoperative evoked potential monitoring, and advanced imaging systems and ideally a multispecialty integrated care approach.

Instrumentation techniques have evolved greatly over the past 2 decades. Newer implant systems offer increased application ease by offering readily adaptable rigid segmental fixation. Nowadays, nonrigid fixation techniques relying on cable and wire fixation play a largely historical role due to their continued reliance on external immobilization with a halo vest or Minerva cast and their need for intact posterior bony structures at the C1 and C2 levels.[100,109-111] The choice of specific fixation/fusion levels depends upon injury variables, such as amount and direction of displacement, fracture location, presence of noncontiguous injuries, and bone quality.[112-114] Although consideration of preservation of motion units, especially in the craniocervical region, may appear to be a noble notion, the primary task of the surgeon in the setting of CCD is to provide definitive treatment at the earliest clinically desirable time for these patients affected by this highly unstable and potentially life-threatening injury.

Multiple posterior fixation techniques have been described for stabilizing the occiput, the atlas, and the axis; however, most of these fixation techniques require some degree of preserved posterior osseous anatomy to anchor the implants and bone graft. Rarely is there a medical indication for anterior atlantoaxial or even atlanto-occipital stabilization for patients with CCD.[115-119] For the exceptional circumstances of major deficiency of posterior craniocervical bone, anterior interarticular screw bridging of either atlantoaxial or anterior or posterior atlanto-occipital joints has been described. Although such techniques of minimalist fixation may hold some theoretical appeal, concerns over ignoring adjacent-ligament injuries affecting the coupled motion unit, which the craniocervical junction after all represents, tend to override the technical aspects of these more limited procedures.[120-123]

To date, there are limited case reports for intraarticular cervicocranial fixation without the use of neutralizing craniocervical rods or plates. In contrast there are multiple studies reporting on high union rates with posterior rods, plates, and combination implants.[124] There appear to be few, if any, meaningful differences between the reported results of the various types of segmental fixation devices, such as Y-, Roy-Camille or reconstruction plates, or rods with a variety of attachments for fixation to the occiput. These devices usually allow for early mobilization of the patient with a simple neck collar worn for a period of 6 weeks to 4 months.[124-130] Occipital fixation of these devices is usually achieved with plates and screw purchase applied parasagittally or along the midline crista of the occiput. In the setting of trauma the use of rigid fixation is clearly preferable over nonrigid fixation, such as described for rheumatoid patients with the use of rectangular rods and wires.[131,132] With the more detailed description of the anatomy of the occiput, cranial screw fixation has become the preferred form of skull fixation.[133-138] Despite all the advancements in implant technology the ultimate treatment goal for injury stabilization has remained a solid arthrodesis with a posterior corticocancellous bone block of autologous or allogeneic sources that can bridge the occipitocervical injury zone.[110,111] Several biomechanical studies have compared posterior occipital–atlantoaxial fixation techniques and have generally concluded that the presence of transarticular or pedicle fixation improves the stability of the construct over that provided by other constructs, such as posterior wiring (**Fig. 24.5**).[139-141] In flexion and extension testing, a posterior plate with transarticular screws provided greater stabilization than posterior wiring or anterior occipitocervical screws. In lateral bending and rotation, the anterior screws were similarly effective to the posterior plate, both of which were more effective than posterior wiring. The anterior screw fixation technique was as stiff as a posterior plate with transarticular screws in stabilizing between the occiput and C2 in axial rotation and lateral bending. In extension and flexion, the anterior screw technique was not as effective as a posterior plate with transarticular screws in providing stability. This anterior screw technique was compared with two commonly used posterior fixation techniques, namely, posterior wiring of a corticocancellous block of bone between the occiput, C1, and C2 and the posterior application of screws applied to C1 and C2 sequentially and bicortical midline screws attaching to the occiput, demonstrating a better biomechanical behavior.[141] Overall presence of a neutralizing plate or rod is a time-honored neutralizing implant that has few or no downsides, whereas isolated intraarticular screws placed from the atlas into the occipital condyles either through anterior or posterior approaches, although clinically possible, have no long-term follow-up and are thus difficult to recommend.

One important aspect of the surgical technique for craniocervical instrumentation is the often overlooked aspect of

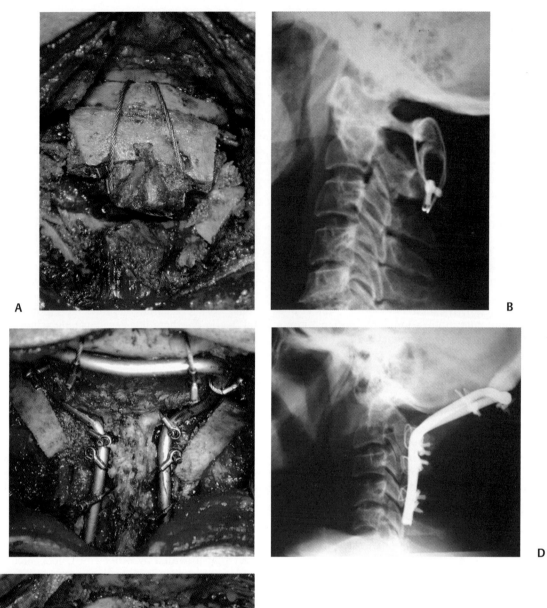

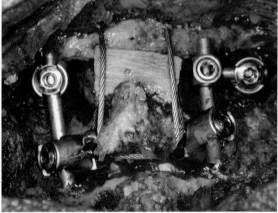

Fig. 24.5 Examples of progression through time of the surgical techniques for occipital–cervical fusion (cases from our department). **(A,B)** C1–C2 fusion with titanium cable and interspinous homograft construction. **(C,D)** Occipital–cervical fusion with titanium rod and cable and postero-lateral homograft. **(E,F)** C1–C2 fusion with screws in lateral mass of C1, sublaminar hooks on C2, and interspinous C1–C2 homograft.

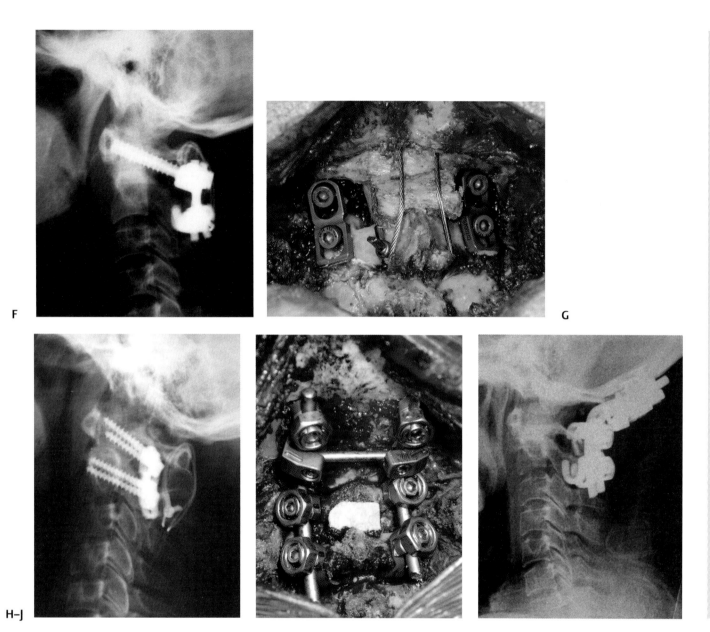

Fig. 24.5 *(Continued)* **(G,H)** C1–C2 fusion (modified Goel technique) with plates, screws in lateral mass of C1 and pedicle of C2 and C1–C2 homograft. **(I,J)** Occipital–cervical fusion with occipital anchors and C1–C2 hooks, rods, crosslink, and interspinous homograft.

postoperative alignment.[45,105] This very important detail and its impact on patient outcomes has received little attention in terms of radiographic and clinical landmarks as well as health-related quality of life outcomes. The basic recommendation is to seek a "neutral" craniocervical alignment and avoid the temptation to fixate the craniocervical junction into a forward flexed position, which would induce compensatory hyperlordosis of the lower cervical spine. In terms of the long-term fate of implants there are no reports on hardware removal being necessary on a routine basis. With proper placement of occipital plates below the level of the inion, posterior occipital soft tissue breakdown should be very uncommon.

◆ Results

Due to factors such as improved patient retrieval, more consistent application of formal resuscitation protocols, and increased injury awareness, more formal long-term observations

of increasing numbers of survivors of CCD have become available.[59,69,88] There remain limitations in the comparability of these studies due to lack of injury severity scales being applied aside form neurological injuries and generalized lack of denominators from whom these injury descriptions arose.

A review of the literature from 1980 to 2007 resulted in 211 documented patients who survived AOD initially and 108 (51%) cases, mainly children and young adults, with reported long-term survival. Of the 196 cases resulting from our recent review, there were 118 surviving patients.

We encountered numerous limitations in our attempt at providing a formal review. As previously stated the key first treatment step following initial resuscitation and patient retrieval consists of timely diagnosis to avoid the high risk of secondary neurological deterioration. As to diagnostic modalities employed, the important factor of delay in diagnosis was difficult to extract due to varying definitions and inconsistent reporting. The actual first diagnostic modality has been addressed in only one study. As to injury classifications used, the Traynelis system is the most popular despite the aforementioned absence of a severity gradient and the possibility to alter the direction of cranial displacement by positioning or manipulation.[9] High-grade neurological injury remains a focal concern of many of the studies available, with a generally unfavorable trend for recovery of high-grade neurological deficits; there are, however, sporadic reports of neurological improvements after AOD.[22,27,31,33,38,41,51,52,54,56,58,66,85,91,93]

Formal review of the literature failed to show any prospectively randomized series comparing conservative and surgical treatment, with the body of literature almost exclusively composed of case series and reports. In the absence of a prospective hypothesis-driven comparison study diagnostic and treatment algorithms remain largely experience or opinion based.

The results of nonoperatively treated occipital condyle and C1 lateral mass fractures have not been addressed in the literature. Of all CCD cases presented, 27% (11 of 41) of those treated with external immobilization alone demonstrated failure of closed management due to either neurological worsening or failure to achieve a stable healing result bony fusion. Results of craniocervical fusion surgery regardless of techniques used seemed to be excellent in terms of bony healing and maintenance or improvement of baseline neurological status. We could find only a single case in which a neurological deterioration occurred after surgery. Based on this cumulative case series comparison we believe that urgent surgical stabilization of CCD at the earliest clinically safe time is the preferred treatment.

◆ Two Key Questions about Craniocervical Dissociation and Evidence-Based-Medicine Answers

What is the Optimal Algorithm for the Timely Diagnosis of Craniocervical Dissociation?

Patients. Patients who sustain traumatic occipital-cervical dissociation, or C1–C2 dissociation

Intervention. Optimal diagnostic algorithm for timely injury detection

Outcomes. CCDs, in the past often fatal, have become increasingly better recognized in trauma patients who survive further than the initial trauma resuscitation. Over the past decade, an increasing number of cases have been reported on the two CCD subtypes, traumatic atlanto-occipital dissociation (AOD) and atlantoaxial dissociation (AAD). This injury entity, if left undiagnosed and undertreated, exposes patients to grave risk of severe complications, with death and high-level tetraplegia being commonly reported adverse events. In contrast, timely diagnosis allows for institution of appropriate treatment with surgery.[1–7] Time to diagnosis of CCD and diagnostic modality that was used to gain the first crucial diagnosis as well as diagnostic modality used to assess stability once the basic injury has been recognized are variables that can be used for discriminatory analysis of the diagnostic pathway.

Evidence summary. Systematic review of 16 articles, which met our inclusion criteria for diagnosis (one class II, four class III, and 11 class IV articles), provided 64 cases, which included case reports due to low primary incidence of cases

and limited survivorship. Primary diagnosis was made primarily with plain x-rays in 18 cases; six cases required plain x-rays + CT scan; one case with flexion-extension plain x-rays + CT scan; and 49 cases with plain x-rays, CT scan, and MRI. Data on delay in diagnosis was identified in one of the larger cohorts to amount to 76% (13 of 17 patients) using strict diagnostic criteria despite availability of all forms of imaging and utilization of a stringent trauma care algorithm. This consecutive case series reported a rate of secondary neurological deterioration of 38% (5 of 13) of patients with delay in diagnosis, which is very similar to previous publications prior to the advent of contemporary imaging modalities.

Quality of evidence. There are no randomized trials. The number of patients is very low due to the low frequency of survivors. With primary outcomes of death and neurological deterioration presenting clearly defined entities, the premise of early diagnosis of CCD with screening plain radiographs continues to remain elusive. Implementation of improved screening parameters and inclusion of the suboccipital region on screening head CT scans used for blunt trauma victims as well as the use of helical CT scans instead of cervical spine plain radiographs in the assessment of at-risk patients remain commonsense measures to decrease delay in diagnosis but await validation in the literature.

Best Estimates. Currently available imaging technology can readily aid in diagnosis of CCD. Inconsistent implementation of these modalities remains a leading cause of missed injuries, which can have devastating effects on injured patients.

Judgment of Benefits versus Risks, Burden, and Costs. Modified imaging protocols and increased disease awareness paired with educational efforts may decrease the incidence of missed injuries for the rare injury incidence of CCD. Routine helical CT and suboccipital imaging obtained on routine head CT in appropriately selected patients may improve the success rate of identifying previously frequently missed injuries, such as CCD. Cost-effectiveness and impact on patient health through different radiation exposure remain to be assessed.

Grade of Recommendation. The quality of evidence to recommend formalized imaging protocols, although mostly based on case reports, can be considered as strong because of the magnitude of adverse impact on a patient if there is a delay in diagnosis. On first suspicion of CCD rapid completion of imaging with CT and MRI is desirable, with additional dynamic testing possibly being necessary in questionable cases to facilitate definitive surgical treatment.

What is the Optimal Treatment with Respect to Health-Related Quality of Life (HRQoL), Neurological Outcomes, and Stability?

Patients. Patients suffering CCD, with variants such as AOD, AAD, or other variants

Intervention. Following timely diagnosis of CCD these usually very unstable injuries should be treated surgically at the earliest clinically feasible time. Nonoperative immobilization of a patient with AAD is recommended at the time of discovery of this injury; however, it provides only limited actual immobilization and incomplete actual reduction capacity. Traction is largely discouraged due to the distractive nature of the injury. Other modalities include collar, halo vest, and taped down head and shoulder pads. For all but incomplete osteoligamentous disruption cases surgical stabilization with rigid stabilization and rapid mobilization are available resources.

Outcomes. Death due to injury or after arrival at the hospital and survivorship with or without neurological deficit are the predominant outcome variables. Neurological deficits can range from isolated cranial nerve deficits to complete or incomplete brain stem and high cord injury patterns. A special subentity of cord injuries presents with those patients who experience a secondary neurological deterioration after arrival at a medical facility. Aspects of long-term function and disability outside of neurological injury are insufficiently documented.

Evidence Summary. Systematic review of 34 articles (one class II, four class III, and 29 class IV articles) allowed extraction of 197 cases that met our inclusion criteria for treatment, with inclusion of case reports due to the low number of surviving patients. We found definitive treatment using nonoperative care documented for five cases (mainly pediatric patients); attempted nonoperative treatment was documented for two patients; and surgical treatment in 178 cases. There is no clear information on the treatment of 19 cases. One patient treated with traction was found to develop overdistraction, with resultant neurological damage. Conservative treatment was reported to have good outcomes with residual atlantoaxial instability in pediatric patients. For surgical cases, 99 patients were considered as having clearly benefited from treatment, however, without specific data on neurological outcomes or in the HRQoL realm. We found reports of 16 cases that were identified to have experienced marked neurological improvement, and seven cases with severe residual neurological sequelae. We found a report of one patient having died. In 78 cases the clinical outcome was not clear.

Quality of evidence. There are no randomized trials and consistent evidence pointing toward large effect size. The serious nature of these life-threatening injuries with the diversity of anatomical lesion site and varying degrees of traumatic comorbidities requires an individualized approach to each patient. Therefore, we decided to include case reports as a source of information. In balance we have rated the quality of the evidence to be high due to the impact a surgical treatment decision has on patients with unstable CCD, and the good results that surviving patients can achieve. In light of unsatisfactory external immobilization means for displaced CCD patients, we found urgent surgical intervention to be increasingly recommended and to be largely a safe and effective intervention. Although preservation of motion is always a desirable goal in terms of selection of fusion levels the potential for overwhelming negative impact of undertreating an injury component in the functional unit formed by the occiput and the upper C-spine usually requires comprehensive fusion of these segments.

Best estimates. Best results can be achieved with stable fusion in anatomical alignment using segmental fixation with adaptability in terms of patient anatomy in regard to HRQoL, neurological outcomes, and stability.

Judgment of benefits versus risks, burden, and cost. Patients who have received stable fixation with anatomical realignment of their craniocervical junction are protected from progression of neurological damage, can be mobilized and rehabilitated immediately, require shorter hospitalization, and may have improved HRQoL. The surgical costs appear lower than attempting to maintain a patient who has an unstable craniocervical spine. There are no comparative data specific to nonsurgical compared with surgical management for patients with unstable CCD.

Grade of recommendation. The quality of the data provided and available for review is graded as moderate. There appear to be clear goals of intervention that can be formulated into five specific entities: (1) decompression of spinal cord or nerves, (2) realignment of injured vertebral segments, (3) permanent stabilization of disrupted ligamentous structures, (4) stop the natural history of the disease, and (5) enable rapid return to functional recovery. We consider this a strong recommendation based in the magnitude of the possible harm to an injured patient and the positive effects attainable by adequate surgical interventions.

◆ Discussion

This systematic review of patients with CCD identified several recurrent themes. Despite readily available diagnostic techniques patients with these injuries continue to be subject to delay in diagnosis. If left untreated, patients with these injuries may be exposed to serious adverse events, such as death or high-grade neurological deterioration. There appears to be a wide spectrum of injury severity, in terms of both skeletal and neurological injury. Prediction of stability in less than obviously disrupted CCD patients remains a major challenge, with nonstandardized assessment strategies being used on an individualized basis. Neurological injury signs are pleomorphic and frequently confusing, thus further increasing chances for delay in diagnosis. Improved screening protocols, such as implementation of routine helical cervical CT scans for spinal clearance or head CT scans with inclusion of the suboccipital region of at-risk patients are promising new approaches that await validation. To enhance full understanding of the CCD injury spectrum, CT scans with sagittal and coronal reformatted views and MRI scans with appropriate imaging sequences are recommended.

Surgical care is largely indicated for unstable injuries with ligamentous disruption and for patients with neurological injury. Stable posteriorly based fusion of the injured segments appears to be associated with favorable recovery. The specific instrumentation technique appears to be of secondary importance, with more recent segmental fixation systems being more user-friendly and offering some biomechanical advantages that may allow for earlier mobilization than previous nonrigid forms of fixation. Their further validation is needed in the form of comparative studies.

References

1. Blackwood III NJ. Atlo-occipital dislocation: a case of fracture of the atlas and axis, and forward dislocation of the occiput on the spinal column, life being maintained for thirty-four hours and forty minutes by artificial respiration, during which a laminectomy was performed upon the third cervical vertebra. Ann Surg 1908;47: 654–658
2. Evarts CM. Traumatic occipitoatlantal dislocation: report of a case with survival. J Bone Joint Surg Am 1970;52:1653–1660
3. Page CP, Story JL, Wissinger JP, Branch CL. Traumatic atlantooccipital dislocation. Case report. J Neurosurg 1973;39:394–397
4. Dvorak J, Panjabi MM. Functional anatomy of the alar ligaments. Spine 1987;12:183–189
5. Dvorak J, Panjabi M, Gerber M, Wichmann W. CT-functional diagnostics of the rotatory instability of upper cervical spine, I: An experimental study on cadavers. Spine 1987;12:197–205

6. Dvorak J, Hayek J, Zehnder R. CT-functional diagnostics of the rotatory instability of the upper cervical spine, II: An evaluation on healthy adults and patients with suspected instability. Spine 1987;12:726–731

7. Dvorak J, Schneider E, Saldinger P, Rahn B. Biomechanics of the craniocervical region: the alar and transverse ligaments. J Orthop Res 1988;6:452–461

8. Adams VI. Neck injuries, I: Occipitoatlantal dislocation: a pathologic study of twelve traffic fatalities. J Forensic Sci 1992;37:556–564

9. Dublin AB, Marks WM, Weinstock D, Newton TH. Traumatic dislocation of the atlanto-occipital articulation (AOA) with short-term survival: with a radiographic method of measuring the AOA. J Neurosurg 1980;52:541–546

10. Bucholz RW, Burkhead WZ. The pathological anatomy of fatal atlanto-occipital dislocations. J Bone Joint Surg Am 1979;61:248–250

11. Alker GJ Jr, Oh YS, Leslie EV. High cervical spine and craniocervical junction injuries in fatal traffic accidents: a radiological study. Orthop Clin North Am 1978;9:1003–1010

12. Patel JC, Tepas JJ III, Mollitt DL, Pieper P. Pediatric cervical spine injuries: defining the disease. J Pediatr Surg 2001;36:373–376

13. Anderson PA, Montesano PX. Morphology and treatment of occipital condyle fractures. Spine 1988;13:731–736

14. Bellis YM, Linnau KF, Mann FA. A complex atlantoaxial fracture with craniocervical instability: a case with bilateral type 1 dens fractures. AJR Am J Roentgenol 2001;176:978

15. Traynelis VC, Marano GD, Dunker RO, Kaufman HH. Traumatic atlanto-occipital dislocation: case report. J Neurosurg 1986;65:863–870

16. Chapman JR, Bellabarba C, Newell DW, Kuntz C IV, West AG, Mirza SK. Craniocervical injuries: atlanto-occipital dissociation and occipital condyle fractures. Semin Spine Surg 2001;13:90–105

17. Grossman MD, Reilly PM, Gillett T, Gillett D. National survey of the incidence of cervical spine injury and approach to cervical spine clearance in U.S. trauma centers. J Trauma 1999;47:684–690

18. Avellino AM, Mann FA, Grady MS, et al. The misdiagnosis of acute cervical spine injuries and fractures in infants and children: the 12-year experience of a level I pediatric and adult trauma center. Childs Nerv Syst 2005;21:122–127

19. Chiu WC, Haan JM, Cushing BM, Kramer ME, Scalea TM. Ligamentous injuries of the cervical spine in unreliable blunt trauma patients: incidence, evaluation, and outcome. J Trauma 2001;50:457–463, discussion 464

20. Fisher CG, Sun JC, Dvorak M. Recognition and management of atlanto-occipital dislocation: improving survival from an often fatal condition. Can J Surg 2001;44:412–420

21. Cohen A, Hirsch M, Katz M, Sofer S. Traumatic atlanto-occipital dislocation in children: review and report of five cases. Pediatr Emerg Care 1991;7:24–27

22. Partrick DA, Bensard DD, Moore EE, Calkins CM, Karrer FM. Cervical spine trauma in the injured child: a tragic injury with potential for salvageable functional outcome. J Pediatr Surg 2000;35:1571–1575

23. Bohlman HH. Acute fractures and dislocations of the cervical spine: an analysis of three hundred hospitalized patients and review of the literature. J Bone Joint Surg Am 1979;61:1119–1142

24. Davis D, Bohlman H, Walker AE, Fisher R, Robinson R. The pathological findings in fatal craniospinal injuries. J Neurosurg 1971;34:603–613

25. Gerrelts BD, Petersen EU, Mabry J, Petersen SR. Delayed diagnosis of cervical spine injuries. J Trauma 1991;31:1622–1626

26. Tepper SL, Fligner CL, Reay DT. Atlanto-occipital disarticulation: accident characteristics. Am J Forensic Med Pathol 1990;11:193–197

27. Davis JW, Phreaner DL, Hoyt DB, Mackersie RC. The etiology of missed cervical spine injuries. J Trauma 1993;34:342–346

28. Zivot U, Di Maio VJ. Motor vehicle–pedestrian accidents in adults: relationship between impact speed, injuries, and distance thrown. Am J Forensic Med Pathol 1993;14:185–186

29. Sun PP, Poffenbarger GJ, Durham S, Zimmerman RA. Spectrum of occipitoatlantoaxial injury in young children. J Neurosurg 2000;93(1, Suppl):28–39

30. Hill SA, Miller CA, Kosnik EJ, Hunt WE. Pediatric neck injuries: a clinical study. J Neurosurg 1984;60:700–706

31. Donahue DJ, Muhlbauer MS, Kaufman RA, Warner WC, Sanford RA. Childhood survival of atlantooccipital dislocation: underdiagnosis, recognition, treatment, and review of the literature. Pediatr Neurosurg 1994;21:105–111

32. Labler L, Eid K, Platz A, Trentz O, Kossmann T. Atlanto-occipital dislocation: four case reports of survival in adults and review of the literature. Eur Spine J 2004;13:172–180

33. DiBenedetto T, Lee CK. Traumatic atlanto-occipital instability: a case report with follow-up and a new diagnostic technique. Spine 1990;15:595–597

34. Ferrera PC, Bartfield JM. Traumatic atlanto-occipital dislocation: a potentially survivable injury. Am J Emerg Med 1996;14:291–296

35. Grabb BC, Frye TA, Hedlund GL, Vaid YN, Grabb PA, Royal SA. MRI diagnosis of suspected atlanto-occipital dissociation in childhood. Pediatr Radiol 1999;29:275–281

36. Kenter K, Worley G, Griffin T, Fitch RD. Pediatric traumatic atlanto-occipital dislocation: five cases and a review. J Pediatr Orthop 2001;21:585–589

37. Przybylski GJ, Clyde BL, Fitz CR. Craniocervical junction subarachnoid hemorrhage associated with atlanto-occipital dislocation. Spine 1996;21:1761–1768

38. Angel CA, Ehlers RA. Images in clinical medicine: Atloido-occipital dislocation in a small child after air-bag deployment. N Engl J Med 2001;345:1256

39. Ohshima T, Kondo T. Forensic pathological observations on fatal injuries to the brain stem and/or upper cervical spinal cord in traffic accidents. J Clin Forensic Med 1998;5:129–134

40. Deliganis AV, Baxter AB, Hanson JA, et al. Radiologic spectrum of craniocervical distraction injuries. Radiographics 2000;20(Spec no):S237–S250

41. Kaufman RA, Dunbar JS, Botsford JA, McLaurin RL. Traumatic longitudinal atlanto-occipital distraction injuries in children. AJNR Am J Neuroradiol 1982;3:415–419

42. Saeheng S, Phuenpathom N. Traumatic occipitoatlantal dislocation. Surg Neurol 2001;55:35–40, discussion 40

43. Mackersie RC, Shackford SR, Garfin SR, Hoyt DB. Major skeletal injuries in the obtunded blunt trauma patient: a case for routine radiologic survey. J Trauma 1988;28:1450–1454

44. Reid DC, Henderson R, Saboe L, Miller JDR. Etiology and clinical course of missed spine fractures. J Trauma 1987;27:980–986

45. Bellabarba C, Mirza SK, West GA, et al. Diagnosis and treatment of craniocervical dislocation in a series of 17 consecutive survivors during an 8-year period. J Neurosurg Spine 2006;4:429–440

46. Chan RNW, Ainscow D, Sikorski JM. Diagnostic failures in the multiple injured. J Trauma 1980;20:684–687

47. Ross SE, Schwab CW, David ET, Delong WG, Born CT. Clearing the cervical spine: initial radiologic evaluation. J Trauma 1987;27:1055–1060

48. Jónsson H Jr, Bring G, Rauschning W, Sahlstedt B. Hidden cervical spine injuries in traffic accident victims with skull fractures. J Spinal Disord 1991;4:251–263

49. Palmer MT, Turney SZ. Tracheal rupture and atlanto-occipital dislocation: case report. J Trauma 1994;37:314–317

50. Lyness SS, Simeone FA. Vascular complications of upper cervical spine injuries. Orthop Clin North Am 1978;9:1029–1038

51. Bell HS. Basilar artery insufficiency due to atlanto-occipital instability. Am Surg 1969;35:695–700

52. Lee C, Woodring JH, Walsh JW. Carotid and vertebral artery injury in survivors of atlanto-occipital dislocation: case reports and literature review. J Trauma 1991;31:401–407

53. Bell HS. Paralysis of both arms from injury of the upper portion of the pyramidal decussation: "cruciate paralysis." J Neurosurg 1970;33:376–380

54. Dickman CA, Hadley MN, Pappas CTE, Sonntag VKH, Geisler FH. Cruciate paralysis: a clinical and radiographic analysis of injuries to the cervicomedullary junction. J Neurosurg 1990;73:850–858

55. Ladouceur D, Veilleux M, Levesque RY. Cruciate paralysis secondary to C1 on C2 fracture-dislocation. Spine 1991;16:1383–1385

56. Schliack H, Schaefer P. Hypoglossal and accessory nerve paralysis in a fracture of the occipital condyle [in German]. Nervenarzt 1965;36:362–364

57. Colnet G, Chabannes J, Commun C, Rigal MC, Alassaf M. Atlanto-occipital luxation and syringomyelia: 2 rare complications of cervical injury. Diagnostic and therapeutic effects. Apropos of a case [in French]. Neurochirurgie 1989;35:58–63

58. Lesoin F, Blondel M, Dhellemmes P, Thomas CE, Viaud C, Jomin M. Post-traumatic atlanto-occipital dislocation revealed by sudden cardiopulmonary arrest. Lancet 1982;2:447–448

59. Naso WB, Cure J, Cuddy BG. Retropharyngeal pseudomeningocele after atlanto-occipital dislocation: report of two cases. Neurosurgery 1997;40:1288–1290, discussion 1290–1291

60. Vakili ST, Aguilar JC, Muller J. Sudden unexpected death associated with atlanto-occipital fusion. Am J Forensic Med Pathol 1985;6:39–43

61. American College of Surgeons. Advanced Trauma Life Support Manual. Chicago: American College of Surgeons; 1992

62. Monu J, Bohrer SP, Howard G. Some upper cervical spine norms. Spine 1987;12:515–519

63. Powers B, Miller MD, Kramer RS, Martinez S, Gehweiler JA Jr. Traumatic anterior atlanto-occipital dislocation. Neurosurgery 1979;4:12–17

64. Wholey MH, Bruwer AJ, Baker HL Jr. The lateral roentgenogram of the neck: with comments on the atlanto-odontoid-basion relationship. Radiology 1958;71:350–356

65. Harris JH Jr, Carson GC, Wagner LK. Radiologic diagnosis of traumatic occipitovertebral dissociation, I: Normal occipitovertebral relationships on lateral radiographs of supine subjects. AJR Am J Roentgenol 1994; 162:881–886

66. Harris JH Jr, Carson GC, Wagner LK, Kerr N. Radiologic diagnosis of traumatic occipitovertebral dissociation, II: Comparison of three methods of detecting occipitovertebral relationships on lateral radiographs of supine subjects. AJR Am J Roentgenol 1994;162:887–892

67. Lee C, Woodring JH, Goldstein SJ, Daniel TL, Young AB, Tibbs PA. Evaluation of traumatic atlantooccipital dislocations. AJNR Am J Neuroradiol 1987;8:19–26

68. Pang D, Nemzek WR, Zovickian J. Atlanto-occipital dislocation, I: Normal occipital condyle–C1 interval in 89 children. Neurosurgery 2007;61:514–521, discussion 521

69. Pang D, Nemzek WR, Zovickian J. Atlanto-occipital dislocation, II: The clinical use of (occipital) condyle–C1 interval, comparison with other diagnostic methods, and the manifestation, management, and outcome of atlanto-occipital dislocation in children. Neurosurgery 2007; 61:995–1015, discussion 1015

70. Wackenheim A. Transversal dislocation of the occipito-cervical joint: a cause of cervico-occipital neuralgia [in Italian]. Radiol Med (Torino) 1966;52:1254–1259

71. Wackenheim A. Roentgen Diagnosis of the Craniovertebral Region. Berlin: Springer-Verlag; 1974

72. Ghatan S, Newell DW, Grady MS, et al. Severe posttraumatic craniocervical instability in the very young patient: report of three cases. J Neurosurg 2004;101(1, Suppl):102–107

73. Dickman CA, Papadopoulos SM, Sonntag VKH, Spetzler RF, Rekate HL, Drabier J. Traumatic occipitoatlantal dislocations. J Spinal Disord 1993;6:300–313

74. Jones DN, Knox AM, Sage MR. Traumatic avulsion fracture of the occipital condyles and clivus with associated unilateral atlantooccipital distraction. AJNR Am J Neuroradiol 1990;11:1181–1183

75. Babbitz JD, Kim KD. Imaging corner: unknown case. Diagnosis and discussion: atlanto-occipital dislocation. Spine 2001;26:1401–1402

76. Blackmore CC, Mann FA, Wilson AJ. Helical CT in the primary trauma evaluation of the cervical spine: an evidence-based approach. Skeletal Radiol 2000;29:632–639

77. Hanson JA, Deliganis AV, Baxter AB, et al. Radiologic and clinical spectrum of occipital condyle fractures: retrospective review of 107 consecutive fractures in 95 patients. AJR Am J Roentgenol 2002;178:1261–1268

78. Scott EW, Haid RW Jr, Peace D. Type I fractures of the odontoid process: implications for atlanto-occipital instability: case report. J Neurosurg 1990;72:488–492

79. Matava MJ, Whitesides TE Jr, Davis PC. Traumatic atlanto-occipital dislocation with survival: serial computerized tomography as an aid to diagnosis and reduction: a report of three cases. Spine 1993;18: 1897–1903

80. Guigui P, Milaire M, Morvan G, Lassale B, Deburge A. Traumatic atlantooccipital dislocation with survival: case report and review of the literature. Eur Spine J 1995;4:242–247

81. Bundschuh CV, Alley JB, Ross M, Porter IS, Gudeman SK. Magnetic resonance imaging of suspected atlanto-occipital dislocation: two case reports. Spine 1992;17:245–248

82. Chaljub G, Singh H, Gunito FC Jr, Crow WN. Traumatic atlanto-occipital dislocation: MRI and CT. Neuroradiology 2001;43:41–44

83. Krakenes J, Kaale BR, Rorvik J, Gilhus NE. MRI assessment of normal ligamentous structures in the craniovertebral junction. Neuroradiology 2001;43:1089–1097

84. Hall AJ, Wagle VG, Raycroft J, Goldman RL, Butler AR. Magnetic resonance imaging in cervical spine trauma. J Trauma 1993;34:21–26

85. Gabrielsen TO, Maxwell JA. Traumatic atlanto-occipital dislocation; with case report of a patient who survived. Am J Roentgenol Radium Ther Nucl Med 1966;97:624–629

86. Kuzma BB, Goodman JM. Diagnosis of atlanto-occipital dislocation. Surg Neurol 1997;48:418–419

87. Gautschi OP, Woodland PR, Zellweger R. Complete medulla/cervical spinal cord transection after atlanto-occipital dislocation: an extraordinary case. Spinal Cord 2007;45:387–393

88. Takayasu M, Hara M, Suzuki Y, Yoshida J. Treatment of traumatic atlanto-occipital dislocation in chronic phase. Neurosurg Rev 1999;22: 135–137

89. Eismont FJ, Bohlman HH. Posterior atlanto-occipital dislocation with fractures of the atlas and odontoid process. J Bone Joint Surg Am 1978;60:397–399

90. Montane I, Eismont FJ, Green BA. Traumatic occipitoatlantal dislocation. Spine 1991;16:112–116

91. Lee AS, MacLean JCB, Newton DA. Rapid traction for reduction of cervical spine dislocations. J Bone Joint Surg Br 1994;76:352–356

92. Steinmetz MP, Verrees M, Anderson JS, Lechner RM. Dual-strap augmentation of a halo orthosis in the treatment of atlantooccipital dislocation in infants and young children: technical note. J Neurosurg 2002;96(3, Suppl):346–349

93. van de Pol GJ, Hanlo PW, Oner FC, Castelein RM. Redislocation in a halo vest of an atlanto-occipital dislocation in a child: recommendations for treatment. Spine 2005;30:E424–E428

94. Anderson PA, Budorick TE, Easton KB, Henley MB, Salciccioli GG. Failure of halo vest to prevent in vivo motion in patients with injured cervical spines. Spine 1991;16(10, Suppl):S501–S505

95. Botte MJ, Garfin SR, Byrne TP, Woo SLY, Nickel VL. The halo skeletal fixator. Principles of application and maintenance. Clin Orthop Relat Res 1989;239:12–18

96. Labbe JL, Leclair O, Duparc B. Traumatic atlanto-occipital dislocation with survival in children. J Pediatr Orthop B 2001;10:319–327

97. Dallek M, Meenen NM, Jungbluth KH, Bentele KH, Grzyska U. Traumatic dislocations of the cranial spine in childhood. Clinical description of 2 cases [in German]. Unfallchirurgie 1995;21:40–44

98. Farley FA, Graziano GP, Hensinger RN. Traumatic atlanto-occipital dislocation in a child. Spine 1992;17:1539–1541

99. Koop SE, Winter RB, Lonstein JE. The surgical treatment of instability of the upper part of the cervical spine in children and adolescents. J Bone Joint Surg Am 1984;66:403–411

100. Sponseller PD, Cass JR. Atlanto-occipital fusion for dislocation in children with neurologic preservation: a case report. Spine 1997;22:344–347

101. Belzberg AJ, Tranmer BI. Stabilization of traumatic atlanto-occipital dislocation. Case report. J Neurosurg 1991;75:478–482

102. Shamoun JM, Riddick L, Powell RW. Atlanto-occipital subluxation/dislocation: a "survivable" injury in children. Am Surg 1999;65:317–320

103. Houle P, McDonnell DE, Vender J. Traumatic atlanto-occipital dislocation in children. Pediatr Neurosurg 2001;34:193–197

104. Chattar-Cora D, Valenziano CP. Atlanto-occipital dislocation: a report of three patients and a review. J Orthop Trauma 2000;14:370–375

105. Hamai S, Harimaya K, Maeda T, Hosokawa A, Shida J, Iwamoto Y. Traumatic atlanto-occipital dislocation with atlantoaxial subluxation. Spine 2006;31:E421–424

106. Horn EM, Feiz-Erfan I, Lekovic GP, Dickman CA, Sonntag VK, Theodore N. Survivors of occipitoatlantal dislocation injuries: imaging and clinical correlates. J Neurosurg Spine 2007;6:113–120

107. Belzberg AJ, Tranmer BI. Stabilization of traumatic atlanto-occipital dislocation. Case report. J Neurosurg 1991;75:478–482

108. Vaccaro AR, Lim MR, Lee JY. Indications for surgery and stabilization techniques of the occipito-cervical junction. Injury 2005;36(Suppl 2): B44–B53

109. Yamaguchi N, Ikeda K, Ishise J, Yamashita J. Traumatic atlanto-occipital dislocation with long-term survival. Neurol Med Chir (Tokyo) 1996; 36:36–39

110. Wertheim SB, Bohlman HH. Occipitocervical fusion: indications, technique, and long-term results in thirteen patients. J Bone Joint Surg Am 1987;69:833–836

111. Hamblen DL. Occipito-cervical fusion: indications, technique and results. J Bone Joint Surg Br 1967;49:33–45

112. Zigler JE, Waters RL, Nelson RW, Capen DA, Perry J. Occipito-cervico-thoracic spine fusion in a patient with occipito-cervical dislocation and survival. Spine 1986;11:645–646

113. Park J-B, Ha K-Y, Chang H. Traumatic posterior atlantooccipital dislocation with Jefferson fracture and fracture-dislocation of C6–C7: a case report with survival. Eur Spine J 2001;10:524–528

114. Junge A, Krueger A, Petermann J, Gotzen L. Posterior atlanto-occipital dislocation and concomitant discoligamentous C3–C4 instability with survival. Spine 2001;26:1722–1725

115. de Andrade JR, Macnab I. Anterior occipito-cervical fusion using an extra-pharyngeal exposure. J Bone Joint Surg Am 1969;51:1621–1626

116. Vaccaro AR, Lehman AP, Ahlgren BD, Garfin SR. Anterior C1–C2 screw fixation and bony fusion through an anterior retropharyngeal approach. Orthopedics 1999;22:1165–1170

117. Lesoin F, Autricque A, Villette L, Franz K, Jomin M. Atlanto-axial arthrodesis by anterior retropharyngeal intermaxillo-hyoidal approach [in French]. Neurochirurgie 1987;33:239–243

118. Vaccaro AR, Ring D, Lee RS, Scuderi G, Garfin SR. Salvage anterior C1–C2 screw fixation and arthrodesis through the lateral approach in a patient with a symptomatic pseudoarthrosis. Am J Orthop 1997;26: 349–353

119. Kandziora F, Kerschbaumer F, Starker M, Mittlmeier T. Biomechanical assessment of transoral plate fixation for atlantoaxial instability. Spine 2000;25:1555–1561

120. Grob D. Transarticular screw fixation for atlanto-occipital dislocation. Spine 2001;26:703–707

121. Grob D, Dvorak J, Panjabi M, Froehlich M, Hayek J. Posterior occipitocervical fusion: a preliminary report of a new technique. Spine 1991;16(3, Suppl):S17–S24

122. Gonzalez LF, Sonntag VK, Dickman CA, Crawford NR. Technique for fixating the atlantooccipital complex with a transarticular screw. Spine 2002;27:219–220

123. Dvorak MF, Sekeramayi F, Zhu Q, et al. Anterior occiput to axis screw fixation, II: A biomechanical comparison with posterior fixation techniques. Spine 2003;28:239–245

124. Chen HJ, Cheng MH, Lau YC. One-stage posterior decompression and fusion using a Luque rod for occipito-cervical instability and neural compression. Spinal Cord 2001;39:101–108

125. Ransford AO, Crockard HA, Pozo JL, Thomas NP, Nelson IW. Craniocervical instability treated by contoured loop fixation. J Bone Joint Surg Br 1986;68:173–177

126. Richter M, Wilke HJ, Kluger P, Neller S, Claes L, Puhl W. Biomechanical evaluation of a new modular rod–screw implant system for posterior instrumentation of the occipito-cervical spine: in-vitro comparison with two established implant systems. Eur Spine J 2000;9: 417–425

127. Kohler H, Vock B, Hochstein P, Wentzensen A. Fusion of the craniocervical transition with "CerviFix" after survived atlanto-occipital dislocation [in German]. Chirurg 1998;69:677–681

128. Lieberman IH, Webb JK. Occipito-cervical fusion using posterior titanium plates. Eur Spine J 1998;7:308–312

129. Lipscomb PR. Cervico-occipital fusion for congenital and post-traumatic anomalies of the atlas and axis. J Bone Joint Surg Am 1957;39-A:1289–1301

130. Roy-Camille R, Benazet JP, Saillant G, Henry P, Mamoudy P, Leonard P. Luxation traumatique occipitoatloidienne: interet de nouveaux signes radiologiques (a propos de deux cas). Rev Orthop Chir Appar Mot 1986;72:303–309

131. Itoh T, Tsuji H, Katoh Y, Yonezawa T, Kitagawa H. Occipito-cervical fusion reinforced by Luque's segmental spinal instrumentation for rheumatoid diseases. Spine 1988;13:1234–1238

132. Sakou T, Kawaida H, Morizono Y, et al. Occipitoatlantoaxial fusión utilizing a rectangular rod. Clin Orthop 1989;(239):136–144

133. Paquis P, Lonjon M, Grellier P. Use of the CCD (Sofamor-Danek) rod plates for instabilities of the craniospinal junction [in French]. Neurochirurgie 1998;44:101–104

134. Abumi K, Takada T, Shono Y, Kaneda K, Fujiya M. Posterior occipitocervical reconstruction using cervical pedicle screws and plate-rod systems. Spine 1999;24:1425–1434

135. Sasso RC, Jeanneret B, Fischer K, Magerl F. Occipitocervical fusion with posterior plate and screw instrumentation: a long-term follow-up study. Spine 1994;19:2364–2368

136. Smith MD, Anderson PA. Occipital cervical fusion. Tech Orthop 1994;9: 37–42

137. Smith MD, Anderson P, Grady MS. Occipitocervical arthrodesis using contoured plate fixation: an early report on a versatile fixation technique. Spine 1993;18:1984–1990

138. Ebraheim NA, Lu J, Biyani A, Brown JA, Yeasting RA. An anatomic study of the thickness of the occipital bone: implications for occipitocervical instrumentation. Spine 1996;21:1725–1729, discussion 1729–1730

139. Richter M, Wilke HJ, Kluger P, Neller S, Claes L, Puhl W. Biomechanical evaluation of a new modular rod–screw implant system for posterior instrumentation of the occipito-cervical spine: in-vitro comparison with two established implant systems. Eur Spine J 2000;9: 417–425

140. Hurlbert RJ, Crawford NR, Choi WG, Dickman CA. A biomechanical evaluation of occipitocervical instrumentation: screw compared with wire fixation. J Neurosurg 1999;90(1, Suppl):84–90

141. Oda I, Abumi K, Sell LC, Haggerty CJ, Cunningham BW, McAfee PC. Biomechanical evaluation of five different occipito-atlanto-axial fixation techniques. Spine 1999;24:2377–2382

142. Eleraky MA, Theodore N, Adams M, Rekate HL, Sonntag VK. Pediatric cervical spine injuries: report of 102 cases and review of the literature. J Neurosurg 2000;92(1 Suppl):12–17

143. Lee SC, Chen JF, Lee ST. Clinical experience with rigid occipitocervical fusion in the management of traumatic upper cervical spinal instability. J Clin Neurosci 2006;13(2):193–198

144. Stulik J, Vyskocil T, Sebesta P, Kryl J. [Harms technique of C1-C2 fixation with polyaxial screws and rods]. Acta Chir Orthop Traumatol Cech 2005;72(1):22–27

145. Harms J, Melcher RP. Posterior C1-C2 fusion with polyaxial screw and rod fixation. Spine 2001;26(22):2467–2471

146. Gautschi OP, Zellweger R. Images in emergency medicine: long-term survival following complete medulla/cervical spinal cord transection. Ann Emerg Med 2007,49(4):540,545

147. Behari S, Kalra SK, Kiran Kumar MV, Salunke P, Jaiswal AK, Jain VK. Chiari I malformation associated with atlanto-axial dislocation: focusing on the anterior cervicomedullary compression. Acta Neurochir 2007;149(1):41–50

148. Anderson AJ, Towns GM, Chiverton N. Traumatic occipitocervical disruption: a new technique for stabilisation. Case report and literature review. J Bone Joint Surg Br 2006;88(11):1464–1468

149. Violas P, Ropars M, Doumbouya N, Bracq H. Case reports: Atlantooccipital and atlantoaxial traumatic dislocation in a child who survived. Clin Orthop Relat Res 2006;446:286–290

150. Yin Q, Ai F, Zhang K, Chang Y, Xia H, et al. Irreducible anterior atlantoaxial dislocation: one-stage treatment with a transoral atlantoaxial reduction plate fixation and fusion. Report of 5 cases and review of the literature. Spine 2005;30(13):E375–381

151. Seibert PS, Stridh-Igo P, Whitmore TA, Dufty BM, Zimmerman CG. Cranio-cervical stabilization of traumatic atlanto-occipital dislocation with minimal resultant neurological deficit. Acta Neurochir 2005; 147(4):435–442

152. Ames CP, Acosta F, Nottmeier N. Novel treatment of basilar invagination resulting from an untreated C-1 fracture associated with transverse ligament avulsion. Case report and description of surgical technique. J Neurosurg Spine 2005;2(1):83–87

153. Ramare S, Lazennec JY, Camelot C, Saillant G, Hansen S, Trabelsi R. Vertical atlantoaxial dislocation. Eur Spine J 1999;8(3):241–243

154. Govender S, Vlok GJ, Fisher-Jeffes N, Du Preez CP. Traumatic dislocation of the atlanto-occipital joint. J Bone Joint Surg Br 2003;85(6):875–878

155. Horn EM, Feiz-Erfan I, Lekovic GP, Dickmen CA, Sonntag VK, Theodore N. Survivors of occipitoatlantal dislocation injuries: imaging and clinical correlates. J Neurosurg Spine 2007;6:113–120

156. Rahimi SY, Stevens EA, Yeh DJ, Flannery AM, Choudhri HF, Lee MR. Treatment of atlantoaxial instability in pediatric patients. Neurosurg Focus 2003;15(6):ECP1

157. Fiore AJ, Haid RW, Rodts GE, Subach BR, Mummaneni PV, et al. Atlantal lateral mass screws for posterior spinal reconstruction: technical note and case series. Neurosurg Focus 2002;12(1):E5

158. Lo PA, Drake JM, Hedden D, Narotam P, Dirks PB. Avulsion transverse ligament injuries in children: successful treament with nonoperative management. Report of three cases. J Neurosurg 2002;96(3 Suppl): 338–342

159. Razif M, Lim HH. Delayed decompression of chronic C1C2 subluxation in a pediatric patient with tetraplegia—is recovery possible? Med J Malaysia 2001;56 Suppl C:76–79

160. Heidecke V, Rainov NG, Burkert W. Occipito-cervical fusion with the cervical Cotrel-Dubousset rod system. Acta Neurochir 1998;140(9): 969–976

161. Dickman CA, Sonntag VK. Posterior C1-C2 transarticular screw fixation for atlantoaxial arthrodesis. Neurosurgery 1998;43(2):275–280

162. Faure A, Bord E, Monteiro da Silva R, Diaz Saldaña A, Robert R. Occipitocervical fixation with a single occipital clamp using inverted hooks. Eur Spine J 1998;7(1):80–83

163. Rainov NG, Heidecke N, Burkert W. Coronally oriented vertical fracture of the axis body: surgical treatment of a rare condition. Minim Invasive Neurosurg 1998;41(2):93–96

164. Schultz KD, Petronio J, Haid RW. Pediatric occipitocervical arthrodesis. A review of current options and early evaluation of rigid internal fixation techniques. Pediatr Neurosurg 2000;33:169–181

165. Song GS, Theodore N, Dickman CA, Sonntag VK. Unilateral posterior atlantoaxial transarticular screw fixation. J Neurosurg 1997;87(6): 851–855

166. Malcom GP, Ransford AO, Crockard HA. Treatment of non-rheumatoid occipitocervical instability. Internal fixation with the Hartshill-Ransford loop. J Bone Joint Surg Br 1994;76:357–366

25

Management of Type II and Type III Odontoid Fractures

Ronald W. Lindsey and Zbigniew Gugala

The axis is a unique second vertebra that plays a critical role in upper cervical spine motion and stability. The specialized anatomy and kinematics of the axis (in combination with the atlas) subjects it to biomechanical loads that can be diverse and considerable. These loads, when excessive, can result in a variety of ligamentous and bony injuries, among which odontoid fractures are the most common.

Fractures of the odontoid can account for up to 20% of all cervical spine injuries. Anderson and D'Alonzo[1] classified these fractures into three types (I, II, and III) based on the level of the fracture (the superior pole/tip, waist, and body, respectively). This classification system has been universally accepted and used to direct treatment.

Type I odontoid fractures do not imperil neurological function or spinal stability; functional outcomes associated with passive, symptomatic treatment have consistently been outstanding. However, the management outcomes of the more threatening type II and III odontoid fractures have proven to be less reliable and, therefore, a vast array of treatment modalities have been advocated, including the following:

- *Nonoperative treatment (passive).* Symptomatic management of the fracture with activity modification and without external supportive devices
- *Nonoperative treatment (active).* Management of the fracture that includes external supportive devices (i.e., braces, halo immobilization, and/or traction)
- *Operative treatment.* It can consist of posterior cervical fixation and fusion (using transarticular screws or sublaminar wires) or anterior fixation (using odontoid screws)

Although the merits and risks associated with these various treatment regimens have been discussed in a plethora of scientific articles over the past several decades, the optimal treatment for type II and III odontoid fractures remains controversial. This systematic review identifies and establishes evidence-based criteria for the management of type II and III odontoid fractures.

◆ Materials and Methods

Literature Search

An exhaustive database search was performed to identify all original published studies pertaining to the topic. The publication database search included the National Library of Medicine and Medline; the search involved all human studies published in English between January 1966 and November 2007. The keywords used in the Boolean search were as follows: (odontoid *OR* dens) *AND* fracture *AND* (treatment *OR* management) *AND* human *AND* adult *AND* English. Papers published prior to the development of the Anderson-D'Alonzo classification in 1974[1] or those that did not use this classification were excluded. The bibliography listed in these papers was evaluated for the presence of additional articles to ensure a thorough and complete literature review.

Evaluating Articles and Weighing Strength of Evidence

The literature selected for review was categorized in accordance with the strength of evidence. The level of evidence format used in the review was defined by Wright et al[2] as follows: level I—prospective randomized clinical trials; level II—nonrandomized prospective cohort studies; level III—retrospective studies, case-control studies; level IV—case series with historical or no control; and level V—expert opinion. All selected articles were assessed by two independent reviewers and categorized in accordance with their level of evidence.

The levels of evidence determined for the odontoid fracture articles selected were then linked to treatment recommendations in accordance with the criteria of the American Medical Association.[3] In these criteria, level I evidence is used to establish practice standards (the strongest recommendation); level II evidence is used to support practice guidelines (suggesting a moderate degree of clinical certainty); and level III evidence is used to establish practice options (reflecting clinical uncertainty). Practice parameters cannot be determined on the basis of level IV or level V evidence, and these studies were excluded from the formulation of treatment recommendations.

Objectives and Paper Selection Criteria

The objective of this systematic review was to address the following four questions:

1. *What provides optimal external immobilization in the nonoperative management of Anderson-D'Alonzo type II and type III odontoid fractures in adults: halo versus brace?*
2. *What is the optimal management for type II odontoid fractures in adults: nonoperative versus operative treatment?*
3. *What produces better outcome in the surgical treatment of Anderson-D'Alonzo type II odontoid fractures in adults: anterior versus posterior fixation?*
4. *What is the optimal treatment of type II and type III odontoid fractures in elderly patients?*

The criteria for identifying the subset of data pertaining to *Question 1* (halo vs brace) of external immobilization in the definitive treatment of odontoid type II and type III fractures consisted of data collected from: (1) clinical studies that compared halo vest versus bracing; (2) clinical studies in which both halo vest and cervical bracing were utilized; and, (3) clinical studies that focused solely on either halo vest or brace immobilization.

The criteria for identifying the subset of data pertaining to *Question 2* (nonoperative vs operative) definitive treatment of type II odontoid fractures consisted of data collected from (1) clinical studies that compared any type of nonoperative treatment with any type of operative treatment; and (2) clinical studies in which both operative and nonoperative treatment modalities were utilized.

The criteria for identifying the subset of data pertaining to *Question 3* (posterior vs anterior fixation) as definitive treatment of type II odontoid fracture consisted of data collected from (1) clinical studies that compared anterior versus posterior operative treatment; (2) clinical studies that included both anterior and posterior fixation; (3) clinical studies that

focused solely on posterior fixation (wiring, clamps, transarticular screws); and (4) clinical studies that focused solely on anterior fixation (single or double screws).

The criteria for identifying the subset of data pertaining to *Question 4* (elderly patients treated for type II and type III odontoid fractures) consisted of data collected from (1) clinical studies that compared treatment of elderly versus nonelderly patients; (2) clinical studies that focused solely on treatment of elderly patients; and (3) clinical studies in which data pertaining to elderly patients could be extracted from a larger series. For the purpose of this review *elderly* was defined as greater or equal to 60 years of age.

◆ Results

The computerized search of the National Library of Medicine and Medline yielded a total of 443 papers published between May 1965 and November 2007. Papers published prior to the advent of the Anderson-D'Alonzo classification[1] (13 papers) were excluded. Among the remaining 430 articles, 227 pertinent papers were selected; all of these reported the treatment of odontoid type II and/or III fractures. The independent reviewers categorized the selected articles in accordance with their level of evidence as follows: level I—0; level II—4; level III—89; level IV—98; level V—36 (**Fig. 25.1**). There was no level I evidence study on odontoid fractures among the selected articles; therefore the authors were unable to establish practice standards in this chapter. There were only four level II evidence studies among the selected articles; therefore this chapter may consider providing some, albeit limited, practice guidelines. Level III evidence studies (89 papers) were used to establish practice options. All level IV and level V evidence studies (134 papers) were reviewed, but they were excluded because they cannot establish practice parameters in accordance with the criteria of the American Medical Association.

A total number of 35 papers pertaining to *Question 1* (halo vest vs brace) were identified following aforementioned criteria. All level II and level III evidence studies are listed in **Table 25.1** with their respective outcomes. Level II evidence was presented in two studies[4,5]; the other 33 studies consisted of level III evidence. Anderson et al prospectively studied

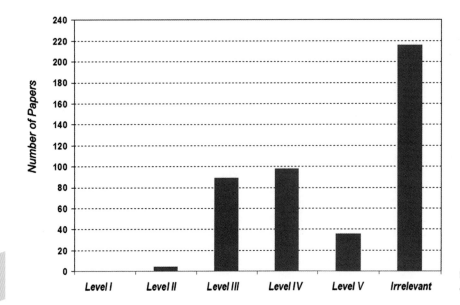

Fig. 25.1 Literature search results and the distribution according to the level of evidence.

Study	Year	Fracture Type	Definitive Therapy	Study Description	Level of Evidence	Outcome
Platzer et al[44]	2007	II	Halo vest	Retrospective review of 90 patients (48 F, 42 M; mean age 69; range 32–91 years) with > 2 year f/u	III	76 patients (84%) healed; 14 (12%) resulted in nonunion; failure to achieve/maintain reduction in 11 patients (12%); satisfaction rate 1.67 (1–4 excellent–poor scale); morbidity 14%; mortality 4%; patient age and initial displacement influenced outcome
Koivikko et al[9]	2004	II	Halo vest	Retrospective review of 69 patients (27 F, 43 M; mean age 57 years) with acute type II fractures to determine risk factors for developing nonunion; patients' follow-up (months): > 24 (10%), 12–24 (14%); 6–12 (36%), 3–6 (33%), < 3 (7%)	III	Union rate was 32 (46%) treated with halo; anterior dislocation, gender, age did correlate with nonunion; fracture gap (> 1 mm), posterior displacement (> 5 mm), delayed treatment (> 4 days, posterior redisplacement (> 2 mm) were risk factors for developing nonunion
Hosssain et al[45]	2004	II/III	Halo vest	Retrospective review of 104 patients (28 F, 76 M; mean age 49; range 32–91 years) with cervical spine injury; 34 injuries involved odontoid	III	Most common complication was loss of reduction and superficial pin-site infection; 17 cases of nonunion/instability; failure rate 10%; 7 patients (18%) resulted in odontoid nonunion
Müller et al[46]	2003	II/III	Brace	Retrospective review of 26 patients (13 F, 13 M; mean age 59; range 15–86 years) with stable odontoid fractures (nondisplaced or minimally displaced); 19 type II; 7 type III	III	Overall complication rate was 11.4%; 20 patients (77%) healed uneventfully; nonunion rate was 15%; and fusion rate 73.7 for type II and 85.7% for type III fractures; 39% of patients were symptom-free at follow-up; 1 pulmonary embolism; 2 loss of reduction requiring internal fixation
Komadina et al[47]	2003	II/III	Halo vest	Retrospective review of 15 patients (2 F; 13 M; mean age 39; range 17–65 years) with type II (10) and type III (5) odontoid fractures	III	Fracture consolidated in 12 (86%) patients; 2 (14%) type II fractures resulted in nonunion; 9 (64%) patients had no complaints; 4 had pain; 9 (64%) patients had normal range of neck motion
Marton et al[48]	2000	I/II/III	Brace Halo vest Surgery	Retrospective review of 29 patients with odontoid type I (1); type II (22) type III (6); 6 type II (mean age 25 years) and 6 type III (mean age 29 years) treated with halo vest; treatment selection based on the fracture displacement	III	5 (83%) type II and 6 (83%) type III resulted in fracture consolidation; 1 type II required halo repositioning; halo vest deemed suitable for young patients with nondisplaced fractures
Cosan TE et al[8]	2001	II	Brace	Retrospective review of 24 upper cervical spine injuries treated with Philadelphia collar for 12 wks; among which were 7 odontoid type II fractures	III	All patients treated successfully with Philadelphia collar alone; those with neurological deficit required decompression surgery
Govender et al[49]	2000	II/III	Brace	Retrospective review of 183 patients (20 F; 163 M; mean age 37; range 18–64 years) with odontoid fractures (109 type II, 74 type III) treated nonoperatively; SOMI brace was used in 120 and a Minerva cast in 63 patients	III	59 (54%) with type II fractures united, 19 (17%) developed fibrous union, 31 (29%) nonunion; all type III fractures united, but in 16 delayed union and 21 malunion occurred; age > 40 and late presentation presented greater risk of nonunion

(Continued on page 232)

Study	Year	Fracture Type	Definitive Therapy	Study Description	Level of Evidence	Outcome
Ziai and Hurlbert[25]	2000	I/II/III	Brace Halo vest Surgery	Retrospective review of 520 patients with cervical spine injury; there were 93 patients (35 F, 58 M; mean age 57, range 16–54 years) with acute (85) and chronic (8) dens fractures; there were 1 type I; 57 type II (67%), and 27 type III (32%) acute dens fractures; 64 were conservatively, and 20 surgically treated	III	In 45 nonsurgically treated patients, overall union was 34 (76%); 8 type II, 3 type III fractures went into nonunion; nonunion rate was 24% for halo, 32% for hard collar; 17% for SOMI brace; and 66% for Guilford brace
Razak et al[50]	1998	II/III	Halo	Cross-sectional study of 53 patients (9 F, 44 M, mean age 33 years) with cervical spine injury treated with halo; there were 4 type II, and 7 type III dens fractures	III	All halo-treated dens fractures united demonstrating clinical union at 11 weeks for type II and 10 weeks for type III dens fractures
Lennarson et al[51]	2000	II	Halo vest	Retrospective review of 33 patients (13 F; 20 M, mean age 49 years) with isolated odontoid type II fracture; included 22 fused (controls) versus 11 nonunion (cases) patients all treated with halo vest were analyzed and compared	III	The only statistically significant difference (*p* = 0.002) between the union and nonunion groups was age (mean 41 vs 66 years, respectively); risk of nonunion for type II dens fracture treated with halo was 21 times greater in patients > 50 years old
Stoney et al[52]	1998	II	Halo vest	Retrospective review of 22 patients with type II odontoid fractures treated with halo vest; 18 patients were assessed radiographically and subjectively at a mean of 40 months postinjury	III	Overall union rate was 82%; posterior malunion had higher incidence of pain, although it did not correlate with cervical stiffness; nonunion patients (18%) did not have neurological sequelae, but they had more pain; nonunion was associated with extension-type injury, age over 65 years, and delayed diagnosis
Greene et al[12]	1997	I/II/III	Brace Halo vest Surgery	Retrospective review of 340 patients (131 F, 209 M; median age 41 years) with acute axis fractures; there were 199 (59%) of dens fractures; 2 were type I; 120 type II, and 77 type III; halo treatment was for 81 type II and 67 type III, SOMI brace for 9 type II and 3 type III with; Philadelphia collar for 5 type II	III	For 88 type II patients treated nonoperatively, overall nonunion rate was in 25 (28%); fracture displacement > 6 mm had 86% nonunion rate; displacement < 6 mm had 18% nonunion rate; for 69 type III patients treated nonoperatively, overall union rate was 1.4%
Chiba et al[13]	1996	I/II/III	Traction Brace Halo cast Minerva cast Surgery	Retrospective review of 104 patients (25 F, 79 M; mean age 35 years) with odontoid fracture; there were 2 type I; 62 type II, and 32 type III dens fractures; 37 patients were managed nonoperatively; patients were divided into 2 groups: fresh (72) treated definitively within 3 weeks; and old (32) delayed treated postinjury (extended time in traction)	III	Type II dens fractures had overall 60% nonunion, 20% malunion, and 10% union rates; type III had overall 6% nonunion, 29% malunion, 65% union rates; device-specific nonunion, malunion, union rates were: Minerva cast, 2, 2, 7; brace 2, 5, 5; halo 2, 0, 6, respectively

Table 25.1 Papers Pertaining to *Question 1* (Halo vs. Brace) Identified in Accordance with the Criteria of the American Medical Association (*Continued*)

Study	Year	Fracture Type	Definitive Therapy	Study Description	Level of Evidence	Outcome
Polin et al[53]	1996	II/III	Philadelphia collar Halo vest	Retrospective review of 54 patients (16 F, 38 M; mean age 50 years) dens fracture; there were 36 type II fractures (20 halo vest; 16 collar); there were 18 type III fractures (18 halo vest; 5 collar)	III	For type II patients, union rate for halo was 74% versus collar 53%, despite age difference (mean age 68 vs 44 years, respectively); 18 (100%) type III patients resulted in union; clinical efficacy of halo and collar was deemed equivalent
Pointillart et al[11]	1994	I/II/III	Minerva brace Surgery	Retrospective review of 150 patients (51 F, 99 M; mean age 54 years) dens fracture; there 3% type I, 52% type II, and 46% type III fractures; 61 patients were treated nonoperatively	III	Overall nonunion rate for polyethylene Minerva cast was 23% (15); most nonunions occurred in elderly patients
Van Holsbeek et al[54]	1993	I/II/III	Halo vest Minerva cast Surgery	Retrospective review of 33 patients (6 F, 27 M; mean age 36 years) dens fracture; there were 1 type I, 28 type II, and 4 type III fractures	III	Nonoperative treatment resulted in 48.5% of type II fractures; all type III fractures united
Anderson et al[4]	1991	II/III	Halo vest	Prospective study of 42 patients (14 F, 28 M; mean age 40, range 2–92) with cervical spine injury treated with halo vest; 39 patients were treated with halo vest primarily; for others halo vest was supplemental stabilization; there were 10 type II and 9 type III odontoid fractures	II	Radiographically determined average fracture site translation and angulation was 1.85 mm and 9 degrees for type II and 1.6 mm and 6.3 degrees for type III fractures, respectively; 13 fractures united, 6 type II lost reduction and produced nonunion
Hadley et al[55]	1989	II/III	Brace Halo vest Surgery	Retrospective review of 229 axis fracture patients; 67 type II odontoid fractures were treated with halo vest (65), SOMI (8), collar (2); type III odontoid fractures were treated with halo vest (46) and SOMI (2)	III	Nonunion rate for type II fractures was 28% (2 treated with halo vest, 1 SOMI, 2 collar); fracture displacement < 6 mm had 10% nonunion rate, whereas > 6 mm had 78% nonunion rate; 14 failed patients were treated surgically
Bucholz and Cheung[10]	1989	II/III	Halo vest Surgery	Retrospective review of 233 patients with cervical spine injury treated with halo versus surgery; there were 17 type II, and 9 type III patients with odontoid fracture treated with halo immobilization	III	13 (88%) type II fractures and 9 (100%) type III fractures united when treated with halo; 3 halo-treated odontoid fracture patients died from cardiopulmonary complications; halo immobilization was deemed as a reliable treatment option for cervical injuries to include type II/III odontoid fractures
Fujii et al[21]	1988	I/II/III	Brace Minerva cast Surgery	Retrospective review of 52 patients with odontoid fractures; there were 2 type I, 31 type II, and 19 type III; 24 patients treated nonoperatively	III	Overall nonunion rate was 21% (5); in type II fractures there were 3 (43%) unions and 4 (57%) nonunions; type III there were 10 union (71%), 3 malunions (21%), 1 (7%) nonunion; 80% nonunions occurred in the elderly (> 60 years)
Govender and Grootboom[56]	1988	II/III	Traction Collar	Retrospective review of 41 patients (6 F, 36 M; median age 32) with odontoid fractures; there were 26 type II and 15 type III; 24 patients treated with traction (1 month) and subsequent (1 month) with rigid collar	III	For type II fusion rate was 73% (19); there were 2 fibrous unions (8%), and 5 nonunions (19%); type III: 15 fusions (100%); complications included 7 tongs pin infections, 3 skin wounds due to halter traction

(Continued on page 234)

Study	Year	Fracture Type	Definitive Therapy	Study Description	Level of Evidence	Outcome
Lind et al[5]	1988	II/III	Halo vest	Prospective study of 83 consecutive patients (27 F, 56 M; mean age 38 years) with unstable spine injury treated with halo vest; 67 patients had follow-up 2–7 years (mean 3 years); there were 11 type II and, 6 type III odontoid fractures	II	Nonunion rate for odontoid fracture was 6% (1 type II); the halo complications for the C-spine series included pin loosening 60%; pin infection 22%; restricted ventilation 8%; pneumonia 5%; pressure sores 4%; redislocation 10%; at long-term follow-up, 24% were symptom-free; 35% had stiffness; 19% pain in subjective evaluation
Schweigel[57]	1987	II/III	Halo vest	Retrospective review of 65 patients (24 F,41 M; mean age 49, range 16–87 years) with odontoid fractures; 28 type II and 19 type III fractures treated with halo-thoracic brace	III	From 47 patients, only 4 (3 type II; 1 type III) developed nonunion after an average of 8 weeks of halo treatment; rate of bony union was 91%; problems with halo were reported as minimal
Hanssen and Cabanela[58]	1987	II/III	Halo vest Halo cast	Retrospective review of 42 consecutive patients (12 F, 30 M; mean age 50, range 14–87 years) with dens fracture; there were 26 type II, 16 type III fractures; 32 patients were followed up	III	Mortality was 19% for type II dens fractures; 75% nondisplaced type II united; all type III fractures united; posterior displacement of type II dens fractures was associated with high mortality and nonunion rate
Lind et al[59]	1987	II/III	Halo vest	Retrospective review of 14 patients (6 F, 8 M; mean age 50, range 22–89) with odontoid fractures; there were 9 type II and, 5 type III	III	Overall union rate was 91% (10) for type II and III combined; complications included skin ulcer, pressure sore, pain at pin sites, neck stiffness
Dunn and Seljeskog[60]	1986	II/III	Halo	Retrospective review of 128 patients (43 F, 85 M; age range 22–89) with odontoid fractures; among 110 acute fractures were 88 type II and 22 type III; 18 chronic injuries were type II; 80 treated with external stabilization	III	For type II union rate was 68% (40), nonunion rate 32% (19); for type III union rate was 100% (15); halo was deemed suitable for all type III and type II with early (< 1 week) diagnosis, < 65 years of age, nondisplaced, displaced anteriorly, or posteriorly (< 2 mm)
Clark and White[6]	1985	II/III	Traction Collar Halo	Multicenter retrospective review of 96 type II dens fx patients (28 F, 68 M; mean age 43 years) and 48 type III dens fx patients (17 F, 31 M, mean age 44 years); 38 type II were treated with halo, and 3 with orthosis; 16 type III were treated with halo and 10 with orthosis	III	Type II union rate was 66% (25) for halo and 0% (3) for orthosis; type III union rate was 100% (16) for halo, and 90% (9 incl. 4 malunion) for orthosis
Hadley et al[61]	1985	II/III	Brace Halo vest	Retrospective review of 107 patients (38 F, 69 M; mean age 40 years) with axis fractures; there were 40 type II and 19 type III; 29 were treated with halo, 6 with SOMI, and 2 with collar	III	Nonunion rate was 26% for minimally displaced (< 6 mm) vs 67% for displaced (> 6 mm) type II fractures regardless of patient age or displacement direction; 6 (25%) halo and 2 (20%) SOMI patients produced nonunion; halo had shorter time to union than SOMI; 100% halo treated type III fractures healed
Wang et al[62]	1984	I/II/III	Brace Halo	Retrospective review of 25 patients (7 F, 18 M, mean 40, range 17–80 years) with odontoid fracture; there were 1 type I, 12 type II, and 12 type III fractures; 15 patients underwent external immobilization	III	Overall union rate was 80% for type II and 100% for type III; halo produced fewer nonunions (20%) compared with brace (57%) of type II patients; displacement strongly affected union in type II but not type III fractures

Table 25.1 Papers Pertaining to *Question 1* (Halo vs. Brace) Identified in Accordance with the Criteria of the American Medical Association (*Continued*)

Study	Year	Fracture Type	Definitive Therapy	Study Description	Level of Evidence	Outcome
Maiman and Larson[7]	1982	II/III	Minerva Surgery	Retrospective review of 51 patients (11 F, 40 M, age range 15–80 years) with odontoid fracture; there were 49 type II, and 2 type III fractures; 15 patients underwent external immobilization	III	100% (15) type II fractures treated conservatively failed to heal; 100% (2) type III fractures united
Ryan and Taylor[63]	1982	I/II/III	Minerva Halo cast	Retrospective review of 23 patients (6 F, 17 M; mean age 44 years) with odontoid fractures; there was 1 type I, 16 type II, 6 type III dens fractures	III	Fusion rates were 60% (9) for type II, 100% (6) for type III; all Minerva-treated patients healed, 66% halo cast treated united
Ekong et al[64]	1981	II/III	Halo	Retrospective review of 22 patients (6 F, 16 M; mean age 53, range 20–86 years) with odontoid fractures treated with halo device for 3 months; there were 15 type II, 6 type III dens fractures; 18 patients had f/u > 6 months	III	Fusion rate was 50% (6) for type II, and 80% (4) for type III fractures; mortality was 16% (4) (3 type II, 1 type III); nonunion was associated with posterior displacement
Anderson and D'Alonzo[1]	1974	I/II/III	Traction Brace	Retrospective review of 60 patients with odontoid fractures; 49 patients (mean age 41 years) had f/u for > 6 months; there were 2 type I, 32 type II, 15 type III	III	Fusion rate for type II was 64% (14); nonunion occurred in 5 nondisplaced in 3 displaced type II; fusion rate for type III was 92% (14); nonunion in 8% (1)

Abbreviations: fx, fracture; SOMI, sterno-occipital-mandibular immobilizer; Tx, treatment.

39 patients with a variety of cervical spine injuries definitively treated with a halo vest. Among these patients were 10 type II and nine type III odontoid fractures. All type III odontoid fractures healed, whereas two thirds (six) lost reduction and produced nonunion. The study suggests that the halo vest can result in a significant amount of angular and translational motion in patients with type II odontoid fractures and increases the risk of nonunion.

Lind et al[5] also prospectively analyzed 83 unstable cervical spine injury patients treated with the halo vest. Among these patients were 11 type II and six type III odontoid fractures. Although the overall nonunion rate was only 6% (one type II), the incidence of halo-related complications was considerable and included pin loosening (60%), pin infection (22%), loss of reduction (10%), restricted ventilation (8%), pneumonia (5%), and pressure sores (4%). Long-term, 35% of patients had neck stiffness and 19% persistent neck pain.

Among the level III studies reviewed, the odontoid type II fracture union rate for bracing varies considerably (0 to 100%).[6–8] It remains unclear, however, which type II injury patients will benefit from this treatment modality. Although the halo vest provides better stability, its reported union rate can vary from 46[9] to 88%.[10] Overall much lower union rate for cervical bracing in select patients may be offset by being better tolerated, whereas the overall high fusion rate for the halo vest may be compromised by the inherent complications associated with the device.

A total number of 14 papers pertaining to *Question 2* (nonoperative vs operative) were identified in accordance with the criteria of the American Medical Association. All studies consisted of level III evidence and are listed in **Table 25.2** with their respective outcomes. Among the larger studies, nonoperative treatment consistently demonstrated a high incidence of nonunion, which ranged from 20 up to 100%.[6,7,11] Nonoperative treatment appeared to be most effective for fractures that were stable or minimally displaced.[12] Operative treatment significantly decreased the incidence of nonunion, and reports range from 0 to 10%[7,13]; moreover, operative treatment has proven successful in salvaging fractures that have failed nonoperative treatment.[14]

A total number of 42 papers pertaining to *Question 3* (anterior vs posterior fixation) were identified in accordance with the criteria of the American Medical Association. All level II and III evidence studies are listed in **Table 25.3** with their respective outcomes. Level II evidence was present in one study[15]; all other studies consisted of level III evidence. ElSaghir and Böhm prospectively studied 30 patients with type II odontoid fractures and a mean age of 45 years (range 21 to 78 years) treated with double anterior screw fixation.[15] All fractures healed without major complications, and the authors concluded that this technique permitted excellent fracture healing with minimal functional compromise.

Among the level III studies reviewed, anterior surgery achieved excellent healing with anterior screw fixation demonstrating union rates ranging from 75 to 100%.[16,17] These excellent results were achieved with a variety of screws (i.e., noncannulated, cannulated, Herbert screws, etc.); furthermore, equally impressive results were realized in studies that specifically compared single versus double anterior screw fixation.[18,19] Compared with younger patients, however, this

Table 25.2 Nonoperative versus Operative Treatment

Study	Year	Definitive Therapy	Study Description	Level of Evidence	Outcome
Marton et al[48]	2000	Collar Halo vest Anterior screw Posterior wiring	Retrospective review of 58 cervical spine injuries; there were 29 odontoid fractures (22 type II, 6 type III); type II treatment: 1 cervical collar, 6 halo vest, 12 anterior screws, 3 posterior wiring, 1 anterior fixation	III	All fractures consolidated with surgical treatment; one patient lost alignment; his halo vest required surgery
Vieweg et al[65]	2000	Brace Halo vest Posterior screws Gallie fusion	Retrospective review of 70 upper cervical spine injuries treated both operatively and nonoperatively; there were fxs treated with odontoid screws (23); posterior fusion (3); halo-vest (3); cervical collar (2)	III	One cervical collar nonunion, 1 halo vest infection, 3 anterior screws instability; all other fractures healed uneventfully
Ziai and Hurlbert[25]	2000	Soft collar Brace Halo vest Anterior screw Posterior fusion	Retrospective review of 93 odontoid patients. There were 57 type II injuries; type II fractures treated halo vests (17), hard collar (13), SOMI brace (5), soft collar (1), anterior screw (11), and anterior screw (11), and posterior cervical fusion/type unknown (4)	III	Anterior screw all healed; posterior fusion all healed (one loss of reduction), eight nonunions with external fixation
Daneyemez et al[66]	1999	Collar Surgery	Retrospective review of 235 patients with cervical spine injuries; 5 odontoid fractures; number of type II unknown; odontoid fractures treated with cervical collar (4), surgery (1)	III	One odontoid fracture treated with cervical collar lost reduction requiring posterior fusion and transoral odontoidectomy
Seybold and Bayley[14]	1998	Hard collar Halo vest Surgery	Retrospective review of 57 patients with odontoid fractures; among were type II; patients treated with posterior fusion (type and number unknown), Philadelphia collar (number unknown), and halo vests (number unknown)	III	Type II halo vests healing 65% (15 of 23), five type II treated with posterior fusion (4 of 6) (1 type III displaced posteriorly); one type II treated in Philadelphia collar and Philadelphia displaced posteriorly
Greene et al[12]	1997	Hard collar Halo vest Surgery	Retrospective review of 340 patients with axis fracture; among them were 120 type II odontoid fractures; type II treated with halo vests (81), SOMI (9), Philadelphia collar (5)	III	Type II treated with halo vest 28% nonunion (25/88), when dense displacement 6 mm or greater nonunion was 86%, 20 type II treated surgically (posterior wiring, anterior odontoid screws) with outcome unclear; this study concludes surgery is indicated when dens displacement > 6 mm
Chiba et al[13]	1996	Plaster cast Brace Halo vest Surgery	Retrospective review of 104 patients with odontoid fractures; there were 62 type II; plaster cast/SOMI/Philadelphia brace (15), halo vests (3), anterior screw fixation (36), transoral anterior fusion (7), posterior fusion Gallie/Brooks (8)	III	Type II fractures failed to heal with cervical collar or brace (2 of 3), halo vests (1 of 3), anterior screw (4 of 46), transoral anterior fusion (2 of 7), posterior arthrodesis (all 9 patients healed)

Table 25.2 Nonoperative versus Operative Treatment (*Continued*)

Study	Year	Definitive Therapy	Study Description	Level of Evidence	Outcome
Pointillart et al[11]	1994	Minerva brace Surgery	Retrospective review of 150 odontoid fractures; there were 81 type II; acute fracture nonunions following (a) traction/Minerva (23%), (b) 19 posterior wirings (20%), and (c) 43 anterior screw(s) (5%)	III	Traction/Minerva (unclear); surgery (anterior screws/ posterior wiring) (unclear). Authors state that anterior screw decreased nonunion from 20% to 5%
Fujii et al[21]	1988	Plaster cast Brace Halo vests Surgery	Retrospective review of 58 odontoid fractures; there were 31 type II treated plaster cast/brace/traction/halo vest (9), surgically (transoral anterior screw, posterior fusion) (19)	III	Outcome 4 of 9 type II treated halo vest nonunion; 4 nonunions postsurgery (type unknown). Authors conclude halo vests appropriate for stable, well-aligned type II fracture.
Clark and White[6]	1985	Nil Traction Brace Halo vest Surgery	Retrospective review 156 odontoid fractures; there were 106 type II fractures received no treatment (18), brace (3), posterior fusion (26), anterior fusion (8), halo casts (38), total traction (3)	III	Nonunion following orthosis (all 21), halo vests (7 of 38 were or 18%), halo vest displacement (2 or 5%), halo vests malunion (3 or 8%), anterior fusion (1 of 8 or 12%) posterior fusion (1 of 25 or 4%). The authors advocate posterior fusion opposed to halo vest.
Hadley et al[61]	1985	Traction Collar Brace Halo vest Surgery	Retrospective review of 107 axis fractures; there were 40 type II; type II fractures were treated posterior surgery (2), and traction/halo vests/ SOMI/collar (38)	III	Nonunion occurred in traction/halo brace (8 of 31 or 26%). The authors recommend early posterior surgery for displacement greater than 6 mm.
Maiman and Larson[7]	1982	Traction Minerva cast Surgery	Retrospective review of 52 odontoid fractures; there were 49 type II; type II treated traction/Minerva cast (15), posterior cervical fusion (34)	III	Nonunion traction/Minerva (all 15 patients), posterior cervical fusion (0). The authors advocated posterior cervical fusion for type II fractures
Anderson and D'Alonzo[1]	1974	Brace Surgery	Retrospective review of 49 odontoid fractures; there were 32 type II fractures; type II fractures were treated in traction/brace (14), posterior wiring (18)	III	Nonunion and traction (5 of 14) surgery (2 of 10). The authors note a 36% nonunion rate with nonoperative treatment and advocate surgery.

Abbreviations: fx, fracture; SOMI, sterno-occipital-mandibular immobilizer; Tx, treatment.

Table 25.3 Papers Pertaining to *Question 3* (Anterior vs. Posterior Fixation) Identified in Accordance with the criteria of the American Medical Association

Study	Year	Definitive Therapy	Study Description	Level of Evidence	Outcome
Platzer et al[36]	2007	Anterior screw	Retrospective review of 110 type II odontoid fx treated with anterior screws (young patients compared with elderly)	III	Nonunion occurred in 3 of 69 younger patients and 5 of 41 patients older then 65 years (4 vs 12%). The authors conclude encouraging results achieved in both groups; anterior screw(s) superior with younger patients.
Stulik et al[67]	2007	Posterior screw	Retrospective review of 28 patients tx with posterior C1–2 screw rod fixation; among were 7 type II fx	III	All cases fused; all 56 C1 screws positioned correctly; 3 of 56 C2 malpositioned

(Continued on page 238)

Study	Year	Definitive Therapy	Study Description	Level of Evidence	Outcome
Lee and Sung[68]	2006	Anterior screw (Herbert)	Retrospective review of 20 consecutive type II and III odontoid fx Tx with anterior Herbert screw; there were 18 type II fx	III	1 fibrous union and 2 unions (all type II)
Moon et al[18]	2006	Anterior screw (single vs double)	Retrospective review of 32 type II and III odontoid fx Tx with 1 vs 2 anterior screw; there were 30 type II	III	All fxs healed. Authors conclude no difference single vs double anterior screws
Bhanot et al[69]	2006	Anterior screw	Retrospective review of 17 displaced type II odontoid fx Tx anterior screw	III	16 of 17 united; 1 nonunion; 2 screws in 3 patients, 1 patient with neurological deficit and 2 malpositioned hardware
Fountas et al[70]	2005	Anterior screw	Retrospective review of 50 type II/type III odontoid fx	III	Union in 38 of 42 patients (90.5%); incidence type II union unknown
Fountas et al[71]	2005	Anterior screw	Retrospective review of 38 consecutive type II/III odontoid fx Tx with anterior screw	III	Union 27(87%); nonunion in 4 (number of type II unknown; ¾ nonunions stable, only ¼ unstable; 96% all fxs stable
Börm et al[16]	2003	Anterior screw (double)	Retrospective review of 27 type II Tx with double anterior screw	III	Union in 11 of 15 (73%) >70-year-old patients; in 9 of 12 <70 years old (75%) complications (medical) 20% (3) elderly patients; 8%(1) young patients. The authors conclude anterior odontoid screw not affected by patient age.
Cornefjord et al[26]	2003	Posterior fusion (Olerud claw)	Retrospective review 26 consecutive patients Tx with posterior C1–C2 fusion; 18 odontoid fx; 14 type II fx	III	20 patients united; 6 patients died from unrelated causes. Authors conclude technique affective.
Alfieri[17]	2001	Halo vest Anterior screw Posterior fusion	Retrospective review of 17 consecutive cases of acute odontoid fx Tx with halo vest, anterior screw (9) and posterior fixation	III	All 9 anterior screw patients healed without complication.
Marton et al[48]	2000	Collar Halo vest Anterior screws Posterior wiring Odontoidectomy	Retrospective review 58 cases of upper cervical spine injuries; there were 22 type II; type II fx were Tx with halo vest (6), anterior screw (11), cervical collar (1), posterior wiring (3)	III	All surgical procedures healed without incident; loss of alignment occurred for type II fx - Tx with halo vest (1) and collar (1)
ElSaghir and Böhm[15]	2000	Anterior screw (double)	Prospective study of 30 type II odontoid fx Tx with double anterior screws	II	All fx healed with no major complications.
Vieweg et al[65]	2000	Halo vest Anterior screw Posterior screws Posterior wiring	Retrospective study of 70 patients with upper cervical spine injuries; there were 23 type II; type II Tx included collar (2) halo vest (3), anterior screw (18), posterior fusion (3)	III	Among type II fx, nonunion with collar with collar (½), infection with halo vest and/or instability with anterior screw (3/18)
Ziai and Hurlbert[25]	2000	Halo vest Collar brace Anterior screw Posterior fusion	Retrospective study of 93 odontoid fx Tx halo vest, collar, brace, anterior screw and posterior fusion; among were 57 type II; type II fx were Tx with halo vest (17), collar (14), brace (7), anterior screw (13), posterior fusion (4)	III	Type II anterior screw union (5; 7 lost to follow up and 1 death); posterior fusion (4 unions; 1 lost to fu; 2 deaths); patients Tx with external fixation experienced 19 unions/8 nonunion/7 lost to fu/ 4 dead. The authors ruled halo immobilization was 70% successful for type II fractures; of all anterior screw patients available for follow-up (9/13) healed.

Study	Year	Definitive Therapy	Study Description	Level of Evidence	Outcome
Apfelbaum et al[22]	2000	Anterior screw	Retrospective review of 147 type II and III odontoid fx Tx with anterior screw; among were 138 type II; 104 double screw; 25 single screw	III	Nonunion occurred in 10 patients (9%) (number of type II unknown) Post operative hardware complications occurred in 10 (9%) (number of type II unknown) 5 patients with screw back out. The authors conclude that anterior screw 85–91% successful in the acute setting.
Henry et al[72]	1999	Anterior screw	Retrospective review of 81 type II and III odontoid fx Tx with anterior screw; there were 29 type II	III	Union 61 patients; nonunion 3 patients (5%); 11 lost to follow-up. The authors conclude anterior screw valid option.
Subach et al[73]	1999	Anterior screw	Retrospective review of 26 consecutive patients with type II odontoid fx Tx with odontoid screw fixation	III	Union occurred in 25 of 26 patients (96%); 2 technical difficulties occurred related to the placement; overall technical difficulties 2 of 26 (8%)
Guiot and Fessler[74]	1999	Halo vest Anterior screw Posterior screws	Retrospective review of 10 cases of complex C1–C2 injuries; series includes 9 complex type II odontoid injuries, type II injuries Tx with anterior screw (6), posterior transarticular screw (2), and transarticular screw in combination with odontoid screw (1)	III	Type II patient died; 8 remaining type II fx healed uneventfully
Morandi et al[75]	1999	Anterior screw	Retrospective review of 17 odontoid fx Tx with anterior screw; number of type II fx unknown	III	1 posteriorly malpositioned screw with loss of dens alignment; significant limitation of cervical rotation in 2 patients, outcome otherwise uneventful
Jenkins et al[19]	1998	Anterior screw (single vs double)	Retrospective review of 42 patients with type II odontoid fx all Tx with anterior screws; single screw 20 patients; double screw 22 patients	III	Union 13/16 single screws; of the 3 failures, 2 experienced screw fracture; adequate union 17/20 double screw patients; nonunion 3 patients (15%); there were no broken screws. The authors conclude anterior screws to be safe but achieve union rate ~83%; no difference between single and double screws.
Greene et al[12]	1997	Collar Brace Halo vest Anterior screw Posterior wiring/ clamps/facet screw	Retrospective review of 340 consecutive cases of acute access fx and their operative or nonoperative management; there were 120 type II fx; 20 Tx with early surgery	III	Of the 95 patients Tx with external immobilization, 88 would be followed and nonunion occurred in 25 (28.4%). The outcome of surgical management is unclear.
Chiba et al[13]	1996	Anterior screw Transoral fusion Posterior fusion	Retrospective review of 104 odontoid fx there were 62 type II; type II fx Tx anterior screw fixation (36), transoral fixation (7), posterior fusion (7)	III	Nonunion 3 cases through extrusion 1 case 2 transoral nonunion (both type II fx), 3 posterior fusions nonunion (2 of 3 type II). The authors advocate anterior screw for type II fx.
Huang and Chen[76]	1996	Posterior Halifax clamp fusion (with halo vest) Anterior screws	Retrospective review 38 patients with atlantoaxial instability; 5 Tx with odontoid screws; 33 Tx with posterior Halifax clamp	III	All fx healed; complications secondary to halo pin loosening and central retinal artery occlusion
Fairholm et al[77]	1996	Posterior screws Transoral decompression	Retrospective review of 51 consecutive patients with undiagnosed or untreated odontoid fx; number of type II unknown; C1 all Tx posterior C1–C2 fusion; 12 with transoral decompression	III	Neurologic recovery excellent in 34 patients; status of fusion union/alignment unclear

(Continued on page 240)

Table 25.3 Papers Pertaining to *Question 3* (Anterior vs. Posterior Fixation) Identified in Accordance with the criteria of the American Medical Association (*Continued*)

Study	Year	Definitive Therapy	Study Description	Level of Evidence	Outcome
Rainov et al[78]	1996	Anterior screw (single)	Retrospective review of 35 cases of odontoid fx Tx with single anterior screws; 30 cases type II	III	Acute fx union 100% (32 patients); anterior screw advocated
Coyne et al[79]	1995	Posterior fusion	Retrospective review of 32 patients with C1–2 instability wiring/fusion; there were 18 type II odontoid fx	III	Among the type II 2 of 18 failed (11%). The authors advocate posterior fusion.
Pointillart et al[11]	1994	Traction Minerva brace, Anterior screw Posterior fusion	Retrospective review of 150 odontoid fx, among which type II (51%) were treated with anterior screw fixation	III	129 patients followed; nonunion occurred in 23% of the 61 external immobilized, 20% of the 19 posterior arthrodesis and 5% of the 43 anterior fixation (number of type II unknown). The authors advocate anterior screw fixation.
Chang et al[80]	1994	Anterior Screw (single, double)	Retrospective review of 12 displaced type II odontoid fx; 7 fx completely reduced and tx with double Herbert screws, 5 fx incompletely reduced and Tx with single Herbert screw	III	All 7 double screw fxs healed w/o loss alignment; all 5 single screw fxs healed, but with mean 0.8 mm anterior displacement and 5-degree anterior angulation
Verheggen et al[81]	1994	Anterior screw	Retrospective review of 18 patients with type II/III odontoid fx Tx with anterior screw fixation; 16 cases were type II	III	Union occurred in 17/18 patients (94%); number of type II unknown; complications include wound infections (1) and loss of alignment with nonunion (1); number of type II unknown; complication rate 11%
Chiba et al[82]	1993	Anterior screw	Retrospective review of 45 patients with odontoid fx Tx with anterior screw; 35 were type II	III	Union occurred in 44 of 45 cases 93%, fx stability and alignment was lost in 2 cases requiring halo vest, and prominent post operative osteophyte occurred in 1 patient for a total of 5 (complications were 11%). The authors advocate anterior screw fixation although they recognize the risk for complication.
Jeanneret and Magerl[83]	1992	Anterior screws Transarticular screws	Retrospective review of 14 patients (6 F, 8 M; mean age 52, range 19–75 years) with type II (4) and III (10) odontoid fractures treated with posterior fusion (2) or transarticular screws (12)		All fractures united; average operative time was comparable for transarticular screws than for Gallie fusion (144 vs 150 minute); there were 2 complications with transarticular screws. Authors recommended transarticular screw fixation to Gallie fusion.
Esses and Bednar[84]	1991	Anterior screw	Retrospective review of 10 patients with acute odontoid fx and nonunion Tx with anterior screw fixation; 8 cases were type II; 4 of the 8 type II were nonunions	III	1 death; the 9 remaining fx healed; 1 complication was a malpositioned screw.
Rodrigues et al[24]	1991	Posterior fusion	Retrospective review of 33 cases of atlantoaxial arthrodesis number of type II unknown	III	100% union; 6 complications to include superficial wound infection (1), loss of fx alignment (1), broken wire (2), and neurological complications (2). The patients with neurological complications had displaced odontoid fx that could not be reduced.
Smith et al[85]	1991	Anterior screw (double)	Retrospective review of 23 patients Tx with anterior screw fixation: number of type II unknown	III	Union achieved in 92%; major complications 4 of 23 (17%); all due to technical issues. The authors advocate this technique, however, note that this is a demanding technique that should be performed only by an experienced surgeon.

Table 25.3 Papers Pertaining to *Question 3* (Anterior vs. Posterior Fixation) Identified in Accordance with the criteria of the American Medical Association (*Continued*)

Study	Year	Definitive Therapy	Study Description	Level of Evidence	Outcome
Montesano et al[86]	1991	Anterior screw	Retrospective review of 13 type II odontoid fx Tx with anterior screw fixation	III	1 death, 11 of 13 united, no neurological complications. The authors note this to be technically demanding and requires extensive preoperative planning.
Jeanneret et al[87]	1991	Anterior screw	Retrospective review of 16 patients (4 F, 12 M; mean age 34, range 14–74 years) treated with double anterior odontoid screws; 13 were followed up for mean 40 (range 7–82) months	III	No operative complications occurred; 100% (13) fractures healed; rotation was preserved in 40% of patients (average bilateral C1–C2 rotation was 25.2 degrees, head rotation 56 degrees. Decrease in rotations was affected by fracture pattern, quality of reduction, and patient's age
Geisler et al[88]	1989	Anterior screw (double)	Retrospective review of 9 type II odontoid patients with 15 mm displacement Tx with anterior screw	III	2 patients died (unrelated to surgery); 100% union in the 7 patients who survived. The authors recommend this procedure for displaced type II odontoid fx.
Fujii et al[21]	1988	Transoral fusion Anterior screw Posterior fusion	Retrospective review of 52 cases with odontoid fx Tx with anteriorly and posteriorly; 31 were type II; 9 type II Tx with traction then halo vest; 19 type II fx Tx surgically (specific technique unclear)	III	Nonunion in 4 of 9 type II Tx with halo vest; nonunion occurred in 2 of 10 anterior screws; 2 of 9 transoral fusions (both type II fractures). Authors recommend anterior screw for acute type II posterior fusion for displaced fractures.
Clark and White[6]	1985	Halo vest Posterior fusion	Retrospective review of 156 type II /III odontoid fx Rx either halo vest or posterior fusion; 106 type II fx; 96 type II fx studied; no Rx (18), brace (3), posterior fusion (26), anterior fusion (8), halo vest (38), traction (3)	III	Nonunion 34% type II Tx with halo; 6 (26%) of the 23 type II fx with significant failed to unite; 96% posterior healed; 7 of 8 (88%) anterior fusions healed. The authors prefer posterior fusion for type II fx, especially in displaced cases.
Waddell and Reardon[23]	1983	Posterior fusion	Retrospective review of 17 patients with odontoid fx; 16 cases type II fx all Tx with Gallie fusion	III	15 of 16 type II fx healed. Authors favor posterior fusion.
Maiman and Larson[7]	1982	Minerva cast Posterior fusion	Retrospective review of 51 patients with odontoid fx were retrospectively reviewed; 49 cases type II fx	III	Nonunion occurred in all (15) type II fx Tx nonoperatively; 25 type II fx Tx posterior fusion and all healed. The authors advocate posterior fusion.
Böhler et al[28]	1982	Anterior screw	Retrospective review of 15 odontoid fx Tx with odontoid screws 12 cases type II fx	III	All fx healed. The authors advocate this technique but only for surgeons experienced with anterior cervical surgery and the use of image of fluoroscopy and bone surgery.

Abbreviations: fx, fracture; Tx, treatment.

technique was reported to be less effective in the elderly with significantly lower union rate[20] and increased complication rate.[21] In a study by Apfelbaum et al,[22] postoperative anterior screw complications occurred in 9% of patients, with the most predominant being screw backout. The anterior screw fixation is demanding and is contraindicated in a setting where an acceptable reduction cannot be achieved.

Prior to the advent of appropriate screw technology, most reports advocated posterior laminar fixation (wiring, camps, claws) with bone graft. This technique also demonstrated a comparable union rate.[6,23–26] More recently, posterior fixation has evolved to include C1–C2 transarticular screw fixation,[27] and the success of this innovation has expanded the indications for posterior surgery to include a variety of complex upper cervical spine injuries. However, posterior fusion has consistently demonstrated greater compromise of neck mobility.[28]

The literature supports the use of both techniques. The anterior screw fixation seems to be preferred in suitable patients (good bone stock, adequate fracture alignment), although posterior fixation is an accepted alternative if the aforementioned criteria cannot be met.

25 Management of Type II and Type III Odontoid Fractures

241

A total number of 18 papers pertaining to *Question 4* (management of type II and III odontoid fractures in elderly patients) were identified in accordance with criteria of the American Medical Association. All level II and III evidence studies are listed in **Table 25.4** with their respective outcomes. Level II evidence was present in one study; all other studies consisted of level III evidence. Bednar et al[29] prospectively studied 11 type II odontoid fractures in patients with a mean age of 74 years (range 68 to 84) to determine the effects of early surgical stabilization on perioperative mortality. They developed and applied a protocol consisting of posterior fixation augmented with a Philadelphia collar following a brief period of bed rest. Apart from achieving a union rate of 91%, the authors were able to significantly decrease the intrahospital mortality (prior to the protocol intrahospital mortality was 27%).

Among the level III studies, halo vest management was associated with an inordinately high mortality rate (greater than 40%).[30,31] Of the elderly patients that survived, the union rate varied from 40 to 80% but was typically associated with a considerable decrease in neck motion and increase in residual neck pain.[20,32,33] More reliable results were achieved with surgical intervention, either with anterior screws[33–36] or with

Table 25.4 Papers Pertaining to *Question 4* (Management of Type II and III Odontoid Fractures in Elderly Patients) Identified in Accordance with the Criteria of the American Medical Association

Study	Year	Fracture Type	Definitive Therapy	Study Description	Level of Evidence	Outcome
Platzer et al[44]	2007	II	Halo vest	Retrospective review of 90 patients (48 F, 42 M; mean age 69, range 32–91 years) patients with 2-year follow-up	III	Union rate was 84% (76); of 14 (16%) nonunion patients 5 were treated with posterior fusion, 9 were symptomatic; 75 (83%) patients returned to preinjury activity level, 15 (17%) had pain and limitation of neck motion
Platzer et al.[36]	2007	II/III	Anterior screw Posterior arthrodesis	Retrospective review of 56 patients (31 F, 25 M; mean age 71.4, range 66–83 years) patients with dens fracture; there were 48 type II (37 treated with anterior and 11 posterior surgery), and 8 type III (all treated with posterior surgery)	III	Overall union rate was 93% (52); 92% for type II and 100% for type III; 4 nonunions were result for anterior screw fixation and had initial displacement > 2 mm; overall morbidity rate was 16%; surgery-related mortality was 6%
Platzer et al.[20]	2007	II	Anterior screw	Retrospective review of dens fracture 110 patients 59 F, 51 M; mean age of 54, range 7–83 years) treated with anterior screw; patients were compared based on age < 65 (mean 37) yrs vs > 65 years (mean 91)	III	Union rate was 93% (102); nongeriatric 4% vs geriatric 12%; overall morbidity was 14%; nongeriatric 8% vs geriatric 22%; overall mortality 4%; nongeriatric 1% vs geriatric 9%; 86% (95) had good functional outcome
Frangen et al[89]	2007	II	Posterior fusion	Retrospective review of 27 patients (17 F, 10 M; median age of 85, range, 63–98) treated with posterior C1/C2 transarticular screws and an additional modified Gallie fusion	III	6 patients died during follow-up (median 40 daysafter trauma), all from cardiopulmonary complications; of 21 surviving patients,20 fused at 3 months after trauma; patients had no long-term symptoms or minor pain
Tashjian et al[30]	2006	II/III	Orthosis halo vest Surgery	Retrospective review of 78 patients > 65 years of age, mean age 81 years) with odontoid fracture; there were 50 type II, 17 type III, and 11 combined fractures; 38 (49%) were treated with halo vest (34 halo primarily, 4 postsurgically); 40 (51%) were treated with hard collar (27 collar primarily, and 13 postsurgically)	III	Intrahospital mortality rate was 31% (24); mortality for halo vest treated patients was 42% vs 20% for non–halo vest; complications were in 66% of halo vest patients vs 36% in non–halo vest patients
Majercik et al[31]	2005		Halo vest	Retrospective review of patients with cervical spine injury treated with halo vest; there were 129 old (mean aged 79.7) and 289 young (mean age 38.3 years) patients	III	Mortality in geriatric was 40% vs 2% in nongeriatric patients; 14 geriatric patients died of pneumonia and 10 of cardiorespiratory arrest

Table 25.4 Papers Pertaining to *Question 4* (Management of Type II and III Odontoid Fractures in Elderly Patients) Identified in Accordance with the Criteria of the American Medical Association (*Continued*)

Study	Year	Fracture Type	Definitive Therapy	Study Description	Level of Evidence	Outcome
Börm et al[16]	2003	II	Anterior screw	Retrospective review of 27 patients with type II odontoid; 15 patients (> 70 years; mean 81) were compared with 12 patients (< 70 years; mean 49); mean follow-up 16.6 months; 15 patients had posterior displacement	III	In >70-year-old patients, fusion rate was 73% and 75% in <70 years patients; additional posterior stabilization was required in 13% vs 17%, respectively; morbidity was 20% vs 8%; overall mortality was 7% (1)
Kuntz et al[90]	2000	II	Orthosis Surgery	Retrospective review of 20 elderly (> 65 years) patients (8 F,12 M; mean age 80 years) treated with orthosis (12) or surgery (11) (anterior screws; posterior screws, or Gallie fusion)	III	Overall morbidity was 20% and mortality 10%; nonsurgical patients failure rate was 50% (6) nonunions and 1 death; surgical patients failure rate was of 9% (11), and 1 death
Harrop et al[35]	2000	II	Anterior screw	Retrospective review of 10 elderly (> 65 years) patients (4 F, 6 M, mean age 80, range 66–92 years) treated with anterior screws fixation; there were 8 posteriorly, and 2 anteriorly displaced (average 6 mm) fractures	III	Union rate was 70% (7); 1 patient with poor screw purchase healed with subsequent halo vest; nonunion occurred in 1 patient and was treated with posterior fusion
Hart et al[40]	2000	II/III	Symptomatic	Retrospective review of 5 elderly (> 70 years) patients with chronic odontoid nonunion without myelopathy were treated nonoperatively; 4 patients had type II, and 1 type III dens nonunion, mean follow-up was 4 years 7 months	III	2 patients had minor neck pain or headache, but no limitation in motion; mean range of motion was 40 degrees in flexion (30–45 degrees), mean extension 26 degrees (20–30 degrees); all patients had no neurological symptoms
Andersson et al[39]	2000	II/III	Orthosis halo vest Surgery	Retrospective review of 29 consecutive (> 65 years) patients (18 F, 18 M, mean age 78, range 66–99 years) with type II (24) and type III (5) dens fractures; 26 were neurologically intact, 3 had neurological symptoms (2 Frankel D, 1 C); 11 were treated with anterior screw; 7 with aposterior C1–C2 fusion; 10 conservatively (9 hard collar, 1 halo vest)	III	Overall mortality rate was 34%; healing rate 100% (7) patients with posterior fusion; 73% (8) for anterior screw fixation; in conservatively treated patients there was 60% (6) nonunions, there was 70% complication rate
Müller et al[91]	1999	II/III	Orthosis Minerva cast Halo vest Surgery	Retrospective review of 23 geriatric (> 70 years) patients (13 F, 10 M; mean age 81, range 71–96 years) with type II (22) and type III (1) odontoid fractures and 54 nongeriatric patients (16 F, 38 M, mean age 48, range 15–69 years) with type II (40) and type III (14) dens fractures	III	Neurological deficits occurred in 13% of both groups of patients and was mainly due to posterior fracture displacement; complication rate was 52.2% in the geriatric vs 32 in nongeriatric patients; associated C1 ring fracture was in 3.4% vs 18% patients, respectively; overall in-hospital mortality of 34.8%, (37% for nonoperative geriatric patients)

(Continued on page 244)

Study	Year	Fracture Type	Definitive Therapy	Study Description	Level of Evidence	Outcome
Campanelli et al[38]	1999	II	Posterior screws	Retrospective review of 7 geriatric patients (age range 63–88 years) with type II displaced odontoid fractures treated with C1–C2 posterior transarticular fixation	III	Union rate was 100% (7); there was 1 death during follow-up, and 2 within 1 year; 4 patients remained active and independent; there was 1 intraoperative vertebral artery injury although no clinical sequelae were observed
Berlemann and Schwarzenbach[33]	1997	II	Anterior screw	Retrospective review of 19 patients (> 65 years of age) with type II dens fractures treated; mean f/u of 4.5 years.	III	Surgery was tolerated well in all patients; union rate was 84% (16) at 3–6 months; there were 10% (20 nonunions that required no treatment; 15 patients became asymptomatic and regained function, 10 had diminished neck rotation
Bednar et al[29]	1995	II	Halo Anterior screw Posterior fusion	Prospective study of 11 geriatric type II dens fracture patients (8 F, 3 M; mean age 74, range 68–84 years) managed with an institutional protocol to determine the effect of early surgical stabilization on perioperative mortality	II	There was no in-hospital mortality; 91% patients achieved bony union at 3 months; 1 (9%) patient (2 mm posterior displacement) had nonunion treated successfully with anterior odontoid screw (union at 6 months)
Ryan and Taylor[32]	1993	II/III	No treatment Traction Soft collar Brace Minerva cast Halo vest/cast Surgery	Retrospective review of 35 geriatric (> 60 years) patients (20 F, 15 M) with 30 type II (60% posteriorly displaced) and 5 III odontoid fractures; treatment for type II and type III included: nil 5, 1; traction 5, 0; collar 6, 1; SOMI brace 4, 1; Minerva halo 9, 1; and surgery 1, respectively	III	Nonunion rate for type II was 77% (80% nil; 100% traction; 100% collar; 50% brace 55% Minerva/halo); overall nonunion rate for type III was 40%; outcome was determined by neurological status at presentation (36% had deficit); myelopathy as a late complication of nonunion was not observed in 9 patients with an average follow-up of 21 months
Hanigan et al[92]	1993	II/III	Hard collar Halo vest Surgery	Retrospective review of 19 geriatric (> 80 years) patients with odontoid fractures; there were 16 type II and 3 type III; 14 patients had mean f/u 28.8 months (range 5–72 months); 8 (< 5 mm posterior displacement) were treated with Philadelphia collar or halo; 5 (> 5 mm displaced) patients were treated with posterior C1–C2 wire fusion	III	Intrahospital mortality was 26% (5 all traction/collar); overall nonunion rate was 37%; 66% patients with external immobilization required surgical treatment; no operative morbidity or mortality occurred in posterior fusion patients (1 died from unrelated cause); prolonged bed rest caused respiratory complications in 33% patients
Pepin et al[37]	1985	I/II/III	Halo vest Surgery	Retrospective review of 41 patients (19 F, 23 M) with type I (1), type II (19), and type III (21) odontoid fractures; 20 patients were < 40, and 19 > 60 of age; 31 fractures were significantly displaced (majority posterior displacement in elderly patients); 26 were treated nonoperatively; 19 with posterior fusion	III	3 patients died (one from a spinal cord transection and two from other injuries); overall nonunion rate was 35% (9) (54% type II, 15% type III); direction of displacement and age did not correlate with nonunion; the halo vest was poorly tolerated in patients > 75 years of age

Abbreviation: SOMI, sterno-occipital-mandibular immobilizer.

posterior fixation.[37-39] Early definitive surgical management resulted in a significant reduction of intrahospital mortality compared with nonoperative approaches. Nonunion is a prevalent outcome in elderly type II odontoid fracture patients, and unlike in the younger patients is less problematic and usually does not require further treatment.[40]

◆ Discussion

Three evidence-based reviews on the management of odontoid fractures currently exist.[41-43] All three classify the strength of evidence in accordance with the evidence class as established by the American Medical Association.[3] The class designation for grading therapeutic studies is less rigorous (i.e., class II studies include those with retrospectively collected data) than the level designation established by Wright et al.[2] This systematic review uses the level designation for grading the management of type II and III odontoid fractures.

Although there appears to be strong agreement among clinicians in regard to odontoid fracture characteristics that affect outcome (fracture type, degree/direction of displacement, angulation, age, delay in diagnosis, and/or definitive treatment), the current literature review demonstrates lack of agreement on the extent to which any one or combination of these factors should influence treatment. The indications for selection of specific treatment modality have not been identified. Moreover, the treatment objectives that constitute acceptable outcome have not been firmly established; anatomical alignment and fusion are typically treatment goals, stability (i.e., a fibrous union in elderly patients), and acceptable alignment (without neurological or functional compromise) may be sufficient.

The symptomatic (no therapy) management of odontoid fractures has yielded abysmal results and, as per consensus of the Cervical Spine Research Society, this management alternative cannot be supported.[6] Because of inherent risks and benefits of all treatment modalities and the absence of specific treatment selection criteria, one can justify the application of a variety of closed or open modalities.

There appears to be significant justification for separating the elderly from younger patients because of the bimodal age distribution and the inferior results for all treatment modalities in the elderly. Pepin et al[37] demonstrated that odontoid fractures type II and III typically occurred in two distinct patient age groups with age range 21 to 30 and 61 to 70 years. Other studies have shown that elderly patients are often incapable of tolerating halo vest immobilization, and due to poor bone stock are unable to achieve stable internal fixation.

The nature of all studies identified constitutes the major limitation of this systematic review. Most of the studies did not separate isolated dens fractures from an assortment of combined cervical spine injuries that included dens fractures. Moreover, many studies consisted of patient groups that were treated with single modalities while only a few were comparative studies. Furthermore, the number of studies reviewed did not clearly delineate the specific treatment or the outcome according to fracture type.

◆ Summary and Recommendations

The major conclusion of this systematic review is that currently there is not sufficient evidence (quality and quantity) to formulate treatment standards or guidelines; the strength of the available evidence cannot exclude any treatment options. This review consists primarily of level III studies and its conclusions are the following:

1. **What provides optimal external immobilization in the nonoperative management of Anderson-D'Alonzo type II and type III odontoid fractures in adults: halo versus brace?**
   - ◆ *Conclusion.* The optimal external immobilization (halo vs brace) in the nonoperative management of adult Anderson-D'Alonzo type II and type III odontoid fractures is age dependent. In the younger patient population, cervical bracing and halo vest immobilization both represent viable treatment options. In the elderly patient population, halo vest immobilization should be used cautiously because of the high incidence of associated mortality; moreover, a stable nonunion/fibrous union of an odontoid type II fracture as a result of cervical bracing may constitute an acceptable outcome in the elderly patient.
   - ◆ *Strength of evidence.* Weak
   - ◆ *Strength of recommendation.* Strong

2. **What is the optimal management for Anderson-D'Alonzo type II odontoid fractures in adults: nonoperative versus operative treatment?**
   - ◆ *Conclusion.* The optimal management for Anderson-D'Alonzo type II odontoid fractures in adults (nonoperative vs operative) is age dependent. In the younger patient population, all closed and open treatment modalities are viable options. In the elderly patient populations, cervical bracing and all open treatment modalities are viable options.
   - ◆ *Strength of evidence.* Weak
   - ◆ *Strength of recommendation.* Strong

3. **What produces better outcomes in the surgical treatment in Anderson–D'Alonzo type II odontoid fractures in adults: anterior versus posterior fixation?**
   - ◆ *Conclusion.* In the adult population (younger and elderly), both anterior screw fixation (single or double) and posterior fusion (wiring and transarticular screws) surgical techniques represent viable treatment options.
   - ◆ *Strength of evidence.* Weak
   - ◆ *Strength of recommendation.* Strong

4. **What is the optimal treatment of Anderson-D'Alonzo type II and type III odontoid fractures in elderly patients?**
   - ◆ *Conclusion.* The optimal treatment of Anderson-D'Alonzo type II and type II odontoid fractures in the elderly patient consists of cervical bracing or surgical stabilization (anterior or posterior).
   - ◆ *Strength of evidence.* Weak
   - ◆ *Strength of recommendation.* Weak

Level I and more level II studies on the management of odontoid fractures are warranted prior to the formulation of treatment standards and guidelines. Currently, the Cochrane group is conducting a study to establish guidelines for the treatment of odontoid fractures (nonoperative vs operative methods) in all patient age groups (including pediatric patients).

References

1. Anderson LD, D'Alonzo RT. Fractures of the odontoid process of the axis. J Bone Joint Surg Am 1974;56:1663–1674
2. Wright JG, Swiontkowski MF, Heckman JD. Introducing levels of evidence to the journal. J Bone Joint Surg Am 2003;85-A:1–3

3. American Medical Association. Attributes to Guide the Development and Evaluation of Practice Parameters/Guidelines. Chicago: American Medical Association; 1996

4. Anderson PA, Budorick TE, Easton KB, Henley MB, Salciccioli GG. Failure of halo vest to prevent in vivo motion in patients with injured cervical spines. Spine 1991;16(10, Suppl):S501–S505

5. Lind B, Sihlbom H, Nordwall A. Halo-vest treatment of unstable traumatic cervical spine injuries. Spine 1988;13:425–432

6. Clark CR, White AA III. Fractures of the dens: a multicenter study. J Bone Joint Surg Am 1985;67:1340–1348

7. Maiman DJ, Larson SJ. Management of odontoid fractures. Neurosurgery 1982;11:471–476

8. Cosan TE, Tel E, Arslantas A, Vural M, Guner AI. Indications of Philadelphia collar in the treatment of upper cervical injuries. Eur J Emerg Med 2001;8:33–37

9. Koivikko MP, Kiuru MJ, Koskinen SK, Myllynen P, Santavirta S, Kivisaari L. Factors associated with nonunion in conservatively-treated type-II fractures of the odontoid process. J Bone Joint Surg Br 2004;86:1146–1151

10. Bucholz RD, Cheung KC. Halo vest versus spinal fusion for cervical injury: evidence from an outcome study. J Neurosurg 1989;70:884–892

11. Pointillart V, Orta AL, Freitas J, Vital JM, Senegas J. Odontoid fractures: review of 150 cases and practical application for treatment. Eur Spine J 1994;3:282–285

12. Greene KA, Dickman CA, Marciano FF, Drabier JB, Hadley MN, Sonntag VK. Acute axis fractures: analysis of management and outcome in 340 consecutive cases. Spine 1997;22:1843–1852

13. Chiba K, Fujimura Y, Toyama Y, Fujii E, Nakanishi T, Hirabayashi K. Treatment protocol for fractures of the odontoid process. J Spinal Disord 1996;9:267–276

14. Seybold EA, Bayley JC. Functional outcome of surgically and conservatively managed dens fractures. Spine 1998;23:1837–1845, discussion 1845–1846

15. ElSaghir H, Böhm H. Anderson type II fracture of the odontoid process: results of anterior screw fixation. J Spinal Disord 2000;13:527–530, discussion 531

16. Börm W, Kast E, Richter HP, Mohr K. Anterior screw fixation in type II odontoid fractures: is there a difference in outcome between age groups? Neurosurgery 2003;52:1089–1092, discussion 1092–1094

17. Alfieri A. Single-screw fixation for acute type II odontoid fracture. J Neurosurg Sci 2001;45:15–18

18. Moon MS, Moon JL, Sun DH, Moon YW. Treatment of dens fracture in adults: a report of thirty-two cases. Bull Hosp Jt Dis 2006;63:108–112

19. Jenkins JD, Coric D, Branch CL Jr. A clinical comparison of one- and two-screw odontoid fixation. J Neurosurg 1998;89:366–370

20. Platzer P, Thalhammer G, Oberleitner G, Schuster R, Vécsei V, Gaebler C. Surgical treatment of dens fractures in elderly patients. J Bone Joint Surg Am 2007;89:1716–1722

21. Fujii E, Kobayashi K, Hirabayashi K. Treatment in fractures of the odontoid process. Spine 1988;13:604–609

22. Apfelbaum RI, Lonser RR, Veres R, Casey A. Direct anterior screw fixation for recent and remote odontoid fractures. J Neurosurg 2000;93(2, Suppl):227–236

23. Waddell JP, Reardon GP. Atlantoaxial arthrodesis to treat odontoid fractures. Can J Surg 1983;26:255–257, 260

24. Rodrigues FA, Hodgson BF, Craig JB. Posterior atlantoaxial arthrodesis: a simplified method. Spine 1991;16:878–880

25. Ziai WC, Hurlbert RJ. A six year review of odontoid fractures: the emerging role of surgical intervention. Can J Neurol Sci 2000;27:297–301

26. Cornefjord M, Henriques T, Alemany M, Olerud C. Posterior atlanto-axial fusion with the Olerud Cervical Fixation System for odontoid fractures and C1-C2 instability in rheumatoid arthritis. Eur Spine J 2003;12:91–96

27. Magerl F, Seemann PS. Stable posterior fusion of the atlas and axis by transarticular screw fixation. In: Kehr P, Weidner A, eds. Cervical Spine. Berlin: Springer-Verlag; 1986:322–327

28. Böhler J. Anterior stabilization for acute fractures and non-unions of the dens. J Bone Joint Surg Am 1982;64:18–27

29. Bednar DA, Parikh J, Hummel J. Management of type II odontoid process fractures in geriatric patients; a prospective study of sequential cohorts with attention to survivorship. J Spinal Disord 1995;8:166–169

30. Tashjian RZ, Majercik S, Biffl WL, Palumbo MA, Cioffi WG. Halo-vest immobilization increases early morbidity and mortality in elderly odontoid fractures. J Trauma 2006;60:199–203

31. Majercik S, Tashjian RZ, Biffl WL, Harrington DT, Cioffi WG. Halo vest immobilization in the elderly: a death sentence? J Trauma 2005;59:350–356, discussion 356–358

32. Ryan MD, Taylor TK. Odontoid fractures in the elderly. J Spinal Disord 1993;6:397–401

33. Berlemann U, Schwarzenbach O. Dens fractures in the elderly: results of anterior screw fixation in 19 elderly patients. Acta Orthop Scand 1997;68:319–324

34. Börm W, Kast E, Richter HP, Mohr K. Anterior screw fixation in type II odontoid fractures: is there a difference in outcome between age groups? Neurosurgery 2003;52:1089–1092, discussion 1092–1094

35. Harrop JS, Przybylski GJ, Vaccaro AR, Yalamanchili K. Efficacy of anterior odontoid screw fixation in elderly patients with type II odontoid fractures. Neurosurg Focus 2000;8:e6

36. Platzer P, Thalhammer G, Ostermann R, Wieland T, Vécsei V, Gaebler C. Anterior screw fixation of odontoid fractures comparing younger and elderly patients. Spine 2007;32:1714–1720

37. Pepin JW, Bourne RB, Hawkins RJ. Odontoid fractures, with special reference to the elderly patient. Clin Orthop Relat Res 1985;(193):178–183

38. Campanelli M, Kattner KA, Stroink A, Gupta K, West S. Posterior C1–C2 transarticular screw fixation in the treatment of displaced type II odontoid fractures in the geriatric population: review of seven cases. Surg Neurol 1999;51:596–600, discussion 600–601

39. Andersson S, Rodrigues M, Olerud C. Odontoid fractures: high complication rate associated with anterior screw fixation in the elderly. Eur Spine J 2000;9:56–59

40. Hart R, Saterbak A, Rapp T, Clark C. Nonoperative management of dens fracture nonunion in elderly patients without myelopathy. Spine 2000;25:1339–1343

41. Traynelis VC. Evidence-based management of type II odontoid fractures. Clin Neurosurg 1997;44:41–49

42. Julien TD, Frankel B, Traynelis VC, Ryken TC. Evidence-based analysis of odontoid fracture management. Neurosurg Focus 2000;8:e6

43. McCormick PC and the Members of the Section on Disorders of the Spine and Peripheral Nerves of the American Association of Neurological Surgeons and the Congress of Neurological Surgeons. Isolated fractures of the axis in adults. Neurosurgery 2002;50(3, Suppl):S125–S139

44. Platzer P, Thalhammer G, Sarahrudi K, et al. Nonoperative management of odontoid fractures using a halothoracic vest. Neurosurgery 2007;61:522–529, discussion 529–530

45. Hosssain M, McLean A, Fraser MH. Outcome of halo immobilisation of 104 cases of cervical spine injury. Scott Med J 2004;49:90–92

46. Müller EJ, Schwinnen I, Fischer K, Wick M, Muhr G. Non-rigid immobilisation of odontoid fractures. Eur Spine J 2003;12:522–525

47. Komadina R, Brilej D, Kosanović M, Vlaović M. Halo jacket in odontoid fractures type II and III. Arch Orthop Trauma Surg 2003;123:64–67

48. Marton E, Billeci D, Carteri A. Therapeutic indications in upper cervical spine instability. Considerations on 58 cases. J Neurosurg Sci 2000;44:192–202

49. Govender S, Maharaj JF, Haffajee MR. Fractures of the odontoid process. J Bone Joint Surg Br 2000;82:1143–1147

50. Razak M, Basir T, Hyzan Y, Johari Z. Halovest treatment in traumatic cervical spine injury. Med J Malaysia 1998;53(Suppl A):1–5

51. Lennarson PJ, Mostafavi H, Traynelis VC, Walters BC. Management of type II dens fractures: a case-control study. Spine 2000;25:1234–1237

52. Stoney J, O'Brien J, Wilde P. Treatment of type-two odontoid fractures in halothoracic vests. J Bone Joint Surg Br 1998;80:452–455

53. Polin RS, Szabo T, Bogaev CA, Replogle RE, Jane JA. Nonoperative management of types II and III odontoid fractures: the Philadelphia collar versus the halo vest. Neurosurgery 1996;38:450–456, discussion 456–457

54. Van Holsbeek E, Stoffelen D, Fabry G. Fractures of the odontoid process. Conservative and operative treatment: prognostic factors. Acta Orthop Belg 1993;59:17–21

55. Hadley MN, Dickman CA, Browner CM, Sonntag VK. Acute axis fractures: a review of 229 cases. J Neurosurg 1989;71(5 Pt 1):642–647

56. Govender S, Grootboom M. Fractures of the dens—the results of non-rigid immobilization. Injury 1988;19:165–167

57. Schweigel JF. Management of the fractured odontoid with halo-thoracic bracing. Spine 1987;12:838–839

58. Hanssen AD, Cabanela ME. Fractures of the dens in adult patients. J Trauma 1987;27:928–934

59. Lind B, Nordwall A, Sihlbom H. Odontoid fractures treated with halo-vest. Spine 1987;12:173–177

60. Dunn ME, Seljeskog EL. Experience in the management of odontoid process injuries: an analysis of 128 cases. Neurosurgery 1986;18:306–310

61. Hadley MN, Browner C, Sonntag VK. Axis fractures: a comprehensive review of management and treatment in 107 cases. Neurosurgery 1985;17:281–290

62. Wang GJ, Mabie KN, Whitehill R, Stamp WG. The nonsurgical management of odontoid fractures in adults. Spine 1984;9:229–230

63. Ryan MD, Taylor TK. Odontoid fractures: a rational approach to treatment. J Bone Joint Surg Br 1982;64:416–421

64. Ekong CE, Schwartz ML, Tator CH, Rowed DW, Edmonds VE. Odontoid fracture: management with early mobilization using the halo device. Neurosurgery 1981;9:631–637

65. Vieweg U, Meyer B, Schramm J. Differential treatment in acute upper cervical spine injuries: a critical review of a single-institution series. Surg Neurol 2000;54:203–210, discussion 210–211

66. Daneyemez M, Kahraman S, Gezen F, Sirin S. Cervical spine injuries and management: experience with 235 patients in 10 years. Minim Invasive Neurosurg 1999;42:6–9

67. Stulik J, Vyskocil T, Sebesta P, Kryl J. Atlantoaxial fixation using the polyaxial screw-rod system. Eur Spine J 2007;16:479–484

68. Lee SH, Sung JK. Anterior odontoid fixation using a 4.5-mm Herbert screw: the first report of 20 consecutive cases with odontoid fracture. Surg Neurol 2006;66:361–366, discussion 366

69. Bhanot A, Sawhney G, Kaushal R, Aggarwal AK, Bahadur R. Management of odontoid fractures with anterior screw fixation. J Surg Orthop Adv 2006;15:38–42

70. Fountas KN, Kapsalaki EZ, Karampelas I, et al. Results of long-term follow-up in patients undergoing anterior screw fixation for type II and rostral type III odontoid fractures. Spine 2005;30:661–669

71. Fountas KN, Machinis TG, Kapsalaki EZ, et al. Surgical treatment of acute type II and rostral type III odontoid fractures managed by anterior screw fixation. South Med J 2005;98:896–901

72. Henry AD, Bohly J, Grosse A. Fixation of odontoid fractures by an anterior screw. J Bone Joint Surg Br 1999;81:472–477

73. Subach BR, Morone MA, Haid RW Jr, McLaughlin MR, Rodts GR, Comey CH. Management of acute odontoid fractures with single-screw anterior fixation. Neurosurgery 1999;45:812–819, discussion 819–820

74. Guiot B, Fessler RG. Complex atlantoaxial fractures. J Neurosurg 1999; 91(2, Suppl):139–143

75. Morandi X, Hanna A, Hamlat A, Brassier G. Anterior screw fixation of odontoid fractures. Surg Neurol 1999;51:236–240

76. Huang CI, Chen IH. Atlantoaxial arthrodesis using Halifax interlaminar clamps reinforced by halo vest immobilization: a long-term follow-up experience. Neurosurgery 1996;38:1153–1156, discussion 1156–1157

77. Fairholm D, Lee ST, Lui TN. Fractured odontoid: the management of delayed neurological symptoms. Neurosurgery 1996;38:38–43

78. Rainov NG, Heidecke V, Burkert W. Direct anterior fixation of odontoid fractures with a hollow spreading screw system. Acta Neurochir (Wien) 1996;138:146–153

79. Coyne TJ, Fehlings MG, Wallace MC, Bernstein M, Tator CH. C1–C2 posterior cervical fusion: long-term evaluation of results and efficacy. Neurosurgery 1995;37:688–692, discussion 692–693

80. Chang KW, Liu YW, Cheng PG, et al. One Herbert double-threaded compression screw fixation of displaced type II odontoid fractures. J Spinal Disord 1994;7:62–69

81. Verheggen R, Jansen J. Fractures of the odontoid process: analysis of the functional results after surgery. Eur Spine J 1994;3:146–150

82. Chiba K, Fujimura Y, Toyama Y, Takahata T, Nakanishi T, Hirabayashi K. Anterior screw fixation for odontoid fracture: clinical results in 45 cases. Eur Spine J 1993;2:76–81

83. Jeanneret B, Magerl F. Primary posterior fusion C1/2 in odontoid fractures: indications, technique, and results of transarticular screw fixation. J Spinal Disord 1992;5:464–475

84. Esses SI, Bednar DA. Screw fixation of odontoid fractures and nonunions. Spine 1991;16(10, Suppl):S483–S485

85. Smith MD, Phillips WA, Hensinger RN. Fusion of the upper cervical spine in children and adolescents: an analysis of 17 patients. Spine 1991;16: 695–701

86. Montesano PX, Anderson PA, Schlehr F, Thalgott JS, Lowrey G. Odontoid fractures treated by anterior odontoid screw fixation. Spine 1991;16(3, Suppl):S33–S37

87. Jeanneret B, Vernet O, Frei S, Magerl F. Atlantoaxial mobility after screw fixation of the odontoid: a computed tomographic study. J Spinal Disord 1991;4:203–211

88. Geisler FH, Cheng C, Poka A, Brumback RJ. Anterior screw fixation of posteriorly displaced type II odontoid fractures. Neurosurgery 1989;25: 30–37, discussion 37–38

89. Frangen TM, Zilkens C, Muhr G, Schinkel C. Odontoid fractures in the elderly: dorsal C1/C2 fusion is superior to halo-vest immobilization. J Trauma 2007;63:83–89

90. Kuntz C IV, Mirza SK, Jarell AD, Chapman JR, Shaffrey CI, Newell DW. Type II odontoid fractures in the elderly: early failure of nonsurgical treatment. Neurosurg Focus 2000;8:e7

91. Müller EJ, Wick M, Russe O, Muhr G. Management of odontoid fractures in the elderly. Eur Spine J 1999;8:360–365

92. Hanigan WC, Powell FC, Elwood PW, Henderson JP. Odontoid fractures in elderly patients. J Neurosurg 1993;78:32–35

26

Management of C2 Traumatic Spondylolisthesis (Hangman's Fracture) and Other Variants

Y. Raja Rampersaud and S. Samuel Bederman

◆ Methods

Eligibility Criteria

We sought to identify all studies that met the following criteria: prospective or retrospective observational or randomized studies; inclusion of separately reported hangman's fractures managed by any two of the following treatments: rigid immobilization, nonrigid immobilization, primary surgical intervention via an anterior approach, or primary surgical intervention via a posterior approach; a minimum number of two patients treated by any single method; and report of any of the following outcomes for a treatment group to allow for direct comparisons: radiographic late displacement, radiographic nonunion, clinical outcome, or secondary surgery.

Study Identification

A systematic search of electronic databases: MEDLINE (1950–09/2007), CINAHL (1982–09/2007), EMBASE (1980–09/ 2007), and Ovid Healthstar (1966–09/2007). For our search strategy, we used the following: (axis/ AND (fractures, bone/ or spinal fractures/ or spinal injuries/ or fracture fixation/ or spondylolisthesis/ or fracture healing/ or immobilization/) AND adult/) OR ((hangman$ fracture$ or traumatic spondylolisthesis or C2 fracture or axis fracture).ti,ab.).

We further hand-searched bibliographies of relevant articles to identify other potentially eligible studies not identified by our electronic search. We independently reviewed the titles and abstracts of all articles identified from our search to determine potential eligibility. All studies that were included by either reviewer were retrieved in full to determine study eligibility and subsequent data abstraction if eligible.

Data Abstraction

Using a standardized data abstraction form, we independently assessed all articles deemed to be potentially eligible. Data were gathered from each article on final eligibility, level of evidence, characteristics of the population, intervention, and outcome. Disagreements about final eligibility were resolved by discussion.

Definitions

To provide a clinically relevant analysis, reported injuries were categorized based on radiographic data (e.g., degree of displacement) or injury classification, into stable and unstable injuries whenever possible. For the purpose of this systematic review, stable injuries were defined as those classified as Effendi or Levine type I or those with up to 3 mm of anterior displacement of C2 on C3 with no or little movement on flexion-extension views, if performed. Unstable injuries were defined as those classified as Effendi type II or III or Levine IIa or those with greater than 3 mm of anterior displacement of C2 on C3 or more than 2 to 3 mm of motion on flexion-extension views. Sufficient data about C2 or C3 angulation was not available from most studies so that an analysis of this parameter was not possible.

Statistical Analysis

All data were entered into electronic form by one author and verified by the second author. Odds ratios for each study were calculated for all outcome measures (late displacement, clinical, nonunions, secondary surgery), comparisons (surgery/no surgery, rigid/nonrigid immobilization, posterior/anterior surgical approach), and fracture groupings (total sample/unstable/ stable fractures). For studies that experienced no outcomes for at least one of the comparison groups, 0.5 was added to each treatment/outcome group to facilitate statistical computation.

Data were pooled across studies using DerSimonian and Laird's random effects model accounting for variation between articles to estimate an overall odds ratio with 95% confidence intervals. We used the Breslow-Day measure to identify the presence of significant heterogeneity across studies.

◆ Traumatic Spondylolisthesis and Other Variants

Epidemiology

The diagnosis and management of traumatic spondylolisthesis of the axis (C2) and associated variants involves knowledge of a spectrum of injuries. Historically these injuries were noted following a submental (i.e., under the chin) knot position used in judicial hanging.[1] In 1965, Schneider et al reported a similar pattern of bony injury at C2 following traumatic injuries and utilized the term *hangman's fractures*.[2] However, unlike judicial hangings where hyperextension is followed by violent distraction and subsequent neurological death, distraction is uncommon after typical traumatic injury, and the majority occur without neurological injury. As such, most authors note that *traumatic spondylolisthesis of the axis (C2)* is the most appropriate term to denote these injuries. Furthermore, given the broad range of reported injuries, most agree that there is also a wide range of injury mechanisms. Consequently, there is considerable variation in the terminology used to describe and classify these injures and little agreement on optimal treatment techniques.[3-5]

Cervical spine injuries occur in 2 to 3% of patients with blunt trauma who undergo imaging studies.[6,7] The best available incidence data regarding cervical injuries can be found from the National Emergency X-Radiography Utilization Study (NEXUS).[6,8] Of 34,069 patients with blunt cervical trauma, 818 (2.4%) had 1496 distinct cervical spine injuries.[8] C2 injures were the most common, accounting for 23.9%. Of 286 C2 fractures, odontoid fractures (32.2%) were the most common followed by traumatic C2 spondylolisthesis and associated variants (20.6%). A similar distribution of C2 odontoid and hangman's type fractures has also been reported in the surgical series by Greene et al (59% vs 22%) and Vieweg et al (44% vs 24%).[9,10]

Traumatic injuries to C2 have a significant incidence of associated minor and major injuries. In particular, closed head injuries (20 to 33%)[11-15] and facial injures (up to 80%)[16] are the most commonly reported. In addition, contiguous and noncontiguous spinal injuries are common (15 to 40%).[11,12,15,16]

◆ Unique Clinical and Diagnostic Features

Due to the high incidence of associated head and neck injuries already noted, the presence of facial injures (lacerations, abrasions, and fractures) or closed head injury (CHI) should raise a high index of suspicion regarding a cervical spine injury, particularly of the upper C-spine. Associated injuries to the head can contribute to the delay in diagnosis of cervical injuries.[15] Specific to C2 traumatic spondylolisthesis, upper cervical neck pain with or with out significant occipital neuralgia is typical.

Associated neurological deficits with traumatic C2 spondylolisthesis are relatively rare, with a reported mean incidence of ~13%, ranging from 0[17-19] up to 36%.[10-12,16,20-24] The majority of published data, however, report a relative paucity of significant or permanent neurological deficits directly related to these injuries. This is in keeping with the nature of these injuries in which the spinal canal is typically expanded rather than compromised. Variants that involve a coronal split through the posterior body of C2 with anterior translations of the remainder of the C2 body on C3 are at higher risk of associated neurological injury.[4,25] In addition, injuries that involve fracture-dislocations of the C2–C3 facet joint (Effendi type III) with an intact or partially intact ring are also associated with a higher incidence of neurological injury.[11]

Classification of C2 traumatic spondylolisthesis has been based on injury morphology or stability as determined by plain radiographs.[26] Although there have been several classification systems, the system proposed by Effendi et al and the subsequent modification by Levine are the most commonly utilized (**Fig. 26.1**).[11,12,26] In general, Effendi type I (injury of the C2 isthmus) injuries are considered to be stable, and type III injuries (that include dislocation of one or both C2–C3 facets) are considered unstable. Type II and IIa (flexion-distraction mechanism) injuries obligatorily have discoligamentous injury through the C2–C3 disk space. As such, they are generally felt to be unstable. However, they demonstrate a wide range of translation and angular deformity and are therefore associated with the most controversy regarding stability and definitive management. It must be noted that these so-called accepted classification systems have never been validated or assessed for reliability. Furthermore, they do not objectively assess instability or discoligamentous injury by dynamic imaging or more contemporary use of magnetic resonance imaging (MRI), the latter of which is the senior author's (YRR) preferred method of investigation.[4,27] As will be described, there is no identifiable superiority between operative and nonoperative treatment for this group of injuries. Consequently, unique case-by-case factors and surgeon preference should play a role in management decisions.

◆ Initial Nonoperative Management

In a broad, qualitative systematic review, Li et al reported that nonoperative management has been utilized in 74% of series (comparative and noncomparative series), with the majority (98%) being type I (46%) and type II injuries (52%) reported in the English language.[26]

Based on the best available evidence (see later discussion), stable injuries, defined as Effendi or Levine type I or those with up to but not more than 3 mm of anterior displacement of C2 on C3 with no or little movement on flexion-extension views or normal discoligamentous signal on MRI, are successfully managed nonoperatively with a short period (6 weeks) of immobilization in a hard cervical orthosis. Upright, plain radiographs should be obtained in the hard collar prior to discharge. These patients should be seen 1 to 2 weeks postinjury with repeat radiographs to rule out any evidence of subluxation.

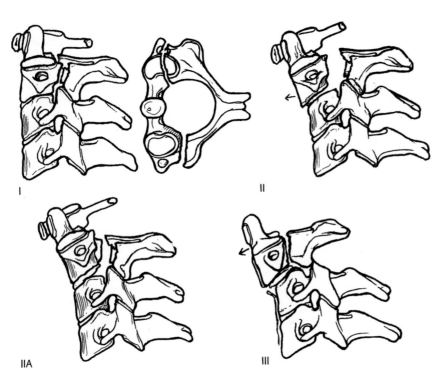

Fig. 26.1 Classification of C2 traumatic spondylolisthesis (Levine and Edwards modification of the Effendi classification system). Type I, minimally displaced with no angulation. Type II, angulated and displaced. Type IIA, minimal displacement with angulation. Type III, severely angulated and displaced with uni/bilateral facet dislocation. (From Anderson DG, Vaccaro AR. Decision Making in Spinal Care. New York, NY: Thieme Medical Publishers; 2007:32. Reprinted with permission.)

Repeat clinical and radiographic assessment is performed at 2, 4, and 6 weeks postinjury.

For unstable injures where nonoperative management is employed, the best available evidence supports reduction with traction followed by halo vest immobilization for 6 to 12 weeks. In our experience, most are treated with 12 weeks in a halo vest. Traction should typically be performed in a monitored setting beginning with 10 pounds in slight neck extension. Occasionally, hyperextension is required to achieve ideal alignment. Serially increasing the weight, typically by 5 lb, up to a maximum weight of 15 to 20 lb, will usually be adequate. Importantly, clinical exam and lateral cervical radiographs or fluoroscopy is frequently performed. However, it must be noted that the majority of the studies that demonstrate successful treatment of type II injuries reported use of traction for 4 to 6 weeks followed by rigid immobilization in a Minerva cast or halo vest in later series.[9,10,12–14,16–19,21–24,28,29] Although prolonged traction and bed rest can certainly be employed, it is less likely to be accepted by today's patients and health care environment.[4] Contemporary recommendations would more appropriately include acute (< 7 days) application of a halo vest and mobilization once reduction is achieved. Because most of these injuries are not associated with neurological injury, low weight reduction over the course of several days as required will typically achieve a good reduction. Upright radiographs prior to discharge and repeat clinical and radiographic assessment are performed at 2, 4, 6, and 12 weeks postinjury. At 12 weeks, controlled flexion/extension views are performed. If the injury is stable on flexion/extension views, the halo vest is discontinued and gentle range of motion and isometric exercises are begun with the use of a cervical collar for as much as an additional 6 weeks. Note, however, radiographic union often lags behind functional union, and bridging bone may not be clearly seen for 6 months.

The literature suggests that a substantial degree of malunion can be well tolerated; however, this commonly held assertion has not been validated by any objective patient-reported outcome measure.

◆ Surgical Management

Primary surgical management of unstable injuries is the recommended treatment for type III injuries and is an acceptable option for type II injuries. In general, operative intervention is more unilaterally recommended for progressive translational or angular displacement during nonoperative treatment, when halo vest application is undesirable or contraindicated, or if prolonged bed rest is not acceptable. For Effendi type III injuries, most authors recommend posterior stabilization. For type II injuries there are proponents of either anterior or posterior surgical stabilization. Based on the best available evidence, there is no clear clinical advantage of one approach over the other and as such this decision is often based on surgeon preference and should optimally incorporate injury- and patient-specific factors. Although some have advocated direct osteosynthesis of C2 via pedicle/isthmic fixation, it is not recommended in the presence of a C2–C3 discoligamentous injury.[4,30–32] Furthermore, the high rate of successful nonoperative treatment of the subgroup of stable injuries that would be amenable to direct osteosynthesis does not support primary surgical management.

For operative treatment of type II injuries, most authors recommend anterior C2–C3 plating (**Fig. 26.2**). This is also the preference of the senior author unless the patient has relative contraindications to a high anterior cervical approach, such as a short neck or nonacceptance of the risk of dysphagia or voice-related complications. For both the anterior and posterior approach, fracture reduction is achieved by traction (see earlier discussion) in the majority of cases.

Anterior Approach

The anterior approach avoids the time and risk involved in rolling the patient to the prone position and avoids the associated muscular morbidity of the posterior approach. In appropriately selected patients, this approach is well tolerated and is a very effective management for this injury. The patient is maintained supine with the head held in an adjustable head holder, such as a Mayfield horseshoe with tong traction. A high medial retropharyngeal approach is utilized to access C2–C3. Once the level is confirmed by intraoperative imaging, the disk is removed and any residual malalignment that was not addressed by traction and head positioning can be reduced by direct translational or levering maneuvers. Placement of a distraction pin at C2 can function as a joystick to help reduction. Adequate lordosis must be confirmed and is usually achieved by extending the patient's neck. A trapezoidal anterior interbody graft and an anterior plate are then placed.

Posterior Approach

The posterior approach is familiar to all spinal surgeons and avoids the potential neurovascular risk associated with the anterior approach. Although not well addressed in the literature, it is our preference to perform a posterior C1–C3 instrumentation using lateral mass fixation if the injury is associated with irreducible C1–C2 intraarticular displacement or significant step deformity (**Fig. 26.3**). For type III injuries the isthmus/pars-interarticularis is typically intact and a C2 "pars" and C3 lateral mass fixation will provide rigid stabilization. For type II injuries, the plane of the isthmus injury is widely variable, and safe passage of screws across the fracture site is not always technically feasible (**Fig. 26.3**). If required, intraoperative imaging is strongly recommended. In this scenario, extension of the instrumentation to C1 is performed. Either lateral mass fixation or a hybrid sublaminar wiring technique can be utilized. Alternatively, it is our preference to perform anterior fixation of C2–C3 to avoid the significant loss of rotational motion associated with fusion across C1–C2. Local autograft is typically adequate for C2–C3 facet fusion; however, structural auto- or allograft may be required when fusing up to C1.

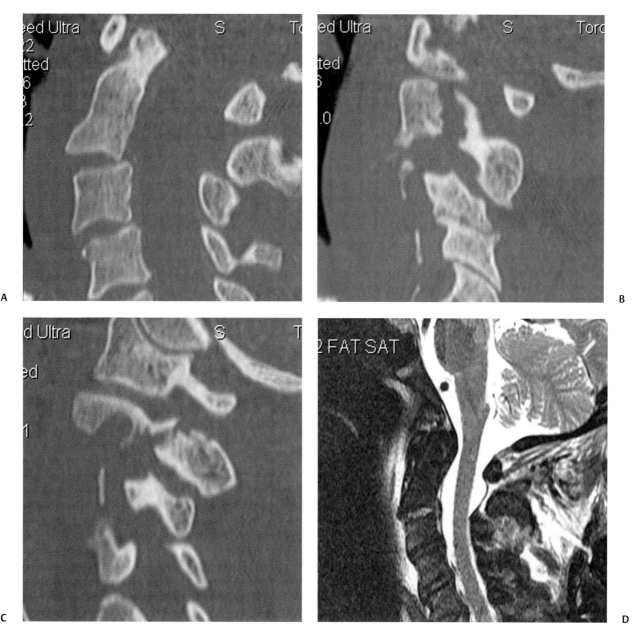

A

B

C

D

Fig. 26.2 (A–C) Sagittal computed tomographic views (midsagittal, left, and right parasagittal) demonstrating a type II traumatic spondylolisthesis of C2. **(D)** Fat-saturated midsagittal magnetic resonance imaging scan demonstrating high signal of the C2–C3 discoligamentous complex. (*Continued on page 252*)

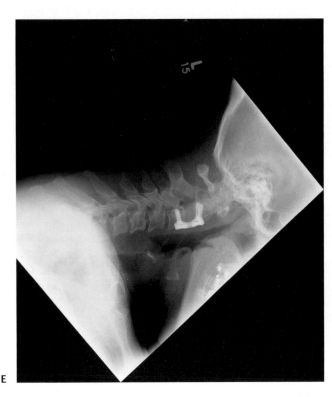

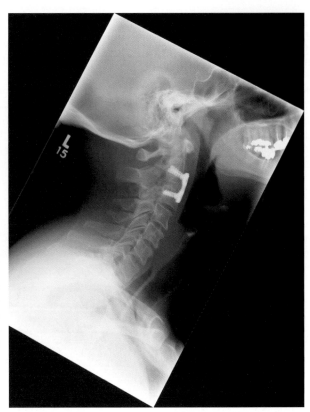

E

F

Fig. 26.2 (*Continued*) **(E,F)** Flexion-extension radiographs at 1 year following anterior reduction, placement of trapezoidal tricortical iliac crest autograft and C2–C3 instrumentation. A solid fusion of the disk space is demonstrated.

◆ Potential Complications and Their Avoidance

Complications associated with traction and halo vest management are best avoided by careful patient selection, particularly in the elderly; patient education and close clinical and radiographic follow-up.[33,34] Assessment for distraction of the

C2–C3 disk space during traction and immediate cessation is paramount to avoiding neurological injury.

Avoidance of neurological or vascular approach-related complications regarding fracture reduction and instrumentation placement requires thorough knowledge of the relevant anatomy as well as instrumentation techniques. For anterior approaches to C2–C3, meticulous identification and protection

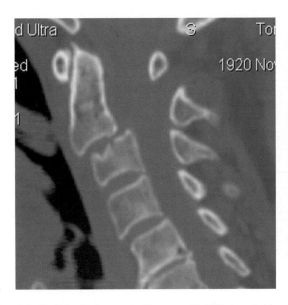

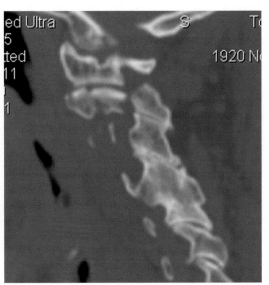

A

B

Fig. 26.3 (A–C) Sagittal computed tomographic (CT) views (midsagittal, left, and right parasagittal) demonstrating a complex traumatic spondylolisthesis of C2 ("variant"). The fracture line is anterior to the

pars on the right, and a segmental fracture of the left pars has occurred. There is also a significant step deformity of the right C1–C2 articulation.

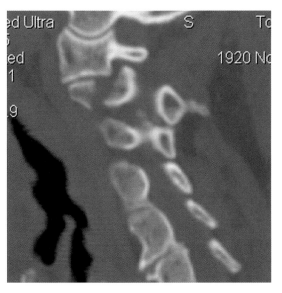

C

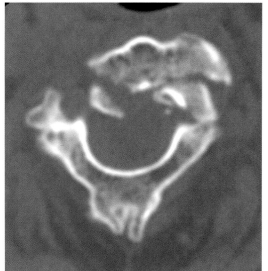

D

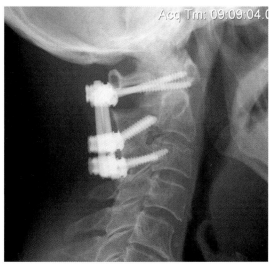

E

Fig. 26.3 (*Continued*) **(D)** Axial CT view demonstrating the oblique coronal orientation of the main fracture plane. **(E)** Lateral radiograph at 1 year following posterior reduction with C1–C3 lateral mass fixation.

of the hypoglossal and superior laryngeal nerve are paramount. For those unfamiliar or early in their experience with this approach, collaboration with an otolaryngologist is recommended.

The use of a rotating spinal frame such as the Jackson table should be utilized to minimize loss of reduction or secondary injury when using the posterior approach. Avoiding vascular or neurological injury during screw placement across the C2 pars or pedicle fracture requires reduction of the fracture, adequate visualization of the orientation of the C2 isthmus/fracture line, and high-quality intraoperative imaging.

◆ Rehabilitation

Associated neurological injuries require aggressive and appropriate neurological rehabilitation. For nonoperative or operative treatment, once injury stability has occurred (6 to 12 weeks), gentle range of motion and isometric strengthening exercises are recommended for 4 to 6 weeks. If rigid operative stabilization has been achieved, gentle exercise can begin as soon as the patient is comfortable. This progresses to more aggressive range of motion and strengthening exercises as tolerated.

◆ Evidence-Based Review

This chapter systematically reviews the available English language literature to answer two questions:

1. What C2 hangman's or associated variant fractures require surgical intervention?
2. When a hangman's fracture is managed operatively or nonoperatively, what is the optimal approach?

◆ Results

From our search, we identified 437 articles. Two of us agreed about the potential relevance of 55 articles based on a review of their titles and abstracts. An additional 34 articles were found to be potentially relevant by a single author (kappa = 0.72) and thus we retrieved 89 articles for full review. Of those published in the English language, 16 articles met our inclusion criteria and contained data relevant to our questions (**Table 26.1**). These 16 studies were published over a long time span that ranged from 1963 to 2005. Five articles were graded to be level 3 and 11 were graded to be level 4. No randomized studies were identified.

Table 26.1 Evidence Summary of Comparative Studies for the Management of Hangman Fractures

Study	Description	Level of Evidence of Primary Question(s)	Topic and Conclusion
Cornish (1968)[20]	Retrospective case series, C2 traumatic spondylolisthesis	IV	12 patients satisfied our inclusion criteria. Treatment was NRI in 4 and ASF in 8. Mean follow-up was unspecified. Outcomes were radiographic and surgeon reported clinical. Three injures were graded stable ("little" movement on controlled flexion-extension view) and managed with NRI. A poor clinical outcome was noted in one. Nine injuries were graded unstable (not clearly defined). One was treated with NRI and required delayed surgery (ASF) with a good final outcome. ASF was performed in the other 8 with poor clinical outcome in 3. All cases achieved radiographic union. CONCLUSION: Primary ASF (noninstrumented) for unstable injuries achieves good outcome. Problem—unclear definition of unstable and poorly defined follow-up.
Francis et al (1981)[16]	Multicentered retrospective case series, C2 traumatic spondylolisthesis	IV	123 patients satisfied our inclusion criteria. Treatment was NRI in 35 and traction (3 day to 12 weeks) + RI in 88. Mean follow-up was 31 months. Outcomes were radiographic and late surgery. Injures were classified based on degree displacement and degree of focal angulation (Francis: I–V). Two of the 35 treated with NRI developed nonunion and had late surgery. Five of the 88 treated with RI developed nonunion and had late surgery. Preference for anterior surgery to preserve C1–C2 rotation (4-ASF and 3-PSF) CONCLUSION: No correlation with degree of displacement was obtained regarding nonunion other than angulation >11 degrees was seen in 6/7 patients with nonunion. Surgery only required for chronic instability. Problem—specific management with respect to grade of injury was not specified.
Grady et al (1986)[17]	Retrospective cohort study, C2 traumatic spondylolisthesis	III	24 patients satisfied our inclusion criteria. Treatment was NRI in 8 [+ short (<2 wks) traction in 3] and RI in 16. Mean follow-up was 14 months. Outcomes were radiographic. Of the 8 patients treated with NRI, 7 were graded stable* and 3 developed late displacement, 2 of which required RI. One patient was graded unstable and had successful treatment with NRI. Of the 16 patients treated with RI, all were graded stable and 3 developed late displacement. All cases achieved radiographic union. CONCLUSION: Presence of subluxation (up to 4 mm in this series) did not preclude successful union in either the collar or halo vest cohort. Problem—no clinical outcomes.
Greene et al (1997)[9]	Retrospective case series, C2 injuries	IV	72 patients satisfied our inclusion criteria. Treatment was NRI in 9, RI in 56, and surgical (nonspecified) in 7. The use of traction was unspecified. Median follow-up was 45 months. Outcomes were radiographic. Injuries were classified according to the Effendi and Francis systems. 53 injuries were considered stable* and treated nonoperatively (unspecified regarding NRI versus RI). 21 were considered unstable, 14 treated nonoperatively (unspecified regarding NRI vs RI) and 7 treated operatively (6 Effendi type II and 1 type III). All cases achieved radiographic union. CONCLUSION: Surgery recommended for "severe," irreducible, injuries. Problem—specific management with respect to grade/severity of injury was not specified. No clinical outcomes.

Table 26.1 Evidence Summary of Comparative Studies for the Management of Hangman Fractures *(Continued)*

Study	Description	Level of Evidence of Primary Question(s)	Topic and Conclusion
Levine and Edwards (1985)[12]	Retrospective cohort study, C2 traumatic spondylolisthesis	III	44 patients satisfied our inclusion criteria. Treatment was NRI in 10, traction (5 days to 6 weeks) + RI in 31 and PSF in 3. Mean follow-up was unclear; "most were followed to 24 months." Outcomes were radiographic. 13 injures were graded stable,* 6 treated with NRI and 7 with RI; no late radiographic displacement. 29 injures were graded unstable, 4 treated with NRI, 24 with RI (2 Effendi type III) and 3 with PSF (3 Effendi type III); late radiographic displacement occurred in 2, 16, and 0, respectively. All cases achieved radiographic union. CONCLUSION: Defined type IIa flexion-distraction injury where traction is relatively contraindicated. Type I and some type II injures can be treated with a collar, otherwise type II and IIa can be treated with halo immobilization. Type III injuries are best treated with reduction (open or closed) and PSF. Problem—nonspecific clinical outcomes.
Lohnert J et al	Retrospective case series, C2 traumatic spondylolisthesis	IV	99 patients satisfied our inclusion criteria. Treatment was NRI in 1, reduction + RI in 77, ASF in 19, and PSF in 2. Mean follow-up was unspecified, but ranged 1–12 years. Outcomes were radiographic. Injuries were classified according to the Levine system. 34 injuries were considered stable and treated with RI; all cases achieved radiographic union. 65 were considered unstable, 1 treated with NRI, 44 with RI, 19 with ASF I and 2 with PSF (C2 pedicle screw); radiographic union was not achieved in 1, 0, 0, and 1, respectively. CONCLUSION: Recommend RI for Levine type I/IIa and ASF for type II. Problem—nondetailed, nonspecific clinical outcomes.
Marar (1975)[21]	Retrospective case series, C2 traumatic spondylolisthesis	IV	14 patients satisfied our inclusion criteria. Treatment was NRI in 10, traction (unspecified duration) + RI in 4. Mean follow-up was unspecified. Outcomes were radiographic and surgeon-reported clinical. Nine injuries were considered stable, 8 treated with NRI (1 poor clinical outcome) and 1 with RI; all cases achieved radiographic union. Five were considered unstable, 2 treated with NRI (2 poor clinical outcome) and 3 with RI (2 poor clinical outcome); all cases achieved radiographic union with no late displacement. CONCLUSION: Recommend RI for Levine type I/IIa and ASF for type II. Problem—nondetailed, nonspecific clinical outcomes.
Moon et al (2001)[18]	Retrospective case series, C2 traumatic spondylolisthesis	IV	42 patients satisfied our inclusion criteria. Treatment was RI in 20, ASF in 16, and PSF in 6. Four weeks of bed rest was used in all patients prior to 1980 (RI 20, ASF 10, and PSF 2). Follow-up ranged 1–7 years. Outcomes were radiographic and surgeon-reported clinical. Injuries were classified according to a modified Effendi system. 19 injuries were considered stable and treated with RI; all cases achieved good radiographic and clinical outcome. 23 injuries were considered unstable, 1 treated with RI, 16 with ASF, and 6 with PSF; all cases, except one (PSF—poor clinical outcome) achieved good radiographic and clinical outcome. CONCLUSION: Recommend ASF for unstable injuries. Problem—with the exception of one case all nonoperative treatment was for stable injuries and all surgical treatment was for unstable injuries.

255

(Continued on page 256)

Study	Description	Level of Evidence of Primary Question(s)	Topic and Conclusion
Muller et al (2000)[13]	Retrospective case series, C2 traumatic spondylolisthesis	IV	26 patients satisfied our inclusion criteria. Treatment was NRI in 11, RI in 11, and operative in 4. Mean follow-up was 44 months for 67% of injuries (26/39). Outcomes were radiographic and surgeon-reported clinical. Injuries were classified according to the Effendi system. Seven injuries were considered stable and treated with NRI; late radiographic displacement occurred in one, and a poor clinical outcome was noted in 4. 19 injuries were considered unstable, 4 treated with NRI, 11 with RI, 1 ASF, and 3 with undefined internal stabilization; late radiographic displacement occurred in 1, 1, 0, and 0, respectively. Clinical outcome was poor in 13 of these 19. CONCLUSION: Recommend ASF for unstable injuries. Problem—67% follow-up. Unable to differentiate clinical outcome with respect to management of unstable injuries.
Pedersen et al (1967)[29]	Retrospective case series, C2 traumatic spondylolisthesis	IV	9 patients satisfied our inclusion criteria. Treatment was traction + RI in 4, ASF in 2, and PSF in 3. Mean follow-up was unspecified. Outcomes were radiographic. Injuries were unclassified. All cases achieved radiographic union. CONCLUSION: High degree of union occurs regardless of type of treatment. Problem—management with respect to grade of injury was not specified. No clinical outcomes.
Pinczewski et al (1983)[22]	Retrospective case series, C2 traumatic spondylolisthesis	IV	10 patients satisfied our inclusion criteria. Treatment was NRI in 3, RI in 6, and PSF in 1. Mean follow-up was 12 months. Outcomes were radiographic and surgeon-reported clinical. Two injuries were considered stable and treated with NRI; poor clinical outcome was noted in one. 8 injuries were considered unstable, 1 treated with NRI, 6 with RI, and 1 with PSF (for facet dislocation); late radiographic displacement, and poor clinical outcome occurred in the 1 patient treated with NRI. All cases achieved radiographic union. CONCLUSION: Uniformly successful outcome of RI was "emphasized." Problem—RI was used for unstable injuries only.
Samaha et al (2000)[14]	Retrospective cohort study, C2 traumatic spondylolisthesis	III	24 patients satisfied our inclusion criteria. Treatment was RI in 15, ASF in 1, and PSF in 8. Mean follow-up was 13 months. Outcomes were radiographic and surgeon-reported clinical. Injuries were classified according to Roy-Camille (modified Effendi). 14 injuries were considered stable and treated with RI; all cases achieved good radiographic outcome, and one had a poor clinical outcome. 10 injuries were considered unstable, 1 treated with RI, 1 with ASF, and 8 with PSF; late radiographic displacement and poor clinical outcome occurred in 1, 1, and 1, respectively. All cases achieved radiographic union. CONCLUSION: Recommend PSF for unstable injuries. Problem—with the exception of one case all nonoperative treatment was for stable injuries and all surgical treatment was for unstable injuries.
Seljeskog and Chou (1976)[23]	Retrospective case series, C2 traumatic spondylolisthesis	IV	23 patients satisfied our inclusion criteria. Treatment was NRI in 5 and traction (up to 6 weeks) + RI in 17. Mean follow-up was unspecified. Outcomes were radiographic. All cases achieved radiographic union. CONCLUSION: Nonoperative treatment resulted in solid union in all cases. Problem—management with respect to grade of injury (11 stable*) was not specified.

Study	Description	Level of Evidence of Primary Question(s)	Topic and Conclusion
Vieweg et al (2000)[10]	Retrospective cohort study, upper cervical injuries	III	17 patients satisfied our inclusion criteria. Treatment was NRI in 3, RI in 1, and ASF in 8. Mean follow-up was 13 months. Outcomes were radiographic and surgeon-reported clinical. Injures were classified according to the Effendi system. 3 injuries were considered stable* and treated with NRI; all cases achieved good radiographic and clinical outcome. 14 injuries were considered unstable, 6 treated with RI, and 8 (all Effendi type III) with ASF; late radiographic displacement occurred in 0 and 1, respectively. All cases achieved radiographic union. Poor clinical outcome occurred in 1 and 1, respectively. CONCLUSION: Recommend primary ASF for Effendi type III injuries. Problem—all surgical treatment was for type III injuries.
Watanabe et al (2005)[19]	Retrospective cohort study, C2 traumatic spondylolisthesis	III	9 patients satisfied our inclusion criteria. Treatment was NRI in 3 and RI in 6. Mean follow-up was 63 months. Outcomes were radiographic and surgeon-reported clinical injures were classified according to the Levine system. Four injuries were considered stable, 1 treated with NRI, and 3 with RI; one case (RI) demonstrated late radiographic displacement and poor clinical outcome. Five injuries were considered unstable, 2 treated with NRI, and 3 with RI; late radiographic displacement occurred in 1 and 2, respectively. Poor clinical outcome occurred in 1 and 2, respectively. CONCLUSION: Long-term outcome with nonoperative treatment is not always benign. All patients with pain had displacement and inferior facet fracture. Problem—surgically treated patients from same institution not included in long-term follow-up.
Zsolczai and Pentelényi (1990)[24]	Retrospective case series, C2 traumatic spondylolisthesis	IV	34 patients satisfied our inclusion criteria. Treatment was closed reduction and RI in 23 and ASF in 11. Mean follow-up was unspecified. Outcomes were radiographic. Thirteen cases treated with RI demonstrated late displacement with no clinical complaints compared with 1 in the ASF-treated group. All cases achieved radiographic union. CONCLUSION: Nonoperative treatment for "stable injuries," RI or ASF for "unstable" injuries. Problem—management with respect to grade or stability of injury was not specified.

Abbreviations: ASF, anterior spinal fusion; NRI, nonrigid immobilization; PSF, posterior spinal fusion; RI, rigid immobilization.

The total number of cases and those with reported outcomes are summarized in **Tables 26.2 and 26.3**. Eighty-three percent of the total number of cases were treated nonoperatively, with 21% treated using nonrigid immobilization (NRI, e.g., cervical collar) and 79% treated with rigid immobilization (RI, e.g., halo vest or Minerva cast). Of the operatively treated cases 65% were treated with an anterior spinal fusion (ASF) compared with posterior spinal fusion (PSF). In 12 of the 16 included studies we were able to categorize injuries as stable and unstable. There were no stable injuries treated surgically in any of the included studies. No validated patient-reported outcome measures were used in any of the studies.

Surgical versus Nonoperative Management

Of the 16 studies included in our systematic review, 10 included comparisons between surgical and nonoperative treatment for hangman's fractures. Of these 10 studies, nine reported on radiographic outcomes (five with unstable fractures), four on clinical outcomes (one with unstable fractures), six on the development of nonunions (three with unstable fractures), and four on the need for secondary surgery (two with unstable fractures).

No significant study heterogeneity was identified in studies that compared surgical with nonoperative treatment. Only a single study, by Zsolczai and Pentelényi,[24] demonstrated a

Table 26.2 Summary of the Total Number of Reported Cases

	Nonoperative (16 studies)			Operative (10 studies)		
	Total	NRI	RI	Total	ASF	PSF
Total	485	101	383	98	64	22
Stable	79	22	57	0	0	0
Unstable	120	12	93	65	43	11

Abbreviations: ASF, anterior spinal fusion; NRI, nonrigid immobilization; PSF, posterior spinal fusion; RI, rigid immobilization.

Note: In 12 of the 16 included studies, we were able to categorize the cases into stable and unstable.

significant benefit of surgical over nonoperative management for late radiographic displacement; however, the pooled analysis of 10 studies did not show any significant benefit (**Fig. 26.4**). No significant benefit of surgical over nonoperative management was identified in our pooled analysis in regard to late displacement, clinical outcome, nonunion, or secondary surgery (**Table 26.4**).

Operative Management: Posterior versus Anterior Surgical Approach

There were three articles that included comparisons between anterior and posterior approaches to surgical management. Of these, all three had radiographic outcomes (two with unstable fractures), one with clinical outcomes (with unstable fractures), three on the development of nonunions (two with unstable fractures), and only one on the need for secondary surgery (with unstable fractures).

No significant heterogeneity was identified in the studies that compared anterior and posterior surgical approaches. A single study (Lohnert and Látal[28]) demonstrated a benefit to an anterior over a posterior surgical approach for the treatment of hangman fractures in preventing late displacement and nonunion in all fractures and those considered unstable. This study, despite showing a statistically significant difference,

Table 26.3 Summary of Reported Outcomes

Radiographic Outcomes—Percentage of Patients with Late Displacement

	Nonoperative (14 /16 studies)			Operative (9 /10 studies)		
	Total	NRI	RI	Total	ASF	PSF
Total	48/358 (13.4) [14]	10/62 (16.1) [9]	38/295 (12.9) [14]	4/90(4.4) [9]	2/56(3.6) [5]	2/22(9.1) [5]
Stable	7/79(8.9) [5]	4/22(18.2) [4]	3/57(5.3) [3]			
Unstable	25/120 (20.8) [7]	5/12 (41.7) [4]	20/93 (21.5) [6]	2/65(3.1) [6]	1/43(2.3) [3]	1/11(9.1) [3]

Radiographic Outcomes—Percentage of Patients with Nonunion

	Nonoperative (10 /16 studies)			Operative (6 /10 studies)		
	Total	NRI	RI	Total	ASF	PSF
Total	8/385(2.1) [10]	3/79(3.8) [7]	5/305(1.6) [9]	1/66(1.5) [6]	0/45(0) [4]	1/14(7.1) [4]
Stable	0/72(0) [4]	0/15(0) [3]	0/57(0) [3]			
Unstable	1/94(1.1) [4]	0/6(0) [2]	0/73(0) [3]	1/53(1.9) [4]	0/35(0) [2]	1/11(9.1) [3]

Clinical Outcomes—Percentage of Patients Requiring Late Surgery

	Nonoperative (5 /16 studies)			Operative (4 /10 studies)		
	Total	NRI	RI	Total	ASF	PSF
Total	6/104(5.8) [5]	1/35(2.9) [4]	5/69(7.2) [4]	0/37(0) [4]	0/24(0) [2]	0/9(0) [2]
Stable	1/20(5.0) [2]	0/13(0) [2]	1/7(14.3) [1]			
Unstable	4/51(7.8) [3]	0/10(0) [3]	4/41(9.8) [3]	1/29(3.4) [3]	0/16(0) [1]	0/9(0) [2]

Clinical Outcomes—Percentage of Patients with Poor Outcome

	Nonoperative (7 /16 studies)			Operative (4 /10 studies)		
	Total	NRI	RI	Total	ASF	PSF
Total	14/80 (17.5) [7]	6/23(26.1) [5]	8/57(14.0) [6]	6/47(12.8) [4]	4/32(12.5) [3]	2/14(14.3) [2]
Stable	5/9(55.6) [2]	5/9(55.6) [2]				
Unstable	8/16(50) [3]	3/4(75) [2]	5/12(41.7) [3]	2/30(6.7) [2]	1/24(4.2) [2]	1/6(16.7) [1]

Abbreviations: ASF, anterior spinal fusion; NRI, nonrigid immobilization; PSF, posterior spinal fusion; RI, rigid immobilization.

Note: Numbers in parentheses represent the percentages and numbers in square brackets represent the number of trials in each grouping.

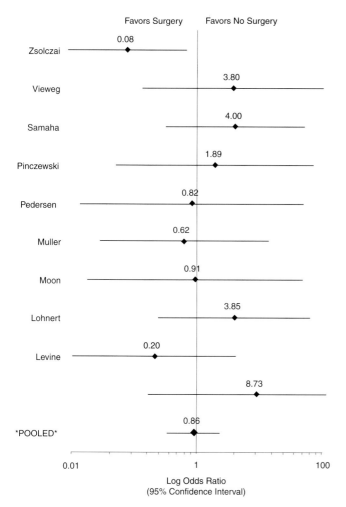

Favors Surgery | Favors No Surgery

Zsolczai 0.08

Vieweg 3.80

Samaha 4.00

Pinczewski 1.89

Pedersen 0.82

Muller 0.62

Moon 0.91

Lohnert 3.85

Levine 0.20

8.73

POOLED 0.86

0.01   1   100

Log Odds Ratio
(95% Confidence Interval)

Fig. 26.4 Late displacement for surgical versus nonoperative treatment for all fracture types. Odds ratios with 95% confidence intervals shown. Left side of unity favors surgical management and right side favors non-operative management.

reported that one of two patients treated with a posterior approach (C2 osteosynthesis) developed late displacement and nonunion of the attempted fusion. The pooled analysis did not show any significant associations. Pooled odds ratios for all other comparisons between the posterior and anterior surgical approach failed to demonstrate any significant differences (**Table 26.5**).

Nonoperative Management: Rigid versus Nonrigid Immobilization

There were 10 articles that included comparisons between rigid and nonrigid immobilization. Of these 10 articles, nine reported on radiographic outcomes (two with stable and four with unstable fractures), four on clinical outcomes (two with unstable fractures), six on the development of nonunions (two with stable and two with unstable fractures), and three on the need for secondary surgery (one with stable and three with unstable fractures).

We found no significant heterogeneity in the variation between studies that compared rigid and nonrigid immobilization of hangman fractures for any of the outcomes.

Pooled analysis did not demonstrate any significant differences in any measure of outcome for rigid versus nonrigid immobilization (**Fig. 26.5**). However, there was a nonsignificant trend in favor of nonrigid immobilization in reducing the rate of secondary surgery. Method of immobilization did not demonstrate any significant association with clinical outcome or secondary surgery (**Table 26.6**).

◆ Discussion

After review of the English literature on the management and outcomes of C2 hangman's fractures, it is apparent that there is a lack of high-quality clinical evidence. Most studies we came across included case reports or reporting only on a single form of treatment. These studies, although providing useful technical information, do not offer us the opportunities for direct treatment comparisons and thus were not included in this review. Our systematic review consisted of retrospective cohort series without the use of any validated measures of outcome (**Table 26.1**).

From our systematic review of comparative observational studies, there was no evidence suggesting which type or types of C2 traumatic spondylolisthesis or variant injuries require surgical intervention or which manner of operative or nonoperative management is optimal.

In general there is a low incidence of nonunion for both stable and unstable C2 traumatic spondylolisthesis regardless of treatment. Although there is a suggestion of a higher incidence of late radiographic displacement with nonsurgical treatment of unstable injuries, this has not been associated with an inferior clinical outcome. All reported clinical outcomes

Table 26.4 Surgical versus Nonsurgical Management of Hangman's Fractures

Group	Outcome	Studies	Odds Ratio	Lower	Upper	P-value
Total	LD	9	0.86	0.29	2.59	0.80
Unstable	LD	5	0.69	0.20	2.36	0.55
Total	Clin	4	1.75	0.49	6.16	0.39
Unstable	Clin	1	0.71	0.04	14.35	0.83
Total	NU	6	2.60	0.44	15.24	0.29
Unstable	NU	3	3.27	0.34	31.11	0.30
Total	SS	4	0.84	0.16	4.48	0.84
Unstable	SS	2	2.37	0.08	66.56	0.61

Abbreviations: Clin, clinical outcome; LD, late displacement; NU, nonunion; SS, secondary surgery.

Note: No significant study heterogeneity identified.

Table 26.5 Posterior versus Anterior Surgical Approach for Treatment of Hangman's Fractures

Group	Outcome	Studies	Odds Ratio	Lower	Upper	P-value
Total	LD	3	8.25	0.23	301.00	0.25
Unstable	LD	2	29.64	0.29	3007.21	0.15
Total	Clin	1	9.00	0.32	254.73	0.14
Unstable	Clin	1	9.00	0.32	254.73	0.14
Total	NU	3	8.25	0.23	301.00	0.25
Unstable	NU	2	29.64	0.29	3007.21	0.15
Total	SS	1	2.54	0.05	141.92	0.65
Unstable	SS	1	2.54	0.05	141.92	0.65

Abbreviations: Clin, clinical outcome; LD, late displacement; NU, nonunion; SS, secondary surgery.

Note: No significant study heterogeneity identified.

were subjective, surgeon-reported measures that suggest a good outcome in the majority of patients treated operatively or nonoperatively. However, two small, long-term studies reported significant residual pain and/or stiffness in 44%[19] and 65%[13] at 5 and 4 years, respectively, for patients treated predominantly by nonoperative means. There is no comparable follow-up among surgical series. Consequently, the generally held position that most of these injuries "do well" is not clearly supported, which should be considered when discussing prognosis with patients.

In this review all injuries categorized as stable were treated nonoperatively. With no demonstrable difference in the reported outcomes, the use of nonrigid immobilization clearly provides minimal burden in all aspects. With low risk and high patient preference, this method of management would be considered optimal management for stable injuries.

Unstable injuries were typically treated by rigid immobilization (50%) or surgery (35%). Unstable injuries treated with nonrigid immobilization (NRI) typically demonstrated inferior radiographic (late displacement) and clinical results (**Table 26.3**). However this represents a very small subgroup, and hence no conclusions can be made regarding the use of NRI for unstable injuries. Dislocation of the C2–C3 facet joints (Effendi type III; total of 23 cases from four of the included studies[10,12,18,22]) was treated surgically in the majority of cases (87%). For all other unstable injuries, conclusions by the authors of the individual studies are contradictory regarding optimal management; hence the treatment of unstable hangman's fractures remains controversial. Although the summary data (**Table 26.3**) from the included comparative studies suggest that rigid immobilization is associated with inferior radiographic and clinical outcomes compared with surgery, the small numbers and variable outcomes in this subgroup do not provide strong evidence in support of operative management.

In this circumstance, we must consider the pros and cons of each treatment. Seven of the 16 reported studies utilized traction for periods ranging from 2 to 6 weeks followed by 6 or more weeks of rigid immobilization. The practical limitations and costs associated with this type of treatment today are unlikely to be acceptable to patients, clinicians, or hospital administrators alike. Contemporary, nonoperative management involves reduction as needed and the use of a halo vest. However, the risk and logistics of halo vest use, particularly in elderly patients, must be weighed against the risk of anterior or posterior surgery. For unstable injuries, comprehensive discussion of operative and nonoperative treatment options, risk:benefit ratios, and patient preference is required.

With the lack of high-level clinical studies and no clear benefit of one treatment over another shown from our systematic review, evidence-based management decisions have to consider multiple factors that include the best level of available evidence that includes expert opinion, relative risk, benefit and burden of the intervention(s), and patient preference. The latter is of greater importance in scenarios of clinical equivalence

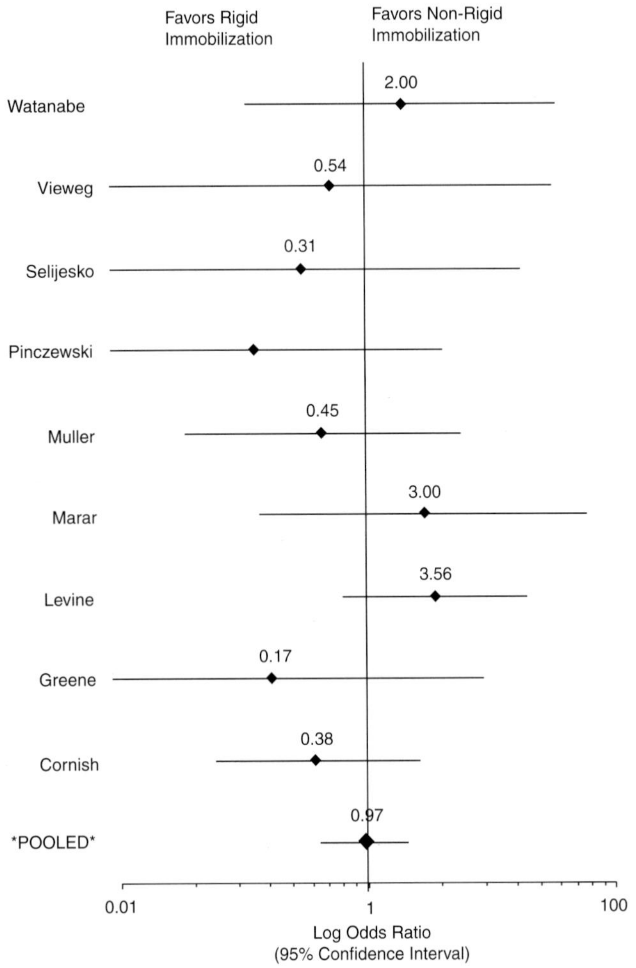

Fig. 26.5 Late displacement for rigid versus non-rigid immobilization for all fracture types. Odds ratios with 95% confidence intervals shown. Left side of unity favors rigid immobilization and right side favors non-rigid immobilization.

Table 26.6 Rigid versus Nonrigid Immobilization of Hangman's Fractures

Group	Outcome	Studies	Heterog	OR	Lower	Upper	*P*-value
Total	LD	9	0.52	0.97	0.42	2.24	0.95
Stable	LD	2	0.64	0.37	0.06	2.19	0.28
Unstable	LD	4	0.82	0.93	0.23	3.77	0.92
Total	Clin	4	0.40	1.00	0.17	5.69	1.00
Unstable	Clin	2	0.53	0.82	0.09	7.63	0.86
Total	NU	6	0.80	0.58	0.17	2.01	0.39
Stable	NU	2	0.81	0.63	0.04	11.16	0.75
Unstable	NU	2	0.48	0.32	0.01	8.03	0.49
Total	SS	3	0.57	3.86	0.82	18.15	0.09
Stable	SS	1	.	3.00	0.10	88.14	0.72
Unstable	SS	3	0.38	1.61	0.26	10.02	0.61

Abbreviations: Clin, clinical outcome; LD, late displacement; NU, nonunion; SS, secondary surgery.

Table 26.7 Clinical Recommendations

	Strength of Recommendation
What C2 hangman's or associated variant fractures require surgical intervention?	• Strong
• Surgical intervention is recommended for Effendi type III injuries (i.e., associated C2–C3 unilateral or bilateral facet dislocation or fracture-dislocation).	• Weak
• Surgical intervention or halo vest immobilization is reasonable treatment option for other unstable hangman's fracture.	
When a hangman's fracture is managed operatively what is the optimal approach?	• Strong
• Anterior or posterior stabilization can be utilized as per surgeon and patient preference. As a note of caution when using posterior approaches, unstable injures treated surgically should include stabilization across C2–C3.	
When a hangman's fracture is managed nonoperatively what is the optimal approach?	• Strong
• For stable injuries, collar immobilization is recommended.	• Strong
• For unstable injuries, rigid immobilization with a halo vest is recommended rather than a collar.	

between two treatment options. Clearly, better-designed high-quality prospective trials are needed to determine the optimal treatment for this condition. Due to the logistic difficulties of such studies for a relatively uncommon surgical condition, it is unlikely that such data will ever be readily available. As such, **Table 26.7** provides graded clinical recommendations based on the best available evidence and expert clinical opinion from the international membership of the Spine Trauma Study Group for the management of C2 traumatic spondylolisthesis.

References

1. Wood-Jones F. The examination of the bodies of 100 men executed in Numbia in Roman times. BMJ 1908;1:736–737
2. Schneider RC, Livingston KE, Cave AJE, Hamilton G. "Hangman's fracture" of the cervical spine. J Neurosurg 1965;22:141–154
3. Hadley MN, Walters BC, Grabb PA, et al. Guidelines for the management of acute cervical spine and spinal cord injuries. Clin Neurosurg 2002;49:407–498
4. Li XF, Dai LY, Lu H, Chen XD. A systematic review of the management of hangman's fractures. Eur Spine J 2006;15:257–269 [comment]
5. Levine AM, Rhyne AL. Traumatic spondylolisthesis of the axis. Semin Spine Surg 1991;3:47–60
6. Hoffman JR, Mower WR, Wolfson AB, Todd KH, Zucker MI; National Emergency X-Radiography Utilization Study Group. Validity of a set of clinical criteria to rule out injury to the cervical spine in patients with blunt trauma. N Engl J Med 2000;343:94–99
7. Lowery DW, Wald MM, Browne BJ, Tigges S, Hoffman JR, Mower WR; NEXUS Group. Epidemiology of cervical spine injury victims. Ann Emerg Med 2001;38:12–16
8. Goldberg W, Mueller C, Panacek E, Tigges S, Hoffman JR, Mower WR; NEXUS Group. Distribution and patterns of blunt traumatic cervical spine injury. Ann Emerg Med 2001;38:17–21
9. Greene KA, Dickman CA, Marciano FF, Drabier JB, Hadley MN, Sonntag VKH. Acute axis fractures: analysis of management and outcome in 340 consecutive cases. Spine 1997;22:1843–1852
10. Vieweg U, Meyer B, Schramm J. Differential treatment in acute upper cervical spine injuries: a critical review of a single-institution series. Surg Neurol 2000;54:203–210, discussion 210–211
11. Effendi B, Roy D, Cornish B, Dussault RG, Laurin CA. Fractures of the ring of the axis: a classification based on the analysis of 131 cases. J Bone Joint Surg Br 1981;63-B:319–327
12. Levine AM, Edwards CC. The management of traumatic spondylolisthesis of the axis. J Bone Joint Surg Am 1985;67:217–226
13. Müller EJ, Wick M, Muhr G. Traumatic spondylolisthesis of the axis: treatment rationale based on the stability of the different fracture types. Eur Spine J 2000;9:123–128
14. Samaha C, Lazennec JY, Laporte C, Saillant G. Hangman's fracture: the relationship between asymmetry and instability. J Bone Joint Surg Br 2000;82:1046–1052
15. Bohlman HH. Acute fractures and dislocations of the cervical spine: an analysis of three hundred hospitalized patients and review of the literature. J Bone Joint Surg Am 1979;61:1119–1142
16. Francis WR, Fielding JW, Hawkins RJ, Pepin J, Hensinger R. Traumatic spondylolisthesis of the axis. J Bone Joint Surg Br 1981;63-B:313–318

17. Grady MS, Howard MA, Jane JA, Persing JA. Use of the Philadelphia collar as an alternative to the halo vest in patients with C-2, C-3 fractures. Neurosurgery 1986;18:151–156

18. Moon MS, Moon JL, Moon YW, Sun DH, Choi WT. Traumatic spondylolisthesis of the axis: 42 cases. Bull Hosp Jt Dis 2001-2002-2002;60:61–66

19. Watanabe M, Nomura T, Toh E, Sato M, Mochida J. Residual neck pain after traumatic spondylolisthesis of the axis. J Spinal Disord Tech 2005; 18:148–151

20. Cornish BL. Traumatic spondylolisthesis of the axis. J Bone Joint Surg Br 1968;50:31–43

21. Marar BC. Fracture of the axis arch. "Hangman's fracture" of the cervical spine. Clin Orthop Relat Res 1975;106:155–165

22. Pinczewski L, Taylor TKF, Ryan MD. Hangman's fracture: nonoperative management with the halocast. Aust N Z J Surg 1983;53:71–76

23. Seljeskog EL, Chou SN. Spectrum of the hangman's fracture. J Neurosurg 1976;45:3–8

24. Zsolczai S, Pentelényi T. The modern approach of hangman's fracture. Acta Chir Hung 1990;31:3–24

25. Starr JK, Eismont FJ. Atypical hangman's fractures. Spine 1993;18: 1954–1957

26. Li X-F, Dai L-Y, Lu H, Chen X-D. A systematic review of the management of hangman's fractures. Eur Spine J 2006;15:257–269

27. Geck MJ, Yoo S, Wang JC. Assessment of cervical ligamentous injury in trauma patients using MRI. J Spinal Disord 2001;14:371–377

28. Lohnert J, Látal J. Fracture of the axis—surgical treatment, II. Axial isthmus [in Slovak]. Acta Chir Orthop Traumatol Cech 1993;60: 47–50

29. Pedersen HE, Roy LJ, Salciccioli GG. Fractures of cervical 2. J Bone Joint Surg Am 1967;49A:1468–1484

30. Arand M, Neller S, Kinzl L, Claes L, Wilke HJ. The traumatic spondylolisthesis of the axis: a biomechanical in vitro evaluation of an instability model and clinical relevant constructs for stabilization. Clin Biomech (Bristol, Avon) 2002;17:432–438

31. Duggal N, Chamberlain RH, Perez-Garza LE, Espinoza-Larios A, Sonntag VK, Crawford NR. Hangman's fracture: a biomechanical comparison of stabilization techniques. Spine 2007;32:182–187

32. Taller S, Suchomel P, Lukás R, Beran J. CT-guided internal fixation of a hangman's fracture. Eur Spine J 2000;9:393–397

33. Tashjian RZ, Majercik S, Biffl WL, Palumbo MA, Cioffi WG. Halo-vest immobilization increases early morbidity and mortality in elderly odontoid fractures. J Trauma 2006;60:199–203

34. Majercik S, Tashjian RZ, Biffl WL, Harrington DT, Cioffi WG. Halo vest immobilization in the elderly: a death sentence? J Trauma 2005;59:350–356, discussion 356–358

VI

Subaxial Cervical Spine Injuries and Their Management

27

The Subaxial Cervical Spine Injury Classification Scale (SLIC)

Usman Zahir, Steven C. Ludwig, Andrew T. Dailey, and Alexander R. Vaccaro

Despite the dramatic advances in cervical spine surgery during the past 2 decades, a well-accepted classification system for subaxial spine fractures has not been developed. Classification systems offer several benefits to the clinician: improved communication between professionals, standardized descriptions of injuries, better insight regarding prognosis, and better guidance for formulating a treatment plan.[1] An ideal classification system for the subaxial spine would incorporate the factors used in treatment decision making, including fracture pattern, mechanism of injury, spinal alignment, neurological injury, and assessment of stability. Traditional classification systems for subaxial spine injuries categorized the injuries on the basis of mechanistic criteria and fracture patterns but did not appropriately assess spinal stability or neurological dysfunction. This chapter discusses a novel classification system for the lower cervical spine, the Subaxial Cervical Spine Injury Classification (SLIC) system. This system evaluates the morphological, neurological, and discoligamentous aspects of lower cervical spine injuries, thus providing both descriptive and prognostic information that will assist in treatment decision making. Additionally, we review the previously described classification systems and the evidence that supports use of the novel system, SLIC.

◆ Epidemiology of Subaxial Spine Injuries

According to the National Spinal Cord Injury Statistical Center,[2] ~12,000 spinal cord injuries occur in the United States per year. The cervical spine is injured in ~2 to 3% of patients who sustain blunt trauma.[2,3] In one review of 818 patients with blunt cervical spine injuries, 60% of fractures and 75% of dislocations occurred in the subaxial spine.[4] Motor vehicle collisions are responsible for the largest proportion (47%) of spinal cord injuries, with falls, gunshot wounds, and sports-related activities being the next most frequent mechanisms.[5] The age distribution for injuries is bimodal. In young adults, motor vehicle collisions are the number one cause. However, in the elderly population, low-energy mechanisms, such as falls, are usually the most common cause. During the past 30 years, the average age at onset for patients with spinal cord injury has increased from 28.7 to 38.0 years. Although 77% of spinal cord injuries occur in male patients, the proportion has decreased slightly during the past 2 decades. Injuries to the cervical spine have the highest average first-year health care cost per patient: $775,567.00 (C1–C4), $500,829.00 (C5–C8), and $283,388.00 (T1 and below). Life expectancy data from the National Spinal Cord Injury Statistical Center are shown in **Table 27.1**.

Table 27.1 Life Expectancy (in years) for Persons Who Survive At Least 1 Year after Spinal Injury

Age at Injury (yr)	No SCI	Motor Functional at Any Level	Para	Low Tetra (C5–C8)	High Tetra (C1–C4)	Ventilator Dependent at Any Level
20	58.4	53.0	45.8	41.0	37.4	23.8
40	39.5	34.5	28.2	24.2	21.2	11.4
60	22.2	18.0	13.2	10.4	8.6	3.2

Abbreviations: SCI, spinal cord injury; Para, paraplegia; Tetra, tetraplegia.

Source: National Spinal Cord Injury Statistical Center. Spinal Cord Injury Facts and Figures at a Glance 2008. http://www.spinalcord.uab.edu/show.asp?durki=116979.

◆ Unique Clinical and Diagnostic Features of Subaxial Spine Injuries

Anatomy of the Subaxial Cervical Spine

The anatomy of the cervical spine allows for greater motion than that in the thoracic and lumbar spine. The cervical spine is therefore more vulnerable to injuries affecting the osseous and ligamentous structures. The subaxial cervical spine consists of five cylindrically shaped vertebral bodies (C3–C7), which form six motion segments. Each motion segment is made up of the vertebral body and the corresponding adjacent soft tissue structures. The vertebral bodies of the subaxial spine share similar morphological conditions yet increase in size caudally. The anterior region includes the anterior vertebral body, annulus fibrosis, and anterior longitudinal ligament. The posterior extension of the vertebra includes the neural arch, spinous process, laminae, and posterior ligamentous structures. The lateral column comprises the superior and inferior facets and the pedicles. The spinal canal, which encloses the spinal cord, is formed from the borders of the four columns. A recent cervical spine injury classification system (Cervical Spine Severity Score system) bases its scoring on the evaluation of the four columns.[1]

The lateral mass is located between the inferior and superior facets along the posterolateral surface of the vertebral body. The subaxial cervical facets are oriented 45 degrees obliquely and play a central role as the load-bearing structures in the cervical spine. The superior and inferior facets of the adjacent vertebrae make up the facet joints, and a second potential articulation (during lateral bending) is the uncovertebral joint, which consists of the lateral surfaces of the vertebral body. The anterior longitudinal ligament (ALL) and posterior longitudinal ligament (PLL) are along the anterior and posterior borders of the vertebral body, respectively. The fibers of the ALL run continuous with the anulus fibrosus. The ligamentum flavum attaches to the laminae and is posterior to the spinal cord within the spinal canal. Interspinous and supraspinous ligaments connect adjacent spinous processes. The ligamentous structures play a role in the stability of the spine and the maintenance of the cervical spine alignment.[6]

Biomechanics of the Subaxial Cervical Spine

One of the most important assessments of the cervical spine in the clinical setting is the determination of stability. During the past 30 years, many biomechanical studies of the cervical spine have been conducted. White and Panjabi[7] studied the cervical spine range of motion and determined the following ranges: flexion-extension, 9 to 20 degrees; lateral bending, 4 to 11 degrees; and axial rotation, 2 to 7 degrees. The load-bearing ability of the cervical spine is shared by the intervertebral disk and the facets. The facets of the cervical spine have a large cross-sectional area compared with the intervertebral disk, and one study showed that 32% of the axial load at C6 (64% total) was carried by each of the facets, whereas 36% was carried by the vertebral body and intervertebral disk.[8]

White and Panjabi[9] defined cervical spine instability as the loss of the ability of the spine to maintain, under physiological loads, its pattern of displacement so that there is no initial or additional neurological deficit, no major deformity, and no incapacitating pain. The ligamentous structures of the cervical spine support tensile forces and resist motions that cause

Table 27.2 Instability in the Cervical Spine

1. All anterior or all posterior elements destroyed or unable to function
2. More than 3.5 mm of horizontal displacement between adjacent vertebrae shown on lateral view radiograph
3. More than 11 degrees of angulation difference between adjacent vertebrae

Source: White AA III, Johnson RM, Panjabi MM, Southwick WO. Biomechanical analysis of clinical stability in the cervical spine. Clin Orthop Relat Res 1975;109:85–96.

tension; flexion is controlled by the posterior ligaments, and extension is affected by the anterior ligaments. Early biomechanical studies showed that as the cervical spine was stressed with physiological loads, instability occurred when all the posterior structures and the PLL were sectioned or when all the anterior structures and the PLL were sectioned, thus showing the crucial role the PLL plays in spinal stability. Studies continue to show that, regarding spinal stability, anterior structures play a less important role.[10]

According to White et al,[11] subaxial cervical spine instability is characterized by a 3.5 mm horizontal displacement of one vertebra in relation to an adjacent vertebra or more than 11 degrees of angulation difference between adjacent vertebrae shown on a lateral view radiograph. The specific findings are described in **Table 27.2**.

A diagnostic checklist of nine categories was formulated by White et al[11] to assess for spinal instability. The checklist is based on biomechanical, anatomical, and experimental data but has not been clinically validated. Each category was assigned a point score, and instability was defined by a total of 5 or more points (**Table 27.3**).

Recently, further attempts have been made to quantify stability in the cervical spine. The Cervical Spine Severity Score system was developed to assess the stability of the cervical spine with the use of an analog-graded scoring system.[1] With that system, the cervical spine is divided into four columns (anterior, posterior, right pillar, and left pillar), and each column is assigned a score (0 to 5) based on the fracture displacement. High scores indicate necessity for surgery (on average, 100% of patients with total scores higher than 7 underwent surgery). For patients with multiple levels of injury, only the most severe level is calculated into the final score. The scoring system was tested for reliability in a blinded retrospective study in which 15 examiners (residents, fellows, radiologists, and attending spine surgeons) reviewed 34 cases of cervical trauma.[12] Results from the study showed excellent intraclass [intraclass correlation coefficient (ICC) 0.977] and interobserver agreement (ICC 0.833). No significant difference in scores was shown based on the experience of the observers (residents and fellows, ICC 0.871; attending surgeons and radiologists, ICC 0.894).

Subaxial Cervical Spine Classification Systems

Traditional classification systems for cervical spine fractures have focused primarily on anatomical, morphological, and mechanistic criteria. The bases for the classification systems have varied from observational studies, retrospective reviews, and cadaver biomechanical studies. Sir Francis

Table 27.3 Diagnostic Checklist for Spinal Instability

	Points
Disruption of anterior elements, with more than 25% loss of height	2
Disruption of posterior elements	2
Sagittal plane translation more than 3.5 mm or more than 20% of anteroposterior diameter of vertebral body	2
Intervertebral sagittal rotation more than 11 degrees	2
Intervertebral distance more than 1.7 mm on stretch test	2
Evidence of cord damage	2
Evidence of root damage	1
Acute intervertebral disk space narrowing	1
Anticipated abnormally large stress	1

Source: White AA III, Johnson RM, Panjabi MM, Southwick WO. Biomechanical analysis of clinical stability in the cervical spine. Clin Orthop Relat Res 1975;109:85–96.

Holdsworth[13] offered a description of spine injuries that used many of the mechanistic and morphological terms for fractures that continue to be used today in cervical spine classification systems. His descriptions were based on a personal observational study of more than 1000 patients who presented at Sheffield Spinal Injuries Centre in Sheffield, England (level IV evidence). His entire research was based on his own personal experiences with fracture patterns and management, and the level of evidence is similar to that of a case series today.

Allen et al[14] developed a formal classification system (the Allen-Ferguson system) that focuses on mechanisms of injury inferred from radiographic images, and it is one of the most widely used systems today. It was developed after the authors reviewed radiographs of 165 patients and formulated categories based on the mechanisms involved. The classification system is based on a descriptive analysis of radiographic images, with level IV evidence. The system divides injuries into six categories: (1) flexion-compression, (2) vertical compression, (3) flexion-distraction, (4) extension-compression, (5) extension-distraction, and (6) lateral-flexion.

Harris et al[15] developed a classification system (the Harris system) similar to the Allen-Ferguson system, with extra emphasis placed on rotational forces instead of distractive forces. Harris et al also divided spine injuries into six categories: (1) flexion, (2) flexion-rotation, (3) hyperextension-rotation, (4) vertical compression, (5) extension, and (6) lateral flexion. The authors categorized injuries based on a review of previously established injury patterns within the cervical spine. This consisted of a retrospective analysis of available clinical and experimental studies and is level IV evidence.

The AO classification (**Table 27.4**) is a comprehensive system that was developed for thoracolumbar spine injuries; however, it is often applied to cervical spine injuries.[16] The system was developed after a retrospective review of 1445 thoracolumbar injuries and assessment of the level of injury, frequency of fracture types/groups, and incidence of neurological deficits (level IV evidence). Categories in the AO system are based on the mechanism of injury and morphology with three general types, A, B, and C, and corresponding subgroups. The classification takes into account injury severity and stability. Type A injuries involve compressive forces on the vertebral body. Type B injuries involve distractive forces on either the anterior or the posterior elements. Type C injuries combine one of the other forces with axial rotation.

Mechanistic classification systems, as already described, classify injuries based on force vectors, with one vector dominating the injury pattern. This results in several challenges that have been identified in the literature. A specific mechanism, for instance, can produce a wide variety of injury patterns and is influenced by preexisting disease states in the spine and associated musculature. Identifying a specific mechanism can be difficult in an unstable spine, where multiple vectors might have been involved in the injury pattern. Morphological classification systems based on analysis of imaging studies have been noted to refer to mechanistic terms in descriptions of injury patterns. The classification systems mentioned thus far do not assess for neurological status or provide adequate emphasis on the role of stability in the fracture patterns.[1] The management of subaxial cervical injuries is based on a well-informed assessment of the fracture pattern, mechanism of injury, spinal stability, and neurological status. An ideal classification system would therefore incorporate all those variables into a unified system for practical use.[17]

◆ SLIC

SLIC is a new classification system that moves away from a purely mechanistic or morphological description of injury patterns for lower cervical spine fractures (**Table 27.5**). It was developed through a literature review and the expert opinion of orthopedic spine surgeons and neurosurgeons. The goal for this new system is not only to classify injuries but also to grade injury patterns based on severity, thus better assisting the clinician in assessing prognosis. By assigning a numerical score, the system will assist the clinician in the decision-making process of whether to pursue an operative or a nonoperative course of action.

SLIC Scoring

SLIC is a novel classification system for lower cervical spine fractures that was developed by the Spine Trauma Study Group (STSG) to focus on three important components to injury: the morphology of the fracture, assessment of the discoligamentous complex, and the neurological status of the patient. Each of these components plays an important role in

Table 27.4 The AO Classification System

A: Compression Injury

  A1: Impaction fracture

    A1.1 End plate impaction

    A1.2 Wedge impaction

    A1.3 Vertebral body collapse

  A2: Split fracture

    A2.1 Sagittal split fracture

    A2.2 Coronal split fracture

    A2.3 Pincer fracture

  A3: Burst fracture

    A3.1 Incomplete burst fracture

    A3.2 Burst-split fracture

    A3.3 Complete burst fracture

B: Distraction injury

  B1: Posterior ligamentary lesion

    B1.1 With disk rupture

    B1.2 With type A fracture

  B2: Posterior osseous lesion

    B2.1 Transverse bicolumn

    B2.2 With disk rupture

    B2.3 With type A fracture

  B3: Anterior disk rupture

    B3.1 With subluxation

    B3.2 With spondylolysis

    B3.3 With posterior dislocation

C: Rotation injury

  C1: Type A with rotation

    C1.1 Rotational wedge fracture

    C1.2 Rotational split fracture

    C1.3 Rotational burst fracture

  C2: Type B with rotation

    C2.1 B1 lesion with rotation

    C2.2 B2 lesion with rotation

    C2.3 B3 lesion with rotation

  C3: Rotational shear

    C3.1 Slice fracture

    C3.2 Oblique fracture

Source: Magerl F, Aebi M, Gertzbein SD, Harms J, Nazarian S. A comprehensive classification of thoracic and lumbar injuries. Eur Spine J 1994;3:184–201.

Table 27.5 SLIC Scale

	Points
Morphology	
No abnormality	0
Compression	1
Burst	2
Distraction	3
Rotation/translation	4
Disco-ligamentous complex	
Intact	0
Indeterminate	1
Disrupted	2
Neurological status	
Intact	0
Root injury	1
Complete cord injury	2
Incomplete cord injury	3
Presence of continued cord compression in the setting of spinal cord injury	+1

Note: Scores ≥5 = surgery; scores ≤ 3 = nonsurgical treatment; score of 4 = equivocal.

Source: Vaccaro AR, Hulbert RJ, Patel AA, Fisher C, Dvorak M, Lehman RA Jr, Anderson P, Harrop J, Oner FC, Arnold P, Fehlings M, Hedlund R, Madrazo I, Rechtine G, Aarabi B, Shainline M, Spine Trauma Study Group. The subaxial cervical spine injury classification system: a novel approach to recognize the importance of morphology, neurology, and integrity of the disco-ligamentous complex. Spine 2007;32:2365–2374.

The SLIC system then assigns a numerical value to each of the components, the sum of which is added to produce a total score. For scores higher than or equal to 5, recommendations are for surgical treatment options; scores less than or equal to 3 are treated nonoperatively. A score of 4 is considered unclear and might be treated operatively or nonoperatively, depending on the clinical circumstances involved.[17] The SLIC system is the first attempt to classify cervical spine fracture by abandoning mechanism and anatomy and instead placing emphasis on injury morphology and clinical status.

1. *Morphology.* Assesses spinal column disruption by diagnostic imaging studies and places fractures into one of three main categories: compression, distraction, and translation/rotation
2. *Discoligamentous complex.* Plays an important role in cervical spine stability; integrity of these structures is assessed by radiographic studies
3. *Neurology.* Neurological status of the patient at the time of injury

Subaxial Cervical Classification Scale: Injury Patterns

The SLIC system divides subaxial cervical spine fractures into three major morphological categories: compression/burst, distraction, translation/rotation. Each of the injuries is discussed, and the importance of the discoligamentous complex and neurological status is incorporated.

prognosis and management and was thought to be an independent predictor of clinical outcome. When classifying an injury, the clinician first describes the level of injury, then the injury morphology, and then a description of particular osseous injuries. Next, soft tissue injury/intervertebral disk findings are described, and then the neurological status of the patient is considered (e.g., C6–C7 translation bilateral facet dislocation with complete disruption of the discoligamentous complex with a herniated disk in the setting of a complete spinal cord injury).

Compression/Burst

Compression and burst fracture patterns usually result from an axial load mechanism to the cervical spine and receive a score of 1 and 2, respectively, on the scoring scale for morphology. The most common levels for compression injuries of the subaxial cervical spine are C6 and C7. This fracture pattern primarily results in bony destruction (loss of vertebral height) caused by axial load, and it is expected that the discoligamentous complex is intact. Compression fractures usually affect the anterior aspect of the vertebral body, with the posterior aspect remaining intact. Pure vertical axial load compression injuries on a straightened cervical spine are rare, and, in most cases, the spine is in slight flexion during the axial load.[14] This is especially true with burst fractures.[18]

Burst fractures are defined as any injury to the vertebral body resulting in fractures extending through the posterior and anterior cortex of the vertebral body. Protrusion of these fracture fragments into the spinal canal can result in varying degrees of neurological dysfunction. Therefore, the presence of neurological dysfunction (especially incomplete injury) plays the predominant role in determining the severity of the fractures based on the SLIC score. A compression fracture in a neurologically intact patient will likely have a low score (morphology = 1, discoligamentous complex = 0, neurology = 0), and a burst fracture in a neurologically intact patient will likely have a SLIC score between 2 and 4 (morphology = 2, discoligamentous complex = 0−2, neurology = 0). **Figure 27.1** shows the use of the SLIC scoring system in assessing a burst fracture in a neurologically intact patient.[19]

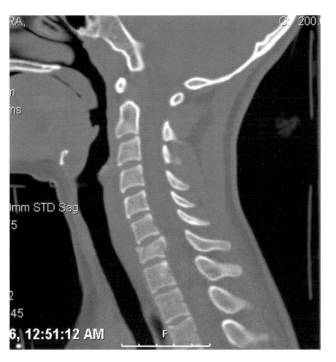

A

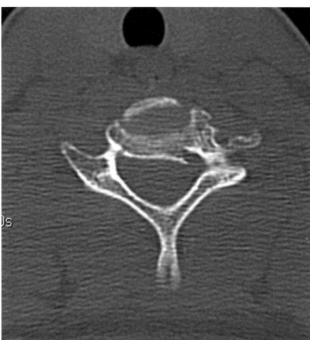

B

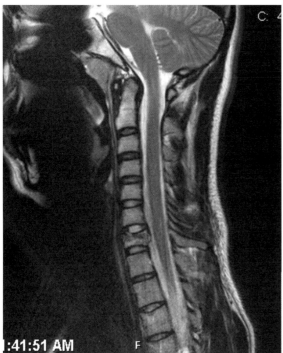

C

Fig. 27.1 Images show C7 burst fracture in a 17-year-old female patient after a fall. Patient was neurologically intact. **(A)** Sagittal view and **(B)** axial view computed tomographic scans show an overall stable alignment. **(C)** Sagittal view T2-weighted magnetic resonance image shows a normal discoligamentous complex. SLIC score of 2 (morphology = 2, discoligamentous complex = 0, neurology = 0). Patient underwent nonoperative treatment. (From Patel AA, Dailey A, Brodke DS, Daubs M, Anderson PA, Hurlbert RJ, Vaccaro AR, Spine Trauma Study Group. Subaxial cervical spine trauma classification: the Subaxial Injury Classification system and case examples. Neurosurg Focus 2008;24:E8. Reprinted with permission.)

Distraction

The physiological movements of flexion and extension are stabilized by the posterior anulus fibrosus and the PLL. Studies have shown the PLL to be one of the most important stabilizers to the spine in both flexion and extension.[20] Distraction injuries result from either hyperextension or a hyperflexion mechanism and involve disruption of the discoligamentous complex that results in dissociation. Distraction injuries receive a score of 3 for morphology, 2 for involvement of the discoligamentous complex, and any additional points for neurological dysfunction.

1. *Hyperflexion.* Hyperflexion injuries result in damage to the posterior ligamentous structures along with trauma to the anterior column of the spine, making hyperflexion a potentially unstable fracture pattern. With hyperflexion forces, a component of compression is often present, resulting in anterior end-plate compression and burst fractures (first category). Yet it is the strain on the posterior ligamentous structures that differentiates compression fractures caused by hyperflexion and those caused by a predominantly axial load mechanism. Depending on the degree of flexion, unilateral or bilateral facet subluxations (less than 25% displacement) can occur. These injury patterns exist along a continuum of severity, depending on the degree of flexion.
2. *Hyperextension.* Hyperextension injuries cause compression of posterior structures with distraction of anterior regions. They often occur classically in spondylotic spines, resulting in disruption of the anterior ligamentous structures, avulsion fractures of the anterior osteophytes, and compression of the posterior elements. Hyperextension injuries also occur along a continuum of severity. Normally, the posterior elements are very stable, and the backward tilt in extension is restricted by the PLL and the facet capsules (in flexion, the facet capsules are free to glide forward); however, when the anterior ligamentous structures are compromised in severe hyperextension, the PLL might be stripped. With these injury patterns, the posterior ligamentous structures of the spine undergo significant strain and tension. Rupture of these structures results in translation of the vertebral bodies. Usually, with a simple hyperextension mechanism in a patient with preexisting spondylosis, the concern is not instability but rather reduced preinjury canal width. The infolding of the ligamentum flavum during hyperextension along with osteophytes can result in significant cord damage with intact ligamentous structures. This is, however, not the case with elderly patients with preexisting ankylosing spondylitis and diffuse idiopathic skeletal hyperostosis who suffer low-energy falls with hyperextension injuries; the presence of cervical spine fractures in those patients should be considered a special case scenario, regardless of the mechanism involved.

Translation/Rotation

Translation/rotation injuries score a 4 for morphology and also involve disruption of the discoligamentous complex, for a total score of 6. Several examples include facet dislocations, unstable teardrop fractures, and advanced-stage flexion-compression injury. Translation/rotation injuries are caused by the same mechanisms as described for the earlier injury patterns and exist along the same continuum but occur after the PLL has torn. Other associated injuries include bilateral lamina and spinous process fractures. The anulus fibrosus is usually disrupted, often with associated disk herniation.[1] Displacements of the vertebral bodies result in significant narrowing of the spinal canal, usually resulting in incomplete or complete spinal cord damage.

1. *Unilateral/bilateral facet fracture dislocations* involve flexion and translation with rotation of one vertebra over another. A pure translational component causes bilateral locked facets; the facets from one vertebra are displaced anteriorly over the inferior vertebra. With a unilateral facet dislocation, a single facet is dislocated and locked; a rotational component is often involved. The rotational component is not necessarily a purely extrinsic force but can be related to intrinsic rotational motions at the facet joint during a unilateral translation.[21]

   Generally, with unilateral facet dislocations, posterior ligamentous structures, joint capsule, and 50% of the anulus fibrosus are disrupted. Yet, consensus regarding what components of the discoligamentous complex are absolutely necessary to create a unilateral facet dislocation is lacking. One experimental cadaver study, for instance, showed that neither the PLL nor the ALL was necessary to create a unilateral facet dislocation but that disruption of the anterior capsule, ipsilateral ligamentum flavum, and more than 50% of the anulus fibrosus were necessary.[21] Although disruption of the ALL and PLL is not absolutely necessary to create a unilateral facet dislocation, both the ALL and the PLL are often disrupted in association with bilateral facet dislocation.[22] It has been shown that bilateral facet dislocations occur most often in the lower vertebrae of the cervical spine.[14] More than 50% displacement of the anteroposterior diameter of the vertebral body on the adjacent body has been thought to indicate bilateral facet dislocation.[23] **Figures 27.2** and **27.3** show the use of the SLIC scoring system in cases of translational spine injuries.[19]
2. *End plate compression fracture with facet fracture/dislocation* occurs when a translation/rotational component involving the facet is associated with a compression fracture of the vertebral body.
3. *Vertebral burst fracture/dislocation (teardrop fracture)* occurs with more severe involvement of the vertebral body. These are often described as quadrangular, teardrop fractures, and burst fracture dislocations; all involve severe disruption of the posterior elements with fragment retropulsion into the spinal canal. Teardrop fractures were first described by Schneider[24] in 1960. The injury has been documented in association with shallow water diving accidents and football injuries involving severe flexion and axial compression forces to the cervical spine.[25] The injury pattern has also been described in association with hyperextension injuries.[15]

   Teardrop fractures occur when a small triangular fragment is detached, usually from the anterior inferior vertebral body. The fracture might involve the full height of the anterior border of the vertebral body. The primary characteristic of teardrop fractures is the detachment of the bone fragment.[26]

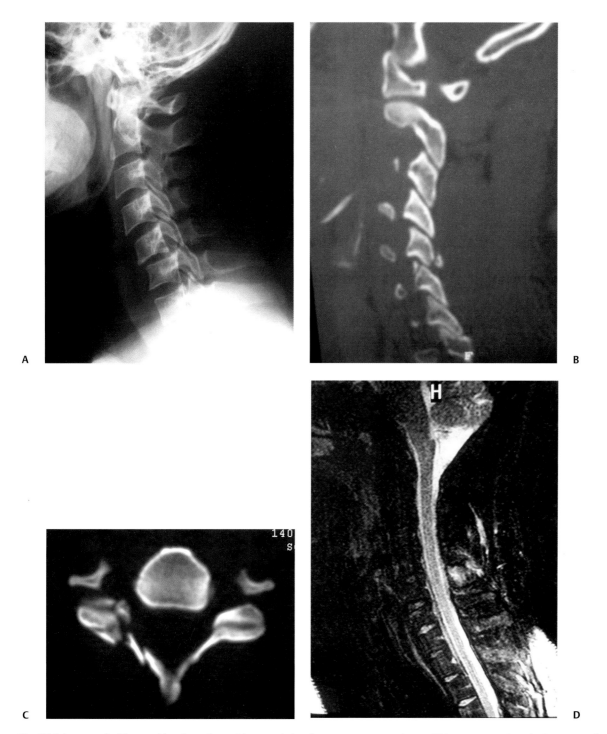

A

B

C

D

Fig. 27.2 Images of a 53-year-old male patient with a translational C5–C6 injury after a motor vehicle accident with subsequent left arm pain, isolated biceps weakness, and index finger sensory deficits. **(A)** Plain radiograph shows the translation of C5. **(B)** Sagittal view and **(C)** axial view computed tomographic scans show left C5 inferior articular facet and C6 superior facet fractures. **(D)** Involvement of the posterior ligamentous structures are highlighted in the magnetic resonance image. This case was assigned a SLIC score of 7 (morphology = 4, disco-igamentous complex = 2, neurology = 1). Patient underwent subsequent operative treatment.(From Patel AA, Dailey A, Brodke DS, Daubs M, Anderson PA, Hurlbert RJ, Vaccaro AR, Spine Trauma Study Group. Subaxial cervical spine trauma classification: the Subaxial Injury Classification system and case examples. Neurosurg Focus 2008;24:E8. Reprinted with permission.)

◆ Reliability and Validity of the Classification Systems[17]

To determine the reliability of the SLIC system, it was compared with the Allen-Ferguson and Harris classification systems. Twenty spine surgeons from the STSG were asked to review 11 cervical trauma cases and apply each of the three classification systems. Interrater reliability, intrarater reliability, and validity were then calculated for each of the classification systems and components of the SLIC system (**Tables 27.6 and 27.7**).

The SLIC score had a high interrater reliability agreement (ICC = 0.71) and an even higher intrarater reliability agreement

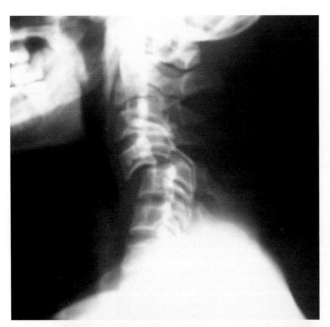

A

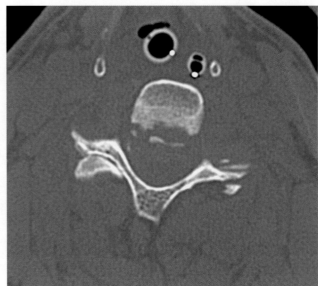

B

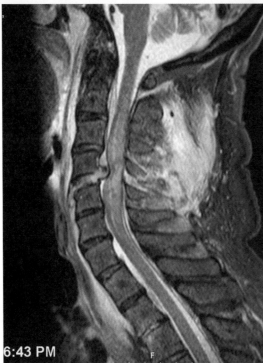

C

6:43 PM

Fig. 27.3 Images of a 32-year-old female patient who was involved in a motor vehicle collision and sustained an anterior C4–C5 dislocation with complete neurological involvement. **(A)** Plain radiograph shows the anterior dislocation of C4, with bilateral facet dislocations noted on **(B)** the computed tomographic scan. **(C)** Magnetic resonance image highlights the involvement of the disk space and the posterior ligamentous structures. Patient was assigned a SLIC score of 8 (morphology = 4, discoligamentous complex = 2, neurology = 2). Patient underwent operative treatment. (From Patel AA, Dailey A, Brodke DS, Daubs M, Anderson PA, Hurlbert RJ, Vaccaro AR, Spine Trauma Study Group. Subaxial cervical spine trauma classification: the Subaxial Injury Classification system and case examples. Neurosurg Focus 2008;24:E8. Reprinted with permission.)

Table 27.6 Interrater Reliability of the SLIC, Allen-Ferguson, and Harris Systems

Measure	Kappa	Rank Order Correlation	Intraclass Correlation	% Agreement
SLIC				
Injury morphology	0.51	0.64	0.57 ± 0.02	63.4
Discoligamentous complex	0.33	0.49	0.49 ± 0.02	57.9
Neurological status	0.62	0.90	0.87 ± 0.01	70.7
Total SLIC	0.20	0.73	0.71 ± 0.01	30.5
Management	0.44	0.57	0.58 ± 0.02	73.9
Allen-Ferguson	0.53	NA	NA	64.6
Harris	0.41	NA	NA	57.3

Source: Vaccaro AR, Hulbert RJ, Patel AA, Fisher C, Dvorak M, Lehman RA Jr, Anderson P, Harrop J, Oner FC, Arnold P, Fehlings M, Hedlund R, Madrazo I, Rechtine G, Aarabi B, Shainline M, Spine Trauma Study Group. The subaxial cervical spine injury classification system: a novel approach to recognize the importance of morphology, neurology, and integrity of the disco-ligamentous complex. Spine 2007;32:2365–2374.

Abbreviation: NA, not applicable.

Table 27.7 Intrarater Reliability of the SLIC, Allen-Ferguson, and Harris Systems

Measure	Kappa	Rank Order Correlation	Intraclass Correlation	% Agreement
SLIC				
Injury morphology	0.65	0.78	0.75 ± 0.07	73.1
Discoligamentous complex	0.50	0.66	0.66 ± 0.09	68.0
Neurological status	0.72	0.91	0.90 ± 0.03	78.8
Total SLIC	0.39	0.83	0.83 ± 0.05	47.0
Management	0.60	0.76	0.77 ± 0.06	80.5
Management by rater's judgment	0.80	NA	NA	93.3
Allen-Ferguson	0.63	NA	NA	71.4
Harris	0.53	NA	NA	67.9

Source: Vaccaro AR, Hulbert RJ, Patel AA, Fisher C, Dvorak M, Lehman RA Jr, Anderson P, Harrop J, Oner FC, Arnold P, Fehlings M, Hedlund R, Madrazo I, Rechtine G, Aarabi B, Shainline M, Spine Trauma Study Group. The subaxial cervical spine injury classification system: a novel approach to recognize the importance of morphology, neurology, and integrity of the disco-ligamentous complex. Spine 2007;32:2365–2374.

(ICC = 0.83). The components of the SLIC system were tested individually. Injury morphology showed moderate interrater agreement (ICC = 0.57, κ = 0.51) and higher intrarater agreement (ICC = 0.75, κ = 0.65), the discoligamentous complex showed fair interrater agreement (ICC = 0.49, κ = 0.33) and moderate intrarater agreement (ICC = 0.66, κ = 0.50), and assessment of neurological status showed the highest interrater agreement (ICC = 0.87, κ =0.62) and the highest intrarater agreement (ICC = 0.90, κ = 0.72). Although the interrater reliability for SLIC management recommendation was moderate (ICC = 0.58, κ = 0.44), the intrarater reliability was much higher (ICC = 0.77, κ = 0.60).

Because the Allen-Ferguson and Harris classification systems are nonordinal in nature, ICC comparisons with the SLIC system could not be conducted; however, the kappa coefficients were compared. The Allen-Ferguson system had moderate interrater agreement (κ = 0.53) and moderate intrarater agreement (κ = 0.63). For the Harris system, interrater and intrarater agreements were lower (κ = 0.41 and 0.53, respectively).

In assessment of validity, raters agreed with the SLIC score in 91.8% of cases regarding operative versus nonoperative scores (nonoperative scores were set at less than 4; operative scores, more than or equal to 5). If the SLIC score of 4 was removed (the score at which no specific recommendation for treatment is made), the rate of agreement rose to 93.8%. Intersystem validity between the SLIC classification and the Allen-Ferguson classification was assessed by approximating the categories for each group. A 71.5% agreement was shown between the SLIC morphology and the Allen-Ferguson system (**Table 27.8**).

Although the surgeons in this study were familiar with both classification systems, this was their first time using the new SLIC system. One might expect that as clinicians become more familiar with the SLIC system and understand its components better, the reliability of the system will increase with future studies. Although this study was limited in that only a small group of surgeons participated, the study was nonetheless a multicenter study.

◆ Summary

Today, classification systems for the cervical spine are largely descriptive in nature. The multitude of descriptive phrases that can be used to describe the same injury pattern and lack

of standardization are areas that need attention. The SLIC system, in addition to being a new classification system for the cervical spine, is the first to link injury patterns to a numerical value that can assist the clinician in determining prognosis and management of the injury.

Based on a review of the current literature, level IV evidence supports the Allen-Ferguson, Harris, and AO classification systems. Much of the literature is focused on observational studies, often involving large case series. A review of the literature shows that critical assessment of these classification systems for reliability or validity has not been attempted. A recently published multicenter study by the STSG is the first to critically analyze the most widely used of these systems (the Allen-Ferguson classification system) and compare it with a new system (the SLIC classification system). The results from that study show, with level III evidence, good validity and moderate interobserver reliability with the use of the SLIC system. The SLIC system also offers the advantage of being simple to use and is the only classification that assists with both diagnosis and treatment management.

Table 27.8 Allen-Ferguson Mechanism of Injury Descriptors Approximately Corresponding to the SLIC Morphology Categories

Homologous Categories between the Allen-Ferguson System and the SLIC Morphology	
Allen-Ferguson Mechanism	**SLIC Morphology Classification**
Compressive flexion	Compression or burst
Vertical compression	Compression or burst
Distractive flexion	Translation or distraction
Compressive extension	Distraction
Distractive extension	Distraction
Lateral flexion	Translation

Source: Allen BL Jr, Ferguson RL, Lehmann TR, O'Brien RP. A mechanistic classification of closed, indirect fractures and dislocations of the lower cervical spine. Spine 1982;7:1–27; Vaccaro AR, Hulbert RJ, Patel AA, Fisher C, Dvorak M, Lehman RA Jr, Anderson P, Harrop J, Oner FC, Arnold P, Fehlings M, Hedlund R, Madrazo I, Rechtine G, Aarabi B, Shainline M, Spine Trauma Study Group. The subaxial cervical spine injury classification system: a novel approach to recognize the importance of morphology, neurology, and integrity of the disco-ligamentous complex. Spine 2007;32:2365–2374.

References

1. Moore TA, Vaccaro AR, Anderson PA. Classification of lower cervical spine injuries. Spine 2006;31(11, Suppl):S37–S43, discussion S61

2. National Spinal Cord Injury Statistical Center. Spinal Cord Injury Facts and Figures at a Glance. 2008. Available at: http://www.spinalcord.uab.edu/show.asp?durki=116979 (accessed February 12, 2009)

3. Lowery DW, Wald MM, Browne BJ, Tigges S, Hoffman JR, Mower WR; NEXUS Group. Epidemiology of cervical spine injury victims. Ann Emerg Med 2001;38:12–16

4. Goldberg W, Mueller C, Panacek E, Tigges S, Hoffman JR, Mower WR; NEXUS Group. Distribution and patterns of blunt traumatic cervical spine injury. Ann Emerg Med 2001;38:17–21

5. Slucky AV, Eismont FJ. Treatment of acute injury of the cervical spine. Instr Course Lect 1995;44:67–80

6. Bass CR, Lucas SR, Salzar RS, et al. Failure properties of cervical spinal ligaments under fast strain rate deformations. Spine 2007;32:E7–E13

7. White AA III, Panjabi MM. Clinical Biomechanics of the Spine. 2nd ed. Philadelphia: Lippincott Williams & Wilkins; 1990

8. Pal GP, Sherk HH. The vertical stability of the cervical spine. Spine 1988;13:447–449

9. White AA III, Panjabi MM. Clinical Biomechanics of the Spine. Philadelphia: JB Lippincott; 1978

10. Nuckley DJ, Konodi MA, Raynak GC, Ching RP, Chapman JR, Mirza SK. Neural space integrity of the lower cervical spine: effect of anterior lesions. Spine 2004;29:642–649

11. White AA III, Johnson RM, Panjabi MM, Southwick WO. Biomechanical analysis of clinical stability in the cervical spine. Clin Orthop Relat Res 1975;109:85–96

12. Anderson PA, Moore TA, Davis KW, et al; Spinal Trauma Study Group. Cervical spine injury severity score: assessment of reliability. J Bone Joint Surg Am 2007;89:1057–1065

13. Holdsworth F. Fractures, dislocations, and fracture-dislocations of the spine. J Bone Joint Surg Am 1970;52:1534–1551

14. Allen BL Jr, Ferguson RL, Lehmann TR, O'Brien RP. A mechanistic classification of closed, indirect fractures and dislocations of the lower cervical spine. Spine 1982;7:1–27

15. Harris JH Jr, Edeiken-Monroe B, Kopaniky DR. A practical classification of acute cervical spine injuries. Orthop Clin North Am 1986;17:15–30

16. Magerl F, Aebi M, Gertzbein SD, Harms J, Nazarian S. A comprehensive classification of thoracic and lumbar injuries. Eur Spine J 1994;3:184–201

17. Vaccaro AR, Hulbert RJ, Patel AA, et al; Spine Trauma Study Group. The subaxial cervical spine injury classification system: a novel approach to recognize the importance of morphology, neurology, and integrity of the disco-ligamentous complex. Spine 2007;32:2365–2374

18. Torg JS, Sennett B, Vegso JJ. Spinal injury at the level of the third and fourth cervical vertebrae resulting from the axial loading mechanism: an analysis and classification. Clin Sports Med 1987;6:159–183

19. Patel AA, Dailey A, Brodke DS, et al; Spine Trauma Study Group. Subaxial cervical spine trauma classification: the Subaxial Injury Classification system and case examples. Neurosurg Focus 2008;25:E8

20. McLain RF, Aretakis A, Moseley TA, Ser P, Benson DR. Sub-axial cervical dissociation: anatomic and biomechanical principles of stabilization. Spine 1994;19:653–659

21. Sim E, Vaccaro AR, Berzlanovich A, Schwarz N, Sim B. In vitro genesis of subaxial cervical unilateral facet dislocations through sequential soft tissue ablation. Spine 2001;26:1317–1323

22. Vaccaro AR, Madigan L, Schweitzer ME, Flanders AE, Hilibrand AS, Albert TJ. Magnetic resonance imaging analysis of soft tissue disruption after flexion-distraction injuries of the subaxial cervical spine. Spine 2001;26:1866–1872

23. Babcock JL. Cervical spine injuries: diagnosis and classification. Arch Surg 1976;111:646–651

24. Schneider RC. Chronic neurological sequelae of acute trauma to the spine and spinal cord, V: The syndrome of acute central cervical spinal-cord injury followed by chronic anterior cervical-cord injury (or compression) syndrome. J Bone Joint Surg Am 1960;42-A:253–260

25. Aito S, D'Andrea M, Werhagen L. Spinal cord injuries due to diving accidents. Spinal Cord 2005;43:109–116

26. Torg JS, Pavlov H, O'Neill MJ, Nichols CE Jr, Sennett B. The axial load teardrop fracture: a biomechanical, clinical and roentgenographic analysis. Am J Sports Med 1991;19:355–364

28

The Cervical Spine Injury Severity Score (CSISS)

Paul A. Anderson and Timothy A. Moore

Classification systems provide a means for communication, assess severity of disease, and serve as a template to base treatment decisions. Additionally, classification systems should foster research. Many systems have been proposed to evaluate subaxial cervical spine injuries but none have been widely accepted. All classification systems are models or approximations with loss of detail. In reality, cervical spine injuries represent a continuous spectrum of injury where categorization in groups causes loss of precision. This loss of precision can be ameliorated by increasing the complexity of the system at the disadvantage of decreasing reliability and increasing confusion.

Cervical spine classifications systems can be divided into morphological systems, mechanistic systems, and systems based on stability of the injury.[1] Morphological systems use pathoanatomical terms, whereas mechanistic systems try to determine the mechanism of injury. Still other systems try to characterize injuries as stable or unstable based on the fracture pattern. Stability continues to be difficult to define clinically. All of these systems fall short of meeting the goals of a functional classification system.

Neurological injury and spinal stability are the two most important factors in planning treatment. Neurological injury can be easily measured with the most reliable and reproducible method documented with the American Spinal Injury Association: International Standards for Neurological Classification of Spinal Cord Injury.[2] Spinal stability was initially described as a dichotomous variable. However, it is in reality a continuous variable and potentially quantifiable. In 2005, the Cervical Spine Injury Severity Score was developed to reliably quantify subaxial cervical spinal stability after trauma.[1] This chapter discusses the medical evidence for the reliability and validity of this system.

Methods

A computerized literature search of the National Library of Medicine from November 15, 2004 to 2009 was performed using keywords "spinal injury" or "spinal fractures" or "spinal injuries." Combinations with the keywords "classification," "diagnosis," or "radiography" were reviewed. All papers focusing on the classification of cervical spine injury were examined. In addition, references obtained from the bibliographies of the manuscripts by Moore and Anderson were included. Four papers discussing the Cervical Spine Injury Severity Score (CSISS) were identified.[1,3–5] The manuscript by Moore was a general overview of classification systems but included the first description of the CSISS and a pilot study of the reliability of a small number of observers. The second publication by Anderson et al measured the reliability of the CSISS, including some of the observers from the study by Moore. A third study examined the reliability in patients with only facet injuries, and the last correlated midterm outcome to classification (**Table 28.1**).

◆ The Cervical Spine Injury Severity Score

The CSISS is based upon a four-column model of the subaxial cervical spine.[3] The four columns include the anterior, right pillar, left pillar, and posterior column (**Fig. 28.1**). The anterior column includes the body, disk and anulus, and the anterior and posterior longitudinal ligaments. Each lateral pillar includes the pedicle, lateral mass, inferior and superior facet articulation, and facet joint capsules. The posterior column includes the lamina, spinous processes, ligamentum flava, and osteoligamentous complex.

Each of the four columns is scored independently using an analog scale ranging from 0 to 5 (**Fig. 28.2**). Zero indicates no injury and 5 the worst possible injury that the column can sustain. Fractional values can be utilized. Scores in between are based on increasing displacement of bone fragments or between bony structures normally held together by ligaments. For instance, a nondisplaced fracture is scored as 1, whereas a 3 mm anterior subluxation of a vertebral body might be scored 2.5. The scores of each column are summed so that the CSISS ranges from 0 to 20.

Table 28.1 Evidentiary Table Evaluating the Cervical Spine Injury Severity Score

Study	Study Type	Subjects	Outcome	Results	Conclusions
Anderson[3]	Reliability	34 Cases 15 Examiners	ICC	Intraobserver ICC = 0.98 Interobserver ICC = 0.88	CSISS reliable Correlates to neurological examination and surgery
Chaput[4]	Decision tree	35 Cases	Surgical approach	CSISS: Anterior 7.5 Posterior 14.1	High CSISS correlates to posterior approach

Abbreviations: CSISS, Cervical Spine Injury Severity Score; ICC, intraclass correlation coefficient.

◆ Results

Anderson et al determined the intraobserver and interobserver reliability of the CSISS in 34 consecutive cases of subaxial cervical spine injury (**Table 28.2**).[3] Plain radiographs and computed tomography (CT) of each case were stored on CD and read in random order using Efilmlite software. Five cases were randomly repeated to assess intraobserver reliability. Fifteen investigators with varying experience scored each case. Reliability was determined using intraclass correlation coefficients (ICCs). Using this metric, reliability can range from -1 to 1, and an excellent test is greater than 0.75.

There was excellent breadth of the distribution of CSISS scores indicating a good spread of injury severity from minimal to severe. The intraobserver and interobserver reliability was excellent with ICCs of 0.98 and 0.88, respectively. No differences of reliability were evident based on the experience of the examiner. Also no differences were present between the four columns.

The worst cases with greatest variation in scores were in patients with subtle ligamentous injury and in patients with fractures in ankylosed spines. The former cases may have improved reliability using magnetic resonance imaging (MRI), which would be expected to improve identification of ligamentous injury. The latter may have been scored differently because some investigators recognized the highly unstable nature of the injury despite minimal fracture displacement.

Validation was done by examining the relationship between treatment, the presence of neurological deficit, and the CSISS score. Neurological deficits were seen in 79% of patients with scores greater than 7 (11/14), whereas in only 15% with scores lower than 7 (3/20). Surgery was performed in all 14 patients with scores greater than 7 compared with only three of 20 patients with lower scores. In the neurologically intact patients again all patients with scores greater than 7 had surgery, whereas only one of 17 neurologically intact patients with scores below 7 had surgery.

Chaput et al investigated the utility of the CSISS to predict surgical approach in cervical trauma.[4] The mean CSISS scores of 35 surgical cases were compared between surgical approaches (anterior, posterior, or combined anterior-posterior). The mean CSISS was 7.5, 14.1, and 15.2 for the anterior, posterior, and combined approaches, respectively. Statistically high CSISS was associated with the use of a posterior or a combined approach (**Fig. 28.3**). These results were independent of surgeon and neurological injury.

Koller et al analyzed outcomes of 28 neurologically intact patients with subaxial injuries treated by an anterior cervical plate (**Fig. 28.4**).[5] They classified injuries according to the AO system (A–C) and the CSISS, correlating these to radiological outcome. The mean CSISS score was 9.6, with a range of 2 to 20. Only five cases had CSISS less than 7. The authors found a good correlation between higher AO and CSISS scores. Further, failure of the anterior plate fixation alone was associated with higher CSISS scores.

◆ Discussion

Anderson's was rigorous and was sufficiently powered to determine the reliability of the CSISS. The results show that the CSISS is reliable with excellent ICCs. It is unknown how MRI would affect the reliability. Validation was performed by

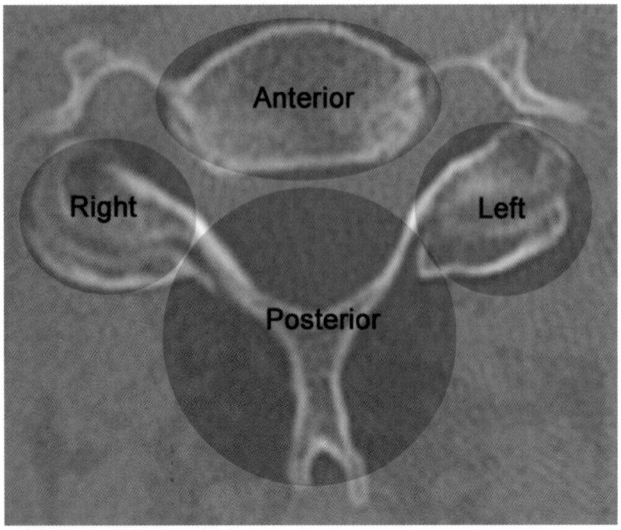

Fig. 28.1 Four-column model to calculate the Cervical Spine Injury Severity Score (CSISS).

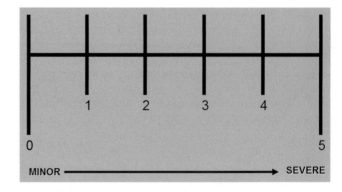

Fig. 28.2 Analog scale of injury severity based on bony and/or ligamentous disruption.

Table 28.2 Reliability of the Cervical Spine Injury Severity Score

	Number of Cases	Number of Observers	Intraclass Correlation Coefficient (ICC)*
	34	15	
Intraobserver			0.98
Interobserver			0.88

*ICC scores greater than 0.75 indicate excellent reliability.

assessing CSISS scores and whether surgery was performed and the presence of neurological deficit (**Table 28.3**). The decision for surgery was made independent of the CSISS. Again the CSISS model was predictive of both confirming the scientific underpinnings of the CSISS that the more severe the injury the greater the CSISS and the more likely a neurological deficit was present and the greater the need for surgery.

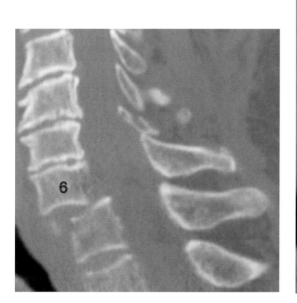

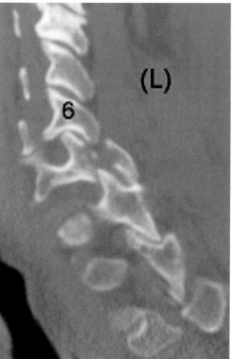

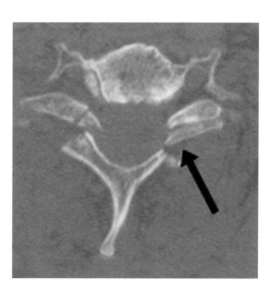

Fig. 28.3 **(A)** A patient with 50% subluxation secondary to bilateral fracture dislocations at C6–C7. Sagittal computed tomography (CT) shows in addition to subluxation a fracture of the body of C7 and comminution of the lamina of C5. No distraction is present posteriorly. The anterior column is graded a 5. **(B)** Left sagittal CT shows comminution of lateral mass and subluxation and is graded a 4. **(C)** A fracture dislocation is seen on the right sagittal CT. This is graded a 5. **(D)** Axial CT shows displaced lamina fractures. The arrow demonstrates the left C6-7 facet fracture dislocation. The posterior column is graded a 2. Total Cervical Spine Injury Severity Score (CSISS) is 16; the patient was treated surgically.

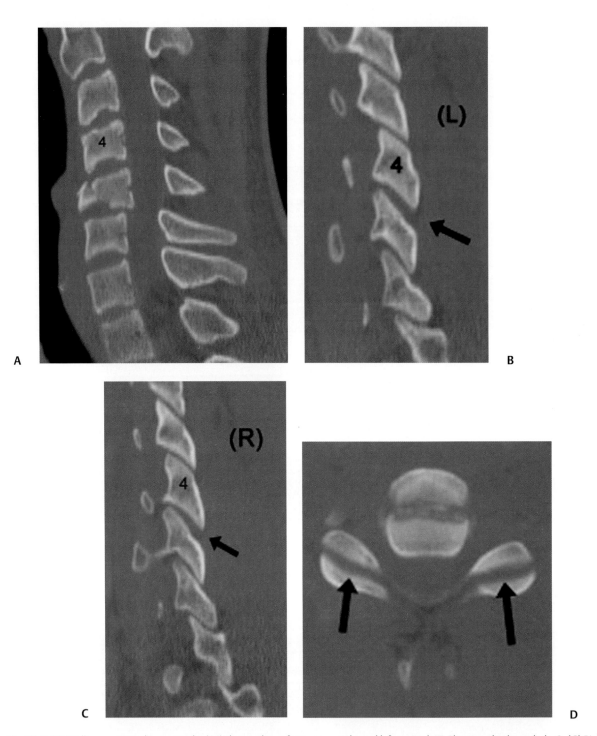

Fig. 28.4 **(A)** Midline computed tomography (CT) shows a burst fracture of C5. The anterior column has a small amount of retropulsion and anterior height loss. It is graded a 3. No posterior distraction is present. **(B)** Facet diastasis (*arrow*) indicating facet capsular injury is seen on both right and left sagittal CT. These are both graded a 2. **(C)** Right sagittal CT. Arrow demonstrates facet diastasis. **(D)** Arrows show bilateral facet diastasis. The posterior column is graded a 0. Total Cervical Spine Injury Severity Score (CSISS) is 6. Patient was treated nonoperatively.

Table 28.3 Validity of the Cervical Spine Injury Severity Score

Author	Neurological Deficit		Surgery	
	CSISS < 7	CSISS ≥ 7	CSISS < 7	CSISS ≥ 7
Anderson[4]	15%	79%	15%	100%
Chaput[5]		**Surgical Approach**		
	Anterior	**Posterior**	**Anteroposterior**	***p*-Value**
CSISS	6.4	11.4	12.1	< 0.002

Abbreviation: CSISS, Cervical Spine Injury Score.

Research Question: What Is the Reliability and Validity of the Cervical Spine Injury Severity Score?

The CSISS has excellent reliability. Validity of the CSISS is suggested but further basic science and clinical research is required.

References

1. Moore TA, Vaccaro AR, Anderson PA. Classification of lower cervical spine injuries. Spine 2006;31(11, Suppl):S37–S43, discussion S61

2. American Spinal Injury Association. American Spinal Injury Association: International Standards for Neurological Classification of Spinal Cord Injury. 6th ed. Chicago: American Spinal Injury Association; 2002:1–24

3. Anderson PA, Moore TA, Davis KW, et al; Spinal Trauma Study Group. Cervical spine injury severity score: assessment of reliability. J Bone Joint Surg Am 2007;89:1057–1065

4. Chaput C, Barber R, Dominguez D, et al. Injury Severity Score (ISS) correlates with surgical approach in subaxial cervical trauma. Spine J 2007; 7:129S–130S

5. Koller H, Reynolds J, Zenner J, et al. Mid- to long-term outcome of instrumented anterior cervical fusion for subaxial injuries. Eur Spine J 2009; 18:630–653

29

Cervical Burst Fractures

David G. Schwartz and Daniel J. Burval

Burst fractures of the subaxial cervical spine are primarily axial load injuries involving the anterior and middle columns of the cervical vertebrae.[1,2] This review focuses on pure axial load burst fractures, which are presumed to occur without posterior ligamentous injury. This enables a critical analysis of the published literature to determine the most efficacious treatment using evidence-based medicine methods.

Cervical burst fractures can have associated injury to the posterior ligamentous structures, especially if there is a combination of axial loading and flexion at the time of injury.[3] Burst fractures of the vertebral body with associated posterior ligamentous injury are more appropriately considered to be flexion-compression injuries, with the burst component being only one part of the fracture. Flexion-compression injuries are discussed in chapter 15 involving injuries to the posterior ligamentous complex.

◆ Epidemiology

A mechanistic classification system was published by Allen and Ferguson and colleagues based on a retrospective review of 165 subaxial cervical spine injuries.[1] In this review, six mechanistic categories were delineated. These categories included flexion-compression, vertical compression, flexion-distraction, extension-compression, extension-distraction, and lateral flexion. As previously stated, vertical compression or axial load is the force responsible for producing a cervical burst fracture. The vertical compression mechanism results most commonly from a direct blow to the head as in diving accidents, spear-tackling injuries, and motor vehicle crashes. According to Allen and Ferguson, these injuries are divided into three stages. Stage I involves both the anterior and the middle columns but is only through one end plate. In stage II, both end plates are involved. If there is retropulsion of the body into the canal, the injury is classified as stage III, which describes a classic burst fracture pattern.[3] The posterior ligamentous complex remains intact. Vertical compression injuries account for ~15% of all subaxial spine injuries.[2,4]

◆ Unique Clinical and Diagnostic Features

The injury force acting axially through the vertebral body can result in simple compression fractures if only the anterior aspect of the bone is involved. A burst fracture results when both the anterior and middle columns (i.e., the anterior and posterior portions of the vertebral body) are involved. Burst fractures are often comminuted with varying degrees of loss of height, kyphosis, and canal retropulsion.[2,5] By definition, there is no posterior interspinous widening as is seen with flexion-compression injuries or teardrop fractures. Neurological injury is common with retropulsion of bone into the canal.

Radiographically, this fracture is evidenced by a vertical fracture line in the frontal projection and by comminution and displacement of vertebral body fragments anteriorly and posteriorly with respect to the contiguous vertebrae in the lateral view. The vertebral body may appear shortened, and the lateral radiograph may reveal posterior protrusion of the middle column extending into the spinal canal. A computed tomographic (CT) scan and magnetic resonance imaging (MRI) will allow for a more precise evaluation with regard to both bone and disk retropulsion into the canal.[6] In addition, these imaging modalities can be used to determine the competence of the end plates immediately adjacent to the burst fracture.

Plain radiographs will often reveal soft tissue swelling. This can be recognized by an increase in the thickness of the prevertebral soft tissues. Retropulsion can be inferred if the anterior vertebral body wedging is coexistent with convexity of the posterior vertebral body as compared with the normal vertebrae, which have a concave posterior surface. When evaluating images of a cervical burst fracture, it is important to determine if there is also an injury to the posterior ligamentous structures, which would make this a much more unstable injury.

To aid in discriminating among these differential diagnoses, we will briefly discuss diagnostic qualities that would suggest an injury to the posterior ligamentous structures. Posterior ligamentous injury can often be inferred by widening of the interspinous distance, distraction or subluxation of the facet joints, and forward subluxation of the superior adjacent vertebral body. Failure of the anterior vertebral body always suggests potential disruption of the discoligamentous complex (DLC).

MRI can play a role in defining injury to the DLC.[7] However, reliable clinical correlation between increased signal in the DLC and mechanical instability has not been demonstrated. MRI also assists in the evaluation of the adjacent disks as well as detection of possible epidural hematoma or other nonbony causes for spinal cord compression. This information is important for weighing treatment options and preoperative planning. MRI is advised in all patients with a neurological deficit unless obtaining the study would lead to a substantial delay in treatment.[6] In the neurologically intact patient or in a patient with a deficit but no facet dislocation, MRI may or may not influence the treatment.

Using the newly developed but validated Subaxial Injury Classification (SLIC) scoring system, typical burst fractures are scored with a 2 for morphology and 0 for an intact DLC.[5] The degree of neurological injury varies and can add up to 4 points to the total score for an incomplete injury with ongoing spinal canal compression. Surgery is typically recommended with SLIC scores greater than or equal to 4.

With either operative or nonoperative treatment, focal cervical kyphosis is to be avoided in the final result. It is measured using the Cobb method and compared with a normal adjacent segment. Without neurological injury, focal kyphosis of 11 degrees or more has historically been used as a criterion for instability, as defined by White et al.[8] This is an indirect attempt to infer incompetency of the posterior ligamentous complex. Unfortunately this value was determined in cadaveric studies without vertebral body fractures. It is only one of many criteria that can be used to determine overall spinal stability. Regardless, it is important to determine if the fractured anterior cervical spine can resist further compressive loads when deciding upon a treatment plan.

Initial Management

Life-threatening issues of airway, breathing, and circulation should be immediately addressed utilizing Advanced Trauma Life Support protocols. A thorough history, physical, and radiographic evaluation is of utmost importance. It is vital to keep a high degree of suspicion and complete frequent exams to correctly identify the extent of any neurological injury. It is also important to avoid missing noncontiguous injuries and deterioration of the neurological status.

The cervical spine should be maintained in a neutral position and immobilized with a hard cervical collar. The patient should initially be placed on a back board, as with all trauma victims. Realignment of a cervical burst fracture with loss of height of more than 25%, focal kyphosis more than 11 degrees, or a neurological deficit is accomplished by applying traction via cervical tongs.[9] Cervical tongs should be affixed, followed by an initial 10 lb applied to counter the weight of the head, and the neck should be gently extended to re-create a lordotic posture. Sequentially, weight is added in 5 lb increments followed by radiographs after each addition. In general, 5 lb of weight is required for each cervical level. For example, 30 lb is needed for a C4 burst fracture, 5 lb each for the C1, C2, C3, and C4 levels plus the initial 10 lb for the head,

although heavier weights can be used. The upper limit of safe weight is unclear because reports in the literature of up to 150 pounds have been used safely for facet reduction. For cervical burst fractures, this amount of weight is almost never required to reduce the kyphosis. It is also unclear in the literature whether a preoperative MRI provides any value with regard to treatment, though it is generally recommended in patients with a neurological injury prior to definitive surgical stabilization. It may help determine stability by evaluating the posterior ligamentous complex, as well as determine structures causing spinal compression.[7] The importance of preventing skin ulceration resulting from a cervical collar or traction cannot be overemphasized.

◆ Nonsurgical Treatment

In those patients who are neurologically intact and there is apparent mechanical stability, a nonoperative course may be attempted. Nonsurgical treatment can be accomplished with initial tong reduction, which historically could be maintained for several weeks prior to placing the patient either in a halo or a rigid cervical orthosis. It is important that acceptable cervical alignment be maintained. Frequent radiographs are obtained to monitor the reduction. Failure to maintain acceptable cervical alignment may lead to late pain or the development of a neurological deficit.[3,9]

◆ Surgical Options

Patients with a neurological deficit generally undergo decompression of retropulsed bone and disk followed by surgical stabilization. Direct decompression of the cervical cord by corpectomy followed by a strut graft for realignment and stabilization has been shown to be the optimal treatment method in most cases.[10–15]

It is not clear what surgical approach should be utilized in the neurologically intact patient. In neurologically intact patients, surgical goals include restoration of mechanical stability and prevention of kyphosis to decrease the possibility of axial neck pain or late neurological deterioration. Unfortunately there are no randomized controlled studies in this patient population of neurologically intact patients. Mechanical instability is suggested by anterior translation, marked kyphosis, facet or posterior arch fractures, and interspinous widening.[5]

◆ Potential Complications and Their Avoidance

The goal of any treatment for cervical burst fractures is to achieve stability and assure neural decompression. All treatments have associated risks and benefits. Halo treatment has reported complications of pin-site loosening (36 to 60%), pin-site infection (20%), loss of reduction (up to 40%), and axial neck pain (18%).[16]

The morbidity after either an anterior or a posterior cervical approach is relatively low. In a 5-year study involving 5356 patients, some of whom were treated for traumatic injuries, the Cervical Spine Research Society studied complications of anterior and posterior approaches. The neurological complication rate involving anterior surgery was 0.64% as compared with 2.18% seen with posterior surgery. A total of nine spinal cord injuries (iatrogenic) were reported in anterior cases and 28 in posterior cases.[17]

Anterior procedures are shown to have a union rate approaching 100%, minimal residual kyphosis, and minimal symptomatic neck pain.[13] Historically, posterior procedures have a higher infection rate and increased residual axial neck pain with elective procedures. However, this was not shown in Brodke et al's comparison of the anterior and posterior approach in 52 patients with subaxial cervical spine fractures, of whom seven had isolated burst fractures and 12 had bursts with facet dislocation.[10]

◆ Rehabilitation

All patients, regardless of treatment, require mechanical stability until fusion. This can be produced by internal fixation, external orthosis, or both. Patients treated with a halo device endure 12 weeks, whereas surgical patients usually wear a hard cervical collar for about 6 weeks or as per surgeon preference. Theoretically, anterior column reconstruction restores mechanical stability, lessening the need for postoperative collars. In practice, however, many surgeons feel that the collar provides feedback to the patient to avoid excessive movements while biological fusion is occurring. Collars may also have a greater role following anterior-alone surgery in the presence of posterior ligamentous injury. Biomechanically, posterior instrumented fusions are more rigid.[18] Questions continue to arise as to how much rigidity is required for successful fusion while minimizing sequelae such as axial neck pain, late instability, and adjacent disk degeneration.[6]

◆ Key Clinical Questions

◆ What is the optimal treatment for subaxial cervical burst fractures?
◆ What is the threshold for surgical intervention with respect to clinical and radiographic findings?

A systematic review was performed to answer the above two questions using the best available evidence in the published literature. MEDLINE (1966–November 2007) was searched for all English language abstracts with the search term "cervical burst fracture." Sixty-one articles were identified. Fifty-five articles were eliminated on review of abstract alone based on topic and methodology. This left six articles comparing the treatment options for cervical burst fractures., including was one level II study (Brodke) and five level III studies.[5,6,10,13,15] Please see **Table 29.1** for further details.

Brodke et al reported the results of a level II prospective randomized study in which anterior and posterior approaches were compared in seven isolated burst fractures with spinal cord injuries. Though there were a total of 19 burst fractures, 12 had a concomitant facet dislocation and thus were excluded from the current analysis. Patients requiring specific approaches, as determined by the surgeons, were excluded from the study. Seventy percent of patients in the anterior group improved at least one Frankel grade, whereas 57% did so in the posterior group. There was no difference between the groups in regard to anterior versus posterior surgery. However, patient numbers were too small to achieve appropriate power or draw meaningful conclusions.

Fehlings et al (level III) retrospectively reviewed 44 patients who underwent posterior fusion with lateral mass plates, 42 of whom had surgery for a traumatic injury.[12] Only seven of the 42 had cervical burst fractures. Surgical indications were instability

Table 29.1 Evidentiary Table

Study	Study Type	Level of Evidence	Outcomes	Summary
Toh et al (2006)[15]	Retrospective comparative	III	Radiological, neurological	11 burst and 20 teardrop (quadrangle) dislocation fxs treated with either anterior decompression/fusion, posterior, or combination. No patient with posterior approach had Frankel improvement. Anterior fusion was preferred.
Koivikko et al (2000)[16]	Retrospective comparative	III	Radiological, neurological	69 consecutive cervical burst or teardrop (quadrangle) fxs (34 traction/halo, 35 anterior fusion/decompression). Anterior preferred with radiological and neurological outcomes
Fisher et al (2002)[13]	Retrospective comparative	III	Radiological, neurological, quality of life	45 teardrop (quadrangle) fxs treated with either anterior decompression/fusion or halo. Improved sagittal balance with surgical arm (3.5 degrees kyphosis vs 11.4) 5 failures in halo,) in anterior. Secondary outcomes not powered enough
Brodke et al (2003)[10]	Prospective randomized	II	Radiological, neurological	52 patients with SCI, Only 19 were burst fxs, patients requiring specific approach were excluded. No difference between groups—N too small for power.
Ripa et al (1991)[14]	Retrospective	III	Radiological	92 subaxial spine fractures (20 burst), no loss of kyphosis, 98.9% fusion rate
Fehlings et al (1994)[12]	Retrospective	III	Radiological, pain	42 subaxial cervical spine fractures (7 burst fractures), posterior instrumented fusion unsuccessful in 3/7 burst fxs.

Abbreviations: fxs, fractures; SCI, spinal cord injury.

that could not be maintained in a halo; this was not defined any further. The authors reported that three cases of burst fractures, which had greater than 25 degrees of sagittal plane kyphosis, were not optimally treated with posterior instrumentation alone. One achieved solid fusion with a residual kyphosis of 19 degrees but was lost to follow-up at 11 months. The second required an anterior strut graft 2 months postoperatively due to kyphosis. The third obtained a solid fusion but had a delayed anterior decompression and strut graft at 13 months by a non-study surgeon for quadriplegia. Further details of this delayed procedure were not reported. Overall mean follow-up was 46 months with a solid fusion obtained in 93% of patients and only two patients complaining of chronic axial neck pain.

Ripa et al (level III) reviewed the records of 92 patients with subaxial cervical spine injuries who underwent anterior decompression, bone graft, and fusion with plate fixation.[14] Twenty of 92 patients had burst fractures. Mean follow-up was 19.3 months. There was no loss of kyphosis as judged on postoperative radiographs. No deep wound infections were reported. The fusion rate was 98.9%. Similar results were reported the same year by Aebi et al, who studied 22 patients with burst or teardrop fractures. However, subgroup analyses of the two injury types were not reported and thus could not be extracted for the current analysis.

Toh et al (level III) reported the results of 31 burst or teardrop fractures treated with either anterior decompression/fusion, posterior surgery, or a combination of techniques.[15] Only 11 patients had burst fractures. The mean follow-up was 23.5 months. No patient who was treated with a posterior approach alone or in combination with anterior surgery had neurological improvement. However, all patients with a burst fracture were treated with anterior surgery; thus a comparison of treatments was not possible.

Koivikko et al (level III) reported the results of a retrospective comparison of 69 neurologically intact and spinal cord injured patients with burst or teardrop fractures treated surgically with anterior decompression and fusion or nonsurgically with skull traction and halo immobilization.[16] The surgical group had markedly better neurological recovery and overall sagittal alignment (2.2 degrees of lordosis vs 12.6 degrees of kyphosis in the halo group).

◆ Summary and Recommendations

Anterior surgery for the cervical spine is superior to the posterior approach in many respects. Anterior surgery employs a simple, relatively atraumatic approach to the spine that directly addresses the pathological anatomy of a burst fracture. Fracture fragments can be removed and spinal cord and nerve roots decompressed under direct visualization. Favorable load distribution following anterior reconstruction is an additional factor that favors an anterior arthrodesis because bone graft can be incorporated under axial compression in a well vascularized bony bed. This is in contrast to posterior fusion, which is under tension and therefore may be less ideal for healing with persistent anterior and middle column incompetence.

◆ What is the optimal treatment for subaxial cervical burst fractures?

The existing literature is confused by its inclusion of a variety of fracture morphologies. Upon careful analysis, however, it becomes clear that burst fractures with neurological injury should be treated with anterior vertebral body resection and stabilization. Despite the weak to moderate evidence, a strong recommendation can be made that operative treatment via corpectomy, strut reconstruction, and plate stabilization via an anterior approach is the optimal treatment for patients with burst fractures and associated neurological injury. Again, despite the paucity of evidence, a strong recommendation can be made that stable fractures in patients without neurological injury can be treated either nonoperatively or operatively through either an anterior or a posterior approach.

◆ What is the threshold for surgical intervention with respect to clinical and radiographic findings?

1. Any neurological deficit
2. Focal kyphosis > 11 degrees or documented progression of kyphosis
3. Loss of vertebral body height > 25%
4. Inability to obtain or maintain reduction to satisfy any of the foregoing criteria

References

1. Allen BL Jr, Ferguson RL, Lehmann TR, O'Brien RP. A mechanistic classification of closed, indirect fractures and dislocations of the lower cervical spine. Spine 1982;7:1–27
2. Reich SM, Cotler JM. Mechanism and patterns of spine and spinal cord injuries. Trauma Q 1993;9:7–28
3. Beiner JM. Flexion-Compression Injuries of the Cervical Spine: Decision Making in Spinal Care. New York, NY: Thieme; 2007
4. Simpson JM, Sutton D, Rizzolo SJ, et al. Traumatic injuries in the adult lower cervical spine. In An HS, Simpson JM, eds. Surgery of the Cervical Spine. London: Martin Dunitz; 1994:267–291
5. Vaccaro AR, Hulbert RJ, Patel AA, et al; Spine Trauma Study Group. The subaxial cervical spine injury classification system: a novel approach to recognize the importance of morphology, neurology, and integrity of the disco-ligamentous complex. Spine 2007;32:2365–2374
6. Vaccaro AR, Cook CM, McCullen G, Garfin SR. Cervical trauma: rationale for selecting the appropriate fusion technique. Orthop Clin North Am 1998;29:745–754
7. Geck MJ, Yoo S, Wang JC. Assessment of cervical ligamentous injury in trauma patients using MRI. J Spinal Disord 2001;14:371–377
8. White AA III, Johnson RM, Panjabi MM, Southwick WO. Biomechanical analysis of clinical stability in the cervical spine. Clin Orthop Relat Res 1975;109:85–96
9. Kwon BK, Vaccaro AR, Grauer JN, Fisher CG, Dvorak MF. Subaxial cervical spine trauma. J Am Acad Orthop Surg 2006;14:78–89
10. Brodke DS, Anderson PA, Newell DW, Grady MS, Chapman JR. Comparison of anterior and posterior approaches in cervical spinal cord injuries. J Spinal Disord Tech 2003;16:229–235
11. Dvorak MF, Fisher CG, Fehlings MG, et al. The surgical approach to subaxial cervical spine injuries: an evidence-based algorithm based on the SLIC classification system. Spine 2007;32:2620–2629
12. Fehlings MG, Cooper PR, Errico TJ. Posterior plates in the management of cervical instability: long-term results in 44 patients. J Neurosurg 1994;81:341–349
13. Fisher CG, Dvorak MF, Leith J, Wing PC. Comparison of outcomes for unstable lower cervical flexion teardrop fractures managed with halo thoracic vest versus anterior corpectomy and plating. Spine 2002;27: 160–166
14. Ripa DR, Kowall MG, Meyer PR Jr, Rusin JJ. Series of ninety-two traumatic cervical spine injuries stabilized with anterior ASIF plate fusion technique. Spine 1991;16(3, Suppl):S46–S55
15. Toh E, Nomura T, Watanabe M, Mochida J. Surgical treatment for injuries of the middle and lower cervical spine. Int Orthop 2006;30:54–58
16. Koivikko MP, Myllynen P, Karjalainen M, Vornanen M, Santavirta S. Conservative and operative treatment in cervical burst fractures. Arch Orthop Trauma Surg 2000;120:448–451
17. Graham JJ. Complications of cervical spine surgery: a five-year report on a survey of the membership of the Cervical Spine Research Society by the Morbidity and Mortality Committee. Spine 1989;14: 1046–1050
18. Do Koh Y, Lim TH, Won You J, Eck J, An HS. A biomechanical comparison of modern anterior and posterior plate fixation of the cervical spine. Spine 2001;26:15–21

30

Flexion and Cervical Distraction Injuries Characterized by the SLIC System

Steven C. Ludwig and Jacqueline E. Karp

The lack of a uniformly accepted classification scheme for subaxial cervical spine injuries has thus far limited the ability to compare the effects of treatments and prognoses reported in many clinical studies. The nonstandardized classification of these injuries has therefore restricted the development of evidence-based recommendations for their treatment. To date, essentially only retrospective clinical studies have addressed the management of subaxial cervical spine injuries; nearly all of them were conducted without case controls. Past subaxial cervical spine injury classification systems, mostly based on injury mechanism, are limited in that they do not reliably measure the degree of spinal instability and have a lack of proven reliability and validity.

The need for a clinically relevant system for classifying subaxial cervical injuries to address the lack of agreement in their management has been met by the newly developed Subaxial Injury Classification (SLIC) scoring system.[1] This user-friendly system attempts to characterize injuries based on morphology and clinical status. Further evaluation of the SLIC system is likely to validate its usefulness in providing prognostic information and treatment guidelines. The SLIC scoring system proposes three major injury characteristics that would direct the treatment of subaxial injuries: (1) injury morphology (as determined by the pattern of spinal column disruption on available imaging studies), (2) integrity of the discoligamentous soft tissue complex (DLC, represented by both anterior and posterior ligamentous structures and the intervertebral disk), and (3) neurological status of the patient (see Chapter 27, Table 27.5). All three characteristics are recognized as major and primarily independent determinants of prognosis and management. Within each of the three categories, subgroups are graded from least to most severe. The system is used to direct treatment options into the broad categories of surgical and nonsurgical. Injuries that score 5 or higher are treated surgically, whereas those scoring 3 or lower are treated nonsurgically. For injury scores of 4, factors such as multisystem trauma and comorbidities need to be considered when deciding whether to treat surgically. If the SLIC scoring system recommends that an injury should be treated operatively, the surgeon must decide which approach or combination of approaches to use. Until recently, no evidence-based algorithm has been available to provide surgical treatment options and identify the optimal approach to be used.[2]

◆ Description of Injuries

Distraction injuries characterized by the SLIC system, which score 3 for injury morphology, occur in two general patterns. One is hyperextension, which usually occurs in elderly persons with spondylotic or stiff spines. Such injuries occur when forces cause hyperextension of the cervical spine with soft tissue failure of the anterior and middle columns (anterior longitudinal ligament and intervertebral disk) or transverse failure of the body without translation.[3] After anterior column failure, a continued distraction-extension force may result in failure of the posterior ligamentous complex and posterior displacement of the body into the canal. Simultaneous compressive forces across the posterior elements can also cause associated posterior element fractures of the lateral masses or pedicles.[4] Posterior infolding of the ligamentum flavum on a spinal canal already narrowed by posterior vertebral osteophytes can cause a severe spinal cord injury (SCI) even in the absence of bony or ligamentous disruption. In ankylosed spines [e.g., diffuse idiopathic skeletal hyperostosis (DISH), ankylosing spondylitis], hyperextension injuries usually occur in the lower cervical spine and might result from seemingly minor trauma. In contrast to highly displaced extension fracture-dislocations, the less displaced injuries that can occur in patients with ankylosed spines can be easily missed, with potentially devastating consequences to neurological status and spinal alignment.[5] The most common neurological deficit associated with hyperextension injuries is central cord syndrome. However, neurological deficits can range from no deficit to a single root level deficit to complete SCI. The major risk in managing patients with hyperextension injuries is failure to identify the injury.

The other pattern of SLIC distraction injuries is hyperflexion. Hyperflexion injuries affect primarily the posterior elements and result in a spectrum of injury ranging from a simple unilateral facet subluxation to bilateral perched facets. The primary mechanism of flexion distraction injuries, as defined by Allen et al,[6] is a flexion-distraction force centered at a mobile cervical spinal unit, most frequently at C5–C6. The mechanism can result from a blow to the head, a fall onto the occiput, or deceleration associated with a motor vehicle collision. Specifically, the mechanism of facet joint injury is attributed to the sliding, stretching, and pinching of the joint[7] that occurs with flexion and distraction forces.

Normally, the facet joints are maintained in a fixed alignment, with minimal movement in flexion and extension. The supraspinous and interspinous ligaments, the ligamentum flavum, and the facet joint capsule maintain this alignment. With a severe flexion-distraction injury, disruption of these ligamentous structures destabilizes the facet joint. The superior vertebra undergoes forward subluxation, with anterior displacement of the corresponding inferior articulating facet on the superior articulating facet of the vertebra below, resulting in uncovering of the articulating facet surfaces (termed the naked facet sign).[8] The degree of facet uncovering might be partial (subluxed facets) or complete (perched facets). With continuation of the injury, the facet may dislocate. Most authors think that for a facet dislocation to occur, rotation with disruption of the interspinous ligament, ligamentum flavum, and facet capsule must occur. Many researchers think that there must also be disruption of the posterior longitudinal ligament and a portion of the intervertebral disk for a facet dislocation to occur.[9] Hyperextension injuries are commonly associated with central cord syndrome, and flexion-distraction injuries can be associated with anterior cord syndrome.

In their retrospective review of 165 subaxial cervical spine injuries, Allen et al[6] grouped injuries into phylogenies according to their radiographic appearance and inferred mechanisms of injury. Injuries were then arranged along a spectrum of anatomical disruption. The phylogenies included flexion-compression, vertical compression, flexion-distraction, extension-compression, extension-distraction, and lateral flexion.

SLIC distraction-extension injuries have been classified by Allen et al[6] as either distraction extension stage 1 (DES 1) (failure of the anterior ligamentous complex, widening of the disk space, and no retrolisthesis) or DES 2 (additional failure of the posterior ligamentous complex and posterior displacement of the cephalad vertebral body on the caudal vertebral body into the canal). The traditional treatment for DES 1 injuries has been either immobilization or anterior instrumented fusion, whereas the traditional treatment for DES 2 injuries has been anterior instrumented fusion. SCIs occur more frequently with DES 2 injuries because of cord compression between the posteroinferior end plate of the displaced vertebral body and anterosuperior lamina of the next caudal vertebrae.[6]

Considering that the system presented by Allen et al[6] does not have a category to describe facet subluxations or perched facets, SLIC flexion-distraction injuries lie somewhere between distraction flexion stage 1 (DFS 1) ("facet sprains" with failure of posterior ligaments, slight widening of facet joints, and interspinous distance) and DFS 2 or DFS 3 (unilateral or bilateral facet dislocation). The traditional treatment for DFS 1 injuries has been immobilization, whereas the traditional treatment for DFS 2 and DFS 3 injuries has been either anterior or posterior instrumented fusion.

◆ Epidemiology

Cervical spine injuries occur in an estimated 150,000 people per year in North America, 11,000 of whom have concomitant SCIs.[10] Cervical spine injuries are more common among the elderly, males, and patients of Caucasian ethnicity. Although the cervical spine is injured in only 2 to 3% of patients who sustain blunt trauma,[10] the potential for instability and catastrophic neurological injury makes timely identification of these injuries critically important. Approximately three fourths of all injuries in patients with blunt cervical spine trauma occur within the subaxial cervical spine (C3–C7).[11] Distraction-extension injuries account for 8 to 22% of subaxial cervical spine injuries.[3] Sufficient reporting of the incidence of specific flexion-distraction injuries, such as facet subluxations and perched facets, is not available.

◆ Unique Clinical and Diagnostic Features of SLIC Distraction Injuries

Initial Evaluation

Initial assessment of any patient with suspected cervical spine injury should begin with the ABCs of resuscitation. Observing the respiratory pattern of patients with cervical spine injuries provides crucial information regarding the level of the injury and the need for ventilatory assistance. Similarly, patients with complete quadriplegia are more likely to require intubation than those with incomplete quadriplegia or paraplegia. Early intubation might be recommended for patients with injury above C5 and complete quadriplegia. Evaluation of the patient's hemodynamic status should occur concomitantly with airway management. Patients with cervical spine injury are at risk for hypovolemic and neurogenic shock because of associated systemic injuries and spinal cord trauma.

After initial resuscitation, the neurological status and spinal column should be assessed. A physical examination should include inspection and palpation of the entire spine with the patient in a logrolled position, with attention to ecchymoses, tenderness, swelling, and gaps between spinous processes. A thorough neurological examination should identify and establish the level of any SCI. To distinguish between complete and incomplete lesions, anal sensation, tone, and contraction must be evaluated. The examination should be repeated frequently to detect any deterioration or improvement. The early neurological examination may be confounded by spinal shock. The duration of spinal shock varies from hours to weeks, although most cases resolve within 48 hours; its termination is marked by return of the bulbocavernosus reflex. Recognition of particular patterns of neurological deficits can help determine prognosis. The American Spinal Injury Association (ASIA) scale is the preferred neurological examination tool because it provides a method to characterize any residual function below the level of the SCI.

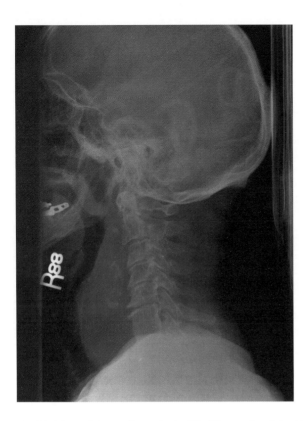

Fig. 30.1 Lateral view radiograph of a C5−C6 extension-distraction injury (distraction extension stage 1). Note anterior retropharyngeal soft tissue swelling and C5−C6 disk space widening.

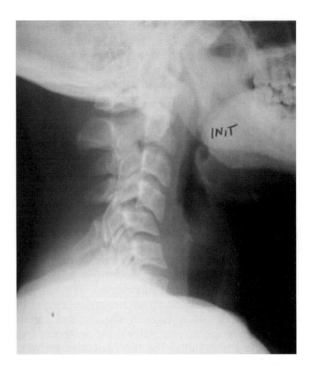

Fig. 30.2 Lateral view radiograph of a C4−C5 flexion-distraction injury. Note facet joint distraction, widening of the interspinous distance, disk space narrowing, and anterolisthesis of C4 on C5. Anterior displacement of the C4 inferior articular facet on the C5 superior articular facet (subluxed facets) can be seen.

Standard Radiographs

Standard radiographic views for evaluating a patient with suspected cervical spine injury include anteroposterior, lateral, and open-mouth odontoid projections to visualize from the occiput to T1. Radiographic findings of extension-distraction injuries (**Fig. 30.1**) may include anterior retropharyngeal soft tissue swelling, disk space widening, and avulsion fractures of anterior osteophytes or the anterosuperior aspect of the caudal vertebral body.

Radiographic findings of flexion-distraction injuries (**Fig. 30.2**) reflect differing degrees of soft tissue and bony disruption and include facet joint widening, widening of the interspinous distance, rotation at the spinous processes, and disk space narrowing. Facets might be fractured, subluxed, or dislocated ("locked") either unilaterally or bilaterally. However, radiographic assessment alone may not be sufficient to exclude damage to the posterior structures of the cervical spine.[12]

The degenerative changes and abnormalities in spinal alignment in patients with ankylosed spines present major diagnostic challenges. It is essential that patients with ankylosed spines be evaluated with computed tomography (CT) and magnetic resonance imaging (MRI) even if no acute injury is visible on initial radiographs.[13]

Computed Tomography

CT is rapidly accessible in most emergency departments and has grown increasingly popular as an initial imaging modality. It is now used for primary screening of high-risk trauma patients and those with neurological deficits or an altered mental status. The potential for missing cervical spine injury

with plain radiography alone is estimated to be 10 to 20%. CT, on the other hand, has a sensitivity and specificity of 98%. Axial view CT scans and sagittal reconstructions are invaluable for defining the bony anatomy of the injury (**Fig. 30.3**). CT scans provide superb visualization of the posterior elements and identification of pedicle or lamina fractures, and sagittal reconstructions provide identification of facet fractures.[14,15] A literature review presented by France et al[16] in 2005 to suggest a standard protocol for initial imaging of the patient with trauma found that, although the mainstay of initial evaluation of the spine after trauma continues to be plain radiography, CT is the best modality to define the bony details of the injury. As such, it should be used to characterize all bony injuries evident on plain radiographs and will likely have a greater role as an initial imaging modality in the patient with trauma. One disadvantage of CT, however, is that it has limited ability to detect ligamentous injuries. CT alone can miss ligamentous injury in up to 30% of cases.[17]

Magnetic Resonance Imaging

MRI, which offers the advantage of directly imaging the soft tissue structures of the disks, ligaments, and spinal cord, is invaluable in assessing the discoligamentous (DLC) injury category of the SLIC system and predicting cervical spine stability (**Figs. 30.4 and 30.5**). Additionally, MRI can show signal change within the spinal cord.[15] MRI can identify soft tissue damage to predict the presence of an unstable flexion-distraction cervical spine injury; MRI findings of patients with facet dislocations have included failure of the posterior musculature, interspinous ligament, ligamentum flavum, and facet capsules.[18] Edema on T2-weighted or fat-suppressed short-tau inversion recovery images (STIR images) allows for diagnosis of the in-

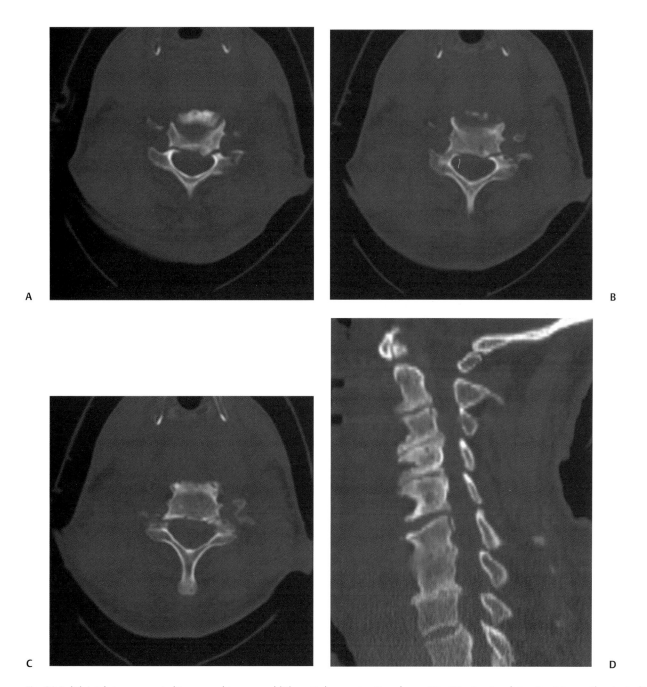

Fig. 30.3 **(A)** Axial view computed tomographic scan and **(B)** sagittal reconstruction show a C5−C6 extension-distraction injury without retrolisthesis (distraction extension stage 1). Note associated C6 left pedicle fracture visible on center axial view image.

jury. MRI is recommended for patients with normal radiographic findings and transient neurological deficits to detect a DLC injury.[19] Normal MRI findings should be considered confirmation of a "cleared" subaxial cervical spine.[20]

◆ Initial Management: Nonoperative Methods with Level of Evidence Determination

Traction and Closed Reduction

Initial management of cervical distraction injuries consists of decompression of the neural elements. This can first be accomplished with cervical traction. Traction plays no role in

the management of extension-distraction injuries with anterior widening because traction would accentuate the deformity. However, traction is used in the management of flexion-distraction injuries.

No medical evidence is currently available to support the use of cervical traction for facet subluxations or perched facets. However, in the analysis of facet subluxations or perched facets within the early spectrum of patients who develop unilateral or bilateral facet dislocations, data support its role. Star et al,[21] in their retrospective review of 53 patients with cervical facet dislocations, provided very low quality evidence that closed reduction can be accomplished in up to 90% of patients with subaxial cervical facet dislocations by a combination of traction, positioning, and occasional manipulation. Sixty-eight percent of patients in this study also showed significant improvement in neurological function.

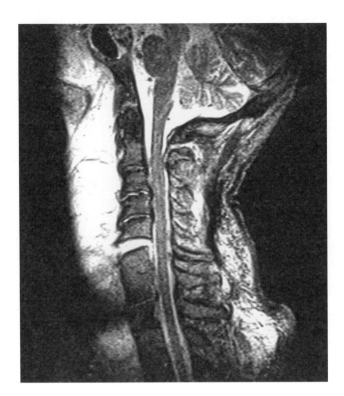

Fig. 30.4 T2-weighted sagittal view magnetic resonance image of a C5–C6 extension-distraction injury. Note increased signal intensity in the C5–C6 interspace, indicating disk disruption.

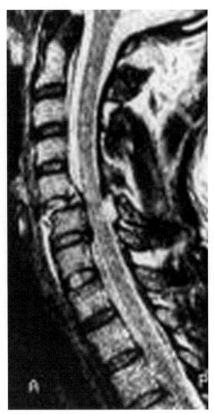

Fig. 30.5 T2-weighted sagittal view magnetic resonance image of a flexion-distraction injury shows slight anterolisthesis of C5 on C6 and disruption of the ligamentum flavum and posterior ligamentous complex.

The role of closed reduction and traction before surgical stabilization of cervical facet dislocations is controversial because intervertebral disk herniation imaged after closed reduction has been implicated as a cause of neurological deterioration in some cases. In their study involving 11 consecutive patients with cervical spine dislocations, Vaccaro et al[22] examined MRI findings before and after closed reduction. Of the nine patients for whom awake closed traction reduction was successful, two had disk herniations before reduction and five had disk herniations after reduction. This study provides very low-quality evidence that closed traction reduction seems to increase the incidence of intervertebral disk herniations. However, the authors observed no relation of these findings to the patients' clinical neurological status.

In their report concerning the methods of reduction of 168 cases of uni- and biarticular subaxial cervical facet dislocations, Vital et al[23] evaluated the efficacy of a particular reduction protocol. The protocol consisted of three successive phases: reduction by traction, reduction by closed maneuvers with the patient under general anesthesia, and open reduction. Of the 168 patients, the protocol failed in five, all of whom had long-standing unilateral dislocation. Of the 91 patients with bilateral dislocation, reduction was achieved by simple traction in 43%, by maneuvers with the patient under general anesthesia in 30%, and by anterior surgery in 27%. Among the patients in the 77 cases of unilateral dislocation, reduction was achieved by traction in 23%, by external maneuvers in 36%, and by anterior surgery in 34%. No neurological deterioration occurred during this protocol. This study provides very low-quality evidence that rapidly progressive traction plus, if necessary, one or two reduction maneuvers under general anesthesia can be attempted to reduce subaxial cervical spine dislocations before open reduction. Although

this study consisted of patients with subaxial cervical dislocations, similar results can be expected with facet subluxations and perched facets.

Bracing

If adequate closed reduction is achieved, it is followed with either external immobilization or internal fixation to provide definitive stabilization. External immobilization may be in the form of a cervical collar, halo vest, or sternal occipital mandibular immobilizer brace. Immobilization is generally required for 6 to 8 weeks, during which upright anteroposterior and lateral view radiographs obtained at frequent intervals should be monitored for loss of reduction and progressive deformity. At the end of immobilization, dynamic flexion-extension radiographs should be scrutinized for any abnormalities in motion to detect continued dynamic instability. If no motion abnormality is shown, the immobilization can be discontinued and physical therapy can be initiated.

No medical evidence is currently available to support the use of bracing specifically for SLIC distraction injuries. However, a retrospective study by Hadley et al[24] of 68 patients with acute traumatic cervical facet fracture-dislocations suggests that external immobilization might provide sufficient stability for facet injuries with minimal (< 1 mm) displacement (very low-quality evidence).

In contrast to purely bony injuries, the ability of external immobilization to provide sufficient stability for ligamentous injuries is less predictable. In general, nonoperative treatment is restricted to bony injuries rather than purely DLC injuries. Persistent pain and instability in patients with cervical spine injury treated with external immobilization have been reported, particularly when the reduction is either not obtained or lost during brace treatment.[24]

Bucholz and Cheung,[25] in their retrospective review of 124 patients with cervical spine injuries treated with halo fixation or cervical fusion, attempted to determine what factors contribute to failure of halo fixation. The overall success rate of halo fixation was 85%, suggesting that the halo vest can be used to treat most patients with cervical spine injuries. However, treatment failed in 13 (23%) of the 57 patients with C3–T1 injuries, nine of whom had locked or perched facets. This study provides low-quality evidence that under certain circumstances (in the presence of old injuries, difficult reduction, or locked or perched facets), cervical fusion may be necessary to avoid unnecessary delay in definitive treatment. Recurrence of deformity is a common complication of closed treatment; almost half of the patients with flexion-distraction injuries treated with a halo vest eventually required surgical stabilization.

Beyer et al,[26] in their retrospective comparative study that included 34 patients with unilateral facet dislocations or fracture-dislocations, provided low-quality evidence that surgical treatment achieves better results than does nonoperative treatment. Ten patients were treated by open reduction and posterior fusion and 24 by nonoperative management. Of the patients managed nonoperatively, 19 underwent halo traction and then halo-thoracic immobilization, four had cervicothoracic orthoses, and one received no treatment. Anatomical reduction was achieved more frequently in the operative group (60% vs 25%). Only 36% of the patients treated by halo traction achieved anatomical alignment; in 25%, halo traction failed to achieve or maintain any degree of reduction.

In their retrospective review of 64 patients with subaxial cervical spine injuries, Lemons and Wagner[27] provided very low-quality evidence that the presence of severe ligamentous injury (as occurs in SLIC distraction injuries), severe vertebral body injury, or both, strongly correlates with failure of nonoperative treatment. However, the authors concluded that injuries without severe ligamentous injury or vertebral body injury can be treated successfully with bracing.

◆ Surgical Options and Postoperative Management with Level of Evidence Determination

Overview

The need for surgical management of subaxial cervical distraction injuries depends on the extent of mechanical instability and neurological compromise. Stabilization with surgical instrumentation and fusion is superior to external immobilization in that it better maintains alignment to promote fusion and imparts immediate stability. In cases that include SCI (complete or incomplete), effective decompression of the spinal canal is a primary goal. SLIC distraction injuries (both extension and flexion) usually score at least 5; therefore, most require surgery according to this system. The choice of a specific surgical technique and approach to treat these injuries, however, is not currently evidence-based.

To determine evidence-based recommendations regarding the surgical treatment of SLIC distraction injuries, a systematic review of the literature was conducted. A comprehensive literature search was performed to identify studies, including any article with an English language abstract. Electronic database searches of MEDLINE (1966 to October 2007) and the Cochrane Database (1980 to October 2007) were performed by using text word searching. Terms used included "subaxial cervical spine injuries," "facet subluxations," "perched facets," "flexion-distraction injuries," and "extension-distraction injuries." Reference lists from relevant articles were also searched for additional citations. To be included in the review, studies had to include adult patients with traumatic SLIC distraction injuries from C3 to T1 and had to have measured the radiographic and/or clinical success of treatment. The most common reason for exclusion was failure to adequately describe injury patterns.

Open Reduction and Stabilization Techniques and Equipment

Facet reduction can be achieved with a posterior approach by placing a narrow curved instrument between the dislocated facets to lever them into a reduced position or, alternatively, by removing the superior part of the more caudal facet to allow the dislocated facet to slip back posteriorly into normal anatomical position. Although burring away part of the superior facet can help disengage the locked facets, it might increase instability once the reduction is achieved.[15] Posterior reduction can also be performed by applying distraction across the spinous processes or across the lamina with the use of a modified laminar spreader.[28] When a pure ligamentous unilateral or bilateral facet subluxation is treated posteriorly, the torn ligamentum flavum and any intervening hematoma or scar tissue should be resected before reducing the posterior elements, considering that immediate quadriparesis after manipulation for bilateral cervical facet subluxation has been reported by Ludwig et al.[29]

Anterior diskectomy can decompress the spinal canal directly. Anterior reduction of the facet subluxation can then be achieved, usually by placing the patient in some degree of cervical extension and intraoperative traction. Reduction can be attempted by various means, such as with weights, with direct manipulation of vertebral bodies with a laminar spreader, or with convergently placed distraction pins inserted into the vertebral bodies.[30] The anteriorly displaced vertebral body can then be pushed or levered back into position once sufficient distraction is achieved to disengage the facets. Ensuring a tight, 100% apposition of the facets will enhance the stability of the anterior approach. Because of the posterior ligament disruption with flexion-distraction injuries and the risk of neurological deficit, it is critical to avoid overdistraction when performing anterior fusion by minimizing the extent of facet distraction.

Anterior stabilization of the subaxial cervical spine involves diskectomy and fusion with an interbody graft and plate fixation (**Fig. 30.6**). Contouring the plate into lordosis enhances the stability of anterior fixation. For posterior stabilization, several fixation choices exist, including interspinous wiring, oblique wiring (between the lateral mass and spinous process), and lateral mass plates and screws (**Fig. 30.7**).

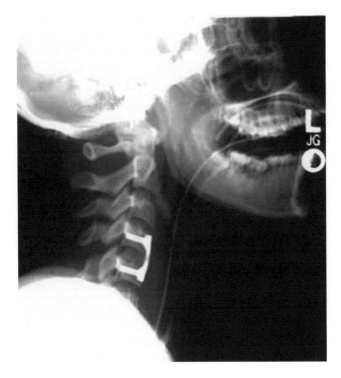

Fig. 30.6 Lateral view upright radiograph obtained after C4–C5 anterior cervical diskectomy and instrumented interbody fusion.

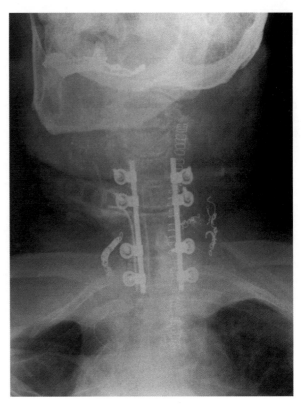

Fig. 30.7 Anteroposterior view radiograph obtained after C4–T1 posterior instrumented fusion.

Evidence Favoring an Anterior Approach for SLIC Distraction Injuries

In their retrospective review of 24 patients with cervical distraction-extension injuries, Vaccaro et al[3] advocated anterior fixation with a cervical graft and plate as a safe and effective method of restoring spinal stability for DES 1 injuries (very low-quality evidence). Of the nine patients in the study treated with anterior fixation for DES 1 injuries, all had stable alignment and none had instrumentation failure.

Henriques et al[31] conducted a retrospective study of 36 patients to evaluate the clinical and radiographic outcomes of anterior fixation for subaxial flexion-distraction injuries. The authors concluded that the use of anterior plate fixation alone for DFS 1 and DFS 2 injuries provides sufficient mechanical stability (very low-quality evidence). Considering that SLIC flexion-distraction injuries lie somewhere between DFS 1 and DFS 2, one can make the same conclusion regarding anterior plate fixation for their treatment.

Elgafy et al[32] conducted a retrospective study of 65 patients with unilateral or bilateral subaxial cervical facet subluxation/dislocations (SLIC flexion-distraction injuries) treated with posterior fixation. Instrumentation failure and subsequent need for anterior revision occurred in two patients, both of whom had bilateral facet subluxations. The authors found that kyphosis at follow-up was significantly correlated with kyphosis on initial films and with bilateral facet subluxations. Because of the high risk of postoperative kyphosis in patients with bilateral facet subluxations and in those with significant preoperative kyphosis, the authors concluded that better results might be obtained with anterior surgery in such patients (very low-quality evidence).

Evidence Favoring a Posterior Approach for SLIC Distraction Injuries

Although anterior reconstruction of the cervical spine with an anterior plate is the ideal treatment for acute distraction-extension injuries, posterior fusion may sometimes be necessary. In their retrospective review of 24 patients with cervical distraction-extension injuries, Vaccaro et al[3] concluded that posterior cervical fusion may be necessary for extension-distraction injuries that are highly unstable and for extension-distraction injuries that require laminectomy (very low-quality evidence).

In their review of 65 patients with unilateral or bilateral subaxial cervical facet subluxation/dislocations treated with posterior fixation, Elgafy et al[32] found that satisfactory alignment was achieved in patients with unilateral injury and in those without significant kyphosis on initial films. The authors thus concluded that posterior instrumentation and fusion is an effective treatment for facet subluxation/dislocations only in patients with unilateral injury and in those without significant preoperative kyphosis (very low-quality evidence).

Evidence That Posterior and Anterior Approaches Are Equivalent

In their prospective randomized clinical trial of anterior versus posterior surgery for unilateral facet injuries, Kwon et al[33] found that acute postoperative morbidity did not differ between anteriorly and posteriorly treated patients. Forty-two patients with unilateral facet injuries were prospectively randomized to undergo either anterior cervical diskectomy and fusion or posterior instrumented fusion. Of the 42 patients, two had unilateral perched facets and four had unilateral subluxed facets (SLIC flexion-distraction injuries). The primary outcome measure was the postoperative time needed to meet a predefined set of discharge criteria. The authors found no significant difference in this measure and thus concluded that both anterior and posterior fixation approaches are valid treatment options. This is the only study to date that provides moderate-quality evidence regarding the surgical treatment of SLIC distraction injuries. However, the number of patients in this study who fulfill this specific injury pattern is extremely small.

Evidence Favoring Circumferential Fixation for SLIC Distraction Injuries

In their retrospective review of 24 patients with cervical distraction-extension injuries, Vaccaro et al.[3] found that certain injury characteristics might necessitate circumferential stabilization (very low-quality evidence). These characteristics include extension-distraction with significant (> 3 mm) translation (DES 2 equivalent injuries). Use of a posterior approach initially, followed by an anterior approach, allows for adequate alignment of the spine in the sagittal plane.

In their retrospective review of 37 patients with ankylosing spondylitis who sustained cervical spine injuries, Einsiedel et al[34] compared the outcomes of patients treated with an anterior approach, posterior approach, and combined anterior-posterior approach. In all five cases in which early implant failure had occurred, the initial stabilization had been anterior only. The authors concluded that combined anterior and posterior stabilization is necessary for treating extension-distraction injuries in patients with DISH or ankylosing spondylitis (low-quality evidence).

◆ Potential Complications and Their Avoidance

Neurological deterioration of either the neurologically intact or SCI patient can occur, and the incidence has been reported to be as high as 6% of patients with cervical SCIs.[35] Potential mechanisms include inadequate immobilization, sustained hypotension, ascending spinal cord necrosis, epidural hematoma, and vertebral artery injury. Treatment includes rapidly identifying and reversing systemic hypotension, optimizing oxygenation, and using imaging studies to determine a structural cause. Plain radiographs can identify problems with alignment that can be corrected with rapid reduction and/or traction. MRI is invaluable for assessing soft tissue injury, and CT myelography can be used when extensive spinal instrumentation prevents adequate MRI visualization. The onset of injury ascension can be categorized into three subsets. Early deterioration (less than 24 hours) is typically related to traction and immobilization, delayed deterioration (between 24 hours and 7 days) is associated with sustained hypotension, and late deterioration (more than 7 days) is associated with vertebral artery injuries.[35]

Intraoperatively, neural element injury can involve the spinal cord or the nerve roots and can result from direct or indirect trauma, traction, or spinal cord ischemia. A minimum systolic blood pressure should be established preoperatively (mean arterial blood pressure > 90 mm Hg) to avoid excessive hypotension and to maintain adequate cord perfusion. Patients with preexisting cord compression are at higher risk of injury.

Nerve root injury has been reported to occur in the cervical spine with both anterior and posterior approaches. Permanent SCI occurring as a result of intraoperative complication is rare. In any patient with segmental instability, quadriplegia can result from manipulation of the neck during intubation, patient positioning, or excessive traction during surgical treatment. Any graft placed for cervical fusion must be contoured, appropriately sized, and positioned to avoid impingement into the spinal canal or excessive distraction.[3]

Complications that are unique to the anterior surgical approach to the cervical spine include dysphagia, esophageal perforation, tracheal injury, and recurrent laryngeal nerve injury with subsequent vocal cord paralysis. Injury to the sympathetic chain, which lies lateral and ventral to the longus colli musculature, might produce Horner syndrome. This can be prevented by avoiding lateral dissection of the longus colli musculature and by careful placement of retractors medial and deep to it. With prolonged pressure or direct trauma caused by surgical instruments, either the carotid artery or esophagus can also be injured. To limit risk of tissue injury, prolonged retraction should be avoided. Although rare, airway obstruction resulting from a hematoma can occur after anterior cervical surgery. It is treated with emergent decompression. Risk factors for airway complications include surgical time of more than 5 hours and exposure of four or more vertebral bodies.

Postoperative wound infections occur more commonly posteriorly than anteriorly. Additionally, they are more common in patients with complete neurological deficits. They are typically diagnosed approximately 2 weeks postoperatively. The most reliable signs are worsening pain with associated wound drainage and fevers. Deep wound infections should be treated aggressively with surgical irrigation and debridement. Although serial debridement procedures might be necessary, many deep wound infections can be successfully managed with suction drainage systems after initial debridement. Long-term antibiotic treatment should be initiated.

◆ Summary

Within the SLIC morphological category of distraction injuries, the nature of DLC disruption often determines whether a posterior or anterior surgical approach is used. Distraction injuries are often best treated by an approach in the direction of maximal soft tissue disruption. For distraction-extension injuries, the pattern of DLC disruption is primarily anterior; thus, most commonly, anterior cervical diskectomy, fusion, and plating are performed. For flexion-distraction injuries with massive posterior ligamentous disruption, a posterior approach is more commonly used. Any injuries with an associated disk herniation are generally treated with an anterior approach. For the remaining majority of SLIC distraction injuries, the surgeon is essentially free to choose either anterior or posterior stabilization, considering that the literature provides only low-quality evidence at best to support one approach over the other in certain cases. The major risk associated with an anterior approach is incomplete reduction intraoperatively and possible posterior ligament infolding. On the other hand, the major risk associated with a posterior approach is progressive disk collapse and the development of segmental kyphosis.

Based on a review of the current literature, evidence-based medicine guidelines for the management of SLIC distraction injuries can be summarized as follows. Only very low-quality evidence exists to support the use of cervical traction and closed reduction maneuvers and to support the use of external immobilization for SLIC distraction injuries. Only low-quality evidence exists to support the operative treatment of SLIC distraction injuries.

Regarding specific approaches, moderate-quality evidence suggests that anterior and posterior fixation approaches are equivalent treatment options for SLIC flexion-distraction injuries. Very low-quality evidence supports anterior surgery for SLIC extension-distraction injuries. Low-quality evidence supports anterior surgery for SLIC flexion-distraction injuries. Additionally, very low-quality evidence supports posterior surgery for extension-distraction injuries for which decompressive laminectomy is required. Currently, no medical evidence supports posterior surgery for the general category of SLIC flexion-distraction injuries. Combined anterior and posterior treatment for extension-distraction injuries with a large (> 3 mm) translational component (DES 2 equivalent) is supported by very low-quality evidence. Combined anterior and posterior treatment for extension-distraction injuries occurring in patients with DISH or ankylosing spondylitis is supported by low-quality evidence. No evidence currently supports the use of combined anterior and posterior treatment for SLIC flexion-distraction injuries.

◆ Clinical Questions (Table 30.1)

Should a surgeon perform anterior or posterior approaches on SLIC distraction injuries?

Evidence-based medicine (EBM) supports an anterior approach for SLIC extension-distraction injuries without a large translational component (DES 1 equivalent) and for SLIC flexion-distraction injuries. EBM supports a posterior approach for

Table 30.1 Evidentiary Table

Study	Description	Quality of Evidence	Topic and Conclusion
Vaccaro et al (2001)[3]	Retrospective case series	Very low	24 patients with subaxial cervical distraction-extension injuries; 16 treated surgically; for DES 1 injuries without significant cervical stenosis (9 patients), anterior fixation performed; for DES 1 injuries with significant anterior thecal sac compression (4 patients), anterior corpectomy and posterior stabilization performed; with significant (> 3 mm) translation (DES 2), circumferential stabilization performed (2 patients); 1 patient treated solely with posterior approach because of need for decompressive laminectomy; outcomes were radiographic; all 16 patients had stable alignment, none had instrumentation failure at last follow-up. CONCLUSION: Anterior fixation is effective method of treating DES 1 injuries. However, posterior fixation might be necessary for DES 1 injuries that require decompressive laminectomy. Injuries with significant (> 3 mm) translation (DES 2 equivalent) might require circumferential stabilization to achieve adequate sagittal alignment.
Henriques et al (2004)[31]	Retrospective case series	Very low	36 patients with subaxial flexion-distraction injuries treated with anterior fixation alone; outcomes were radiographic and clinical (records reviewed for "clinical remarks and complications"); solid union seen in 6 of 6 patients with DFS 1 injury and 15 of 17 patients with DFS 2 injury; in patients with DFS 3 injury, 7 of 13 anterior fixations failed. CONCLUSION: Use of anterior plate fixation alone for DFS 1 and DFS 2 injuries provides sufficient mechanical stability and acceptable clinical outcomes.
Elgafy et al (2006)[32]	Retrospective case series	Very low	65 patients with unilateral or bilateral cervical facet subluxation/dislocations treated with posterior fixation; outcomes were radiographic; 2 patients (both with bilateral facet subluxations) experienced instrumentation failure and ultimately required anterior revision; kyphosis at follow-up was significantly correlated with kyphosis shown on initial films and bilateral facet subluxation. CONCLUSION: Posterior instrumentation and fusion results in satisfactory alignment. However, high risk of postoperative kyphosis in patients with bilateral facet subluxations and in those with significant preoperative kyphosis. In such patients, better results might be obtained with anterior or combined anterior and posterior surgery.
Einsiedel et al (2006)[34]	Retrospective observational with control group	Low	37 patients with ankylosing spondylitis who suffered cervical extension-distraction injuries treated surgically; 24 treated circumferentially, 11 anteriorly, and 2 posteriorly; outcomes were radiographic; in all 5 cases in which implant failure required revision surgery, initial stabilization had been anterior only.

Table 30.1 Evidentiary Table *(Continued)*

Study	Description	Quality of Evidence	Topic and Conclusion
			CONCLUSION: Extension-distraction injuries in patients with DISH or ankylosing spondylitis should be treated with anterior decompression and fusion and anterior-posterior stabilization.
Kwon et al (2007)[33]	Randomized clinical trial	Moderate	42 patients with unilateral facet injuries of cervical spine randomized to undergo anterior diskectomy and fusion or posterior instrumented fusion; only 6 patients had SLIC flexion-distraction injuries specifically, 2 with perched facets and 4 with subluxed facets; primary outcome was postoperative time needed to meet set of discharge criteria; no significant difference in measure between 2 groups (no difference in acute postoperative morbidity). CONCLUSION: Both anterior and posterior fixations are valid treatment options for unilateral cervical facet injuries.

Abbreviations: DES, distraction-extension stage; DISH, diffuse idiopathic skeletal hyperostosis.

SLIC extension-distraction injuries that are highly unstable or that require an extensive decompressive laminectomy.

Should a surgeon perform a circumferential approach on SLIC distraction injuries?

EBM supports a circumferential approach for SLIC extension-distraction injuries with a large (> 3 mm) translational component (DES 2 equivalent) and extension-distraction injuries occurring in patients with ankylosing spondylitis or DISH.

Acknowledgment We thank Senior Editor and Writer Dori Kelly, MA, University of Maryland, for her expertise in the preparation of this chapter.

References

1. Vaccaro AR, Hulbert RJ, Patel AA, et al; Spine Trauma Study Group. The subaxial cervical spine injury classification system: a novel approach to recognize the importance of morphology, neurology, and integrity of the disco-ligamentous complex. Spine 2007;32:2365–2374

2. Dvorak MF, Fisher CG, Fehlings MG, et al. The surgical approach to subaxial cervical spine injuries: an evidence-based algorithm based on the SLIC classification system. Spine 2007;32:2620–2629

3. Vaccaro AR, Klein GR, Thaller JB, Rushton SA, Cotler JM, Albert TJ. Distraction extension injuries of the cervical spine. J Spinal Disord 2001; 14: 193–200

4. White AA, Panjabi MM. The problem of clinical instability in the human spine: a systematic approach. In: White AA, Panjabi MM, eds. Clinical Biomechanics of the Spine. 2nd ed. Philadelphia: JB Lippincott; 1990: 277–378

5. Simmons EH. The surgical correction of flexion deformity of the cervical spine in ankylosing spondylitis. Clin Orthop Relat Res 1972;86:132–143

6. Allen BL Jr, Ferguson RL, Lehmann TR, O'Brien RP. A mechanistic classification of closed, indirect fractures and dislocations of the lower cervical spine. Spine 1982;7:1–27

7. Yoganandan N, Knowles SA, Maiman DJ, Pintar FA. Anatomic study of the morphology of human cervical facet joint. Spine 2003;28:2317–2323

8. Lingawi SS. The naked facet sign. Radiology 2001;219:366–367

9. Whitley JE, Forsyth HF. The classification of cervical spine injuries. Am J Roentgenol Radium Ther Nucl Med 1960;83:633–644

10. Lowery DW, Wald MM, Browne BJ, Tigges S, Hoffman JR, Mower WR ; NEXUS Group. Epidemiology of cervical spine injury victims. Ann Emerg Med 2001;38:12–16

11. Goldberg W, Mueller C, Panacek E, Tigges S, Hoffman JR, Mower WR ; NEXUS Group. Distribution and patterns of blunt traumatic cervical spine injury. Ann Emerg Med 2001;38:17–21

12. Brown T, Reitman CA, Nguyen L, Hipp JA. Intervertebral motion after incremental damage to the posterior structures of the cervical spine. Spine 2005;30:E503–E508

13. Davis SJ, Teresi LM, Bradley WG Jr, Ziemba MA, Bloze AE. Cervical spine hyperextension injuries: MR findings. Radiology 1991;180:245–251

14. LeBlang SD, Nuñez DB Jr. Helical CT of cervical spine and soft tissue injuries of the neck. Radiol Clin North Am 1999;37:515–532, v–vi.

15. Kwon BK, Vaccaro AR, Grauer JN, Fisher CG, Dvorak MF. Subaxial cervical spine trauma. J Am Acad Orthop Surg 2006;14:78–89

16. France JC, Bono CM, Vaccaro AR. Initial radiographic evaluation of the spine after trauma: when, what, where, and how to image the acutely traumatized spine. J Orthop Trauma 2005;19:640–649

17. Stassen NA, Williams VA, Gestring ML, Cheng JD, Bankey PE. Magnetic resonance imaging in combination with helical computed tomography provides a safe and efficient method of cervical spine clearance in the obtunded trauma patient. J Trauma 2006;60:171–177

18. Vaccaro AR, Madigan L, Schweitzer ME, Flanders AE, Hilibrand AS, Albert TJ. Magnetic resonance imaging analysis of soft tissue disruption after flexion-distraction injuries of the subaxial cervical spine. Spine 2001; 26:1866–1872

19. Geck MJ, Yoo S, Wang JC. Assessment of cervical ligamentous injury in trauma patients using MRI. J Spinal Disord 2001;14:371–377

20. Benzel EC, Hart BL, Ball PA, Baldwin NG, Orrison WW, Espinosa MC. Magnetic resonance imaging for the evaluation of patients with occult cervical spine injury. J Neurosurg 1996;85:824–829

21. Star AM, Jones AA, Cotler JM, Balderston RA, Sinha R. Immediate closed reduction of cervical spine dislocations using traction. Spine 1990;15: 1068–1072

22. Vaccaro AR, Falatyn SP, Flanders AE, Balderston RA, Northrup BE, Cotler JM. Magnetic resonance evaluation of the intervertebral disc, spinal ligaments, and spinal cord before and after closed traction reduction of cervical spine dislocations. Spine 1999;24:1210–1217

23. Vital JM, Gille O, Sénégas J, Pointillart V. Reduction technique for uni- and biarticular dislocations of the lower cervical spine. Spine 1998;23:949–954, discussion 955

24. Hadley MN, Fitzpatrick BC, Sonntag VK, Browner CM. Facet fracture-dislocation injuries of the cervical spine. Neurosurgery 1992;30: 661–666

25. Bucholz RD, Cheung KC. Halo vest versus spinal fusion for cervical injury: evidence from an outcome study. J Neurosurg 1989;70:884–892

26. Beyer CA, Cabanela ME, Berquist TH. Unilateral facet dislocations and fracture-dislocations of the cervical spine. J Bone Joint Surg Br 1991; 73:977–981

27. Lemons VR, Wagner FC Jr. Stabilization of subaxial cervical spinal injuries. Surg Neurol 1993;39:511–518

28. Fazl M, Pirouzmand F. Intraoperative reduction of locked facets in the cervical spine by use of a modified interlaminar spreader: technical note. Neurosurgery 2001;48:444–445, discussion 445–446

29. Ludwig SC, Vaccaro AR, Balderston RA, Cotler JM. Immediate quadriparesis after manipulation for bilateral cervical facet subluxation: a case report. J Bone Joint Surg Am 1997;79:587–590

30. de Oliveira JC. Anterior reduction of interlocking facets in the lower cervical spine. Spine 1979;4:195–202

31. Henriques T, Olerud C, Bergman A, Jónsson H Jr. Distractive flexion injuries of the subaxial cervical spine treated with anterior plate alone. J Spinal Disord Tech 2004;17:1–7

32. Elgafy H, Fisher CG, Zhao Y, et al. The radiographic failure of single segment posterior cervical instrumentation in traumatic cervical flexion distraction injuries. Top Spinal Cord Inj Rehabil 2006;12:20–29

33. Kwon BK, Fisher CG, Boyd MC, et al. A prospective randomized controlled trial of anterior compared with posterior stabilization for unilateral facet injuries of the cervical spine. J Neurosurg Spine 2007;7:1–12

34. Einsiedel T, Schmelz A, Arand M, et al. Injuries of the cervical spine in patients with ankylosing spondylitis: experience at two trauma centers. J Neurosurg Spine 2006;5:33–45

35. Harrop JS, Sharan AD, Vaccaro AR, Przybylski GJ. The cause of neurologic deterioration after acute cervical spinal cord injury. Spine 2001;26: 340–346

31

Distraction Injuries and Ankylosing Spondylitis in Cervical Trauma

Jean-Charles Le Huec, Richard Meyrat, Richard J. Bransford, Robert A. Morgan, and Stephane Aunoble

Distraction injuries of the subaxial cervical spine may include lesions resulting from either excessive flexion or extension movements. They make up ~28% of all subaxial spine injuries.[1] Distraction injuries are caused by compression in one column accompanied by compensatory distraction in the opposite column and are predominantly soft tissue injuries, with only 20% of cases resulting in a fracture. In distraction-flexion injuries (**Fig. 31.1**), forced flexion results in compression of the anterior column and distraction of the posterior column. Radiographic studies reveal varying degrees of anterior translation of the affected segment with varying degrees of facet subluxation. Distraction-extension injuries (**Fig. 31.2**) occur after a forced extension movement produces compression of the posterior column and distraction of the anterior column. Radiographic studies usually demonstrate widening of the affected disk space and varying degrees of posterior column fractures. Clinical series demonstrate that most distraction injuries of the subaxial cervical spine occur at C6–C7.[2,3] Distraction-flexion injuries are more common than hyperextension injuries (12% vs 2%).[1,4–6]

◆ Morphology

An understanding of the mechanism of cervical injury of the subaxial spine is crucial in developing a correct diagnosis and formulating an appropriate treatment plan. Fractures and dislocations of the subaxial spine are generally the result of a combination of force vectors including flexion, rotation, extension, and vertical compression. In the case of distraction-extension injuries, the dominant force vector is extension followed by distraction of the anterior column. In distraction-flexion injuries, the dominant force vector is flexion followed by distraction of the posterior column. Several classification systems have been created to define subaxial injuries. Among these, the Allen and Ferguson classification system has been the most commonly used scheme to differentiate and characterize subaxial injury mechanisms. Its incorporation into the recently developed Subaxial Cervical Spine Injury Classification (SLIC) system, as

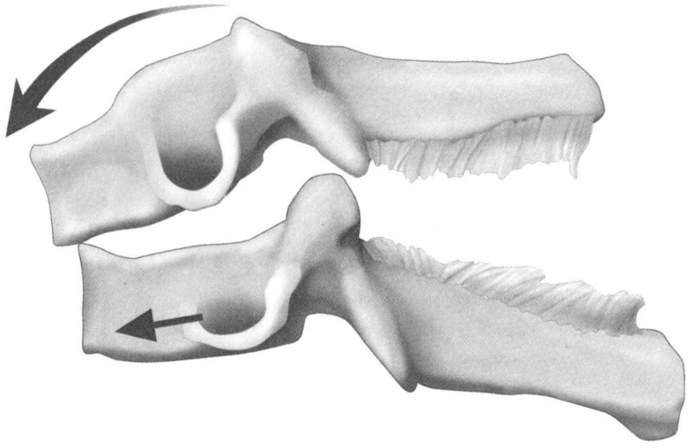

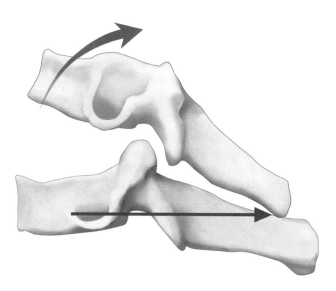

Fig. 31.1 Distraction-flexion subaxial cervical injury.

Fig. 31.2 Distraction-extension subaxial cervical injury.

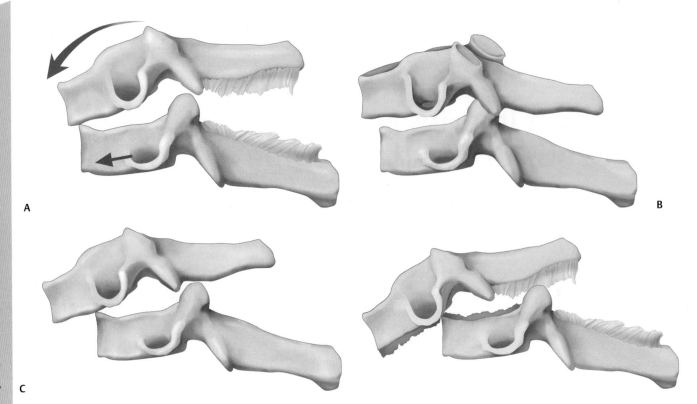

Fig. 31.3 Four stages of distraction-flexion injuries. **(A)** Stage I, facet subluxation (less than 25% anterolisthesis). **(B)** Stage II, unilateral facet dislocation (25% anterolisthesis). **(C)** Stage III, bilateral facet dislocation (50% anterolisthesis). **(D)** Stage IV, complete disruption of all three columns (> 50% anterolisthesis).

discussed in Chapter 27, reflects its continuing relevance in cervical trauma.

The Allen and Ferguson classification system, presented in 1982, is a mechanistic classification system of injuries to the subaxial cervical spine.[7] It defines six phylogenies, each based on the direction of the major force vector resulting in the initial injury. These include compressive flexion, vertical compression, compressive extension, distractive flexion, distractive extension, and lateral flexion. Distraction-flexion injuries are further broken into four stages, each stage representing increasing severity of injury (**Fig. 31.3**). Distraction-extension injuries are divided into two stages in the same manner (**Fig. 31.4**). Each of these stages (or subtypes) of distraction injuries is discussed in more detail in a following section.

◆ Distraction-Flexion Injuries

Distraction-flexion injuries result in compressive trauma of the anterior column and in a distraction injury of the posterior column. With the exception of unilateral facet dislocation, the primary force vector in these injuries is flexion resulting in distraction of the posterior elements. Unilateral facet dislocation is produced by an element of a rotational force vector.[1,3] A varying degree of posterior ligamentous injury is present, and in more severe cases, the middle column structures are involved. Allen and Ferguson classified distraction-flexion injuries (phylogeny) under four subtypes. Each subtype represents varying degrees of facet displacement.

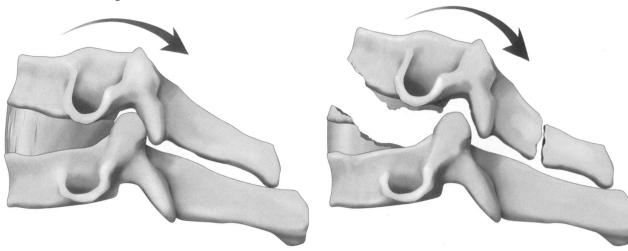

Fig. 31.4 Two stages of distraction-extension injuries. **(A)** Stage I, intact posterior longitudinal ligament without posterior translation. **(B)** Stage II, disruption of all three columns with posterior translation

Stage I represents facet subluxation (**Fig. 31.3A**), stage II unilateral facet dislocation (**Fig. 31.3B**), stage III bilateral facet dislocation with 50% displacement of anterolisthesis (**Fig. 31.3C**), and stage IV complete dislocation of all three columns (**Fig. 31.3D**). Each subtype represents progressive severity of ligamentous and bony injury from a posterior to anterior direction.[8] Magnetic resonance imaging (MRI) has shed light on specific soft tissue structures thought to be involved in these injuries.[9,10]

Distraction-flexion stage I injuries are generally limited to the posterior ligamentous complex, including the posterior cervical musculature, the superspinous and interspinous ligaments, and the ligamentum flavum. Varying degrees of the facet joint capsules can be involved, resulting in facet subluxation. Stage II injuries (unilateral facet dislocation) are characterized by disruption of the ipsilateral facet capsule and ipsilateral disk space in addition to the posterior structures involved in stage I injuries. The posterior longitudinal ligament (PLL) is usually preserved, limiting the extent of anterior translation between the involved vertebrae to 25% (**Fig. 31.5**). Stage III injuries (bilateral facet dislocation) result from bilateral disruption of the supporting structures in all three columns including the PLL and varying degrees of the anterior longitudinal ligament (ALL) (**Fig. 31.6**). By definition, the PLL must be disrupted for complete dislocation of both facet joints to occur. The increased instability allows greater

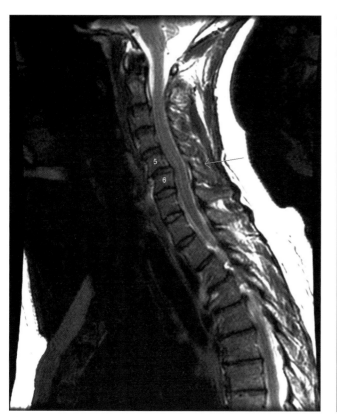

A

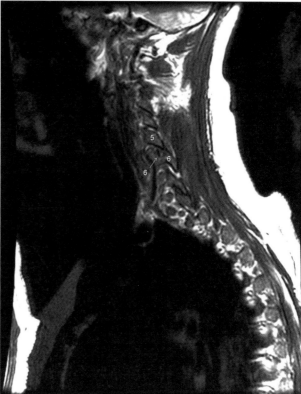

B

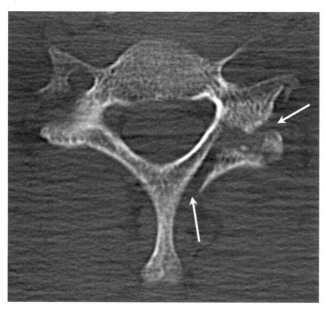

C

Fig. 31.5 Unilateral dislocated left C5–C6 facets. **(A)** Magnetic resonance imaging (MRI) T2 sagittal view showing 25% anterior translation. **(B)** MRI T2 sagittal cut demonstrating left C5–C6 jumped facets. **(C)** Computed tomographic axial cuts demonstrating left C5–C6 jumped facets.

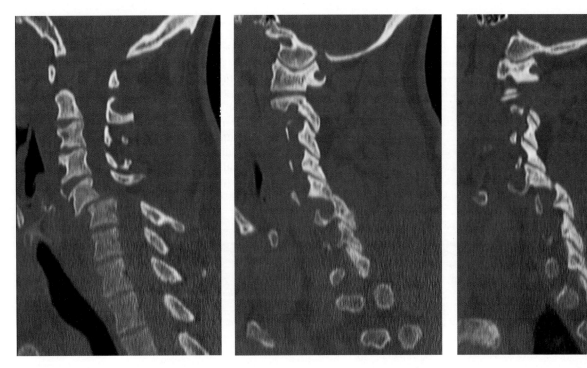

A–

Fig. 31.6 C5–C6 bilateral facet dislocation. **(A)** Computed tomographic sagittal cut demonstrating 50% anterior translation; **(B)** left C5–C6 jumped facets; **(C)** right C5–C6 jumped facets.

anterior displacement, usually 50%. Stage IV represents the most severe flexion-extension injury subtype with all three columns completely severed and anterior subluxation of over 50% (**Fig. 31.7**). The extensive ligamentous injury can sometimes result in a phenomenon known as floating vertebra, representing the most severe form of cervical instability.[11]

The incidence of vertebral artery injury is 11% in patients with cervical injury with a predilection for distraction-flexion injuries. One should have a high index of suspicion for such an injury, even in the absence of any clinical signs or symptoms, prompting an evaluation with magnetic resonance angiography (MRA) or computed tomographic (CT) angiogram (**Fig. 31.8**). The causative factors responsible for vertebral artery disruption appear to be a combination of a high-velocity distraction-flexion and rotational shear forces coupled with vertebral malalignment. Sim et al showed that occlusion of the vertebral artery injury was proportional to the severity of vertebral rotation, translation, and distraction.[12]

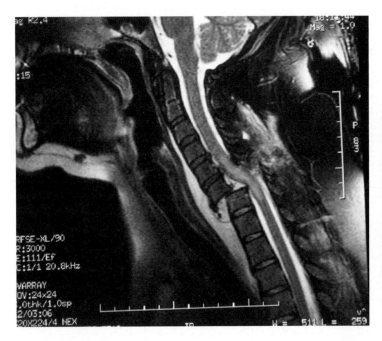

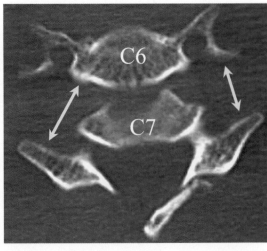

A   B

Fig. 31.7 Stage IV distraction-flexion injury. **(A)** Magnetic resonance imaging T2 sagittal cut showing complete disruption of all three columns with over 50% anterior translation. **(B)** Computed tomographic axial cut showing similar findings.

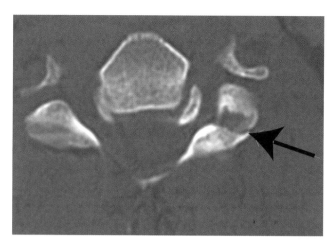

A

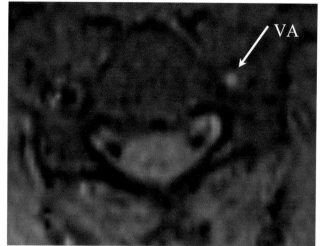

VA

B

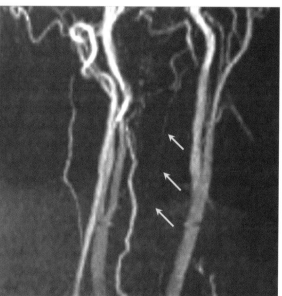

C

Fig. 31.8 Magnetic resonance angiography (MRA) demonstrating left vertebral artery dissection from type II distraction-flexion injury. **(A)** Computed tomographic axial cut showing left C5–C6 facet dislocation. **(B)** MRA axial cut showing flow void of left vertebral artery (VA). **(C)** MRA showing absence of left vertebral artery.

Both vertebral arteries are at risk in stage III and IV injuries. These findings support recommendations for immediate closed reduction and stabilization of advanced distraction-flexion deformities. Correction of vertebral displacement can reopen a potentially occluded vertebral artery, greatly reducing the possibility of a future cerebral ischemic event. Anticoagulation therapy and a neurointerventional consult should be considered in patients with known vertebral artery injury.

Neurological Damage

About 40% of all cervical spine injuries result in neurological damage. About a third of all spinal cord injuries (SCIs) are complete.[13] The majority is due to bilateral facet fracture dislocation and burst fractures of the cervical spine. In one series, 84% of bilateral facet fractures were associated with complete SCI.[14] This startling finding is supported by the fact that an anterior translation of 50% results in 40 to 50% canal occlusion, often aggravated by the presence of a traumatic herniation (up to 54% of patient with distraction-flexion injuries[15]). Seventy percent of unilateral locked facets (stage II) present with radiculopathy, whereas only 10% of unilateral locked facets are associated with cord

injuries.[16] The dislocated facet is wedged into the intervertebral foramen leading to foraminal stenosis and compression of the exiting nerve root. The anterior cord syndrome is usually seen in burst fractures (classically, flexion teardrop injuries) and bilateral facet fracture-dislocations. It results from direct injury to the anterior spinal cord or to the anterior spinal artery by protrusion of bony fragments or herniated disks into the spinal canal. Injury, thrombosis, or laceration of the anterior spinal artery (**Fig. 31.9A**) can also result in anterior cord syndrome (**Fig. 31.9B**). Brown-Séquard syndrome can result from flexion injuries, although a series by Braakman and Penning showed hyperextension injuries as a common cause.[17] Brown-Séquard syndrome results from unilateral hemisection of the cord (**Fig. 31.9C**). This rare injury usually results from penetrating injuries but can be seen following lateral mass fractures of the cervical spine.[18]

Imaging

The interested reader is referred to Chapter 12 for a detailed discussion on radiological findings of the acutely injured cervical spine.

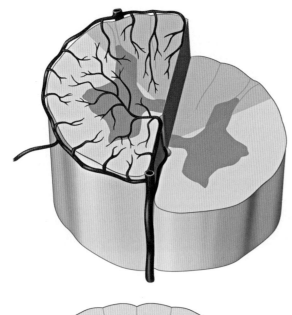

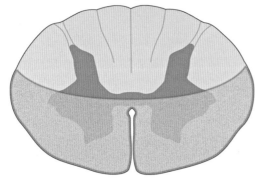

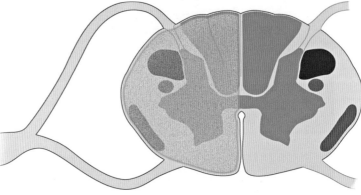

Fig. 31.9 Spinal cord injuries. **(A)** Anatomy of cervical spinal cord demonstrating anterior distribution of anterior spinal artery and distribution of right posterior spinal artery. Ischemic injury to anterior spinal artery can lead to **(B)** anterior cord syndrome. **(C)** Hemisection of cord, or Brown-Séquard syndrome.

Plain Films

Lateral

Anterior Column   The alignment of the anterior and posterior cortices of the cervical spine can be helpful in discerning dislocation. The alignment of the posterior cortices is more sensitive in discerning different types of dislocation. Less than 25% of anterolisthesis of the affected level may signify facet fractures. A 25% shift is often consistent with unilateral facet dislocation (**Fig. 31.5**). Anterolisthesis of 50% or above signifies facet dislocation (**Fig. 31.6**).

Posterior Column   Facet subluxation is the hallmark sign of distraction-flexion injuries, evidenced by the lack of parallel alignment of the facet joint. Uncovering of > 50% of the superior facet of the vertebra below the lesion (the "bowtie" sign) is seen in bilateral dislocation injuries, whereas a "double-sail" sign can be seen in unilateral dislocations. Fanning of the spinous processes may be observed, implying posterior column disruption. Horizontal avulsion fractures of the spinous process are a common feature in distraction-flexion injuries.

Anteroposterior   Interspinous distance of 1.5 times above or below an affected level may indicate a dislocation or subluxation. Unilateral facet dislocation may result in lateral rotation of one spinous process with respect to the others, toward the affected side.

Oblique   The neural foramina are best seen on this view. A dislocated facet occluding the foramen is seen in dislocations.

Computed Tomography

Most of the foregoing findings can be seen on two- and three-dimensional (2-D and 3-D) CT reconstruction. In addition, fractures of the articular facets, lateral mass, pedicles, and laminae are very well delineated in axial cuts.

Magnetic Resonance Imaging

MRI is useful in revealing blood, soft tissue edema, and discoligamentous disruption. A flow void signal can represent an occluded vertebral artery. High signal intensity of the soft tissue of the posterior column (interspinous ligament, supraspinous ligament, flavum, and paraspinous muscles) is a hallmark of distraction-flexion injuries. With increasing severity of injury, tear in the PLL, avulsion of the disk space, and compromise of the ALL are observed. An epidural hematoma or a ruptured disk compressing the ventral dural sac is sometimes seen. Intramedullary lesions such as cord edema or cord contusion can be differentiated by their different signal characteristics on MRI. Central hemorrhage may expand peripherally.

Evidence-Based Review of Treatment Options

Is Closed Reduction Safe and Effective for Distraction-Flexion Injuries?

Closed reduction has been demonstrated in multiple clinical studies to be both safe and effective for a variety of distraction-flexion injuries (**Table 31.1**).[3,4,6,14,16,19–36] This subject is

Table 31.1 Evidenciary Table for Distraction-Flexion Injuries of the Subaxial Cervical Spine

Study	Description of Study	Quality of Evidence	Topic and Conclusion
Dvorak et al (2007)[38]	Retrospective outcomes study of 90 unilateral facet injuries	Low	Health-related quality of life instruments are used to assess operative versus nonoperative treatment of these injuries. CONCLUSION: Operative management should be strongly considered in this group.
Elgafy 2007[108]	Retrospective case-control study of 65 patients with cervical fracture dislocations treated with posterior instrumentation	Very low	Instrumentation was 47.6% lateral mass plating, 46.2% interspinous process wiring, combined 6.2%. Iliac crest autograft was used in 57/65 patients. Solid fusion was achieved in 96.7%. Bilateral facet injuries with initial segmental kyphosis was strongly associated with late kyphosis. CONCLUSION: Consider anterior-posterior procedure in bilateral facet subluxations/dislocations to prevent late kyphosis.
Harrington and Park (2007)[52]	Prospective consecutive case series of 22 distraction-flexion injury patients treated with operative reduction and stabilization	Very low	12 patients with single-level unilateral facet subluxation underwent open anterior reduction and plating. 10 patients with single-level bilateral facet subluxation underwent open anterior reduction and plating followed by posterior plating. CONCLUSION: Anterior reduction and plating is safe and effective for single-level unilateral facet subluxations. A combined anterior-posterior approach is safe and effective for single-level bilateral facet subluxations.
Mizuno et al (2007)[19]	Retrospective case series of 11 patients with locked facets treated operatively	Very low	3 of 5 bilateral locked facets were able to be reduced closed, whereas 2 of 6 unilateral locked facets were able to be reduced closed. 5 were anterior only, 3 were posterior only, and 3 were combined procedures. CONCLUSION: Both anterior and posterior procedures are safe and effective in treating distraction-flexion injuries.
Johnson et al (2004)[53]	Retrospective case series of 87 distraction-flexion injuries treated with anterior diskectomy and plating	Very low	65 patients had bilateral facet injuries, 22 had unilateral injuries. 15 patients had evidence of vertebral end plate fracture. 11 patients had radiographic progression of deformity, and 9 of these 11 demonstrated pseudarthrosis. CONCLUSION: Anterior diskectomy and plating is safe and effective for distraction-flexion injuries not involving end plate or facet fractures.
Anderson et al (2004)[109]	Retrospective observational study of 45 patients with facet dislocations	Very low	Timing of reduction did not correlate with neurological recovery, whereas younger age and better initial motor scores did correlate with improved neurological outcomes. CONCLUSION: Late recovery of motor function in young, incomplete spinal cord injured patients can be expected.
Koivikko et al (2004)[2]	Retrospective study of 106 distraction flexion injuries with operative arm and nonoperative control group	Low	Operative management consisted of posterior Rogers wiring in 51 patients. 16 nonoperatively treated patients subsequently underwent operative management for late instability or neurological decline. Operatively treated patients had improved radiographic parameters and less neck pain. CONCLUSION: Operative management with posterior wiring was safe and effective. Patients had improved radiographic parameters and less neck pain.
Brodke et al (2003)[49]	Randomized prospective study of 52 patients with spinal cord injuries and subaxial instability	Moderate	24 distraction-flexion injuries total were treated with 6 anterior diskectomy and plating procedures and 18 posterior instrumented fusions. There was no statistically significant difference in complications or neurological or radiographic outcomes between the two groups. CONCLUSION: Both anterior diskectomy and plating as well as posterior instrumented fusion are safe and effective in treating distraction-flexion injuries.
Do Koh et al (2001)[43]	Biomechanical study evaluating posterior versus anterior instrumentation	Moderate	Posterior instrumentation was significantly stiffer than anterior instrumentation in distraction-flexion model. CONCLUSION: Anterior only procedures may not be adequate for highly unstable injuries.
Ordonez et al (2000)[42]	Retrospective case series of 10 patients with distraction-flexion injuries treated with anterior reduction and plating	Very low	Satisfactory reduction was obtained in 9 patients, with one patient requiring an additional posterior procedure to achieve reduction. Risk factors for failed reduction include significant posterior element disruption and facet fracture comminution. CONCLUSION: Anterior diskectomy and plating is safe and effective in distraction-flexion injuries that are not highly unstable or involve facet fractures.
Shapiro et al (1999)[20]	Retrospective case series of 51 consecutive patients with unilateral locked facets	Very low	10/37 patients with radiculopathy resolved with closed reduction, 9/37 improved to "near normal" prior to open reduction, 18/37 improved to "near normal" after open reduction. Lateral mass

(Continued on page 302)

Study	Description of Study	Quality of Evidence	Topic and Conclusion
			plates and spinous process wiring was significantly better at obtaining and maintaining cervical lordosis. CONCLUSION: Lateral mass plating was superior to wiring procedures in obtaining and maintaining cervical lordosis. Anterior approaches are occasionally necessary for canal decompression.
Shanmuganathan et al (1996)[60]	Retrospective radiological review of 21 patients with traumatic isolation of the articular pillar	Very low	The most common mechanisms for this injury were distraction-flexion and hyperflexion-rotation. In only one of 21 cases was this injury due to an extension mechanism. CONCLUSION: Traumatic isolation of the articular pillar is a radiographic finding associated with distraction-flexion injuries.
Fehlings et al (1994)[46]	Retrospective case series of 44 consecutive patients treated with posterior lateral mass plating	Very low	22 patients with distraction-flexion injuries followed for an average of 36 months demonstrated 16 solid fusions, 1 failure, 3 lost to follow-up, two late deaths. CONCLUSION: Posterior lateral mass plating is safe and effective in treating distraction-flexion injuries.
Lieberman and Webb (1994)[4]	Retrospective case series of 41 patients age greater than 65 with cervical spine fractures	Very low	14 patients with distraction-flexion injuries, 12 bilateral and 2 unilateral. 2/12 bilateral facet dislocation patients were treated with a posterior fusion, 1/12 with a halo vest, 3/12 with traction/bed rest, 4/12 died. CONCLUSION: Closed management of distraction-flexion injuries may be successful. There is a high mortality in the elderly patient who sustains this injury pattern.
Lukhele (1994)[41]	Retrospective case series of 43 patients with facet fractures treated with posterior wiring	Very low	12 patients had associated laminar fractures, 5 of which went on to develop deformity and increased neurological deficit. These were subsequently treated with anterior diskectomy and plating. CONCLUSION: Intact posterior elements are necessary for successful posterior wiring.
Pasciak and Doniec (1993)[110]	Retrospective case series of 32 patients with unilateral facet dislocations	Very low	15/23 dislocations were able to be reduced and held in traction up to 3 weeks. Instability was demonstrated in 7 patients with subsequent unspecified fusion. 8 patients failed closed reduction and underwent posterior reduction and fusion. CONCLUSION: Failure of closed reduction and late instability is common in unilateral facet injuries.
Shapiro (1993)[16]	Retrospective case series of 24 patients with unilateral locked facets	Very low	5 patients underwent successful closed reduction, with two thirds having resubluxation in halo. 1 of 24 patients posteriorly reduced and wired resubluxed and subsequently underwent an anterior fusion with plating. CONCLUSION: Posterior reduction and wiring was more effective than halo management for unilateral locked facet injuries.
Hadley et al (1992)[14]	Retrospective case series of 68 patients with facet fracture dislocations	Very low	28 patients failed closed reduction. 7/31 closed reduced patients treated in halo developed late instability. CONCLUSION: Posterior reduction and wiring was more effective than halo management for unilateral and bilateral facet fracture dislocations.
Mahale and Silver (1992)[22]	Retrospective case series of 13 patients with missed bilateral facet dislocation.	Very low	10/13 patients were able to be reduced, only 1/13 patients developed late instability. 5/13 patients had insignificant improvement in paralysis after reduction. CONCLUSION: Bilateral facet dislocations are unstable and at risk for severe neurological injury
Anderson et al (1991)[5]	Retrospective case series of 30 patients treated with posterior cervical plating	Very low	19 patients treated with otherwise unspecified subluxations of the subaxial cervical spine demonstrated solid fusion at a mean 17.8-month follow-up. CONCLUSION: Posterior cervical plating is safe and effective for treatment of distraction-flexion injuries.
Beyer et al (1991)[47]	Retrospective case series of 34 patients with unilateral facet dislocations and fracture dislocations	Very low	Adjacent segment instability found at levels around nonanatomical arthrodesis regardless of operative or nonoperative treatment. CONCLUSION: Posttraumatic kyphosis predisposes patients to adjacent segment degeneration. Posterior arthrodesis is safe and effective in treatment of distraction-flexion injuries but may place the patient at risk of fusion extension beyond the instrumented level.
Nazarian and Louis (1991)[48]	Retrospective case series of 23 distraction-flexion injuries treated with posterior instrumentation	Very low	11 unilateral fracture dislocations, 4 bilateral fracture dislocations, and 5 fracture separations of the articular pillar. Solid arthrodesis was achieved without loss of reduction using a plate–screw construct.

Study	Description of Study	Quality of Evidence	Topic and Conclusion
			CONCLUSION: Posterior instrumented fusion is safe and effective for this injury pattern.
Wolf et al (1991)[23]	Retrospective case series of 52 patients with bilateral facet dislocations	Very low	49/52 patients were treated operatively and subsequently followed. Operative procedures included 3 anterior fusion and plating, 2 combined, 44 posterior wiring. Closed reduction by traction alone was successful in 31 patients. CONCLUSION: Anterior, posterior, and combined procedures are safe and effective in treatment of distraction-flexion injuries.
Aebi et al (1990)[54]	Retrospective case series of 86 patients who sustained a cervical spine injury and were treated with anterior cervical plating	Very low	64 patients had predominantly posterior lesions including discoligamentous or osseoligamentous injuries and were treated with single-level diskectomy and plating. One patient redislocated at 10 days postoperatively requiring reoperation. No pseudarthroses identified at mean follow-up of 40 months. CONCLUSION: Anterior cervical diskectomy and plating is safe and effective for the treatment of distraction-flexion injuries that are not highly unstable.
Rockswold et al (1990)[6]	Retrospective case series of 140 patients with cervical spine injuries	Very low	57 patients had distraction-flexion injuries including 36 anterior subluxation, 11 bilateral locked facets, 10 unilateral locked facets. Halo management was successful in 10/36 anterior subluxations, 9/11 bilateral locked facets, and 4/10 unilateral locked facets. CONCLUSION: Halo management of distraction-flexion injuries is prone to treatment failure in anterior subluxations and unilateral locked facets.
Sears and Fazl (1990)[24]	Retrospective case series of 173 patients with cervical spine injuries treated in halo	Very low	38 patients sustained unilateral facet dislocations, 32 sustained bilateral facet dislocations. 39/70 patients either failed reduction or resubluxed in the halo. 16/31 patients definitively treated in halo achieved stability with good alignment. CONCLUSION: Halo management of distraction-flexion injuries is prone to treatment failure in distraction-flexion injuries.
Benzel and Kesterson (1989)[25]	Retrospective case series of 50 consecutive patients treated with posterior interspinous compression wiring	Very low	Two patients underwent additional anterior diskectomy and fusion, 1 due to postoperative noted spinous process fracture, one due to neurological deterioration from reduction-induced disk herniation. 9 patients were treated in a Minerva brace, 5 patients treated in a halo, 3 were treated with bed rest, the remainder in cervical collars. There was one death. CONCLUSION: Posterior wiring is safe and effective in treating distraction-flexion injuries.
Bucholz and Cheung (1989)[65]	Retrospective case series of 124 cervical spine injuries	Very low	20 distraction-flexion injuries included in the series with 3 treated with operative reduction due to failure of closed reduction. 9/13 halo treatment failures were in patients with bilateral facet subluxation or dislocation. CONCLUSION: Bilateral facet subluxation or dislocation is a predictor of halo treatment failure
Ostl et al (1989)[111]	Retrospective case series of 167 patients with distraction-flexion injuries of the subaxial cervical spine	Very low	20 anterior subluxations, 101 facet fracture-dislocations, 46 bilateral facet dislocations. 2/95 patients treated with closed reduction under general anesthesia had a transient neurological loss. 14/85 patients treated closed developed late instability. 6/91 patients failed closed reduction and underwent posterior reduction and wiring. CONCLUSIONS: Bilateral facet dislocations are at risk for late instability when treated in halo. Closed reduction under general anesthesia is a risk for postoperative neurological deficit.
Argenson et al (1988)[1]	Retrospective case series of 47 patients with displacement of the subaxial cervical spine	Very low	41 patients treated with anterior cervical fusion and plating, 6 patients treated with posterior plating. Reduction maintained in 22 of 26 unilateral facet dislocations treated anteriorly. CONCLUSION: Anterior reduction and plating is safe and effective for treatment of unilateral facet dislocations.
Lind et al (1988)[26]	Prospective observational study of 83 patients with cervical spine injuries	Low	31 patients had distraction-flexion injuries with 10 unilateral and 7 bilateral facet dislocations. 2 unilateral facet injuries demonstrated late instability as did 2 of the bilateral facet injuries. CONCLUSION: Bilateral facet dislocations are at high risk of treatment failure in halo.

31 Distraction Injuries and Ankylosing Spondylitis in Cervical Trauma

(Continued on page 304)

Table 31.1 Evidenciary Table for Distraction-Flexion Injuries of the Subaxial Cervical Spine *(Continued)*

Study	Description of Study	Quality of Evidence	Topic and Conclusion
Rorabeck et al (1987)[27]	Retrospective case series of 26 patients with unilateral facet dislocations	Very low	20/26 patients failed closed reduction. 10/26 patients were treated with operative reduction and posterior wiring with 8/10 maintaining anatomical alignment. CONCLUSION: Patients with unreduced facet dislocations are at risk for late pain
Rorabeck et al (1987)[27]	Retrospective case series of 26 patients with unilateral facet dislocations	Very low	20/26 patients failed closed reduction. 10/26 patients were treated with operative reduction and posterior wiring with 8/10 maintaining anatomical alignment. CONCLUSION: Patients with unreduced facet dislocations are at risk for late pain
Glaser et al (1986)[30]	Retrospective case series of 245 cervical spine injuries	Very low	17 distraction-flexion injuries were included in this series. 3/12 unilateral facet dislocations and 1/5 bilateral facet dislocations failed treatment. CONCLUSION: Distraction-flexion injuries are at increased risk of treatment failure with closed management in halo.
Ersmark and Kalén (1986)[29]	Retrospective case series of 36 subaxial cervical spine injuries treated in a halo vest	Very low	29 dislocations not otherwise specified were stable after halo treatment. CONCLUSION: Nonoperative management of subaxial cervical spine dislocations may be successful.
Chan et al (1983)[28]	Retrospective case series of 188 cervical spine injuries treated in a halo	Very low	150 subaxial cervical spine fractures and fracture dislocations treated in halo. 13/53 unilateral or bilateral facet dislocations failed treatment. CONCLUSION: Distraction-flexion injuries have a high treatment failure rate with closed management in a halo.
O'Brien et al (1982)[3]	Retrospective case series of 34 patients with distraction flexion injuries	Very low	20 bilateral locked facets, 15 unilateral locked facets. 18 successful closed reductions with subsequent halo treatment, 3 of which developed late instability and went on for operative management. CONCLUSION: Closed treatment of these injuries with a halo can be successful, but late instability is a possible outcome.
Sonntag (1981)[32]	Retrospective case series of 15 patients with bilateral locked facets	Very low	All patients were reduced either closed or operative. 4/6 closed reduced patients were treated successfully nonoperatively. Nine patients were operatively treated with posterior wiring. CONCLUSION: Posterior stabilization is safe and effective. Closed reduction under general anesthesia is associated with risk of neurological deficit.
Bohlman (1979)[31]	Retrospective case series of 300 patients with cervical spine injuries	Low	158 patients had distracion-flexion injuries. 5 arterial occlusions identified at autopsy in patients with facet dislocations, 4 radicular and one vertebral. CONCLUSIONS: Distraction-flexion injuries are associated with late instability and failure of nonoperative management.
De Oliveira 1979[112]	Retrospective case series of 10 patients treated with anterior reduction of locked facets	Very low	10 unilateral and 2 bilateral locked facets successfully reduced via anterior approach with subsequent bone grafting and supine traction for 4 weeks followed by halo placement. No late instability. CONCLUSION: Acute instability can be treated through an anterior approach with prolonged postoperative traction.
Burke and Tiong (1975)[35]	Retrospective case series of 176 patients with cervical spine injuries	Very low	51 distraction-flexion injuries, all treated nonoperatively. 1/14 anterior subluxation and 2/14 unilateral facet injuries demonstrated late instability and were treated operatively via anterior approach. CONCLUSION: late instability can be effectively treated through an anterior approach.
Cheshire (1969)[36]	Retrospective case series of 257 patients with cervical spine injuries	Very low	95 distraction-flexion injuries with 6 patients treated with early operative reduction, 4 posteriorly, 2 anteriorly. Late instability occurred in 4/19 anterior subluxations, 3/41 unilateral facet dislocation, 2/35 bilateral facet dislocation. CONCLUSION: Late instability is a complication of nonoperative management.
Beatson (1963)[33]	Retrospective case series of 59 patients with additional anatomic and biomechanical study	Very low	20 patients had unilateral facet dislocations, 23 patients had bilateral facet dislocations. 2/20 bilateral dislocations were diagnosed after onset of tetraplegia. CONCLUSION: Bilateral facet dislocations are unstable and at risk for catastrophic neurological complications

treated in more detail in Chapter 22; the interested reader is referred there to review the techniques, nuances, and evidence-based review of closed reduction. There is one important caveat to closed reduction of distraction-flexion injuries. The use of traction in stage IV distraction-flexion injuries, facet fracture dislocations, and three-column cervical injury in patients with ankylosing spondylitis[37] can precipitate neurological deterioration due to stretching of the spinal cord (**Fig. 31.10**). The aforementioned cervical injuries are considered some of the most unstable in spine trauma.

Is Nonoperative Management Ever Indicated for Distraction-Flexion Injuries of the Subaxial Cervical Spine?

Facet dislocation injuries are more likely to fail closed reduction than other types of subaxial cervical injuries. In addition, they are less likely to maintain closed reduction when successful.[26,28–30] Failure to maintain reduction appears to be related to the extensive ligamentous injury in dislocation injuries. Unlike fractures, ligaments do not heal well, and as a result, distraction-flexion injuries often fail conservative management,

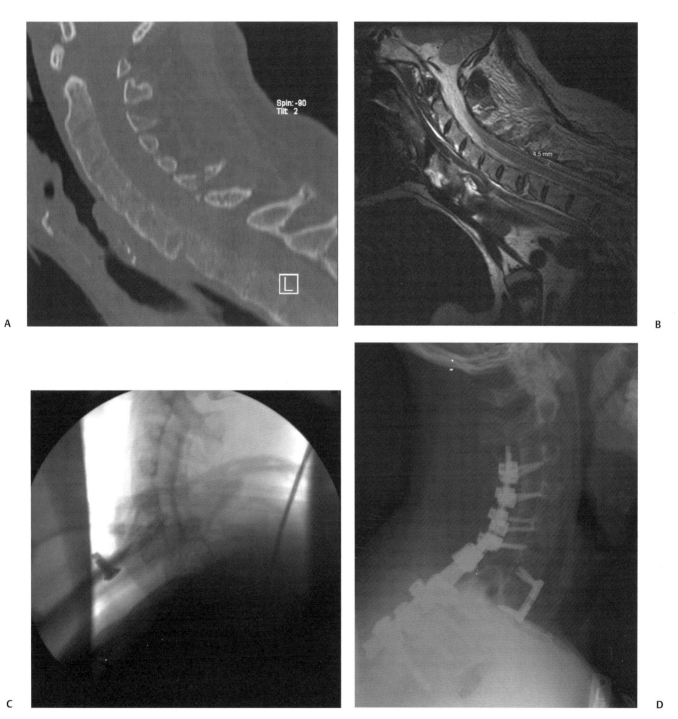

Fig. 31.10 A 32-year-old man with ankylosing spondylitis (AS) presenting with C6–C7 three-column injury after a motor vehicle accident. **(A)** Computed tomographic sagittal view. **(B)** Magnetic resonance imaging T2 sagittal view demonstrating posterior epidural hematoma. **(C)** Lateral x-ray showing inappropriate closed reduction with halo (note severe anterior translation). Patient began complaining of paresthesia of all extremities and was taken immediately for surgery for anterior and posterior stabilization. **(D)** Postoperative lateral C-spine x-ray. Patient regained baseline neurological status.

requiring surgical stabilization. With these important caveats in mind, the halo vest has been used successfully in many very low quality studies for many years. The early series that demonstrated very high success rates also relied on prolonged periods of bed rest in traction prior to allowing upright posture in the halo vest. Late kyphosis, instability, and pain are common in even stage I and II injuries.[2,3,26,28,31]

The most rigorous study looking at the use of the halo vest for nonoperative treatment of cervical spine injuries is the low-quality study by Lind et al in 1988, which was a prospective observational study of 83 patients with assorted cervical spine injuries. Thirty-one patients had distraction-flexion injuries, with 10 being unilateral and seven being bilateral facet dislocations. Two of the 10 unilateral facet injuries demonstrated late instability as did two of the seven bilateral facet injuries. One patient required operative treatment for redislocation while in the halo.[26]

In patients who will not tolerate operative intervention, it is a weak recommendation that bed rest with cervical traction may be a treatment option. In selected patients who otherwise refuse operative intervention, it is a weak recommendation that treatment of stage I and stage II distraction-flexion injuries in a halo vest may be successful in closely monitored circumstances.

Is Posterior Instrumentation Effective for Treating Distraction-Flexion Injuries of the Subaxial Cervical Spine?

The longest history of internal fixation for distraction-flexion injuries derives from posteriorly based approaches (**Table 31.1**). Early operative treatment consisted of either anterior or posterior reductions and bone grafting with continued bed rest and eventually a halo vest. The highest-quality study looking at posterior wiring is a low-quality study by Bohlman in 1979, which was a retrospective case series of 300 patients with assorted cervical spine injuries. One hundred fifty-eight patients had distraction-flexion injuries. Of note, five patients had arterial occlusions identified at autopsy in patients with facet dislocations, four of which were radicular and one vertebral. Posterior wiring when coupled with bone grafting and halo vest immobilization was demonstrated to be safe and effective. Other studies from that era also demonstrate the safety and efficacy of posterior wiring techniques.[25,27,32] Studies have also demonstrated the superiority of posterior wiring techniques over halo vest treatment for the treatment of stage I and stage II injuries.[2,14,16] More recent studies have demonstrated the superiority of operative compared with nonoperative management strategies for unilateral facet fractures.[38]

The later development of lateral mass screw and pedicle screw fixation techniques has in some sense limited the role for wiring. Lateral mass fixation is mechanically more stable and does not require the same level of intact posterior elements to be efficacious.[20,39,40] Failure of wiring techniques has been associated with facet fractures, lamina fractures, spinous process fractures, as well as highly unstable distraction-flexion injuries.[25,39–41] More recent series have demonstrated the efficacy of wiring techniques.[2,23,42] The most rigorous study evaluating the efficacy of posterior wiring compared with nonoperative management with a halo vest for distraction-flexion injuries was the low-quality study by Koivikko et al in 2004, which was a retrospective study of 106 distraction-flexion injuries with an operative arm and an appropriate nonoperative control group.[2] In this study,

operative management consisted of posterior Rogers wiring in 51 patients, of which six patients subsequently required revision for loss of reduction. Sixteen nonoperatively treated patients subsequently underwent operative management for late instability or neurological decline. Operatively treated patients had improved radiographic parameters and less neck pain. There was no difference in neurological outcomes.

In patients with a stage I or stage II distraction-flexion injury without fracture who have undergone successful closed reduction and who have a preoperative MRI demonstrating no evidence of ventral disk herniation, it is a weak recommendation that posterior wiring is safe and effective when coupled with bone graft and external immobilization.

Is a Posterior-Only Approach Safe and Effective for Treating Distraction-Flexion Injuries of the Subaxial Cervical Spine?

The posterior approach is a logical choice to an injury caused by disruption of the posterior ligamentous structures. Posterior fixation immediately restores the posterior tension band and has been shown to be more biomechanically stable when compared with anterior fixation, particularly in flexion.[43] Fixation screws and rods are biomechanically superior to other types of posterior fixation techniques.[39,44] In addition, open reduction can be done under direct visualization once posterior decompression of the injured segment is completed (flavotomy, removal of fractured lamina, and evacuation of hematoma). With few exceptions, the posterior approach can be used to treat all distraction-flexion injuries in the absence of a herniated disk if the posterior bony structures are reasonably intact.[45]

Presumably, injury to the disk during acute distraction leads to rapid degeneration of the disk space resulting in disk collapse over time.[46] The decrease in height of the anterior column forces the cervical spine into kyphosis, even in the presence of posterior fixation. These kyphotic deformities have been shown to cause cervical pain and are associated with adjacent segment degeneration in trauma patients.[47] For this reason, supplementing posterior fixation with an anterior cervical diskectomy and fusion may be appropriate.

Although the posterior approach avoids complications related to the anterior approach such as dysphagia, hoarseness, and possible injury to the esophagus, it is associated with a higher infection rate and more extensive muscle dissection. Clinical studies have demonstrated the safety and efficacy of posterior only solutions utilizing lateral mass screw fixation[5,23,46,48] as well as their superiority to wiring.[20,49] The most rigorous study comparing anterior to posterior solutions was the moderate-quality study by Brodke et al in 2003, which was a randomized prospective study of 52 patients with spinal cord injuries and subaxial instability.[49]

In this study, 24 distraction-flexion injuries were treated with six anterior diskectomy and plating procedures and 18 posterior instrumented fusions. There was no statistically significant difference in complications and neurological or radiographic outcomes between the two groups.

In stage I and stage II distraction-flexion injuries, it is a strong recommendation that posterior-only solutions are safe and effective. In stage III and stage IV distraction-flexion injuries, it is a weak recommendation that posterior-only solutions are safe and effective.

Is an Anterior-Only Approach Safe and Effective for Treating Distraction-Flexion Injuries of the Subaxial Cervical Spine?

The anterior approach allows decompression of the disk space and decompression of the spinal cord and nerve roots. It often allows superior realignment compared with the posterior approach and involves a single-level fusion construct. A trapezoidal interbody graft produces a lordotic curve, creating tight apposition of the facets. Failure of open reduction is equivalent to the posterior approach (~4%). The anterior approach is less traumatic, requires less manipulation during positioning, results in less postoperative pain, and is technically simple. The bone graft is under direct compression enhancing optimal fusion. Because of the excellent outcome of the anterior approach and the fact that many distraction-flexion injuries present with traumatic hernias, many authors advocate it as a primary surgical approach to the unstable subaxial spine.[50]

The integrity of the PLL appears to have important implications in the stability of a motion segment. As the degree of posterior soft tissue injury increases, the instantaneous axes of rotation shift anteriorly.[8,43,51] The PLL provides a crucial posterior band mechanism that prevents the instantaneous axes of rotation from going beyond the end plates. In the cases of distraction-flexion injuries stage I and II, the PLL is intact and an anterior fixation can sufficiently stabilize the motion segment. Very low quality clinical studies have demonstrated the safety and efficacy of anterior-only approaches for stage I and stage II distraction-flexion injuries that do not involve end plate, body, or facet fractures.[1,19,23,42,49,52–54]

It is a strong recommendation for stage I and stage II distraction-flexion injuries without associated end plate or facet fractures that anterior diskectomy and plating is safe and effective.

What Is the Treatment Recommendation for Treating Stage III and Stage IV Distraction-Flexion Injuries of the Subaxial Cervical Spine?

In stage III and IV, the posterior longitudinal ligament is disrupted and the instantaneous axis of rotation moves anteriorly to involve the vertebral end plates. In this situation, an anterior fixation is inadequate because no posterior tension band mechanism exists. Do Koh et al demonstrated biomechanically that anterior-only instrumentation was inadequate in this environment.[43] Henriques showed a 50% failure rate of anterior fixation in patients with stage 3 distraction-flexion injuries.[51] Very low quality clinical studies have demonstrated increased failure rates of anterior-only solutions in these highly unstable injuries, particularly when they are associated with either end plate or facet fractures.[42,53,54] A very low quality prospective consecutive case series by Harrington and Park demonstrated the safety and efficacy of combined anterior-posterior instrumentation for these highly unstable injuries.[52] Also published the same year was a retrospective study by Mizuno et al demonstrating the safety and efficacy of combined anterior-posterior procedures for these types of injuries.[19]

Additionally, they demonstrated that posterior only solutions are at risk for requiring an anterior additional procedure for late disk herniation. These two studies expanded on the earlier work by Wolf et al, which also demonstrated the safety and efficacy of the combined approach in treating these highly unstable injuries.[23]

It is a weak recommendation that stage III and IV distraction-flexion injuries should be treated with both anterior fixation and posterior fixation.

What Are Other Indications for Combined Procedures?

It is a strong recommendation that failure of open reduction during the anterior approach necessitates an additional posterior approach. This may necessitate an anterior-posterior-anterior procedure.

It is a strong recommendation that distraction-flexion injuries of the subaxial cervical spine with evidence of vertebral fracture (even when subtle) and/or facet fracture not be fixed by anterior-only methods.

It is a strong recommendation that combined procedures begin with the anterior approach to decompress neural elements prior to attempted reduction in the case of failed closed reduction.

It is a strong recommendation that posterior instrumentation be supported with an anterior graft in a situation where the vertebral body is fractured.

◆ Distraction-Extension Injuries

Distraction-extension injuries occur after compressive trauma of the posterior and middle column of the spine and distraction of the anterior discoligamentous structures (**Fig. 31.2**). Typically, the face directly strikes a hard surface, resulting in posterior recoil of the head and neck. Facial trauma points toward this type of injury. Hyperextension injuries tend to involve the lower subaxial spine (C5–C7) and are more common in the elderly. A stiff, spondylotic spine and high risk for falls (e.g., stairs) predispose this population to this pattern of injury. One study sited a mortality rate as high as 42% with an average age of 72, reflecting the susceptibility of the elderly.[55] Spivak et al demonstrated a 60 times higher mortality rate in older patients with spinal cord injuries.[56]

Like distraction-flexion injuries, the integrity of the posterior anulus and PLL has important implications in the severity of the structural injury. As hyperextension force continues to be applied, the ALL and anterior anulus is disrupted, followed by the destruction of the posterior anulus and PLL. The anterior discoligamentous structures are avulsed, followed by posterior horizontal translation of the vertebral segment. The PLL is stripped off, further destabilizing the segment (**Fig. 31.11A**). Compression of the posterior elements results in fractures of the articular joints and spinous processes (**Figs. 31.4B, 31.11B,C**). Unilateral or bilateral fractures of the laminae with varying degrees of displacement result from contact between the suprajacent and the subjacent neural arch during forced extension.

According to the Allen and Ferguson classification distraction-extension injuries are divided into two types: stage I and stage II. Stage I distraction-extension injuries are limited by an intact middle column. Posterior translation of the superior vertebra is not seen (**Fig. 31.4A**). There is predominantly soft tissue injury including prevertebral edema, disrupted ALL, and a widened disk space. In stage II injuries, all three columns are compromised resulting in retrolisthesis of the superior vertebra into the spinal canal (**Fig. 31.4B**). The prevertebral edema is much more

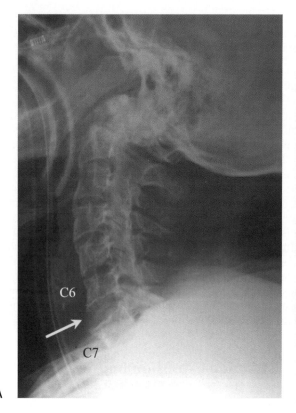

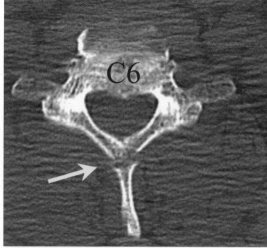

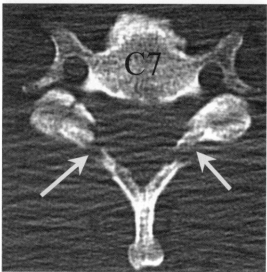

Fig. 31.11 Distraction-extension subaxial cervical injury. **(A)** Lateral C-spine x-ray showing widened disk space due to avulsion of the anterior discoligamentous complex resulting in posterior translation at C6–C7 interspace. **(B,C)** Fractures of bilateral laminae and spinous process as a result of forced extension.

pronounced and highly suggestive of significant discoligamentous complex disruption, even in a well-aligned cervical spine.[57] Neurological sequelae are more severe as a result of spinal cord compression between the posteroinferior edge of the cephalad vertebral body and the subjacent lamina.[58] An anteroinferior avulsion fracture fragment is characteristically seen, with its transverse dimension greater than its vertical dimension. In contrast to a flexion teardrop fracture, the ALL is ruptured.

An extension teardrop fracture (not to be confused with a flexion teardrop fracture) results from avulsion of the

anteroinferior aspect of the affected vertebral body by the intact ALL (**Fig. 31.12**). The vertical dimension of the triangular fragment is greater than its transverse dimension. The anterior third of the disk is intact, whereas the posterior two thirds is torn horizontally.[1] Hyperextension teardrop fracture involving C2 is seen in the brittle, spondylotic spine of the elderly and results from a low-impact trauma. Neurological impairment and soft tissue swelling are usually absent. In contrast hyperextension teardrop fractures of the subaxial cervical spine usually occur in young patients and are the result of high-velocity impact.[52,57] This very severe injury

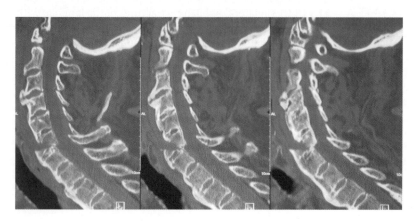

Fig. 31.12 Reverse teardrop fracture.

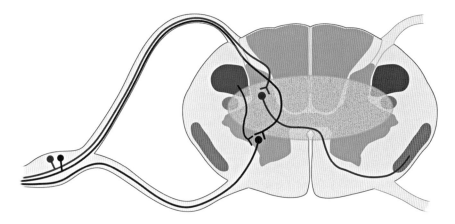

Fig. 31.13 Central cord syndrome, classically related to hyperextension injuries in the presence of cervical stenosis.

results in extensive soft tissue swelling, and acute central cord syndrome (**Fig. 31.13**) is present in 80% of patients.[59]

Distraction-extension with a rotational force vector is thought to produce bilateral fracture-dislocation, an extremely unstable condition. Some authors believe it may actually be caused by a hyperflexion–lateral rotation mechanism[1,60] These fractures occur when the inferior articular mass is fractured by the one above under axial compression during rotation.[1] A double fracture line or "double outline sign" sets the entire articular pillar free.[59] The anterior line passes through the pedicle, and the posterior one goes through the junction between the articular mass and the lamina, a condition also known as pedicolaminar fracture-separation injury. This sets the stage for a "free-floating" articular pillar fragment to dissociate, disengaging the posterior column.[60] Bilateral free-floating articular fragments in combination with the initial disruption of the anterior and middle column during force extension result in a highly mobile segment.

Neurological Damage

Mild hyperextension injuries are notorious for producing disproportionately severe neurological complications compared with the structural damage incurred. This characteristic is due to the narrowing of the spinal canal during extension. The narrowing of the canal in the subaxial cervical spine during extension is three times greater than that during flexion.[61,62] The sagittal dimension of the cervical spinal canal plays an important role in determining the degree of neurological deficit resulting in hyperextension injuries.[63] The predilection of acquired cervical stenosis in the elderly population explains the higher rate and severity of neurological complications in this group.

Despite its notorious association with neurological injury, distraction-extension injuries are less likely to result in complete cord injury compared with hyperflexion injuries. Further, incomplete cord lesions resulting from hyperextension injuries often spare the anterolateral aspect of the spinal cord, greatly improving prognosis for recovery of motor function. Of the incomplete cord injuries, central cord syndrome (CCS) (**Fig. 31.13**) is by far the most common and has become synonymous with hyperextension injuries. It represented 35% of all spinal cord injuries in a Canadian study.[13] Posterior cord syndrome (**Fig. 31.14**), an injury isolated to the posterior column, can rarely occur. It presents with loss of proprioception and varying degrees of sensation with preservation of motor function.

Imaging

The hallmarks of distraction-extension injuries include anterior retropharyngeal soft tissue swelling, widening of the disk space, high fluid signal in an otherwise degenerative disk space, avulsion fractures of the anteroinferior corner of a vertebral body, and fractures of the neural arch, facets, and spinous processes.[57] The extent of ligamentous damage in distraction-extension injuries is often underestimated on radiographs.[64] Not infrequently, severe distraction-extension injuries can present with a normally aligned cervical spine despite disruption of the ALL, intervertebral disk, ligamentum flavum, and paraspinal muscles. In these cases, an MRI can be helpful in assessing the extent of ligamentous damage.

Plain Films

Lateral

Prevertebral soft tissue swelling is consistently observed in distraction-extension injuries. Extensive prevertebral soft tissue swelling implies extensive disruption of the anterior discoligamentous complex. In more severe injuries, widening of the disk space anteriorly (over 1.7 mm) and posterior translational displacement of the adjacent vertebra can be seen. Narrowing of the interspinous space is also seen. A triangular avulsion fracture fragment of the anteroinferior end plate of the suprajacent vertebra whose vertical height exceeds its transverse length is characteristic of a hyperextension teardrop fracture. The avulsion fragment remains attached to the disk, whereas the remaining portion of the vertebral body

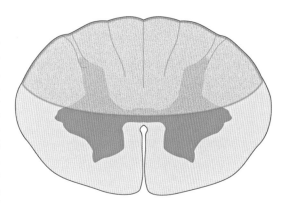

Fig. 31.14 Posterior cord syndrome.

is tilted backward, sometimes called a reverse teardrop fracture (**Fig. 31.12**).

Anteroposterior

Disruption of the lateral margin of the cervical spine represents an articular pillar fracture.

Oblique

This view can show facet fracture lines as well as facet disarticulation.

Computed Tomography

Isolated fractures of one or both laminae may be seen on axial cuts. Facet fractures are easily observed on both axial and reconstructed images.

Magnetic Resonance Imaging

MRI often shows a typical injury pattern of the anterior soft tissues. Retropharyngeal swelling with rupture of the anterior ligament and anterior disk is almost always seen. Stripping of the PLL from the posterior border of the inferior vertebra is characteristic of hyperextension injuries. Disk extrusion can occur.

Evidence-Based Review of Treatment Options

As in the case for distraction-flexion injuries, the treatment strategy is aimed at decompressing the neural structures, realigning the spine, and stabilizing an unstable motion segment. However, the surgeon must also take into account the overall medical condition of the patient. In contrast to patients with distraction-flexion injuries, patients with distraction-extension injuries are significantly older (mean 65 years) and are more susceptible to the morbidities of surgical intervention. The high mortality rate in this group is well documented.[4,55] The surgeon must weigh the risks and benefits of operative intervention against less invasive forms of treatment.

What Is the Role of Closed Reduction in Distraction-Extension Injuries of the Subaxial Cervical Spine?

Closed reduction before surgery has been recommended for all patients with distraction-extension injuries for reasons already previously discussed in Chapter 22. Distraction-extension injuries are notorious for failing closed reduction maneuvers, especially in cases with facet fractures. Some authors do not recommend closed reduction in distraction-extension injuries complicated by facet fractures because the risk for neurological injury from overdistraction is increased.[1] Closed reduction has been successful in several clinical studies.[6,35,65,66] It is a strong recommendation that closed reduction be considered in distraction-extension injuries of the subaxial cervical spine (**Table 31.2**).

Is There a Role for Nonoperative Management of Distraction-Extension Injuries of the Subaxial Cervical Spine?

Risks associated with halo immobilization such as pin loosening, pin tract infection, inner calvarium penetration, ring migration, pressure sores, nerve injury, dysphagia, and cervical

malalignment must be considered. In spite of this, several very low quality retrospective series have demonstrated the safety and efficacy of closed reduction followed by halo vest immobilization for this injury pattern.[6,35,65] The study by Rockswold et al is particularly important because it highlights an increased mortality related to maintaining a cervical flexion posture for reduction.[6]

It is a weak recommendation that halo vest management of these injuries is safe and effective if a neutral cervical flexion posture can be maintained and flexion avoided.

Is There a Role for Anterior-Only Management of Distraction-Extension Injuries of the Subaxial Cervical Spine?

As previously mentioned, the surgical approach and the choice of fixation technique are dictated by the anatomical and biomechanical nature of the cervical injury. Distraction-extension stage I injuries result in disruption of the anterior column and varying degrees of the middle column. Anterior cervical decompression and fusion with an anterior cervical plate is a logical solution because it directly reconstructs the anterior tension band. Vacarro et al showed excellent alignment without instrumentation failure on follow-up in all distraction-extension stage I patients treated with ACDF.[55] Great care should be taken to avoid overdistraction of the spine during placement of the interbody graft. Placement of an excessively large spacer has been shown to cause changes in electrophysiological signals, presumably due to cord lengthening and vascular ischemia in an edematous cord whose vascular supply is already compromised by the original injury vector.[55] Therefore it is very important to have electrophysiological monitoring when performing surgery in distraction-extension injuries.

Distraction-extension type II injuries are more complex and more unstable. These injuries involve all three columns and require a robust fixation construct. A stand-alone cervical decompression and fusion with an anterior cervical plate is insufficient because the instantaneous axis has moved anteriorly to involve the vertebral end plates.[55]

It is a weak recommendation that anterior-only management of stage I distraction-extension injuries of the subaxial cervical spine is safe and effective.

It is a strong recommendation that anterior-only management of stage II distraction-extension injuries of the subaxial cervical spine be avoided and that a combined procedure utilizing posterior stabilization with a screw–rod construct be added to any anterior procedure in these highly unstable injuries.

Is There a Role for Posterior-Only Management of Distraction-Extension Injuries of the Subaxial Cervical Spine?

The posterior approach is particularly attractive because open reduction is often easier to perform, and posterior fixation alone provides adequate stability for distraction-extension type II injuries. For these reasons, the posterior approach is recommended for patients who have failed closed reduction. Posterior fixation must extend at least two segments to decrease the risk of kyphosis. In the setting of extensive damage to the posterior elements, one should consider a 360-degree stabilization construct. There are limited clinical studies looking at this rare injury.[5,55]

It is a strong recommendation based on limited evidence that posterior-only solutions utilizing screw–rod constructs

Table 31.2 Evidenciary Table for Distraction-Extension Injuries of the Subaxial Cervical Spine

Paper Author	Description of Study	Quality of Evidence	Topic and Conclusion
Vaccaro et al (2001)[55]	Retrospective consecutive case series of 24 patients with distraction-extension injuries	Very low	16 injuries were treated operatively, 8 nonoperatively. 9 patients were treated anteriorly only, 6 patients were treated with combined anterior and posterior procedures, one patient was treated posteriorly only. CONCLUSION: Anterior fusion with plating was safe and effective if overdistraction was avoided. Combined procedures were often necessary. Closed reduction and treatment with halo was successful. Mortality in this patient population is high.
Lieberman and Webb (1994)[4]	Retrospective case series of 41 patients with cervical spine fractures	Very low	3 patients with distraction-extension injuries. 1 died, one was treated with a collar, one quadriparetic patient was treated with operative reduction, anterior fusion. CONCLUSION: This was an uncommon injury pattern in this series.
Anderson et al (1991)[5]	Retrospective case series of 30 patients treated with posterior cervical plating	Very low	One patient with an extension type injury at C5–C6 was quadriparetic and treated with posterior plating to solid fusion despite a screw loosening in a C4-C7 construct. CONCLUSION: Posterior plating is safe and effective in this uncommon injury.
Rockswold et al (1990)[6]	Retrospective case series of 140 patients with cervical spine injuries	Very low	7 patients sustained unstable extension injuries, 3 were successfully treated in a halo vest, 3 were successfully treated operatively. CONCLUSION: Nonoperative management may be successful if flexion positioning can be avoided.
Bucholz and Cheung (1989)[65]	Retrospective case series of 124 cervical spine injuries	Very low	12 extension injuries, all treated initially in halo. 1/12 failed halo treatment and subsequently underwent posterior wiring with successful result. CONCLUSION: Halo treatment of these injuries may be safe and effective in the treatment of distraction-extension injuries.
Dorr et al (1982)[66]	Retrospective review of 115 cervical spine injuries	Very low	45 extension injuries. Two patients had posterior fusions with failure of bed rest/traction, three patients had late laminectomies. CONCLUSION: Nonoperative management of these injuries can be successful.
Burke and Tiong (1975)[35]	Retrospective case series of 176 patients with cervical spine injuries	Very low	22 patients sustained distraction-extension injuries. 4 patients died within 3 months and were excluded from the study. The remaining 18 patients were treated with bed rest and cervical traction for 8 weeks. CONCLUSION: Nonoperative management of these injuries can be successful.

are safe and effective in the operative management of distraction-extension injuries of the subaxial cervical spine.

Ankylosing Spondylitis and Diffuse Idiopathic Skeletal Hyperostosis

Definitions

Ankylosing spondylitis (AS) is a degenerative inflammatory arthritis that primarily affects the spine and sacroiliac joints. It has an incidence of 1.4% and a male predominance (3:1).[67] About 90% of patients express the human leukocyte antigen (HLA)-B27 genotype thus placing it in the systemic rheumatoid category. AS eventually leads to complete fusion of the spine with bridging syndesmophytes, producing a condition known as bamboo spine. However, the spine is very brittle as a consequence of the osteoporotic process of the disease.

Diffuse idiopathic skeletal hyperostosis (DISH) is similar to AS in that it causes autofusion of the spine yet is of unknown etiology. It is not associated with other clinical manifestations as are found in AS, and radiographical features are unique in that the fusion is more osteodense with flowing ossifications, giving the appearance of dripping wax.

Demographics

Though different in etiology, the two most common types of ankylosing spinal diseases (ASDs) share important clinical features: functional spinal ankylosis, poor bone quality, advanced age, mechanism of injury, and multiple comorbidities. This has led to a similar approach in the treatment and evaluation of spine fractures in patients affected by these two conditions.[68] Oftentimes it is difficult to fully differentiate AS from DISH, and occasionally both pathological entities exist simultaneously. Spinal fractures are 3.5 times more common in this population compared with the general population.[68,69] Of these fractures, 75% are located in the cervical spine, with a predilection for the subaxial spine and the cervicothoracic junction.[70-72] The most common mechanism is hyperextension occurring in as many as 90%,[68] usually the result of low-energy trauma such as a simple fall. With both DISH and AS, long lever arms produced by stiffness of the spine exert large forces across the fracture site, with the effect of rendering even harmless-appearing fractures highly unstable.[73–75] In contrast to distraction injuries in the healthy spine, the ligaments in a spine affected by ASD are ossified and are usually completely severed in even minimally displaced fractures. As a result, fractures in patients with ASD are highly unstable. The fracture is usually transverse-oriented usually involving a partially ossified disk or the anterior vertebral body.[68,76] The fracture can often extend 1 to 2 levels cranially posteriorly. Patients with both AS and DISH are susceptible to noncontiguous spine fractures in as high as 10% of injuries[68] due to the stiffened spine and weakened bone.

Spinal Cord Injury and Epidural Hematomas

Cervical fractures in ASD patients are associated with a very high incidence of SCI and of mortality.[72,77] The incidence of SCI is ~11.4 times higher than that found in the general population.[72] Epidural hematomas are frequently found in these patients and lend credence to obtaining MRI scans, which are more likely to identify this problem (**Fig. 31.10B**).[68] The associated likelihood of neurological compromise in those with epidural hematomas is 88%. Although the risk of epidural hematoma in AS patients who sustain fractures of the spine has been well established in the literature,[78,79] the risk in DISH patients has been thought to be much lower.[74,75,77,78,80,81] Often these patients are quadriplegic and are especially prone to pulmonary complications given the associated morbidities in these already compromised patients.

Morbidity and Mortality

Morbidity and mortality rates in this patient population are near 50% and 20 to 30%, respectively.[69,71,75,77,80–82] Over 80% of the patients in some series had at least one significant adverse event related to their spine injury or its treatment.[68] Among the most severe were those that resulted in neurological compromise. The primary determinant of mortality is the patient's age, which also correlates with the number of comorbidities. The threefold higher likelihood of death in patients with low-energy injuries is attributed to their significantly older age and greater number of comorbidities. That the risk of death increases significantly in patients 70 years of age or older probably reflects a progressive decline in the patient's overall health, which created the environment leading to fracture of the ankylosed spine under low-energy conditions.[68] The fracture itself is probably one of the final manifestations of impending demise, albeit one that is likely to accelerate the process.

Diagnostics

In assessing these patients, one must maintain a very high index of suspicion and generally assume there is an injury until proven otherwise, even with very low mechanism injuries. Opacity and anatomical distortion of the osteoporotic spine can cause difficulties in detection of nontranslated fractures on plain radiographs.[83] As such, plain radiographs are unacceptable as a diagnostic modality, and at a minimum, these patients require fine-cut CT and possibly MRI (**Fig. 31.10**).[75,83–90] Unstable spine fractures in patients with ASD are unrecognized for days to weeks in up to 65% of cases, which may further compromise the patient's neurological condition.[81,86] In the largest series reported, almost one fifth of patients with ASD had a delay in diagnosis of their spine fracture (**Fig. 31.15**), affecting most commonly patients with AS and patients transferred from outside community facilities.[68] Patients with unrecognized fractures typically reported only axial pain until abrupt neurological deterioration occurred. Delay in diagnosis has been reported to be associated with neurological complications in 19 to 100% of patients.[91,92] Because of the challenges in identifying minimally displaced fractures with plain films and CT, recommended protocols in evaluating patients with ASD who report back or neck pain, or who have had a fracture identified in a specific region of the spine, include mandatory MRI of the entire spine, unless contraindicated or not feasible due to severe kyphotic deformity or other medical comorbidities.[74,78,81,86,88,93,94]

Management

Surgeons managing cervical fractures in ASD must exert great caution because treatment failure can have devastating consequences. Although there are reports of conservative management of ASD patients with fractures,[70,76,86] it is generally agreed that an aggressive approach is warranted in this fragile population. Rowed found that four of 21 patients placed in a halo had recurrent dislocation, one with onset of new deficits due to secondary dislocation.[95] Harrop et al reported two AS patients with 3-column injury who experienced acute neurological worsening after initial halo vest or traction immobilization (**Fig. 31.10**).[89]

Because of the similarities between fractures in an ankylosed spine and osteoporotic long bone fractures, most recommend the use of multilevel posterior segmental instrumentation for stabilizing spine fractures in patients with ASD with multiple points of fixation balanced equally across both sides of the fracture (**Fig. 31.10C**).[68,73,75,96–102] In these cases anterior fixation alone is biomechanically inadequate with higher rates of failure.[68,75] Precise placements of fixation screw can be challenging because joint spaces such as anterior disk space and facet joints are usually fused, blurring anatomical landmarks. Intraoperative imaging guidance is recommended, but even this can prove challenging given the body habitus of some of these patients in combination with diffuse osteopenia. The surgeon must choose between either a posterior approach or a combined approach to achieve adequate biomechanical stability. Short-segment constructs are unacceptable due to osteopenia and the long lever arms, and ideal constructs will include three levels of pedicle or lateral mass screw fixation bilaterally, above and below the fracture. No patient in the largest series had failure of fixation when instrumented in this manner.[68] Because of the absence of comparison groups within the literature, no specific conclusions can be reached about the minimum number of fixation points required in spine-injured patients with ASD. Secondary anterior column reconstruction may be necessary to achieve fracture healing if there is a large anterior column defect resulting from correction of the patient's preinjury kyphotic alignment. Both AS and DISH patients have pathological processes that form bone, and nonunions in these patients do not occur provided stability is achieved.

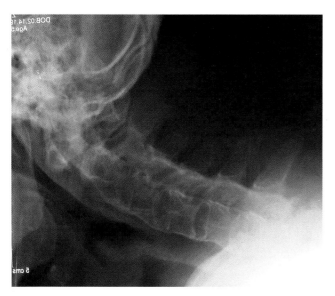

A

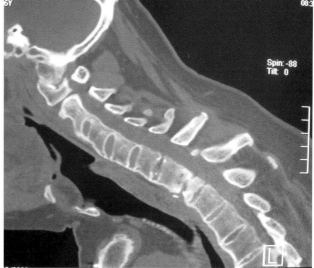

B

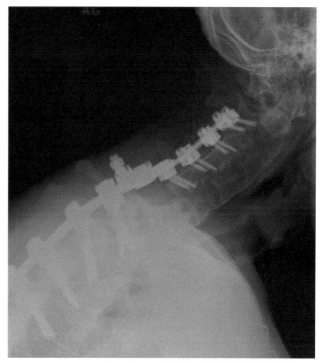

C

Fig. 31.15 A 56-year-old man with ankylosing spondylitis and chronic neck pain suffered a fall at work. Despite severe neck pain, appropriate workup was delayed 2 months after the incident. Patient's fracture had begun to heal from the delay requiring a more aggressive intervention. **(A)** Lateral C-spine x-ray showing splaying of C6 and C7 spinous process secondary to fracture through C7 resulting in severe chin-on-chest deformity. **(B)** Computed tomographic sagittal view showing early ankylosing of fracture-deformity. **(C)** Postoperative lateral C-spine x-ray after C7 posterior subtraction osteotomy with excellent correction of chin-on-chest deformity.

Outcomes and Quality of Evidence

AS and DISH are two unique pathological processes that can occur in the face of trauma, changing the nature of management. Given the nature of these diseases, recommendations related to the fractures themselves do not necessarily apply to these specialized patients. Despite numerous articles in the literature related to these particular entities, there are no prospective studies with respect to management or diagnostic assessment; the majority of the literature includes case reports, case series, or retrospective reviews providing at best low to very low quality of evidence when it comes to recommendations. There are two main questions related to this patient subpopulation with fractures: Should all patients who present with a low-mechanism injury and pain undergo an aggressive diagnostic workup? Should all patients with a fracture in the face of AS or DISH undergo operative management of their injury?

Should All Patients Who Present With a Low-Mechanism Injury and Pain Undergo an Aggressive Diagnostic Workup?

There is no literature with quality of evidence stronger than low to very low with respect to this question; however, the numerous reports and limited series suggest that plain radiographs are insufficient in this patient subpopulation. These patients frequently have minimally displaced injuries in the setting of osteopenia and distorted anatomy, and the consequences of a missed injury can have devastating neurological repercussions. Epidural hematomas are much more common in AS patients than the general population, and if unrecognized, this can cause a progressive neurological decline (**Fig. 31.10B**).

Koivikko et al concluded in their assessment of 18 patients that for any suspected cervical spine injuries, multidetector computed tomography (MDCT) is the imaging modality of choice.[83] In a later study, Koivikko et al concluded that MRI can visualize unstable fractures of the cervical and upper thoracic spine. Paravertebral hemorrhages and any ligamentous injuries should alert radiologists to seek transverse fractures.[99] Michel et al emphasized the importance of MRI in demonstrating posterior element signal abnormalities in a retrospective review of nine cases.[103] Nakstad et al, Pedrosa et al, Shih et al, and Wang et al have all emphasized that MRI was a key part of any radiological protocol in patients with AS and neck trauma.[104–107] Despite the numerous, repeated reports, this is at best low-grade evidence. In Caron et al's study of 112 patients with fractures, 21 patients had a delay in diagnosis secondary to an inadequate diagnostic workup, with 81% having a decline in neurological status.[71] Unlike the regular population, the onus is on the clinician in this patient subpopulation to prove there is *not* an injury as opposed to proving that there *is* an injury.

The strong recommendation of the Spine Trauma Study Group (STSG) is that any patient with a diagnosis of AS and DISH ought to undergo a CT scan at a minimum and, unless contraindicated, an MRI as well. These patients are at very high risk, and a delay in diagnosis of a missed fracture can have serious repercussions on the neurological outcome and can potentially impact survival.

Should All Patients With a Fracture in the Face of AS or DISH Undergo Operative Management of Their Injury?

There are certainly reports in the literature of patients being treated conservatively with successful outcomes and solid union (**Table 31.3**); however, none of these studies have been conducted in the last 20 years. Given the generally highly unstable nature of these injuries, the overwhelming recommendation from most modern reports is surgical management though still at best with low-grade evidence. Most

Table 31.3 Ankylosing Spondylitis/Diffuse Idiopathic Skeletal Hyperostosis Evidenciary Table

Paper Author	Description of Study	Quality of Evidence	Topic and Conclusion
Caron et al (2009)[71]	Retrospective review of 112 patients with AS or DISH and fractures	Low	CONCLUSION: Patients with spine fractures and ankylosing conditions are at high risk for complications and death and should be counseled accordingly. Multilevel posterior segmental instrumentation allows effective fracture healing. AS and DISH patients represent similar patient populations for the purpose of treatment and future research.
Kanter et al (2008)[96]	Retrospective review of 13 patients.	Very low	CONCLUSION: Patients with AS are highly susceptible to extensive neurological injury and spinal deformity after sustaining cervical fractures from even minor traumatic forces. These injuries are uniquely complex in nature.
Koivikko et al (2008)[99]	Retrospective review of 20 patients with AS undergoing MRI	Very low	CONCLUSION: MRI can visualize unstable fractures of the cervical and upper thoracic spine. Paravertebral hemorrhages and any ligamentous injuries should alert radiologists to seek transverse fractures. Diagnostic images can be obtained with a flexible multipurpose coil if the use of standard spine array coil is impossible due to a rigid collar or excessive kyphosis.
Thumbikat et al (2007)[113]	Retrospective review of 18 cases of AS with SCI	Very low	CONCLUSION: Neurological deficits were often subtle on initial presentation, resulting in many injuries being missed because of a low index of suspicion and poor visualization of lower cervical fractures on conventional radiographs. Extension of the ankylosed kyphotic cervical spine during conventional immobilization or for radiological procedures resulted in neurological deficits.
Einsiedel et al (2006)[81]	Retrospective Review of 37 patients with AS and fractures	Very low	CONCLUSION: The authors have performed only posterior and anterior procedures since 1997. Diagnostic investigations include CT scanning or MRI of the whole spine. Because additional injuries are common. In cases in which diagnosis is delayed, patients present with more severe neurological deficits. Because of postoperative pulmonary and ischemic complications, the mortality rate is high.
Feldtkeller et al (2006)[82]	Review of questionnaire sent to 1,071 patients with AS	Low	CONCLUSION: A considerable proportion of AS patients will experience a vertebral fracture during the course of the disease, in particular if peripheral joints are also involved.
Cornefjord et al (2005)[76]	Retrospective chart review of 19 patients.	Very low	CONCLUSION: The results indicate that using both pedicle screws and lateral mass screws rigidly connected to a rod is suited for treating subaxial cervical spine fractures in patients with ankylosing spondylitis, allowing high healing rates.
Wang et al (2005)[107]	Retrospective review of 12 patients with AS and fracture	Very low	CONCLUSIONS: MRI shows abnormalities in AS that may not be clear or even detectable by using other imaging methods. MRI can serve to evaluate AS patients with spinal fracture for the possibility of three-column involvement.

Table 31.3 Ankylosing Spondylitis/Diffuse Idiopathic Skeletal Hyperostosis Evidenciary Table (*Continued*)

Paper Author	Description of Study	Quality of Evidence	Topic and Conclusion
Koivikko et al (2004)[98]	Retrospective review of 18 patients with AS	Very low	CONCLUSION: MDCT is superior to plain radiographs or MRI, showing significantly more injuries and yielding more information on fracture morphology. In these patients, for any suspected cervical spine injuries, MDCT is therefore the imaging modality of choice.
Nakstad et al (2004)[104]	Retrospective review of 11 patients with AS	Very low	CONCLUSION: A protocol is presented that consists of lateral conventional x-ray, CT with reformatted images, and MRI. MRI is recommended as part of the radiological protocol following neck traumas in all patients with AS.
Vosse et al (2004)[115]	15,097 questionnaires to AS patients with 59 patients reporting 66 fractures	Low	CONCLUSION: 0.4% of patients with AS reported confirmed vertebral fracture at a mean age of 50 years, occurring after 2 decades of disease, mainly without trauma or after minimal trauma, with frequent neurological complications mostly followed by incomplete neurological recovery.
Alaranta et al (2002)[67]	Retrospective cohort review of 1103 patients with SCI	Low	The incidence rate of patients with AS for traumatic SCI was found to be 11.4 times greater than expected for the population at large. The neurological injury was at the cervical level in 84% of the patients with AS, but only in 48% of the patients with traumatic SCI in general. CONCLUSION: Patients with AS seem to run a higher risk of traumatic SCI than the population at large.
Mitra et al (2000)[116]	66 men with AS were assessed for BMD and compared with 39 healthy subjects.	Low	CONCLUSION: There was no correlation between BMD and vertebral fractures in these patients. AS patients with mild disease had a higher risk of fractures compared with the normal population.
Finkelstein et al (1999)[83]	Retrospective review of 21 patients	Very low	CONCLUSION: A high index of suspicion and an appreciation of the extreme instability of a fracture in AS must be present.
Meyer (1999)[117]	Retrospective study of 29 patients with DISH	Very low	CONCLUSION: All elderly patients with diffuse idiopathic skeletal hyperostosis-like pathology, history of trivial trauma, and complaint of neck pain should be examined carefully for fractures because mortality rates increase sharply in patients with decreased neurological function.
Olerud et al (1999)[118]	Retrospective review of 65 patients with cervical spine fractures	Very low	CONCLUSION: Severe comorbidity, neurological injury, high age, and AS proved to be significant risk factors for death. Patients having AS run a higher than normal risk of sustaining a cervical spine fracture.
Olerud et al (1996)[119]	Retrospective review of 31 patients with AS and spinal fractures	Very low	CONCLUSION: Minor trauma can cause fracture in an ankylosed spine. The risk of late neurological deterioration is substantial. Because the condition is very rare and the treatment is demanding and associated with a very high risk of complications, the treatment of these patients should be centralized in special spinal trauma units.
Apple and Anson (1995)[69]	Multicenter study of 59 patients	Low	CONCLUSION: Patients in the nonoperative group had a significantly shorter length of stay and a significantly lower cost of care. No other differences between operative and nonoperative groups were identified in regard to other outcome variables.
Colterjohn and Bednar (1995)[75]	Retrospective prevalence study of 281 cases.	Low	CONCLUSION: Cervical traumatized patients with flexural injury or chronic multilevel spinal arthritis with ankylosis are at increased risk of having secondary motor neurological deterioration.
Donnelly et al (1994)[79]	BMD assessments in 87 patients with AS and fractures and compared with control population.	Low	CONCLUSION: Vertebral fractures that result from osteoporosis are a feature of longstanding AS. BMD used as a measure of osteoporosis of the spine in advanced AS is unreliable, probably as a result of syndesmophyte formation and does not predict the risk of vertebral fracture. Alternative sites such as the neck of the femur should be used for sequential assessment of BMD in AS.
Hendrix et al (1994)[91]	Retrospective review of 15 cases of DISH	Very low	CONCLUSION: Trivial trauma was the most common cause of fracture in the spine ankylosed by diffuse idiopathic skeletal hyperostosis. The severity of SCI in these patients was greater than in previous reports. Patients with shorter ankylosed segments had less severe cord injuries.

(Continued on page 316)

Paper Author	Description of Study	Quality of Evidence	Topic and Conclusion
Rowed (1992)[95]	Retrospective review of 21 patients with AS and spine injuries	Very low	CONCLUSION: Fracture/dislocations of the cervical spine should be managed initially by halo vest immobilization, without prior traction and with careful incremental correction of flexion deformity. Decompression is performed as required for extradural hematoma or intervertebral disk herniation, and internal fixation is performed for recurrent dislocation.
Detwiler et al (1990)[78]	Retrospective review of 11 patients.	Very low	CONCLUSION: The initiation of axial traction as initial therapy for cervical injuries followed by early surgical stabilization in patients with AS is supported. The difficulty of maintaining spinal alignment and the devastating pulmonary problems attendant on conservative management may be obviated by early fusion.
Graham and Van Petegehem (1989)[86]	Retrospective review of 15 patients.	Very low	CONCLUSION: Conservative management is associated with a high rate of fracture union and low rate of complications. Surgical management may be indicated for neurologically impaired individuals or unstable fractures.
Hunter and Dubo (1983)[94]	Retrospective review of 20 patients	Very low	CONCLUSION: Bony union can be achieved with nonoperative management. Difficulties in diagnosis make management difficult.
Weinstein et al (1982)[120]	Retrospective review of 13 patients with fractures out of 105 patients	Very low	CONCLUSION: The study emphasizes the value of computerized tomography scanning of the spine for diagnosis, and halo vest application as a nonoperative treatment for cervical immobilization. Nonoperative immobilization is the recommended treatment unless spinal dislocation or bone fragment displacement has occurred at the fracture site.

Abbreviations: AS, ankylosing spondylitis; DISH, diffuse idiopathic skeletal hyperostosis; MDCT, multidetector computed tomographic; MRI, magnetic resonance imaging; SCI, spinal cord injury.

agree that a long posterior construct is sufficient with possibly anterior supplemental support if there is a remaining defect after posterior instrumentation. Anterior instrumentation alone is unacceptable and has a higher risk of failure.[71] Unlike most patients, these patients are already fused over multiple segments; therefore, long segment fixation does not have any impact on the ultimate mobility of their spine. Given the long lever arms associated with their inflexible spine, multiple points of fixation are mandated. Nonoperative management should only be utilized in those in whom surgical management is contraindicated because the risks of displacement and neurological decline are much higher in this patient group. Although this treatment protocol is well supported by the limited retrospective reviews and case series, there is only low to very low support from the literature.

References

1. Argenson C, Lovet J, Sanouiller JL, de Peretti F. Traumatic rotatory displacement of the lower cervical spine. Spine 1988;13:767–773
2. Koivikko MP, Myllynen P, Santavirta S. Fracture dislocations of the cervical spine: a review of 106 conservatively and operatively treated patients. Eur Spine J 2004;13:610–616
3. O'Brien PJ, Schweigel JF, Thompson WJ. Dislocations of the lower cervical spine. J Trauma 1982;22:710–714
4. Lieberman IH, Webb JK. Cervical spine injuries in the elderly. J Bone Joint Surg Br 1994;76:877–881
5. Anderson PA, Henley MB, Grady MS, Montesano PX, Winn HR. Posterior cervical arthrodesis with AO reconstruction plates and bone graft. Spine 1991;16(3, Suppl):S72–S79
6. Rockswold GL, Bergman TA, Ford SE. Halo immobilization and surgical fusion: relative indications and effectiveness in the treatment of 140 cervical spine injuries. J Trauma 1990;30:893–898
7. Allen BL Jr, Ferguson RL, Lehmann TR, O'Brien RP. A mechanistic classification of closed, indirect fractures and dislocations of the lower cervical spine. Spine 1982;7:1–27
8. Sim E, Vaccaro AR, Berzlanovich A, Schwarz N, Sim B. In vitro genesis of subaxial cervical unilateral facet dislocations through sequential soft tissue ablation. Spine 2001;26:1317–1323
9. Vaccaro AR, Madigan L, Schweitzer ME, Flanders AE, Hilibrand AS, Albert TJ. Magnetic resonance imaging analysis of soft tissue disruption after flexion-distraction injuries of the subaxial cervical spine. Spine 2001;26:1866–1872
10. O'Brien PJ, Schweigel JF, Thompson WJ. Dislocations of the lower cervical spine. J Trauma 1982;22:710–714
11. Leventhal MR. Fractures, dislocations, and fracture-dislocations of the spine. In: Canale ST, ed. Campbell's Operative Orthopaedics. St Louis: Mosby 2003:1597–1690
12. Sim E, Vaccaro AR, Berzlanovich A, Pienaar S. The effects of staged static cervical flexion-distraction deformities on the patency of the vertebral arterial vasculature. Spine 2000;25:2180–2186
13. Pickett GE, Campos-Benitez M, Keller JL, Duggal N. Epidemiology of traumatic spinal cord injury in Canada. Spine 2006;31:799–805
14. Hadley MN, Fitzpatrick BC, Sonntag VK, Browner CM. Facet fracture-dislocation injuries of the cervical spine. Neurosurgery 1992;30:661–666
15. Rizzolo SJ, Piazza MR, Cotler JM, Balderston RA, Schaefer D, Flanders A. Intervertebral disc injury complicating cervical spine trauma. Spine 1991;16(6, Suppl):S187–S189
16. Shapiro SA. Management of unilateral locked facet of the cervical spine. Neurosurgery 1993;33:832–837, discussion 837
17. Braakman R, Penning L. Mechanisms of injury to the cervical cord. Paraplegia 1973;10:314–320
18. Wang MY, Prusmack CJ, Green BA, Gruen JP, Levi AD. Minimally invasive lateral mass screws in the treatment of cervical facet dislocations: technical note. Neurosurgery 2003;52:444–447, discussion 447–448

19. Mizuno J, Nakagawa H, Inoue T, Nonaka Y, Song J, Romli TM. Spinal instrumentation for interfacet locking injuries of the subaxial cervical spine. J Clin Neurosci 2007;14:49–52

20. Shapiro S, Snyder W, Kaufman K, Abel T. Outcome of 51 cases of unilateral locked cervical facets: interspinous braided cable for lateral mass plate fusion compared with interspinous wire and facet wiring with iliac crest. J Neurosurg 1999;91(1, Suppl):19–24

21. Paeslack V, Frankel H, Michaelis L. Closed injuries of the cervical spine and spinal cord: results of conservative treatment of flexion fractures and flexion rotation fracture dislocation of the cervical spine with tetraplegia. Proc Veterans Adm Spinal Cord Inj Conf 1973; 19:39–42

22. Mahale YJ, Silver JR. Progressive paralysis after bilateral facet dislocation of the cervical spine. J Bone Joint Surg Br 1992;74:219–223

23. Wolf A, Levi L, Mirvis S, et al. Operative management of bilateral facet dislocation. J Neurosurg 1991;75:883–890

24. Sears W, Fazl M. Prediction of stability of cervical spine fracture managed in the halo vest and indications for surgical intervention. J Neurosurg 1990;72:426–432

25. Benzel EC, Kesterson L. Posterior cervical interspinous compression wiring and fusion for mid to low cervical spinal injuries. J Neurosurg 1989;70:893–899

26. Lind B, Sihlbom H, Nordwall A. Halo-vest treatment of unstable traumatic cervical spine injuries. Spine 1988;13:425–432

27. Rorabeck CH, Rock MG, Hawkins RJ, Bourne RB. Unilateral facet dislocation of the cervical spine: an analysis of the results of treatment in 26 patients. Spine 1987;12:23–27

28. Chan RC, Schweigel JF, Thompson GB. Halo-thoracic brace immobilization in 188 patients with acute cervical spine injuries. J Neurosurg 1983;58:508–515

29. Ersmark H, Kalén R. A consecutive series of 64 halo-vest-treated cervical spine injuries. Arch Orthop Trauma Surg 1986;105:243–246

30. Glaser JA, Whitehill R, Stamp WG, Jane JA. Complications associated with the halo-vest: a review of 245 cases. J Neurosurg 1986;65:762–769

31. Bohlman HH. Acute fractures and dislocations of the cervical spine: an analysis of three hundred hospitalized patients and review of the literature. J Bone Joint Surg Am 1979;61:1119–1142

32. Sonntag VK. Management of bilateral locked facets of the cervical spine. Neurosurgery 1981;8:150–152

33. Beatson TR. Fractures and dislocation of the cervical spine. J Bone Joint Surg Br 1963;45:21–35

34. Burke DC, Berryman D. The place of closed manipulation in the management of flexion-rotation dislocations of the cervical spine. J Bone Joint Surg Br 1971;53:165–182

35. Burke DC, Tiong TS. Stability of the cervical spine after conservative treatment. Paraplegia 1975;13:191–202

36. Cheshire DJ. The stability of the cervical spine following the conservative treatment of fractures and fracture-dislocations. Paraplegia 1969;7:193–203

37. De Barros Filho TEP, De Haidar Jorge HM, Oliveira RP, et al. Risk of excessive traction on distraction-flexion type injuries of the low cervical spine. Acta Ortop Bras 2006;14:75–77

38. Dvorak MF, Fisher CG, Aarabi B, et al. Clinical outcomes of 90 isolated unilateral facet fractures, subluxations, and dislocations treated surgically and nonoperatively. Spine 2007;32:3007–3013

39. Roy-Camille R, Saillant G, Mazel C. Internal fixation of the unstable cervical spine by posterior osteosynthesis with plates and screws. In: Cervical Spine Research Society, eds. The Cervical Spine. Philadelphia: JB Lippincott; 1989:390–403

40. Roy-Camille R, Saillant G, Laville C, Benazet JP. Treatment of lower cervical spinal injuries—C3 to C7. Spine 1992;17(10, Suppl):S442–S446

41. Lukhele M. Fractures of the vertebral lamina associated with unifacet and bifacet cervical spine dislocations. S Afr J Surg 1994;32:112–114

42. Ordonez BJ, Benzel EC, Naderi S, Weller SJ. Cervical facet dislocation: techniques for ventral reduction and stabilization. J Neurosurg 2000; 92(1, Suppl):18–23

43. Do Koh Y, Lim TH, Won You J, Eck J, An HS. A biomechanical comparison of modern anterior and posterior plate fixation of the cervical spine. Spine 2001;26:15–21

44. Gill K, Paschal S, Corin J, Ashman R, Bucholz RW. Posterior plating of the cervical spine: a biomechanical comparison of different posterior fusion techniques. Spine 1988;13:813–816

45. Levine AM, Mazel C, Roy-Camille R. Management of fracture separations of the articular mass using posterior cervical plating. Spine 1992;17(10, Suppl):S447–S454

46. Fehlings MG, Cooper PR, Errico TJ. Posterior plates in the management of cervical instability: long-term results in 44 patients. J Neurosurg 1994;81:341–349

47. Beyer CA, Cabanela ME, Berquist TH. Unilateral facet dislocations and fracture-dislocations of the cervical spine. J Bone Joint Surg Br 1991; 73:977–981

48. Nazarian SM, Louis RP. Posterior internal fixation with screw plates in traumatic lesions of the cervical spine. Spine 1991;16(3, Suppl): S64–S71

49. Brodke DS, Anderson PA, Newell DW, Grady MS, Chapman JR. Comparison of anterior and posterior approaches in cervical spinal cord injuries. J Spinal Disord Tech 2003;16:229–235

50. Ulrich C, Arand M, Nothwang J. Internal fixation on the lower cervical spine—biomechanics and clinical practice of procedures and implants. Eur Spine J 2001;10:88–100

51. Henriques T. Biomechanical and clinical aspects on fixation techniques in the cervical spine. In: Comprehensive Summaries of Uppsala Dissertations from the Faculty of Medicine. 2003:1–37

52. Harrington JF Jr, Park MC. Single level arthrodesis as treatment for midcervical fracture subluxation: a cohort study. J Spinal Disord Tech 2007;20:42–48

53. Johnson MG, Fisher CG, Boyd M, Pitzen T, Oxland TR, Dvorak MF. The radiographic failure of single segment anterior cervical plate fixation in traumatic cervical flexion distraction injuries. Spine 2004;29: 2815–2820

54. Aebi M, Zuber K, Marchesi D. Treatment of cervical spine injuries with anterior plating. Indications, techniques, and results. Spine 1991;16(3, Suppl):S38–S45

55. Vaccaro AR, Klein GR, Thaller JB, Rushton SA, Cotler JM, Albert TJ. Distraction extension injuries of the cervical spine. J Spinal Disord 2001;14:193–200

56. Spivak JM, Weiss MA, Cotler JM, Call M. Cervical spine injuries in patients 65 and older. Spine 1994;19:2302–2306

57. Rao SK, Wasyliw C, Nunez DB Jr. Spectrum of imaging findings in hyperextension injuries of the neck. Radiographics 2005;25:1239–1254

58. Taylor AR. The mechanism of injury to the spinal cord in the neck without damage to vertebral column. J Bone Joint Surg Br 1951;33-B:543–547

59. Lee JS, Harris JH, Mueller CF. The significance of prevertebral soft tissue swelling in extension teardrop fracture of the cervical spine. Emerg Radiol 1997;4:132–139

60. Shanmuganathan K, Mirvis SE, Dowe M, Levine AM. Traumatic isolation of the cervical articular pillar: imaging observations in 21 patients. AJR Am J Roentgenol 1996;166:897–902

61. Panjabi MM, White AA III. Basic biomechanics of the spine. Neurosurgery 1980;7:76–93

62. Louis R. Spinal stability as defined by the three-column spine concept. Anat Clin 1985;7:33–42

63. Eismont FJ, Clifford S, Goldberg M, Green B. Cervical sagittal spinal canal size in spine injury. Spine 1984;9:663–666

64. Jónsson H Jr, Bring G, Rauschning W, Sahlstedt B. Hidden cervical spine injuries in traffic accident victims with skull fractures. J Spinal Disord 1991;4:251–263

65. Bucholz RD, Cheung KC. Halo vest versus spinal fusion for cervical injury: evidence from an outcome study. J Neurosurg 1989;70:884–892

66. Dorr LD, Harvey JP Jr, Nickel VL. Clinical review of the early stability of spine injuries. Spine 1982;7:545–550

67. Alaranta H, Luoto S, Konttinen YT. Traumatic spinal cord injury as a complication to ankylosing spondylitis: an extended report. Clin Exp Rheumatol 2002;20:66–68

68. Altenbernd J, Bitu S, Lemburg S, et al. Vertebral fractures in patients with ankylosing spondylitis: a retrospective analysis of 66 patients [in German]. Rofo 2009;181:45–53

69. Apple DF Jr, Anson C. Spinal cord injury occurring in patients with ankylosing spondylitis: a multicenter study. Orthopedics 1995;18:1005–1011

70. Broom MJ, Raycroft JF. Complications of fractures of the cervical spine in ankylosing spondylitis. Spine 1988;13:763–766

71. Caron T, Nguyen Q, Agel J, Chapman JR, Bellabarba C. Spine fractures in patients with ankylosing disorders. Spine 2009; In press

72. Bernini PM, Floman Y, Marvel JP Jr, Rothman RH. Multiple thoracic spine fractures complicating ankylosing hyperostosis of the spine. J Trauma 1981;21:811–814

73. Chapman J, Bransford R. Geriatric spine fractures: an emerging healthcare crisis. J Trauma 2007;62(6, Suppl):S61–S62

74. Cooper C, Carbone L, Michet CJ, Atkinson EJ, O'Fallon WM, Melton LJ III. Fracture risk in patients with ankylosing spondylitis: a population based study. J Rheumatol 1994;21:1877–1882

75. Colterjohn NR, Bednar DA. Identifiable risk factors for secondary neurologic deterioration in the cervical spine-injured patient. Spine 1995;20:2293–2297

76. Cornefjord M, Alemany M, Olerud C. Posterior fixation of subaxial cervical spine fractures in patients with ankylosing spondylitis. Eur Spine J 2005;14:401–408

77. de Peretti F, Sane JC, Dran G, Razafindratsiva C, Argenson C. Ankylosed spine fractures with spondylitis or diffuse idiopathic skeletal hyperostosis: diagnosis and complications [in French]. Rev Chir Orthop Repar Appar Mot 2004;90:456–465

78. Detwiler KN, Loftus CM, Godersky JC, Menezes AH. Management of cervical spine injuries in patients with ankylosing spondylitis. J Neurosurg 1990;72:210–215

79. Donnelly S, Doyle DV, Denton A, Rolfe I, McCloskey EV, Spector TD. Bone mineral density and vertebral compression fracture rates in ankylosing spondylitis. Ann Rheum Dis 1994;53:117–121

80. Duhem-Tonnelle V, Duhem R, Allaoui M, Chastanet P, Assaker R. Fracture luxation of the cervical spine in patients with ankylosing spondylitis: six cases [in French[. Neurochirurgie 2008;54:46–52

81. Einsiedel T, Kleimann M, Nothofer W, Neugebauer R. Special considerations in therapy of injuries of the cervical spine in ankylosing spondylitis (Bechterew disease) [in German]. Unfallchirurg 2001;104(12):1129–1133

82. Feldtkeller E, Vosse D, Geusens P, van der Linden S. Prevalence and annual incidence of vertebral fractures in patients with ankylosing spondylitis. Rheumatol Int 2006;26:234–239

83. Finkelstein JA, Chapman JR, Mirza S. Occult vertebral fractures in ankylosing spondylitis. Spinal Cord 1999;37:444–447

84. Geusens P, Vosse D, van der Linden S. Osteoporosis and vertebral fractures in ankylosing spondylitis. Curr Opin Rheumatol 2007;19:335–339

85. Grisolia A, Bell RL, Peltier LF. Fractures and dislocations of the spine complicating ankylosing spondylitis: a report of six cases. 1967. Clin Orthop Relat Res 2004;(422):129–134

86. Graham B, Van Peteghem PK. Fractures of the spine in ankylosing spondylitis. Diagnosis, treatment, and complications. Spine 1989;14:803–807

87. Hanson CA, Shagrin JW, Duncan H. Vertebral osteoporosis in ankylosing spondylitis. Clin Orthop Relat Res 1971;74:59–64

88. Hanson JA, Mirza S. Predisposition for spinal fracture in ankylosing spondylitis. AJR Am J Roentgenol 2000;174:150

89. Harrop JS, Sharan A, Anderson G, et al. Failure of standard imaging to detect a cervical fracture in a patient with ankylosing spondylitis. Spine 2005;30:E417–E419

90. Harun S. Delayed spinal cord compression in ankylosing spondylitis. J Accid Emerg Med 1998;15:336

91. Hendrix RW, Melany M, Miller F, Rogers LF. Fracture of the spine in patients with ankylosis due to diffuse skeletal hyperostosis: clinical and imaging findings. AJR Am J Roentgenol 1994;162:899–904

92. Heyde CE, Fakler JK, Hasenboehler E, et al. Pitfalls and complications in the treatment of cervical spine fractures in patients with ankylosing spondylitis. Patient Saf Surg 2008;2:15

93. Hunter T, Dubo H. Spinal fractures complicating ankylosing spondylitis. Ann Intern Med 1978;88:546–549

94. Hunter T, Dubo HI. Spinal fractures complicating ankylosing spondylitis: a long-term followup study. Arthritis Rheum 1983;26:751–759

95. Rowed DW. Management of cervical spinal cord injury in ankylosing spondylitis: the intervertebral disc as a cause of cord compression. J Neurosurg 1992;77:241–246

96. Kanter AS, Wang MY, Mummaneni PV. A treatment algorithm for the management of cervical spine fractures and deformity in patients with ankylosing spondylitis. Neurosurg Focus 2008;24:E11

97. Karasick D, Schweitzer ME, Abidi NA, Cotler JM. Fractures of the vertebrae with spinal cord injuries in patients with ankylosing spondylitis: imaging findings. AJR Am J Roentgenol 1995;165:1205–1208

98. Koivikko MP, Kiuru MJ, Koskinen SK. Multidetector computed tomography of cervical spine fractures in ankylosing spondylitis. Acta Radiol 2004;45:751–759

99. Koivikko MP, Koskinen SK. MRI of cervical spine injuries complicating ankylosing spondylitis. Skeletal Radiol 2008;37:813–819

100. Kubiak EN, Moskovich R, Errico TJ, Di Cesare PE. Orthopaedic management of ankylosing spondylitis. J Am Acad Orthop Surg 2005;13:267–278

101. Madsen OR. Bone mineral density and fracture risk in patients with ankylosing spondylitis. Ugeskr Laeger 2008;170:3956–3960

102. May PJ, Raunest J, Herdmann J, Jonas M. Treatment of spinal fracture in ankylosing spondylitis [in German]. Unfallchirurg 2002;105:165–169

103. Michel JL, Souteyrand AC, Kabre M, Dubost JJ, Soubrier M, Ristori JM. Fractures of the ankylosed spine: MRI features [in French] J Radiol 2007;88(11 Pt 1):1703–1706

104. Nakstad PH, Server A, Josefsen R. Traumatic cervical injuries in ankylosing spondylitis. Acta Radiol 2004;45:222–226

105. Pedrosa I, Jorquera M, Mendez R, Cabeza B. Cervical spine fractures in ankylosing spondylitis: MR findings. Emerg Radiol 2002;9:38–42

106. Shih TT, Chen PQ, Li YW, Hsu CY. Spinal fractures and pseudoarthrosis complicating ankylosing spondylitis: MRI manifestation and clinical significance. J Comput Assist Tomogr 2001;25:164–170

107. Wang YF, Teng MM, Chang CY, Wu HT, Wang ST. Imaging manifestations of spinal fractures in ankylosing spondylitis. AJNR Am J Neuroradiol 2005;26:2067–2076

108. Johnson MG, Fisher CG, Boyd M, Pitzen T, Oxland TR, Dvorak MF, et al. The radiographic failure of single segment anterior cervical plate fixation in traumatic cervical flexion distraction injuries. Spine 2004;29:2815–2820

109. Anderson DG, Voets C, Ropiak R, et al. Analysis of patient variables affecting neurologic outcome after traumatic cervical facet dislocation. Spine J 2004;4:506–512

110. Pasciak M, Doniec J. Results of conservative treatment of unilateral cervical spine dislocations. Arch Orthop Trauma Surg 1993;112:226–227

111. Ostl OL, Fraser RD, Griffiths ER. Reduction and stabilisation of cervical dislocations: an analysis of 167 cases. J Bone Joint Surg Br 1989;71:275–282

112. de Oliveira JC. Anterior reduction of interlocking facets in the lower cervical spine. Spine 1979;4:195–202

113. Thumbikat P, Hariharan RP, Ravichandran G, McClelland MR, Mathew KM. Spinal cord injury in patients with ankylosing spondylitis: a 10-year review. Spine 2007;32:2989–2995

114. Zdichavsky M, Blauth M, Knop C, Lange U, Krettek C, Bastian L. Ankylosing spondylitis. Therapy and complications of 34 spine fractures [in German]. Chirurg 2005;76:967–975

115. Vosse D, Feldtkeller E, Erlendsson J, Geusens P, van der Linden S. Clinical vertebral fractures in patients with ankylosing spondylitis. J Rheumatol 2004;31:1981–1985

116. Mitra D, Elvins DM, Speden DJ, Collins AJ. The prevalence of vertebral fractures in mild ankylosing spondylitis and their relationship to bone mineral density. Rheumatology (Oxford) 2000;39:85–89

117. Meyer PR Jr. Diffuse idiopathic skeletal hyperostosis in the cervical spine. Clin Orthop Relat Res 1999;(359):49–57

118. Olerud C, Andersson S, Svensson B, Bring J. Cervical spine fractures in the elderly: factors influencing survival in 65 cases. Acta Orthop Scand 1999;70:509–513

119. Olerud C, Frost A, Bring J. Spinal fractures in patients with ankylosing spondylitis. Eur Spine J 1996;5:51–55

120. Weinstein PR, Karpman RR, Gall EP, Pitt M. Spinal cord injury, spinal fracture, and spinal stenosis in ankylosing spondylitis. J Neurosurg 1982;57:609–616

32

Traumatic Central Cord Syndrome Secondary to Cervical Spondylosis

Jeremy Reynolds and Marcel F. Dvorak

The management of spinal cord injury (SCI) associated with a fracture or dislocation is often overwhelmingly guided by the pattern of injury to the spinal column. Reduction, decompression and stabilization have long been the goals of surgical treatment. Achieving stability of the column is often a goal complementary to that of optimizing neurological recovery. Patients with traumatic central cord syndrome (TCCS) provide some of the most dramatic opportunities for neurological improvement when compared with other subgroups of SCI,[1–3] particularly evident in young patients with TCCS.[4]

TCCS is an incomplete SCI that disproportionately affects the upper extremities more than the lower extremities and occurs in two general populations. The first population group is the relatively young individual with a high-energy injury that leads to either a fracture/subluxation or a dislocation. The second category is the older individual who, due to a low-energy fall or cervical hyperextension injury (**Fig. 32.1**) presents with a TCCS that occurs in the presence of cervical spondylosis and spinal canal stenosis but without obvious injury to the spinal column.[5–7] Patients in this second group present with often profound incomplete neurological impairment and have no fracture or subluxation. Management decisions in these cases can be particularly complex.

The first contributor to this therapeutic complexity is the generally favorable neurological prognosis whereby the patient may have already experienced significant motor improvement between the time of injury and the moment of initial neurological evaluation in the emergency department. Next is the fact that in this cervical spondylosis subgroup there is no radiographically identifiable pattern of instability; with no fracture or subluxations to encourage the surgeon to operate (**Fig. 32.2**). The presence of cervical spondylosis and the concomitant stenosis has frequently been longstanding and in most cases has been asymptomatic. Finally, there is some degree of spinal cord swelling, edema, and possibly also hematoma, which may extend within the spinal cord over one or several vertebral segments. These features present a fairly complex set of management variables, all of which have therapeutic impact.

The definition of a TCCS is that of an incomplete neurological syndrome and involves motor and/or sensory sparing in the lowest sacral segments (more thoroughly discussed in Chapter 4). Differentiating TCCS from other incomplete neurological syndromes is the disproportionate motor dysfunction affecting the upper extremities more than the lower extremities, the presence of the most profound motor and

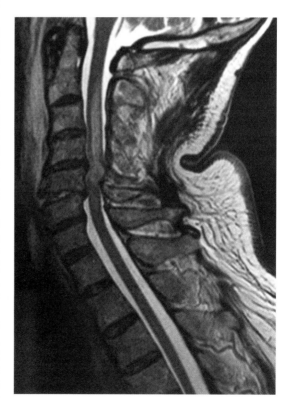

Fig. 32.1 T2 midsagittal magnetic resonance imaging section of the cervical spine of a 63-year-old male with a profound incomplete central cord syndrome due to a cervical hyperextension injury.

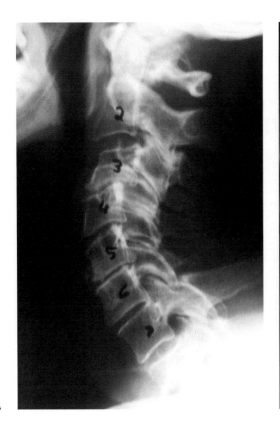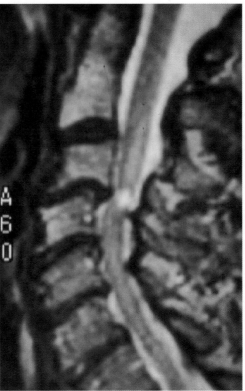

A   B

Fig. 32.2 **(A)** A plain radiograph and **(B)** a T2 sagittal magnetic resonance imaging scan of a 72-year-old male with severe cervical spondylosis and an incomplete traumatic central cord syndrome secondary to "pincer" spinal cord compression at the C3–C4 level.

sensory deficits in the distal upper extremities, the variable sensory deficits in the upper and lower extremities, and initially profound bowel and bladder dysfunction. Furthermore, we are limiting the scope of this chapter to the subgroup of TCCS patients who do not have radiographic instability of their spine; no fractures, no subluxations, and no dislocations. We include within this chapter those patients with cervical spondylosis, cervical spinal canal stenosis, and acute traumatic cervical disk protrusions (**Fig. 32.3**).

There are multiple variables that are proposed as contributors to the functional outcome of these individuals, and the most overwhelming of these is the patients' initial neurological impairment and their subsequent motor recovery.[8] With more than 80% of patients achieving functionally independent ambulation and urinary and bowel continence, the overall prognosis for functional recovery is very favorable. With such a favorable overall prognosis, the influence of various therapeutic options on the eventual outcome is not easily determined. This is particularly the case when one considers the role, timing, and technique of surgical intervention.

This chapter, therefore, assists the surgeon in answering two questions that arise in the early management of these TCCS patients: (1) What is the optimal treatment for an acute central cord injury without fracture or instability with respect to neurological recovery? (2) If surgical treatment is selected, what is the optimal surgical approach for decompressing a spondylotic cervical spine that has sustained a TCCS? We will use the methodology of a systematic review to identify the literature's contribution to these two questions. We will then add the components of expert opinion, risk:benefit, patient preference, and costs to generate a final summary recommendation.

The extent of spinal cord compression may extend over an individual level or multiple levels; may involve ventral and/or dorsal impingement on the spinal canal; and may be superimposed on a lordotic, neutral, or kyphotic cervical spine. For our defined population single-level pathology will usually be secondary to an acute cervical disk herniation[6,9] but may also be the result of a very focal single level spinal stenosis. Although cervical spondylosis and ossified posterior longitudinal ligament (OPLL) may cause a localized encroachment, multisegment involvement is more common as either continuous or segmental disease.[7] The role of cervical alignment is yet another factor that is relevant to consideration of surgery in this patient group. The importance of restoring sagittal cervical alignment has gained increasing credence in the multilevel cervical decompression literature.[10] We have attempted to extract data regarding this component of management where possible.

◆ **Methodology**

We have performed a thorough literature search based upon the following two questions:

1. What is the optimal treatment for an acute central cord syndrome (CCS) without fracture or instability with respect to neurological recovery?
2. What is the optimal surgical approach and surgical timing for decompressing a spondylotic cervical spine that has sustained an incomplete spinal cord injury?

A comprehensive literature search was performed to identify potential studies including any article with an English

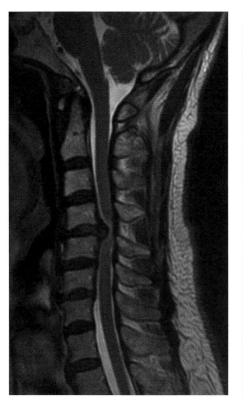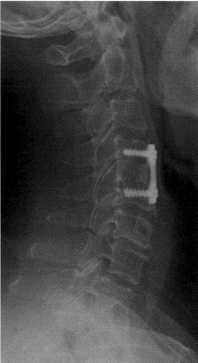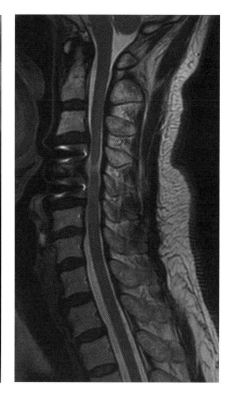

A–C

Fig. 32.3 Acute traumatic cervical disk herniation at the C4–C5 level in a 48-year-old female who presented with a moderate traumatic central cord syndrome that improved from an initial American Spinal Injury Association motor score of 42 preoperatively to a follow-up motor score of 88 at 1 year post–anterior diskectomy, fusion, and plating. **(A)** Initial and **(B)** postoperative T2 sagittal magnetic resonance imaging and **(C)** lateral radiograph.

language abstract. Electronic database searches of MEDLINE (1966 to January 2008) and EMBASE (1980 to January 2008) were performed using both medical subject headings (MeSH) and text word searching. Terms used included "spinal cord injury," "incomplete, cervical, central cord syndrome," "cervical trauma," and "cervical spondylosis." A search of the electronic database of CINAHL (1982 to January 2008) was conducted using the same text word search. Both the Database of Abstracts of Reviews of Effects and the Cochrane Database of Systematic Reviews were searched using text words. Reference lists from relevant articles were hand searched for additional citations. Content experts from the Spine Trauma Study Group were sought and questioned as to possible additional references. We reviewed the scientific literature independently of each other and graded according to levels of evidence as described by Schünemann et al.[11] When we had a disagreement, we met and reviewed the manuscript in question and came to a conclusion regarding the appropriate level of evidence.

◆ Review of Evidence

The fundamental question that the treating surgeon has to answer is whether to operate acutely or to consider an initial period of nonsurgical treatment. This question has two components, the first relating to whether there is a benefit to surgical decompression in this population and the second to the potential timing of this intervention. If the timing of surgery is not relevant, then it would be most reasonable to observe the patients' motor and sensory function for as long as they continue to make neurological gains, and to reserve surgery for those patients whose spontaneous neurological improvement ceases or plateaus at a nonfunctional level. These two fundamental issues relate to the first question posed in this chapter and have been the subject of nine papers.[5,8,12–18] See **Table 32.1**.

This chapter's ability to address question 1 has been compromised by the tendency on the part of treating surgeons to choose to operate upon those subjects in whom neurological injury is profound, those in which early spontaneous recovery is absent, those whose neurology has reached an unsatisfactory plateau, and those in which there is a radiographically proven substantial degree of bony or soft tissue compression of the spinal cord. Clearly, despite the presence of an acutely injured spinal cord, not all patients presenting with acute CCS require surgical decompression. There are several selection biases, many of which are difficult to quantify. Patients tend to be selected for surgery after a period of "neurological plateau" or failure to spontaneously recover; however, there is no recognized definition of the length of time or allowable neurological variability that would be consistent with a lack of spontaneous recovery. Generally, the patients with the more profound initial deficit or the deficit that fails to spontaneously recover are selected for surgery, and this results in a significant disadvantage for the surgical group outcomes because this group is functionally worse at the time of selection.

There are several observational cohort studies that do not attempt to compare therapeutic alternatives and simply assess the outcome of TCCS with the goal of identifying variables that predict outcome regardless of whether the patient is treated nonoperatively or operatively. Although observational cohort

321

Table 32.1 References in Which the Primary Conclusion or a Major Component of the Conclusion Relates to Question 1: What Is Optimal Treatment for an Acute Central Cord Syndrome without Fracture or Instability with Respect to Neurological Recovery?

Study	Primary Question Study Type	N	Assessment Tool	Secondary Question	Summary	Quality of Evidence Supporting Summary
Guest et al (2002)[16]	Retrospective case series	50	ASIA/PSIMFS, length of stay	Timing of surgery	Patients benefitted from early (< 24 h) surgery with respect to ICU/hospital length of stay. Only those patients without spondylosis/stenosis had improved motor recovery resulting from early surgery. No adverse events from early surgery	Moderate
Yamazaki et al (2005)[17]	Retrospective comparative	47	JOA	Timing of surgery	No benefit from surgical intervention unless performed within 2 weeks	Low
Chen et al (1998)[5]	Retrospective comparative	37	PSIMFS		Reduced length of stay in both ICU and rehabilitation in the surgical group. Earlier neurological recovery trends in surgical group but convergence at 2 years.	Low
Saruhashi et al (1998)[18]	Retrospective case series	33	JOA and ASIA	Compares TCCS with incomplete transverse	Supports the role of surgery in the presence of compressive lesion on MRI and recovery plateau. Poorer outcome with multilevel compression. TCCS patients outperform transverse incomplete in JOA/ASIA recovery	Low
Dvorak et al (2005)[8]	Retrospective case series	70	ASIA, NASS, FIM, SF-36		Improvement in Functional Independence Measurement score in operative group but no significant motor improvement versus nonoperative	Low
Chen et al (1997)[15]	Retrospective comparative	28	Activities of daily living		Improved outcomes with surgery and potential and functional hand grasping for prevention of late myelopathy	Very low
Asazuma et al (1996)[12]	Retrospective case series	35	Frankel grade	Timing of surgery	Recommends surgery if TCCS in the presence of compressive lesion and no improvement within 4 weeks	Very low
Brodkey et al (1980)[14]	Retrospective case series	7	MRC muscle grading		Neurological recovery seen following surgery despite recovery plateau preop in all patients	Very low
Bose et al (1984)[13]	Retrospective comparative	28	ASIA		Good neurological recovery following surgery on patients in whom recovery has plateaued with imaging evidence of compression	Very low

Abbreviations: ASIA, American Spinal Injury Association; FIM, Functional Independence Measure; ICU, intensive care unit; JOA, Japanese Orthopaedic Association; NASS, North American Spine Society; MRC, Medical Research Council; PSIMFS, post-spinal injury motor function scale; TCCS, traumatic central cord syndrome; SF-36, Short Form-36.

studies are generally a weaker form of evidence, these studies may be valuable if they provide adequate follow-up; use sound, validated outcome instruments; and report results that are generally consistent across multiple similar studies.[1,7,14,19]

The studies that relate to the second question of this chapter; the choice of surgical approach, are generally case series that describe the selection criteria of the surgeons who are retrospectively describing the treatment of a heterogeneous group of patients. These papers will be presented together with those that address the first question because there is significant overlap with the papers that are pertinent to both questions. There are six low-quality studies[5–7,9,17,18] that contain information relevant specifically to the second question (see **Table 32.2**).

The study by Yamazaki et al[17] recruited 47 patients. Twenty-three patients were selected for surgery due to inadequate

Study	Primary Question Study Type	N	Assessment Tool	Secondary Question	Summary	Quality of Evidence Supporting Summary
Chen et al (1998)[5]	Retrospective comparative	37	PSIMFS	See Table 32.1	16/37 patients treated operatively 7 with 1-or 2-level pathology treated with anterior surgery. 9 with multilevel (> 3 levels) pathology: 2 3-level corpectomy and 7 laminectomies Both patients with 3-level corpectomy had surgical complications: 1 with dysphagia the other neurological deterioration. Favors anterior surgery if 3+ level involvement	Very low
Saruhashi et al (1998)[18]	Retrospective case series	33	JOA and ASIA	See Table 32.1	Supports the role of a directed surgical approach with 14 anterior only, 5 posterior only and 2 combined procedures without major surgical complication.	Very low
Yamazaki et al (2005)[17]	Retrospective comparative	47	JOA	See Table 32.1	20 expansive laminoplasty, 3 ACDF No major drawbacks seen with posterior approach in multilevel disease	Very low
Song et al (2005)[6]	Retrospective comparative	22	Frankel	Timing of surgery	All patients underwent surgery with improvement by at least 1 Frankel grade and no deleterious issues from early surgery (< 72 h) 12 anterior procedures for 1- to 2-level cord compression and 10 posterior for multilevel involvement. This study illustrates a selective approach to the surgical plan.	Very low
Dai and Jia (2000)[9]	Retrospective case series	24	ASIA		All patients presenting with TCCS secondary to HNP undergoing ACDF had good neurological recovery.	Very low
Uribe et al (2005)[7]	Retrospective case series	15	ASIA	Timing of surgery	All patients underwent posterior open door laminoplasty with good neurological recovery. Early surgery is safe.	Very low

Abbreviations: ACDF, anterior cervical discectomy and fusion; ASIA, American Spinal Injury Association; HNP, herniated nucleus pulposus; JOA, Japanese Orthopaedic Association; TCCS, traumatic central cord syndrome.

recovery or deterioration of neurological function or persistent dysesthetic pain. Twenty-four were treated nonoperatively. There were similar numbers in each group with associated diseases (OPLL, stenosis, disk herniation, and spur formation), although specifically there were four OPLL patients in the surgical group compared with only one in the nonoperative group. There were two disk herniations in each group. A tendency toward a narrower canal anteroposterior (AP) diameter was seen in the surgical cohort (8.9 mm vs 10.3 mm). The surgical patients also had a lower admission Japanese Orthopaedic Association (JOA) cervical myelopathy score (8.8 vs 13.1). The patients were followed up for a minimum of 6 months with a mean follow-up of 40 months. Both cohorts had a very similar JOA recovery rate (66% surgical vs 68% nonoperative).

When the surgical cohort was further stratified into early (within 2 weeks; mean 8 days) and late (after 2 weeks; mean 30 days) intervention, the patients in the early surgery group, despite having worse JOA score (8.7) and a narrower AP

diameter (8.8 mm), exhibited greater recovery (80%) than the late surgery group (48%) and was interpreted by the authors as a compelling argument for early surgery. This retrospective comparative study is likely underpowered and provides low-quality evidence. This study additionally reports good results for 20 multilevel expansive laminoplasty as well as three anterior cervical decompression and fusions. This provides very low quality support for the posterior approach when considering multilevel disease.

Chen et al authored two studies, the first of which[15] reports on a series of 114 retrospectively reviewed cases of CCS admitted to a Taiwanese neurosurgical department with only 17 acute CCS patients without spinal instability or fracture included in a 28-strong surgical group and 11 patients with spondylosis in the nonoperative group. The author reported on upper limb function and activities of daily living but did not use validated outcome instruments. It was not possible to compare early recovery postsurgery versus nonoperatively managed cases. Functional hand grasping at 30 days appeared to favor the surgical group, but there was no statistical analysis. All patients did well from a lower limb perspective, and bladder function improved in most patients. The paper concludes that surgery has a role in improving outcomes for CCS and preventing late myelopathic change secondary to compression. The quality of supporting evidence for this statement is very low.

The second paper by Chen et al[5] assesses 37 patients with cervical spondylosis presenting with TCCS and reports on the post–spinal injury motor score (PSIMS), a value that is derived from the American Spinal Injury Association (ASIA) motor score. The patients are a combination of specific cases from the Taiwanese hospital in the original paper and a further dataset from Phoenix, Arizona. The principal criterion for surgery was failure to improve more than 1 motor grade within 2 weeks (mean 9.3 days). All seven patients with single-level pathology, and two of the nine patients with multilevel pathology, underwent anterior surgery. Seven patients with multilevel compression had posterior procedures. Other than a failure of the surgical group to improve neurologically following admission the two groups were well matched. The authors of this study concluded that the surgically treated patients enjoyed a significantly reduced hospital stay (13 vs 21 days) and rehabilitation period (39 vs 68 days) despite initially appearing to have less spontaneous recovery. The motor outcomes, although trending lower in the nonoperative group at 1 month and 6 months, did not achieve statistical significance, but this study is underpowered to assess this accurately. What is clear, however, is that both groups converge at 2 years with a mean motor improvement of 2.75 PSIMS (SD = 1.33) and 2.0 PSIMS (SD = 1.12) for the surgical and nonsurgical groups, respectively. The most significant surgical complications occurred in the multisegment anterior surgery group, where one patient deteriorated neurologically and one had hoarseness. With regard to the first question, this paper provides low-quality evidence in favor of surgery primarily due to the reduction of hospital stay and rehabilitation requirement but not based on long-term neurological or functional outcome. This paper provides very low quality evidence that three-level corpectomy may not be the best approach for multilevel disease; however, this does not allow for assessment of the complexity or the sagittal alignment of the specific cases.

Asazuma et al,[12] in a retrospective case series, reported on 19 nonoperative and 26 surgical patients. Although the average time from injury to surgery was over 6 months, a small cohort of early surgery patients (< 4 weeks) showed better neurological improvement. The lack of improvement in the surgical group (early and late) as compared with the nonoperative group may be due to the very long average time between injury and intervention. This paper provides very low quality support for early surgical intervention in the presence of spinal cord compression. There is no discussion in this paper regarding the choice of surgical approach.

Saruhashi et al[18] reported on 33 patients with CCS and no evidence of fracture or subluxation. Twelve patients were treated conservatively both initially and throughout their course. The remaining 21 patients all reached a neurological plateau after initial nonsurgical treatment and had magnetic resonance imaging (MRI) evidence of cord compression and thus were treated surgically. Specific anatomical criteria (one or multiple levels of compression) were used to determine surgical approach. This study is significantly underpowered to make any conclusions; however, it does provide low-quality evidence for surgery when there is MRI evidence of spinal cord compression and a failure to improve neurologically.

Brodkey[14] was one of the first to suggest surgical treatment of CCS. In a case series of only seven patients, all treated surgically, Brodkey et al remarked on the rapid neurological improvement following surgery despite the relatively static clinical course immediately prior to surgery. This very low quality study heralded the onset of future studies of surgical decompression for this patient population.

Bose et al[13] reviewed 28 patients and compared the half that was treated surgically with the half treated nonoperatively. Although underpowered, Bose et al reported good neurological improvement following surgery, the indication for which included a lack of neurological improvement and imaging evidence of spinal cord compression. The quality of evidence in support of surgery is very low in this study due to the small number of patients analyzed.

Dai and Jia[9] retrospectively reviewed 24 patients with disk herniations causing acute CCS. All patients had anterior decompression and good neurological improvement thus supporting, with very low quality evidence, anterior surgery for this subgroup of patients.

Uribe et al,[7] in a paper that presents the results of posterior laminoplasty in a group of patients with TCCS and cervical spondylosis, reported on the results of early (mean 3 days postinjury) surgery in 15 patients. By reporting early postoperative neurological improvement in all patients, the paper by Uribe et al has provided very low quality evidence in support of early surgery.

Guest et al[16] retrospectively reviewed 50 patients with TCCS specifically to analyze the outcomes of those operated on early (< 24 h) as opposed to those operated on later. The authors' report improved (shortened) length of hospital and intensive care unit (ICU) stay in the early group. In a subgroup of patients with spondylosis or stenosis, there was no difference in motor outcome between early and late surgery. The inclusion of some patients with fractures (10 patients) makes it difficult for us to draw conclusions specific to the spondylotic and stenotic patients that are the primary focus of this chapter. Nevertheless, Guest et al's paper does provide moderate-quality evidence for the safety and efficacy of surgery and particularly of early surgical treatment for these patients.

Song et al[6] described 22 patients, 12 of which had anterior decompression for one and two levels of cord compression and 10 had posterior surgery for multilevel compression. All patients were operated on within the first month and all improved neurologically. This study provides low-quality evidence in support of using the number of levels of compression to inform the choice of surgical approach.

Dvorak et al[8] performed long-term cross-sectional outcomes on a group of 70 patients and analyzed surgery as one of multiple variables that were thought to influence outcome. The surgically treated patients reported significantly better functional outcome scores [Functional Independence Measure (FIM)] than those treated nonoperatively. Although significant motor improvement was not demonstrated in the surgical group, this study does provide low-quality evidence of the beneficial effects of surgery.

Guidelines

With respect to the first question, there are several studies which suggest that surgically treated patients with cervical spondylosis and TCCS have improved neurological outcomes when compared with those treated nonoperatively. In fact, there is not a single study showing that surgery results in anything less than immediate neurological improvement, despite a period of no improvement prior to surgical intervention.

The literature is consistent in suggesting that prior to surgical intervention, MRI or CT-myelographic evidence of continued bony or soft tissue compression of the spinal cord must be demonstrated. The literature is consistent in that many authors will allow early spontaneous recovery to occur; however, in its absence surgical decompression appears to be the treatment course with the best early outcomes and perhaps the best long-term outcomes.[8]

The issue of the timing of surgical intervention is inextricably linked to the first question. If the timing of surgery had no effect on outcome, then all patients could be treated nonoperatively, and surgery could be delayed till weeks or even months after the injury without compromising the patient's recovery or outcome. The literature provides low-quality evidence that there is no deleterious neurological effect of early (within 1 week of injury) surgery in these patients as compared with delayed or late surgery. Quite the contrary, there is some evidence (though very low quality) of a neurological benefit to early decompression, though this benefit may be more difficult to measure at longer follow-up. Several authors have made the observation that their patients who are operated on late do not have the same neurological improvement as those who have early decompression.[5,8,16,17] Apart from the neurological consequences of early surgery, the literature reports other reasons to favor early decompression, namely shorter hospital and ICU lengths of stay.[5,16]

With respect to the second question, the optimal surgical approach to decompress the patient with cervical spondylosis, the literature provides some general guiding principles. First of all, most papers treat acute disk protrusions causing one- and two-level cord compression with an anterior approach, either diskectomy or corpectomy and plating.[5,6,9] Other anterior pathologies, such as spondylotic bars and bone spurs, when they occur at one or two levels, appear to be fairly consistently approached anteriorly.

The literature is also consistent in recommending a posterior approach when multiple levels contribute to the cord compression, particularly when the underlying condition is OPLL, congenital, or developmental multilevel stenosis, or diffuse idiopathic skeletal hyperostosis (DISH).[5–7,18]

◆ The Consensus of Experts

When this systematic review of the literature was presented to the members of the Spine Trauma Study Group, there were several consistent recommendations that were based upon the consensus expert opinion of the surgeons. With respect to the question of the relative role of surgery and nonoperative care, the experience of the surgeons reflected the often immediate and progressive neurological improvement that often follows surgical decompression. Based upon experience and the results of ongoing prospective studies on the timing of surgical decompression in all spinal cord injury patients, there were some surgeons whose practice it is to recommend early (as soon as technically feasible) surgical decompression for any patient with a significant neurological deficit secondary to cord compression due to cervical spondylosis and acute TCCS.

Furthermore, the STSG surgeons identified that, unlike the elective patient who is weighing a variety of treatment options for a degenerative condition, the acutely injured TCCS patient is already admitted to hospital and is facing what is often a significant acute hospital stay and potentially prolonged rehabilitation requirement. The evidence that surgical treatment may in fact reduce hospital stay and ICU stay when combined with the fact that the patient is already hospitalized and surgery would potentially be performed within hours of the decision being made are factors that significantly influence the risk–benefit analysis as well as the costs and the burden on the patient of the therapeutic decision-making process. The generally acceptable risk profile of the proposed surgical procedures (very few reports of neurological worsening), as well as the potential benefits of surgery, combine to influence both the patient and the surgeon's preferred treatment.

Following a discussion of the literature, reflection on the issues of risk, benefit, burden, and cost, and including the consensus of the expert members of the STSG, several recommendations were put forward by the members of the STSG:

- There was a strong recommendation based on low-quality evidence that early (as soon as feasible) surgical decompression should be recommended for patients with TCCS and spondylosis when their initial neurological impairment is significant, they fail to demonstrate spontaneous neurological recovery, and there is radiographic evidence of bony or soft tissue cord compression.
- Furthermore, a strong recommendation could be made, based on low-quality evidence that nonsurgical treatment is appropriate initial treatment for patients with TCCS and spondylosis when their initial neurological impairment is minimal, or their initial neurological impairment is significant and there is early spontaneous recovery, and when there is minimal or no evidence of bony or soft tissue cord compression.
- With respect to the second question, the group produced a strong recommendation, based on low-quality evidence that anterior surgical treatment with diskectomy and/or corpectomy is the optimal surgical approach for patients with TCCS due to acute traumatic disk herniation.
- Based on poor-quality evidence there is a weak recommendation to support anterior surgical treatment with diskectomy and/or corpectomy as the optimal surgical approach for patients with TCCS due to one- or two-level spinal cord compression due to focal stenosis.
- There was a strong recommendation, based on poor-quality but consistent evidence that posterior surgical treatment with laminoplasty or laminectomy and fusion is the optimal surgical approach for patients with TCCS due to multilevel (two or more spinal levels) spinal cord compression due to multifocal stenosis.

Although the literature was not clear on this last point, the surgeons' expert opinion was consistent in the recommendation that posterior surgery be reserved as well for those with lordotic cervical spines. A dorsal decompression in the presence of a focal or global kyphosis seen not to correct to neutral on dynamic radiographs was felt unlikely to be successful.

◆ Outstanding Issues

These recommendations are intended to ease the decision-making burden of the clinician notwithstanding the individual nature of each case. The obvious "absentee" from these recommendations is the patient with multilevel compression and a fixed kyphotic cervical spine. It seems likely that in these cases there will be a requirement for a combined surgical procedure. The emphasis should remain on adequate decompression and this should not be compromised by the selected deformity correction solution.

There are three main options when planning for such cases, and the selected strategy will be influenced by the underlying pathology. The most obvious solution is the multilevel corpectomy either as a stand-alone procedure or, if in the presence of a damaged posterior tension band, in combination with posterior instrumentation. This approach has been shown to present with considerable risk of major complication. An alternative in patients with long-segment anterior compressive pathology as a result of either spondylosis or OPLL is a wide posterior decompression, facetectomy, and fusion combined, where required, with a corrective osteotomy to allow the cord to "float back," thus facilitating decompression.[10]

Finally, in patients whose anterior pathology is related purely to the disk at multiple levels it would seem very reasonable to address these multiple foci with contoured interbody grafts to decompress locally and gain partial deformity correction. This could then be combined with a posterior fusion and facetectomy to improve lordosis and lock down the grafts. Additionally, if there are concerns regarding ligamentum flavum thickening or in-folding this could be addressed with a laminectomy. Two adjuncts to such complex cases are intraoperative ultrasound to assess for adequacy of decompression and the use of neuromonitoring. The latter would be especially useful at the time of intubation, positioning, and deformity correction.

◆ Conclusions and Recommendations

In contrast with complete cord injury, patients with central cord injury are generally perceived as having a good potential for meaningful functional recovery. It has become apparent over the last 2 decades that there may well be a role for surgery in these patients solely to decompress without the need to correct spinal column instability.

We can confidently recommend that surgical decompression be considered in appropriately selected patients with acute TCCS in the knowledge that this mode of treatment is safe and effective at optimizing neurological recovery. The trend among surgeons is to perform the decompression as early as technically feasible in the patient with high-grade cord compression on the MRI and a significant neurological deficit.

In contrast with the elective spine patient considering treatment options for an elective degenerative condition,

these patients are already hospitalized and the incremental risk and burden on the patient to undergo surgical decompression (a relatively safe procedure) is much less daunting and more likely to present a therapeutic alternative that is viewed favorably by the patient.

References

1. Ishida Y, Tominaga T. Predictors of neurologic recovery in acute central cervical cord injury with only upper extremity impairment. Spine 2002;27:1652–1658, discussion 1658
2. Maynard FM, Reynolds GG, Fountain S, Wilmot C, Hamilton R. Neurological prognosis after traumatic quadriplegia: three-year experience of California Regional Spinal Cord Injury Care System. J Neurosurg 1979;50:611–616
3. Merriam WF, Taylor TK, Ruff SJ, McPhail MJ. A reappraisal of acute traumatic central cord syndrome. J Bone Joint Surg Br 1986;68:708–713
4. Penrod LE, Hegde SK, Ditunno JF Jr. Age effect on prognosis for functional recovery in acute, traumatic central cord syndrome. Arch Phys Med Rehabil 1990;71:963–968
5. Chen TY, Dickman CA, Eleraky M, Sonntag VK. The role of decompression for acute incomplete cervical spinal cord injury in cervical spondylosis. Spine 1998;23:2398–2403
6. Song J, Mizuno J, Nakagawa H, Inoue T. Surgery for acute subaxial traumatic central cord syndrome without fracture or dislocation. J Clin Neurosci 2005;12:438–443
7. Uribe J, Green BA, Vanni S, Moza K, Guest JD, Levi AD. Acute traumatic central cord syndrome—experience using surgical decompression with open-door expansile cervical laminoplasty. Surg Neurol 2005;63:505–510, discussion 510
8. Dvorak MF, Fisher CG, Hoekema J, et al. Factors predicting motor recovery and functional outcome after traumatic central cord syndrome: a long-term follow-up. Spine 2005;30:2303–2311
9. Dai L, Jia L. Central cord injury complicating acute cervical disc herniation in trauma. Spine 2000;25:331–335, discussion 336
10. Levi L, Wolf A, Mirvis S, Rigamonti D, Fianfaca MS, Monasky M. The significance of dorsal migration of the cord after extensive cervical laminectomy for patients with traumatic central cord syndrome. J Spinal Disord 1995;8:289–295
11. Schünemann HJ, Jaeschke R, Cook DJ, et al; ATS Documents Development and Implementation Committee. An official ATS statement: grading the quality of evidence and strength of recommendations in ATS guidelines and recommendations. Am J Respir Crit Care Med 2006;174:605–614
12. Asazuma T, Satomi K, Suzuki N, Fujimura Y, Hirabayashi K. Management of patients with an incomplete cervical spinal cord injury. Spinal Cord 1996;34:620–625
13. Bose B, Northrup BE, Osterholm JL, Cotler JM, DiTunno JF. Reanalysis of central cervical cord injury management. Neurosurgery 1984;15:367–372
14. Brodkey JS, Miller CF Jr, Harmody RM. The syndrome of acute central cervical spinal cord injury revisited. Surg Neurol 1980;14:251–257
15. Chen TY, Lee ST, Lui TN, et al. Efficacy of surgical treatment in traumatic central cord syndrome. Surg Neurol 1997;48:435–440, discussion 441
16. Guest J, Eleraky MA, Apostolides PJ, Dickman CA, Sonntag VK. Traumatic central cord syndrome: results of surgical management. J Neurosurg 2002;97(1, Suppl):25–32
17. Yamazaki T, Yanaka K, Fujita K, Kamezaki T, Uemura K, Nose T. Traumatic central cord syndrome: analysis of factors affecting the outcome. Surg Neurol 2005;63:95–99, discussion 99–100
18. Saruhashi Y, Hukuda S, Katsuura A, Asajima S, Omura K. Clinical outcomes of cervical spinal cord injuries without radiographic evidence of trauma. Spinal Cord 1998;36:567–573
19. Shrosbree RD. Acute central cervical spinal cord syndrome—aetiology, age incidence and relationship to the orthopaedic injury. Paraplegia 1977;14:251–258

33

Surgical Approach to Rotational/Translational Injuries Using the SLIC System

Brian K. Kwon and Marcel F. Dvorak

The Subaxial Injury Classification (SLIC) scoring system incorporates a score for the morphology of the injury (0 to 4), the status of the discoligamentous complex (0 to 2), and the status of the neurological elements (0 to 3).[1] A sum of these three scores equaling 5 or greater represents an injury that possesses a strong rationale for surgical intervention. Within this framework, rotation/translation injuries score the highest number of points on the morphology scale (4 points) and are almost always associated with significant discoligamentous disruption (2 points). Hence these injuries already score 6 on the SLIC scale and accordingly warrant surgical fixation, even without the neurology status being considered. This chapter addresses the question: *What is the optimal surgical approach for these injuries?*

◆ Injury Types

All of the injuries within the morphological subset of "rotation/translation" exhibit pure translation or translational rotation of one vertebra relative to an adjacent vertebra. Within this subset, however, exists a spectrum of different injuries, including unilateral or bilateral facet fracture subluxations/dislocations (**Fig. 33.1**), and fractures of the anterior vertebral body in association with disruption to the posterior elements. In addition to multiple configurations of facet joint disruption (**Fig. 33.2**), posterior element injuries also include fractures of the spinous process, lamina, lateral masses. Anteriorly, the vertebral body can be fractured in several different configurations, including burst fractures or sagittal and coronal plane fractures leading to the so-called teardrop or quadrangular fracture patterns (**Fig. 33.3**). Although these seem to be a heterogeneous complex of injuries, they are unified within this morphological subset fundamentally by the presence of translation or translational rotation of one vertebra relative to its adjacent vertebra. To this end, the presence of translation implies that the anterior and posterior osteoligamentous structures of the spinal column have been grossly disrupted, albeit in a heterogeneous manner. The high degree of mechanical instability shared among these injury patterns provides the rationale within a treatment-oriented algorithm to view them as a single morphological entity.

◆ Surgical Approaches

The subaxial cervical spine can be approached either anteriorly or posteriorly, with both approaches being very familiar to spine surgeons. Anterior surgery typically involves a structural reconstruction of the disk or vertebral body and anterior plate fixation. Posterior surgery typically includes lateral mass screw–rod fixation and possibly interspinous wiring/cabling (the latter being a technique that has largely been supplanted by the former).

The anterior approach allows for direct decompression of the spinal cord from bone or disk material and for reconstruction of the anterior column using structural bone graft or a prosthetic implant (e.g., mesh cage). The anterior approach is an anatomical one that avoids the painful stripping and denervation of dorsal musculature off the spine in the posterior approach. Additionally, approaching the spine anteriorly obviates the need to turn the patient with an unstable cervical spine prone, potentially reducing the risk of neurological injury. However, the anterior approach may lead to swallowing and airway problems (particularly in elderly individuals), that can result in pulmonary complications. The posterior approach allows for dorsal decompression of the spinal cord and restoration of the posterior tension band. Realignment of the spine is more easily performed from the posterior approach (although techniques for doing so from the anterior approach are well described). Posterior fixation in the form of lateral mass screws–rods has a biomechanical advantage to anterior fixation in the form of anterior plating. However, posterior fixation may need to be extended to include additional motion segments, depending on the extent and pattern of posterior element fractures.

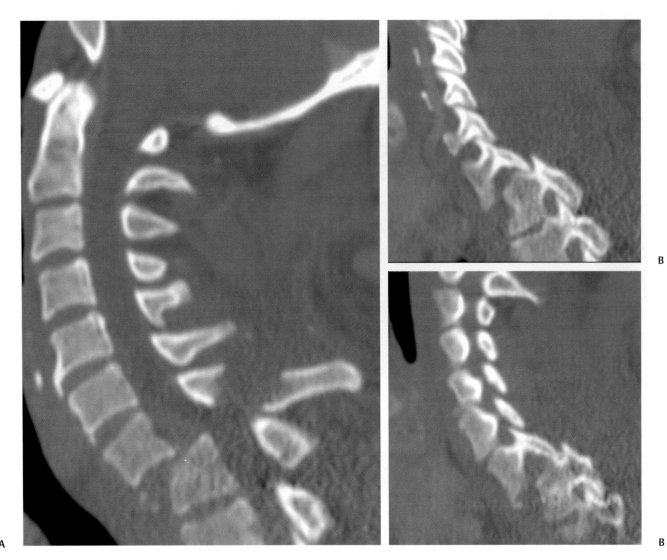

Fig. 33.1 (A–C) This 58-year-old male sustained a bilateral facet dislocation at C7/T1. Note the anterior translation of C7 on T1, and the anterior end plate/body fracture of T1. Also note that the posterior element injury consists of **(B,C)** both facet joints dislocating, and the spinous process and lamina fracturing.

With these considerations in mind, the decision surgeons are faced with in addressing a SLIC rotation/translation injury is determining which approach is most appropriate: anterior fixation alone, posterior fixation alone, or a combined/circumferential fixation.

A comprehensive English literature search was performed to answer the question, *What is the optimal surgical approach to SLIC rotation/translation injuries?* Prior to performing this search, criteria for defining a study that was relevant to this question were established. To be included in this literature review the study had to have adult patients (age > 16 years) with subaxial cervical traumatic injuries considered to be SLIC rotation/translation injuries treated surgically with anterior, posterior, or combined anterior and posterior surgical approaches. The study had to measure the radiographic and/or clinical success of the treatment utilizing validated outcome measures and/or radiographic measures and must have described the surgical approach utilized. Studies were excluded if they failed to define the surgical approach or were describing either traumatic injuries outside the subaxial cervical spine or nontraumatic conditions within it. Additionally, studies describing surgical stabilization with techniques that are no longer utilized were excluded (e.g., Cloward procedure anteriorly, or sublaminar wiring posteriorly).

◆ Literature Review

A comprehensive literature search was performed to identify potential studies including any article with an English language abstract. Electronic database searches of MEDLINE (1966 to January 2008) and EMBASE (1980 to January 2008) were performed using both medical subject headings (MeSH) and text word searching. Terms used included "fracture," "cervical, spine fractures," "fracture fixation—internal," and "cervical vertebra." A search of the electronic database of CINAHL (1982 to January 2008) was conducted using the same text word search. Both the Database of Abstracts of Reviews of Effects and the Cochrane Database of Systematic Reviews were searched using text words. Reference lists from relevant articles were hand searched for additional citations. Content experts from the Spine Trauma Study Group (STSG) were sought and questioned as to possible additional references. The scientific literature was then graded,

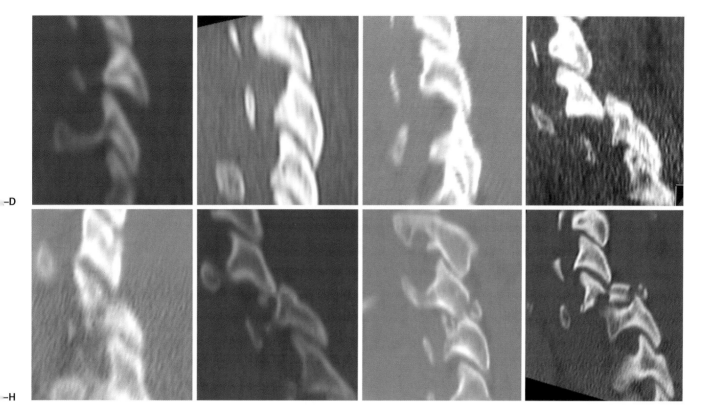

Fig. 33.2 (A–H) The facet joints are important posterior stabilizers and can be disrupted in multiple different configurations. **(A–C)** The disruption may be primarily through the soft tissue/capsule with varying levels of subluxation or **(D)** frank dislocation. Alternatively, the facets can be fractured, with either the **(E)** inferior or **(F)** superior facet or **(G,H)** both being fractured in association with varying degrees of translation.

and recommendations were made regarding the strength of the evidence based on the American Thoracic Society guidelines after presenting a summary of this literature to a group of over 30 surgeons at the STSG.[2]

◆ Results

The literature search performed in January 2008 revealed 727 papers of potential relevance. The study selection process eliminated 580 papers by a review of the abstracts alone. An additional 117 papers were excluded after a review of their methodology and results sections. Most of these were excluded due to relevance and methodological issues. This left a total of 30 papers that met all inclusion criteria. Of these 29 papers, three were considered to provide level 2 evidence based on their prospective or systematic methodology and applicability to the primary question. Three papers were considered to provide level 3 evidence as retrospective comparative studies. The remaining 23 papers were considered to provide level 4 evidence as retrospective case series.

◆ Discussion and Recommendations

Tables 33.1, **33.2**, and **33.3** demonstrate that high-quality studies addressing the question of which surgical approach to take (anterior, posterior, or combined) are lacking. Few comparative studies exist, and the majority of studies that were reviewed were of a retrospective, case series nature with a single approach applied to a heterogeneous set of injuries. It is, however, acknowledged that these injuries are, by their very nature, fairly heterogeneous from a morphological standpoint. What unifies these injuries is the pure translation or translational rotation of one vertebra relative to an adjacent vertebra. The principal features that subcategorize and differentiate injuries within the translation/rotation group are the presence or absence of fractures affecting the vertebral body and the presence, severity, and location of residual compression of the neural elements.

Based on the evidence described in **Tables 33.1**, **33.2**, and **33.3**, the following proposals were made to the spine surgeons of the STSG to incorporate this layer of clinical experience and expertise into a recommendation for treatment:

1. Based on published clinical evidence that is weak *and* the expert opinion of the members of the STSG, *it is strongly recommended* that unilateral and bilateral facet injuries can be treated via anterior or posterior fixation alone, provided that there is no end plate or vertebral body fracture and that there is no displaced disk causing ventral cord compression. The decision of choosing anterior or posterior fixation can therefore be reasonably based on surgeon preference and patient preference. This recommendation stems largely from the moderate-quality evidence from Kwon et al[3] and Brodke et al[4] that demonstrated no apparent difference in outcome between anteriorly or posteriorly treated patients who suffered these injuries, and additionally, the very low quality evidence of acceptable clinical and radiographic results being achieved with either approach. In Kwon's prospective, randomized study of anterior or posterior surgery for unilateral facet injuries the time to achieving discharge criteria postoperatively (the primary outcome measure) did not differ significantly

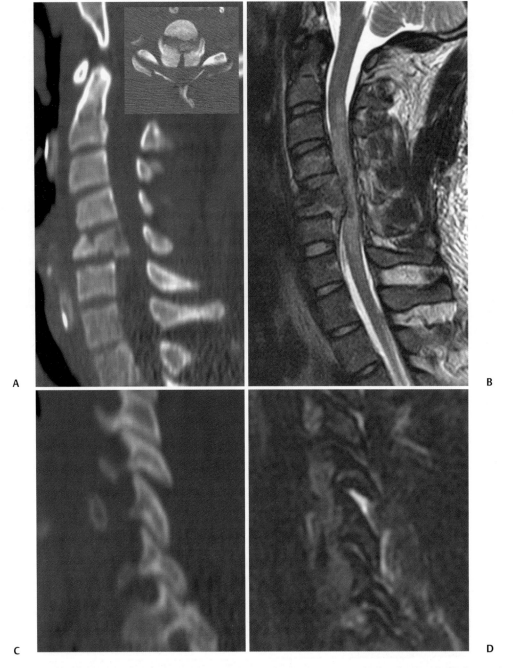

A

B

C

D

Fig. 33.3 (A–D) Teardrop/quadrangular fracture pattern. In association with disruption of the posterior elements, varying degrees of anterior vertebral body failure can occur. **(A)** In this case, a "teardrop" fragment anteriorly is fractured off of C5, with severe kyphosis and posterior translation of the remainder of C5 into **(B)** the canal due to the disruption of **(C,D)** the facets posteriorly.

between the two groups. However, in the analysis of secondary outcomes, posteriorly treated patients had a much higher wound infection rate and fell into greater segmental kyphosis as the injured disk collapsed anteriorly. Concerns expressed about the anterior approach include complications of dysphagia, hoarse voice, and early radiographic failure when utilized in the presence of end plate compression fractures (see later discussion) and very comminuted or large facet fracture fragments.[5]

2. Based on published clinical evidence that is weak *and the* expert opinion of the members of the STSG, *it is weakly recommended* that unilateral and bilateral facet injuries in the presence of an end plate fracture but in the absence of a disk herniation should be treated posteriorly. This

recommendation stems from the very low quality evidence from Johnson et al,[6] who demonstrated that these injuries treated with anterior fixation alone had a high radiographic failure rate. This was postulated to occur due to the fractured end plate not being able to support an interbody graft. Because surgeons are very comfortable with both anterior and posterior approaches and there would be little risk to opting for a posterior approach in the presence of an end plate fracture, it was felt that a recommendation could be made to support performing this stabilization posteriorly. The recommendation is weak due to the lack of unanimous consensus within the STSG membership.

With respect to bilateral facet subluxations specifically, Elgafy et al demonstrated that patients with bilateral facet

Table 33.1 Studies Considered to Provide Moderate Quality Evidence (Prospective Clinical Studies or Systematic Reviews of the Literature)

Study	Description	Topic and Conclusion
Dvorak et al (2007)[9]	Systematic review of literature on surgical or nonsurgical treatment of subaxial trauma up to November 2006	A systematic review of papers on surgical management of subaxial injuries, which were evaluated and consensus achieved with expert opinion to establish treatment algorithms for SLIC translation/rotation injuries. - Considered moderate quality due to its systematic methodology. CONCLUSIONS: Facet injuries can be effectively treated with either an anterior or a posterior approach alone, although the presence of an end plate fracture leads to high failure rate with anterior fixation alone. The presence of severe vertebral body injury with significant translation should be addressed with combined fixation.
Kwon et al (2007)[3]	Prospective, randomized trial of anterior versus posterior stabilization of unilateral facet injuries without SCI; appropriately powered for the primary outcome (time required to achieve standard prospective discharge criteria)	42 patients were randomized to anterior or posterior fusion for unilateral facet injuries without SCI. There was no significant difference in the 1° outcome (time to discharge postoperatively). 2° outcomes revealed better sagittal alignment (8.8° lordosis vs 1.6° kyphosis) in anterior patients, and fewer wound infections (0 vs 4). - While prospective and randomized, this is considered moderate quality because of the difficulty postoperative in determining the extent of translation/displacement within the cohort of patients. CONCLUSIONS: Anterior and posterior surgical stabilization result in similar acute postoperative morbidity.
Brodke et al (2003)[4]	Prospective, randomized (by day of admission) trial of anterior versus posterior stabilization of subaxial injuries with SCI; no power analysis performed, no primary outcome measure identified	52 patients were randomized to anterior or posterior approaches. 36 patients had bilateral facet dislocations with or without a burst component. Higher rate of fusion with posterior surgery (100% vs 90%, NS); no difference in neurological recovery or postoperative complications. - Considered moderate quality due to the inability to distinguish the results of the SLIC translation/rotation injuries from others (although they represented the majority of the patients) and the lack of a primary outcome measure or power analysis. CONCLUSIONS: Anterior and posterior surgical stabilization result in similar fusion rates, neurologic recovery, and post-operative complications.

Abbreviations: NS, non-significant; SCI, spinal cord injury; SLIC, Subaxial Cervical Spine Injury Classification.

Table 33.2 Studies Considered to Provide Low-Quality Evidence (Retrospective Comparative Clinical Studies)

Song and Lee (2008)[10]	Retrospective comparative study of anterior fixation versus circumferential fixation for unilateral and bilateral facet injuries	50 patients retrospectively reviewed, with 38 receiving anterior alone, and 12 receiving combined approaches. All patients fused, though fusion time was greatest for bilateral facet injuries treated with anterior surgery alone. No differences in sagittal alignment, neurological recovery, or complications among the groups. - Considered low quality due to its retrospective nature and inability to determine exactly how much translation existed in the unilateral injuries, which represented most of these injuries (32). CONCLUSIONS: Anterior and anterior + posterior surgical stabilization had similar clinical and radiographic outcomes.
Toh et al (2006)[11]	Retrospective comparative study of anterior versus posterior fixation for burst and teardrop injuries	Retrospective review of 11 burst fractures and 21 teardrop fracture dislocations treated posteriorly (prior to 1992) and anteriorly after 1992. All burst fractures were treated anteriorly. For teardrop fracture dislocations, the anteriorly treated injuries had a much better "bone fragment reduction rate" (indicative of the completeness of spinal canal decompression) than posteriorly treated injuries (61% vs 6%). - Considered low quality due to the heterogeneity of the injury patterns (burst fractures with a pure axial component and the absence of posterior injury are not considered to be included in this rotation/translation morphology), and the outdated posterior fixation system (Luque rods or Mizuno plates). CONCLUSIONS: Anterior decompression and fixation is preferred over posterior fixation for teardrop fracture dislocations. Again, this conclusion should be considered carefully due to the older posterior fixation techniques.
Lifeso and Colucci (2000)[8]	Retrospective comparative study of unilateral facet injuries (anterior vs posterior vs conservative treatment)	29 retrospective controls and 18 prospectively evaluated patients with unilateral facet injuries and 3–5 mm anterior translation. The retrospective controls were treated with hard collar (12), halo (6), or posterior fusion (11, variety of methods). The prospective patients all had single-level ACDF. Posterior fusion had a success rate of 55% (6/11), whereas anterior fusion had a success rate of 100% - Considered low quality due to its retrospective nature and heterogeneous cohort.

(Continued on page 332)

Table 33.2 Studies Considered to Provide Low-Quality Evidence (Retrospective Comparative Clinical Studies) *(Continued)*

	CONCLUSIONS: Anterior fusion was more successful at achieving fusion and maintaining alignment than posterior fusion, although in the posterior group only 5 of 11 had lateral mass screws, whereas the others had wiring techniques. Hence it is a weak comparison between anterior and posterior approaches, and this should be considered when drawing conclusions from this study.

Abbreviations: ACDF, anterior cervical discectomy and fusion.

Table 33.3 Studies Considered to Provide Very Low Quality Evidence (Retrospective Clinical Case Series or Biomechanical In Vitro Studies)

Rabb et al (2007)[12]	Retrospective case series	Retrospective review of 25 patients with unilateral facet fracture/-subluxations treated surgically. 21 were treated with single-level ACDF and plate fixation, 3 with lateral mass screws, 1 combined. No comparisons drawn. All fused. No characterization of the actual injury (translation or kyphosis) was described. CONCLUSIONS: Anterior fixation alone provides sufficient stability for fusion of unilateral facet fractures with subluxation.
Mizuno et al (2007)[13]	Retrospective comparative study of anterior versus posterior versus combined fixation for unilateral and bilateral facet lock injuries	Retrospective review of 6 unilateral and 4 bilateral facet lock injuries with associated SCI treated with anterior (5), posterior (3), and combined (2) fixation. One patient treated with posterior fixation had delayed neurological deterioration secondary to traumatic disk herniation (and hence required anterior fixation). - Considered very low quality despite its comparative nature due to its small numbers and lack of outcome measures (clinical or radiographic) to distinguish the anterior from posterior and combined approaches. CONCLUSIONS: Anterior or posterior fixation alone are sufficient to stabilize unilateral or bilateral fact injuries, although the small numbers make it difficult to place a great deal of weight on this conclusion.
Elgafy et al (2006)[7]	Retrospective case series	Radiographic review of 27 unilateral and 38 bilateral facet injuries treated with single-level posterior segmental fixation (lateral mass plates, interspinous wiring, or both). Mean translation and kyphosis of 5 mm and 9.8 degrees were reduced to 0 mm and 3.7 degrees lordosis at a follow-up of at least 12 months. Fusion was achieved in 97%, although healing in more than 5 degrees of kyphosis was associated with significant preoperative kyphosis ($>$ 5 degrees), and advanced age. CONCLUSIONS: Posterior fusion alone for unilateral and bilateral facet injuries results in a high fusion rate; elderly patients with significant preoperative kyphosis are high risk of healing in significant kyphosis.
Ianuzzi et al (2006)[14]	Biomechanics study comparing anterior and posterior fixation	Biomechanical study of cervical flexion teardrop fracture with complete DLC disruption. Single-level fixations with anterior, posterior, or combined approaches were compared, and then a corpectomy model compared anterior versus combined fixation. All fixation constructs were stiffer than the intact spinal segment. In general, combined fixation provided greater reduction in motion than anterior or posterior alone. - Considered very low quality because even though it is a comparative study, it is an in vitro experiment CONCLUSIONS: the greatest reduction in intervertebral motion is achieved with combined anterior/posterior fixation, although either approach alone provides greater stiffness than the intact segment.
Kotani et al (2005)[15]	Retrospective case series	Retrospective review of 23 lateral mass fractures and 8 facet joint fractures treated with posterior pedicle screws (and 4 with additional anterior stabilization). All fused, and the need to fuse an additional level was obviated in about half of the cases due to the use of pedicle fixation. Alignment was well maintained. CONCLUSIONS: Pedicle screw fixation provides good fixation and high union rate and can obviate the need for extending the fusion to an additional level. It should be noted that this fixation technique (pedicle screws in the subaxial spine above C7) is not widely used outside of Japan.
Johnson et al (2004)[6]	Retrospective case series	Radiographic review of 22 unilateral and 65 bilateral facet injuries treated with ACDF with locking plate. Mean translation and kyphosis of 4.6 mm and 7.5 degrees were reduced to 0.9 mm and 3.6 degrees of lordosis at follow-up of at least 9 months. Radiographic failure occurred in 11 patients (13%), and was highly associated with the presence of an end plate fracture of the subjacent vertebra. No correlation between radiographic failure and injury type (unilateral or bilateral) was found.

		CONCLUSIONS: Anterior fusion alone for unilateral and bilateral facet injuries usually results in good realignment and solid fusion but has a high rate of failure in the presence of an end plate fracture.
Henriques et al (2004)[16]	Retrospective case series	Retrospective review of ACDF with plate fixation alone for 36 patients with distractive flexion injuries (6 flexion sprain, 17 unilateral, and 13 bilateral facet dislocation). 15 of 17 unilateral facet patients and 6 of 13 bilateral facet patients healed without loss of alignment. CONCLUSIONS: Anterior fixation alone leads to a high fusion rate for unilateral facet injuries but has a very high rate of failure for bilateral facet injuries.
Lambiris et al (2003)[17]	Retrospective case series	Retrospective review of 53 patients undergoing ACDF for a variety of subaxial cervical injuries. Radiographic fusion was observed in all patients and none had local kyphosis > 10 degrees, although 15% had screw malposition, 1 patient had translation > 2.5 mm. CONCLUSIONS: Anterior fixation alone provides a high fusion rate with acceptable maintenance of alignment.
Hadley[18] Clin. Neurosurg. 49: 407–98, March 2002	Qualitative systematic review of low and very low quality studies	Review of reports (predominantly retrospective case series) of surgical and nonsurgical treatment of a heterogeneous group of either subaxial cervical injuries, distractive flexion injuries, or compressive flexion injuries. - Considered very low quality because a primary question was not asked, and it did not attempt to address the question of this chapter (which surgical approach is better). CONCLUSIONS: The literature would indicate that both anterior and posterior fixation are valid treatment options for facet injuries or flexion-teardrop injuries.
Fisher et al (2002)[19]	Retrospective comparative study (Surgery versus Halo)	Retrospective review of 17 teardrop fractures treated with anterior fusion, versus 22 treated with halo vest. Anterior fusion led to a significantly higher fusion rate (100%) and better sagittal alignment than halo vest immobilization. - Considered very low quality because the primary question of this chapter is not whether to treat surgically or nonoperatively, but which surgical approach is better CONCLUSIONS: Anterior fusion results in a high fusion rate and better sagittal alignment for teardrop fractures than halo vest immobilization.
Koh et al (2001)[20]	Biomechanics study comparing anterior and posterior fixation	Biomechanical comparison of anterior cervical plating versus posterior lateral mass screw–plate fixation (either alone or in combination) for fixation of a single-level flexion distraction injury or fixation of a single-level corpectomy (for burst fracture). In both models, posterior fixation was better than anterior fixation at controlling motion, with a combination of the two providing the most stability. - Considered very low quality because even though it is a comparative study, it is an in vitro experiment. CONCLUSIONS: Posterior lateral mass screw–plate fixation is superior to anterior fixation alone in cadaveric modeling of flexion-distraction injuries.
Razack et al (2000)[21]	Retrospective case series	Retrospective review of 22 patients with bilateral facet dislocations treated with single-level ACDF and plate fixation alone. All 22 patients fused, although one sustained a plate fracture at 7 months postop (but eventually healed). CONCLUSIONS: Anterior fixation alone provides sufficient stability for bilateral facet dislocations.
Koivikko[22] Arch Orthop Trauma Surg 2000	Retrospective case series	Retrospective comparison between 34 burst/teardrop fractures treated with halo vs 35 treated with anterior cervical fusion. Of the group treated surgically, one had screw loosening. Alignment was significantly better in surgically treated patients than halo treated. Alignment showed 7.4% translation and 2.2 degrees lordosis in anterior fixation patients, 21.5% and 12.6 degrees kyphosis in halo. - Similar to the Fisher et al paper, this is a comparison between surgery and nonop care and so for the purposes of this chapter (which asks which surgical approach is better) this study represents a retrospective case series CONCLUSIONS: Anterior surgery provides better alignment than halo immobilization.
Shapiro et al (1999)[23]	Retrospective case series	Retrospective review of 46 cases of unilateral facet dislocation treated with interspinous and facet wiring versus interspinous braided cable and lateral mass plates. In the first 24 patients with interspinous and facet wiring, one required anterior fusion for fixation failure. In the second 22 patients with braided cable and lateral mass plates, 5 had supplemental ACDFs (due to disk herniation)—fusion was seen in all patients. They report that 46% of the wiring and 64% of the cable–plate

(*Continued on page 334*)

		patients had "perfect" anatomical realignment, suggesting that the cable–plate fixation provides better sustained alignment. CONCLUSIONS: Interspinous braided cable with lateral mass plate fixation provides a high fusion rate with good sagittal alignment.
Ebraheim et al (1995)[24]	Retrospective case series	Retrospective review of 30 patients, among which there were 12 unilateral facet dislocations, 2 bilateral facet dislocations, 7 ligamentous instabilities, 3 burst fractures, and 2 teardrop fractures treated with posterior lateral mass screws/plates. Fusion was obtained reliably, although 6 patients had screw loosening - Weaknesses of this study include the heterogeneity of the cohort—some with tumor or cervical myelopathy—and the poor radiographic characterization of the injuries. CONCLUSIONS: Posterior fixation provides a high union rate with acceptable maintenance of alignment.
Fehlings et al (1994)[25]	Retrospective case series	Retrospective review of 44 patients treated with posterior lateral mass screw–plate constructs. 29 had unilateral and bilateral facet injuries with a variety of posterior element fractures, 10 had burst/teardrop fractures. Three patients required revision (2 posterior, 1 anterior). CONCLUSIONS: Posterior stabilization results in a high union rate for these fractures.
Levine et al (1992)[26]	Retrospective case series	Retrospective review of 24 fracture/separations of the lateral mass ("floating lateral mass") treated with posterior lateral mass plating. All eventually fused. 16 had anatomical reductions, 8 healed in kyphosis (4 with ≤5 degrees, 3 with ≤10 degrees, ≤1 with 30 degrees of kyphosis). CONCLUSIONS: Posterior fusion provides a high fusion rate with reliable maintenance of alignment in most patients.
Cybulski et al (1992)[27]	Retrospective case series	Retrospective review of 21 patients with subaxial cervical injuries who required circumferential fixation after persistent instability was noted following posterior interspinous or facet wiring with bone grafting. 9 had "locked facets" and 7 had teardrop injuries. - Weaknesses of this study include the heterogeneity of the cohort and the older fixation techniques (posterior wiring or anterior fusion without plating) CONCLUSIONS: The authors conclude that anterior interbody fusion (without plating) or posterior fixation alone is insufficient to stabilize the spine in the presence of a three-column injury.
Ripa et al (1991)[28]	Retrospective case series	Retrospective review of 92 patients with subaxial injuries treated with anterior fixation alone—48 with "grossly unstable three-column injuries," 20 with anterior vertebral body fracture with kyphosis, and 13 with posterior ligament disruption with anterior disk herniation. Fusion was achieved in 98.9% by 3.1 months; 13% had evidence of "less than ideal hardware position" and one had loss of spinal alignment with translation > 2.5 mm. - Weaknesses of this study include the heterogeneity of the cohort and the older anterior plate technology (nonlocking plate) CONCLUSIONS: Anterior fusion provides a high rate of fusion with reliable maintenance of alignment.
Aebi et al (1991)[29]	Retrospective case series	22 burst/teardrop injuries and 64 DLC or osteoligamentous injuries (unilateral/bilateral facet dislocations, fracture-separations of the lateral masses), all treated with anterior fixation with nonlocking plates. All patients went on to fuse by 3–4 months, though there was one screw loosening and one plate fracture. No patients had translation greater than 2 mm or kyphosis of more than 10 degrees upon healing. - Weaknesses of this study include the older plate technology, heterogeneity of injuries, and only briefly characterized radiographic data on fusion and alignment) CONCLUSIONS: Anterior fusion (even with a nonlocking plate) provides a high union rate with acceptable alignment.
Anderson et al (1991)[30]	Retrospective case series	Retrospective review of 9 burst fractures and 19 subluxations treated with posterior AO reconstruction plates and ICBG. All patients had solid unions. Between surgery and final follow-up there was an average 1.1 degree increase in kyphosis, but no translation greater than 0.5 mm. CONCLUSIONS: Posterior fixation provides a high union rate with acceptable maintenance of alignment.
Beyer et al (1991)[31]	Retrospective case series	Retrospective review of 36 patients with unilateral facet injuries 10 of whom were treated with posterior interspinous wiring, 26 of whom were treated nonoperatively. The patients who were treated with posterior fusion had better clinical and radiographic outcomes. - Weaknesses include small patient sample and older fixation techniques (interspinous wiring).

Table 33.3 Studies Considered to Provide Very Low Quality Evidence (Retrospective Clinical Case Series or Biomechanical In Vitro Studies) (*Continued*)

		CONCLUSIONS: Posterior fixation provides better clinical and radiographic results than halo immobilization for unilateral facet injuries.
Cooper et al (1988)[32]	Retrospective case series	Retrospective review of 19 patients with "fractures and/or subluxations" from C3–C7. Two patients (one with ankylosing spondylitis) had failure of fixation, whereas the remaining healed. - Weakness includes the lack of characterization of the type of injury. CONCLUSIONS: Posterior fixation alone provides a reliable method of stabilizing the cervical spine.
Goffin et al (1989)[33]	Retrospective case series	Retrospective review of 41 patients with a variety of injuries (7 bilateral facet dislocations, 5 unilateral facet dislocations, 9 anterior subluxations, 9 vertebral body compression fractures, 5 hangman's fractures, and 6 hyperextension injuries. All but two patients had "excellent immediate postoperative stability"—two required revision due to loosening. No comment on long-term radiographic outcome. - Weaknesses include the patient heterogeneity, older fixation, poor description of results. CONCLUSIONS: Anterior fixation provides good immediate stability (providing a rationale for surgical treatment over prolonged traction and halo immobilization).

Abbreviations: ACDF, anterior cervical discectomy and fusion; AO, Arbeitgemeinschaft für Osteosynthesefragen; DLC, discoligamentous complex; ICBG, iliac crest bone graft; SCI, spinal cord injury.

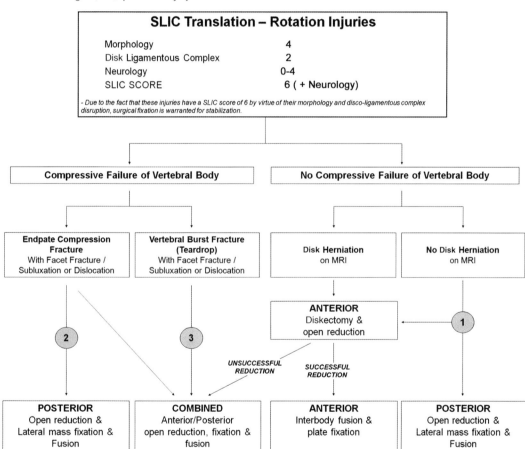

Recommendation 1. Based on published clinical evidence that is weak and the expert opinion of the members of the Spine Trauma Study Group, it is **strongly recommended** that unilateral and bilateral facet injuries can be treated via either anterior or posterior fixation alone, provided that there is no endplate or vertebral body fracture and that there is no displaced disk causing ventral cord compression. The decision of choosing anterior or posterior fixation can therefore be reasonably based on surgeon preference and patient preference.

Recommendation 2. Based on published clinical evidence that is weak and the expert opinion of the members of the Spine Trauma Study Group, it is **weakly recommended** that unilateral and bilateral facet injuries in the presence of an endplate fracture but in the absence of a disk herniation should be treated posteriorly.

Recommendation 3. Based on published clinical evidence that is WEAK and the expert opinion of the members of the Spine Trauma Study Group, it is **weakly recommended** that unilateral and bilateral facet injuries in the presence of a vertebral body fracture (i.e., Teardrop/burst) should be treated with circumferential stabilization (particularly when the facets are fractured).

Fig. 33.4 Recommendations for treatment of Subaxial Cervical Spine Injury Classification (SLIC) rotation/translation injuries.

subluxations (perched facets without fracture) developed higher degrees of kyphosis following posterior instrumented fusion.[7] It was postulated (similar to Kwon et al[3]) that the disruption of the disk that occurs with these distraction injuries leads to progressive disk space collapse which the posterior fixation is unable to overcome, thus allowing the spinal segment to drift into kyphosis. This tendency of posterior fusions to lead to kyphosis has been identified by Lifeso, who recommended anterior plating for these injuries.[8] The long-term clinical significance of segmental kyphosis remains to be seen.

3. Based on published clinical evidence that is weak *and* the expert opinion of the members of the STSG, *it is weakly recommended* that unilateral and bilateral facet injuries in the presence of a vertebral body fracture (i.e., teardrop/burst) should be treated with circumferential stabilization (particularly when the facets are fractured). This recommendation was made with concern expressed about the nature of the vertebral body fracture and posterior injury and the influence that this has on decision making. It is recognized that an axial burst fracture which does not have significant posterior element injury is conceptually different from the rotation/translation injury (and is represented differently in the SLIC scale), but that the distinction may not always be clear.

The recommendations for treatment of SLIC rotation/translation injuries can be summarized in the algorithm depicted in **Fig. 33.4.**

References

1. Vaccaro AR, Hulbert RJ, Patel AA, et al; Spine Trauma Study Group. The subaxial cervical spine injury classification system: a novel approach to recognize the importance of morphology, neurology, and integrity of the disco-ligamentous complex. Spine 2007;32:2365–2374
2. Schünemann HJ, Jaeschke R, Cook DJ, et al; ATS Documents Development and Implementation Committee. An official ATS statement: grading the quality of evidence and strength of recommendations in ATS guidelines and recommendations. Am J Respir Crit Care Med 2006;174:605–614
3. Kwon BK, Fisher CG, Boyd MC, et al. A prospective randomized controlled trial of anterior compared with posterior stabilization for unilateral facet injuries of the cervical spine. J Neurosurg Spine 2007;7:1–12
4. Brodke DS, Anderson PA, Newell DW, Grady MS, Chapman JR. Comparison of anterior and posterior approaches in cervical spinal cord injuries. J Spinal Disord Tech 2003;16:229–235
5. Spector LR, Kim DH, Affonso J, Albert TJ, Hilibrand AS, Vaccaro AR. Use of computed tomography to predict failure of nonoperative treatment of unilateral facet fractures of the cervical spine. Spine 2006;31:2827–2835
6. Johnson MG, Fisher CG, Boyd M, Pitzen T, Oxland TR, Dvorak MF. The radiographic failure of single segment anterior cervical plate fixation in traumatic cervical flexion distraction injuries. Spine 2004;29:2815–2820
7. Elgafy H, Fisher CG, Zhao Y, et al. The radiographic failure of single segment posterior cervical instrumentation in traumatic cervical flexion distraction injuries. Top Spinal Cord Inj Rehabil 2006;12:20–29
8. Lifeso RM, Colucci MA. Anterior fusion for rotationally unstable cervical spine fractures. Spine 2000;25:2028–2034
9. Dvorak MF, Fisher CG, Fehlings MG, et al. The surgical approach to subaxial cervical spine injuries: an evidence-based algorithm based on the SLIC classification system. Spine 2007;32:2620–2629
10. Song KJ, Lee KB. Anterior versus combined anterior and posterior fixation/fusion in the treatment of distraction-flexion injury in the lower cervical spine. J Clin Neurosci 2008;15:36–42
11. Toh E, Nomura T, Watanabe M, Mochida J. Surgical treatment for injuries of the middle and lower cervical spine. Int Orthop 2006;30:54–58
12. Rabb CH, Lopez J, Beauchamp K, Witt P, Bolles G, Dwyer A. Unilateral cervical facet fractures with subluxation: injury patterns and treatment. J Spinal Disord Tech 2007;20:416–422
13. Mizuno J, Nakagawa H, Inoue T, Nonaka Y, Song J, Romli TM. Spinal instrumentation for interfacet locking injuries of the subaxial cervical spine. J Clin Neurosci 2007;14:49–52
14. Ianuzzi A, Zambrano I, Tataria J, et al. Biomechanical evaluation of surgical constructs for stabilization of cervical teardrop fractures. Spine J 2006;6:514–523
15. Kotani Y, Abumi K, Ito M, Minami A. Cervical spine injuries associated with lateral mass and facet joint fractures: new classification and surgical treatment with pedicle screw fixation. Eur Spine J 2005;14:69–77
16. Henriques T, Olerud C, Bergman A, Jónsson H Jr. Distractive flexion injuries of the subaxial cervical spine treated with anterior plate alone. J Spinal Disord Tech 2004;17:1–7
17. Lambiris E, Zouboulis P, Tyllianakis M, Panagiotopoulos E. Anterior surgery for unstable lower cervical spine injuries. Clin Orthop Relat Res 2003;(411):61–69
18. Hadley MN, Fitzpatrick BC, Sonntag VK, Browner CM. Facet fracture-dislocation injuries of the cervical spine. Neurosurgery 1992;30:661–666
19. Fisher CG, Dvorak MF, Leith J, Wing PC. Comparison of outcomes for unstable lower cervical flexion teardrop fractures managed with halo thoracic vest versus anterior corpectomy and plating. Spine 2002;27:160–166
20. Do Koh Y, Lim TH, Won You J, Eck J, An HS. A biomechanical comparison of modern anterior and posterior plate fixation of the cervical spine. Spine 2001;26:15–21
21. Razack N, Green BA, Levi AD. The management of traumatic cervical bilateral facet fracture-dislocations with unicortical anterior plates. J Spinal Disord 2000;13:374–381
22. Koivikko MP, Myllynen P, Santavirta S. Fracture dislocations of the cervical spine: a review of 106 conservatively and operatively treated patients. Eur Spine J 2004;13:610–616
23. Shapiro S, Snyder W, Kaufman K, Abel T. Outcome of 51 cases of unilateral locked cervical facets: interspinous braided cable for lateral mass plate fusion compared with interspinous wire and facet wiring with iliac crest. J Neurosurg 1999;91(1, Suppl):19–24
24. Ebraheim NA, Rupp RE, Savolaine ER, Brown JA. Posterior plating of the cervical spine. J Spinal Disord 1995;8:111–115
25. Fehlings MG, Cooper PR, Errico TJ. Posterior plates in the management of cervical instability: long-term results in 44 patients. J Neurosurg 1994;81:341–349
26. Levine AM, Mazel C, Roy-Camille R. Management of fracture separations of the articular mass using posterior cervical plating. Spine 1992;17(10, Suppl):S447–S454
27. Cybulski GR, Douglas RA, Meyer PR Jr, Rovin RA. Complications in three-column cervical spine injuries requiring anterior-posterior stabilization. Spine 1992;17:253–256
28. Ripa DR, Kowall MG, Meyer PR Jr, Rusin JJ. Series of ninety-two traumatic cervical spine injuries stabilized with anterior ASIF plate fusion technique. Spine 1991;16(3, Suppl):S46–S55
29. Aebi M, Zuber K, Marchesi D. Treatment of cervical spine injuries with anterior plating. Indications, techniques, and results. Spine 1991;16(3, Suppl):S38–S45
30. Anderson PA, Henley MB, Grady MS, Montesano PX, Winn HR. Posterior cervical arthrodesis with AO reconstruction plates and bone graft. Spine 1991;16(3, Suppl):S72–S79
31. Beyer CA, Cabanela ME, Berquist TH. Unilateral facet dislocations and fracture-dislocations of the cervical spine. J Bone Joint Surg Br 1991;73:977–981
32. Cooper PR, Cohen A, Rosiello A, Koslow M. Posterior stabilization of cervical spine fractures and subluxations using plates and screws. Neurosurgery 1988;23:300–306
33. Goffin J, Plets C, Van den Bergh R. Anterior cervical fusion and osteosynthetic stabilization according to Caspar: a prospective study of 41 patients with fractures and/or dislocations of the cervical spine. Neurosurgery 1989;25:865–871

34

Management of Cervical Thoracic Junctional Injuries

Christopher I. Shaffrey and Justin S. Smith

Traumatic injuries at the cervicothoracic junction are a relatively rare event compared with injury to other areas of the cervical spine. This injury has been reported in between 2% and 9% of all cervical fractures and dislocations.[1–4] Complete or incomplete neurological deficits are quite common with injuries in this location.[1,2,5,6] Missed or delayed diagnosis is common at the cervicothoracic region on standard lateral cervical spine radiographs.[7] Evaluation by lateral radiographs is particularly compromised in muscular or obese patients and in cases of polytrauma.[1,2,8] A range of injures can occur, including vertebral body fractures, unilateral and bilateral facet dislocations, fracture-dislocations, and isolated fractures of the posterior elements.[1–4,9]

Unique anatomical and biomechanical forces are present where the lordotic and highly mobile cervical spine joins the kyphotic and relatively immobile thoracic spine. Historically, treatment of cervicothoracic injuries has included the use of external orthoses and halo immobilization with limited success. With the introduction of modern spinal instrumentation, the management approach has shifted to surgical treatment with reduction, instrumentation, and fusion.[6,9] Due to the relative rarity of these injuries, the ideal surgical approach for management has not been clearly defined. There is debate over whether the vast majority of these injures can be treated with a posterior only approach or if anterior or combined approaches have clearly defined roles for these injuries. The roles for plain radiographs, computed tomography (CT), and magnetic resonance imaging (MRI) for the diagnosis of cervicothoracic injury are undecided.

◆ Epidemiology and Classification Systems

Traumatic injury to the cervicothoracic junction is relatively uncommon. Evans demonstrated an incidence of 2.4% for fracture or fracture-dislocation at the C7–T1 level in 587 cervical injuries accumulated over a 26-year period.[2] Amin and Saifuddin found a 4.49% incidence of cervicothoracic fracture-dislocations in a retrospective review of 156 spine injuries.[1] Nichols et al reported an incidence of 9% of cervicothoracic junction injuries in 397 cervical spine injuries.[4] Motor vehicle accidents are the most common cause of injury, followed by falls from a height.[5,9] Burst fractures, unilateral and bilateral facet dislocations, fracture-dislocations, lateral mass fractures, and neural arch fractures have all been reported. The reported incidence of fracture-dislocations ranges from 26 to 86%.[1,5,6]

Multiple classification systems have been proposed to categorize injuries to both the cervical and thoracic spine but none are unique to the cervicothoracic junction.[10–12] A mechanistic classification as proposed by Allen and Ferguson and colleagues for subaxial cervical spine injuries has been occasionally used for cervicothoracic trauma.[13] Six categories of injury have been described, including compressive flexion, vertical compression, distractive flexion, compressive extension, distractive extension, and lateral flexion.[13] The majority of recent reports use descriptive terminology for the classification of injury, similar to that recently proposed by Vaccaro and associates based on injury severity.[12] In the Subaxial Injury Classification (SLIC) and Severity Scale injury morphology is categorized as compression, burst fracture, distraction injuries, and rotation/translation injuries based on progressive instability.[12] Lenoir et al used both descriptive and the AO classification.[5] The AO classification is based on principles for long bone fracture classification and was originally proposed by Magerl et al and subsequently modified by Gertzbein.[14,15] The overall AO classification is based on three basic fracture types: A (compression injuries), B (distraction injuries), and C (torsion injuries).[14,15]

◆ Clinical and Diagnostic Features

The cervicothoracic junction is a difficult area to image using plain radiographs. Rethnam recently reported a series 100 swimmer's view radiographs randomly selected over a 2-year period in trauma patients.[16] The radiographs were assessed for adequate visualization of the C7 body and C7–T1 junction. Only 55% of the radiographs were adequate. None of the inadequate radiographs provided satisfactory visualization of the C7 body and the C7–T1 junction.[16] In a prospective study of 73 severely injured patients, Jelly and associates found 12 patients with fractures of the cervicothoracic junction using spiral CT.[17] Conventional radiography demonstrated injury in only five of these 12 patients (42%). Because of these imaging difficulties, delays in diagnosis are not uncommon. Evans in 1991 reported on 14 dislocations at the cervicothoracic junction, with nearly two thirds not properly diagnosed on admission.[2] More recently, Amin reported a delay in diagnosis in three of seven (43%) patients with cervicothoracic injury.[1]

Tan et al reported a series of 360 blunt trauma patients in whom the C7–T1 level was not adequately visualized on plain radiographs.[18] Using CT, 11 injuries to the cervicothoracic junction were discovered. The cost-effectiveness of CT for averting potential sequelae was $9192 for each fracture identified, $16,852 for each potentially or definitely unstable fracture identified, and $50,557 for each definitely unstable fracture identified.[18] CT imaging is also useful for surgical planning by providing an assessment of the integrity of osseous structures adjacent to the injury site and by enabling measurement for implants, particularly in this area where anatomical variability exists.[19]

The role for MRI in cervicothoracic junction injury has been poorly defined. Several recent publications have recommended the use of MRI when the presence and severity of cervicothoracic injury have not been clearly defined.[1,5,8] MRI may be helpful to characterize the severity of injury to the neural elements and to identify evidence of hematoma, as well as to assess for the presence of disk herniation or ligamentous injury that may contribute to ongoing neural compromise or result in spinal instability. The role for MRI in incomplete neurological deficits prior to reduction and fixation has not been defined for cervicothoracic injury.

Neurological deficits are common with these injuries. Nichols found neurological deficits occurred in 22 of 37 patients (59%) with cervicothoracic injury.[4] Twelve of the 22 patients (54.5%) had paraplegia or quadriplegia and 10 of 22 (45.5%) had less substantial neurological deficits. In a series of six patients with cervicothoracic injury, Sapkas et al demonstrated some form of neurological deficit in each patient, with one patient having a Frankel A deficit, one each having a Frankel B and C grade, and three having nerve root injuries.[6] Amin and Saifuddin found neurological deficits in six of seven patients, with three of seven patients presenting with Frankel A neurological deficits and three with Frankel D deficits.[1] Lenoir et al evaluated 30 patients who underwent surgery for unstable cervicothoracic injury and also found on initial clinical examination neurological deficits in every patient.[5] Sixteen of the patients were classified Frankel A with a spectrum of incomplete deficits occurring (6 Frankel B, 2 Frankel C, and 6 Frankel D).[5]

Because of the mechanisms involved in cervicothoracic junctional injury, injuries to other organ systems are common. Lenoir et al used American Society of Anesthesiologists (ASA) scoring to evaluate preoperative condition of 30 patients with cervicothoracic junction injuries and found nine patients with an initial ASA score of 3 or 4, indicating substantial preoperative comorbidity.

◆ Nonoperative Management

Historically, nonoperative treatment, including prolonged bed rest with immobilization or bracing, was utilized as the primary treatment for cervicothoracic injuries.[2] Evans reported on 14 patients with cervicothoracic injury with the majority treated with manipulation or skeletal traction. Four patients died within 7 weeks from pulmonary emboli. One patient developed a cerebral abscess from skeletal tongs that resulted in temporary hemiparesis.[2] Neurological recovery with nonoperative management was poor. Each patient with a complete neurological injury either died (four patients) or had no improvement in neurological status (seven patients). However, all three patients with incomplete neurological deficits became ambulatory.[2] Successful treatment of compression fractures, lateral mass fractures, and spinous process fractures has been demonstrated using either external orthosis or halo immobilization.[1]

◆ Surgical Treatment

The treatment goals for the surgical management of cervicothoracic injuries include reduction of the fracture and/or dislocation, direct or indirect decompression of the neural elements (when applicable), and achievement of rigid fixation to permit rapid mobilization without the use of a halo vest immobilization. Evolution of surgical techniques and spinal instrumentation has profoundly influenced the management of these injuries. Application of anterior and posterior spinal instrumentation is complicated by poor visualization of the cervicothoracic junction using standard intraoperative radiographic techniques.[19]

Isolated anterior instrumentation and fusion are commonly performed in the subaxial cervical spine for fractures and dislocations. However, for cervicothoracic junction fractures and dislocations, anterior approaches are used less commonly due to the presence of the sternum, clavicle, and great vessels inhibiting access to this region of the spine.

The transition from cervical lordosis to thoracic kyphosis causes significant variation in wound depth.[9] The mediastinal structures substantially complicate placement of anterior spinal instrumentation and may necessitate a medial clavicle resection, partial or complete sternotomy, or high thoracotomy to achieve adequate access.[8] Relatively poorer bone quality of the upper thoracic vertebral bodies and the biomechanical shortcoming of anterior-only instrumentation have limited the use of anterior only techniques.[20] Although several articles have reported successful outcomes for anterior-only decompression and instrumentation for pathological fractures of the cervicothoracic junction, the reported use for fractures and dislocations is extremely limited.[21]

Prior to the advent of rigid posterior fixation techniques, circumferential procedures were routinely recommended by some authors. Sapkas et al performed a retrospective review of 10 patients treated with cervicothoracic pathology.[6] Six of these patients had cervicothoracic fractures or fracture-dislocations. Five of the 10 patients were managed with circumferential procedures. There were three excellent, five good, and two fair results. Two cases that were treated with spinous process wiring and one that was treated with Hartshill frame–rod with wires had imperfect reduction with subsequent loss of the reduction. In contrast, those patients treated with screw–plate fixation had no loss of reduction or complications.[6]

Most posterior instrumentation techniques used at the cervicothoracic junction are modifications of techniques used for subaxial cervical and thoracic fixation. Historically, spinous process and sublaminar wiring were the principle method of fixation despite biomechanical shortcomings. An evolution from wire–rod techniques to screw–plate and finally to screw and hook–rod techniques has occurred over the past 20 years.[22]

Chapman et al reported a consecutive series of 23 patients treated for cervicothoracic instability (19 with fractures or ligamentous instability caused by trauma) treated with an AO reconstruction plate and screw fixation of the cervical and thoracic spine.[9] The number of motion segments fused ranged from two to nine with an average of four. All patients obtained a solid fusion and there were few complications. More recently Lenoir evaluated 30 patients who underwent posterior reduction, instrumentation, and fusion for cervicothoracic trauma.[5] Satisfactory fracture injury reduction was achieved in almost all patients. One patient had residual lateral translation when evaluated by CT scan. Fusion occurred in all patients but there were two cases of instrumentation loosening prior to arthrodesis occurring.

Although there are several reports describing use of screw–rod instrumentation systems for management of instability caused by tumors of the cervicothoracic junction, the number of reports detailing use in cervicothoracic trauma is limited.[23,24] Screw–rod systems provide flexibility in correcting deformity, result in immediate rigid internal fixation, and result in high rates of fusion. Rods accommodate a range of cervical and thoracic fixation options, including lateral mass screws, cervical pedicle screws, thoracic pedicle screws, and thoracic hooks.[22] Tapered rods, dual-diameter rods, and domino (rod–rod) connectors permit joining cervical lateral mass and pedicle screws with thoracic pedicle screws or hooks.[25]

A challenge in optimizing fixation at the cervicothoracic junction is created by the unique bony morphology of C7. This vertebra commonly has a smaller lateral mass compared with the rest of the subaxial cervical spine limiting adequate lateral mass screw fixation. A C7 pedicle screw has biomechanical advantages compared with a lateral mass screw but has increased risk of neurological injury with imprecise placement. Rhee et al demonstrated in biomechanical testing in a cadaver model that when stabilizing C7–T1 with T1 pedicle screws, a C7 pedicle screw construct provides significantly greater normalized stiffness than a C7 lateral mass screw construct in axial compression, torsion, bending, and flexion.[26] However, if lateral mass fixation is extended to include both C6 and C7, a construct with similar normalized stiffness to that using C7 pedicle screws can be achieved except in axial compression. Supplemental spinous wiring by the triple wire method did not significantly increase the normalized stiffness of the lateral mass constructs tested.[26]

Accurate placement of pedicle screws at the cervicothoracic junction is complicated by greater medial angulation of the pedicles at the cervicothoracic junction compared with the lower thoracic spine and difficulty with intraoperative imaging. Lee and associates assessed for pedicle breach on postoperative CT in 60 consecutive patients who underwent a variety of posterior spinal procedures, including pedicle screw placement at C7, T1, and T2.[19] A total of 86, 63, and 45 screws were placed using open (laminoforaminotomy), two-dimensional (2-D) fluoroscopy and three-dimensional (3-D) computer-assisted techniques. Independent review of the CT imaging demonstrated that screws were completely within the pedicle in 70.9% with open placement, 81% with 2-D placement, and 89% with 3-D placement. No screws required revision in any group.[19]

Neurological recovery is principally dictated by neurological function at the time of injury. Lenoir et al documented that all 16 patients with Frankel A injuries remained unchanged. Complete or partial neurological recovery was recorded in nine or 14 patients with an initial neurological status of Frankel B, C, or D. Only one patient deteriorated in this series (Frankel C to

Frankel B).[5] Similarly, Amin and Saifuddin recently found each patient with a Frankel A deficit did not recover, whereas all patients with incomplete injuries (Frankel D) recovered to grade E.[1] Chapman et al documented better neurological recovery. Of seven patients with complete spinal cord injury (Frankel A), five remained unchanged, one improved to grade B, and one to grade C. All incomplete quadriplegics improved at least one Frankel grade. All three grade D patients improved to grade E. Of the four patients with grade C incomplete spinal cord injury, two improved to grade D, and two improved to grade E.[9]

◆ Potential Complications

Complications are common after surgical management of cervicothoracic injury. Lenoir et al documented 23 of 30 patients remained in the intensive care unit an average of 33 days. Ten patients developed pulmonary infections, including a case of adult respiratory distress syndrome. Eight patients required temporary tracheostomy. One case of pulmonary embolus resulting in patient death was noted. Two cases of wound infection and two cases of instrumentation failure were detailed. Other smaller series demonstrated a similar spectrum of complications.[5]

◆ Recommendations

Can most cervicothoracic junction injures be treated with a posterior only approach or are there clearly defined roles for anterior or combined approaches for specific categories of injury?

Recommendation (Strength)

The literature provides no consensus on the optimal surgical approach (**Table 34.1**). There is no established fundamental strategy for the application of instrumentation for the treatment of an unstable cervicothoracic spine. The two largest series document satisfactory management of these injures utilizing exclusively a posterior reduction, instrumentation, and fusion procedure (weak). Biomechanical data demonstrate deficiencies in flexion/extension of very unstable injuries with posterior instrumentation alone, even with fixation from C5–T3.[27] Circumferential reconstruction improved stability in models with great instability (weak).[27,28] In cases of substantial ventral decompression caused by bone or disk material, the option of ventral decompression (± instrumentation) followed by posterior instrumentation is supported by a limited number of reported cases (weak).

Are there clearly defined roles for plain radiographs, CT, and MRI for the diagnosis of cervicothoracic injury?

Recommendation (Strength)

Plain radiographs have deficiencies as the sole radiographic method of evaluating cervicothoracic injury in high-energy blunt trauma and multitrauma patients (strong) (**Table 34.1**). The literature supports the use of CT for the evaluation of the cervicothoracic junction in cases of high-energy blunt trauma, in trauma cases where the cervicothoracic junction is poorly visualized, in cases where injury is suspected on

Table 34.1 Results of Systematic Review

Study	Description	Quality of Evidence	Topic and Conclusion
Chapman et al (1996)[9]	Retrospective case series	Very low	Assessment of neurological and radiological outcomes, as well as complications, following posterior instrumentation for instability of the cervicothoracic region (23 patients). CONCLUSIONS: No neurovascular or pulmonary complications associated with surgery. All patients achieved solid arthrodesis without instrumentation complications requiring reoperation. One case of wound infection. No patient's neurological status deteriorated after surgery. Five patients with radiculopathy all improved to asymptomatic at follow-up. All incomplete quadriplegics improved at least one Frankel grade. Of seven Frankel grade A patients, five remained unchanged and one each improved to grades B and C. Authors concluded that posterior fixation is a satisfactory method of treatment.
Lenoir T et al (2006)[5]	Retrospective case series	Very low	Assessment of neurological and functional outcomes following posterior reduction and instrumentation for unstable injury of the cervicothoracic region (30 patients). CONCLUSIONS: Satisfactory reductions in 27 patients (two mechanical failures with delayed mobilization of implants and one with persistent lateral translation in frontal plane). Bony fusion documented by computed tomography in all cases. Complete or partial neurological recovery in nine of 14 patients with Frankel grade B, C, or D. None of 16 patients initially graded Frankel A recovered neurological function. Authors concluded that choice of posterior approach was appropriate as a one-stage procedure.
Sapkas et al (1999)[6]	Retrospective case series	Very low	Assessment of neurological and radiographic outcomes following posterior-only (five patients) or combined anterior and posterior (five patients) surgical stabilization in patients with unstable injuries of the cervicothoracic junction (10 patients) CONCLUSIONS: Patients with incomplete cord injury improved their Frankel grades by at least one grade. All patients with root deficits improved. No improvement in neurological function in any Frankel grade A patient. No cases of instrumentation complications requiring reoperation. All patients had significant pain relief. Complications included temporary vocal cord paralysis, dysphagia, and Horner syndrome in one patient, one wound infection, and five medical complications. Authors conclude that surgical approach should be dictated by the injury, with anterior approaches included for decompression and/or reconstruction of the failed anterior column.
Amin and Saifuddin (2005)[1]	Retrospective case series	Very low	Assessment of injury patterns and neurological and radiological outcomes in patients with fractures and dislocations of the cervicothoracic junction (seven patients). CONCLUSIONS: Injury initially missed in three patients based on either no imaging (one case) or plain x-rays only (two cases). Neurological deficit was related to the degree of anterior of C7 on T1. All three patients with complete neurological deficit did not improve. Remaining four patients had either no or mild deficit at presentation, and all four had normal examination at follow-up.

clinical evaluation, and in cases of neurological deficit without a fracture or dislocation clearly identified elsewhere (strong). The value of MRI for evaluating cervicothoracic junction trauma is less clear, but numerous reports recommend use particularly in cases with incomplete neurological deficits or where questions exist regarding spinal stability.

References

1. Amin A, Saifuddin A. Fractures and dislocations of the cervicothoracic junction. J Spinal Disord Tech 2005;18:499–505
2. Evans DK. Dislocations at the cervicothoracic junction. J Bone Joint Surg Br 1983;65:124–127
3. Gisbert VL, Hollerman JJ, Ney AL, et al. Incidence and diagnosis of C7-T1 fractures and subluxations in multiple-trauma patients: evaluation of the advanced trauma life support guidelines. Surgery 1989;106:702–708, discussion 708–709
4. Nichols CG, Young DH, Schiller WR. Evaluation of cervicothoracic junction injury. Ann Emerg Med 1987;16:640–642
5. Lenoir T, Hoffmann E, Thevenin-Lemoine C, Lavelle G, Rillardon L, Guigui P. Neurological and functional outcome after unstable cervicothoracic junction injury treated by posterior reduction and synthesis. Spine J 2006;6:507–513
6. Sapkas G, Papadakis S, Katonis P, Roidis N, Kontakis G. Operative treatment of unstable injuries of the cervicothoracic junction. Eur Spine J 1999;8:279–283
7. Vanden Hoek T, Propp D. Cervicothoracic junction injury. Am J Emerg Med 1990;8:30–33
8. An HS, Vaccaro A, Cotler JM, Lin S. Spinal disorders at the cervicothoracic junction. Spine 1994;19:2557–2564

9. Chapman JR, Anderson PA, Pepin C, Toomey S, Newell DW, Grady MS. Posterior instrumentation of the unstable cervicothoracic spine. J Neurosurg 1996;84:552–558

10. Dvorak MF, Fisher CG, Fehlings MG, et al. The surgical approach to subaxial cervical spine injuries: an evidence-based algorithm based on the SLIC classification system. Spine 2007;32:2620–2629

11. Mirza SK, Mirza AJ, Chapman JR, Anderson PA. Classifications of thoracic and lumbar fractures: rationale and supporting data. J Am Acad Orthop Surg 2002;10:364–377

12. Vaccaro AR, Hulbert RJ, Patel AA, et al; Spine Trauma Study Group. The subaxial cervical spine injury classification system: a novel approach to recognize the importance of morphology, neurology, and integrity of the disco-ligamentous complex. Spine 2007;32:2365–2374

13. Allen BL Jr, Ferguson RL, Lehmann TR, O'Brien RP. A mechanistic classification of closed, indirect fractures and dislocations of the lower cervical spine. Spine 1982;7:1–27

14. Gertzbein SD. Scoliosis Research Society. Multicenter spine fracture study. Spine 1992;17:528–540

15. Magerl F, Aebi M, Gertzbein SD, Harms J, Nazarian S. A comprehensive classification of thoracic and lumbar injuries. Eur Spine J 1994;3: 184–201

16. Rethnam U, Yesupalan RS, Bastawrous SS. The swimmer's view: does it really show what it is supposed to show? A retrospective study. BMC Med Imaging 2008;8:2

17. Jelly LM, Evans DR, Easty MJ, Coats TJ, Chan O. Radiography versus spiral CT in the evaluation of cervicothoracic junction injuries in polytrauma patients who have undergone intubation. Radiographics 2000;20(Spec No):S251–S259, discussion S260–S262

18. Tan E, Schweitzer ME, Vaccaro L, Spetell AC. Is computed tomography of nonvisualized C7–T1 cost-effective? J Spinal Disord 1999;12: 472–476

19. Lee GY, Massicotte EM, Rampersaud YR. Clinical accuracy of cervicothoracic pedicle screw placement: a comparison of the "open" laminoforaminotomy and computer-assisted techniques. J Spinal Disord Tech 2007;20:25–32

20. Bueff HU, Lotz JC, Colliou OK, et al. Instrumentation of the cervicothoracic junction after destabilization. Spine 1995;20:1789–1792

21. Kaya RA, Türkmenoğlu ON, Koç ON, et al. A perspective for the selection of surgical approaches in patients with upper thoracic and cervicothoracic junction instabilities. Surg Neurol 2006;65:454–463, discussion 463

22. Smucker JD, Sasso RC. The evolution of spinal instrumentation for the management of occipital cervical and cervicothoracic junctional injuries. Spine 2006;31(11, Suppl):S44–S52, discussion S61

23. Albert TJ, Klein GR, Joffe D, Vaccaro AR. Use of cervicothoracic junction pedicle screws for reconstruction of complex cervical spine pathology. Spine 1998;23:1596–1599

24. Mazel C, Hoffmann E, Antonietti P, Grunenwald D, Henry M, Williams J. Posterior cervicothoracic instrumentation in spine tumors. Spine 2004;29:1246–1253

25. Deen HG. Cervicothoracic fusion performed using dual-diameter rods and polyaxial lateral mass screws: case illustration. J Neurosurg 2002; 97(1, Suppl):148

26. Rhee JM, Kraiwattanapong C, Hutton WC. A comparison of pedicle and lateral mass screw construct stiffnesses at the cervicothoracic junction: a biomechanical study. Spine 2005;30:E636–E640

27. Prybis BG, Tortolani PJ, Hu N, Zorn CM, McAfee PC, Cunningham BW. A comparative biomechanical analysis of spinal instability and instrumentation of the cervicothoracic junction: an in vitro human cadaveric model. J Spinal Disord Tech 2007;20:233–238

28. Ames CP, Bozkus MH, Chamberlain RH, et al. Biomechanics of stabilization after cervicothoracic compression-flexion injury. Spine 2005;30: 1505–1512

VII

Thoracolumbar Spine Injuries and Their Management

35

The Thoracolumbar Injury Classification and Severity Score (TLICS)

Joseph L. Petfield, Michael M. Vosbikian, Peter G. Whang, and Alexander R. Vaccaro

Physicians have developed classification systems for several medical conditions to facilitate communication between health care professionals, to allow for an accurate assessment of patient prognosis, and to standardize descriptions of a particular illness or injury for the purpose of guiding treatment and conducting clinical research. The ideal spine fracture classification system should be reliable and easy to use while simultaneously providing a precise, detailed description of injury pathogenesis that may be used to direct subsequent treatment decisions. In the past century, no less than seven classification systems have been developed to describe thoracolumbar spinal injuries,[1-7] Despite these considerable efforts, none of these classification systems has been uniformly adopted. As a result of recent advances in the surgical care of thoracolumbar spinal injuries, the ideal strategy for the classification and treatment of these injuries remains a matter of significant debate. The current literature does not clearly define the indications for operative versus nonoperative management of these fractures, especially for patients without neurological deficits.[8-11] Moreover, as noted by Audigé and colleagues, most fracture classification schemes have not been validated using proven scientific methodology.[12] The Thoracolumbar Injury Classification and Severity Score (TLICS) represents the cumulative efforts of the Spine Trauma Study Group to develop a scientifically validated thoracolumbar injury classification system that may be employed to guide the treatment of these injuries.[13-15] This chapter provides an in-depth discussion of the TLICS system and reviews the evidence that supports the reliability of this classification system.

◆ The Evolution of Thoracolumbar Injury Classification Systems

Historically, the most widely used thoracolumbar fracture classification system in North America is the Denis system, which breaks down the thoracolumbar spine into three columns.[5] This system consists of four major types of spinal injuries: compression, burst, seat-belt-type injuries, and fracture

dislocation; each fracture is then further classified into 1 of 16 subtypes. The AO (Arbeitsgemeinschaft für Osteosynthesefragen) system pioneered by Magerl et al[6] is based on a scale of progressive morphological damage and consists of three primary fracture types: A (compression), B (distraction), and C (translation/rotation), in conjunction with a total of 27 possible subcategories.

Several recent studies have evaluated the reliability and reproducibility of the AO and Denis classification systems. In 1999, Blauth et al[16] examined the interobserver agreement of spinal surgeons at 22 spine trauma centers using the AO system following evaluation of plain x-rays and computed tomographic (CT) images of 14 lumbar spine fractures. The average interobserver agreement for injury mechanism (i.e., A, B, or C) was 67%, ranging from 41 to 91%. Moreover, the κ coefficient indicative of interobserver reliability was 0.33, which corresponded to fair reliability; this value was observed to decrease even further as more subcategories were included. In a survey of five observers involving 53 thoracolumbar spinal injuries, Oner et al[17] compared the reliability of the AO to the Denis system. The authors found the reliabilities of both systems to be fair to moderate. The interobserver agreement of the Denis system was greater than that of the AO classification, which demonstrated suboptimal reproducibility. Wood et al[18] also compared the inter- and intraobserver reliabilities of the Denis and AO systems via a survey of 31 fractures that were reviewed by 19 spine surgeons on two separate occasions 3 months apart. According to this investigation, both systems exhibited only moderate reliability, with the intraobserver agreements decreasing substantially with the inclusion of greater levels of subclassification. The authors expressed some concern that the excessive complexity of the AO system may make it unreliable for practical use, whereas the Denis system may be incomplete because it does not place adequate emphasis on imaging and the assessment of the posterior ligamentous complex (PLC).

Recognizing the limitations of these contemporary thoracolumbar fracture classification systems, the members of the Spine Trauma Study Group (STSG) developed a novel system through a validation process of three steps described by

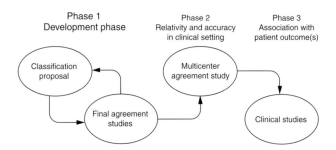

Fig. 35.1 The three-phase validation process outlined by Audigé. (From Audigé L, Bhandari M, Hanson B, Kellam J. A concept for the validation of fracture classifications. Journal of Orthopaedic Trauma 2005;19:401–406.)

Audigé et al (**Fig. 35.1**).[12] Following an exhaustive review of the literature, acquisition of expert opinions, and numerous face to face meetings, the STSG conceived a preliminary point-based classification system known as the Thoracolumbar Injury Severity Score (TLISS).[19] This system incorporates variables that were thought most critical in determining the choice of operative or nonoperative treatment for a given traumatic spinal injury. The TLISS features a scoring algorithm based upon three factors: the mechanism of injury as interpreted by the observer of available imaging studies, the integrity of the posterior ligamentous complex (PLC), and the neurological status of the patient. Point values are allocated according to the radiographic and clinical findings, which are used to calculate a total score. Patients with a score of 3 or less may be candidates for nonoperative treatment, whereas surgical intervention is considered for injuries scoring 5 or higher. A total of 4 is indeterminate, in which case the exact method of treatment is largely dictated by the surgeon's clinical expertise and patient preference.

The reliability of the TLISS was established by two studies; both of which demonstrated this system to be reasonably reliable.[14,20] Although the TLISS demonstrated excellent interrater agreement with regard to neurological scoring and treatment recommendations, the mechanism of injury, was associated with only a fair level of agreement. To address this potential limitation, the STSG modified the original format of the TLISS so that the interpretation of the traumatic mechanism was replaced by a description of injury morphology as one of the three principal scoring categories.[14] Furthermore, the practice of assigning points to every assumed mechanism of injury was adjusted so that only the most severe morphological class is considered in the total score. Once these modifications were integrated into the algorithm, the TLISS was renamed the Thoracolumbar Injury Classification and Severity Score (TLICS).

◆ Discussion

What are the principal domains used to characterize a thoracolumbar spinal injury and are they predictive of outcome?

The Thoracolumbar Injury Classification and Severity Score

The TLICS system takes into account three major variables that have been identified as being important for accurately characterizing a traumatic injury to the thoracolumbar spine: (1) the morphological appearance of the fracture evident on imaging studies; (2) the integrity of the PLC; and (3) the neurological status of the patient.[14] Additional subgroups have also been created within each of these categories to describe the injury in greater detail.[13] Like the TLISS system, the TLICS system also includes an injury severity score derived from the points allocated to each of the three main categories, which may be valuable for determining the most suitable treatment for each thoracolumbar fracture.

Morphology[13]

Injury morphology is typically assessed using several different modalities such as plain radiographs, CT, and magnetic resonance imaging (MRI). The predominant fracture pattern is classified as one of three basic types: (1) compression, (2) translation/rotation, or (3) distraction (**Fig. 35.2**).

Compression injuries occur when the vertebral body fails as a result of an axial load. In its most benign form, only the anterior portion of the vertebral body is involved. With greater axial forces, the entire vertebral body may be disrupted, which may be accompanied by retropulsion of bone into the spinal canal (i.e., a burst fracture). Reflecting the relative instability of these injuries, compression and burst fractures are allotted 1 and 2 points, respectively.[13]

The application of torsional and shear forces to the spine may give rise to a rotation or translational type injury, which generally results following a high-energy impact load. These injuries are usually more unstable than a compression type injury. On an anteroposterior (AP) x-ray as well as axial or coronal CT reconstructions, rotational injuries will often demonstrate increased horizontal separation of the spinous processes, malalignment of the pedicles above and below the level of injury, or evidence of medial-lateral displacement. Conversely, AP translation may be apparent on a lateral radiograph or sagittal CT images. Given its greater severity, this morphological pattern is allocated a score of 3 points.

A distraction injury may actually bring about a complete dislocation of the spinal column which fails as a result of supraphysiological tensile stresses, which are sufficient to damage many of the osseous and/or ligamentous structures across the anterior and posterior spinal elements. Depending on the position of the spine at the time of the injury, angulation in the sagittal or coronal planes may also be present at the fracture site. Due to the inherent instability of this fracture pattern, a distraction injury is given a score of 4 points.

For more complex fracture patterns, these morphological descriptors may also be combined (e.g., a distraction-compression fracture). Nevertheless, in these situations, points are only assigned to the most severe injury pattern.

Integrity of the Posterior Ligamentous Complex

The PLC includes the supraspinous and interspinous ligaments, ligamentum flavum, and bilateral facet joint capsules, all of which contribute to the stability of the spinal column by resisting excessive flexion, rotation, translation, and distraction. Due to its poor healing potential in adults, any injury to the PLC typically necessitates surgical intervention. The integrity of the PLC may be examined clinically by palpating the posterior elements, as well by evaluating a battery of imaging studies, which may exhibit splaying of the spinous processes, subluxation of the facet joints, or vertebral body translation. The condition of the PLC is classified as intact (0 points), indeterminate (2 points), or disrupted (3 points).[13]

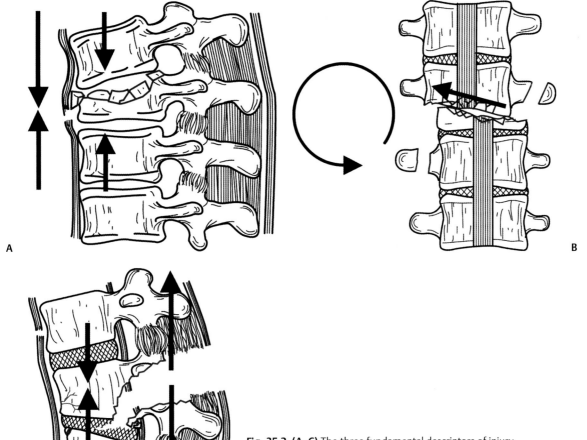

Fig. 35.2 (A–C) The three fundamental descriptors of injury morphology incorporated by the Thoracolumbar Injury Classification and Severity Score (TLICS) system. (From Vaccaro AR, Lehman Jr. RA, Hurlbert RJ, et al. A new classification of thoracolumbar injuries: the importance of injury morphology, the integrity of the posterior ligamentous complex, and neurologic status. Spine 2005;30:2325–2333. Reprinted with permission.)

Neurological Status

The neurological function of a patient who has sustained a thoracolumbar fracture is an essential factor for assessing spinal stability, determining the need for a surgical procedure, and estimating the long-term prognosis of the injury. In an increasing order of surgical acuity, the neurological status of the patient is categorized as intact (0 points), nerve root or complete spinal cord injury [American Spinal Injury Association A (ASIA A), 2 points], and incomplete spinal cord or cauda equina injury (ASIA B, C, or D, 3 points).[13]

Using these three classes of TLICS system, the clinician can easily, yet precisely, stratify a specific thoracolumbar injury. For example, a flexion-distraction burst fracture (4 points) with disruption of the PLC (3 points) in the setting of an incomplete spinal cord injury (3 points) would result in a total score of 10 points (**Table 35.1**).

Surgical Decision Using TLICS

The Injury Severity Score (ISS) not only serves to define the severity of a thoracolumbar injury but it may also be utilized as a reference for directing subsequent treatment. An ISS of 3 or less suggests that the injury may be addressed nonoperatively, whereas a patient with a score of 5 or greater may benefit from a surgical intervention. An ISS of 4 points is regarded as a "gray

Table 35.1 The Thoracolumbar Injury Classification Severity Score (TLICS) Algorithm

Morphology Type	Qualifier	Points
Compression	Compression fracture	1
	Burst fracture	1
Translational/rotational		3
Distraction		4
Neurological involvement:		0
Intact		2
Nerve root		
Cord, conus medullaris	Incomplete	3
	Complete	2
Cauda equina		3
Posterior ligamentous complex		0
integrity:		2
Intact		3
Injury suspected/indeterminate		
Injured		

Source: Bono CM, Vaccaro AR, Hurlbert RJ, et al. Validating a newly proposed classification system for thoracolumbar spine trauma: looking to the future of the thoracolumbar injury classification and severity score. Journal of Orthopaedic Trauma. 2006;20:567–572. Reprinted with permission.

35 The Thoracolumbar Injury Classification and Severity Score (TLICS)

347

zone" in which the fracture may be treated in either fashion depending on the surgeon's clinical opinion and patient issues such as the presence of other medical comorbidities.[13,19]

If an injury is treated with an operation, the TLICS system is indispensable for determining which surgical approach may be preferable. The integrity of the PLC and neurological status are two of the most important factors that influence whether a patient should be managed with an anterior, posterior, or circumferential procedure.[13] Compression of the spinal cord from anterior bony fragments in association with an incomplete neurological injury generally indicates the need for an anterior approach to facilitate an adequate decompression. In contrast, disruption of the PLC may require posterior fixation to restore stability to the spinal column. An injury spanning all three columns of the spinal column in conjunction with an incomplete neurological deficit may justify a combination of anterior and posterior techniques (**Table 35.2**).

Although these recommendations may be helpful for deciding whether a patient possibly needs surgery and the optimal surgical approach, it is important to recognize that each of these injuries represents a unique clinical situation. The most appropriate therapeutic regimen may not be obvious until a comprehensive assessment of the fracture has been completed. Other traumatic injuries and systemic comorbidities such as rib fractures, burns affecting the tissues overlying the spine, ankylosing spondylitis, or osteoporosis may also influence the treatment plans that are instituted for these individuals. Although these additional clinical data may be too cumbersome to include in any classification scheme, clinicians must be cognizant of these issues when treatment decision making is necessary.[13,19]

◆ Discussion

Has the TLICS system been validated in clinical practice as a useful means of managing a thoracolumbar spinal injury?

As discussed in the preceding sections, the TLICS was initially developed in an attempt to improve on the previously validated TLISS by embracing the idea that the mechanism of injury may represent a more significant source of variation than fracture morphology. Harrop et al[14] presented 56 thoracolumbar injuries to a group of 48 spine trauma specialists trained in either orthopedic or neurological surgery. Each case was scored using the TLISS scale along with treatment recommendation. After 3 months, the cases were again reviewed in a different order so that the validity and reliability of the system could be established. The intrarater reliabilities for the mechanism of injury, integrity of the PLC, and neurological status were 59.4%, 68.4%, and 91.0%, respectively. Similarly, the interrater reliabilities for these same variables were 50.7%, 59.4%, and 96.3%, respectively. In this study, 91% of the surgeons agreed with the treatment plans that were suggested by the TLISS scale (i.e., a total score >4 is an indication for operative management). Despite only moderate agreement between the surgeons regarding the mechanism of injury and the integrity of the PLC, the overall validity of the TLISS was found to be very high. However, to address these potential weaknesses of the TLISS system, the STSG replaced fracture mechanism with morphology, which was thought to be a more objective assessment of injury severity. The STSG recommended careful scrutiny of all MRI sequences[20]

Table 35.2 Determining the Optimal Surgical Approach as Predicted by Thoracolumbar Injury Classification and Severity Score (TLICS) Descriptors

Neurological Status	Posterior Ligamentous Complex	
	Intact	Disrupted
Intact	Posterior approach	Posterior approach
Root injury	Posterior approach	Posterior approach
Incomplete spinal cord injury or cauda equina	Anterior approach	Combined approach
Complete spinal cord injury or cauda equina	Posterior (anterior)* approach	Posterior (combined)* approach

Source: Vaccaro AR, Lehman Jr. RA, Hurlbert RJ, et al. A new classification of thoracolumbar injuries: the importance of injury morphology, the integrity of the posterior ligamentous complex, and neurologic status. Spine 2005;30:2325–2333. Reprinted with permission.

*Aggressive decompression in American Spinal Injury Association A (ASIA A) patients is practiced in many institutions to optimize any potential for neurological recovery, reconstruct the vertebral support column, restore cerebrospinal fluid flow to prevent syringomyelia, and allow for short-segment fixation.

(T1, T2, and fat-suppressed T2) to get a better understanding of the integrity of the PLC. These changes and suggestions to the classification scheme were designed to further enhance the validity of the TLISS algorithm, which had already been shown to yield a high level of agreement (>90%) among surgeons. Whang et al[21] directly compared the TLISS and TLICS models. In this prospective investigation, 25 thoracolumbar injuries were initially scored by five groups of surgeons with disparate levels of training using the TLISS scheme; 3 months later, these same cases were graded with the TLICS system. The results of this analysis confirmed that both systems demonstrated excellent reproducibility and validity (>90%). However, in contrast to the hypothesis set forth by Harrop et al[14] and Vaccaro et al,[20] the interrater reliability of the TLISS scheme was actually higher than that of the TLICS system. Nevertheless, since the mechanism of the injury is intimately related to its morphology, it may be assumed that both of these factors should be taken into account during the evaluation and subsequent management of thoracolumbar fractures (**Fig. 35.3**).

Bono et al[22] noted that any classification system must comply with the three phases outlined by Audigé et al.[12] First of all, the algorithm must employ universal "clinically relevant diagnostic terms"[12] that are based on clinical findings and relevant imaging studies. The second phase requires an assessment by different surgeons at multiple centers that allows appropriate adjustments to be made to the system so that a sufficient level of agreement may be achieved. At this time, the first and second phases have been completed for the TLICS scheme. Finally, the third phase entails scientific validation of the classification system. To satisfy this condition, the TLICS must be thoroughly evaluated by a series of prospective, randomized studies to estimate its utility for clinical practice and to resolve any remaining controversies (e.g., injury mechanism versus morphology, the optimal modality for imaging the PLC, etc.). These clinical trials are currently being conducted by the STSG, the results of which may determine

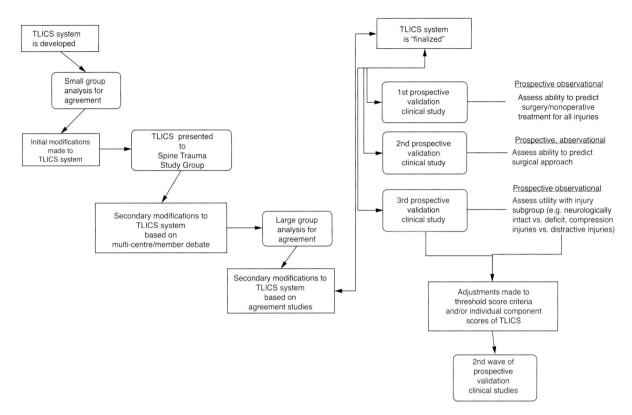

Fig. 35.3 The evolution of the Thoracolumbar Injury Classification and Severity Score (TLICS) system proposed by the Spine Trauma Study Group, which is currently being validated by several large, prospective, randomized, multicenter studies. (From Bono CM, Vaccaro AR, Hurlbert RJ, et al. Validating a newly proposed classification system for thoracolumbar spine trauma: looking to the future of the thoracolumbar injury classification and severity score. Journal of Orthopaedic Trauma 2006;20:567–572. Reprinted with permission.)

whether the TLICS system will ultimately gain widespread acceptance among spine surgeons for the classification and treatment of thoracolumbar fractures.

◆ Recommendations and Summary

Clearly, the accurate classification and effective management of thoracolumbar spinal injuries are currently topics of considerable debate. However, the TLICS system appears to be a promising system for achieving these objectives. Its excellent reliability and validity reported by various studies demonstrates that the TLICS system has improved user friendliness and usefulness compared with other popular classification systems such as the Denis and AO classification systems. The TLICS scoring algorithm is both logical and simple so that it is able to be used by surgeons and nonsurgeons alike yet is also comprehensive enough to describe complex fractures with great precision. Given its myriad advantages, which have been corroborated by the existing literature, the TLICS system may have the potential to become the "gold standard" for evaluating and directing the subsequent treatment of thoracolumbar injuries (**Table 35.3**).

Table 35.3 Relevant Results of the Systematic Review

Study	Description	Level of Evidence of Primary Question	Topic and Conclusion
Whang et al (2007)[21]	Prospective cohort study	II	25 patients with thoracolumbar injuries were analyzed on 2 separate occasions separated by 3 months. The TLISS was used on admission of the patient and the TLICS was used later. Both systems were shown to be quite reproducible and valid, yet the TLISS was shown be more reliable in each of the 3 classifications, but none were deemed statistically significant by Cohen's kappa. However, with respect to interrater correlation, the TLISS system showed a statistically significant difference with respect to mechanism versus morphology ($P < 0.01$), the PLC evaluation ($P < 0.01$), and the appropriate management ($P < 0.0001$). As far as the validity is concerned, the TLICS has a higher percentage of correctly predicting treatment modalities (95.4), a higher specificity (0.971), and a higher PPV (0.951); however, these are not statistically significant with respect to the scores in the TLISS (92.7, 0.953, and 0.930)

(Continued on page 350)

Table 35.3 Relevant Results of the Systematic Review *(Continued)*

Study	Description	Level of Evidence of Primary Question	Topic and Conclusion
			CONCLUSION: The TLISS seems to be more dependable with respect to interobserver reliability, but both systems have excellent validity.
Harrop et al (2006)[14]	Prospective cohort study	II	56 clinical vignettes were given to 48 spine surgeons to determine the reliability and validity of the TLISS. It was shown that with respect to agreement about the mechanism of injury, integrity of the PLC, and neurological status, the intrarater agreements were 59.4%, 68.4%, and 91.0%, respectively. The intrarater agreements were 50.7%, 59.4%, and 96.3%, respectively. The study also showed that the surgeons agreed with the recommendations of the TLISS score >90% of the time.
			CONCLUSION: The TLICS/TLISS are both valid models for thoracolumbar injury due to the high agreement with the treatment recommendation, yet there is less reliability than anticipated; hence the modification of mechanism of injury (TLISS) to morphology (TLICS).
Vaccaro et al (2006)[20]	Prospective cohort study	II	71 cases were given to 5 spine surgeons who were to evaluate the cases via the TLISS and report whether they agreed or disagreed with the recommendations associated with the score. The study showed an agreement of over 90% and rather good reliability but points out that reliability may be able to be improved with the change of evaluating the mechanism of injury to the morphology of the injury as well as utilizing MRI (T1, T2, and fat-suppressed T2) to better focus on the integrity of the PLC in the injury.
			CONCLUSION: The TLISS has proven to be a reliable and valid classification system thus far, and the use of more sophisticated imaging along with substitution of morphology for mechanism (TLICS) may prove to make the system even more reliable and valid through better objectivity.
Vaccaro et al (2005)[13]	Systematic literature review	III	Illustrates that the TLICS was developed based on the results of 2 validation literature surveys, the first at a single institution using 71 cases and another by the STSG using 56 cases. Proposes that the TLICS not only aids the decision as to whether surgery is appropriate but also aids in planning the surgical approach based on the integrity of the PLC and the neurological status of the patient. Reinforces that comorbidities and patient variability will still play a major role despite the use of a classification system like the TLICS.
			CONCLUSION: The TLICS, building off the TLISS model, creates a system for the assessment of thoracolumbar injuries and aids in planning the surgical approach based on the incorporation of the integrity of the PLC and the neurological status of the patient, thus making it comprehensive as well.
Lee (2005)	Systematic review/ instructional literature	V	Proposes that the TLICS is both simple and reliable so that both surgeons and nonsurgeons can objectively assess and manage thoracolumbar spine injuries. Proposes that the TLICS will be an improvement over the Denis system in that, although the Denis system has good inter- and intraobserver reliability (kappa = 0.6), the simplicity of the system may lead to misclassifications of management (surgical vs nonsurgical). Proposes that the TLICS will be an improvement over the AO system's inter- and intraobserver reliability (kappa = 0.33) because the new system is simpler.
			CONCLUSION: The TLICS should be a simpler and more straightforward system so that there is better reliability than is seen in the AO system with better management recommendations than the Denis system.
Bono et al (2006)[15]	Expert opinion	V	Proposes that the TLICS was developed based on the analysis of previous systems and will be an improvement once validated with respect to reliability and predicting management and outcomes associated with thoracolumbar injuries. States that the TLICS system has passed through the first 2 phases of validation as delineated by Audigé, et al (phase 1: using variables that can be detected in a clinical setting; phase 2: multicenter, multisurgeon assessment for reliability) and is ready for the third and final stage of validity, which is where a prospective observational study is appropriate to fine-tune and validate the system.
			CONCLUSION: The TLICS system has passed through 2 of the 3 stages of validation outlined by Audigé et al and should prove to be a successful clinical assessment tool for thoracolumbar spinal injuries.

Abbreviations: AO, Arbeitsgemeinschaft für Osteosynthesefragen; TLICS, Thoracolumbar Injury Classification Severity Score; TLISS, Thoracolumbar Injury Severity Score; PLC, posterior ligamentous complex; PPV, positive predictive value.

VII Thoracolumbar Spine Injuries and Their Management

References

1. Böhler L. Die techniek deknochenbruchbehandlung imgrieden und im kreigen. 1930
2. Nicoll EA. Fractures of the dorso-lumbar spine. J Bone Joint Surg Br 1949;31:376–394
3. Holdsworth F. Fractures, dislocations, and fracture-dislocations of the spine. J Bone Joint Surg Am 1970;52:1534–1551
4. Louis R. Unstable fractures of the spine, III: Instability. A. Theories concerning instability [in French]. Rev Chir Orthop Repar Appar Mot 1977; 63:423–425
5. Denis F. The three column spine and its significance in the classification of acute thoracolumbar spinal injuries. Spine 1983;8:817–831
6. Magerl F, Aebi M, Gertzbein SD, Harms J, Nazarian S. A comprehensive classification of thoracic and lumbar injuries. Eur Spine J 1994;3: 184–201
7. McCormack T, Karaikovic E, Gaines RW. The load sharing classification of spine fractures. Spine 1994;19:1741–1744
8. Willén J, Lindahl S, Nordwall A. Unstable thoracolumbar fractures: a comparative clinical study of conservative treatment and Harrington instrumentation. Spine 1985;10:111–122
9. Jacobs RR, Nordwall A, Nachemson A. Reduction, stability, and strength provided by internal fixation systems for thoracolumbar spinal injuries. Clin Orthop Relat Res 1982;(171):300–308
10. Wood K, Buttermann G, Mehbod A, et al. Operative compared with nonoperative treatment of a thoracolumbar burst fracture without neurological deficit: a prospective, randomized study. J Bone Joint Surg Am 2003;85-A:773–781
11. Yi L, Jingping B, Gele J, Baoleri X, Taixiang W. Operative versus nonoperative treatment for thoracolumbar burst fractures without neurological deficit. Cochrane Database Syst Rev 2006;(4):CD005079
12. Audigé L, Bhandari M, Hanson B, Kellam J. A concept for the validation of fracture classifications. J Orthop Trauma 2005;19:401–406
13. Vaccaro AR, Lehman RA Jr, Hurlbert RJ, et al. A new classification of thoracolumbar injuries: the importance of injury morphology, the integrity of the posterior ligamentous complex, and neurologic status. Spine 2005;30:2325–2333
14. Harrop JS, Vaccaro AR, Hurlbert RJ, et al; Spine Trauma Study Group. Intrarater and interrater reliability and validity in the assessment of the mechanism of injury and integrity of the posterior ligamentous complex: a novel injury severity scoring system for thoracolumbar injuries. Invited submission from the Joint Section Meeting On Disorders of the Spine and Peripheral Nerves, March 2005. J Neurosurg Spine 2006;4: 118–122
15. Bono CM, Vaccaro AR, Hurlbert RJ, et al. Validating a newly proposed classification system for thoracolumbar spine trauma: looking to the future of the thoracolumbar injury classification and severity score. J Orthop Trauma 2006;20:567–572
16. Blauth M, Bastian L, Knop C, Lange U, Tusch G. Inter-observer reliability in the classification of thoraco-lumbar spinal injuries [in German]. Orthopade 1999;28:662–681
17. Oner FC, Ramos LM, Simmermacher RK, et al. Classification of thoracic and lumbar spine fractures: problems of reproducibility: a study of 53 patients using CT and MRI. Eur Spine J 2002;11:235–245
18. Wood KB, Khanna G, Vaccaro AR, Arnold PM, Harris MB, Mehbod AA. Assessment of two thoracolumbar fracture classification systems as used by multiple surgeons. J Bone Joint Surg Am 2005;87:1423–1429
19. Vaccaro AR, Zeiller SC, Hulbert RJ, et al. The thoracolumbar injury severity score: a proposed treatment algorithm. J Spinal Disord Tech 2005;18: 209–215
20. Vaccaro AR, Baron EM, Sanfilippo J, et al. Reliability of a novel classification system for thoracolumbar injuries: the Thoracolumbar Injury Severity Score. Spine 2006;31(11, Suppl):S62–S69, discussion S104
21. Whang PG, Vaccaro AR, Poelstra KA, et al. The influence of fracture mechanism and morphology on the reliability and validity of two novel thoracolumbar injury classification systems. Spine 2007;32:791–795
22. Bono C, Parke W, Garfin S. Development of the spine. In: Herkowitz H, Garfin S, Eismont F, Bell G, Balderston R, eds. Rothman-Simeone the Spine. Vol 1. 5th ed. Philadelphia: Saunders Elsevier; 2006:3
23. Lee JY, Vaccaro AR, Lin MR, et al. Thoracolumbar injury classification and severity score: a new paradigm for the treatment of thoracolumbar spine trauma. J Ortho Sci 2005;10(6):671–675

36

Management of Thoracolumbar Compression Fractures

Todd McCall and Andrew T. Dailey

Vertebral body compression fractures are caused by axial compression with or without flexion. The morphological term *compression fracture* can encompass a variety of vertebral body injuries, which Magerl and Aebi[1] subdivided into impaction fractures (A1), split fractures (A2), and burst fractures (A3). This chapter specifically addresses impaction (A1) fractures, which can be further subdivided into end plate impaction (A1.1), wedge impaction (A1.2), and vertebral body collapse (A1.3). All of these impaction fractures are considered stable, owing to an intact posterior column and absence of spinal canal narrowing. End plate and wedge impaction fractures both have an intact posterior wall, with end plate fractures having up to 5 degrees of wedging, whereas wedge fractures have greater than 5 degrees of wedging. Vertebral body collapse is distinguished by symmetrical collapse of vertebral body height without compromise of the spinal canal. To clarify, *compression fractures* in this chapter refers specifically to Magerl type A1 fractures and not burst fractures.

◆ Etiology and Epidemiology

Compression fractures occur in three distinct patient populations defined by the cause of the fracture: young men in traumatic events, elderly women with osteoporosis, and individuals with spinal column involvement of a neoplastic process including metastasis or multiple myeloma. Compression injuries are the most common fractures of the thoracolumbar spine.[2] In the series of 1445 patients analyzed by Magerl et al,[3] 66.1% of fractures were type A, with type A1 fractures encompassing 34.7% of all fractures. The Scoliosis Research Society performed a prospective study of 1019 traumatic spinal fractures, which encompassed both stable and unstable fractures, and found that 66.8% of patients were male, with a mean age of 31.7 years.[4] Together, motor vehicle accidents and falls accounted for 85% of injuries, with the T11 to L1 levels accounting for 52% of afflicted vertebrae.

The leading cause of vertebral compression fractures is osteoporosis. The National Osteoporosis Foundation has reported that osteoporosis afflicts 10 million individuals,[5] with an estimated annual incidence of 700,000 osteoporotic vertebral body compression fractures.[6] Twenty-six percent of women older than 50 years have a vertebral compression fracture,[7] and the prevalence increases to 40% by the age of 80 years.[8]

Pathological compression fractures are also fairly frequent. The spine is the most common site of skeletal metastases,[9] and ~30% of patients with a neoplastic process develop spinal metastases.[10,11] Multiple myeloma has a particularly high predisposition to involve bone, with skeletal involvement in 60 to 80% of cases.[12]

◆ Clinical Features

Irrespective of the cause, the principal symptom of a compression fracture is focal pain. An estimated 84% of vertebral compression fractures are associated with pain.[6] Acute pain typically lasts ~4 to 6 weeks, with the pain occurring axially and correlating with the level of fracture. Activity aggravates the pain, whereas lying down or sitting alleviates it. Point tenderness is a common finding on examination but is not present in 10% of cases.[13]

Chronic pain is common after traumatic compression fractures. Young[14] retrospectively reviewed a cohort of 116 patients with primarily wedge compression fractures and found that after 3 to 8 years only 26% of patients were pain free, whereas 52% of patients had pain that was not incapacitating, and 22% of subjects had incapacitating pain necessitating a job change. The author found no correlation between the severity or longevity of pain and degree of deformity. In another retrospective review, Folman and Gepstein[15] evaluated 85 patients with wedge compression fractures and found that 69.4% of patients had pain, with a mean score of 2.94 on a 10-point scale at a mean 8.9 years of follow-up. In this study, pain intensity correlated with the degree of local kyphosis but not anterior column deformity.

One third of osteoporotic vertebral compression fractures also result in chronic pain, which is more likely to ensue when one level is severely collapsed or multiple levels are involved.[16,17] Other side effects of osteoporotic compression fractures include impaired mobility, limited exercise tolerance, chronic depression, and an increased likelihood of death.[18] Loss of vertebral body height, thoracic kyphosis, and pain can contribute to impaired pulmonary function, with the severity of pulmonary function decline correlating with the severity of spinal column deformity.[19,20]

◆ Nonoperative Management

Potential conservative therapies for vertebral compression fractures include analgesic medications, bed rest, bracing, and rehabilitation.[5,21] Very low quality evidence suggests that traumatic thoracolumbar compression fractures can be treated with a short period of bed rest alone, and bracing is not required. In the retrospective cohort of Folman and Gepstein[15] patients were treated with a combination of bed rest, bracing, and physical therapy. Bracing and intensive physical therapy had no effect on outcome, and the authors thought only a single session of physical therapy was useful to reinitiate ambulation. Similarly, a group of 127 patients with stable compression fractures were treated successfully with an average of 8 days of bed rest and no bracing.[22] Finally, in the retrospective cohort by Young[14] in which the most common treatment was bed rest, there was no tendency for deformity to progress.

In patients with osteoporosis, physical therapy is critical to educate the patient on new ways to perform daily activities in a manner that does not exacerbate pain and also to perform strengthening exercises. The results of a randomized, controlled trial of postmenopausal women demonstrated that patients randomized to resistive back-strengthening exercises had significantly stronger back extensor strength and fewer compression fractures than patients in the control group at 10 years of follow-up.[23] Because weight-bearing exercises are crucial in the prevention of disease progression, bed rest in the long run can be counterproductive.[24] Narcotic medications can be considered for short-term pain control, but their use should be closely regulated. Nonsteroidal antiinflammatory medications can also provide symptomatic relief, and cyclooxygenase (COX)-2 inhibitors are favored by some to minimize gastrointestinal side effects.[5] Braces may help by reducing pain, improving posture, and providing additional support when muscles are weak. Three-point braces, such as the Jewitt or Cash orthoses, are usually preferable to encourage spinal extension. Medical treatment of osteoporosis includes calcium supplements, vitamin D, hormone replacement, and bisphosphonates.[25] Of note, none of these conservative therapies helps restore loss of height or reduce kyphotic deformity.[26]

Moderate quality studies suggest that patients treated with conservative therapies alone for osteoporotic compression fractures do not have acute improvement in pain but can appreciate significant improvement in discomfort and function in the long term. Nakano et al[27] performed a matched case-control study in which patients with osteoporotic compression fractures were treated with either vertebroplasty or conservative measures. In the conservative treatment group, the initial mean pain visual analogue scale (VAS) score of 7.5 significantly declined to 2.6 at 6 months and 2.0 at 12 months. Although the 6- and 12-month scores were still higher than the mean VAS score of the surgical treatment group at the same time points, a reduction of the mean VAS score that is greater than 3, as was found with the control group, is generally considered clinically relevant. In another nonrandomized trial comparing vertebroplasty and nonoperative treatment, Diamond et al[28] also found that conservative therapy alone led to significant reduction in pain scores at 6 weeks and 6 to 12 months, but not 24-hour follow-up compared with pretreatment scores. There was not a significant difference between the treatment and control groups at the 6-week and 6- to 12-month time points. Physical function, measured by the Barthel index, also significantly improved in the conservative treatment group at 6 weeks and 6 to 12 months.

Besides the usual conservative measures, symptomatic relief from pathological fractures can possibly be achieved with radiotherapy. For example, in a retrospective review of 108 patients who received radiation therapy for breast cancer spinal metastases, 83% of patients noted a complete or almost complete analgesic effect.[29] In cases of multiple myeloma, treatment with bisphosphonates should also be considered to help deter bone destruction.

◆ Surgical Treatment: Vertebroplasty and Kyphoplasty

In the past 2 decades, vertebroplasty (**Table 36.1**) and kyphoplasty (**Table 36.2**) have emerged as surgical options that play a central role in the treatment of osteoporotic vertebral compression fractures. Before the common use of vertebroplasty and kyphoplasty, the principal surgical option for treatment of compression fractures was decompression and fusion; however, surgical fixation frequently failed in elderly patients because of the common problem of osteopenia.[30] Vertebroplasty was first introduced in 1987 by Galibert et al,[31] who successfully treated seven patients who had painful vertebral angiomas. Since then, the use of vertebroplasty has expanded to include treatment of traumatic, osteoporotic, and pathological compression fractures. Osteoporotic compression fractures are now the most common indication for these procedures.

Vertebroplasty involves the percutaneous injection of cement, such as polymethylmethacrylate (PMMA), directly into the cancellous bone of a vertebral body, with the goal of alleviating pain associated with a vertebral compression fracture and preventing further loss of vertebral body height or progression of kyphotic deformity. Kyphoplasty was introduced later as a modification of vertebroplasty in which a balloon (tamp) is inflated in the vertebral body to compress the cancellous bone and create a cavity. Theoretically, the cavity allows the cement to be injected under less pressure and minimizes extravasation. Additional goals of kyphoplasty include restoring vertebral body height and reducing kyphosis (**Fig. 36.1**).[32]

Indications

A prospective cohort of 28 patients treated with kyphoplasty for 33 Magerl type A compression fractures, including 24 type A1 fractures, provided low-quality evidence on the potential use of kyphoplasty for traumatic compression fractures.[33] After a mean follow-up of 30 months, VAS scores were significantly reduced to a mean of 0.8 from a preoperative level of 8.7. The mean Roland-Morris disability score also significantly declined. All active patients returned to work within 3 months, which compares favorably with conservative treatment

Table 36.1 Evidence Summary of Comparative Studies of Vertebroplasty

Study	Quality Rating	Description of Study	Comments and Conclusions
Diamond et al (2003)[28]	Moderate	Prospective, nonrandomized trial comparing vertebroplasty treatment ($N = 55$) with a control group of conservative management ($N = 24$) for osteoporotic VCFs. Mean follow-up 215 days. Patients failed conservative treatment for 1 to 6 weeks. VAS and Barthel physical functioning index scores were significantly better in the vertebroplasty group 24 hours after treatment. At 6-week and 6- to 12-month follow-up, there was no significant difference in pain scores.	Vertebroplasty offered more improvement in VAS and physical functioning scores immediately, but clinical outcomes at longer follow-up were similar compared with those seen after conservative treatment.
Nakano et al (2006)[27]	Moderate	Matched case-control study comparing treatment of osteoporotic VCFs treated with vertebroplasty ($N = 30$) or conservative treatment alone ($N = 30$). Mean follow-up of 17 months. Patients failed conservative treatment for at least 4 weeks. The vertebroplasty group had significant improvement in mean VAS scores from a preoperative mean of 7.9 to 0.7 at 6 months and 0.7 at 12 months. The control also had significant improvement in mean VAS scores, reducing from 7.5 preoperatively to 2.6 at 6 months and 2.0 at 12 months. The vertebroplasty scores were significantly lower at both time points. Mean recovery rate of the deformity index was significantly better in the vertebroplasty group ($+3.7\%$) compared with the control group (-13.2%). 20% rate of spinal canal cement leakage, and 7% rate of leakage into the intervertebral disk.	While both vertebroplasty and conservative treatment significantly reduced VAS scores compared with preoperative values, pain scores in the vertebroplasty patients were significantly less than those in the control group at 6- and 12-month follow-up. Deformity index was also better in the treatment group.
Voormolen et al (2007)[80]	Moderate	Prospective randomized trial comparing vertebroplasty ($N = 18$) and optimal pain medication ($N = 16$). Follow-up at 1 day and 2 weeks after treatment. Patients failed conservative treatment for 6 weeks to 6 months. At 1 day the vertebroplasty group had significantly better VAS scores and less analgesic use than the control group. However, at 2 weeks the VAS scores did not differ significantly between groups. At 2 weeks QUALEFFO and RMD scores were significantly better in the treatment group.	Compared with a control group, vertebroplasty significantly improved quality of life and disability. Vertebroplasty also significantly reduced pain scores at 1 day but not 2 weeks. At 2 weeks, pain scores were lower, but the study may have been underpowered to find a significant difference.
Heini et al (2000)[108]	Low	Prospective cohort of 17 patients with 45 osteoporotic VCFs treated with vertebroplasty. Minimum follow-up of 1 year. VAS scores significantly decreased compared with preoperative levels on the first postoperative day. Median VAS scores unchanged at 12-week and 1-year follow-up. 20% rate of cement extravasation.	Vertebroplasty resulted in immediate reduction of VAS scores, which remained low 1 year postoperatively.
Kobayashi et al (2005)[109]	Low	Prospective cohort of 175 patients with 250 osteoporotic VCFs treated by vertebroplasty. Mean follow-up of 18 days. Significant decrease in the mean VAS score from 7.2 preoperatively to 2.1 at 1 day postoperatively. Cement leakage rate of 75.6%, with no symptomatic cases.	Vertebroplasty leads to immediate pain relief of osteoporotic VCFs.
Legroux-Gérot (2004)[90]	Low	Prospective cohort of 16 patients with 21 osteoporotic VCFs treated with vertebroplasty. Mean follow-up of 35 months. Significant decrease in average Huskisson's VAS (71 to 39) and MGM (3.0 to 1.6) scores for pain assessment at time of last follow-up. 75% of patients with long-term pain reduction. With the NHP only the pain dimension showed a significant decrease. Cement leakage rate of 87.5%, with one asymptomatic PE.	Vertebroplasty improves VAS and MGM pain scores long term.
McGraw et al (2002)[86]	Low	Prospective cohort of 100 patients with VCFs secondary to either osteoporosis ($N = 92$), neoplasm ($N = 5$), or other causes ($N = 3$) underwent 156 vertebroplasty procedures. Mean follow-up of 21.5 months. Significant reduction in mean VAS score (8.9 to 2.0) compared with preoperative levels. 97% reported significant pain relief 24 hours after treatment. 93% of patients noted improved ambulation. Complications included a sternal fracture and a transient radiculopathy.	Vertebroplasty for VCFs significantly improves VAS scores.
McKiernan et al (2003)[103]	Low	Prospective cohort of 41 patients with 65 VCFs treated with vertebroplasty. Postoperative imaging done 2 weeks after surgery. Mean anterior and middle vertebral body heights improved by 8.4 and 8.7 mm, or 52% and 59% restoration of lost height, respectively.	Vertebroplasty improved vertebral body height. Cause of fractures not reported.

Study	Quality Rating	Description of Study	Comments and Conclusions
McKiernan et al (2003)[54]	Low	Prospective radiographic analysis of 41 patients treated with vertebroplasty for 65 VCFs, 23 (35%) of which were mobile. Mobile fracture anterior height significantly increased an average of 106% compared with initial fracture height, with an absolute increase of 8.4 mm. Kyphotic angle in mobile fractures decreased by 40%. 7.7% rate of asymptomatic cement leakage.	Vertebroplasty significantly increased the vertebral body height of mobile VCFs.
McKiernan et al (2004)[98]	Low	Prospective cohort of 46 patients with 49 osteoporotic VCFs treated with vertebroplasty. Follow-up of 6 months. Significant improvement in the mean VAS score (7.7 to 2.8) on postoperative day 1 and stayed improved through follow-up period. All five domains of OQLQ also significantly improved. 15% cement leakage rate.	Vertebroplasty for treatment of osteoporotic VCFs improves pain and quality of life scores.
Pérez-Higueras et al (2002)[91]	Low	Prospective cohort of 13 patients with 27 VCFs treated with vertebroplasty. Average follow-up of 65 months. Significant decline in the mean VAS score from 9.1 preoperatively to 2.2 at last follow-up. Also improvement with the short MPQ. 59% rate of cement extravasation.	Decline in VAS scores after treatment of VCFs with vertebroplasty can last at least 5 years.
Prather et al (2006)[89]	Low	Prospective cohort of 50 patients with 103 osteoporotic VCFs treated with vertebroplasty. 80% of patients with 1 year of follow-up. Significant improvement in the mean VAS score from 7.8 preoperatively to 3.1 immediately postoperatively and remained significantly decreased at 1 year. Also significant in ODI and RMD scores at 1-month and 1-year follow-up.	Vertebroplasty significantly improves pain and functional scores at least 1 year postoperatively in the treatment of osteoporotic VCFs.
Voormolen et al (2006)[51]	Low	Prospective cohort of 112 patients with 168 osteoporotic VCFs treated with vertebroplasty. Mean follow-up of 10 months. The mean VAS score significantly reduced from 8.8 preoperatively to 3.3 at 24 hours after surgery, 2.5 at 12 months, and 2.8 at 1–3 years. Clinically significant complication rate of 2.7%.	Vertebroplasty significantly reduced VAS scores over 12 months.
Zoarski et al (2002)[97]	Low	Prospective cohort of 30 patients with 54 osteoporotic VCFs treated with vertebroplasty. Follow-up ranged from 15 to 18 months. Significant improvement in all 4 modules of the MODEMS questionnaire, which includes the SF-36, at 2 weeks postoperatively. Verbal pain scores significantly reduced at long-term follow-up. 1 asymptomatic epidural cement leak.	Vertebroplasty for VCFs significantly improves pain long term.
Amar et al (2001)[41]	Very low	Retrospective cohort of 97 patients with either osteoporosis ($N = 93$) or neoplasm ($N = 4$) who underwent vertebroplasty for 258 VCFs. Mean follow-up of 14.7 months. A majority of patients had decrease in analgesic use (63%), improved ambulation (51%), improved sleep comfort (50%), and improved quality of life (74%). Complications included PE ($N = 3$), radiculopathy ($N = 3$), dural tear ($N = 1$), and cement leakage into the epidural space ($N = 4$).	Vertebroplasty improved pain and quality of life in most patients. No defined scales for outcome measures and no statistical analysis.
Anselmetti et al (2007)[110]	Very low	Retrospective cohort of 283 patients with osteoporosis ($N = 211$), metastasis ($N = 50$), lymphoproliferative disorder ($N = 16$), or other benign lesion ($N = 6$) treated for 749 VCFs with vertebroplasty. Median follow-up of 7 months. PI-NRS scores were significantly reduced, with 86% of patients noting a clinically relevant level of pain reduction, defined by a reduction of at least 2 points.	Vertebroplasty significantly reduced pain due to VCFs.
Barr et al (2000)[42]	Very low	Retrospective cohort of 46 patients with either osteoporosis ($N = 38$) or neoplasm ($N = 8$) who underwent vertebroplasty on 84 vertebrae. Follow-up ranged from 3 weeks to 42 months. Of patients with osteoporosis, 63% had marked or complete pain relief, and another 32% noted moderate pain relief. Patients with neoplasm experienced pain relief in 50% of cases, and one case required subsequent fusion at the treated level. 6.4% complication rate.	Vertebroplasty consistently decreased pain from compression fractures secondary to osteoporosis. Fractures due to neoplasm were usually stabilized, but pain relief was inconsistent.
Brown et al (2004)[85]	Very low	Retrospective cohort of 90 patients with osteoporotic VCFs treated with vertebroplasty divided into 3 groups defined by age of the fracture: <1 year ($n = 49$), 1–2 years	Vertebroplasty can improve pain in VCFs greater than 1 year of age. Arbitrary pain and mobility scales.

(Continued on page 356)

Study	Quality Rating	Description of Study	Comments and Conclusions
		(N = 16), or >2 years (N = 25). Median 12-month follow-up. 80% of patients with fractures older than 1 year had reduction in pain. No significant difference in clinical benefit based on age of fracture. Patients with fractures less than 1 year old had significantly improved mobility compared with older fractures. Complications not reported.	
Brown et al (2005)[92]	Very low	Retrospective cohort of 45 patients with 94 osteoporotic VCFs older than 1 year treated by vertebroplasty. Mean follow-up of 13.1 months. 100% of the 15 patients with preoperative bone marrow edema on T2-weighted MRI had improvement in pain. In patients with no edema, 80% had improvement of symptoms. The difference between these groups was not significant. Complications not reported.	Vertebroplasty can improve pain in VCFs greater than 1 year of age. Arbitrary pain and mobility scales. Bone marrow edema not a significant predictor of clinical response.
Carlier et al (2004)[111]	Very low	Prospective cohort of 30 patients with 46 osteoporotic VCFs treated with vertebroplasty. VAS scores reduced in 91% of patients after 24 hours. Mean reduction of 6.4 degrees when preoperative estimated reducibility > 5 degrees. Cement leakage in 37% of cases.	Vertebroplasty reduced pain in first 24 hours in most patients. No statistical analysis of VAS scores.
Chung et al (2002)[112]	Very low	Cohort of 7 patients with osteoporotic VCFs associated with severe lumbar radicular pain treated with vertebroplasty. Mean follow-up of 9.1 months. All patients noted marked pain relief at time of discharge, from preoperative scores of 9–10 to postoperative scores ≤ 3. Two patients had recurrent pain during the follow-up period.	Vertebroplasty may be an effective treatment for lumbar radicular pain secondary to osteoporotic VCFs. No statistical analysis of pain scores.
Cyteval et al (1999)[113]	Very low	Cohort of 20 patients with osteoporotic VCFs treated with vertebroplasty. Significant decrease in VAS scores 24 hours postoperatively, with all patients improving. Pain recurred in one patient at 1 month. At 6 months, 4 patients with new VCFs. No general complications. 40% cement leakage rate.	Vertebroplasty resulted in immediate postoperative decrease in VAS scores.
Dublin et al (2005)[104]	Very low	Retrospective cohort of 30 patients with 40 osteoporotic VCFs treated with vertebroplasty. Follow-up time not stated. Significant improvement in the pretreatment vertebral height, with a mean improvement of 47.6%. Kyphotic angle also significantly improved with mean correction of 5 degrees. Complications not mentioned.	Vertebroplasty can improve vertebral body height and kyphotic deformity.
Evans et al (2003)[52]	Very low	Retrospective cohort of 245 patients with osteoporotic VCFs treated with vertebroplasty. Median follow-up of 7 months by telephone. Pain, graded on a 10-point scale, significantly decreased from mean preoperative level of 8.9 to 3.4 after vertebroplasty. Impairment of ambulation and activities of daily living also significantly decreased. 4.9% rate of symptomatic complications including rib fracture (N = 7) and radiculopathy (N = 2).	Vertebroplasty significantly improved pain, ambulation, and activities of daily living.
Gangi et al (1994)[114]	Very low	Cohort of 10 patients with osteoporosis (N = 4), hemangioma (N = 5), or metastasis (N = 1) treated for VCFs with vertebroplasty. Follow-up ranged from 4 to 17 months. All patients had a reduction of pain, with no recurrences. Reported no complications.	Pain not measured by a scale, with no statistical analysis comparing preoperative and postoperative levels.
Gaughen et al (2002)[49]	Very low	Retrospective cohort of 48 patients with 84 osteoporotic VCFs treated with vertebroplasty. Follow-up up to 1 month. 95% of patients had an improvement of ≥3 points on an 11-point scale. Mobility also improved. Antecedent venography did not significantly improve effectiveness or safety of vertebroplasty. 71% cement extravasation rate. One postoperative CSF leak.	Vertebroplasty improved pain in most patients. No statistical analysis comparing preoperative and postoperative pain scores.
Gaughen et al (2002)[13]	Very low	Retrospective cohort of 100 patients either with (N = 90) or without (N = 10) spinous process tenderness associated with VCFs treated with vertebroplasty. Follow-up of 1 month. Overall, 91% of patients with reduction of 3 or more points on an 11-point pain scale, with no significant difference between groups. Also an overall improvement of mobility in 88% of patients with no significant difference between groups. No clinical complications.	Vertebroplasty improves pain and mobility problems associated with VCFs irrespective of spinal process tenderness.

Study	Quality Rating	Description of Study	Comments and Conclusions
Gaughen et al (2002)[115]	Very low	Retrospective cohort of 6 patients who underwent repeat vertebroplasty on a previously treated level with 1 month of follow-up. $5/6$ (83%) of patients at least a 3-point improvement in an 11-point pain scale. Mean pain reduction of 6.5 points. 4/4 patients with preoperative mobility impairment had postoperative improvement.	Repeat vertebroplasty on previously treated level is feasible and may offer therapeutic benefit. No statistical analysis of pain scores.
Grados et al (2000)[77]	Very low	Retrospective cohort of 25 patients treated with vertebroplasty for 34 osteoporotic VCFs. Mean follow-up of 48 months. Significant decrease in the mean VAS score at 1 month (37 mm) and time of maximum follow-up (34 mm) compared with preoperative scores (80 mm). Seven cases of cement extravasation into the disc space, 2 cases of nerve root pain, and 1 PE. Significant increase in new fracture adjacent to cemented level (OR 2.27, 95% CI 1.1–4.56), whereas odds ratio of fracture next to uncemented level 1.44 (0.82–2.55).	Vertebroplasty significantly decreased VAS scores 1 month postoperatively for osteoporotic VCFs.
Hiwatashi et al (2003)[116]	Very low	Cohort of 37 patients with osteoporosis ($N = 30$), metastasis ($N = 3$), MM ($N = 2$), lymphoma ($N = 1$), or myelodysplasia ($N = 1$) underwent vertebroplasty for treatment of 85 VCFs. Postoperative imaging performed immediately after the procedure. Mean anterior (2.5 mm), middle (2.7 mm), and posterior (1.4 mm) vertebral body height significantly increased. Complications not reported.	Vertebroplasty can increase vertebral body height.
Hodler et al (2003)[68]	Very low	Retrospective cohort of 152 patients with either osteoporosis ($N = 121$), malignant disease ($N = 30$), or hemangioma ($N = 1$) treated for 363 VCFs with vertebroplasty. Mean follow-up of 8.8 months. Pain scores improved in 86% of patients immediately after treatment, and at last follow-up 88% had improved pain scores. Only predictor of outcome at last follow-up was immediate postoperative pain relief. Cement leakage occurred at 258 levels. Major complications included PE ($N = 10$), rib fracture ($N = 4$), and pneumothorax ($N = 2$).	Vertebroplasty improved pain in most patients. Pain was graded on an arbitrary scale with no statistical analysis comparing preoperative and postoperative scores.
Jang et al (2003)[105]	Very low	Retrospective cohort of 16 patients with intravertebral pseudarthrosis of a vertebral body secondary to avascular necrosis treated with vertebroplasty. Mean follow-up 11 months. The immediate postoperative average VAS score reduced to 4.3 from preoperative level of 9.0. Significant improvement of 8.5 degrees of mean kyphotic deformity and 7.0 mm of mean anterior vertebral height. 2 asymptomatic cases of cement leakage.	Vertebroplasty may be used to treat intravertebral pseudarthrosis secondary to avascular necrosis. No statistical analysis of VAS scores.
Jensen et al (1997)[117]	Very low	Cohort of 29 patients with 47 osteoporotic VCFs treated with vertebroplasty. Immediate clinical results reported. 90% of patients "described pain relief and improved mobility" within 24 hours after treatment. 9 patients with cement leakage, 2 patients with cement leakage into the inferior vena cava, and 2 patients with nondisplaced rib fractures.	Vertebroplasty can improve pain within a day of surgery.
Kaufmann et al (2001)[118]	Very low	Retrospective cohort of 75 patients with 122 osteoporotic VCFs treated with vertebroplasty. Mean follow-up of 7 days. Pain was significantly reduced, as measured on an 11-point scale, from a mean of 9.4 preoperatively to 1.9 postoperatively. Activity and analgesic use also significantly improved. Fracture age did not significantly correlate with clinical outcome. No complications mentioned.	Vertebroplasty significantly reduced pain, improved activity, and reduced analgesic use.
Kim et al (2002)[45]	Very low	Retrospective cohort of 49 patients treated for 75 VCFs with either unipedicular or bipedicular vertebroplasty. Average follow-up of 6.5 weeks. Mean pain scores, based on an 11-point scale, decreased in both the unipedicular (6.6) and bipedicular (7.3) groups, with no significant difference between the groups. Complications not reported.	Uni- and bipedicular approaches for vertebroplasty provide similar pain relief. No statistical analysis of pain scores comparing preoperative and postoperative levels.
Kim et al (2004)[95]	Very low	Retrospective cohort of 70 osteoporotic VCFs with IVVP in 67 patients treated with vertebroplasty. On initial assessment 48 hours postoperatively, marked to complete pain relief (VAS 0–3) occurred in 63% of patients, and	Vertebroplasty reduced initial postoperative pain levels in VCFs with IVVP. No change in vertebral body height.

(*Continued on page 358*)

Study	Quality Rating	Description of Study	Comments and Conclusions
		another 33% had moderate pain relief. No significant change in vertebral body height. At last follow-up (mean 16.4 months), outcomes were excellent in 14%, good with 67%, and fair or poor in 19%. Cement extravasation rate of 14.3%, with no symptomatic cases.	
Krauss et al (2006)[93]	Very low	Cohort of 144 patients with 192 VCFs treated with vertebroplasty. 23% of vertebral bodies with intravertebral clefts. Follow-up up to 24 months. VAS scores significantly reduced, with no difference between fractures with and without clefts. VCFs with clefts had a significantly better mean kyphotic reduction of 3.7 degrees compared with 0.6 degrees for noncleft VCFs. Also a significantly lower rate of cement leakage in the cleft group (18%) compared with the noncleft group.	No difference in VAS score reduction by vertebroplasty between VCFs with and without clefts. VCFs with clefts have better kyphotic reduction and a lower cement leakage rate.
Lane et al (2002)[119]	Very low	Retrospective cohort of 125 patients with 236 osteoporotic VCFs treated with vertebroplasty. 12-month follow-up. Significant improvement in pain scores, as determined on an 11-point scale. No significant clinical difference in efficacy between VCFs with or without intravertebral clefts.	Vertebroplasty reduces pain at 1 year postoperatively.
Layton et al (2007)[120]	Very low	Retrospective review of cohort of 552 patients treated with vertebroplasty for VCFs secondary to osteoporosis (84%), neoplasm (11%), hemangiomas, or trauma. Follow-up of 2 years. VAS and RMD scores significantly improved immediately after the procedure and remained improved at 2-year follow-up. 1.8% rate of clinically significant complications, with rib fractures (1%) being the most common. 5 cases of radiculopathy, 1 case of central spinal canal compromise, and 1 PE.	Vertebroplasty significantly reduced VAS and RMD scores for 2 years in this large series.
Lee and Chen (2004)[106]	Very low	Cohort of 200 patients with single-level osteoporotic VCFs that underwent closed reduction vertebroplasty by restoring the table to restore vertebral body height and reduce kyphosis. Radiographs measured preoperatively and immediately postoperatively. Significant restoration of mean anterior (46%), middle (47%), and posterior (35%) vertebral body height. Kyphotic deformity improved a mean of 6.6 degrees or 43%. 14.5% rate of PMMA leakage, which were all symptomatic.	Closed reduction vertebroplasty successfully improved vertebral body height and reduced kyphotic deformity.
Maynard et al (2000)[121]	Very low	Retrospective cohort of 27 patients with 28 osteoporotic VCFs treated with vertebroplasty. Mean follow-up of 5.7 months. Pain scores improved an average of 7.4 points on a 10-point scale. No discussion of complications.	Vertebroplasty improved pain scores. No statistical analysis of pain scores. Bone scan activity was predictive of treatment success.
Moreland et al (2001)[63]	Very low	Retrospective cohort of 35 patients with 53 VCFs treated with vertebroplasty. Maximum follow-up at 3 months. 89% of patients experienced pain relief. 3 asymptomatic cases of cement leakage, with 2 resulting in a PE. 2 other cases of cement leakage requiring surgical decompression and 1 possible CSF leak.	Vertebroplasty can result in serious complications. No formal pain score or statistical analysis.
Mousavi et al (2003)[53]	Very low	Retrospective cohort of 21 patients with either osteoporosis (N = 12) or metastatic disease (N = 9) who underwent vertebroplasty for 33 VCFs. One week after surgery VAS scores were significantly reduced. No significant difference in pain scores in patients with less than 10% cement extravasation compared with those with greater than 10% extravasation. Cement leakage in 87.9% of cases. One case of cement extravasation led to a painful extruded disk, and another case resulted in central canal compromise requiring surgical decompression.	Vertebroplasty resulted in significantly reduced VAS scores, although they were only presented in a graph. High cement extravasation rate, with two clinically significant cases.
Nakano et al (2002)[122]	Very low	Retrospective cohort of 16 patients that underwent treatment of 12 osteoporotic VCFs, 3 osteoporotic burst fractures, and 1 case of pseudarthrosis with vertebroplasty. Final follow-up at 12–18 months. Improvement of VAS scores in all patients immediately, which was maintained at last follow-up. Significant improvement of the deformity index in patients with VCFs immediately and at 6 months postoperatively. 24% cement leakage rate.	Vertebroplasty provided immediate pain relief that lasted at least 6 months. No statistical analysis of VAS scores. Deformity index significantly improved in VCFs.

Table 36.1 Evidence Summary of Comparative Studies of Vertebroplasty (*Continued*)

Study	Quality Rating	Description of Study	Comments and Conclusions
Nirala et al (2003)[123]	Very low	Prospective cohort of 22 patients with either osteoporosis (*N* = 20) or metastasis (*N* = 2) leading to 31 VCFs treated with vertebroplasty. Mean follow-up of 1 year. Within 24 hours, 57% of patients had complete pain relief and 38% obtained notable pain relief. No return of pain or further loss of vertebral body height at last follow-up. 1 case of epidural cement extravasation.	Small cohort of vertebroplasty cases with no clear pain scale used and no statistical analysis reported.
Peh et al (2002)[96]	Very low	Cohort of 37 patients with 48 severe osteoporotic VCFs, defined by less than one third of original vertebral height, treated with vertebroplasty. Mean follow-up of 11 months. At follow-up, 97% of patients had pain relief. 8% rate of cement leakage with no major complications.	Vertebroplasty effectively reduces pain due to severe osteoporotic VCFs. No statistical analysis comparing preoperative and postoperative pain levels.
Peh et al (2003)[94]	Very low	Cohort of 18 patients with 19 osteoporotic VCFs and intraosseous vacuum phenomena treated with vertebroplasty. Mean follow-up of 9.9 months. Pain relief, assessed with the VAS, was complete in 44.4% of cases, partial in 33.3%, and unchanged in 22.2%. Vertebral body height improved in 95% of cases. Cement extravasation occurred into the disk in 79% of cases and paravertebral soft tissues in 42% of cases.	Vertebroplasty is an effective treatment of VCFs with intraosseous vacuum phenomena. No absolute values or statistics reported for VAS scores of vertebral body heights.
Ryu et al (2002)[60]	Very low	Retrospective cohort of 159 patients with 347 osteoporotic VCFs treated with vertebroplasty. 1 day postoperative VAS scores improved in 95 patients, worsened in 3, and were unchanged with 61. At 3 months, of 102 patients evaluated with VAS scores, 89 patients had improvement and 13 were unchanged compared with preoperative scores. PMMA leakage in 26.5% of treated vertebrae. A larger amount of PMMA used correlated with a higher rate of leakage. Cement leakage led to significantly higher VAS scores immediately after treatment, but not at 3 months.	Vertebroplasty reduced VAS scores 3 months after the procedure, at which time cement leak did not change the therapeutic effect. However, immediately after treatment cement leakage led to significantly higher VAS scores.
Teng et al (2003)[124]	Very low	Cohort of 53 patients with 73 osteoporotic VCFs treated with vertebroplasty. Radiographs obtained with 14 days of the procedure. Significant improvement in mean kyphotic angle (4.3°) and restoration of anterior (29%) and middle (27%) vertebral body height. No mention of complications.	Vertebroplasty increases vertebral body height and reduces kyphotic deformity.
Yu et al (2004)[84]	Very low	Retrospective cohort of 68 patients with single-level osteoporotic VCFs treated with vertebroplasty. Mean follow-up of 13 months. Fractures classified as acute (within 2 weeks), subacute (2 weeks to 2 months), or chronic (after 2 months for analysis). Overall 94.1% of patients with good or excellent results at 1-week follow-up, defined by progress of 2 grades on the Denis pain scale. No significant difference between the 3 groups at 1-day or 1-week follow-up. Overall 11.8% rate of cement leakage, with the acute group having a significantly higher rate (27.3%). 10.3% adjacent level fracture rate. One case of infection.	Vertebroplasty results in a high rate of pain control for acute, subacute, and chronic VCFs.

Abbreviations: CI, confidence interval; CSF, cerebrospinal fluid; IVVP, intravertebral vacuum phenomenon; MGM, McGill-Melzack; MM, multiple myeloma; MODEMS, Musculoskeletal Outcomes Data Evaluation and Management Scale; MPQ, McGill questionnaire; NHP, Nottingham Health Profile; ODI, Oswestry Disability Index; OR, odds ratio; OQLQ, Osteoporosis Quality of Life Questionnaire; PE, pulmonary embolism; PI-NRS, pain intensity numeric rating scale; PMMA, polymethylmethacrylate; QUALEFFO, Quality of Life Questionnaire of the European Foundation for Osteoporosis; RMD, Roland-Morris Disability score; SF-36, Short Form-36; VAS, Visual Analogue Scale; VCF, vertebral compression fracture.

alone.[14] However, no firm conclusions can be reached regarding the efficacy of kyphoplasty for treatment of traumatic compression fractures because there was no control group, and the results may simply reflect the natural history of the fractures in the treated patient population.

Several studies of low or very low quality have provided evidence that vertebroplasty or kyphoplasty for treatment of pathological compression fractures can reduce pain acutely[34,35] and long term[36] increase mobility[37] and improve Short Form-36 or Oswestry disability index scores.[38–40] Still, higher-quality data are needed to specifically define the indications for these procedures in the setting of pathological fractures. In general, vertebroplasty or kyphoplasty may be considered for patients who have painful vertebral compression fractures with at least 3 months of life expectancy. Often patients with a vertebral deformity are otherwise poor surgical candidates, in which case vertebroplasty or kyphoplasty can offer a minimally invasive option that potentially reduces pain and prevents progression of deformity.

The surgical indications for vertebroplasty and kyphoplasty in the treatment of osteoporotic compression fractures are discussed in the following evidence-based review.

Table 36.2 Evidence Summary of Comparative Studies of Kyphoplasty

Study	Class	Description of Study	Comments and Conclusions
Grohs et al (2005)[55]	Moderate	Prospective nonrandomized trial comparing vertebroplasty (N = 23 patients, 29 procedures) and kyphoplasty (N = 28 patients, 35 procedures) for osteoporotic VCFs. Follow-up performed 1 day, 4 months, and 2 years postoperatively. Median duration of 8 weeks of pain prior to treatment. Both the vertebroplasty and kyphoplasty groups had a significant reduction in VAS scores at all time points postoperatively. The kyphoplasty group had significant improvements in ODI scores at 4 months and 1 year (but not 2 years) along with kyphotic wedge and vertebral height measurements while the vertebroplasty group did not. Cement leakage rate into critical areas (epidural space and segmental vessels) was higher in vertebroplasty group (25%) than the kyphoplasty group (0%).	Vertebroplasty and kyphoplasty both had significant reduction in VAS scores at all time points of follow-up. ODI scores were significantly reduced after kyphoplasty alone at 4 months and 1 year but not 2 years. Kyphoplasty resulted in improved kyphotic wedge and vertebral body height, unlike vertebroplasty.
Kasperk et al (2005)[81]	Moderate	Prospective nonrandomized trial comparing kyphoplasty (N = 40) with conservative management (N = 20) for treatment of osteoporotic VCFs. Follow-up of 6 months. Kyphoplasty significantly improved middle vertebral body height 12.1%, compared with a 8.2% decline in the control group. Significant improvement in kyphoplasty group for VAS and EVOS scores, compared with the control group.	Kyphoplasty was superior to conservative treatment of osteoporotic VCFs with regard to vertebral body height, pain (VAS), and daily activity (EVOS) measurements.
Berlemann et al (2004)[82]	Low	Prospective cohort of 24 patients with 27 osteoporotic VCFs treated with kyphoplasty. Follow-up of 1 year. All but one patient with reduction in VAS scores at 1 year compared with preoperative scores. Mean kyphosis reduction of 48%. Potential for reduction was related to age of the fracture. Pain relief was not related to amount of reduction. 15 patients with asymptomatic cement leaks.	Kyphoplasty reduced VAS scores in most patients, and this effect lasted at least one year. No statistical analysis of pain scores.
Coumans et al (2003)[87]	Low	Prospective cohort of 78 patients with either osteoporosis (N = 63) or MM (N = 15) who underwent 188 kyphoplasty procedures. Significant improvement in 7 scores of SF-36 inventory at 18 months. Significant improvements postoperatively compared with preoperatively in mean VAS (7 to 3.2) and ODI (48 to 33) scores. Improvements in VAS and ODI maintained throughout follow-up period. 5 cases of asymptomatic cement extravasation.	Benefits obtained from kyphoplasty in SF-36, VAS, and ODI scores occur at initial postoperative evaluation and last for at least one year.
Crandall et al (2004)[83]	Low	Prospective cohort of 47 patients with 86 osteoporotic VCFs treated with kyphoplasty. At 2-week postoperative follow-up there was a significant decrease in the mean VAS score (7.3 to 4.3) in both acute (<10 weeks) and chronic (>4 months) fractures. Most patients with improvement in ODI, with no difference between acute and chronic groups. Kyphotic angle had significant improvement in both the acute (7 degree) and chronic (5 degree) groups. Both groups also with significant improvement in vertebral body height, although acute fractures with significantly more height restoration.	Kyphoplasty more effectively reduces acute fractures, although improvement in pain is similar in acute and chronic fractures.
Garfin et al (2006)[99]	Low	Prospective cohort of 155 subjects with 214 VCFs treated with kyphoplasty. One patient had MM, but the rest had osteoporosis. 65% of patients with 24-month follow-up. Significant improvement in mean VAS and SF-36 scores at first follow-up and at 24 months. Mean percent midvertebral lost height restored was 32%. 10% rate of cement extravasation.	Kyphoplasty improves VAS and SF-36 scores for at least 2 years postoperatively. Vertebral body height is also improved.
Lieberman et al (2001)[32]	Low	Prospective cohort of 30 patients with painful fractures due to osteoporosis (N = 24) or MM (N = 6) who underwent 70 kyphoplasty procedures. Mean follow-up 6.7 months. Height was improved in 70% of treated vertebral bodies, with an average restoration of 47% of lost height. Significant improvement in SF-36 scores. No major complications.	Kyphoplasty resulted in early improvements of SF-36 scores and vertebral body height.
Maestretti et al (2007)[33]	Low	Prospective cohort of 28 patients with 33 traumatic compression fractures (Magerl type A) without neurological deficit treated with kyphoplasty. Mean follow-up of 30 months. Significant reduction in the mean VAS score at last follow-up (0.8) compared with preoperative scores (8.7). Also noted significant improvement in mean segmental kyphosis and Roland-Morris disability scores.	Kyphoplasty effectively restores vertebral body height, improves segmental kyphosis, and reduces VAS scores in treatment of traumatic compression fractures.

Table 36.2 Evidence Summary of Comparative Studies of Kyphoplasty (*Continued*)

Study	Class	Description of Study	Comments and Conclusions
		Mean height restoration (Beck index) significantly improved from 0.7 preoperatively to 0.87 at 24 hours and 0.84 at last follow-up. 6 cases of cement leakage.	
Phillips et al (2003)[16]	Low	Prospective cohort of 29 patients with 61 osteoporotic compression fractures treated with kyphoplasty. Follow-up was up to 1 year. VAS scores improved significantly from the preoperative mean (8.6) at 1 week (2.6) and 1 year (0.6) after the procedure. 96.5% of patients satisfied or very satisfied. Sagittal alignment improved a mean of 14.2 degrees, with a mean of 8.8 degrees of correction of local spinal kyphosis. Extravertebral cement leak rate of 9.8%	Kyphoplasty significantly improved kyphotic deformity. Also reduced pain 1 week and 1 year after the procedure. At 1 year VAS data available on 19 of 36 patients.
Stoffel et al (2007)[102]	Low	Prospective cohort of 74 patients with 118 osteoporotic compression (32%) or burst (62%) fractures. Mean follow-up of 15 months. Kyphotic deformity significantly reduced a mean of 5 degrees. Also significant improvement in mean VAS, KPS, and SF-36 scores, with the changes being durable. 28% rate of cement leakage per treated level. Complications included a monoparesis secondary to cement leakage requiring surgical decompression in a case of a compression fracture, along with 2 transient radiculopathies.	Kyphoplasty is an effective and safe treatment of both compression and burst fractures. Significant improvement in VAS, KPS, and SF-36 scores along with kyphotic deformity.
Atalay et al (2005)[125]	Very low	Retrospective cohort of 57 patients with 77 VCFs due to osteoporosis, trauma, lytic disease, or hemangioma treated with kyphoplasty. Follow-up of 6.5 months. Decrease in the mean VAS score from 91 preoperatively to 11 at follow-up. No serious complications	Kyphoplasty significantly improved VAS scores for the treatment of VCFs.
Feltes et al (2005)[88]	Very low	Retrospective cohort of 13 patients with 20 osteoporotic VCFs treated with kyphoplasty. Follow-up of 1 month. The mean VAS score was significantly decreased from 7.8 preoperatively to 2.4 immediately postoperatively and 1.4 one month after surgery. No significant improvement in vertebral body height. No major complications reported.	Kyphoplasty significantly improved VAS scores for the treatment of osteoporotic VCFs immediately and 1 month postoperatively.
Ledlie and Renfro (2003)[56]	Very low	Retrospective cohort of 96 patients with either osteoporosis ($N = 90$) or metastatic cancer ($N = 6$) underwent kyphoplasty for 133 VCFs. Follow-up up to 1 year. VAS scores improved significantly from the preoperative mean (8.6) at 1 week (2.7) and 1 year (1.4) after the procedure. Significant anterior (25%) and middle (27%) vertebral body height improvement, which was still present at 1 year. 12 cases of cement leak and one PE.	Kyphoplasty significantly improved vertebral height. Also reduced pain 1 week and 1 year after the procedure. At 1 year VAS data available on 29 of 96 cases.
Ledlie and Renfro (2005)[126]	Very low	Retrospective cohort of 100 patients with 138 VCFs, which were 98% osteoporotic, treated with kyphoplasty. Mean follow-up of 16.9 months. Significant improvement in the number of fractures with wedge, biconcave, or crush deformity.	Kyphoplasty resulted in significant normalization of vertebral body deformities.
Ledlie and Renfro (2006)[100]	Very low	Retrospective cohort of 117 patients with 151 VCFs, of which 97% were associated with osteoporosis, treated with kyphoplasty. A subgroup of 77 patients with 97 VCFs had 2 years of follow-up. Mean VAS scores significantly decreased from 8.9 preoperatively to 2.8 at 1 week and 1.5 at 2 years after surgery. Ability to ambulate significantly improved at 1-week and 2-year follow-up. At 2-year follow-up, vertebral body height was still significantly improved compared with preoperative measurements.	Kyphoplasty results in improved VAS scores, ambulation, and vertebral body height for at least 2 years after surgery.
Majd et al (2005)[107]	Very low	Retrospective cohort of 222 patients with 360 osteoporotic VCFs treated with kyphoplasty. Mean follow-up of 21 months. 78% of patients with complete pain relief, and 11% with partial pain reduction. Significant height restoration in anterior (30%) and middle (50%) vertebral body height, with no relationship to fracture age. Mean of 7 degrees improvement in angulation of fractured vertebral bodies. 10.6% rate of cement extravasation, with one case of radiculopathy.	Kyphoplasty significantly improves vertebral body height secondary to osteoporotic VCFs. No formal pain scale, and no statistical analysis of pain or vertebral body angulation improvement.

(*Continued on page 362*)

36 Management of Thoracolumbar Compression Fractures

Table 36.2 Evidence Summary of Comparative Studies of Kyphoplasty *(Continued)*

Study	Class	Description of Study	Comments and Conclusions
Rhyne et al (2004)[101]	Very low	Retrospective cohort of 52 patients with 82 osteoporotic VCFs treated with kyphoplasty. Mean follow-up of 9 months. Significant increase in mean anterior (4.6 mm) and middle (3.9 mm) vertebral height, along with the Cobb angle (14%). Significant improvement was also seen, compared with preoperative scores with the mean VAS score (9.2 to 2.9) and the Roland-Morris Disability survey (19.3 to 8.1). 9.8% rate of cement leaking. 13.5% rate of reoccurrence.	Kyphoplasty significantly improved vertebral body height, Cobb angle, pain, and patient disability.

Abbreviations: EVOS, European Vertebral Osteoporosis Study; KPS, Karnofsky Performance Scale; MM, multiple myeloma; ODI, Oswestry Disability Index; PE, pulmonary embolism; SF-36, Short Form-36; VAS, visual analogue scale; VCF, vertebral compression fracture.

Potential contraindications to surgery include uncorrected coagulopathy, active infection, spinal canal compromise, radiculopathy, posterior vertebral body cortical fractures, and severe (> 75%) vertebral body collapse.[35,41–44]

Technical Aspects

Kyphoplasty is performed in an operating room under general anesthesia, with the patient in a prone position. The principal concerns when performing a vertebroplasty or kyphoplasty are proper placement of the needle or trocar for injection of the cement and avoiding extravasation of the cement, which can lead to compression of neural elements or venous embolism. Therefore, two fluoroscopic C-arms are used simultaneously to provide both lateral and anterior–posterior views when inserting the trocar and injecting the cement. The trajectory of the trocar should enter the pedicle in the lateral superior quadrant and traverse the pedicle into the vertebral body, with a goal of the trocar being placed in the anteromedial portion of the vertebral body. The results of both clinical[45] and ex vivo biomechanical studies[46,47] suggest that a unipedicular approach can be as effective as a bipedicular approach. A transpedicular approach is reasonable if the pedicles are at least 4 to 5 mm wide. If the pedicles are too small to cannulate, as frequently occurs above T8, a lateral extrapedicular trajectory can be used. Once the location of the trocar is deemed satisfactory, an inflatable balloon tamp is expanded with radiopaque medium to a maximum PSI of 400. After inflation of the balloon, some authors prefer to use antecedent venography with contrast before the injection of cement to avoid a venous embolism,[48] whereas others have concluded that this maneuver does not help avoid complications.[49,50] If there is concern about venous or transcortical extravasation, the trocar may be moved or the cement may be allowed to solidify before more is injected. The cement should be injected under live fluoroscopy, and the injection should be halted once the cement enters the posterior third of the vertebral body.

Complications

The rate of clinically significant, or symptomatic, complications for vertebroplasty ranges from 2.7 to 6.4%.[42,51,52] More serious complications of vertebroplasty result from extravasation of cement into the epidural space. Reported rates of cement leakage for vertebroplasty range from 7.7 to 87.9%[53,54] but fortunately most incidents remain asymptomatic.

Several studies suggest that kyphoplasty has a lower rate of cement extravasation than vertebroplasty. Reported rates of cement leakage with kyphoplasty generally range from 0 to 12.5%.[55,56] The authors of one prospective, nonrandomized trial reported a 25% rate of cement leakage with vertebroplasty but

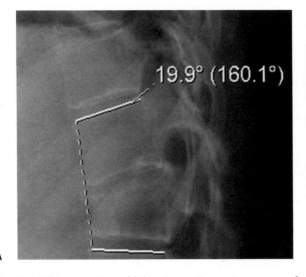
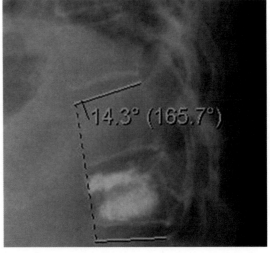

A   B

Fig. 36.1 **(A)** Preoperative and **(B)** postoperative roentgenograms of a 63-year-old patient who underwent kyphoplasty of a T12 compression fracture. The anterior vertebral height increased 4 mm and the kyphotic deformity decreased 5.6 degrees.

0% for kyphoplasty.[55] The results of an in vivo study demonstrated significantly less vascular and transcortical extravasation of injected contrast with kyphoplasty than with vertebroplasty.[57] In a systematic review by Taylor et al,[58] cement leakage was significantly higher with vertebroplasty (40%) than with kyphoplasty (8%), and 3% of vertebroplasty leaks were symptomatic, whereas no kyphoplasty leaks were reported to be symptomatic. In another systematic review of 69 studies, Hulme et al[59] found similar rates of extravasation for vertebroplasty (41%) and kyphoplasty (9%), with subsequent clinical complications occurring in 3.9% and 2.2% of vertebroplasty and kyphoplasty cases, respectively.

An increased rate of cement extravasation with vertebroplasty compared with kyphoplasty may have clinical consequences beyond an increased risk of complications. In a retrospective study of a cohort of 159 patients treated with vertebroplasty, patients with epidural cement leakage realized significantly worse VAS scores than patients without leakage immediately after the procedure but not at 3 months of follow-up.[60] Only 30% of patients who clinically improved initially had epidural leakage, and all patients with aggravated symptoms had cement extravasation. Thus, if kyphoplasty results in a lower incidence of cement extravasation, better short-term clinical outcomes may be expected.

Compression of neural elements can lead to paralysis with involvement of the spinal cord[61] or radiculopathy with compromise of a neural foramen,[41,62] necessitating surgical decompression.[53,63,64] Hulme et al[59] reported neurological complications were seen in 0.6% of vertebroplasty cases and 0.03% of kyphoplasty cases. Cement may also flow into venous channels and ultimately lead to a pulmonary embolism,[65–67] which is reported to occur in 0.6% and 0.01% of vertebroplasty and kyphoplasty cases, respectively.[59] Other complications include infections, epidural hematomas, dural tears, and rib fractures or pneumothorax in thoracic cases.[41,68,69] Pedicle fractures may be a more frequent complication of kyphoplasty because of the larger trocar size.[70] Osteomyelitis is a rare complication that may require corpectomy.[71]

The reported risk of developing an adjacent-level fracture after these procedures varies widely for both vertebroplasty (8 to 52%) and kyphoplasty (3 to 29%).[72–77] It is interesting that the occurrence of new fractures after vertebroplasty or kyphoplasty is weighted toward the first 30 postoperative days,[72,74] making extrapolation of normalized annual fracture rates from data generated by short follow-up periods problematic. The higher incidence of fractures in the early postoperative period could potentially be explained by increased patient activity and higher stress secondary to a diminished level of pain. Furthermore, the presence of one osteoporotic fracture can increase the risk of developing another fracture up to 12.6-fold,[78] and therefore fractures occurring after treatment may reflect the natural history of the disease. A retrospective review of 25 patients showed that new fractures were significantly more likely to occur adjacent to a cemented level [odds ratio (OR) 2.27, 95% confidence interval (CI) 1.1 to 4.56], but not adjacent to an uncemented fractured vertebrae (OR 1.44, 95% CI 0.82 to 2.55).[77] On the other hand, the authors of a prospective review of 16 patients did not find a significant odds ratio for fractures occurring adjacent to cemented (OR 3.18, 95% CI 0.51 to 19.64) or uncemented fractures (OR 2.14, 95% CI 0.17 to 26.31). Other potential risk factors for developing adjacent-level fractures include cement extravasation into a disk[76] and osteoporosis secondary to steroid use.[79] Overall, the current data are inconsistent, and

no firm conclusions can be reached concerning the risk of adjacent-level fractures after vertebroplasty or kyphoplasty.

◆ Questions for Discussion

What are the indications for vertebroplasty or kyphoplasty after a compression fracture of osteoporotic spine?

Since vertebroplasty was first introduced for the treatment of hemangiomas, the use of vertebroplasty and kyphoplasty has evolved to encompass a wide spectrum of patients. Even within the subset of patients with osteoporosis, these procedures have been applied to patients with very heterogeneous clinical and radiographic characteristics. Regardless of the indication, the primary outcome for assessing the efficacy of these procedures is pain reduction.

One of the biggest variables among studies of vertebroplasty and kyphoplasty is the duration of symptoms prior to treatment or, as a correlate, the age of the fracture. Voormolen et al[80] performed a prospective, randomized, controlled trial with 34 patients in which they compared vertebroplasty with optimal pain medication (control group) in the treatment of subacute and chronic painful osteoporotic fractures, defined as greater than 6 weeks but less than 6 months old. Patients in the surgical treatment group had significantly improved VAS scores compared with the control group 1 day after treatment but not 2 weeks later. At 1 day, the treatment group had a reduction in mean VAS scores of 2.3, compared with 0.5 for the control group, which is of questionable clinical value. Roland-Morris disability scores were significantly better for the treatment group at both time points. This study was graded as moderate-quality evidence, instead of good quality, for several issues. First, there were relatively few subjects, which raises concerns about the study design being underpowered. Second, the follow-up was only for 2 weeks. Third, defining the "gold standard" of treatment for osteoporotic compression fractures to be optimal pain medication without other treatments such as bracing and physical therapy is debatable.

Diamond et al[28] provided moderate-quality evidence with a prospective, nonrandomized trial comparing vertebroplasty with conservative management in patients with symptoms ranging in duration from 1 to 6 weeks and a mean follow-up of 215 days. Twenty-four hours after treatment the vertebroplasty group had a significant 53% reduction in the mean pain score from 19 to 9 on a 25-point scale, which was also significantly better than the control group's mean pain score of 19 at the same time point. At the 6-week and 6- to 12-month follow-up points, both groups had significant improvement compared with preoperative pain scores, with no difference between groups. Physical function (Barthel index) scores followed a similar trend, with only the vertebroplasty group improving at 24 hours but both groups recognizing similar improvement at 6 weeks and 6 to 12 months.

Nakano et al[27] presented more moderate quality evidence with a matched case-control study, comparing vertebroplasty with conservative treatment. This study consisted of 60 patients with symptoms of at least 4 weeks duration and a mean follow-up of 17 months. Patients in the vertebroplasty group had a significant reduction in their mean VAS score from 7.9 preoperatively to 0.7 at 6 months and 0.7 at 12 months. The control group also realized a significant reduction in a mean VAS score from 7.5 preoperatively to 2.6 at 6 months and 2.0 at 12 months. Compared with patients in the control group, pain scores for those in the vertebroplasty group were significantly lower at both postoperative time points, although the clinical significance is questionable since the difference between groups is small.

Kasperk et al[81] performed a prospective, nonrandomized, controlled trial comparing kyphoplasty with conventional medical management, which generated moderate-quality evidence. A total of 60 patients were enrolled in the study after at least 12 months of symptoms, with follow-up at 3 and 6 months. VAS scores improved in the kyphoplasty group from a preoperative mean of 26.2 to 42.4 at 3 months and 44.2 at 6 months. The mean VAS scores at 3 and 6 months for the kyphoplasty group were significantly better than those for the conservative treatment group.

Together, these four trials offer moderate-quality evidence that vertebroplasty and kyphoplasty, compared with conservative therapy, can improve pain control when symptoms have been present from 1 week to greater than 12 months. Low and very low quality evidence from several other studies suggest that the age of fracture does not influence clinical outcome after vertebroplasty or kyphoplasty.[82–84] The authors of a retrospective cohort study of 90 patients treated with vertebroplasty found that 92% of patients with fractures less than 1 year old had complete or partial pain relief, compared with 87% of patients with fractures 1 to 2 years old and 76% of patients with fractures greater than 2 years old.[85] There was no statistically significant difference between the three groups.

The results of the studies by Voormolen et al[80] and Diamond et al[28] demonstrated that pain scores improve in 24 hours after vertebroplasty, coinciding with several other studies that provide low or very low quality evidence that pain scores significantly improve in the first 24 hours after vertebroplasty or kyphoplasty.[68,86–89] The results of the studies by Nakano et al[27] and Kasperk et al[81] also suggest these procedures are superior to conservative treatment for reducing pain a year after treatment, although the results of the studies by Voormolen et al[80] and Diamond et al[28] did not. Other studies provide low-quality evidence that the benefits of vertebroplasty can last even longer. Legroux-Gérot et al[90] found that 75% of patients had improved pain scores at last follow-up (mean 35 months), whereas Pérez-Higueras et al[91] demonstrated that the mean VAS score significantly declined from 9.1 preoperatively to 2.2 at last follow-up (mean 65 months).

Spinous process tenderness on physical examination is frequently considered an inclusion criterion when selecting vertebral levels for treatment with vertebroplasty or kyphoplasty. However, in a retrospective cohort, Gaughen et al[13] provided very low quality evidence suggesting the contrary. Overall, 91% of 100 patients noted at least a three-point reduction in pain with an 11-point scale. The 10 patients who had no spinous process tenderness before treatment did not have a significantly different clinical result than those individuals with point tenderness.

Several radiographic findings have been evaluated with regard to the efficacy of vertebroplasty. The authors of a retrospective cohort of 45 patients treated with vertebroplasty demonstrated that 100% of patients with increased T2 signal on magnetic resonance imaging, indicative of bone edema at the treated level had improvement in pain, whereas 80% of patients without increased T2 signal noted reduced pain.[92] The difference between groups was not significant, providing

very low quality evidence that increased T2 signal on magnetic resonance imaging is not predictive of vertebroplasty efficacy. Very low quality evidence does suggest that osteoporotic compression fractures associated with intravertebral clefts[93] and intraosseous vacuum phenomena[94,95] are amenable to treatment with vertebroplasty. In a cohort study providing very low quality evidence, Peh et al[96] looked at whether vertebroplasty is beneficial with severe compression fractures. Thirty-seven patients were identified with vertebrae collapsed to one third or less of their original height. Sixty-five percent of fractures were classified as gibbus, 27% as vertebra plana, and 8% as H-shaped. At a mean follow-up of 11 months, 97% of patients had complete or partial pain relief.

In summary, moderate-quality evidence suggests that vertebroplasty or kyphoplasty is indicated for fractures with ages varying from 1 week to greater than 12 months. Low and very low quality evidence provides additional support that fracture age does not influence clinical outcome and that fractures greater than 2 years of age can be effectively treated. Very low quality evidence suggests that spinous process tenderness is not a prerequisite for treatment with vertebroplasty or kyphoplasty. Low and very low quality evidence also suggests that vertebra plana fractures and fractures with clefts or intraosseous vacuum phenomena are candidates for these treatments. Finally, very low quality evidence indicates that T2 hyperintensity on magnetic resonance imaging is not required for vertebroplasty or kyphoplasty to successfully reduce pain.

Are kyphoplasty and vertebroplasty equivalent treatments for osteoporotic compression fractures?

As with assessing the indications for these procedures, the primary outcome of interest for comparing vertebroplasty and kyphoplasty is pain control. Secondary measures include patient function and correction of deformity. Grohs et al[55] provided moderate-quality evidence with a prospective, nonrandomized trial directly comparing vertebroplasty and kyphoplasty. This study included a total of 51 patients with osteoporotic vertebral compression fractures and follow-up at 1 day, 4 months, and 2 years postoperatively. The mean postoperative VAS scores for the kyphoplasty group 1 day (3.5), 4 months (3.2), and 2 years (2.0) after surgery were significantly lower than the mean preoperative score (7.4). Likewise, the mean VAS scores for the vertebroplasty group at 1 day (3.0), 4 months (5.7), and 2 years (4.6) were all significantly lower than the preoperative score (7.8). Although both treatment groups provided significant improvement in VAS scores, the authors concluded that "a long-lasting effect on pain was found only after balloon kyphoplasty" and that "kyphoplasty was superior in decreasing pain." On the basis of the data presented, these conclusions appear unjustified. First, the vertebroplasty group had a significant reduction in pain scores at all time points, showing there was a long-lasting effect on pain. Second, there was no statistical analysis directly comparing vertebroplasty and kyphoplasty scores to support the statement that kyphoplasty is superior. Although the vertebroplasty VAS scores were higher at the 4-month and 2-year follow-up times, there were no statistics to confirm that this difference was significant. Therefore, we conclude from these data that both kyphoplasty and vertebroplasty significantly reduced VAS scores from 1 day to 2 years postoperatively.

Any further comparisons between vertebroplasty and kyphoplasty with respect to pain reduction can only be done indirectly between different studies. Several studies already described provide moderate-quality evidence suggesting that both vertebroplasty and kyphoplasty effectively reduce pain,[27,28,80,81] although the duration of efficacy is variable between studies. Low and very low quality evidence suggests that both vertebroplasty[86,95] and kyphoplasty[16,82] have the potential to reduce pain in up to ~90% of patients. The major caveat with these studies is that there is no control group and, as previously discussed, conservative treatment can also have significant long-term results. Therefore, it is unclear whether these results reflect the efficacy of treatment or the natural history of osteoporotic fractures.

Data on functional outcomes after vertebroplasty and kyphoplasty are often difficult to compare because they involve a variety of different measures, including the Oswestry Disability Index (ODI), Short Form-36 questionnaire (SF-36), and Roland-Morris disability (RMD) score. In one study, Grohs et al[55] provided data on functional outcome with the ODI at all follow-up points. The kyphoplasty group had a significant improvement in ODI scores at 4 months and 1 year, but not 2 years, whereas the vertebroplasty group did not have a significant improvement at any time. However, other moderate-quality data showed that vertebroplasty can improve functional outcomes, measured by the RMD[80] and Barthel physical functioning[28] scores at short-term follow-up. The trial by Kasperk et al[81] also supplied moderate-quality evidence that kyphoplasty can improve patient daily activity, measured by the European Vertebral Osteoporosis Study (EVOS) questionnaire, 6 months after treatment. Several other studies provide evidence of low and very low quality that both vertebroplasty[52,89,97,98] and kyphoplasty[32,87,99–102] can significantly improve patient functioning, with some of these studies providing long-term follow-up.

One of the purported advantages of kyphoplasty over vertebroplasty is that kyphoplasty reduces kyphotic deformity. Two questions need to be addressed when evaluating this issue: First, does kyphoplasty actually reduce deformity better than vertebroplasty? Second, does the reduction of kyphotic deformity have clinical relevance pertaining to pain improvement? As with functional outcome, reported studies have involved use of a wide variety of measures to evaluate correction of deformity, including absolute increase of vertebral body, percent height restoration, change of kyphotic angulation, and varying indices. Because of this wide variety of measurements, a direct comparison between studies is difficult.

Again, Grohs et al[55] provided moderate-quality data concerning deformity correction for both kyphoplasty and vertebroplasty. The local kyphosis significantly decreased to 6 degrees from 13 degrees for fractures treated with kyphoplasty, whereas there was no change in the vertebroplasty group. Nakano et al[27] evaluated deformity after vertebroplasty and found that the deformity index and kyphosis rate were significantly better with vertebroplasty than the control group at follow-up. On the basis of the data presented in the study, the difference between groups appears to be due to a worsening of deformity in the control group, whereas deformity in the treatment group was stabilized over time but not appreciably improved. A similar trend was found for kyphoplasty by Kasperk et al[81]; in their study, the kyphotic angle was relatively stable in patients 6 months after kyphoplasty, whereas patients in the control group had significant worsening of the kyphotic angle. Low and very low quality evidence from several studies has demonstrated a significant improvement in vertebral body height and kyphotic angle after vertebroplasty,[54,103–106] although these findings are not universal.[95] Similarly, the majority of low and very low quality evidence shows that kyphoplasty can increase vertebral body height and decrease kyphotic deformity,[32,56,100–102,107] but not all studies support these findings.[88]

Only low-quality data were identified that address the issue of whether pain relief is related to the extent of deformity correction. Berlemann et al[82] prospectively examined a cohort of 24 patients with osteoporotic fractures treated by kyphoplasty and found that the magnitude of pain relief was not related to the degree of kyphosis reduction. Interestingly, reduction of kyphosis was related to the age of fracture, which Crandall et al[83] also found to be true, but Majd et al[107] did not.

To summarize, direct comparisons between vertebroplasty and kyphoplasty are difficult because of a paucity of data. Moderate-quality evidence demonstrates that both vertebroplasty and kyphoplasty reduce pain, although the durability of vertebroplasty results over time has been less consistent across studies. Low and very low quality data suggest that the degree of pain relief is comparable between procedures. Moderate-quality data also show that both vertebroplasty and kyphoplasty improve patient functional scores, although we found no moderate class evidence that vertebroplasty improves patient functioning long term. Low and very low quality evidence indicates that both procedures improve patient function with a variety of measures in short-term and long-term follow-up. Moderate-quality evidence shows that vertebroplasty consistently stabilizes the progression of deformity, whereas kyphoplasty either improves or stabilizes deformity. The majority of low and very low quality evidence demonstrated that both procedures can improve deformity. However, data do not support the perception that deformity correction improves clinical outcome.

◆ Summary

Magerl type 1A compression fractures can be caused by acute trauma, osteoporosis, and neoplastic processes. These fractures are relatively common, and osteoporotic fractures are expected to become more frequent with an aging population. Conservative treatments appear to reduce pain but are not effective for rapid symptomatic relief. The age of a fracture is not a critical factor in patient selection for vertebroplasty or kyphoplasty. Moderate-quality evidence suggests that vertebroplasty and kyphoplasty are fairly equivalent treatments for the reduction of pain and improvement of patient function, although the improvements seen with vertebroplasty have not been shown to be as robust over time. Kyphoplasty appears to have a lower rate of cement extravasation, and consequently a lower complication rate.

References

1. Magerl F, Aebi M. A comprehensive classification of thoracic and lumbar injuries. In: Aebi M, Thalgott JS, Webb JK, eds. AO ASIF Principles in Spine Surgery. Berlin: Springer; 1998:20–41
2. Whitesides TE Jr. Traumatic kyphosis of the thoracolumbar spine. Clin Orthop Relat Res 1977;(128):78–92

3. Magerl F, Aebi M, Gertzbein SD, Harms J, Nazarian S. A comprehensive classification of thoracic and lumbar injuries. Eur Spine J 1994;3:184–201

4. Gertzbein SD. Scoliosis Research Society. Multicenter spine fracture study. Spine 1992;17:528–540

5. Prather H, Watson JO, Gilula LA. Nonoperative management of osteoporotic vertebral compression fractures. Injury 2007;38(Suppl 3):S40–S48

6. Cooper C, Atkinson EJ, O'Fallon WM, Melton LJ III. Incidence of clinically diagnosed vertebral fractures: a population-based study in Rochester, Minnesota, 1985-1989. J Bone Miner Res 1992;7:221–227

7. Silverman SL. The clinical consequences of vertebral compression fracture. Bone 1992;13(Suppl 2):S27–S31

8. Melton LJ III, Kan SH, Frye MA, Wahner HW, O'Fallon WM, Riggs BL. Epidemiology of vertebral fractures in women. Am J Epidemiol 1989;129:1000–1011

9. Hammerberg KW. Surgical treatment of metastatic spine disease. Spine 1992;17:1148–1153

10. Cobb CA III, Leavens ME, Eckles N. Indications for nonoperative treatment of spinal cord compression due to breast cancer. J Neurosurg 1977;47:653–658

11. Wong DA, Fornasier VL, MacNab I. Spinal metastases: the obvious, the occult, and the impostors. Spine 1990;15:1–4

12. Katzel JA, Hari P, Vesole DH. Multiple myeloma: charging toward a bright future. CA Cancer J Clin 2007;57:301–318

13. Gaughen JR Jr, Jensen ME, Schweickert PA, Kaufmann TJ, Marx WF, Kallmes DF. Lack of preoperative spinous process tenderness does not affect clinical success of percutaneous vertebroplasty. J Vasc Interv Radiol 2002;13:1135–1138

14. Young MH. Long-term consequences of stable fractures of the thoracic and lumbar vertebral bodies. J Bone Joint Surg Br 1973;55:295–300

15. Folman Y, Gepstein R. Late outcome of nonoperative management of thoracolumbar vertebral wedge fractures. J Orthop Trauma 2003;17:190–192

16. Phillips FM, Ho E, Campbell-Hupp M, McNally T, Todd Wetzel F, Gupta P. Early radiographic and clinical results of balloon kyphoplasty for the treatment of osteoporotic vertebral compression fractures. Spine 2003;28:2260–2265, discussion 2265–2267

17. Burton AW, Rhines LD, Mendel E. Vertebroplasty and kyphoplasty: a comprehensive review. Neurosurg Focus 2005;18:e1

18. Kado DM, Browner WS, Palermo L, Nevitt MC, Genant HK, Cummings SR; Study of Osteoporotic Fractures Research Group. Vertebral fractures and mortality in older women: a prospective study. Arch Intern Med 1999;159:1215–1220

19. Schlaich C, Minne HW, Bruckner T, et al. Reduced pulmonary function in patients with spinal osteoporotic fractures. Osteoporos Int 1998;8:261–267

20. Leech JA, Dulberg C, Kellie S, Pattee L, Gay J. Relationship of lung function to severity of osteoporosis in women. Am Rev Respir Dis 1990;141:68–71

21. Rapado A. General management of vertebral fractures. Bone 1996;18(3, Suppl):191S–196S

22. Weitzman G. Treatment of stable thoracolumbar spine compression fractures by early ambulation. Clin Orthop Relat Res 1971;76:116–122

23. Sinaki M, Itoi E, Wahner HW, et al. Stronger back muscles reduce the incidence of vertebral fractures: a prospective 10 year follow-up of postmenopausal women. Bone 2002;30:836–841

24. Palombaro KM. Effects of walking-only interventions on bone mineral density at various skeletal sites: a meta-analysis. J Geriatr Phys Ther 2005;28:102–107

25. Khosla S, Riggs BL. Treatment options for osteoporosis. Mayo Clin Proc 1995;70:978–982

26. Reginster J, Minne HW, Sorensen OH, et al; Vertebral Efficacy with Risedronate Therapy (VERT) Study Group. Randomized trial of the effects of risedronate on vertebral fractures in women with established postmenopausal osteoporosis. Osteoporos Int 2000;11:83–91

27. Nakano M, Hirano N, Ishihara H, Kawaguchi Y, Watanabe H, Matsuura K. Calcium phosphate cement-based vertebroplasty compared with conservative treatment for osteoporotic compression fractures: a matched case-control study. J Neurosurg Spine 2006;4:110–117

28. Diamond TH, Champion B, Clark WA. Management of acute osteoporotic vertebral fractures: a nonrandomized trial comparing percutaneous vertebroplasty with conservative therapy. Am J Med 2003;114:257–265

29. Prié L, Lagarde P, Palussière J, et al. Radiotherapy of spinal metastases in breast cancer. Apropos of a series of 108 patients [in French] Cancer Radiother 1997;1:234–239

30. Dickman CA, Fessler RG, MacMillan M, Haid RW. Transpedicular screw-rod fixation of the lumbar spine: operative technique and outcome in 104 cases. J Neurosurg 1992;77:860–870

31. Galibert P, Deramond H, Rosat P, Le Gars D. Preliminary note on the treatment of vertebral angioma by percutaneous acrylic vertebroplasty [in French]. Neurochirurgie 1987;33:166–168

32. Lieberman IH, Dudeney S, Reinhardt MK, Bell G. Initial outcome and efficacy of "kyphoplasty" in the treatment of painful osteoporotic vertebral compression fractures. Spine 2001;26:1631–1638

33. Maestretti G, Cremer C, Otten P, Jakob RP. Prospective study of stand-alone balloon kyphoplasty with calcium phosphate cement augmentation in traumatic fractures. Eur Spine J 2007;16:601–610

34. Cotten A, Dewatre F, Cortet B, et al. Percutaneous vertebroplasty for osteolytic metastases and myeloma: effects of the percentage of lesion filling and the leakage of methyl methacrylate at clinical follow-up. Radiology 1996;200:525–530

35. Weill A, Chiras J, Simon JM, Rose M, Sola-Martinez T, Enkaoua E. Spinal metastases: indications for and results of percutaneous injection of acrylic surgical cement. Radiology 1996;199:241–247

36. Fourney DR, Schomer DF, Nader R, et al. Percutaneous vertebroplasty and kyphoplasty for painful vertebral body fractures in cancer patients. J Neurosurg 2003;98(1, Suppl):21–30

37. Alvarez L, Pérez-Higueras A, Quiñones D, Calvo E, Rossi RE. Vertebroplasty in the treatment of vertebral tumors: postprocedural outcome and quality of life. Eur Spine J 2003;12:356–360

38. Dudeney S, Lieberman IH, Reinhardt MK, Hussein M. Kyphoplasty in the treatment of osteolytic vertebral compression fractures as a result of multiple myeloma. J Clin Oncol 2002;20:2382–2387

39. Lane JM, Hong R, Koob J, et al. Kyphoplasty enhances function and structural alignment in multiple myeloma. Clin Orthop Relat Res 2004;(426):49–53

40. Pflugmacher R, Beth P, Schroeder RJ, Schaser KD, Melcher I. Balloon kyphoplasty for the treatment of pathological fractures in the thoracic and lumbar spine caused by metastasis: one-year follow-up. Acta Radiol 2007;48:89–95

41. Amar AP, Larsen DW, Esnaashari N, Albuquerque FC, Lavine SD, Teitelbaum GP. Percutaneous transpedicular polymethylmethacrylate vertebroplasty for the treatment of spinal compression fractures. Neurosurgery 2001;49:1105–1114, discussion 1114–1115

42. Barr JD, Barr MS, Lemley TJ, McCann RM. Percutaneous vertebroplasty for pain relief and spinal stabilization. Spine 2000;25:923–928

43. Cotten A, Boutry N, Cortet B, et al. Percutaneous vertebroplasty: state of the art. Radiographics 1998;18:311–320, discussion 320–323

44. Peters KR, Guiot BH, Martin PA, Fessler RG. Vertebroplasty for osteoporotic compression fractures: current practice and evolving techniques. Neurosurgery 2002;51(5, Suppl):S96–S103

45. Kim AK, Jensen ME, Dion JE, Schweickert PA, Kaufmann TJ, Kallmes DF. Unilateral transpedicular percutaneous vertebroplasty: initial experience. Radiology 2002;222:737–741

46. Steinmann J, Tingey CT, Cruz G, Dai Q. Biomechanical comparison of unipedicular versus bipedicular kyphoplasty. Spine 2005;30:201–205

47. Molloy S, Riley LH III, Belkoff SM. Effect of cement volume and placement on mechanical-property restoration resulting from vertebroplasty. AJNR Am J Neuroradiol 2005;26:401–404

48. McGraw JK, Heatwole EV, Strnad BT, Silber JS, Patzilk SB, Boorstein JM. Predictive value of intraosseous venography before percutaneous vertebroplasty. J Vasc Interv Radiol 2002;13(2 Pt 1):149–153

49. Gaughen JR Jr, Jensen ME, Schweickert PA, Kaufmann TJ, Marx WF, Kallmes DF. Relevance of antecedent venography in percutaneous vertebroplasty for the treatment of osteoporotic compression fractures. AJNR Am J Neuroradiol 2002;23:594–600

50. Vasconcelos C, Gailloud P, Beauchamp NJ, Heck DV, Murphy KJ. Is percutaneous vertebroplasty without pretreatment venography safe? Evaluation of 205 consecutives procedures. AJNR Am J Neuroradiol 2002;23:913–917

51. Voormolen MH, Lohle PN, Lampmann LE, et al. Prospective clinical follow-up after percutaneous vertebroplasty in patients with painful osteoporotic vertebral compression fractures. J Vasc Interv Radiol 2006;17:1313–1320

52. Evans AJ, Jensen ME, Kip KE, et al. Vertebral compression fractures: pain reduction and improvement in functional mobility after percutaneous polymethylmethacrylate vertebroplasty retrospective report of 245 cases. Radiology 2003;226:366–372

53. Mousavi P, Roth S, Finkelstein J, Cheung G, Whyne C. Volumetric quantification of cement leakage following percutaneous vertebroplasty in metastatic and osteoporotic vertebrae. J Neurosurg 2003;99(1, Suppl):56–59

54. McKiernan F, Jensen R, Faciszewski T. The dynamic mobility of vertebral compression fractures. J Bone Miner Res 2003;18:24–29

55. Grohs JG, Matzner M, Trieb K, Krepler P. Minimal invasive stabilization of osteoporotic vertebral fractures: a prospective nonrandomized comparison of vertebroplasty and balloon kyphoplasty. J Spinal Disord Tech 2005;18:238–242

56. Ledlie JT, Renfro M. Balloon kyphoplasty: one-year outcomes in vertebral body height restoration, chronic pain, and activity levels. J Neurosurg 2003;98(1, Suppl):36–42

57. Phillips FM, Todd Wetzel F, Lieberman I, Campbell-Hupp M. An in vivo comparison of the potential for extravertebral cement leak after

vertebroplasty and kyphoplasty. Spine 2002;27:2173–2178, discussion 2178–2179

58. Taylor RS, Taylor RJ, Fritzell P. Balloon kyphoplasty and vertebroplasty for vertebral compression fractures: a comparative systematic review of efficacy and safety. Spine 2006;31:2747–2755

59. Hulme PA, Krebs J, Ferguson SJ, Berlemann U. Vertebroplasty and kyphoplasty: a systematic review of 69 clinical studies. Spine 2006;31: 1983–2001

60. Ryu KS, Park CK, Kim MC, Kang JK. Dose-dependent epidural leakage of polymethylmethacrylate after percutaneous vertebroplasty in patients with osteoporotic vertebral compression fractures. J Neurosurg 2002; 96(1, Suppl):56–61

61. Lee BJ, Lee SR, Yoo TY. Paraplegia as a complication of percutaneous vertebroplasty with polymethylmethacrylate: a case report. Spine 2002;27:E419–E422

62. Ratliff J, Nguyen T, Heiss J. Root and spinal cord compression from methylmethacrylate vertebroplasty. Spine 2001;26:E300–E302

63. Moreland DB, Landi MK, Grand W. Vertebroplasty: techniques to avoid complications. Spine J 2001;1:66–71

64. Patel AA, Vaccaro AR, Martyak GG, et al. Neurologic deficit following percutaneous vertebral stabilization. Spine 2007;32:1728–1734

65. Chen HL, Wong CS, Ho ST, Chang FL, Hsu CH, Wu CT. A lethal pulmonary embolism during percutaneous vertebroplasty. Anesth Analg 2002;95:1060–1062 table of contents.

66. Jang JS, Lee SH, Jung SK. Pulmonary embolism of polymethylmethacrylate after percutaneous vertebroplasty: a report of three cases. Spine 2002;27:E416–E418

67. Tozzi P, Abdelmoumene Y, Corno AF, Gersbach PA, Hoogewoud HM, von Segesser LK. Management of pulmonary embolism during acrylic vertebroplasty. Ann Thorac Surg 2002;74:1706–1708

68. Hodler J, Peck D, Gilula LA. Midterm outcome after vertebroplasty: predictive value of technical and patient-related factors. Radiology 2003;227:662–668

69. Garfin SR, Yuan HA, Reiley MA. New technologies in spine: kyphoplasty and vertebroplasty for the treatment of painful osteoporotic compression fractures. Spine 2001;26:1511–1515

70. Nussbaum DA, Gailloud P, Murphy K. A review of complications associated with vertebroplasty and kyphoplasty as reported to the Food and Drug Administration medical device related web site. J Vasc Interv Radiol 2004;15:1185–1192

71. Walker DH, Mummaneni P, Rodts GE Jr. Infected vertebroplasty: report of two cases and review of the literature. Neurosurg Focus 2004;17:E6

72. Fribourg D, Tang C, Sra P, Delamarter R, Bae H. Incidence of subsequent vertebral fracture after kyphoplasty. Spine 2004;29:2270–2276, discussion 2277

73. Kim SH, Kang HS, Choi JA, Ahn JM. Risk factors of new compression fractures in adjacent vertebrae after percutaneous vertebroplasty. Acta Radiol 2004;45:440–445

74. Uppin AA, Hirsch JA, Centenera LV, Pfiefer BA, Pazianos AG, Choi IS. Occurrence of new vertebral body fracture after percutaneous vertebroplasty in patients with osteoporosis. Radiology 2003;226:119–124

75. Cortet B, Cotten A, Boutry N, et al. Percutaneous vertebroplasty in the treatment of osteoporotic vertebral compression fractures: an open prospective study. J Rheumatol 1999;26:2222–2228

76. Lin EP, Ekholm S, Hiwatashi A, Westesson PL. Vertebroplasty: cement leakage into the disc increases the risk of new fracture of adjacent vertebral body. AJNR Am J Neuroradiol 2004;25:175–180

77. Grados F, Depriester C, Cayrolle G, Hardy N, Deramond H, Fardellone P. Long-term observations of vertebral osteoporotic fractures treated by percutaneous vertebroplasty. Rheumatology (Oxford) 2000;39: 1410–1414

78. Melton LJ III, Atkinson EJ, Cooper C, O'Fallon WM, Riggs BL. Vertebral fractures predict subsequent fractures. Osteoporos Int 1999;10: 214–221

79. Harrop JS, Prpa B, Reinhardt MK, Lieberman I. Primary and secondary osteoporosis' incidence of subsequent vertebral compression fractures after kyphoplasty. Spine 2004;29:2120–2125

80. Voormolen MH, Mali WP, Lohle PN, et al. Percutaneous vertebroplasty compared with optimal pain medication treatment: short-term clinical outcome of patients with subacute or chronic painful osteoporotic vertebral compression fractures. The VERTOS study. AJNR Am J Neuroradiol 2007;28:555–560

81. Kasperk C, Hillmeier J, Nöldge G, et al. Treatment of painful vertebral fractures by kyphoplasty in patients with primary osteoporosis: a prospective nonrandomized controlled study. J Bone Miner Res 2005;20:604–612

82. Berlemann U, Franz T, Orler R, Heini PF. Kyphoplasty for treatment of osteoporotic vertebral fractures: a prospective non-randomized study. Eur Spine J 2004;13:496–501

83. Crandall D, Slaughter D, Hankins PJ, Moore C, Jerman J. Acute versus chronic vertebral compression fractures treated with kyphoplasty: early results. Spine J 2004;4:418–424

84. Yu SW, Lee PC, Ma CH, Chuang TY, Chen YJ. Vertebroplasty for the treatment of osteoporotic compression spinal fracture: comparison of remedial action at different stages of injury. J Trauma 2004;56: 629–632

85. Brown DB, Gilula LA, Sehgal M, Shimony JS. Treatment of chronic symptomatic vertebral compression fractures with percutaneous vertebroplasty. AJR Am J Roentgenol 2004;182:319–322

86. McGraw JK, Lippert JA, Minkus KD, Rami PM, Davis TM, Budzik RF. Prospective evaluation of pain relief in 100 patients undergoing percutaneous vertebroplasty: results and follow-up. J Vasc Interv Radiol 2002;13(9 Pt 1):883–886

87. Coumans JV, Reinhardt MK, Lieberman IH. Kyphoplasty for vertebral compression fractures: 1-year clinical outcomes from a prospective study. J Neurosurg 2003;99(1, Suppl):44–50

88. Feltes C, Fountas KN, Machinis T, et al. Immediate and early postoperative pain relief after kyphoplasty without significant restoration of vertebral body height in acute osteoporotic vertebral fractures. Neurosurg Focus 2005;18:e5

89. Prather H, Van Dillen L, Metzler JP, Riew KD, Gilula LA. Prospective measurement of function and pain in patients with non-neoplastic compression fractures treated with vertebroplasty. J Bone Joint Surg Am 2006;88:334–341

90. Legroux-Gérot I, Lormeau C, Boutry N, Cotten A, Duquesnoy B, Cortet B. Long-term follow-up of vertebral osteoporotic fractures treated by percutaneous vertebroplasty. Clin Rheumatol 2004;23:310–317

91. Pérez-Higueras A, Alvarez L, Rossi RE, Quiñones D, Al-Assir I. Percutaneous vertebroplasty: long-term clinical and radiological outcome. Neuroradiology 2002;44:950–954

92. Brown DB, Glaiberman CB, Gilula LA, Shimony JS. Correlation between preprocedural MRI findings and clinical outcomes in the treatment of chronic symptomatic vertebral compression fractures with percutaneous vertebroplasty. AJR Am J Roentgenol 2005;184:1951–1955

93. Krauss M, Hirschfelder H, Tomandl B, Lichti G, Bär I. Kyphosis reduction and the rate of cement leaks after vertebroplasty of intravertebral clefts. Eur Radiol 2006;16:1015–1021

94. Peh WC, Gelbart MS, Gilula LA, Peck DD. Percutaneous vertebroplasty: treatment of painful vertebral compression fractures with intraosseous vacuum phenomena. AJR Am J Roentgenol 2003;180:1411–1417

95. Kim DY, Lee SH, Jang JS, Chung SK, Lee HY. Intravertebral vacuum phenomenon in osteoporotic compression fracture: report of 67 cases with quantitative evaluation of intravertebral instability. J Neurosurg 2004;100(1, Suppl Spine):24–31

96. Peh WC, Gilula LA, Peck DD. Percutaneous vertebroplasty for severe osteoporotic vertebral body compression fractures. Radiology 2002; 223:121–126

97. Zoarski GH, Snow P, Olan WJ, et al. Percutaneous vertebroplasty for osteoporotic compression fractures: quantitative prospective evaluation of long-term outcomes. J Vasc Interv Radiol 2002;13(2 Pt 1):139–148

98. McKiernan F, Faciszewski T, Jensen R. Quality of life following vertebroplasty. J Bone Joint Surg Am 2004;86-A:2600–2606

99. Garfin SR, Buckley RA, Ledlie J; Balloon Kyphoplasty Outcomes Group. Balloon kyphoplasty for symptomatic vertebral body compression fractures results in rapid, significant, and sustained improvements in back pain, function, and quality of life for elderly patients. Spine 2006;31:2213–2220

100. Ledlie JT, Renfro MB. Kyphoplasty treatment of vertebral fractures: 2-year outcomes show sustained benefits. Spine 2006;31:57–64

101. Rhyne A III, Banit D, Laxer E, Odum S, Nussman D. Kyphoplasty: report of eighty-two thoracolumbar osteoporotic vertebral fractures. J Orthop Trauma 2004;18:294–299

102. Stoffel M, Wolf I, Ringel F, Stüer C, Urbach H, Meyer B. Treatment of painful osteoporotic compression and burst fractures using kyphoplasty: a prospective observational design. J Neurosurg Spine 2007; 6:313–319

103. McKiernan F, Faciszewski T, Jensen R. Reporting height restoration in vertebral compression fractures. Spine 2003;28:2517–2521, 3

104. Dublin AB, Hartman J, Latchaw RE, Hald JK, Reid MH. The vertebral body fracture in osteoporosis: restoration of height using percutaneous vertebroplasty. AJNR Am J Neuroradiol 2005;26:489–492

105. Jang JS, Kim DY, Lee SH. Efficacy of percutaneous vertebroplasty in the treatment of intravertebral pseudarthrosis associated with noninfected avascular necrosis of the vertebral body. Spine 2003;28:1588–1592

106. Lee ST, Chen JF. Closed reduction vertebroplasty for the treatment of osteoporotic vertebral compression fractures. Technical note. J Neurosurg 2004;100(4, Suppl Spine):392–396

107. Majd ME, Farley S, Holt RT. Preliminary outcomes and efficacy of the first 360 consecutive kyphoplasties for the treatment of painful osteoporotic vertebral compression fractures. Spine J 2005;5:244–255

108. Heini PF, Wälchli B, Berlemann U. Percutaneous transpedicular vertebroplasty with PMMA: operative technique and early results: a prospective study for the treatment of osteoporotic compression fractures. Eur Spine J 2000;9:445–450

109. Kobayashi K, Shimoyama K, Nakamura K, Murata K. Percutaneous vertebroplasty immediately relieves pain of osteoporotic vertebral compression fractures and prevents prolonged immobilization of patients. Eur Radiol 2005;15:360–367

110. Anselmetti GC, Corrao G, Monica PD, et al. Pain relief following percutaneous vertebroplasty: results of a series of 283 consecutive patients treated in a single institution. Cardiovasc Intervent Radiol 2007; 30:441–447

111. Carlier RY, Gordji H, Mompoint DM, Vernhet N, Feydy A, Vallée C. Osteoporotic vertebral collapse: percutaneous vertebroplasty and local kyphosis correction. Radiology 2004;233:891–898

112. Chung SK, Lee SH, Kim DY, Lee HY. Treatment of lower lumbar radiculopathy caused by osteoporotic compression fracture: the role of vertebroplasty. J Spinal Disord Tech 2002;15:461–468

113. Cyteval C, Sarrabère MP, Roux JO, et al. Acute osteoporotic vertebral collapse: open study on percutaneous injection of acrylic surgical cement in 20 patients. AJR Am J Roentgenol 1999;173:1685–1690

114. Gangi A, Kastler BA, Dietemann JL. Percutaneous vertebroplasty guided by a combination of CT and fluoroscopy. AJNR Am J Neuroradiol 1994;15:83–86

115. Gaughen JR Jr, Jensen ME, Schweickert PA, Marx WF, Kallmes DF. The therapeutic benefit of repeat percutaneous vertebroplasty at previously treated vertebral levels. AJNR Am J Neuroradiol 2002;23:1657–1661

116. Hiwatashi A, Moritani T, Numaguchi Y, Westesson PL. Increase in vertebral body height after vertebroplasty. AJNR Am J Neuroradiol 2003;24:185–189

117. Jensen ME, Evans AJ, Mathis JM, Kallmes DF, Cloft HJ, Dion JE. Percutaneous polymethylmethacrylate vertebroplasty in the treatment of osteoporotic vertebral body compression fractures: technical aspects. AJNR Am J Neuroradiol 1997;18:1897–1904

118. Kaufmann TJ, Jensen ME, Schweickert PA, Marx WF, Kallmes DF. Age of fracture and clinical outcomes of percutaneous vertebroplasty. AJNR Am J Neuroradiol 2001;22:1860–1863

119. Lane JI, Maus TP, Wald JT, Thielen KR, Bobra S, Luetmer PH. Intravertebral clefts opacified during vertebroplasty: pathogenesis, technical implications, and prognostic significance. AJNR Am J Neuroradiol 2002;23:1642–1646

120. Layton KF, Thielen KR, Koch CA, et al. Vertebroplasty, first 1000 levels of a single center: evaluation of the outcomes and complications. AJNR Am J Neuroradiol 2007;28:683–689

121. Maynard AS, Jensen ME, Schweickert PA, Marx WF, Short JG, Kallmes DF. Value of bone scan imaging in predicting pain relief from percutaneous vertebroplasty in osteoporotic vertebral fractures. AJNR Am J Neuroradiol 2000;21:1807–1812

122. Nakano M, Hirano N, Matsuura K, et al. Percutaneous transpedicular vertebroplasty with calcium phosphate cement in the treatment of osteoporotic vertebral compression and burst fractures. J Neurosurg 2002;97(3, Suppl):287–293

123. Nirala AP, Vatsal DK, Husain M, et al. Percutaneous vertebroplasty: an experience of 31 procedures. Neurol India 2003;51:490–492

124. Teng MM, Wei CJ, Wei LC, et al. Kyphosis correction and height restoration effects of percutaneous vertebroplasty. AJNR Am J Neuroradiol 2003;24:1893–1900

125. Atalay B, Caner H, Gokce C, Altinors N. Kyphoplasty: 2 years of experience in a neurosurgery department. Surg Neurol 2005;64(Suppl 2):S72–S76

126. Ledlie JT, Renfro MB. Decreases in the number and severity of morphometrically defined vertebral deformities after kyphoplasty. Neurosurg Focus 2005;18:e4

37

Nonoperative and Surgical Management of Thoracolumbar Burst Fractures: A Systematic Review

Lali H. S. Sekhon

Spinal cord injury (SCI) occurs in various countries throughout the world with an annual incidence of 15 to 40 cases per million, with the causes of these injuries ranging from motor vehicle accidents and community violence to recreational activities and workplace-related injuries. Thoracolumbar injuries in association with SCI occur in 30% of cases. Of these, 80% are from T10 to L2.[1] Of the thoracolumbar fractures, burst fractures comprise 45% of all major thoracolumbar trauma.[2] Even though these fractures are common, their precise management is controversial, with both conservative and surgical options available. The precise kind of conservative management is variable and the optimal surgical approach is also open to conjecture with advocates of anterior, posterior, and combined approaches.

This chapter systematically reviews the available English-speaking literature to answer two questions:

1. What is the optimal surgical approach when considering surgical morbidity, risk, and long-term outcomes with respect to pain and disability in neurologically intact burst fractures?
2. What is the optimal nonoperative treatment for stable burst fractures?

◆ Definitions

Burst fractures typically involve breach of the posterior cortical wall of the vertebral body with some degree of encroachment of the spinal canal with possible compromise of the neural elements (**Fig. 37.1**). Burst fractures have been referred to as "stable" or "unstable" depending on whether or not the posterior elements are intact or compromised (**Fig. 37.2**) and whether or not there is neurological deficit, particularly spinal cord, conus medullaris, or cauda equina. Unstable burst fractures are thought to more likely drift into kyphosis and have a greater risk of new or worsening neurological deficit with conservative care and immobilization.

Denis proposed a classification of thoracolumbar fractures based upon the three-column model.[3] The anterior column comprised the anterior longitudinal ligament and anterior half of the vertebral body, the middle column comprised the posterior half of the vertebral body and posterior longitudinal ligament, and the posterior column comprised the facet joints, lamina, and spinous processes and their ligaments. Denis suggested that fractures involving the anterior and middle columns could be classified as burst fractures, with simple crush fractures involving the anterior column alone (**Fig. 37.3**).

Whang et al developed a classification system for thoracolumbar injuries that reflected a review of the literature and opinions of experienced spine trauma surgeons.[4] The Thoracolumbar Injury Classification and Severity Score (TLICS) is a modification of a previously described Thoracolumbar Injury Severity Score (TLISS)[5] to guide surgeons on optimal management of fractures (**Table 37.1**). The TLICS score is based on scoring three different parameters, namely morphology of the fracture, neurological status, and posterior ligamentous complex status. A score up to 10 is derived with burst fractures automatically scoring 2 for morphology. A score less than 3 is suggested to be ideal for conservative management, and a score > 5 generally suggests the need for surgery. The validity and reliability of the TLICS score have been established.

◆ Management Options

Bracing and Conservative Care

Conservative care has comprised a combination of bed rest and bracing for an extended period of time. Bed rest may be unavoidable because of concomitant injuries or pain. Although prolonged bed rest was initially popular, this is increasingly less used because the potential complications associated with recumbency such as pneumonia and

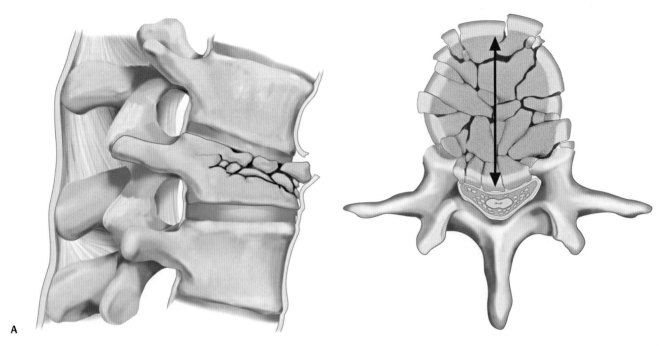

A   B

Fig. 37.1 **(A)** A simple crush fracture with involvement of the anterior column alone. **(B)** A typical axial image of a burst fracture where the middle column is violated in addition to the anterior column with bony retropulsion into the spinal canal.

thromboembolism have been increasingly recognized. Bracing, if used, typically involves some form of thoracolumbar orthosis such as a thoracolumbosacral orthosis (TLSO) plastic molded jacket or extension brace worn for 6 to 12 weeks to allow fracture healing.

Surgery

Surgical management of thoracolumbar burst fractures is typically advocated when either neurological deficit is present or when actual or potential instability is thought to be

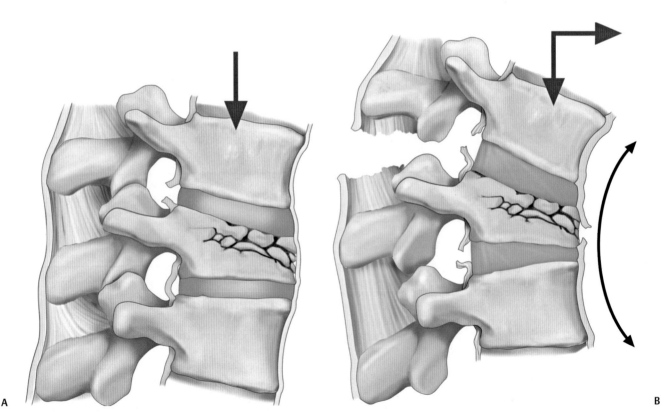

A   B

Fig. 37.2 **(A)** A stable burst fracture. The anterior and middle columns are breached with axial loading but the posterior column is intact. **(B)** An unstable burst fracture, where the posterior ligamentous structures are compromised in addition to the anterior and middle columns.

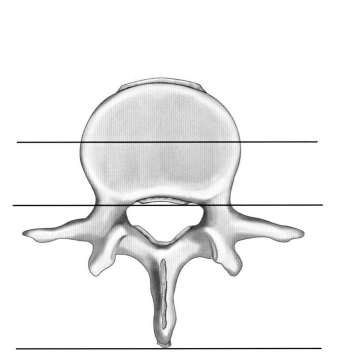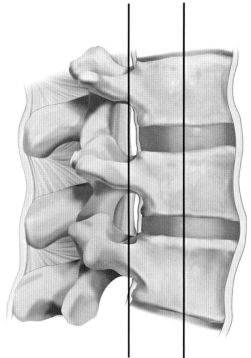

Fig. 37.3 **(A)** Axial and **(B)** sagittal drawings to illustrate the three-column concept proposed by Denis et al. Note that the anterior column is the anterior longitudinal ligament and anterior half of the vertebral body. The middle column is the posterior half of the vertebral body and posterior longitudinal ligament. The posterior column is the facet joint complex and the supra- and interspinous ligaments.

Table 37.1 Thoracolumbar Injury Classification and Severity Score (TLICS)

Parameter	Points
Morphology	
Compression	1
Burst	2
Translational/rotational	3
Distraction	4
Neurological status	
Intact	0
Nerve root injury	2
Spinal cord/conus medullaris injury	
Complete	2
Incomplete	3
Cauda equina	3
Posterior ligamentous complex	
Intact	0
Indeterminate	2
Disrupted	3
Treatment Recommendations:	

Total score < 3—Nonoperative treatment

Total score = 4—Nonoperative versus operative treatment

Total score > 5—Operative treatment

present. Surgical approaches typically involve some form of acute stabilization involving instrumentation, commonly with the aim of long-term fusion across damaged motion segments. Decompression, either directly or indirectly, is also usually performed (**Fig. 37.4**).

Posterior Approaches

Posterior approaches typically involve either long- or short-segment pedicle screw or hook (or combined) constructs. Decompression can be obtained indirectly with ligamentotaxis or with direct approaches using transpedicular and posterolateral techniques in addition to the stabilization. Most posterior approaches involve spanning several levels above and below the injured level, and typically it is thought to be more difficult to restore vertebral body height and correct kyphosis with posterior approaches (**Fig. 37.5**).

Anterior Approaches

Anterior approaches have gained popularity because they theoretically allow for more direct decompression of neural elements with the potential to reduce kyphosis more easily as well as minimize the number of levels that are arthrodesed (**Fig. 37.6**).

Other Approaches

Combined anterior/posterior approaches have been described for particularly unstable burst fractures as well as posterior approaches using an extracavitary or other approach (**Figs. 37.7**

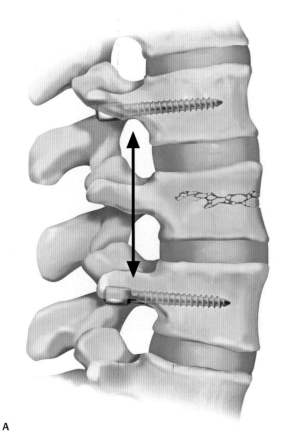

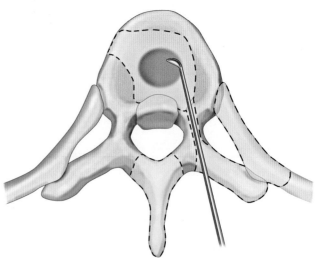

Fig. 37.4 Common methods of decompression for thoracolumbar burst fractures. **(A)** Indirect decompression through ligamentotaxis. Pedicle screws are placed above and below the fractured segment with distraction effected across the fractured segment. An intact posterior longitudinal ligament can facilitate reduction of the retropulsed fragment. **(B)** All methods for direct neural decompression with anterior approaches, simple laminectomy, transpedicular decompression, and posterolateral costotransversectomy approaches.

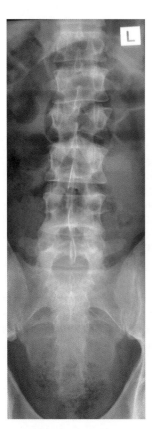

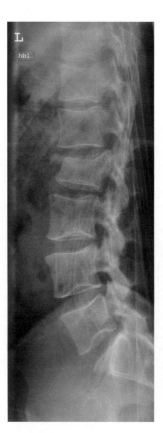

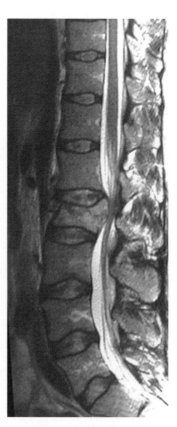

Fig. 37.5 Posterior stabilization for a lumbar burst fracture. This 40-year-old male fell from a motorcycle. He was neurologically intact. **(A)** Anteroposterior (AP) and **(B)** lateral lumbar x-rays show an L2 burst fracture with retropulsion but no significant kyphosis. **(C)** shows a sagittal T2-weighted magnetic resonance scan of the lumbar spine with significant retropulsion compressing the cauda equina. He was managed via a posterior laminectomy and pedicle screw instrumentation and fusion.

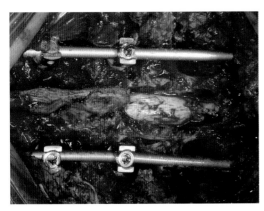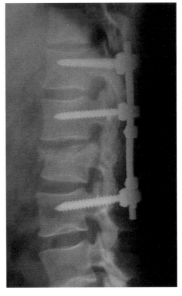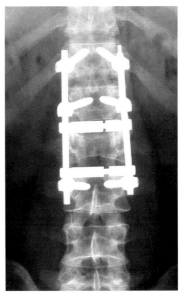

D–F

Fig. 37.5 *(Continued)* **(D)** Intraoperative view. The final construct is shown, with **(E)** lateral and **(F)** AP x-rays showing the instrumented T12–L3 fusion.

and 37.8). The utility of newer techniques such as vertebroplasty and kyphoplasty for these fractures is not clear.

Potential Complications

The common potential complications that may occur with the management of burst fractures include worsening of neurological deficit (which is thankfully rare and may be related to unaddressed or progressive instability) or worsening kyphosis with associated risks of neurological deficit, deformity, and/or pain. Surgical stabilization (either anterior or posterior), decompression (either direct or indirect), and realignment (whether postural or open) attempt to avoid the aforementioned complications. Surgical management does expose patients to risks of an intervention, which include general risks of infection, bleeding, and the like. The precise relationship between postoperative or persistent kyphosis and persistent or new pain and disability is not defined. The efficacy of correction

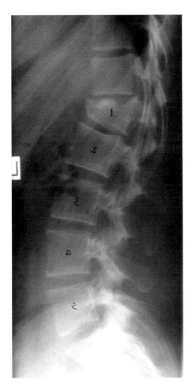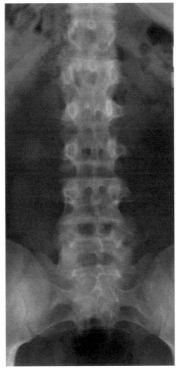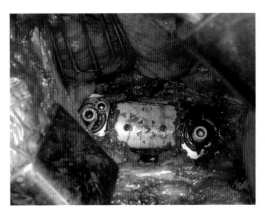

A, B   C

Fig. 37.6 Anterior decompression and stabilization of lumbar burst fracture: **(A)** Anteroposterior (AP) and **(B)** lateral x-rays of a 23-year-old male who suffered an incomplete conus injury after a skiing injury. Note the kyphosis and significant retropulsion visible on the lateral x-ray with the splaying of the L1 pedicles on the AP lumbar spine x-ray.
(C) Intraoperative view of the reconstruction after a left thoracotomy and L1 vertebrectomy. Staples are visible in place in the T12 and L2 vertebral bodies. A polyethylether ketone (PEEK) cage packed with autograft spans the L1 vertebrectomy segment. **(D)** The same view after securing the anterior segmental plate fixation. The final construct is shown, *(Continued on page 374)*

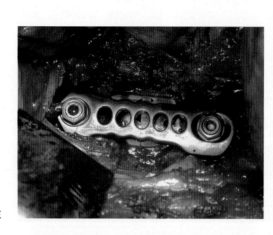
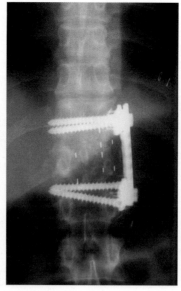
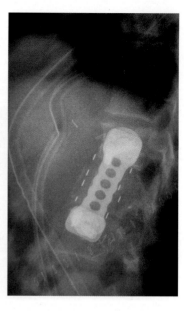

D, E

F

Fig. 37.6 (*Continued*) **(E)** AP and **(F)** lateral, with the radiolucent PEEK cages in place. A partial correction of the kyphosis has been obtained.

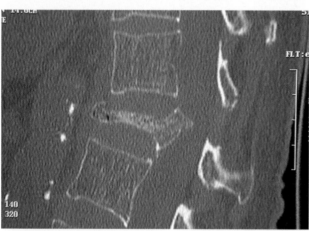

A

Fig. 37.7 Posterior transpedicular decompression and vertebroplasty of an L1 traumatic insufficiency fracture. This 78-year-old woman with known osteoporosis suffered an incomplete spinal cord injury after a fall. **(A)** A reconstructed sagittal helical computed tomographic scan showing the relative osteopenia with a significant crush fracture with severe retropulsion and loss of height. **(B)** Sagittal T2-weighted magnetic resonance imaging confirms cord deformation. The patient underwent posterior decompression via a transpedicular approach, open vertebroplasty, and segmental fixation. **(C)** Postoperative lateral and **(D)** anteroposterior x-rays with a good decompression and restoration of height.

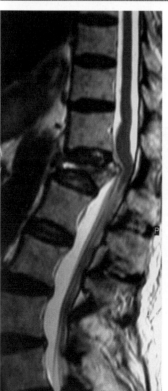
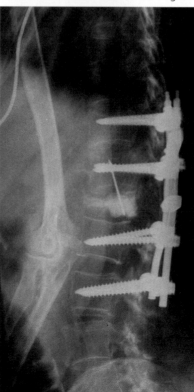
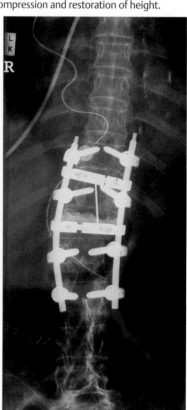

B–D

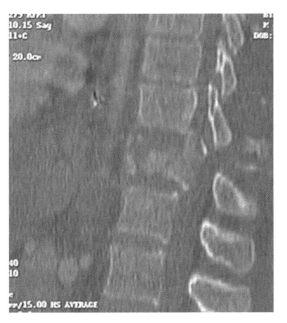

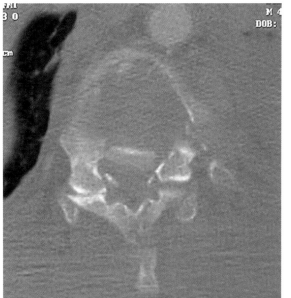

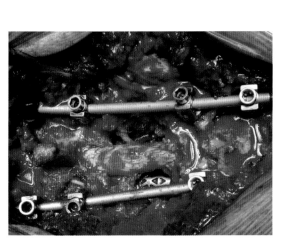

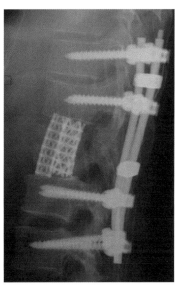

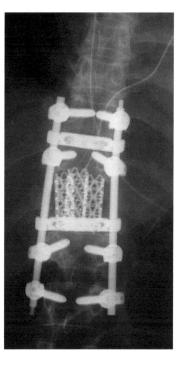

Fig. 37.8 Posterior transpedicular decompression and three-column reconstruction through a single-stage transpedicular approach. This 34-year-old male was involved in a motor vehicle accident and sustained a severe T12 burst fracture with incomplete deficit and three-column injury. **(A)** Sagittal reconstructed helical computed tomographic (CT) scan showing severe three-column disruption at the level of the injury. **(B)** This is also shown in the axial CT scan. **(C)** The intraoperative view with a bilateral transpedicular decompression effected, segmental fixation placed two levels above and one level below the fracture, and the anterior column reconstructed with three titanium cages filled with autograft. The postoperative appearance is confirmed by the **(D)** lateral and **(E)** anteroposterior x-rays, which show good restoration of alignment with three-column reconstruction.

of persisting deformity is unclear. Mitigating factors that may affect the incidence of potential complications include polytrauma and patients with preexisting poor bone quality.

◆ Material and Methods

A systematic review of the literature published from 1966 to 2007 was performed using MEDLINE. The search terms "burst," "fracture," "nonoperative," "operative," and "surgery" were used. The term "cervical" was used as an exclusionary item. Only articles in English were included. Only articles that included a full abstract were included. Studies in pediatric patients were excluded. Case reports were excluded. Specific points of interest were the types of interventions offered, clinical and radiological outcomes, and complications. Focus was placed on patients with isolated injuries without significant polytrauma. The level of evidence of included articles was assessed according to the guidelines proposed by the Center for Evidence Based Medicine (www.cebm.net). All studies that discussed nonoperative management were then analyzed. Studies reporting surgery were subclassified depending on whether approaches were ventral or dorsal.

In conclusion, the strength of the final recommendation was determined according to the guidelines proposed by Guyatt et al.[6] Recommendations were made for T10–L2 burst fractures in adult patients with isolated vertebral column injuries and good bone quality. Special consideration would be suggested for polytrauma or the elderly.

◆ Results

A total of 399 peer-reviewed papers were used for the final analysis. **Tables 37.2** and **37.3** summarize the relevant studies.

The Optimal Surgical Approach in Neurologically Intact Burst Fractures

The initial series of papers was narrowed according to the previous criteria to a total of 36 studies that specifically looked at the outcome of the surgical approach. Three studies were class I randomized, controlled studies (but for the purposes of the questions here would be downgraded to class II

or III), two studies were prospective cohort studies classified as class II evidence, with 11 studies regarded as class III.

Wood et al[7] is one of three randomized, controlled studies reviewed. In their study, 53 of 55 consecutive patients were recruited from one of three sites. Twenty-seven patients were randomized to conservative care, which involved either a postural reduction and cast or a hyperextension custom-molded jacket TLSO worn for 12 to 16 weeks. Twenty-six patients underwent the placement of a posterior screw–hook construct and fusion or an anterior vertebrectomy, rib strut graft, and instrumentation. The patients were randomized and then treatment tailored by the treating physician. A mean follow-up of 44 months (minimum 24 months) was obtained. Medical Outcomes Study Short Form-36 (SF-36), modified Roland-Morris Disability Score (RMDS), Oswestry Disability Index (ODI), visual analogue scale (VAS), and radiographic evaluation were performed. Three patients from each group were lost to follow-up, and one was excluded when he crossed over from the nonoperative to the operative treatment arm. This study was randomized, but treatment was not consistent. This and other methodological concerns led to the publishing journal classifying it as level II evidence. The authors found that there was no difference in kyphosis or pain between the two groups but better physical outcome and function in the nonoperated group.

Table 37.2 Summary of Studies Looking at Surgical Approach and Effect on Outcome in Surgery for Burst Fractures

No.	Study	Country of Origin	Summary of Study	Conclusion	Study Design	Grade
1	Wood et al (2003)[7]	USA	47 patients with stable burst fx; 24 had surgery (anterior or posterior); 23 nonop. Average 44 months follow-up	More complications with surgery. No difference in kyphosis or clinical outcome	Randomized controlled study	I (downgraded to level II)
2	Alanay et al (2001)[8]	Turkey	20 patients had posterior surgery with or without transpedicular grafting	No effect on kyphosis	Randomized controlled study	I
3	Shen et al (2001)[9]	Taiwan	80 patients: 47 hyperextension brace; 33 posterior 3-segment fixation	Sl. Better kyphotic correction with surgery. Otherwise no difference.	Randomized controlled study	I (downgraded to level III)
4	Andreychik et al (1996)[10]	USA	55 patients, 79 months follow-up. Anterior and posterior surgery with follow-up	Anterior approaches gave better anatomical alignment. No clinical sequelae of residual kyphosis.	Prospective cohort study	II
5	Tezeren and Kuru (2005)[11]	Turkey	18 consecutive patients; 9 posterior short (PS) segment fixation; 9 posterior long (LS) fusion	PS had 55% failure rate; LS better at last follow-up. Clinical outcome was the same.	Prospective cohort study	II
6	Jodoin et al (1985)[12]	France	108 patients over 10 years, op and nonop Mx	Laminectomy: more complications. Fusion: earlier ambulation and discharge and less pain. Increased residual deformity with laminectomy, short fusion, and by nonsurgical modality. The neurological recovery same with or without decompression. Less deformity if fusion long or laminectomy not done with fusion	Retrospective cohort study	III

Table 37.2 Summary of Studies Looking at Surgical Approach and Effect on Outcome in Surgery for Burst Fractures *(Continued)*

No.	Study	Country of Origin	Summary of Study	Conclusion	Study Design	Grade
7	Dewald (1984)[22]		31 L3–L5 burst fx, 46 months follow-up	Nonop Mx does well. Long fusions and flat back associated with low back pain	Retrospective cohort study	III
8	An et al (1992)[16]	USA	22 L3–L5 fx, surgery and no surgery 3- to 5-year follow-up	Both did well. Short fusions better than long	Retrospective cohort study	III
9	Briem et al (2004)[23]	Germany	20 patients, 10 with front/back fusion; 10 with posterior alone	No difference between two groups in outcome. Kyphosis did not affect outcome, worse than preop	Retrospective cohort study	III
10	Sasso et al (2006)[24]	USA	53 patients, 40 anterior only versus 13 short-segment posterior	Posterior only lost 8.1 deg; ant only lost 1.8 deg of kyphosis. Better realignment with anterior	Retrospective cohort study	III
11	Thomas et al (2006)[14]	Canada	Literature review. Op versus nonop Mx	No evidence to support one approach. No evidence that kyphosis matters	Literature review of class III evidence	III
12	Chen and Lee. (2004)[25]	Taiwan	6 patients neurologically intact had vertebroplasty for burst fx	Vertebroplasty plays a role in very selective cases	Prospective case series	III
13	Been and Bouma. (1999)[26]	The Netherlands	46 patients having anterior or posterior surgery. 6-year follow-up	Same clinical outcome. No difference in kyphosis	Retrospective cohort study	III
14	Seybold et al (1999)[18]	USA	42 patients L3–L5 fx follow-up 46 months	Op versus nonop Mx did not affect outcome	Retrospective cohort study	III
15	Kaneda et al (1997)[27]	Japan	150 consec patients, anterior op 8 years follow-up	Good neurological outcome	Case series consec pts	III
16	Kraemer et al (1996)[19]	Canada	24 patients, 2 years after op or nonop Mx SF-36 R compared	No difference in functional outcome op versus nonop	Retrospective cohort study	III
17	McAfee et al (1982)[28]	USA	16 patients with burst fx had posterior decompression and fusion. No controls. CT and neurological follow-up	Good outcomes. One-stage decompression-stabilization reduces the incidence of progressive kyphosis, neurological deterioration, and mechanical back pain common in both conservative treatment and with wide laminectomy.	Case series	IV
18	Kaneda et al (1984)[29]	Japan	24 patients with neurological deficit treated via anterior approach.	All 24 improved	Case series	IV
19	Garfin et al (1985)[30]	USA	9 patients, posterolateral decompression and fusion. CT follow-up	Allowed for realignment and decompression	Case series	IV
20	Riska et al (1987)[31]	Finland	905 patients 37% had deficit. All unstable fx had posterior fusion. 79 anterior fusion. 4-year follow-up	Of 78: 53 better, 18 neuro normal, 25 no change. Possibly suggests anterior approach best if solitary bone fragment	Retrospective case series	IV
21	Highland and Salciccioli (1985)[32]		60 patients Posterior fusions	Laminar fractures with deficit and neural tissue entrapment common. Suggest a posterior approach	Retrospective case series	IV

37 Nonoperative and Surgical Management of Thoracolumbar Burst Fractures

(Continued on pgae 378)

Table 37.2 Summary of Studies Looking at Surgical Approach and Effect on Outcome in Surgery for Burst Fractures (*Continued*)

No.	Study	Country of Origin	Summary of Study	Conclusion	Study Design	Grade
22	Crutcher et al (1991)[33]		13 patients. Posterior indirect decompression and fusion	Posterior distraction instrumentation can achieve ~50% reduction in canal stenosis and that results will be influenced by fracture morphology.	Retrospective case series	IV
23	Starr and Hanley (1992)[34]	USA	22 patients underwent posterior fusion: indirect decompression via ligamentotaxis	Patients did well. No relationship between neuro status and x-rays.	Retrospective case series	IV
24	Stephens et al (1992)[35]	USA	17 patients, posterior transpedicular decompression and fusion. 19 months follow-up	Excellent clinical results. Kyphosis worse by 11 degrees	Retrospective case series	IV
25	Akalan and Ozgen (1994)[36]	Turkey	44 burst fractures treated by posterior approach	Better realignment and good results	Retrospective case series	IV
26	Akbarnia (1994)[37]	USA	13 patients, long rods and short arthrodesis with removal of hardware at 6 months	Good results. 12 fused. Most facet joints spanned not fused.	Retrospective case series	IV
27	Sanderson et al (1999)[13]	Australia	24 patients who underwent posterior fusion	Good or excellent outcome in 62% with slight correction of kyphosis	Retrospective case series	IV
28	Mahar et al (2007)[38]	USA	Retrospective review and cadaveric analysis. 12 patients. Short segment fixation	At follow-up radiological parameters acceptable treatment option.	Retrospective case series	IV
29	Payer (2006)[39]	Switzerland	20 patients. Stage back/front. 2-year follow-up	Neurologically improved. Kyphosis improved.	Retrospective case series	IV
31	Andress et al (2002)[40]	Germany	50 patients, posterior op	Worse than preinjury state; no kyphosis	Retrospective case series	IV
32	Razak et al (2000)[41]	Malaysia	26 patients with short segment fixation. 24.4 months follow-up	Good clinical results with some kyphosis correction. 100% fused. Some screw loosening	Retrospective case series	IV
33	Shen and Shen (1999)[42]	Taiwan	Retrospective review 38 patients with emphasis posterior elements	Less restrictive nonop Mx did not affect outcome; no effect of spinous process/laminar fx	Retrospective case series	IV
34	Okuyama et al (1996)[43]	Japan	Retrospective review 45 patients with anterior op 54 months follow-up	Anterior operation restores alignment, earlier return to work, earlier rehab	Retrospective case series	IV
35	Limb et al (1995)[2]	England	Retrospective review 20 patients admitted over 2 years with burst fx	No correction between degree of stenosis and neurological injury	Retrospective case series	IV
36	Weyns et al (1994)[44]	Belgium	Retrospective review of 93 cases treated with posterior fusion	Excellent neurological outcome at mean 26 months	Retrospective case series	IV

Abbreviations: fx, fracture; op, operative; nonop, nonoperative; Mx, management.

Alanay et al[8] was also classified as class I evidence. The authors looked at 20 patients with burst fractures and no neurological deficit. All had surgery via posterior short-segment pedicle instrumentation (defined as one level above and below the fracture). Half had addition of a transpedicular bone graft; half did not. The authors specifically looked at kyphosis and found no difference in their radiological outcomes.

Shen et al[9] compared nonoperative management with posterior stabilization in 80%. The study was class I in that it was randomized and controlled but no comparison was made between differing surgical arms, which for this review would downgrade the level of evidence. Forty-seven patients had a hyperextension brace, whereas the remainder underwent three-level posterior fixation. The surgical groups had better

Table 37.3 Summary of KMK Studies on Nonoperative Management of Burst Fractures

No.	Study	Country of Origin	Summmary of Study	Conclusion	Study Design	Grade
1	Reid et al (1988)[15]	Canada	21 of 404 patients 1-year follow-up. Neurologically intact. Braced in full-contact orthosis for 6 months	Patients did well. None reoperated upon. Brace ok if: neurologically intact; kyphosis <35 deg; 3 degree of retropulsion not an issue	Prospective case series	III
2	An et al (1992)[16]	USA	22 L3–L5 fx, surgery and no surgery 3- to 5-year follow-up. Conservative Rx: body cast 3 months	Both groups did well. Short fusions better than long.	Retrospective cohort study	III
3	Knight et al (1993)[17]	USA	22 2 and 3-column injuries patients. 12 op, 10 nonop	No difference between 2 groups. Nonop Mx did well.	Retrospective cohort study	III
4	Thomas et al (2006)[14]	Canada	Literature review. Op versus nonop Mx	No evidence to support one approach. No evidence that kyphosis matters	Literature review of class III evidence	III
5	Seybold et al (1999)[18]	USA	42 patients L3–L5 fx follow-up 46 months looked at type of nonoperative management	Op versus nonop Mx did not affect outcome	Retrospective cohort study	III
6	Kraemer et al (1996)[19]	Canada	24 patients, 2 years after op or nonop Mx SF-36 and RM score compared	No difference in functional outcome op versus nonop	Retrospective cohort study	III
7	Moller et al (2007)[21]	Sweden	27 patients with burst fractures eval clinically and radiologically 23–41 years after injury	Patients did well. Adjacent discs did not degenerate prematurely	Retrospective case series	IV
8	Fredrickson et al (1982)[45]	USA	Review of 4 patients with L5 burst fx	Conservative care works ok.	Case series	IV
9	Willen et al (1990)[46]		54 patients, nonop Mx	>50% compression, >50% stenosis, rotational and L1 fx do worse	Retrospective case series	IV
10	Braakman et al (1991)[47]		71 patients with deficit. Surgical and nonsurgical	Outcomes the same. Surgery mobilized quicker.	Retrospective case series	IV
11	Finn and Stauffer (1992)[20]		7 patients with L5 burst fractures. Nonop Mx. They were treated conservatively by immobilization for 6 to 8 weeks in a body-jacket cast that included one lower extremity to the knee. The patients were allowed to walk 10 to 14 days after the injury. A thoracolumbosacral orthosis was worn for an additional 3 months.	Did well with nonop Mx.	Retrospective case series	IV
12	Kinoshita et al (1993)[48]	Japan	23 patients, nonop Mx, 10 intact	8 had full recovery. 1 late operation. Conservative Rx plays a role.	Retrospective case series	IV
13	Mumford et al (1993)[49]	USA	41 patients; nonop Mx	Nonop Mx works well. Kyphosis does worsen.	Retrospective case series	IV
14	Shen and Shen (1999)[42]	Taiwan	Retrospective review 38 patients with emphasis posterior elements; 9 had Jewett braces, nil for remainder	Less restrictive nonop Mx did not affect outcome; no effect of spinous process/laminar fx	Retrospective case series	IV
15	Andreychik et al (1996)[10]	USA	L2–L5 fx, 55 pts, 79 months follow-up, Op and nonop. 30 nonop with bed rest and brace	Nonop is ok if no deficit; otherwise anterior op	Retrospective cohort series	IV

Abbreviations: fx, fracture; op, operative; nonop, nonoperative; Mx, management.

kyphotic correction but with no clinical correlate. This study was a class I randomized, controlled study, but because only one treatment arm was used the level of evidence was downgraded to level III.

Of the remaining studies, three were classified as class II.[10,11] Andreychik et al[10] looked at 55 patients, 30 of whom were braced and 25 of whom had surgery. Of the surgical group, eight had long posterior fusions, eight had short posterior constructs, six had anterior decompression and fusions, and three had initial posterior fusions then anterior procedures. Mean follow-up was 39 months. No neurological deteriorations occurred. No differences in pain or functional outcomes occurred between groups. Multi-root involvement patients seem to benefit from anterior approaches. Short posterior constructs lost alignment more readily than longer constructs. Overall, there was no difference in outcomes.

Tezeren and Kuru[11] compared two groups of a total of 18 consecutive patients with neurologically intact burst fractures and compared long instrumentation (hooks two levels above and pedicle screws two levels below) to short segment fixation (pedicle screws one level above and one level below). At follow-up the short segment fixation had a 55% implant failure rate, whereas the long constructs had longer operating times and blood loss. There was no difference in clinical outcome measures or kyphosis.

Eleven of the 36 studies were classified as level III evidence, and 20 studies as level IV. Overall the studies did not favor either an anterior or a posterior approach with stabilization in terms of overall outcome or morbidity. Jodoin et al[12] found laminectomy alone had poorer neurological outcome. Sanderson et al[13] looked at short posterior segment fixation without fusion in 28 patients. Patients had good clinical outcome at 2 years with a 14% implant failure rate. The authors suggested fusion was not necessary to achieve good outcomes. Thomas et al[14] provided an extensive review of the literature looking at operative and nonoperative management of thoracolumbar burst fractures. They concluded that persistent kyphosis did not appear to affect clinical outcome, and there was no good evidence to favor one surgical approach over another.

The Optimal Nonoperative Treatment for Stable Burst Fractures

When assessing the literature for evidence to support the optimal nonoperative management of stable lumbar burst fractures, the 399 publications were narrowed to 15 studies that focused on the results of conservative management. There was no class I or class II evidence. Six papers were classified as class III, with the remaining nine publications classified as class IV. Almost all studies used some form of orthosis for at least 3 months after injury. All papers suggested conservative management for neurologically intact patients. There were no controls in any study that were not braced. The specifics of the conservative care protocols when compared with surgical series have already been discussed. In this group, the precise type of orthosis, duration of bed rest, or bracing was not delineated. Restrictions such as when the orthosis was not worn were also not typically discussed, so it was unclear if the orthosis had been worn continually, when out of bed, or with some other concession. Similarly, it was not clear if any advice was given to patients with respect to restriction of activities and for how long such

restrictions applied. No advice with respect to smoking or antiinflammatory use was presented.

Reid et al[15] looked at 21 patients who were neurologically intact and placed into a full-contact thoracolumbar orthosis. They reported that with greater than 1 year follow-up neurological outcome was satisfactory and progression into kyphosis did not occur.

An et al[16] reported 7 low lumbar burst fractures placed in a body cast for 3 months. These patients did well.

Knight et al[17] reported 10 patients with burst fractures managed conservatively. They specifically stated that various modes of external immobilization were used, again with no consistent pattern.

The other class III studies[14,18,19] were not specific on the type of nonoperative treatment initiated. Most of these studies used 3 months as the benchmark. The duration of bed rest prior to mobilization was not clear.

Of the class IV studies, Finn and Stauffer[20] reported seven patients with low lumbar burst fractures treated conservatively by immobilization for 6 to 8 weeks in a body-jacket cast that included one lower extremity to the knee.

Moller et al[21] reported on 27 patients with thoracolumbar burst fractures managed conservatively with a mean follow-up of 27 years. Primary treatment had included direct mobilization, with or without a soft brace, in 16 patients. Five patients had been mobilized in a stiff brace, as soon as the pain allowed, for a mean of 8 weeks (range, 3 to 14 weeks), and six had been immobilized in bed for a mean of 3 weeks (range, 2 to 4 weeks), in three patients partly because of associated extremity injuries. After immobilization, two of these six patients had worn a stiff brace for 8 and 24 weeks, respectively.

Overall, when reviewing these studies for the optimal nonoperative treatment for stable burst fractures, most studies consistently braced in some fashion for a duration of at least 6 to 8 weeks, and typically for up to 12 to 14 weeks. As stated earlier, no class I or II studies were found.

◆ Discussion

After reviewing the literature on the optimal surgical approach for managing neurologically intact patients with thoracolumbar burst fractures, in terms of clinical and radiological outcome, morbidity, and risk, it is apparent that only three studies approached level 1 evidence. None definitively suggested superiority of one surgical approach over another. The literature did not support the notion that postoperative kyphosis had any clinical sequelae, and the incidence of new or progressive neurological deficit was similar. Short segment posterior constructs did appear to have a higher failure rate. The studies labeled as class 1 in this study did suffer from methodological concerns as previously discussed. The studies as a whole suffered from a lack of uniformity in definitions of outcomes, variable outcome measures, variable follow-up times, and nonrandomization or only single surgical treatment arms. In short, no clear consensus could be reached on the optimal surgical approach for thoracolumbar burst fractures in neurologically intact patients.

The literature review on the optimal modality of nonoperative management was fraught with a paucity of data and no class I or II data, and little could definitely be recommended. Bracing was universally used. The role/duration of bed rest could not be delineated. The duration of bracing could not be categorically defined, although for most studies this was in the range of 2 to 4 months. In neurologically intact patients conservative care did not seem to be fraught with a high incidence of catastrophic neurological deterioration.

◆ Summary and Recommendation

After reviewing all the available evidence with respect to the optimal nonoperative management and the optimal surgical approach in the management of thoracolumbar burst fractures in the neurologically intact patient, it is evident that the two questions posed in the introduction cannot be conclusively answered on the basis of available published literature. After reviewing 36 papers relating to surgical management, the quality of evidence was moderate, and no definitive recommendation could be made to support one type of surgical approach over another in terms of long-term outcome or morbidity. After review of 15 papers that analyzed nonsurgical care of thoracolumbar burst fractures, the quality of evidence was poor, and no consensus could be made on the basis of the literature as to optimal nonoperative management.

Using the criteria outlined by Schünemann et al,[6] the Spine Trauma Study Group gave a strong recommendation that for T10–L2 burst fractures in neurologically intact patients anterior and/or posterior approaches would be reasonable. It was emphasized that in cases of polytrauma anterior approaches may be advocated more cautiously, and in the elderly with poor bone quality consideration should be given for posterior approaches. The group made a weak recommendation for a thoracolumbar orthosis for 6 to 12 weeks with a limited period of bed rest as the optimal treatment paradigm if conservative care was advocated.

References

1. Sekhon LH, Fehlings MG. Epidemiology, demographics, and pathophysiology of acute spinal cord injury. Spine 2001;26(24, Suppl):S2–S12
2. Limb D, Shaw DL, Dickson RA. Neurological injury in thoracolumbar burst fractures. J Bone Joint Surg Br 1995;77:774–777
3. Denis F. The three column spine and its significance in the classification of acute thoracolumbar spinal injuries. Spine 1983;8:817–831
4. Whang PG, Vaccaro AR, Poelstra KA, et al. The influence of fracture mechanism and morphology on the reliability and validity of two novel thoracolumbar injury classification systems. Spine 2007; 32:791–795
5. Vaccaro AR, Baron EM, Sanfilippo J, et al. Reliability of a novel classification system for thoracolumbar injuries: the Thoracolumbar Injury Severity Score. Spine 2006;31(11, Suppl):S62–S69, discussion S104
6. Schünemann HJ, Jaeschke R, Cook DJ, et al; ATS Documents Development and Implementation Committee. An official ATS statement: grading the quality of evidence and strength of recommendations in ATS guidelines and recommendations. Am J Respir Crit Care Med 2006; 174:605–614
7. Wood K, Buttermann G, Mehbod A, et al. Operative compared with nonoperative treatment of a thoracolumbar burst fracture without neurological deficit: a prospective, randomized study. J Bone Joint Surg Am 2003;85-A:773–781
8. Alanay A, Acaroglu E, Yazici M, Oznur A, Surat A. Short-segment pedicle instrumentation of thoracolumbar burst fractures: does transpedicular intracorporeal grafting prevent early failure? Spine 2001;26:213–217
9. Shen WJ, Liu TJ, Shen YS. Nonoperative treatment versus posterior fixation for thoracolumbar junction burst fractures without neurologic deficit. Spine 2001;26:1038–1045
10. Andreychik DA, Alander DH, Senica KM, Stauffer ES. Burst fractures of the second through fifth lumbar vertebrae: clinical and radiographic results. J Bone Joint Surg Am 1996;78:1156–1166
11. Tezeren G, Kuru I. Posterior fixation of thoracolumbar burst fracture: short-segment pedicle fixation versus long-segment instrumentation. J Spinal Disord Tech 2005;18:485–488
12. Jodoin A, Dupuis P, Fraser M, Beaumont P. Unstable fractures of the thoracolumbar spine: a 10-year experience at Sacré-Coeur Hospital. J Trauma 1985;25:197–202
13. Sanderson PL, Fraser RD, Hall DJ, Cain CM, Osti OL, Potter GR. Short segment fixation of thoracolumbar burst fractures without fusion. Eur Spine J 1999;8:495–500
14. Thomas KC, Bailey CS, Dvorak MF, Kwon B, Fisher C. Comparison of operative and nonoperative treatment for thoracolumbar burst fractures in patients without neurological deficit: a systematic review. J Neurosurg Spine 2006;4:351–358
15. Reid DC, Hu R, Davis LA, Saboe LA. The nonoperative treatment of burst fractures of the thoracolumbar junction. J Trauma 1988;28:1188–1194
16. An HS, Simpson JM, Ebraheim NA, Jackson WT, Moore J, O'Malley NP. Low lumbar burst fractures: comparison between conservative and surgical treatments. Orthopedics 1992;15:367–373
17. Knight RQ, Stornelli DP, Chan DP, Devanny JR, Jackson KV. Comparison of operative versus nonoperative treatment of lumbar burst fractures. Clin Orthop Relat Res 1993;(293):112–121
18. Seybold EA, Sweeney CA, Fredrickson BE, Warhold LG, Bernini PM. Functional outcome of low lumbar burst fractures: a multicenter review of operative and nonoperative treatment of L3-L5. Spine 1999;24:2154–2161
19. Kraemer WJ, Schemitsch EH, Lever J, McBroom RJ, McKee MD, Waddell JP. Functional outcome of thoracolumbar burst fractures without neurological deficit. J Orthop Trauma 1996;10:541–544
20. Finn CA, Stauffer ES. Burst fracture of the fifth lumbar vertebra. J Bone Joint Surg Am 1992;74:398–403
21. Moller A, Hasserius R, Redlund-Johnell I, Ohlin A, Karlsson MK. Nonoperatively treated burst fractures of the thoracic and lumbar spine in adults: a 23- to 41-year follow-up. Spine J 2007;7:701–707
22. DeWald RL. Burst fractures of the thoracic and lumbar spine. Clin Orthop Relat Res 1984;(189):150–161
23. Briem D, Lehmann W, Ruecker AH, Windolf J, Rueger JM, Linhart W. Factors influencing the quality of life after burst fractures of the thoracolumbar transition. Arch Orthop Trauma Surg 2004;124:461–468
24. Sasso RC, Renkens K, Hanson D, Reilly T, McGuire RA Jr, Best NM. Unstable thoracolumbar burst fractures: anterior-only versus short-segment posterior fixation. J Spinal Disord Tech 2006;19:242–248
25. Chen JF, Lee ST. Percutaneous vertebroplasty for treatment of thoracolumbar spine bursting fracture. Surg Neurol 2004;62:494–500, discussion 500
26. Been HD, Bouma GJ. Comparison of two types of surgery for thoracolumbar burst fractures: combined anterior and posterior stabilisation vs. posterior instrumentation only. Acta Neurochir (Wien) 1999;141: 349–357
27. Kaneda K, Taneichi H, Abumi K, Hashimoto T, Satoh S, Fujiya M. Anterior decompression and stabilization with the Kaneda device for thoracolumbar burst fractures associated with neurological deficits. J Bone Joint Surg Am 1997;79:69–83
28. McAfee PC, Yuan HA, Lasda NA. The unstable burst fracture. Spine 1982;7:365–373
29. Kaneda K, Abumi K, Fujiya M. Burst fractures with neurologic deficits of the thoracolumbar-lumbar spine: results of anterior decompression and stabilization with anterior instrumentation. Spine 1984; 9:788–795
30. Garfin SR, Mowery CA, Guerra J Jr, Marshall LF. Confirmation of the posterolateral technique to decompress and fuse thoracolumbar spine burst fractures. Spine 1985;10:218–223
31. Riska EB, Myllynen P, Böstman O. Anterolateral decompression for neural involvement in thoracolumbar fractures: a review of 78 cases. J Bone Joint Surg Br 1987;69:704–708
32. Highland TR, Salciccioli GG. Is immobilization adequate treatment of unstable burst fractures of the atlas? A case report with long-term follow-up evaluation. Clin Orthop Relat Res 1985;(201):196–200
33. Crutcher JP Jr, Anderson PA, King HA, Montesano PX. Indirect spinal canal decompression in patients with thoracolumbar burst fractures treated by posterior distraction rods. J Spinal Disord 1991;4:39–48
34. Eaton RG. Excision and fascial interposition arthroplasty in the treatment of Kienböck's disease. Hand Clin 1993;9:513–516
35. Stephens GC, Devito DP, McNamara MJ. Segmental fixation of lumbar burst fractures with Cotrel-Dubousset instrumentation. J Spinal Disord 1992;5:344–348
36. Akalan N, Ozgen T. Infection as a cause of spinal cord compression: a review of 36 spinal epidural abscess cases. Acta Neurochir (Wien) 2000; 142:17–23
37. Akbarnia BA. Pediatric spine fractures. Orthop Clin North Am 1999;30: 521–536, x
38. Mahar A, Kim C, Wedemeyer M, et al. Short segment fixation of lumbar burst fractures using pedicle fixation at the level of the fracture. Spine 2007;32(14):1503–1507
39. Payer M. Unstable burst fractures of the thoraco-lumbar junction: treatment by posterior bisegmental correction/fixation and staged anterior

corpectomy and titanium cage implantation. Acta Neurochir (Wien) 2006;148:299–306, discussion 306

40. Andress HJ, Braun H, Helmberger T, Schürmann M, Hertlein H, Hartl WH. Long-term results after posterior fixation of thoraco-lumbar burst fractures. Injury 2002;33:357–365

41. Razak M, Basir T, Hyzan Y, Johari Z. Halovest treatment in traumatic cervical spine injury. Med J Malaysia 1998;53(Suppl A):1–5

42. Shen WJ, Shen YS. Nonsurgical treatment of three-column thoracolumbar junction burst fractures without neurologic deficit. Spine 1999;24: 412–415

43. Okuyama K, Abe E, Chiba M, Ishikawa N, Sato K. Outcome of anterior decompression and stabilization for thoracolumbar unstable burst fractures in the absence of neurologic deficits. Spine 1996;21:620–625

44. Weyns F, Rommens PM, Van Calenbergh F, Goffin J, Broos P, Plets C. Neurological outcome after surgery for thoracolumbar fractures: a retrospective study of 93 consecutive cases, treated with dorsal instrumentation. Eur Spine J 1994;3:276–281

45. Fredrickson BE, Yuan HA, Miller H. Burst fractures of the fifth lumbar vertebra: a report of four cases. J Bone Joint Surg Am 1982;64:1088–1094

46. Willén J, Anderson J, Toomoka K, Singer K. The natural history of burst fractures at the thoracolumbar junction. J Spinal Disord 1990;3:39–46

47. Braakman R, Fontijne WP, Zeegers R, Steenbeek JR, Tanghe HL. Neurological deficit in injuries of the thoracic and lumbar spine: a consecutive series of 70 patients. Acta Neurochir (Wien) 1991;111:11–17

48. Kinoshita H, Nagata Y, Ueda H, Kishi K. Conservative treatment of burst fractures of the thoracolumbar and lumbar spine. Paraplegia 1993; 31:58–67

49. Mumford J, Weinstein JN, Spratt KF, Goel VK. Thoracolumbar burst fractures: the clinical efficacy and outcome of nonoperative management. Spine 1993;18:955–970

38

Thoracolumbar Flexion-Distraction Injuries

Stephen P. Kingwell and Charles G. Fisher

Thoracolumbar distraction injuries are common in spine referral centers and represent between 5 and 15% of total thoracolumbar spinal trauma.[1-5] The unique radiographic findings associated with bony distraction injuries have been recognized for over 60 years and were first described by Chance in 1948 as "flexion fractures of the spine."[6] The pathomechanics of Chance fractures and their ligamentous counterparts have been further clarified since their initial description, and they represent a distinct group of thoracolumbar injuries.[1,4,7-10]

◆ Background

Etiology

The most common mechanisms causing thoracolumbar distraction injuries are high-velocity motor vehicle collisions, but they may also occur with falls from a height.[5,11,12] Historically, the injury pattern has been associated with the use of lap belts.[12-14]

Biomechanics

When the thoracolumbar spine is subjected to a distractive force and flexed around a fulcrum, a flexion-distraction injury occurs.[1,7,9] The posterior and middle columns fail in tension while the anterior column may fail in tension or compression. Axial loading of the spine is known to occur with sudden deceleration, and this may contribute to compression of the anterior column.[15] Others have suggested that the injury pattern can occur with compression to the flexed spine.[16,17] According to Denis, the anterior part of the anterior column maintains its role as a hinge in seat-belt-type injuries, and when this is disrupted a fracture-dislocation results.[4] The pattern of injury, whether ligamentous or bony, depends on the direction and magnitude of the load applied, the degree of spinal flexion, the bone mineral density, and the presence and location of a fulcrum.[15,17,18]

Clinical Presentation

Examination

A thorough Advanced Trauma Life Support (ATLS) approach should be adhered to when evaluating a trauma patient with an injury to the spinal column.[19] Specific to thoracolumbar distraction injuries, the abdomen must be inspected for contusions or ecchymoses (seat belt sign).[20] The spine should be palpated for interspinous gaps and noncontiguous fractures.

Neurology

The incidence of neurological deficits in patients with flexion-distraction injuries ranges from 11 to 32%.[1,3,7,12,13] This is lower than for patients with burst fractures or fracture-dislocations[2] because the mechanism "decompresses" as the spine distracts from a posterior to anterior direction.

Associated Injuries

The association between seat-belt fractures and concomitant abdominal injuries is well described.[10,13] The incidence of abdominal trauma in this patient group is reported to be 44 to 67%. This is often life-threatening intraabdominal trauma, and the diagnosis may be delayed.[1,11-13,21,22] A high index of suspicion, particularly for hollow viscus injury, in addition to solid organ and vascular trauma is critical.[13,23]

Classification

Numerous classification systems exist for thoracolumbar fractures. A clinically relevant classification system must be concise, utilize clear and consistent radiographic and clinical characteristics, and help guide treatment.[7] Furthermore, the classification should assist the surgeon in predicting potential outcomes from various treatments.[23] A summary of existing classifications for thoracolumbar flexion-distraction injuries

Table 38.1 Classification of Thoracolumbar Flexion-Distraction Injuries

Denis (1983)	McAfee (1983)	Gertzbein (1987)	Magerl (1994)	TLICS (2005)
Compression	Wedge-compression	Specific for flexion-distraction injuries	Type A. Vertebral body compression	Injury morphology
Burst	Stable burst	Posterior fracture	Type B. Anterior and posterior element injury with distraction	Compression (1)/burst (1)
Seat-belt type	Unstable burst	I—bone		Translational/rotational (3)
One-level: through bone (Chance)-A or ligaments and disk-B	Chance fracture (distraction of anterior column)	II—ligamentous	B1. Posterior disruption ligamentous	Distraction (4)
Two-level:	Flexion-distraction injury (compression of anterior column)	III—oblique	B1.1. With transverse disruption of the disk	Integrity of posterior ligamentous complex
Middle column through bone-C or ligaments-D	Translational injury	Anterior fracture	B1.2. With type A fracture of the vertebral body	Intact (0)
Fracture-dislocation (includes flexion rotation, shear, and flexion distraction)		A—disk	B2. Posterior disruption osseous	Suspected/indeterminate (2)
		B—anterior body		Injured (3)
		C1—superior end plate	B2.1. Transverse bicolumn fracture	Neurological status
		C2—inferior end plate	B2.2. With transverse disruption of the disk	Intact (0)
		State of body		Nerve root (2)
		D—compression	B2.3. With A type fracture of the vertebral body	Cord, conus
		E—burst		Complete (2)
		F—intact	Type C. Anterior and posterior element injury with rotation	Incomplete (3)
				Cauda equina (3)
				Surgery recommended for score of 5 or more

Abbreviation: TLICS, Thoracolumbar Injury Classification and Severity Score.

is found in **Table 38.1**. A novel Thoracolumbar Injury Classification and Severity Score (TLICS) has recently been developed by consensus opinion of the Spine Trauma Study Group (STSG). The three critical variables in this classification system are the injury morphology, the integrity of the posterior ligamentous complex, and the neurological status of the patient.

Imaging

Plain Radiographs

The classic findings on plain radiographs include widening of the interspinous distance and horizontal fractures of the transverse processes, pedicles, or pars interarticularis. Loss of height of the anterior vertebral body or an increase in posterior vertebral body height and the disk space may occur.[4] Thirty percent of AO B-type fractures are missed with plain x-rays and computed tomography (CT) with two-dimensional (2-D) reconstructions.[24]

Computed Tomography

The use of spiral CT scans with reformatted images in the sagittal and coronal planes allows for thorough assessment of the injury morphology and subsequent treatment planning (**Figs. 38.1 and 38.2**).

Magnetic Resonance Imaging

Magnetic resonance imaging (MRI) allows for a detailed assessment of the posterior osteoligamentous complex (**Fig. 38.3**). Although variable sequences can be used to assess the bony injury, short-tau inversion recovery (STIR) and fat-suppressed T2-weighted images are most useful to delineate the soft tissue injury.[25] Typically, edema and hemorrhage are seen in the subcutaneous fat over contiguous levels and in

the posterior ligamentous structures. Contiguous anterosuperior vertebral body compression fractures are not uncommon and are readily seen on MRI.[26]

Treatment

Nonoperative Treatment

Reduction of the fracture is achieved with positioning and is maintained with the use of a custom-molded thoracolumbosacral orthosis (TLSO) or hyperextension brace. Maintenance of reduction is confirmed with upright x-rays in the brace.

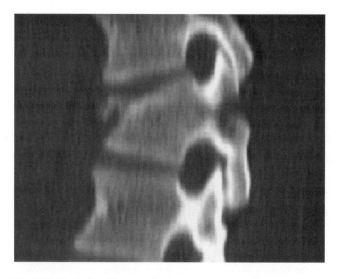

Fig. 38.1 Sagitally reformatted computed tomographic image demonstrating anterior body compression and distraction through posterior elements. Transverse fracture through pedicle without facet subluxation.

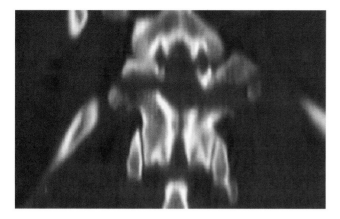

Fig. 38.2 Coronally reformatted computed tomographic image demonstrating transverse fracture through both pedicles.

Operative Technique

Patients are positioned prone, and a postural reduction is obtained. Decompression is performed to ensure that no soft tissue compression (infolding of the ligamentum flavum) occurs during the instrumented reduction. Commonly, four points of segmental instrumentation are all that is required for stability (**Fig. 38.4**). A compression maneuver is used to reduce the fracture. A formal fusion is performed if the injury is primarily ligamentous and may or may not be performed if it is a bony injury. Instrumentation is generally removed if a formal fusion is not performed.

◆ Outcomes and Rationale for Systematic Review

Thoracolumbar distraction fractures represent a distinct injury from compression or translational injuries. Despite this fact there have been few attempts to analyze patients with this pattern of injury outside of large heterogeneous cohorts of thoracolumbar fractures. As with all thoracolumbar fractures, outcomes have historically been surgeon driven with an emphasis on radiological parameters, complications, or non-validated outcome measures. However, in patients with thoracolumbar trauma, radiographic results may not correlate with clinical results.[27] It behooves surgeons to evaluate their interventions with patient-centered, validated outcome measures.

The traditional approach to the treatment of thoracolumbar flexion-distraction injuries has been dictated by patient factors, including associated injuries and neurological deficits. Importantly, the characteristics of the injury, specifically the degree of soft tissue disruption is a key piece of information required for decision making.[4,5,11,12,16,21,28–32] Considering these factors, most thoracolumbar flexion-distraction injuries are treated surgically. In a multicenter study of 1019 spinal fractures 81% of 99 flexion-distraction injuries were treated surgically.[2] The goals of treatment include obtaining spinal stability, prevention of neurological deficit, and return to pain-free function.

This chapter provides definitive, evidence-based answers to two key questions related to the management of thoracolumbar distraction injuries. This process will synthesize the best available evidence, utilize the consensus expert opinion of the STSG, and consider the concept of patient preference[33] in offering clinically relevant grades of recommendations for surgeons who treat thoracolumbar distraction injuries. The grades of

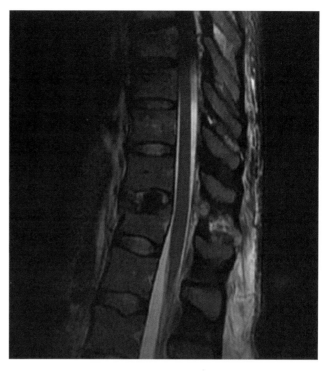

Fig. 38.3 T2-weighted magnetic resonance imaging demonstrating vertebral body compression and increased signal in posterior ligamentous complex.

recommendation, whether strong or weak, are based on the quality of evidence in conjunction with the balance of the benefits and harms of the intervention.[34] Specifically, a focused, qualitative, systematic review was performed to investigate the two pertinent questions regarding thoracolumbar distraction injuries.

> **Question 1:** Does surgery improve outcomes in patients with a thoracolumbar flexion-distraction injury without neurological deficit as compared with nonoperative treatment?
>
> **Question 2:** Should a formal fusion be performed or not in the operative reduction and stabilization of "bony flexion distraction injuries"?

Theoretically, "bony" flexion-distraction injuries should not require a formal fusion. An adequate fracture reduction would allow for bony healing and the possibility to maintain spinal segment motion. In fact, this rationale is used to justify the treatment of Chance fractures with a brace.[23]

◆ Systematic Review

To answer the specific questions in this systematic review our inclusion and exclusion criteria were determined a priori to define our population of interest. Specifically, we included neurologically intact adult patients ($>$ 16 years of age), with an injury defined as flexion-distraction/Chance/seat-belt/AO type B1 or B2, and involving the thoracolumbar spine (T10–L3). To maximize the validity of our results, studies evaluated in the review had to include a minimum of 10 patients,[35] adequately describe the treatment rendered, and use a functional assessment to evaluate the patient outcomes (reports of pain and function were considered acceptable).

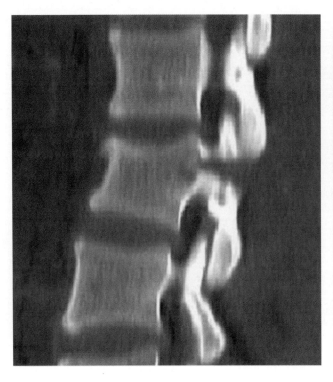

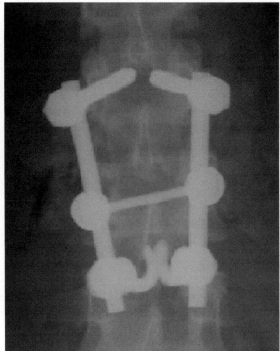

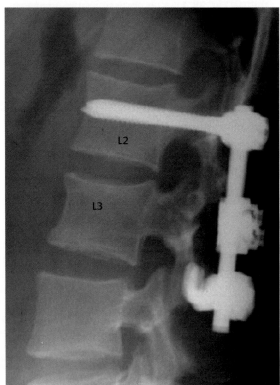

Fig. 38.4 (A) Bony flexion-distraction injury through L3. **(B,C)** L3 Flexion-distraction injury reduced and stabilized with instrumentation over one level. Alternate method would include pedicle screws at L2 and L4.

On occasion, if all the necessary data were available, selected patient data were extracted from larger study populations of patients with flexion-distraction injuries. This was done to include as many patients as possible that met our inclusion criteria even if they were analyzed together with patients whom we had excluded (neurological deficit or injury outside of T10–L3).

A qualitative synthesis of the published literature was planned because we hypothesized from the outset that there would not be a sufficient number of randomized, controlled trials to make a quantitative analysis worthwhile.

The quality of evidence of the selected studies was then assigned a score of high, moderate, low, or very low based on the GRADE approach.[34] Subsequently, a decision was made based on the benefits, harms, and costs of the proposed interventions (surgery or brace). From this analysis, a grade of recommendation was determined for the treatment of patients with thoracolumbar distraction injuries.

Six studies were accepted for qualitative analysis based on the inclusion criteria. There was only one prospective study, which was a cohort design, and five retrospective studies. The methodological quality of the studies was low and very

Table 38.2 Results of Systematic Review

Study	Description	Quality of Evidence	Topic and Conclusion
Finkelstein et al (2003)[16]	Prospective cohort study	Low	Single-level fixation of bony and ligamentous FDIs (11 patients) CONCLUSIONS: Significant abdominal injury was associated with greater disability on Oswestry but kyphosis was not. Single-level fixation resulted in good outcomes in patients with bony and ligamentous injuries.
Miyanji et al (2006)[21]	Retrospective cohort study with cross-sectional outcome analysis	Low	Assessment of long-term radiographic and quality of life outcomes in thoracolumbar FDIs (25 operative, 15 nonoperative) CONCLUSIONS: Surgical treatment had worse HRQoL and NASS score compared with controls (normative data) but nonoperative patients no different from controls. No association between radiographic sagittal alignment and functional outcome. Associated injury independent predictor of worse outcome.
Liu et al (2003)[5]	Retrospective case series	Very low	Review of surgical treatment for thoracolumbar FDIs if ligamentous or initial kyphosis > 15 degrees (17 patients). CONCLUSIONS: All patients had a "good" result according to the criteria of Anderson and Henley such that there was no or occasional back pain, full function, and no medication.
Anderson et al (1991)[11]	Retrospective case series	Very low	Review of surgical and nonoperative treatment of thoracolumbar FDIs (11 patients). CONCLUSIONS: All operatively treated patients had "good" result according to Anderson and Henley criteria. Nonoperatively treated patients had one third good, fair, and poor results, respectively. Inferior radiographic results in nonoperative group.
LeGay et al (1990)[12]	Retrospective case series	Very low	Review of surgical and nonoperative treatment of lumbar FDIs (13 patients). CONCLUSIONS: Facet involvement, whether subluxation or dislocation, led to treatment failure in most patients treated initially with bed rest and bracing.
Gumley et al (1982)[3]	Retrospective case series	Very low	Review of surgical and nonoperative treatment of lumbar bony FDIs (13 patients) CONCLUSIONS: Nonoperatively treated Chance fractures may go on to nonunion if reduction not achieved or maintained.

Abbreviation: FDI, flexion-distraction injury; HRQoL, health-related quality of life; NASS, North American Spine Society.

low. The indications for surgery were variable or not discussed. Older studies, which utilized outdated surgical techniques, were included to avoid bias in excluding studies that investigated the outcomes of nonoperative treatments. The nonoperative treatment protocols generally consisted of periods of bed rest that are considered unacceptable by today's standards.[12,28] As such, data were not pooled but the relevant results were summarized (**Table 38.2**).

◆ Evidence

Surgical Versus Nonoperative Treatment of Thoracolumbar Distraction Injuries

In the study by Miyanji et al,[21] nonoperatively treated patients with flexion-distraction injuries had similar functional outcome scores on a disease-specific scale as well as health-related quality of life (HRQoL) compared with matched controls. Surgically treated patients were found to have statistically significant lower Short Form-36 (SF-36) and North American Spine Society (NASS) outcome instrument scores compared with age- and sex-matched normative data. Regression analysis demonstrated that associated other system injury independently influenced the SF-36 physical component score, but the degree of kyphosis at follow-up did not affect outcome. Importantly, the type of treatment had an influence on the SF-36 mental component score and the NASS pain/disability score, with lower scores more likely in the surgically treated group.

There are several potential explanations for these findings. Traditional indications for nonoperative treatment in the setting of a thoracolumbar distraction injury are the presence of a bony injury, ability to obtain and maintain the fracture reduction, absence of neurological deficit, and absence of associated injuries, which would contraindicate the use of an orthosis. The decision to treat nonoperatively selects for patients with less severe injuries and avoids fusion-related motion loss and surgical complications. Finally, the NASS lumbar spine assessment instrument is not specifically designed for spine trauma, and despite potential content validity the instrument may not accurately reflect spine trauma functional outcomes.

Adequate radiographic outcomes have been demonstrated in patients with flexion-distraction injuries treated nonoperatively if the fracture kyphosis is adequately reduced and maintained.[12,32] If residual kyphosis is significant (> 30 degrees) the incidence of pain may be increased in the medium term in all thoracolumbar fractures[2]; however, this has not been demonstrated specifically in patients with thoracolumbar flexion-distraction injuries.

Finkelstein et al[16] conducted a prospective study on patients with flexion-distraction injuries. Eleven patients satisfied our inclusion criteria. Treatment was single-level fixation of the thoracolumbar distraction injury irrespective of whether the injury was primarily ligamentous or bony. The outcomes used were radiographic and the Oswestry Functional Assessment Questionnaire. The average preoperative kyphosis was 11.4 and at latest follow-up was 0.3 of lordosis. The average Oswestry score was 11.4 (normative population mean is 10.14). For their whole series of 21 patients significant abdominal injury was associated with greater disability on the Oswestry but kyphosis was not. They concluded that single-level fixation resulted in good outcomes in patients with bony and ligamentous injuries. Although this was prospectively collected data, without a control group of nonoperatively treated patients it is difficult to determine whether certain patients with bony flexion-distraction injuries were overtreated. Certainly, their results suggest that single-level fixation can be performed with good results and minimal morbidity.

Liu et al[5] found similar results with operative treatment of bony and ligamentous flexion-distraction injuries; however, their study was retrospective and the outcome measure used was not validated. Seventeen patients satisfied our inclusion criteria. Treatment consisted of fixation one level above and below the injury. The surgical indications included posterior column ligamentous disruption or initial kyphosis > 15 degrees. The average preop kyphosis was 15.5 and final kyphosis was 3.8. All patients had a "good" result according to the criteria of Anderson et al[11] such that there was occasional or a complete absence of back pain, full function, and no medication. They concluded that the results of surgery are good in patients with flexion-distraction injuries; however, there was no control group and their outcome measure is not validated nor is it patient driven.

LeGay et al[12] reviewed 18 patients with flexion-distraction injuries. Thirteen patients satisfied our inclusion criteria. Although a validated outcome measure was not used, the authors attempted to characterize the patients' functional outcome by quantifying pain and activity. The authors classified the fractures according to the method of Gumley et al.[3] Twelve of 13 patients were treated with prolonged bed rest followed by a brace. Nonoperative treatment resulted in fair or poor results in 60% of patients with "facet involvement." Good or excellent results were found in six of seven patients without facet involvement who were treated nonoperatively. The authors suggested that initial kyphosis of 17 degrees may portend a poor prognosis, and this has been demonstrated in vitro.[36] Based on this retrospective series, one can conclude that nonoperative treatment is viable in certain patients. No definitive conclusion can be made regarding the specific patient or injury factors that led to an acceptable outcome with nonoperative treatment; however, facet involvement, whether subluxation or dislocation, likely leads to treatment failure.

The duration of bed rest would not be considered acceptable by today's standards.

Gumley et al[3] had similar good results in neurologically intact patients with Chance fractures treated with extension casting or spinal fusion. Treatment decisions were based on the authors' interpretation of fracture "stability" and as such, meaningful conclusions are difficult. However, the authors did surgically treat three patients with nonunions who were initially managed with bed rest at a different institution. This reinforces the principal that bony reduction must be achieved and maintained for nonoperative treatment to be successful.

In the retrospective series by Anderson et al,[11] better results were reported with surgical treatment. Eleven patients satisfied our inclusion criteria. Treatment consisted of surgery with Harrington rods, whereas nonoperative treatment was extension casting and bracing for 3 to 6 months. Indications for nonoperative treatment included bony injury, less than 10 degrees kyphosis, and no neurological deficit. Six patients were treated nonoperatively and five operatively. Initial kyphosis in the nonoperative group was 9.2 degrees and at follow-up 14.8. Initial kyphosis in the operative group was 22.4 and at final follow-up was 1 degree. According to their back pain rating scale nonoperative treatment resulted in 2 good, 2 fair, and 2 poor results, whereas operative treatment resulted in five good results. In the setting of small numbers and nonvalidated outcomes the only conclusion that can be made is that inferior radiographic results were seen in the nonoperative group.

There are limitations of our systematic review. Including only studies with functional outcome measures inherently eliminates older studies that generally focused on radiographic outcomes. Consequently, a greater proportion of nonoperative studies may have been excluded but at the benefit of excluding studies that utilized outdated surgical techniques. Nevertheless, to accurately answer the primary question only studies with functional outcome measures were deemed appropriate. It was felt that the inclusion of nonvalidated functional outcome scores such as pain and assessment of "function" would be acceptable to attempt to answer the primary question accurately and be representative of the literature. Furthermore, the two studies with a validated outcome measure would suggest that radiographic kyphosis does not impact the function of patients with thoracolumbar distraction injuries.[16,21]

There are a large number of patients with flexion-distraction injuries that could not be analyzed because they are grouped within "unstable thoracolumbar fractures." With the small numbers of patients in this systematic review it is possible that they do not represent thoracolumbar distraction injuries as a whole. However, the patients analyzed do represent the best available evidence, and when combined with consensus expert opinion, meaningful conclusions can be made.

An analysis of the quality of evidence must be combined with estimates of benefit, harm, and costs to the patient and/or society.[34] Patients with thoracolumbar distraction injuries represent a diverse group, and treatment decisions should be individualized. For example, bony flexion-distraction injuries may be adequately treated with a brace; however, considerations include the costs of the brace, the orthotist, follow-up visits, and serial x-rays. Furthermore, brace utilization may not be acceptable to a patient based on other factors such as a delay in treatment secondary to abdominal injuries or tube thoracostomies or even rehabilitation time and occupational considerations.

The costs of a surgical procedure include the instrumentation, operating room (OR) time, and changes in the hospital length of stay (more or less), and this cost may be significantly affected by the treatment approach. Percutaneous treatment of bony flexion-distraction injuries may allow patients to mobilize quicker with smaller hospital costs and may be preferable to patients rather than brace treatment depending on the perceived risks. The overriding consideration, however, is that the balance of all these factors is not clear.

Is Formal Fusion Necessary in Bony Flexion-Distraction Injuries?

There are no comparative studies on flexion-distraction injuries in the literature to answer this question, nor are there any substantial retrospective data. In fact, the issue of whether a formal fusion was performed or not is rarely reported in the various surgical techniques described for flexion-distraction injuries. The question of whether to perform a posterolateral fusion is critical because it adds operating time, increases blood loss, limits segmental motion, and has been reported to have long-term donor site morbidity as high as 37%.[37]

Liu et al[5] instrumented but did not formally fuse two patients with Chance fractures. Green et al[13] instrumented and performed a posterolateral fusion on all patients in their series with flexion-distraction injuries. Iliac crest autograft harvest and posterolateral fusion were standard surgical techniques in the series reported by Finkelstein et al.[16]

The question of whether a formal fusion is required has been investigated in patients with thoracolumbar burst fractures, and the results should be applicable to patients with bony flexion-distraction injuries. Sanderson et al[38] reported on the clinical and radiographic results of 28 patients with unstable burst fractures treated with instrumentation but no fusion and demonstrated results comparable to patients treated with fusion. Wang et al,[39] in a randomized study, found that the short-term results in 58 patients with surgically treated burst fractures were the same on the low back outcome score whether they had fusion or not. Furthermore, the nonfusion group had less intraoperative blood loss, less operative time, and more segmental motion.

Thoracolumbar distraction injuries represent an ideal patient group for percutaneous stabilization techniques.[40] First, these injuries do not usually require a formal decompression, although some authors advocate removing the ligamentum flavum prior to reduction. Flexion-distraction injuries generally only require segmental instrumentation at two levels; the injury level and one level cranially or one level above and below depending on the pedicle fracture morphology. Therefore, percutaneous rod passage is easier than in patients requiring multiple fixation points. Finally, in the setting of a purely bony injury, one should expect fracture healing without a formal fusion. Early implant removal may allow for preservation of segmental motion. Two case reports have documented good results with percutaneous stabilization of bony flexion-distraction injuries without fusion and early implant removal.[41,42]

Equally important is the determination of the number of levels to fuse when a significant discoligamentous disruption has occurred. Because a significant proportion of flexion-distraction injuries are two-level injuries (Denis C and D type)[4] instrumenting one level above and below the injury

sacrifices two motion segments. Adjacent two-level instrumentation, which sacrifices one motion segment, may be indicated when the pedicles and the middle column are intact.[5]

◆ Spine Trauma Study Group Recommendations

It is difficult to compare surgical and nonsurgical treatment of thoracolumbar distraction injuries because historically nonoperative treatment has been reserved for patients with osseous injuries, less severe deformities, an absence of neurological deficit, and a lack of associated injuries. The concept that ligamentous flexion-distraction injuries cannot heal without a formal fusion has been the basis for operative treatment for many years, and as such there is no high-quality study definitively proving it. The necessity of a formal fusion in the operative treatment of bony flexion-distraction injuries has been equally dogmatic, but this should be challenged. Three separate recommendations can be made after careful analysis of the systematic review and relevant considerations by the STSG representing clinical expertise.

1A. For patients with bony thoracolumbar flexion-distraction injuries and no contraindication to brace treatment, nonoperative and operative treatments provide similar outcomes. Patient preference and clinical circumstances and experience should dictate treatment. This is a strong recommendation in a setting of low-quality evidence.

1B. For patients with ligamentous or irreducible bony thoracolumbar flexion-distraction injuries, operative treatment consisting of fixation above and below (or at the injury level) is suggested. This is a strong recommendation in a setting of very low quality evidence.

2. Stabilization of bony flexion-distraction injuries without fusion is an acceptable treatment. This is an important consideration because bony flexion-distraction injuries may prove to be an ideal indication for temporary minimally invasive stabilization techniques. This is a weak recommendation in a setting of very low quality evidence.

Ultimately, patient preference must be incorporated into the decision-making process because it represents a key component of the evolving concept of evidence-based medicine, and treatment recommendations must continue to be individualized to the clinical scenario.

References

1. Gertzbein SD, Court-Brown CM. Flexion-distraction injuries of the lumbar spine. Mechanisms of injury and classification. Clin Orthop Relat Res 1988;227:52–60
2. Gertzbein SD. Scoliosis Research Society. Multicenter spine fracture study. Spine 1992;17:528–540
3. Gumley G, Taylor TK, Ryan MD. Distraction fractures of the lumbar spine. J Bone Joint Surg Br 1982;64:520–525
4. Denis F. The three column spine and its significance in the classification of acute thoracolumbar spinal injuries. Spine 1983;8:817–831
5. Liu YJ, Chang MC, Wang ST, Yu WK, Liu CL, Chen TH. Flexion-distraction injury of the thoracolumbar spine. Injury 2003;34:920–923
6. Chance GQ. Note on a type of flexion fracture of the spine. Br J Radiol 1948;21:452–453

7. Magerl F, Aebi M, Gertzbein SD, Harms J, Nazarian S. A comprehensive classification of thoracic and lumbar injuries. Eur Spine J 1994;3: 184–201

8. McAfee PC, Yuan HA, Fredrickson BE, Lubicky JP. The value of computed tomography in thoracolumbar fractures: an analysis of one hundred consecutive cases and a new classification. J Bone Joint Surg Am 1983; 65:461–473

9. Rennie W, Mitchell N. Flexion distraction fractures of the thoracolumbar spine. J Bone Joint Surg Am 1973;55:386–390

10. Smith WS, Kaufer H. Patterns and mechanisms of lumbar injuries associated with lap seat belts. J Bone Joint Surg Am 1969;51:239–254

11. Anderson PA, Henley MB, Rivara FP, Maier RV. Flexion distraction and chance injuries to the thoracolumbar spine. J Orthop Trauma 1991;5: 153–160

12. LeGay DA, Petrie DP, Alexander DI. Flexion-distraction injuries of the lumbar spine and associated abdominal trauma. J Trauma 1990;30:436–444

13. Green DA, Green NE, Spengler DM, Devito DP. Flexion-distraction injuries to the lumbar spine associated with abdominal injuries. J Spinal Disord 1991;4:312–318

14. Howland WJ, Curry JL, Buffington CB. Fulcrum fractures of the lumbar spine. Transverse fracture induced by an improperly placed seat belt. JAMA 1965;193:240–241

15. Willén J, Lindahl S, Irstam L, Aldman B, Nordwall A. The thoracolumbar crush fracture: an experimental study on instant axial dynamic loading: the resulting fracture type and its stability. Spine 1984;9:624–631

16. Finkelstein JA, Wai EK, Jackson SS, Ahn H, Brighton-Knight M. Single-level fixation of flexion distraction injuries. J Spinal Disord Tech 2003;16:236–242

17. Hoshikawa T, Tanaka Y, Kokubun S, Lu WW, Luk KD, Leong JC. Flexion-distraction injuries in the thoracolumbar spine: an in vitro study of the relation between flexion angle and the motion axis of fracture. J Spinal Disord Tech 2002;15:139–143

18. Neumann P, Osvalder AL, Hansson TH, Nordwall A. Flexion-distraction injury of the lumbar spine: influence of load, loading rate, and vertebral mineral content. J Spinal Disord 1996;9:89–102

19. Harris MB, Sethi RK. The initial assessment and management of the multiple-trauma patient with an associated spine injury. Spine 2006; 31(11, Suppl):S9–S15, discussion S36

20. Garrett JW, Braunstein PW. The seat belt syndrome. J Trauma 1962; 2: 220–238

21. Miyanji F, Fisher CG, Keynan O, Wing PC, Boyd M, Dvorak MF. Flexion-distraction injuries of the thoracolumbar spine: health-related quality of life and radiographic outcomes. Top Spinal Cord Inj Rehabil 2006;12: 58–69

22. Vaccaro AR, Kim DH, Brodke DS, et al. Diagnosis and management of thoracolumbar spine fractures. Instr Course Lect 2004;53:359–373

23. Vaccaro AR, Lehman RA Jr, Hurlbert RJ, et al. A new classification of thoracolumbar injuries: the importance of injury morphology, the integrity of the posterior ligamentous complex, and neurologic status. Spine 2005;30:2325–2333

24. Leferink VJ, Veldhuis EF, Zimmerman KW, ten Vergert EM, ten Duis HJ. Classificational problems in ligamentary distraction type vertebral fractures: 30% of all B-type fractures are initially unrecognised. Eur Spine J 2002;11:246–250

25. Lee HM, Kim HS, Kim DJ, Suk KS, Park JO, Kim NH. Reliability of magnetic resonance imaging in detecting posterior ligament complex injury in thoracolumbar spinal fractures. Spine 2000;25: 2079–2084

26. Groves CJ, Cassar-Pullicino VN, Tins BJ, Tyrrell PN, McCall IW. Chance-type flexion-distraction injuries in the thoracolumbar spine: MR imaging characteristics. Radiology 2005;236:601–608

27. Weinstein JN, Collalto P, Lehmann TR. Thoracolumbar "burst" fractures treated conservatively: a long-term follow-up. Spine 1988;13:33–38

28. Gertzbein SD, Court-Brown CM. Rationale for the management of flexion-distraction injuries of the thoracolumbar spine based on a new classification. J Spinal Disord 1989;2:176–183

29. McGuire RA, Freeland AE. Flexion-distraction injury of the thoracolumbar spine. Orthopedics 1992;15:379–381

30. Triantafyllou SJ, Gertzbein SD. Flexion distraction injuries of the thoracolumbar spine: a review. Orthopedics 1992;15:357–364

31. Vanichkachorn JS, Vaccaro AR. Nonoperative treatment of thoracolumbar fractures. Orthopedics 1997;20:948–953, quiz 954–955

32. Yu WY, Siu CM. Seat belt injuries of the lumbar spine—stable or unstable? Paraplegia 1989;27:450–456

33. Fisher CG, Wood KB. Introduction to and techniques of evidence-based medicine. Spine 2007;32(19, Suppl):S66–S72

34. Schünemann HJ, Jaeschke R, Cook DJ, et al; ATS Documents Development and Implementation Committee. An official ATS statement: grading the quality of evidence and strength of recommendations in ATS guidelines and recommendations. Am J Respir Crit Care Med 2006;174:605–614

35. Verlaan JJ, Diekerhof CH, Buskens E, et al. Surgical treatment of traumatic fractures of the thoracic and lumbar spine: a systematic review of the literature on techniques, complications, and outcome. Spine 2004;29:803–814

36. Neumann P, Nordwall A, Osvalder AL. Traumatic instability of the lumbar spine: a dynamic in vitro study of flexion-distraction injury. Spine 1995;20:1111–1121

37. Frymoyer JW, Howe J, Kuhlmann D. The long-term effects of spinal fusion on the sacroiliac joints and ilium. Clin Orthop Relat Res 1978; 134:196–201

38. Sanderson PL, Fraser RD, Hall DJ, Cain CM, Osti OL, Potter GR. Short segment fixation of thoracolumbar burst fractures without fusion. Eur Spine J 1999;8:495–500

39. Wang ST, Ma HL, Liu CL, Yu WK, Chang MC, Chen TH. Is fusion necessary for surgically treated burst fractures of the thoracolumbar and lumbar spine?: a prospective, randomized study. Spine 2006; 31:2646–2652, discussion 2653

40. Rampersaud YR, Annand N, Dekutoski MB. Use of minimally invasive surgical techniques in the management of thoracolumbar trauma: current concepts. Spine 2006;31(11, Suppl):S96–S102, discussion S104

41. Beringer W, Potts E, Khairi S, Mobasser JP. Percutaneous pedicle screw instrumentation for temporary internal bracing of nondisplaced bony Chance fractures. J Spinal Disord Tech 2007;20:242–247

42. Eichinger JK, Arrington ED, Kerr GJ, Molinari R. Bony flexion-distraction injury of the lower lumbar spine treated with instrumentation without fusion and early implant removal: a method of treatment to preserve lumbar motion: two-year follow-up of a teenage patient. J Spinal Disord Tech 2007;20:93–96

39

Thoracolumbar Hyperextension Injuries in the Stiff Spine

Rune Hedlund and Jorrit-Jan Verlaan

Patients with ankylosing disorders of the spine such as ankylosing spondylitis (AS) and diffuse idiopathic skeletal hyperostosis (DISH) are disproportionally prone to hyperextension fractures of the spine.[1] It is estimated that patients with ankylosing spine disorders such as AS and DISH sustain a four- to eightfold fracture risk.[2] In both ankylosing disorders, minor trauma may result in fractures, which typically tend to go unrecognized, are unstable, and are associated with permanent neurological deficits and high mortality.[1] The ankylosed spine is vulnerable to fractures because energy from traumatic impacts cannot be easily absorbed by elastic deformation as in the healthy flexible spine. Moreover, multiple fused segments may cause the spine to behave like a long bone (e.g., a femur) and when failure loads are exerted it may fracture with displacements similar to long bones, leading to disastrous neurological and vascular damage (**Figs. 39.1 and 39.2**).[3]

In general, hyperextension fractures of the spine are rare instances and are considered to occur predominantly in the cervical spine.[4] In a series of 154 hyperextension injuries Burke found only four of these type of fractures to occur in the thoracic region.[5] In Bedbrook and Clark's series of 54 hyperextension fractures, only one occurred in the thoracic spine.[6] In Magerl et al's series of thoracolumbar fractures only three out of 1445 (0.21%) were type B3 extension injuries, and when Matejka analyzed a total of 965 admitted patients with thoracolumbar fractures, he also found only four hyperextension fractures.[7,8] Because three of these four patients had preexistent ankylosed spines (two patients had DISH, one had AS) the study hypothesized that thoracolumbar hyperextension fractures were highly unusual but would predominantly occur in patients with ankylosed spines.[8]

From the literature it can be learned that hyperextension-type fractures occurring in the ankylosed spine are indeed highly unstable and are frequently accompanied by permanent neurological deficit.[1] These two characteristics currently represent key elements for the decision to treat surgically or nonoperatively. A recent concept developed by the Spine Trauma Study Group called the Thoracolumbar Injury Classification and Severity Score (TLICS) incorporates three major spine trauma characteristics: basic fracture morphology, presence of neurological deficit, and integrity of the posterior ligamentous complex to guide treatment and predict clinical prognosis by assigning points to each of the three variables.[9] The total number of points correlates with injury severity. When TLICS is applied to hyperextension fractures associated with AS or DISH, the combined scores of the three parameters will sum up to at least 7 points (4 points for the obligatory extension/distraction morphology and 3 points for the posterior ligamentous complex disruption) strongly suggesting surgery, 4 points being the cutoff point, even in the absence of neurological deficit.[10] The concept of TLICS has, however, not yet been validated for patients with AS or DISH, and thoracolumbar hyperextension fractures and therefore the suggestion for surgical treatment can be debated.[11] From the literature it becomes clear that nonoperative treatment has frequently been performed for patients with AS or DISH and hyperextension fractures, although with variable success.[1] Robust evidence for the decision to treat either operatively or nonoperatively is presently nonexistent. Therefore, the research question for the present review was: Does surgical treatment improve the outcome of patients with ankylosing spondylitis or diffuse idiopathic skeletal hyperostosis with hyperextension fractures of the thoracolumbar spine?

In this systematic review the treatment, complications, and outcome of patients with ankylosing spinal disorders suffering hyperextension fractures of the thoracolumbar spine are presented in two distinct parts, the first of which describes the cohort of patients with AS, and the second of which describes the cohort of patients with diffuse idiopathic skeletal hyperostosis.

◆ Hyperextension Fractures of the Thoracolumbar Spine in Ankylosing Spondylitis

AS is an autoimmune spondylarthropathy in which the sacroiliac joints and spinal segments become fused after recurrent inflammatory processes.[12] The etiology of AS is

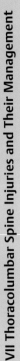

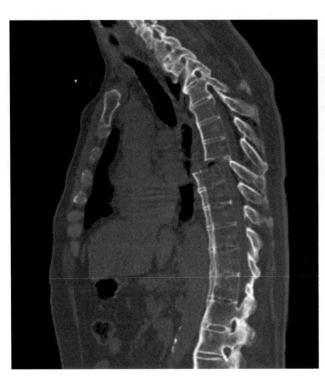

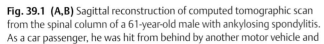

A

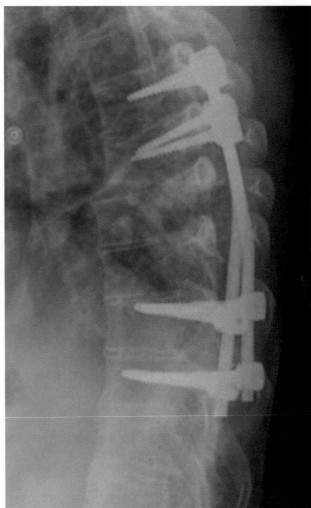

B

Fig. 39.1 (A,B) Sagittal reconstruction of computed tomographic scan from the spinal column of a 61-year-old male with ankylosing spondylitis. As a car passenger, he was hit from behind by another motor vehicle and became instantly paraplegic. A Th7–Th8 hyperextension fracture was diagnosed and treated with pedicle screw fixation.

mostly speculative, and current treatment is directed at decreasing symptoms, which include back pain, stiffness, and progressive deformation.

The risk of highly unstable hyperextension thoracolumbar fractures with severe neurological deficit of the spine is increased in patients with AS (**Fig. 39.1**).[2] The present systematic review addresses the question: Does surgical treatment improve the outcome of hyperextension fractures of the thoracolumbar spine in ankylosing spondylitis?

Material and Methods

A systematic review of the literature published from 1980 to 2007 was performed using a PubMed and EMBASE search on AS in combination with thoracolumbar fracture. Search parameters were "ankylosing spondylitis" AND "trauma" and their respective synonyms. Articles in languages other than English, French, or German were excluded, as were articles without abstract or articles published before 1980. The initial selection of references was by title and abstract; full-text papers were included after meeting all inclusion criteria: the article is from an international peer reviewed journal; AS and

hyperextension fractures are present in adults; there is a sufficiently detailed description of fracture type and trauma mechanism and an adequate description of neurological status, complications, and period of follow-up. Excluded were articles describing cervical or cervicothoracic hyperextension injuries. Case reports fulfilling all criteria were included also, to obtain as much information as possible on this subject. Cross-referencing was finally used to identify and retrieve the remaining eligible articles. In case of overlap of papers from the same author or institution, the least informative paper was excluded. The level of evidence of included articles was assessed according to the guidelines proposed by the Center for Evidence Based Medicine (www.cebm.net). Data were extracted according to predefined and generally accepted criteria and subsequently pooled to increase estimates of treatment effect (see **Table 39.1** for the list of criteria). The first 3 months after admission were defined as the posttreatment period; thereafter it was defined as the follow-up period. The clinical and neurological outcomes were assessed separately for both operative and nonoperative treatment strategies. The strength of the final recommendation was determined according to the guidelines proposed by Guyatt et al.[13]

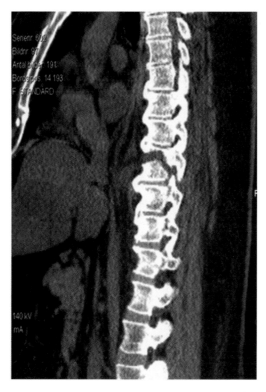
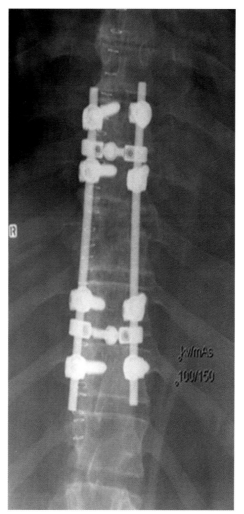

Fig. 39.2 (A,B) Sagittal reconstruction of computed tomographic scan from a 40-year-old male weighing 145 kg (BMI 50). The patient was expelled from a boat run aground and landed on his back resulting in pain and immediate paraplegia. Diffuse idiopathic skeletal hyperostosis (DISH) was observed on at least five levels and a Th9 hyperextension/distraction fracture in an ankylosed segment was diagnosed. The patient was operated on with fixation from Th7 to Th11; postoperatively he remained paraplegic.

Table 39.1 Parameters Extracted from Papers and Definitions

Parameter	Definition
Author(s)	
Institution(s)	
Journal	International peer reviewed
Language	English, German, French
Mean year of treatment	Average of first and last year of patient treatment
Study design	Randomized, controlled trial, prospective/retrospective series, case reports
Number of individuals	
Mean age (range)	Years
Number of males	
Follow-up	Months
Level of evidence	According to Center for Evidence Based Medicine (www.cebm.net)
Fracture level	Thoracic, lumbar
Basic fracture type	Compression, distraction, rotation/translation

(Continued on page 394)

Table 39.1 Parameters Extracted from Papers and Definitions (*Continued*)

Parameter	Definition
Trauma mechanism	Hyperextension
Low-energy impact	Fall from standing/sitting position
High-energy impact	Fall from height (> 2 m), motor vehicle accidents, etc.
Delayed diagnosis	Diagnosis established > 24 hours
Neurological status	According to ASIA classification
Surgical treatment	Posterior, anterior, combined AP, laminectomy
Postoperative immobilization	Plaster jacket, brace
Nonoperative treatment	Bed rest, plaster jacket, brace
Fusion	Yes/no
Complications	As described by authors

Results

The literature search and subsequent cross-referencing resulted in 104 international peer reviewed references on "ankylosing spondylitis and trauma" based on abstract and title. Twenty references were excluded because of insufficient detail and/or overlap from same author/institution. Another 59 papers were excluded because they described cervical or cervicothoracic injuries in combination with AS. The results from this review are therefore based on 25 references (three in the German and 22 in the English language) describing a total of 65 patients with AS suffering hyperextension fractures.[8,14–37] The eligible articles were descriptions of retrospective case series (*n* = 10 papers) or case reports (*n* = 15 papers); the level of evidence was grade IV for all.

The mean age of the patients was 60.5 ± 11.4 years with a range of 34 to 92 years; 46 patients were male and 19 female (male/total ratio: 0.71). The average duration of follow-up was 6 months (median: 4 months; range 0 to 78 months). In 39 patients the fracture was located in the thoracic spine, and in 26 patients it was located in the lumbar spine. Low-energy impacts were endured by 48 patients, whereas high-energy impacts were involved in the remaining 17 patients. At admission 20.0% of the 65 patients presented with American Spinal Injury Association A (ASIA A) neurological deficit, 4.6% with ASIA B, 9.2% with ASIA C, and 9.2% with ASIA D, and 57.0% were neurologically intact (ASIA E). A rationale for the decision to treat surgically (46 patients = 70.8%) or nonoperatively (19 patients = 29.2%) was usually not provided explicitly. In the group treated

surgically, a total of 23 ASIA levels were lost between admission and surgery (representing 0.5 ASIA scale on average for each patient). No short-term (< 3 to 4 days) neurological deterioration was described after admission in the conservatively treated group.

Surgical treatment consisted of posterior fixation (long segment with Luque/Harrington instrumentation or short segment with pedicle screw constructs) in the majority of cases (41/46 = 89.1%), sometimes in combination with decompression. An anterior stabilization was performed in two patients, a combined anteroposterior stabilization was performed in another two patients, and laminectomy only in one patient. Nonoperative treatment consisted of bed rest, plaster jackets, or braces. The motivation behind each individual treatment strategy and the total intended period of (postsurgical) immobilization were typically not provided.

The number of patients lost to follow-up within 3 months posttrauma was 20 (43.5%) for the surgical group and five (26.3%) for the nonoperatively treated group. The reasons for this high number of patients lost to follow-up included: transfer to paraplegia center or rehabilitation center, early death, or unknown. The neurological status of the patients from admission through the treatment period to follow-up is presented in **Table 39.2** and **Table 39.3**. The preoperative versus postoperative data for surgically treated patients suggest an improvement for patients with ASIA C, often converting to ASIA D, a change less obvious in the pretreatment versus posttreatment group of conservatively treated patients. Complications were numerous in this relatively small cohort of patients. A delayed (> 24 hours) diagnosis of the fracture was

Table 39.2 Neurological Status of Patients Treated Surgically (in %)

ASIA	Admission *n* = 46	Preoperative *n* = 46	Postoperative *n* = 46	Follow-Up *n* = 26
A	19.5	26.1	28.3	15.4
B	6.5	6.5	6.5	0.0
C	10.9	21.8	13.0	7.7
D	10.9	13.0	19.6	30.8
E	52.2	32.6	32.6	46.1
Total	100.0%	100.0%	100.0%	100.0%

Abbreviation: ASIA, American Spinal Injury Association.

Table 39.3 Neurological Status of Patients Treated Nonoperatively (in %)

ASIA	Admission n = 19	Pretreatment n = 19	Posttreatment n = 19	Follow-Up n = 14
A	21.0	26.3	26.3	28.6
B	0.0	0.0	0.0	0.0
C	5.3	5.3	5.3	0.0
D	5.3	15.8	15.8	7.1
E	68.4	52.6	52.6	64.3
Total	100.0%	100.0%	100.0%	100.0%

Abbreviation: ASIA, American Spinal Injury Association.

noted in 15 patients (23.1%). Deterioration of neurological deficit before onset of treatment was observed in nine patients (13.8%); all these patients underwent subsequent surgical stabilization. After treatment, deterioration of neurological deficit was observed in two patients treated surgically (2/46 = 4.3%) and in three patients treated nonoperatively (3/19 = 15.8%). In the surgically treated group, four patients (4/46 = 8.7%) died in the posttreatment period; in the nonoperatively treated group two patients (2/19 = 10.5%) died. During follow-up, another three surgically treated patients died. Perioperative and postoperative complications were numerous and are listed in **Table 39.4**.

Discussion

Although patients with AS and thoracolumbar hyperextension fractures are currently considered by many spine surgeons to perform better in terms of functional and neurological outcome when stabilized surgically, there is no consensus on the optimal treatment.[1] In this systematic review we tried to find evidence for the hypothesis that surgical treatment would offer benefits over nonoperative treatment. The first and foremost conclusion that can be drawn from this work is the absence of any robust prospective medium- to long-term follow-up study on this subject. The prevalence of AS is known to be ~0.1 to 0.2% in the general population.[12] This number may be too small for spine traumatologists to be regularly confronted with patients suffering this disease. Although many case reports and small series have already been published, studies with larger numbers of

Table 39.4 Miscellaneous Complications in Patients with AS and Thoracolumbar Hyperextension Fractures

Complications Reported	Surgical Treatment	Nonoperative Treatment
Aortic rupture (at admission)	3	1
Cerebrovascular accident	1	0
Deep infection	4	0
Hemothorax	0	1
Material failure	2	0
Pneumonia	0	1
Pseudarthrosis	0	1
Secondary operation	2	1

patients seem too difficult to initiate and propagate by single-center efforts.

Because thoracolumbar hyperextension-type fractures are often highly unstable and frequently lead to neurological deficit, the optimal treatment is likely to differ from "regular" fractures sustained by the general trauma population.[38] In the case of AS, the long and stiff mechanical lever arms render the spine at risk for secondary dislocation during nursing/manipulation until sufficient bony fusion of the fracture has been established. Immediate and rigid stabilization may help the patient to get mobile quickly and start rehabilitation early.[1] The current consensus is therefore to treat hyperextension fractures of the thoracic and lumbar spine with internal stabilization.

From the neurological data obtained in this review some interesting phenomena were observed. None of the conservatively treated patients deteriorated neurologically in the period up to immobilization therefore it is suggested that these patients had relatively stable injuries. On the other hand, in the group of 46 surgically treated patients, 23 ASIA scales were lost in nine patients from the moment of admission until surgery. It is reasonable to suggest less stable fracture configurations were present more often in this group of patients. Moreover, it can be suggested that this rapid and sometimes severe decline in neurological function forced surgeons to immediately and aggressively stabilize these spines by surgical intervention. Considering the difference in neurological status from admission until definite treatment, the two groups under study (surgical and conservative) were probably not comparable from the start. When examining the neurological results from the pretreatment versus posttreatment period it can be suggested that no immediate neurological improvement was observed in the nonoperative group. In the surgical group a small improvement was noticed especially with reference to the ASIA C and D categories. Again, it must be stressed that the groups may not have been comparable considering the relatively large number of acutely deteriorating patients in the surgical group preoperatively. Extracting valid conclusions from the period from posttreatment to follow-up is difficult due to the profound influence of number of patients lost to follow-up. Complications reported were numerous and included four aortic ruptures representing a remarkably high number compared with data from a recent systematic review on the outcome and complications of over 5000 patients with "regular" traumatic thoracolumbar fractures.[38] Presumably, the dislocation of the hyperextended and fractured thoracolumbar AS spine is severe enough to overstretch (and/or puncture) the aorta, causing it to rupture.

Conclusion and Recommendation

Notwithstanding the limited level of evidence available we suggest the following conclusions can be drawn from the systematic review:

♦ Most hyperextension fractures in AS are caused by low-energy impacts.
♦ Patients with AS and hyperextension fractures frequently present with neurological deficits.
♦ Neurological deficits at admission may easily deteriorate in the absence of definite and rigid stabilization of the spine.
♦ Surgical stabilization may provide a better prospective for neurological recovery.

The research question: Does surgical treatment improve the outcome of hyperextension fractures of the thoracolumbar spine in ankylosing spondylitis? cannot be answered convincingly when only 25 papers of grade IV level of evidence, representing 65 patients, are available for study. For an individual patient with AS suffering a hyperextension fracture, however, initiation of the optimal treatment is of great importance because unstable fracture configurations can lead to catastrophic and irreversible neurological deterioration. In this respect immediate and aggressive surgical stabilization may represent the preferable treatment option when the risks (complications of surgery) and benefits (halt or reversal of neurological deterioration) of this strategy are balanced. Therefore, despite the low level of evidence, the results of this systematic review leads to a recommendation for surgical treatment of hyperextension fractures in patients with ankylosing spondylitis. Among the members of the Spine Trauma Study Group, this recommendation is unanimously supported.

♦ Hyperextension Fractures of the Thoracolumbar Spine in Diffuse Idiopathic Skeletal Hyperostosis

DISH was first described by Forestier and Rotes-Querol in the 1950s.[39] The three distinct ankylosing disorders of the spine: DISH, AS, and ossification of the posterior longitudinal ligament (OPLL) can lead to grossly unstable fractures after minor trauma with severe neurological compromise.[1] The diagnosis of DISH is based solely on radiographic abnormalities using the Resnick criteria: flowing bulky ossification of the anterolateral aspect of the anterior longitudinal ligament over at least four contiguous vertebrae combined with preserved disk heights, absence of ankylosis of facet joints and lack of erosion, sclerosis, or ankylosis of the sacroiliac joints.[40] DISH may also affect ligamentous and tendinous structures often leading to calcifications of, for example, pelvic ligaments, Achilles tendon insertions, triceps insertions, and patellar tendon insertions.[41]

The range of spinal motion is relatively well preserved, most likely because the facet joints are, by definition, spared.[42] Resnick reported a ~50% reduction of range of motion in the cervical and thoracolumbar spine.[43] Interestingly, Goethe's skeleton has been preserved and was found to show signs of DISH with eight thoracic vertebrae (T5–T12) and five right ribs ankylosed, possibly explaining his well

known stiff posture and gait.[44] Similar to AS, fractures in DISH can be difficult to assess on plain radiographs due to excess ossifications in addition to degenerative changes. A computed tomographic (CT) scan or magnetic resonance imaging (MRI) should be performed if inconclusive radiographs are obtained in DISH patients with pain after trivial trauma (**Fig. 39.2**).[45] The prevalence and expression of DISH increase with age and it is more common in men.[46] Prevalence rates between 2.9% and 25% have been reported.[47,48] DISH is associated with diabetes type 2 and obesity and has been suggested to be a phenotypic expression of the metabolic syndrome.[49] In a study on human remains excavated from an abbey court in Maastricht, 40% of the skeletons showed evidence of DISH at a relatively young age, and the authors suggested that "a monastic way of life" could predispose to DISH.[50] No drugs are specifically effective in the treatment of DISH. Surgical treatment becomes an issue only in case of spinal fracture, myelopathy, or dysphagia.[1,51] Currently, there is no general agreement whether hyperextension fractures of the ankylosed spine in patients with DISH should be operated on or treated conservatively. The research question in the present review therefore was: Does surgical treatment improve the outcome of hyperextension fractures of the thoracolumbar spine in diffuse idiopathic skeletal hyperostosis?

Material and Methods

Because it was obvious that level I studies were not available for this topic, a quantitative systematic review or meta-analysis was not considered. A qualitative systematic review with no intention of quantification was chosen with categorization of appropriate studies according to their level of evidence.

Inclusion/Exclusion Criteria

Studies were included that fulfilled the following inclusion criteria:

♦ Written in English, German, or French
♦ Describing patients with a diagnosis of DISH and hyperextension fracture of the thoracolumbar spine with fracture in or immediately adjacent to the ankylosed segment
♦ Providing a detailed description of conservative or operative treatment
♦ Describing outcome in terms of neurological status, complications of treatment, and patient survival

Exclusion criteria were failure to identify injury pattern and only cervical or cervicothoracic fracture.

Literature Review

Potential studies were identified by searches on Google, Scirus, Sumsearch, eMedicine, TRIP, Cochrane reviews including Cochrane Central Register of Controlled Trials, EMBASE, Medline, and PubMed (**Table 39.5**). The reference lists from relevant articles were hand searched for additional citations (cross referencing). Articles were included or excluded based on abstract review. Articles not excluded were subsequently assessed using complete reports.

Table 39.5 Search Results from Various Sources

Database	Hits in All Text	Possibly Relevant	Definitely Relevant
Scirus	109	1	1
Sumsearch	1	1	0
eMedicine	1	1	0
TRIP	13	13	0
Cochrane Review	438	0	0
Cochrane Central	65	2	0
PubMed	40	31	8
Embase	23	13	2
Medline	101	1	0

Results

In the literature (searched until September 2007), 67 potentially relevant papers in English, German, or French were identified. Following assessment of abstracts 60 studies were excluded, the great majority because of lack of treatment details on the mechanism of trauma. In five papers identified from PubMed and one paper from a reference list, the criteria for inclusion were fully met.[52–57] An additional paper by Le Hir and coworkers was included separately by virtue of describing the largest series of DISH patients with thoracolumbar hyperextension fractures ($n = 6$) to date.[58] Because the paper did not meet all inclusion criteria it was solely used for discussion purposes in the present study. All studies had retrospective designs with variable documentation on the type of fracture, treatment applied, and outcome. All studies were case series or single-case presentations with level of evidence grade IV. The seven papers described 16 patients, 12 males/4 females, with a mean age of 69 years (ranging from 58 to 82 years) (**Table 39.6**). A low energy trauma was endured in seven patients; a high energy trauma in nine patients. The mechanism of injury was not always fully documented but could be inferred from the radiographs with reasonable certainty in all cases. When excluding the paper by Le Hir, the selection process left us with just 10 patients to address the research question, five patients were treated surgically, and five were treated conservatively.

Paley et al reported on two patients with thoracolumbar hyperextension fractures, located at Th11 and at L1, in patients with DISH.[57] The mechanisms of trauma were not described, but the description of the fracture implied hyperextension injuries. The patient with the Th11 fracture also had an undisplaced fracture through the Th5–Th6 disk space. Both patients were treated conservatively with bed rest followed by unprotected ambulation and body jacket, respectively. The combined Th11 and Th5–Th6 fractures healed without deformity or neurological sequelae, whereas the L1 fracture developed a nonsymptomatic pseudarthrosis. Israel et al published a case of a 70-year-old woman with DISH who suffered a hyperextension fracture-dislocation of Th10 with complete paraplegia immediately after undergoing a right-sided thoracotomy (for an elective tumor resection) with the patient positioned on her side.[55] She was subsequently treated with Cotrel Dubousset instrumentation and demonstrated partial neurological recovery postoperatively but died 9 months later.

Corke reported on a 71-year-old woman weighing 105 kg with diet-controlled diabetes mellitus who was admitted after a fall.[54] After initiating ambulation she developed severe low back pain followed by complete paraplegia. The radiographs showed a hyperextension fracture of the upper lumbar spine, and she was subsequently treated with spinal traction. Her condition deteriorated rapidly, and she died of pneumonia 8 days after admission. Bernini et al reported on a 63-year-old male who fell from his tractor and suffered immediate complete paraplegia.[52] The initial radiographs revealed no fracture. Repeated radiographs and tomograms 2 weeks after trauma showed DISH and a compression-burst fracture of Th3 and Th4 and a hyperextension fracture at Th10. He underwent posterior spinal fusion and Harrington rod instrumentation. There was no improvement in neurological status at 4 months. Burkus and Denis reported on four males (59 to 64 years of age); all had DISH and suffered hyperextension fractures of the thoracic spine, without neurological deficits, following motor vehicle accidents.[53] Radiographs revealed widening of the anterior disk space without translation in all four cases without involvement of the vertebral bodies. After obtaining MRI and CT scans all cases showed fractures of the posterior column, which were not detected on the plain radiographs. Three patients were operated on by posterior fusion with Cotrel Dubousset instrumentation, one patient was treated with a brace. All surgically treated patients went on to heal without complications, whereas the braced patient lost alignment of the spine and developed progressive neurological

Table 39.6 Demographics, Trauma, Treatment, and Outcome of the Patients Included

Study	N	M/F	Age	Level	Trauma	Mechanism	ASIA at Admission	Treatment	Outcome
Burkus and Denis (1994)[53]	4	4 M	58–69	T	MVA	Hyperextension	E	3 surgery 1 conserv	No complications Paraplegia
Paley et al (1991)[57]	2	2 M	65, 80	TL	Fall	Not reported	E	2 conserv	One pseudarthrosis
Bernini et al (1981)[52]	1	M	63	T	Fall	Hyperextension	A	Surgery	Healed with paraplegia
Corke (1981)[54]	1	f	71	TL	Fall	Hyperextension	E	Conserv	Paraplegia and death
Israel et al (1994)[55] death	1	f	70	T	Surgery	Hyperextension	A	Surgery	Partial recovery and
McKenzie et al (1991)[56]	1	M	63	T	MVA	Hyperextension	E	Conserv	Probably healed

Abbreviations: ASIA, American Spinal Injury Association; T, thoracic; TL, thoracolumbar; MVA, motor vehicle accident.

deterioration. Although his fracture healed, he remained paraplegic. Based on this experience, Burkus and Denis recommended operative treatment of thoracolumbar hyperextension fractures in patients with DISH. McKenzie et al reported a case of successful conservative treatment in a patient with DISH and a hyperextension fracture of Th10, showing only disruption of the anterior longitudinal ligament, and argued that in case of isolated anterior column injury, conservative treatment may be sufficient.[56]

In the predominantly radiological paper by Le Hir et al six patients with hyperextension spine fractures (five in the thoracolumbar spine and one in the cervical spine) were reported.[58] At admission one patient had an L1 radiculopathy, the other patients were neurologically intact. Three patients developed progressive paraplegia within 10 to 30 days after the traumatic event, and 2 months posttrauma four patients had died. Clinical data were unfortunately sparse and the history of treatment received could not be linked to individual patients.

Summary of Outcome According to Treatment

Operatively treated patients (n = 5): Three patients with no neurological deficit immediately operated on with Cotrel Dubousset instrumentation healed without complications; all three were from the Burkus and Denis paper. One paraplegic patient treated, after a delay, by Harrington rod instrumentation showed a healed fracture but remained paraplegic. One further patient who was treated with Cotrel Dubousset instrumentation showed some neurological improvement but died 9 months postoperatively.

Conservatively treated patients (n = 5): Two patients developed paraplegia during treatment; one developed a pseudarthrosis; one healed his fracture, and the last one probably healed his fracture.

Discussion

The research question, Does surgical treatment improve the outcome of patients with ankylosing spondylitis or diffuse idiopathic skeletal hyperostosis with hyperextension fractures of the thoracolumbar spine? cannot be answered conclusively due to the very limited number of studies and patients reported. This systematic review only identified 10 patients with DISH and reasonably well documented thoracolumbar hyperextension injuries, their treatment, and outcome. The results of the present systematic review showed that hyperextension fractures of the thoracolumbar spine in patients with DISH predominantly occur in older males; a situation similar to AS.[1] In all cases the fracture involved both the anterior and posterior spinal column. This type of injury has been described by all current classification systems as highly unstable with considerable risk of severe neurological consequences. Patients with DISH and hyperextension fractures almost invariably score 7 points or more in the TLICS system (4 points for a distraction fracture and 3 for posterior column disruption), strongly suggesting the need for surgical intervention.[9]

From theoretical considerations as well as from the current systematic review it seems clear that hyperextension fractures of the thoracolumbar spine in patients with DISH are unstable injuries with a high potential for catastrophic neurological injury as a result of primary (due to the traumatic impact) and secondary (due to manipulation and unthoughtful transfers) fracture dislocation. Therefore, definite stabilization by means of surgical reduction and fixation should be seriously considered in this category of patients.

In the series by de Peretti et al, treatment was unfortunately not reported, and although the patients in this study could not be included in the present work, they still contribute to our understanding of the nature of this type of fracture. De Peretti et al retrospectively described 28 patients, 23 of them with spinal cord injury.[59] Twenty-two out of 28 patients died within 3 months posttrauma, mainly due to complications associated with recumbency.

Conclusion and Recommendation

It can be concluded that, although this systematic review identified only a few papers of low levels of evidence, the conclusion that immediate operative stabilization should be seriously considered seems appropriate. Among the members of the Spine Trauma Study Group, this opinion is unanimously supported.

◆ Summary

Despite the limited number of reports and low levels of evidence found during the conduction of this systematic review on the treatment of thoracolumbar hyperextension fractures in ankylosing spondylitis and diffuse idiopathic skeletal hyperostosis, the results seem to favor surgical stabilization of these types of injuries over nonoperative treatment. The recommendation for surgical treatment is widely supported by all members of the Spine Trauma Study Group but urgently needs scientific confirmation in well-executed larger clinical studies.

References

1. Westerveld LA, Verlaan JJ, Oner FC. Spinal fractures in patients with ankylosing spinal disorders: a systematic review of the literature on treatment, neurological status and complications. Eur Spine J 2008;18: 146–156

2. Cooper C, Carbone L, Michet CJ, Atkinson EJ, O'Fallon WM, Melton LJ III. Fracture risk in patients with ankylosing spondylitis: a population based study. J Rheumatol 1994;21:1877–1882

3. Apple DF Jr, Anson C. Spinal cord injury occurring in patients with ankylosing spondylitis: a multicenter study. Orthopedics 1995;18:1005–1011

4. Rao SK, Wasyliw C, Nunez DB Jr. Spectrum of imaging findings in hyperextension injuries of the neck. Radiographics 2005;25:1239–1254

5. Burke DC. Hyperextension injuries of the spine. J Bone Joint Surg Br 1971;53:3–12

6. Bedbrook G, Clark WB. Thoracic spine injuries with spinal cord damage. J R Coll Surg Edinb 1981;26:264–271

7. Magerl F, Aebi M, Gertzbein SD, Harms J, Nazarian S. A comprehensive classification of thoracic and lumbar injuries. Eur Spine J 1994;3: 184–201

8. Matejka J. Hyperextension injuries of the thoracolumbar spine [in German]. Zentralbl Chir 2006;131:75–79

9. Rihn JA, Anderson DT, Harris E, et al. A review of the TLICS system: a novel, user-friendly thoracolumbar trauma classification system. Acta Orthop 2008;79:461–466

10. Lee JY, Vaccaro AR, Lim MR, et al. Thoracolumbar injury classification and severity score: a new paradigm for the treatment of thoracolumbar spine trauma. J Orthop Sci 2005;10:671–675

11. Bono CM, Vaccaro AR, Hurlbert RJ, et al. Validating a newly proposed classification system for thoracolumbar spine trauma: looking to the future of the thoracolumbar injury classification and severity score. J Orthop Trauma 2006;20:567–572

12. Braun J, Sieper J. Ankylosing spondylitis. Lancet 2007;369:1379–1390

13. Guyatt G, Schünemann HJ, Cook D, Jaeschke R, Pauker S. Applying the grades of recommendation for antithrombotic and thrombolytic therapy: the Seventh ACCP Conference on Antithrombotic and Thrombolytic Therapy. Chest 2004;126(3, Suppl):179S–187S

14. Boriani S, Romano B. Spinal lesions due to hyperextension in ankylosing spondylitis. Ital J Orthop Traumatol 1983;9:365–368

15. Fast A, Parikh S, Marin EL. Spine fractures in ankylosing spondylitis. Arch Phys Med Rehabil 1986;67:595–597

16. Fazl M, Bilbao JM, Hudson AR. Laceration of the aorta complicating spinal fracture in ankylosing spondylitis. Neurosurgery 1981;8:732–734

17. Finkelstein JA, Chapman JR, Mirza S. Occult vertebral fractures in ankylosing spondylitis. Spinal Cord 1999;37:444–447

18. Gelineck J, De Carvalho A. Fractures of the spine in ankylosing spondylitis. Rofo 1990;152:307–310

19. Graham B, Van Peteghem PK. Fractures of the spine in ankylosing spondylitis: diagnosis, treatment, and complications. Spine 1989;14:803–807

20. Graham GP, Evans PD. Spinal fractures in patients with ankylosing spondylitis. Injury 1991;22:426–427

21. Grisolia A, Bell RL, Peltier LF. Fractures and dislocations of the spine complicating ankylosing spondylitis: a report of six cases. 1967. Clin Orthop Relat Res 2004;(422):129–134

22. Hanson JA, Mirza S. Predisposition for spinal fracture in ankylosing spondylitis. AJR Am J Roentgenol 2000;174:150

23. Hitchon PW, From AM, Brenton MD, Glaser JA, Torner JC. Fractures of the thoracolumbar spine complicating ankylosing spondylitis. J Neurosurg 2002;97(2, Suppl):218–222

24. Hunter T, Dubo HI. Spinal fractures complicating ankylosing spondylitis: a long-term followup study. Arthritis Rheum 1983;26:751–759

25. Juric G, Coumas JM, Giansiracusa DF, Irwin RS. Hemothorax—an unusual presentation of spinal fracture in ankylosing spondylitis. J Rheumatol 1990;17:263–266

26. May PJ, Raunest J, Herdmann J, Jonas M. Treatment of spinal fracture in ankylosing spondylitis [in German]. Unfallchirurg 2002;105:165–169

27. Olerud C, Frost A, Bring J. Spinal fractures in patients with ankylosing spondylitis. Eur Spine J 1996;5:51–55

28. Peh WC, Chu FS, Ho TK. Case of the month: a nasty shock on awakening. Br J Radiol 1994;67:1141–1142

29. Samartzis D, Anderson DG, Shen FH. Multiple and simultaneous spine fractures in ankylosing spondylitis: case report. Spine 2005;30: E711–E715

30. Savolaine ER, Ebraheim NA, Stitgen S, Jackson WT. Aortic rupture complicating a fracture of an ankylosed thoracic spine: a case report. Clin Orthop Relat Res 1991;(272):136–140

31. Schaberg FJ Jr. Aortic injury occurring after minor trauma in ankylosing spondylitis. J Vasc Surg 1986;4:410–411

32. Straiton N. Fractures of the lower vertebral column in ankylosing spondylitis. Br J Clin Pract 1987;41:933–934

33. Tetzlaff JE, Yoon HJ, Bell G. Massive bleeding during spine surgery in a patient with ankylosing spondylitis. Can J Anaesth 1998;45:903–906

34. Thorngren KG, Liedberg E, Aspelin P. Fractures of the thoracic and lumbar spine in ankylosing spondylitis. Arch Orthop Trauma Surg 1981;98:101–107

35. Tiesenhausen K, Thalhammer M, Koch G, Schleifer P. Traumatic aortic rupture in ankylosing spondylitis—a fatal complication [in German]. Unfallchirurg 2001;104:1101–1103

36. Trent G, Armstrong GW, O'Neil J. Thoracolumbar fractures in ankylosing spondylitis: high-risk injuries. Clin Orthop Relat Res 1988;227:61–66

37. Upadhyay SS, Ho EK, Hsu LC. Positioning for plain spinal radiography producing paraplegia in a patient with ankylosing spondylitis. Br J Radiol 1991;64:549–551

38. Verlaan JJ, Diekerhof CH, Buskens E, et al. Surgical treatment of traumatic fractures of the thoracic and lumbar spine: a systematic review of the literature on techniques, complications, and outcome. Spine 2004;29:803–814

39. Resnick D, Shapiro RF, Wiesner KB, Niwayama G, Utsinger PD, Shaul SR. Diffuse idiopathic skeletal hyperostosis (DISH) [ankylosing hyperostosis of Forestier and Rotes-Querol]. Semin Arthritis Rheum 1978;7:153–187

40. Resnick D, Niwayama G. Radiographic and pathologic features of spinal involvement in diffuse idiopathic skeletal hyperostosis (DISH). Radiology 1976;119:559–568

41. Maat GJR, Mastwijk RW, Van der Velde EA. Skeletal distribution of degenerative changes in vertebral osteophytosis, vertebral osteoarthritis and DISH. Int J Osteoarchaeol 1995;5:289–298

42. Schlapbach P, Beyeler C, Gerber NJ, et al. Diffuse idiopathic skeletal hyperostosis (DISH) of the spine: a cause of back pain? A controlled study. Br J Rheumatol 1989;28:299–303

43. Resnick D, Shaul SR, Robins JM. Diffuse idiopathic skeletal hyperostosis (DISH): Forestier's disease with extraspinal manifestations. Radiology 1975;115:513–524

44. Ullrich H. Goethe's skull and skeleton [in German] Anthropol Anz 2002;60:341–368

45. Chong CF. Fracture of the delicate bamboo: a diagnostic pitfall. Ann Emerg Med 2004;44:88–89

46. Westerveld LA, van Ufford HM, Verlaan JJ, Oner FC. The prevalence of diffuse idiopathic skeletal hyperostosis in an outpatient population in the Netherlands. J Rheumatol 2008;35:1635–1638

47. Kim SK, Choi BR, Kim CG, et al. The prevalence of diffuse idiopathic skeletal hyperostosis in Korea. J Rheumatol 2004;31:2032–2035

48. Weinfeld RM, Olson PN, Maki DD, Griffiths HJ. The prevalence of diffuse idiopathic skeletal hyperostosis (DISH) in two large American Midwest metropolitan hospital populations. Skeletal Radiol 1997;26:222–225

49. Denko CW, Malemud CJ. Body mass index and blood glucose: correlations with serum insulin, growth hormone, and insulin-like growth factor-1 levels in patients with diffuse idiopathic skeletal hyperostosis (DISH). Rheumatol Int 2005;26:292–297

50. Verlaan JJ, Oner FC, Maat GJ. Diffuse idiopathic skeletal hyperostosis in ancient clergymen. Eur Spine J 2007;16:1129–1135

51. Eviatar E, Harell M. Diffuse idiopathic skeletal hyperostosis with dysphagia (a review). J Laryngol Otol 1987;101:627–632

52. Bernini PM, Floman Y, Marvel JP Jr, Rothman RH. Multiple thoracic spine fractures complicating ankylosing hyperostosis of the spine. J Trauma 1981;21:811–814

53. Burkus JK, Denis F. Hyperextension injuries of the thoracic spine in diffuse idiopathic skeletal hyperostosis: report of four cases. J Bone Joint Surg Am 1994;76:237–243

54. Corke CF. Spinal fracture and paraplegia after minimal trauma in a patient with ankylosing vertebral hyperostosis. Br Med J (Clin Res Ed) 1981;282:2035

55. Israel Z, Mosheiff R, Gross E, Muggia-Sullam M, Floman Y. Hyperextension fracture-dislocation of the thoracic spine with paraplegia in a patient with diffuse idiopathic skeletal hyperostosis. J Spinal Disord 1994;7:455–457

56. McKenzie MK, Bartal E, Pay NT. A hyperextension injury of the thoracic spine in association with diffuse idiopathic skeletal hyperostosis. Orthopedics 1991;14:895–898

57. Paley D, Schwartz M, Cooper P, Harris WR, Levine AM. Fractures of the spine in diffuse idiopathic skeletal hyperostosis. Clin Orthop Relat Res 1991;267:22–32

58. Le Hir PX, Sautet A, Le Gars L, et al. Hyperextension vertebral body fractures in diffuse idiopathic skeletal hyperostosis: a cause of intravertebral fluidlike collections on MR imaging. AJR Am J Roentgenol 1999;173:1679–1683

59. de Peretti F, Sane JC, Dran G, Razafindratsiva C, Argenson C. Ankylosed spine fractures with spondylitis or diffuse idiopathic skeletal hyperostosis: diagnosis and complications [in French]. Rev Chir Orthop Repar Appar Mot 2004;90:456–465

40

Thoracolumbar Injury Classification for Fracture-Dislocations

Justin S. Smith and Christopher I. Shaffrey

Fracture-dislocations are among the most unstable spinal injuries and have the highest rate of complete neurological injury.[1] These fractures are frequently associated with other injuries that may complicate the management plan. Historically, these fractures were treated with attempts at postural reduction and prolonged bed rest. However, with the introduction of modern spinal instrumentation, the management approach has shifted to surgical treatment with reduction, instrumentation, and fusion. Whether the optimal surgical approach is posterior or anterior only or a combination of the two approaches and whether the neurological status of the patient should influence this decision remain controversial issues. Also unsettled is the optimal timing for surgical treatment and whether this should be influenced by the neurological status of the patient.

◆ Epidemiology and Classification Systems

In reported series of spinal injuries, thoracolumbar fracture-dislocations typically represent a relatively small but significant subset of injuries.[2–4] In a retrospective study by Denis, of 412 thoracolumbar spinal injuries, fracture-dislocations represented ~16% of the injuries, whereas nearly two thirds were compression or burst fractures.[2] In a multicenter series of 1019 consecutive thoracolumbar fractures reported by Gertzbein and the Scoliosis Research Society, 16% were fracture-dislocations, 63% were burst fractures, and 10% each were compression or flexion-distraction fractures.[3]

Thoracolumbar fracture-dislocations are typically associated with a violent shearing force, most commonly from motor vehicle accidents, falls, or direct blows. In a series of 24 cases reported by Convery et al, 15 (63%) were due to motor vehicle accidents, five (21%) were due to recreational vehicles, and two (8%) each were due to "flying vehicles" and falls.[5] A recent report by Inamasu and Guiot emphasized the importance of using three-point seat belt systems in motor vehicles, reporting that among 39 patients with

thoracolumbar junction injury from motor vehicle collision, the incidence of flexion-distraction/fracture-dislocation injuries among restrained and unrestrained front seat occupants was 0% versus 33% ($p < 0.01$).[6]

Fracture-dislocations can occur at any point along the spine; however, there is a distinct predilection for the thoracolumbar region (T10–L3).[2,7–9] Although the first through ninth thoracic vertebrae may suffer fracture-dislocations, they are relatively protected by the rigidity of the rib cage. In contrast, the lower thoracic and upper lumbar vertebrae constitute a transition zone from kyphosis to lordosis that renders this region more vulnerable to fracture-dislocation with high impact injury. In a series of 67 thoracic, lumbar, and lumbosacral fracture-dislocation injuries reported by Denis, the five levels between T10 and L3 accounted for nearly two thirds of the cases.[2]

Multiple classification systems have been proposed to define and subclassify spinal fracture-dislocation injuries.[10] Among the most widely recognized and simplistic is the Denis three-column model of spinal injury (**Fig. 40.1**).[2] The primary distinguishing feature of fracture-dislocations in the Denis classification is failure of all three columns under compression, tension, rotation, or shear that results in subluxation or dislocation. This system distinguishes three subtypes of fracture-dislocation, including flexion-rotation, shear, and flexion-distraction.

Another commonly used classification system for spinal fractures was based on AO principles for long-bone fracture classification and was originally proposed by Magerl et al[11] and subsequently modified by Gertzbein.[12] The overall AO classification is based on three basic fracture types: A (compression injuries), B (distraction injuries), and C (torsion injuries). Each of these types has three subtypes, providing nine major groups (**Fig. 40.2**). Each of these major groups also has multiple subtypes, producing in excess of 50 distinct injury patterns. Based on this system, groups that would reflect fracture-dislocation injuries would include B3 and C1–C3. This classification system, although richly descriptive, suffers from poor interobserver agreement.[13,14] A recent report by Wood et al demonstrates that both the Denis and the AO system for classification of thoracolumbar fractures had only moderate reliability and repeatability even among well-trained spine surgeons.[15] The intraobserver agreement was only 82% and 79% for the AO and Denis types, respectively, and was only 67% and 56% for the AO and Denis subtypes, respectively.[15]

Vaccaro et al recently reported a new classification system for thoracolumbar injuries that not only aims to provide a simple and reliable means of categorizing injuries but also to aid in clinical management.[16] The authors also reported an algorithm to suggest surgical approach based on neurological status and the integrity of the posterior

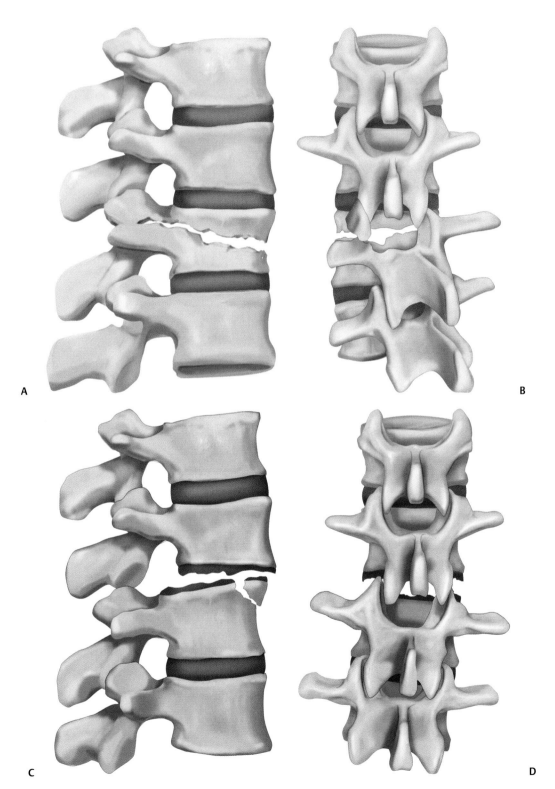

A

B

C

D

Fig. 40.1 Fracture-dislocation injuries as classified by Denis. **(A,B)** Flexion-rotation fractures (type A) demonstrate complete disruption of the three columns through bone or **(C,D)** through disk.   (*Continued on page 402*)

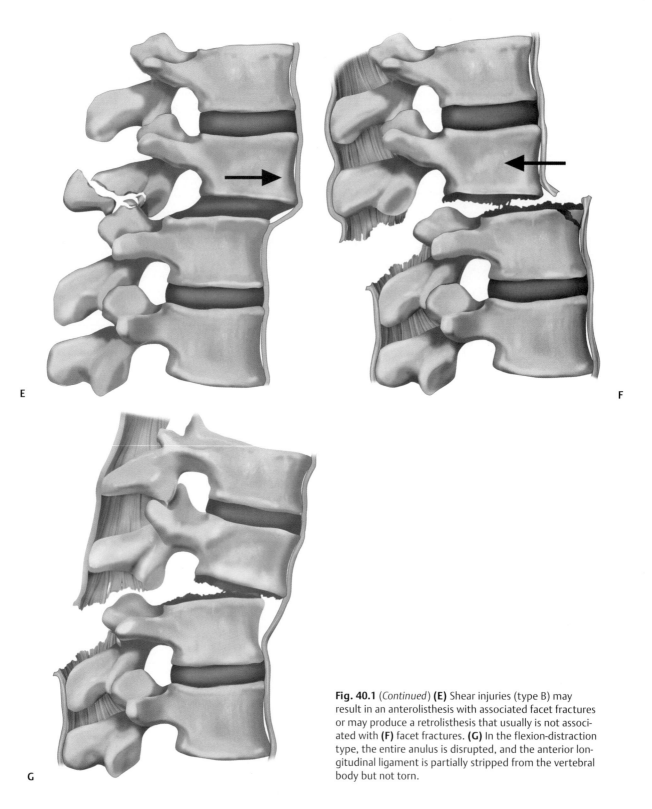

E

F

G

Fig. 40.1 (*Continued*) **(E)** Shear injuries (type B) may result in an anterolisthesis with associated facet fractures or may produce a retrolisthesis that usually is not associated with **(F)** facet fractures. **(G)** In the flexion-distraction type, the entire anulus is disrupted, and the anterior longitudinal ligament is partially stripped from the vertebral body but not torn.

ligamentous complex (PLC). Given the severe radiographic morphology, disruption of the PLC, and often compromised neurological status of patients suffering a thoracolumbar fracture-dislocation, these cases almost invariably receive a score of 5 or greater in the Thoracolumbar Injury Classification and Severity Score (TLICS) system recommending surgical intervention.

◆ **Clinical and Diagnostic Features**

Patients presenting with a thoracolumbar fracture-dislocation injury have typically suffered a high-impact injury, and a significant majority have neurological deficits. For example, Dickson et al reported on the neurological status of 95 patients presenting with thoracolumbar fracture-dislocation injuries.[7]

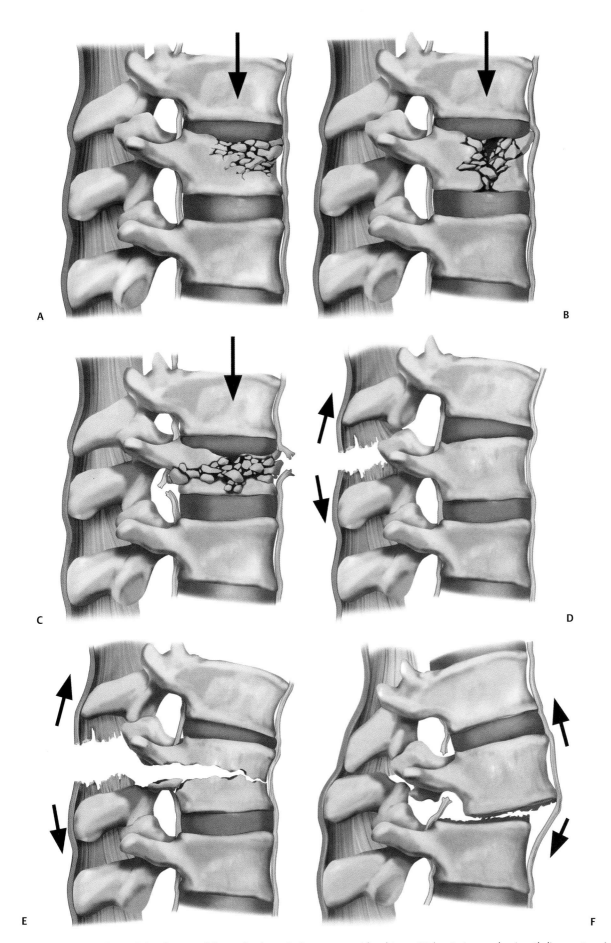

Fig. 40.2 (A–C) AO/Magerl classification of thoracolumbar spinal injuries. "A" indicates compression injuries, with subtype A1 (impaction), A2 (split), and A3 (burst). **(D–F)** "B" indicates distraction injuries, with subtypes B1 (posterior, predominantly ligamentous injury), B2 (posterior, predominantly osseous injury), and B3 (anterior, through the disk). (Continued on page 404)

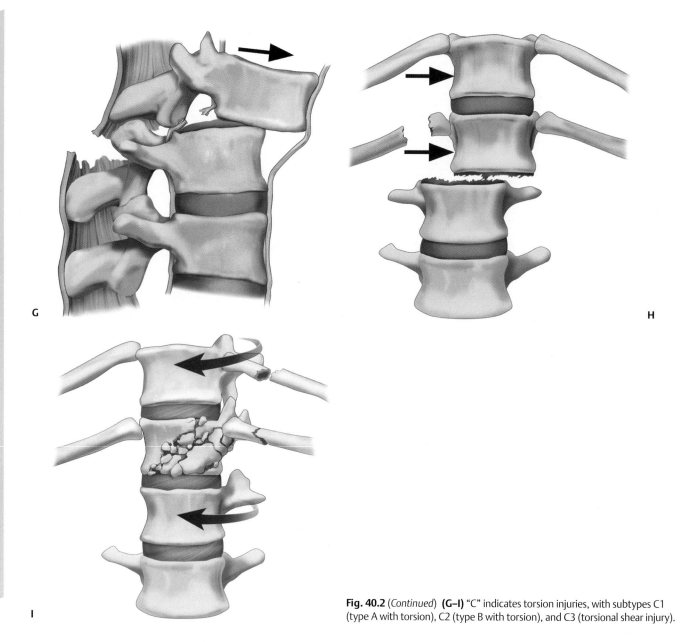

G

H

I

Fig. 40.2 (*Continued*) **(G–I)** "C" indicates torsion injuries, with subtypes C1 (type A with torsion), C2 (type B with torsion), and C3 (torsional shear injury).

Of the 93 patients who survived, 45% were Frankel grade A (complete motor and sensory deficit below level of injury) at presentation, and only 4% were Frankel grade E (normal sensory and motor function).[7,17] In a series of 24 patients presenting with acute lumbar fracture-dislocation reported by Convery et al, 38% had complete paraplegia, 33% had incomplete paraplegia (8% cord, 13% conus, 13% cauda), and 29% were neurologically intact.[5] Among 158 patients with thoracic or lumbar fracture-dislocations, Gertzbein reported that 74% had absent or impaired bladder function at presentation.[3] Other studies have also reported high incidences of significant neurological deficits associated with thoracolumbar fracture-dislocations.[18,19]

The high-impact injuries associated with generation of thoracolumbar fracture-dislocations also produce a high incidence of other associated injuries. In the series of 95 patients reported by Dickson et al, associated injuries occurred in 46 (48%), with 33 of these patients having multiple associated injuries.[7] The high incidence of associated injuries underscores the need to carefully and completely evaluate patients

who have suffered a fracture-dislocation and may complicate the surgical management of these fractures.

Evaluation of spinal trauma typically includes anteroposterior and lateral radiographs of the cervical, thoracic, and lumbar spine, although the use of whole-body spinal spiral computed tomography (CT) is replacing radiographs in certain centers. Thoracolumbar fracture-dislocations are usually readily apparent on plain radiographs and should be suspected if any translation or rotation through the injury level(s) is present (**Fig. 40.3A**). Suspicion of a fracture-dislocation injury should prompt further evaluation with CT, including axial fine cuts and sagittal reconstructions (**Fig. 40.3B,C,D**). These images can help define the fracture pattern and identify levels of canal compromise. CT imaging is also useful for surgical planning by providing an assessment of the integrity of osseous structures adjacent to the injury site and by enabling measurement for implants.

For cases of incomplete neurological injury, magnetic resonance imaging (MRI) may be helpful to characterize the nature of injury to the neural elements and to identify

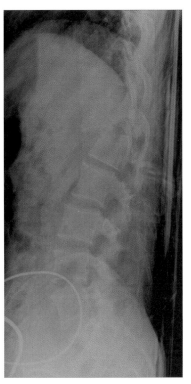
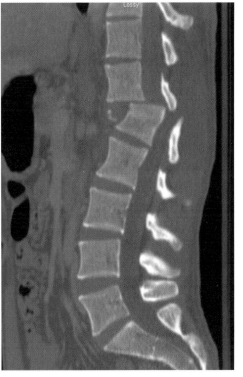
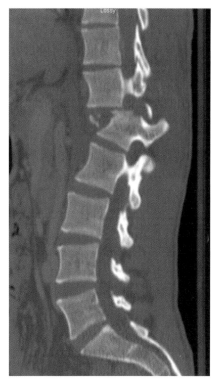

A-C

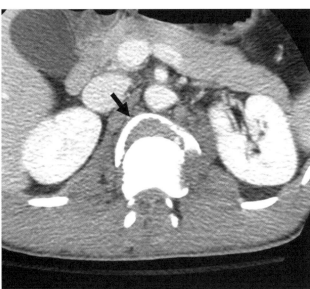

D

Fig. 40.3 Imaging of a 23-year-old man's status after a severe crushing injury. **(A)** Lateral radiograph and **(B)** midline and **(C)** off midline computed tomographic (CT) sagittal reconstructions showing a fracture-dislocation of the T12–L1 vertebrae. **(D)** Axial CT image at the level of the fracture-dislocation showing both the T12 (*arrow*) and L1 vertebral bodies.

evidence of hematoma and disk herniation that may contribute to ongoing compromise. MRI may also be useful to clarify injury stability. In addition, for the few patients with thoracolumbar fracture-dislocation who are neurologically intact, MRI prior to reduction and fixation may be helpful to identify herniated disk material that may compromise neural structures with reduction. The utility of MRI in patients with complete neurological deficits is less clear, and the literature lacks specific studies addressing the application of MRI in this setting. Depending on the management plan and the overall stability of the patient, MRI may help identify compression of neural elements due to hematoma or disk herniation and the status of the posterior ligamentous complex. However, the additional yield of MRI in the setting of fracture-dislocations may be limited, with the severity of the injury readily evident on CT imaging.

◆ Nonoperative Management

Historically, nonoperative treatment, including prolonged bed rest with immobilization or bracing, was recommended as the primary treatment for thoracolumbar fractures.[17,20–24] However, studies favoring nonoperative over surgical treatment for thoracolumbar fractures typically did not distinguish the outcomes of fracture-dislocation injuries from the outcomes of the group as a whole.[25,26] Thus the reported favorable outcomes with nonoperative treatment for thoracolumbar fractures did not necessarily reflect the outcomes of fracture-dislocation injuries, but rather were obscured by a disproportionately larger number of the more prognostically favorable burst and compression fractures,[22,23] which in many cases continue to be effectively treated nonoperatively.

Case reports and reports of very small series have suggested the use of halo-bifemoral traction for the reduction of thoracolumbar fracture-dislocations.[27–29] Although these authors did not encounter any apparent complications related to this technique, there exists potential risk of neurological injury, especially in the setting of incomplete neural injury. Patient acceptance of this technique is also questionable.

Few reports that detail nonoperative care for thoracolumbar fractures provide a discussion of the medical complications associated with the extended period of bed rest, and even fewer detail these findings specifically for the fracture-dislocation injuries. In addition, the length of hospital stay, rehabilitation time, and overall cost are not clearly detailed in the literature. Jones et al reported a 6% incidence of deep venous thrombosis associated with a 24-week course of bed rest and bracing for thoracic and lumbar spine fractures.[23] Davies et al reported a 6% incidence of pulmonary embolism among 34 patients treated non-operatively for thoracolumbar fractures.[25] Convery et al reported on 24 patients treated with early surgery for lumbar spine fracture-dislocation and performed an analysis indicating that, had these patients been treated nonoperatively, both the length of hospitalization and overall cost would have been twice as high.[5]

Based on available literature, there are no studies that compare the outcomes of nonoperative and operative treatment specifically for thoracolumbar fracture-dislocation. Instead, recommendations must be based on expert opinion. For patients who are neurologically intact or who have incomplete neurological injury, nonoperative treatment measures should not be the first line of treatment if the patient is adequately stable to tolerate surgical treatment (strong recommendation). For patients with a complete neurological injury, surgical treatment should be favored over nonoperative treatment to minimize the potential for further loss of spinal alignment and to minimize the chances of developing a painful spinal deformity (strong recommendation).

◆ Surgical Treatment

The treatment goals for fracture-dislocation of the thoracolumbar spine are to reduce the fracture, stabilize the spine, decompress the neural elements, and allow rapid mobilization. Until the application of Harrington instrumentation, efforts to achieve these goals were primarily based on prolonged bed rest following either postural reduction or open reduction, with the latter occasionally including a decompression. In the 1970s, multiple retrospective reviews of case series were published on stabilization of thoracolumbar fracture-dislocations using Harrington rod instrumentation. Flesch et al evaluated 40 patients with unstable thoracolumbar fractures, with 34 of these injuries being rotatory fracture-dislocations, with the remaining fractures being burst or compression injuries that subsequently became unstable following laminectomy.[30] However, the authors did not clearly distinguish outcomes specifically for the fracture-dislocation patients. All 40 patients underwent Harrington rod instrumentation and fusion, and a subset of these patients also underwent laminectomy for decompression. Instrumentation and fusion were performed on average 46 days following injury (range of 7 days to 11 months). At follow-up all patients had a stable spine without evidence of deformity and with one exception all had a solid fusion. Although there was no neurological improvement in the cases with complete deficit

at presentation ($n = 12$), 90% of the patients with incomplete cord or cauda equina lesions regained some neural function. Based on historical comparisons, the authors argued that Harrington instrumentation also produced earlier mobilization, rehabilitation, and hospital discharge.

Dickson et al evaluated 95 patients, all with thoracolumbar fracture-dislocations, who were treated with open reduction and stabilization with Harrington instrumentation and fusion.[7] Mean time from injury to spinal instrumentation was 16 days (range of 0 to 90 days). The authors reported earlier mobilization and rehabilitation but noted that the recovery rate was no better than prior reports that relied on postural reduction and prolonged bed rest.[17,31]

Convery et al also reported on the use of Harrington instrumentation to achieve stabilization in patients with thoracolumbar fracture-dislocation in 24 patients.[5] The authors demonstrated a 50% reduction in both the total hospital stay and cost compared with historical series in which operative intervention was avoided. The functional results were at least comparable to the results of other series, and the complication rates were similar to prior series, with the exception of postoperative pain in two patients.

Although instrumentation systems have evolved substantially beyond the Harrington system, the literature describing the application of more modern instrumentation to thoracolumbar fracture-dislocation injuries is extremely limited. In 1993, Sasso and Cotler retrospectively compared three posterior instrumentation systems (Harrington rods and hooks, Luque rods with sublaminar wires, and AO dynamic compression plates with pedicle screws) in 70 patients with unstable fractures of the thoracic and lumbar spine, only 14 of which were thoracolumbar fracture-dislocations.[9] The authors noted similar neurological recovery among the three groups but demonstrated the need to fuse fewer levels with pedicle screws (mean 3.3, range 2 to 6), compared with Harrington rods (mean 6.0, range 5 to 9) and Luque rods (mean 6.3, range 4 to 8). Other reports describing the use of posterior segmental instrumentation for thoracolumbar fractures also provide favorable results; however, either specific outcomes for fracture-dislocations were not provided or very few fracture-dislocation cases were included.[19,32–40]

Anterior decompression and reconstruction following reduction and posterior instrumentation is a relatively common treatment technique and is described in a subset of patients with thoracolumbar fracture-dislocations. Riska et al reported a retrospective review of a series of 905 patients with fracture or fracture-dislocation of the thoracolumbar spine that had been treated with reduction and posterior instrumentation.[41] In 79 of these patients, an anterolateral decompression was subsequently performed due to persistent neurological deficit and demonstration of "encroachment" into the spinal canal. Of these 79 patients, 19 had initially presented with a fracture-dislocation injury, and six (32%) demonstrated neurological improvement with the subsequent anterior decompression.

A lateral extracavitary approach (LECA) for thoracic and thoracolumbar spine trauma has been reported in a study by Resnick and Benzel,[42] in which 33 patients underwent LECA for anterior column reconstruction in conjunction with posterior segmental instrumentation. Notably, the proportion of patients with fracture-dislocations was not specified. The authors reported no cases of neurological worsening and no mortality associated with the procedure. They did report a high incidence of complications, part of which they attributed to the effects of the injury. They concluded that the biomechanical advantages that may be obtained with a combined anterior and posterior construct must be balanced against the added morbidity of such a procedure.

The literature lacks data defining optimal timing of surgery for patients with thoracolumbar fracture-dislocation. Gaebler et al reported a retrospective series of 88 patients with thoracolumbar fracture ($n = 77$) or fracture-dislocation ($n = 11$).[34] The authors' management approach was to perform pedicle stabilization, transpedicular disk resection, and autologous cancellous bone grafting on an urgent basis. They concluded that the earlier operative decompression and spine stabilization take place, the better is the recovery rate for patients with neurological deficits and that the highest recovery rate occurs if patients are operated on within 8 hours of injury.

Although focused on the cervical region, Vaccaro et al offer the only available randomized, prospective study in humans of the neurological outcome of early versus late surgery for spinal cord injury.[43] Patients with acute cervical spine injury due to a traumatic event without progressive worsening of neurological status were randomized to undergo surgical treatment within 72 hours ($n = 34$) or at least 5 days ($n = 28$) from the time of injury. The authors noted no significant difference in length of intensive care unit stay, length of inpatient rehabilitation, or improvement in American Spinal Injury Association grade or motor score between the early and late surgery groups. They concluded that there appears to be no significant neurological or functional benefit to early versus delayed surgery after spinal cord injury. It remains unclear whether the results of this study can be extrapolated to the thoracic spinal cord, conus, or cauda equina.[44]

The literature does not clearly define optimal timing of surgery for thoracolumbar fractures based on the presence of other significant injuries, such as injuries to the head, pelvis, chest, intraabdominal contents, and spine. Kerwin et al reported a retrospective review of 361 traumatic spine injuries and assessed outcome based on whether surgery to address the spine fracture was performed early (< 48 hours after injury) or late (> 48 hours after injury).[45] A significantly greater mortality was identified among patients in the early surgery group (7.6% vs 2.5%, $p = 0.03$). They did note a shorter length of hospitalization in the early surgery group but attributed this to the increased mortality. Although the majority of deaths were associated with cervical fractures, this study does underscore the need to ensure that patients are properly resuscitated before surgery.

Thus the overall strength of evidence in the literature with regard to the surgical treatment of thoracolumbar fracture-dislocations is weak. Instead, expert opinion must be relied upon in making recommendations. Based on expert opinion, patients with thoracolumbar fracture-dislocation who are neurologically intact or who have incomplete deficits have the potential for neurological deterioration and should be treated surgically on an urgent basis (strong recommendation). Patients with thoracolumbar fracture-dislocation with a complete neurological injury should also undergo early surgical stabilization with segmental instrumentation and fusion due to the potential for further loss of spinal alignment, to prevent potentially painful deformity and to reduce medical complications (strong recommendation). In general, the posterior approach with segmental instrumentation and fusion enables reduction, stabilization, fusion, and potentially decompression if indicated and is the technique of choice for treating these injuries (strong recommendation). Pedicle screw fixation systems should be used for posterior fixation

to minimize the number of spinal levels that must be fused to achieve stabilization (strong recommendation). Reduction may be aided by partial or complete facetectomy and through the use of instrumentation systems with reduction screws. Both short- and long-segment posterior instrumented fusions are treatment options (weak recommendation). A supplemental anterior approach may be indicated to enable further decompression of the neural elements and/or to provide additional anterior column support, particularly in cases with incomplete neurological deficits (weak recommendation). Neuromonitoring should be performed during surgical treatment of thoracolumbar fracture-dislocations in the setting of incomplete neurological injury. Use of a brace following surgical stabilization is a reasonable treatment option. Early mobilization and rehabilitation should be encouraged as indicated and permitted.

◆ Potential Complications

In cases of thoracolumbar fracture-dislocation, the spine is highly unstable. There is a significant risk of worsening neurological injury in patients without complete neurological injuries if appropriate spinal precautions are not followed at all times, including when transferring the patient to the gantry for imaging studies and when positioning the patient for surgery. Although limited reports suggest the use of halo-bifemoral traction to aid in the reduction of thoracolumbar fracture-dislocations,[27–29] such an approach requires extreme caution to prevent additional neurological injury in the setting of incomplete neurological injury. It is important to perform open reduction in a well controlled fashion to prevent further neurological injury.

In addition to potential complications related to spinal instability, operative treatment of acute spinal trauma may be associated with significant blood loss, and if feasible, equipment to recycle lost blood should be used. Traumatic dural tears should be identified and repaired to minimize the chances of a postoperative cerebrospinal fluid (CSF) leak.

◆ Rehabilitation

Thoracolumbar fracture-dislocation injuries are frequently associated with neurological deficits. Early stabilization with instrumentation enables earlier mobilization and initiation of rehabilitation. A substantial number of patients have complete spinal cord, conus, or cauda equina lesions that may require extensive inpatient rehabilitation.

◆ Case Example

A 23-year-old man presented, after suffering a severe crushing injury, with a near-complete neurological deficit with minimal left lower extremity sparing along the left anterior thigh [American Spinal Injury Association grade B (ASIA B)]. Plain radiographic and CT imaging showed a fracture-dislocation of the T12–L1 vertebrae (AO type C injury) (**Fig. 40.3**). He underwent urgent open reduction of the dislocation with T10 through L3 posterior segmental instrumentation and T10 through L3 arthrodesis using a combination of iliac crest bone graft and local bone graft (**Figs. 40.4A,B**). Postoperative MRI demonstrates

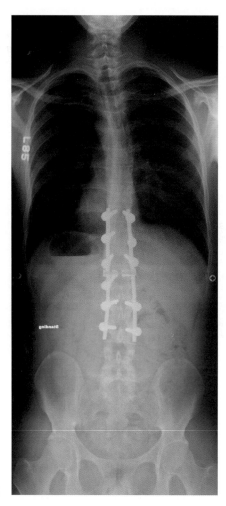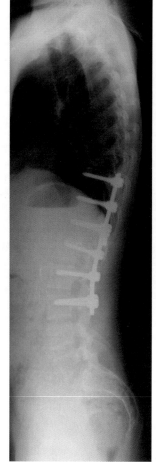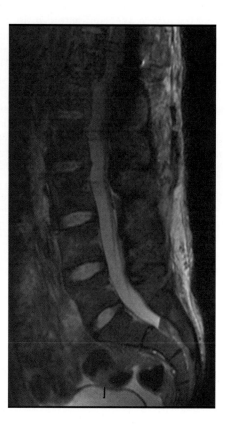

A–C

Fig. 40.4 Postoperative imaging of a patient presenting with a fracture-dislocation of the T12–L1 vertebrae. **(A)** Anteroposterior and **(B)** lateral radiographs showing reduction of the fracture-dislocation and T10 through L3 posterior segmental instrumentation. **(C)** Postoperative T2 sagittal magnetic resonance imaging scan showing decompression of the neural elements.

decompression of the neural elements (**Fig. 40.4C**). On clinical follow-up, he has regained 5/5 lower extremity strength, except for 3/5 right plantar flexion and 4/5 left plantar flexion. In addition he has regained bowel control but still catheterizes.

◆ Recommendations

Question 1: What is the optimal surgical approach with regard to surgical morbidity, risk, and long-term outcomes in patients with thoracolumbar fracture-dislocation and does the optimal surgical approach differ based on the neurological status of the patient (intact, incomplete deficit, or complete deficit)?

Recommendation (strength): Although the literature provides no consensus on the optimal surgical approach (**Table 40.1**), expert opinion suggests that either posterior (intact or complete injury) or combined posterior and then anterior approaches (incomplete deficits) are reasonable surgical options for the management of

patients with thoracolumbar fracture-dislocation (weak recommendation).

Question 2: What is the optimal timing of surgical treatment with regard to surgical morbidity, risk, and long-term outcomes in patients with thoracolumbar fracture-dislocation and does the optimal surgical timing differ based on the neurological status of the patient (intact, incomplete deficit, or complete deficit)?

Recommendation (strength): The literature provides no consensus on the optimal timing of surgery for thoracolumbar fracture-dislocation patients (**Table 40.1**). Based on expert opinion, for patients who are either neurologically intact or demonstrate incomplete deficit, urgent surgical reduction, stabilization, and appropriate decompression are suggested to prevent worsening neurological status and to expedite rehabilitation (strong recommendation). For patients with a complete neurological deficit, early surgical reduction, stabilization, and appropriate decompression constitute an acceptable treatment to maximize chances of neurological recovery, reduce the chances of developing a painful deformity, and expedite rehabilitation (strong recommendation).

Table 40.1 Results of Systematic Review

Study	Description	Quality of Evidence	Topic and Conclusion
Dickson et al (1978)[7]	Retrospective case series	Very Low	Assessment of neurological outcome and length of hospital stay for patients with thoracolumbar FDI treated with ORIF (Harrington rods) at mean time from injury of 15.7 days (95 patients) CONCLUSIONS: Overall improvement in Frankel grade comparable to that in prior reports of treatment with postural reduction and bed rest. Improvement in Frankel grade not significantly different between those having early surgery (day of injury) and those having delayed surgery (8 to 35 days later). Mean hospital stay of 107 days (including rehabilitation).
Flesch et al (1977)[30]	Retrospective case series	Very low	Assessment of neurological outcome and length of hospital stay for patients with thoracolumbar FDI treated acutely with ORIF (Harrington rods) (34 patients) CONCLUSIONS: Some neural recovery occurred in over 90% of patients with incomplete cord or cauda equina lesions, but there was no recovery in any patient with a complete lesion. Mean hospital stay of 115 days (including rehabilitation).
Convery et al (1978)[5]	Retrospective case series	Very low	Assessment of neurological outcome, length of hospital stay and cost for patients with thoracolumbar FDI treated acutely with ORIF (Harrington rods) (24 patients) CONCLUSIONS: Compared with prior reported series not treating with acute ORIF, there was at least 50% reduction in total hospitalization stay and costs. Functional results based on criteria of Barthel comparable to other series. Mean hospital stay of 105 days (including rehabilitation).
Riska et al (1987)[41]	Retrospective case series	Very low	Assessment of anterolateral decompression for thoracolumbar FDI patients with persistent severe neural involvement and canal narrowing following posterior instrumentation (Meurig Williams plates or Harrington rods) without laminectomy (19 patients) CONCLUSIONS: One third of patients had improvement of neurological status based on Frankel grade. Earlier surgery associated with greater improvement. Anterolateral decompression may benefit a subset of FDI patients.
Sasso and Cotler (1993)[9]	Retrospective case series	Very low	Comparison of three posterior instrumentation systems (Harrington rods and hooks, Luque rods with sublaminar wires, compression plates with pedicle screws) for acute treatment of thoracolumbar FDI (14 patients) CONCLUSIONS: No significant difference in neurological improvement (Frankel grade) among treatment groups. Hospital stay (excluding rehabilitation) was shorter for pedicle screw group (12 days) compared with Luque rod (52 days) and Harrington rod groups (23 days). Mean number of instrumented levels was less in the pedicle screw group (3.3 levels) compared with the Luque rod (6.3 levels) and the Harrington rod (6.0 levels) groups.

Abbreviations: FDI, fracture-dislocation injury; ORIF, open reduction and internal fixation.

References

1. Vaccaro AR, Kim DH, Brodke DS, et al. Diagnosis and management of thoracolumbar spine fractures. Instr Course Lect 2004;53:359–373

2. Denis F. The three column spine and its significance in the classification of acute thoracolumbar spinal injuries. Spine 1983; 8:817–831

3. Gertzbein SD. Scoliosis Research Society. Multicenter spine fracture study. Spine 1992;17:528–540

4. Lifeso RM, Arabie KM, Kadhi SK. Fractures of the thoraco-lumbar spine. Paraplegia 1985;23:207–224

5. Convery FR, Minteer MA, Smith RW, Emerson SM. Fracture-dislocation of the dorsal-lumbar spine: acute operative stabilization by Harrington instrumentation. Spine 1978;3:160–166

6. Inamasu J, Guiot BH. Thoracolumbar junction injuries after motor vehicle collision: are there differences in restrained and nonrestrained front seat occupants? J Neurosurg Spine 2007;7:311–314

7. Dickson JH, Harrington PR, Erwin WD. Results of reduction and stabilization of the severely fractured thoracic and lumbar spine. J Bone Joint Surg Am 1978;60:799–805

8. Roberts JB, Curtiss PH Jr. Stability of the thoracic and lumbar spine in traumatic paraplegia following fracture or fracture-dislocation. J Bone Joint Surg Am 1970;52:1115–1130

9. Sasso RC, Cotler HB. Posterior instrumentation and fusion for unstable fractures and fracture-dislocations of the thoracic and lumbar spine: a comparative study of three fixation devices in 70 patients. Spine 1993;18:450–460

10. Mirza SK, Mirza AJ, Chapman JR, Anderson PA. Classifications of thoracic and lumbar fractures: rationale and supporting data. J Am Acad Orthop Surg 2002;10:364–377

11. Magerl F, Aebi M, Gertzbein SD, Harms J, Nazarian S. A comprehensive classification of thoracic and lumbar injuries. Eur Spine J 1994;3:184–201

12. Gertzbein SD. Spine update: classification of thoracic and lumbar fractures. Spine 1994;19:626–628

13. Blauth M, Bastian L, Knop C, Lange U, Tusch G. Inter-observer reliability in the classification of thoraco-lumbar spinal injuries [in German]. Orthopade 1999;28:662–681

14. Verlaan JJ, Diekerhof CH, Buskens E, et al. Surgical treatment of traumatic fractures of the thoracic and lumbar spine: a systematic review of the literature on techniques, complications, and outcome. Spine 2004; 29:803–814

15. Wood KB, Khanna G, Vaccaro AR, Arnold PM, Harris MB, Mehbod AA. Assessment of two thoracolumbar fracture classification systems as used by multiple surgeons. J Bone Joint Surg Am 2005;87:1423–1429

16. Vaccaro AR, Lehman RA Jr, Hurlbert RJ, et al. A new classification of thoracolumbar injuries: the importance of injury morphology, the integrity of the posterior ligamentous complex, and neurologic status. Spine 2005;30:2325–2333

17. Frankel HL, Hancock DO, Hyslop G, et al. The value of postural reduction in the initial management of closed injuries of the spine with paraplegia and tetraplegia, I. Paraplegia 1969;7:179–192

18. Braakman R, Fontijne WP, Zeegers R, Steenbeek JR, Tanghe HL. Neurological deficit in injuries of the thoracic and lumbar spine: a consecutive series of 70 patients. Acta Neurochir (Wien) 1991;111:11–17

19. Tasdemiroglu E, Tibbs PA. Long-term follow-up results of thoracolumbar fractures after posterior instrumentation. Spine 1995; 20:1704–1708

20. Guttmann L. Initial treatment of traumatic paraplegia. Proc R Soc Med 1954;47:1103–1109

21. Guttmann L. Spinal deformities in traumatic paraplegics and tetraplegics following surgical procedures. Paraplegia 1969;7:38–58

22. Guttmann L. Surgical aspects of the treatment of traumatic paraplegia. J Bone Joint Surg Am 1949;31B:399–403

23. Jones RF, Snowdon E, Coan J, King L, Engel S. Bracing of thoracic and lumbar spine fractures. Paraplegia 1987;25:386–393

24. Lewis J, McKibbin B. The treatment of unstable fracture-dislocations of the thoraco-lumbar spine accompanied by paraplegia. J Bone Joint Surg Br 1974;56-B:603–612

25. Davies WE, Morris JH, Hill V. An analysis of conservative (non-surgical) management of thoracolumbar fractures and fracture-dislocations with neural damage. J Bone Joint Surg Am 1980;62:1324–1328

26. Osti OL, Fraser RD, Cornish BL. Fractures and fractures-dislocations of the lumbar spine: a retrospective study of 70 patients. Int Orthop 1987;11:323–329

27. Hutchinson MR, Dall BE. Fracture-dislocation of the thoracic and lumbar spine: advantages of halo-bifemoral traction. J Spinal Disord 1993;6: 482–488

28. Uriarte E, Elguezabal B, Tovio R. Fracture-dislocation of the thoracic spine without neurologic lesion. Clin Orthop Relat Res 1987; (217): 261–265

29. Wang GJ, Whitehill R, Stamp WG, Rosenberger R. The treatment of fracture dislocations of the thoracolumbar spine with halofemoral traction and Harrington rod instrumentation. Clin Orthop Relat Res 1979;(142): 168–175

30. Flesch JR, Leider LL, Erickson DL, Chou SN, Bradford DS. Harrington instrumentation and spine fusion for unstable fractures and fracture-dislocations of the thoracic and lumbar spine. J Bone Joint Surg Am 1977;59:143–153

31. Burke DC, Murray DD. The management of thoracic and thoraco-lumbar injuries of the spine with neurological involvement. J Bone Joint Surg Br 1976;58:72–78

32. Carl AL, Tromanhauser SG, Roger DJ. Pedicle screw instrumentation for thoracolumbar burst fractures and fracture-dislocations. Spine 1992; 17(8, Suppl):S317–S324

33. Chavda DV, Brantigan JW. Technique of reduction and internal fixation of thoracolumbar fracture-dislocation using pedicle screws and variable screw placement plates. Orthop Rev 1994;(Suppl):25–31

34. Gaebler C, Maier R, Kutscha-Lissberg F, Mrkonjic L, Vècsei V. Results of spinal cord decompression and thoracolumbar pedicle stabilisation in relation to the time of operation. Spinal Cord 1999;37:33–39

35. Inamasu J, Guiot BH, Nakatsukasa M. Posterior instrumentation surgery for thoracolumbar junction injury causing neurologic deficit. Neurol Med Chir (Tokyo) 2008;48:15–21, discussion 21

36. Korovessis PG, Baikousis A, Stamatakis M. Use of the Texas Scottish Rite Hospital instrumentation in the treatment of thoracolumbar injuries. Spine 1997;22:882–888

37. Moon MS, Choi WT, Moon YW, Kim YS, Moon JL. Stabilisation of fractured thoracic and lumbar spine with Cotrel-Dubousset instrument. J Orthop Surg (Hong Kong) 2003;11:59–66

38. Parker JW, Lane JR, Karaikovic EE, Gaines RW. Successful short-segment instrumentation and fusion for thoracolumbar spine fractures: a consecutive 41/2-year series. Spine 2000;25:1157–1170

39. Ruan DK, Shen GB, Chui HX. Shen instrumentation for the management of unstable thoracolumbar fractures. Spine 1998;23: 1324–1332

40. Weyns F, Rommens PM, Van Calenbergh F, Goffin J, Broos P, Plets C. Neurological outcome after surgery for thoracolumbar fractures: a retrospective study of 93 consecutive cases, treated with dorsal instrumentation. Eur Spine J 1994;3:276–281

41. Riska EB, Myllynen P, Böstman O. Anterolateral decompression for neural involvement in thoracolumbar fractures: a review of 78 cases. J Bone Joint Surg Br 1987;69:704–708

42. Resnick DK, Benzel EC. Lateral extracavitary approach for thoracic and thoracolumbar spine trauma: operative complications. Neurosurgery 1998;43:796–802, discussion 802–803

43. Vaccaro AR, Daugherty RJ, Sheehan TP, et al. Neurologic outcome of early versus late surgery for cervical spinal cord injury. Spine 1997;22: 2609–2613

44. Fehlings MG, Perrin RG. The role and timing of early decompression for cervical spinal cord injury: update with a review of recent clinical evidence. Injury 2005;36(Suppl 2):B13–B26

45. Kerwin AJ, Frykberg ER, Schinco MA, Griffen MM, Murphy T, Tepas JJ. The effect of early spine fixation on non-neurologic outcome. J Trauma 2005;58:15–21

41

Confounders and Their Influence on the Thoracolumbar Injury Classification and Severity Score (TLICS)

Allister R. Williams and Jonathan N. Grauer

Throughout history, clinicians have been in search of tools that allow them to more efficiently understand the clinical problems that they face. In modern medicine, injury classification systems have been an example of such a tool. They provide a means for clinicians to effectively describe clinical findings to their colleagues in a consistent and informative manner, develop treatment algorithms, and assess outcomes.

Regardless of the medical specialty involved, all good classification systems share the same intrinsic qualities. They should be simple to understand and apply in order to allow rapid and efficient implementation into the clinical practice of the majority of the members of a specialty. In addition, a classification system should provide excellent reliability so that its application among individual specialists is consistent, essentially high inter- and intraobserver reliability. Lastly, and of greatest importance is that the classification system aids the clinician in determining the most appropriate treatment modality for a particular patient.

The thoracolumbar injury classification and severity score (TLICS) has proven to have the characteristics that are desirable in a medical classification system.[1] The scoring system is simple and can be easily implemented by the majority of spine surgeons. TLICS has good reliability and compares favorably with other thoracolumbar injury classifications in this regard. TLICS also aids the spine surgeon in determining if a particular injury requires surgical stabilization or can be treated nonoperatively. Although TLICS possesses the qualities that make a classification system effective, it, like other classification systems, is susceptible to unusual patient characteristics that make the classification less reliable. It is essential that the spine surgeon understand these confounders and their influence on treatment.

◆ Elderly Patients

The elderly population, defined as those in the population 65 or older, has significantly increased. To that point, this population increased 21% from 1980 to 1990 alone. In 2004 the United States census bureau reported that the elderly represented 12% of the US population and that number was expected to increase to 21% by the year 2050. Due to the population growth of the elderly and their increased desire to engage in a more active lifestyle, the number of elderly trauma patients that the spine surgeon sees has increased and will continue to increase during the foreseeable future.

The elderly population presents unique challenges for the spine surgeon. This group has in general a higher incidence of comorbidities that may have a negative effect on outcomes. This may lead one to avoid surgery where the TLICS system suggests an operative treatment. It has been estimated that the mortality rate from geriatric trauma with or without surgical intervention increases 7% for each 1-year increment after age 65.[2]

Along with the other comorbidities in the elderly, there is an increased prevalence of vascular pathologies such as atherosclerosis. This may be a consideration if an anterior approach is to be used. In such a situation, the surgeon may choose to avoid an anterior thoracolumbar approach due to the relative morbidity even though it might be preferred in a younger patient.

Further, the incidence of osteoporosis rises in older population groups. Not only does this increase the risk of fracture in the elderly, but it also makes spinal instrumentation more challenging and more likely to fail.[3] As with other comorbidities, this might lead one to use different surgical techniques (such as wires or hooks as opposed to screws) or avoid surgery altogether if sufficient stability cannot be achieved with traditional instrumentation. Mackey et al found that for each standard deviation reduction in bone mineral density the multivariate relative hazard ratio increased significantly for the incidence of high-energy fracture.[4] This factor has led to the use of cement augmentation by some spinal surgeons as a means of increasing screw pullout strength in the osteoporotic spine.[5]

Alternatively, if an elderly patient cannot be mobilized due to an injury or brace intolerance, the threshold for surgery may be lowered to avoid the complications of prolonged bed rest. This certainly has to be weighed against the morbidity of operating on this population.

Overall, the geriatric patient presents a significant challenge. The TLICS classification proposes a decision algorithm to optimize risk/benefit considerations. However, the surgeon must recognize that the variables already noted may alter these relative considerations and treatment recommendations, and counseling must be adjusted accordingly.

◆ Pediatric Patients

The pediatric patient also requires special considerations. In general, pediatric patients have more tolerance for injury, and an injury that would require a surgical intervention according to the TLICS classification system can be treated nonoperatively in this population. For example, fractures involving the vertebral apophyseal end plate are injuries unique to the developing spine. In pediatric spinal fractures this relatively weak cartilaginous interface can separate from the end plate, causing a unique fracture type. The injury to the posterior ligamentous complex is usually in the form of a periosteal sleeve-type fracture. Although this flexion-distraction injury pattern (score 4) with injury to the posterior ligamentous complex (score 3) would require surgical intervention under the TLICS system these fractures often heal rapidly with closed reduction and orthosis application.

◆ Obese Patients

Obesity has become a commonly encountered medical condition in the spine trauma patient. As a result, the comorbidities that are associated with obesity are of great concern when determining appropriate treatment algorithms. Given that ~33% of men and women were obese in the United States in 2005, surgical planning may be significantly affected by this variable.

There are several ways that obesity may alter treatment plans. First of all, the risks of anesthesia, positioning, and postoperative care are significantly increased. A recent study by Patel et al found that having a body mass index (BMI) above 30 increased the risk of complication by 20%, and a BMI above 40 increased the risk of complications by 36%.[6] Further, anterior approaches in particular may become more challenging. Conversely, braces are clearly of less utility in the obese patient, affording less stability than in the more slender patient.

As an example is the case of an intact patient (neuro 0) with an axial burst fracture pattern (2 points) with an intact posterior ligamentous complex (PLC) (0 points) for a total score of 2 points would generally be treated nonoperatively with a hyperextension orthosis. It is well known that hyperextension orthoses are minimally effective in obese patients. As an alternative this patient might benefit from a short-segment posterior instrumentation with or without fusion if there is concern of kyphosis.

◆ Stiff Spines

Injuries to the stiff or ankylotic spine present unique challenges. Patients with ankylosing spondylitis, diffuse idiopathic skeletal hyperostosis (DISH), or severe arthrosis require specific evaluation. The long moment arm of forces around such fractures significantly increases their risk of displacement.[7] Further, such fractures are often transverse in nature and may be difficult to visualize on standard imaging. Therefore, patients with evidence of these conditions require more extensive imaging modalities such as computed tomography and magnetic resonance imaging and low thresholds for surgical intervention if fractures are identified.

◆ Polytrauma Patients

The polytrauma patient also presents specific concerns. Injuries that would usually be treated nonoperatively may require surgical intervention to allow for faster mobilization or provide spinal stability in a patient that due to other injuries cannot tolerate an orthosis. A common example of this is a polytrauma patient that has a lumbar spine burst fracture without PLC disruption or neurological injury. This patient could be treated with an orthosis under the TLICS system, but multiple concurrent injuries such as chest wall or abdominal injuries might preclude this, making operative intervention preferable.

◆ Summary

The thoracolumbar injury classification and severity score provides an excellent descriptive tool for clinicians to describe injury patterns in a consistent and reproducible manner while also providing insight into the most effective method of clinical treatment, whether it be surgical or non-surgical, and the most appropriate surgical approach.

Although TLICS provides an excellent tool for the treatment of thoracolumbar spine injuries there are several confounders, some of which are mentioned in this chapter, that clinicians must be aware of and consider as important variables that will influence what method should be used to provide optimal treatment for their patients.

References

1. Vaccaro AR, Lehman RA Jr, Hurlbert RJ, et al. A new classification of thoracolumbar injuries: the importance of injury morphology, the integrity of the posterior ligamentous complex, and neurologic status. Spine 2005;30:2325–2333
2. Grossman MD, Miller D, Scaff DW, Arcona S. When is an elder old? Effect of preexisting conditions on mortality in geriatric trauma. J Trauma 2002;52:242–246

3. Yuan HA, Garfin SR, Dickman CA, Mardjetko SM. A historical cohort study of pedicle screw fixation in thoracic, lumbar, and sacral spinal fusions. Spine 1994;19(20, Suppl):2279S–2296S

4. Mackey DC, Lui LY, Cawthon PM, et al; Study of Osteoporotic Fractures (SOF) and Osteoporotic Fractures in Men Study (MrOS) Research Groups. High-trauma fractures and low bone mineral density in older women and men. JAMA 2007;298:2381–2388

5. Frankel BM, Jones T, Wang C. Segmental polymethylmethacrylate-augmented pedicle screw fixation in patients with bone softening caused by osteoporosis and metastatic tumor involvement: a clinical evaluation. Neurosurgery 2007;61:531–537, discussion 537–538

6. Patel N, Bagan B, Vadera S, et al. Obesity and spine surgery: relation to perioperative complications. J Neurosurg Spine 2007;6:291–297

7. Olerud C, Frost A, Bring J. Spinal fractures in patients with ankylosing spondylitis. Eur Spine J 1996;5:51–55

42

Surgical Management of Osteoporotic Thoracolumbar Spinal Fractures

Oliver I. Schmidt, Yohan Robinson, Ralf H. Gahr, and Marcel F. Dvorak

◆ Pathology of Osteoporosis

Osteoporosis is defined as a disease state with reduced bone mass and bone stability and associated increased fracture risk.[1,2] Osteoporosis is defined by the World Health Organization as a bone mineral density (BMD) measurement more than 2.5 standard deviations (*t*-score) below peak bone mass (PBM),[3] resembling less than 120 mg/mL in the osteopenic and less than 80 mg/mL in the osteoporotic spine.[4] The peak bone mass is highest between the ages of 25 and 35 and the greater the peak bone mass, the lower the chance of developing osteoporosis later in life.[5,6]

Osteoporosis is classified as either primary or secondary osteoporosis. Primary osteoporosis consists of two types: type I (postmenopausal), characterized by rapid bone loss over an 8- to 10-year period of time; and type II (age-associated idiopathic), affecting both males and females, due to the inevitable physiological changes and environmental factors associated with aging. It is important to remember that the prevalence of osteoporosis increases with age in both sexes. Secondary osteoporosis is the result of an identifiable agent or disease process that accounts for the change in BMD.

The measurement of BMD verifies the diagnosis and allows the treatment response to be monitored. Numerous methods to measure BMD have been developed and tested over the years. Based on accuracy, precision error, and practicality, dual-energy x-ray absorptiometry (DXA) is the current gold standard.[7,8] Various national guidelines for diagnosis and treatment of osteoporosis have been established based on the highest level of evidence available (e.g., www.guideline.gov, www.dv-osteologie.de).

Often osteoporosis is diagnosed first from vertebral compression fractures (VCFs) following minor trauma.[9,10] Over 700,000 osteoporotic vertebral fractures occur each year, worldwide, with only one third being symptomatic.[11] With growing life expectancy, osteoporosis-associated fractures represent a socioeconomic challenge.[12] Nowadays osteoporosis is generally accepted as a multifactorial process of diverse pathogenetic mechanisms leading to loss of bone mass and microarchitecture.[13,14]

Bone homeostasis is under the influence of endogenous changes as well as external mechanical loads from physical activity.[15] Bone consists of cells (15%, osteoblasts, osteoclasts) and extracellular matrix, that is divided into mineralized (40%, calcium hydroxyapatite) and nonmineralized (45%, predominantly collagen type I) components.[16] The more the bone is mineralized, the more it can withstand compressive forces. Whereas cortical (cancellous) bone of, for example, the femur is best at bending and torsional forces, trabecular bone of the vertebral body is best at resisting compressive loads.

Bone remodeling balances osteoclast resorption and osteoblast formation of skeletal bone.[17,18] Remodeling takes place in trabecular bone, predominantly. Phases of osteolytic activity are followed by osteoblast-related bone formation. In osteoporosis, the reaction of osteoblasts is inadequate, leading to an imbalance in bone homeostasis with secondary loss of bone mass.[19] Bone microarchitecture in the vertebral body is weakened, leading to impaired interconnections between horizontal and vertical beams of bone.[20] Hence the capacity of the vertebral body to bear weight is impaired. As a consequence, microfractures occur with microcallus formation, representing signs of instability and overuse.[21]

It was shown that in estrogen-related osteoporosis, remodeling favors and prolongs the osteolytic phase,[19] and physiological bone formation under stress is impaired in the estrogen-deprived osteoblasts.[22] Fracture risk is inversely associated with the circulating levels of estrogen.

In contrast, osteoporosis in the elderly population is primarily associated with decreased calcium resorption from intestinal disease and vitamin D deficiency, leading to secondary hyperparathyroidism.[23] Type II osteoporosis affects trabecular and cortical bone, whereas postmenopausal osteoporosis is restricted to the trabecular bone predominantly, resulting in a greater risk for both spinal fractures and wrist and hip fractures.[1] Because active vitamin D (calcitriol) inhibits synthesis of parathormon (PTH), lower levels of calcitriol can worsen hyperparathyroidism in a feedback loop.[24] In addition to the loss of bone mass, decreased vitamin D and PTH levels impair neuromotor function and potentially increase the risk of falls.[25] Altered trunk dimensions may also worsen progressive dietary calcium deficiency by causing early satiety.[26] Supplementation of vitamin D and calcium is effective treatment for hyperparathyroidism, serves to reduce the loss of bone mass, increases bone formation, and leads to a reduced fall and fracture risk.[24]

Mechanisms of intercellular communication of bone resorption in osteoclasts and formation in osteoblasts have been described.[27,28] Ligands and receptors of the Tumor Necrosis Factor (TNF)-family (RANK, RANKL, OPG) control and balance bone mass at the cellular level. Disturbed remodeling in postmenopausal women is linked to increased activation of the RANK/RANKL pathway, and clinical studies using antibodies against the ligand show promising results.[29] Transcription factors are also known to control the differentiation of stem cells into osteoblasts and osteoclasts. The hypothalamic axis also influences bone homeostasis, as is seen in Chronic Regional Pain Syndrome (CRPS)-associated osteopenia and traumatic brain injury–related heterotopic ossifications.[30,31]

◆ Diagnosis and Treatment of Osteoporotic Fractures

Millions of elderly people worldwide suffer from osteoporosis and pathological osteoporotic fractures. The annual incidence of VCF is 1.21% in women and 0.68% in men, increasing markedly with age.[32] With the continued aging of our population, VCFs represent an important cause of disability and a significant source of health care resource utilization.[33] For decades nonsurgical management with pain control and physical therapy–assisted mobilization has been the only treatment option and has proven successful in many cases. However, many patients remain immobilized due to chronic back pain.[34] The obvious functional and physical consequences of VCFs lead to anxiety and depression and have a devastating impact on interpersonal relationships and social roles.[35] One should be aware of the fact that untreated VCFs are correlated with significantly shorter life expectancy both in women ($p < 0.01$) and in men ($p < 0.0001$) within 1 year of the onset of symptoms.[36] It is not known whether the VCF is simply a sign of frailty in the elderly or if it actually contributes to mortality.

Osteoporotic microfractures in vertebrae lead to micromovement in the trabecular bone and induce pain and discomfort from nearby periosteal nerve fibers.[37,38] This pain resides only from fracture healing or when the status of the vertebra plana is reached. Usually an osteoporotic fracture is regarded as healed around 12 months postinjury.[39]

The rationale behind vertebroplasty (VP) and balloon kyphoplasty (BKP) in the osteoporotic spine is to immediately restore anterior column support by injecting nonresorbable polymethylmethacrylate (PMMA) or resorbable calcium phosphate cement (CaP) and thus prevent posttraumatic kyphosis and associated pain.[39–42] Long-term follow-up (36 months) in these prospective controlled, nonrandomized trials shows significant better results regarding pain relief in those patients treated by BKP compared with conservative treatment only.

Imaging Role of Magnetic Resonance Imaging

The diagnosis of osteoporosis is made with DXA, the gold-standard, as well as quantitative computed tomographic (CT) scan. Although new experimental approaches such as microcomputed CT and high-resolution and quantitative magnetic resonance imaging (MRI), are capable of imaging trabecular bone changes in osteoporotic and aging bone, there is so far no significant role for the MRI in the diagnostic workup of osteoporosis.[43–47]

In contrast, MRI is used to evaluate the osteoporosis-related fracture of the spine. Osteoporotic fractures are diagnosed for the most part by anteroposterior and lateral plane x-rays.[48,49] Plain radiographs are usually sufficient to identify a fracture, whereas in the cervicothoracic junction or in a highly osteoarthritic spine additional CT scanning is needed to verify the presence of a fracture. CT scanning is capable of generating slices of less than 1 mm with the highest level of bone contrast available and computer-generated reconstructions in axial and sagittal planes. MRI delivers the highest rate of soft tissue contrast and demonstrates edema and marrow signal changes in normal and pathological vertebrae. The standard protocol consists of T1- and T2-weighted sequences at 2 to 4 mm slices. Because up to 50% of the elderly population appear to have silent VCFs and noncontiguous, multilevel injury is reported in 4 to 24%,[4] it is difficult to determine which fracture is acute without bone scan or MRI confirmation.[50] MRI is the ideal diagnostic procedure in separating acute from old osteoporotic vertebral fractures.[51–53] Bone bruises and edema are seen in fat-suppressed and short-tau sequences. If local tenderness and pain are associated with x-ray- and MRI-demonstrated injuries to the vertebral body, an acute (osteoporotic) VCF is diagnosed.[54] In contrast to previous knowledge, bone bruise and edema are not prerequisites for successful and pain-reducing BKP in the osteoporotic VCF.[39,55] Instead the restoration of vertebral height is better in those vertebrae presenting with bone edema.

When faced with several VCFs, MRI can be helpful in identifying the painful vertebrae. Just recently, it was reported that whole spine MRI is capable of identifying secondary spinal fractures in up to 77% of patients, thus illustrating the greater sensitivity of whole spine MRI compared with radiography for identification of secondary fractures.[50] MRI signal intensity changes can also assist in selecting levels for cement augmentation and has been reported to improve outcomes in patients with multiple-level VCFs.[56]

MRI is also helpful in differentiating benign osteoporotic VCFs from those due to a malignant etiology.[57–59] Despite several reports claiming MRI findings that can aid in differentiating benign from malignant lesions, the best way to ensure that a metastatic or primary malignant lesion is not missed, is to perform a biopsy either at the time of a VP or BKP or as a separate diagnostic procedure.

Indications for Cement Augmentation

Despite the dramatic improvements in the medical treatment of osteoporosis, the timely restoration of quality of life has grown into a major issue in VCF treatment. Galibert et al presented the first cases of successful vertebral augmentation by intravertebral injection of PMMA in patients with vertebral hemangiomas.[60] Later, VP was successfully introduced for the management of osteoporotic VCFs.[61] The primary goal of VP is pain relief by stabilization of the continuously symptomatic VCF. VP compared with optimal pain medication results in immediate pain relief and improvement of mobility as demonstrated in the VERTOS study.[55] In addition, it was shown that even after failed initial conservative treatment of VCFs, VP is a safe and effective treatment in the short and long term.[62] A significant drawback of VP is the fact that apart from whatever postural correction occurs during positioning for the VP, kyphosis cannot be corrected through this procedure. The biomechanical understanding of progressive kyphosis leading to increased anterior column load and then leading to subsequent VCF led to the basic rationale for BKP. With this technique, reduction of the anterior vertebral body collapse and resultant kyphosis is achieved by a transpedicular intracorporal balloon expansion and is maintained by injecting PMMA cement.[63] Up to the present, the concept of BKP has been successfully applied in thousands of patients with VCF. Although both VP and BKP are equally effective at decreasing fracture-related pain, it is BKP that claims to improve the biomechanics of the spine, as well as improving pulmonary function and quality of life.[64,65] Furthermore it is still unclear whether the benefits of BKP outweigh its complications.[66] The results of the ongoing multicenter randomized, controlled trials will give us further evidence.[64]

Based on the fact that all osteoporotic fractures have some underlying medical disease, an interdisciplinary forum was established with radiologists, surgeons, endocrinologists, oncologists, and nuclear medicine specialists reviewing clinical and diagnostic results as well as discussing all potential aspects of conservative and surgical therapies. From more than 3900 individual cases treated according to this approach since 2001, the authors defined indications, contraindications, and standardized protocols for BKP that made their way into national guidelines.[69] Indications for BKP include (1) painful osteoporotic VCFs, (2) pathological/metastatic painful or unstable VCFs as well as stable painful VCFs, (3) painful vertebral lesions from multiple myeloma and osteolytic lesions, and (4) vertebral hemangioma.[39]

Decision-Making Vertebroplasty versus Balloon Kyphoplasty

Although both VP and BKP report pain relief in over 90% of patients, and both techniques reportedly provide "stability" to the fractures' vertebral segments, there are substantial differences in the two techniques. VP may be performed under local anesthetic and can be performed through a relatively small cannula, thus making it more amenable to small pedicles and those upper thoracic vertebrae. VP is also relatively inexpensive relative to BKP. The difficulties with VP, however, include the necessity to insert cement under high pressure, thus leading to an increased risk of cement leaks. Although it might sound obvious, a high amount of injected cement is not associated with a better clinical result,[70] and experimental studies show that cement arrangement in highly osteoporotic bone is more local, whereas in stronger trabecular bone diffuse dispersion will prevail.[71] VP will not create a void in the fractured vertebra and will not correct the kyphotic deformity, elevate the end plate, or restore anterior vertebral body height.

BKP, on the other hand, will actively restore anterior vertebral body height and correct kyphosis. Only 10% of osteoporotic fractures can be reduced from hyperlordotic posture prior to surgery. In addition, 60% of anterior vertebral column height can be restored from BKP only, in contrast to simple injection of cement as performed in VP.[72] This in part may be related to general anesthesia influencing fracture reduction

through muscle relaxation in contrast to VP under local anesthesia. Because the posttraumatic kyphotic angle is suggested to be a risk factor for adjacent fractures in the osteoporotic spine,[73] BKP is favored due to its higher potential for restoration of a physiological sagittal profile in comparison to VP. This is in line with a systematic review on BKP including 26 studies with primary clinical data, demonstrating effectiveness and safety of BKP for the treatment of VCFs of osteoporotic and tumor origin, also highlighting the fact that some data (height restoration, kyphotic deformity, leakage rate) indicate greater benefit of BKP over VP.[74]

Following balloon expansion, the cement is injected through a larger cannula and is injected into a void that has been created by the balloon. The cement is thus injected under much lower pressure, and there is less of a risk of cement leakage, extravasation, and resultant complications. This is favored in particular for metastatic VCFs, which tend to have increased bony osteolysis and neoplastic vessels.[75]

In a prospective cohort of 56 patients at 1-year follow-up no difference regarding pain relief was found between VP and BKP.[76] Similar results were documented for short-term follow-up at 6 months[77] and 12 months.[78] Grohs et al found that only BKP is capable of maintaining significant pain reduction over 2 years versus VP, and increased general health featured by Oswestry score was seen in the BKP and not VP group at 1 year postintervention.[79]

General evidence-based recommendations on where to do VP or BKP cannot be given.[80,81] In a position statement on percutaneous vertebral augmentation, it was stated that there is no proven advantage of either vertebro- or kyphoplasty with regard to pain relief, vertebral height restoration, and complication rate, and both options should be reimbursed by payors as safe and effective treatment for painful VCFs.[82] However, based on the current literature, VP could be useful in low-grade VCFs due to the limited potential to restore anterior vertebral body height. In higher posttraumatic kyphotic angles of more than 15 degrees or one third of height loss, BKP seems more appropriate.[83] There is level III evidence for both procedures resulting in equivalent pain relief in recent systematic reviews.[84,85] There is some suggestion, however, that the risk of cement extravasation and adjacent-segment fracture is lower with the deformity correction that occurs with BKP. The results of the KAVIAR study (NCT00323609), which directly compares VP and BKP, will help resolve these issues and is expected to be available in 2011.

Indications for Combined Cement Augmentation and Posterior Instrumentation

Due to the often severe comorbidity of elderly patients suffering VCF, BKP has been discussed as an alternative therapy of burst fractures instead of surgical stabilization.[86] In these cases further displacement of the posterior vertebral body fragment into the spinal canal or extravasation of cement into the spinal canal through the middle column fracture line are both feared complications and have been reported before.[66,87] To protect the posterior wall several surgeons perform posterior instrumentation of the adjacent vertebrae.[88] This can be done using percutaneous posterior instrumentation or with a conventional open technique. Verlaan et al investigated the use of BKP after posterior instrumentation in burst fractures in 20 patients (mean age 41.8 years).[89,90] No bone fragment displacement was found. Asymptomatic cement leakage occurred in five cases. Vertebral anterior height could be restored to 91% of the estimated intact height. Nöldge et al performed BKP with posterior instrumentation in nine patients with burst fractures.[88] They found a reduction of mean Visual Analogue Pain Scores of 6.2 preoperatively to 2.0 after 1 year.

Another indication for instrumentation is the use of CaP cement injection, as it is favored in the young patient. In the effort to not use exogenous PMMA in the young patient, resorbable CaP cement can be injected, that after time gets integrated into the trabecular bone via appositional bone formation.[67,91] A prerequisite for this approach is a stable environment devoid of micromovement in the injured vertebral body. Percutaneous implant insertion and its later removal could produce the stable conditions required for this technique. Feasibility of this approach has been successfully demonstrated by Maestretti et al in a prospective consecutive series with compression and burst fractures.[92]

Indications for Open Reduction and Stabilization

The aforementioned cement augmentation method with balloon-assisted VCF reduction addresses segmental kyphosis. If multiple VCFs lead to significant kyphosis and fixed sagittal imbalance, then cement augmentation alone will reduce the fracture pain but will not improve the global spinal imbalance. Gross spinal imbalance may be disabling itself and may lead to a significantly reduced quality of life. Increased kyphosis may cause subsequent VCF due to an increased anterior load.[93] Furthermore fixed sagittal imbalance may lead to falls with further fractures and morbidity. Therefore the theoretical urge to correct global sagittal imbalance may be reasonable in some very carefully selected cases. Due to advanced age and the multiple comorbidities of these patients spinal surgeons are not at all eager to surgically correct these global deformities, knowing that both opening and closing wedge procedures are associated with complications leading to disabling morbidity.[94] The prevalent osteopenic bone quality requires long instrumentations, which have the risk of adjacent VCF and pedicle fractures.[95]

Kim et al investigated the results of anterior-posterior correction in 32 patients with global sagittal imbalance (mean age 64.6 years).[96] They found an improvement of 54% in Oswestry Disability Index (ODI) ($p < 0.001$) and of 70% in the VAS after two years ($p < 0.001$). Subsequent compression fractures occurred in four cases and screw loosening in two cases. Suk et al. compared the anterior-posterior opening-wedge ($n = 11$) to the pedicle subtraction closing-wedge osteotomy ($n = 15$) and found significantly larger correction of the deformity with pedicle subtraction osteotomy ($p < 0.05$).[97] Additionally less operation time and mean blood loss ($p < 0.05$) was seen with pedicle subtraction osteotomies. Cho et al. compared two closing-wedge osteotomies – the Smith-Petersen versus the pedicle subtraction osteotomy – for the correction of global sagittal imbalance.[98] They found similar rates of correction, but higher rates of coronal decompensation with Smith-Peterson osteotomies ($p < 0.02$). Furthermore they found higher blood loss in pedicle subtraction osteotomies ($p < 0.001$). In another study the authors showed that with pedicle subtraction osteotomy the Oswestry Disability Index improved significantly after 5 years ($p < 0.001$).[99] The available results favor

the posterior-only pedicle subtraction osteotomy because of the higher potential of correction and lesser operation time.

Nonsurgical Therapy

Regardless of whether the osteoporotic VCF is treated with or without surgical stabilization or injection techniques, all patients require optimal medical treatment of their osteoporosis. Medical comorbidities, general frailty, and severe osteoporosis that preclude any form of vertebral fixation are all relative contraindications for surgical treatment. A rough guideline is a T-score on bone mineral density testing of less than −3.5 or −4 will make any fixation difficult. Surgical treatment will not influence the degree of the osteoporosis itself and is only successful if in addition to the surgical treatment, optimal medical management of the osteoporosis is initiated.[100]

One pillar of treatment is pain control. VCFs cause severe pain, requiring a multimodal pain management.[101] Physical therapy plays a major role in mobilization and rehabilitation after VCF. By improving spinal extensor strength, load can be taken away from the anterior column. Getting the patient out of bed is a major task to prevent pneumonia and further physical deterioration.[102] There are patients who benefit from bracing to reduce spinal flexion, especially those with poor muscular endurance and gross thoracic kyphosis. Most commonly used are three-point contact braces (e.g., Jewitt- or Cash-braces).

For treatment of osteoporosis, calcium supplementation[103] and bisphosphonates have been proven successful in VCF reduction.[104]

◆ Operative Technique of Balloon Kyphoplasty

In contrast to VP, where reduction can only be achieved through positioning, a balloon is used in BKP to additionally improve vertebral height and to form a cavity, which is surrounded by compressed bone structure reducing the risk of cement leakage. Four possible approaches for BKP are known, of which the transpedicular access is most commonly used.

Percutaneous Bilateral Transpedicular Balloon Kyphoplasty

In the thoracolumbar spine mostly a bilateral transpedicular approach is chosen to enable a symmetric reposition and augmentation of the VCF. After positioning under fluoroscopic control biopsy needles are used to enter the pedicles on both sides of the fractured vertebra. A K-wire is placed through the biopsy needle into the vertebral body close to the anterior wall. Then using the K-wire a Seldinger technique is used to widen the pedicular entrance with the introducer. Then empty bone-fillers are used to form a cavity for the placement of the balloons. Two balloons are positioned into the vertebral body under fluoroscopic control, and controlled inflation of the balloons is performed. After successful reduction the cavity is filled with bone cement from both pedicles. One should be careful that the viscosity of the cement is high enough to avoid cement leakage. After successful cement application the introducers are removed and skin closure is performed (**Fig. 42.1**).

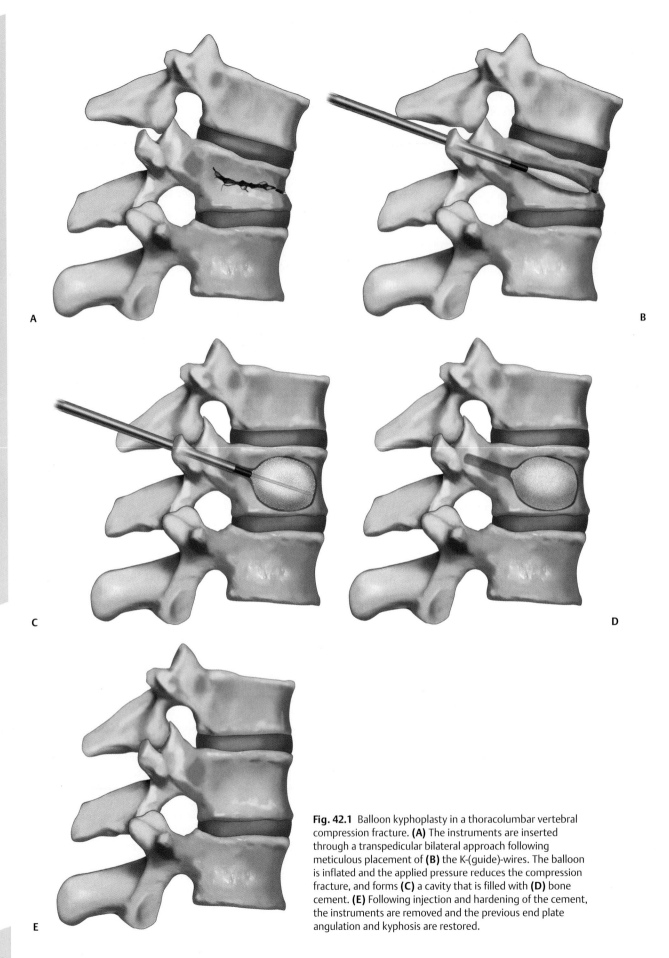

A

B

C

D

E

Fig. 42.1 Balloon kyphoplasty in a thoracolumbar vertebral compression fracture. **(A)** The instruments are inserted through a transpedicular bilateral approach following meticulous placement of **(B)** the K-(guide)-wires. The balloon is inflated and the applied pressure reduces the compression fracture, and forms **(C)** a cavity that is filled with **(D)** bone cement. **(E)** Following injection and hardening of the cement, the instruments are removed and the previous end plate angulation and kyphosis are restored.

Percutaneous Unilateral Extrapedicular Balloon Kyphoplasty

In the thoracic spine pedicles become narrower, and placement of the balloons with enough convergency is difficult. Therefore extrapedicular accesses have been successfully developed to avoid pedicle perforation and neurological damage or intraspinal cement leakage. Widely used is the transcostovertebral access from far lateral.[105,106] From posterior the needle passes above the transverse process and meets the pedicle at the lateral body wall. The lateral view confirms the placement of the tip of the needle close to the base of the pedicle. To allow optimal placement in the vertebral body enough convergence has to be sought. A single balloon is then used for reduction and the cavity then filled with cement as described earlier. Boszczyk et al performed successfully extrapedicular transcostovertebral BKP in 55 high and midthoracic vertebrae.[106] One epidural cement leakage and one perforation of the lateral cortical wall were described, both without clinical significance. Ryu et al performed extrapedicular single-BKP in 37 vertebrae with results comparable to a bipedicular approach (**Fig. 42.2**).[105]

Open Unilateral Interlaminary Balloon Kyphoplasty

In cases of burst fractures with neurological compromise some authors perform an open interlaminary BKP.[107] After a median incision and paramedian access through the thoracolumbar fascia the paravertebral muscles are retracted unilaterally. Then the interlaminary space is cleared by lateral flavectomy and laminotomy. Then the lateral dural sac is cautiously retracted and the posterior wall of the fractured vertebra is exposed, and BKP can be performed with a single balloon positioned into the center of the vertebral body. After BKP the spinal canal has to be investigated for cement leakage (**Fig. 42.3**).

Open Anterior Balloon Kyphoplasty

BKP may be performed using anterior access.[108] The biopsy needle may be placed directly on the anterior wall of the fractured vertebra, and a single balloon can be placed into the vertebral body. After reduction cement is applied through the introducer. The application of the thoracoscopically assisted anterior BKP is technically limited to the length of the applicators compared with the size of the patient.

Special Technical Notes

Navigation

To increase balloon placement accuracy and to reduce the radiation exposure during BKP, computer-assisted fluoroscopic navigation may be used.[109] Through navigation the radiation exposure can be reduced by 76%, whereas accuracy of placement can be increased dramatically.[110]

Eggshell Procedure

To avoid cement leakage the eggshell procedure can be applied.[111] For this procedure after reduction with the BKP balloon a small amount of doughy cement is injected and then the balloon reinserted and reinflated. Once the cement hardens the cavity can be filled with cement, with the "eggshell" preventing cement leakage.

Types of Cement

A variety of injectable radiopaque cements have been developed and are available from different companies.[112,113] All can be divided into nonresorbable cements relying on PMMA or resorbable CaP. In contrast to PMMA, injected CaP cement can be digested by osteoclasts and integration of CaP results from

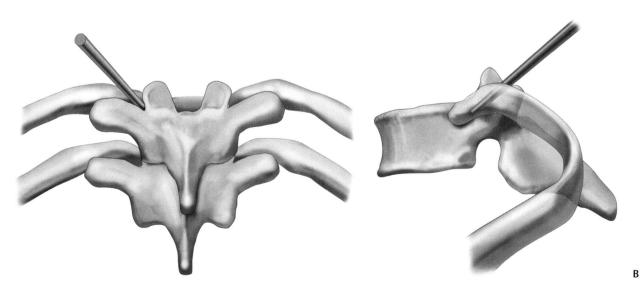

A   B

Fig. 42.2 (A,B) Balloon kyphoplasty in the upper thoracic spine using an extrapedicular, unilateral approach. Decreasing pedicle diameter in the upper thoracic spine does not allow safe transpedicular passage to the vertebral body; hence the extrapedicular transcostovertebral approach has been developed. From a more lateral entry point the guidewire enters the pedicle at the level of the posterior wall of the vertebral body. Consecutively, the balloon is placed more centrally inside the vertebral body, allowing an optimized reduction and thereby limiting the procedure to the use of one single balloon only.

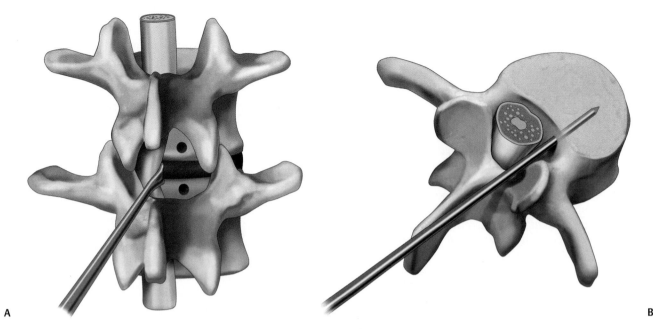

Fig. 42.3 (A,B) Open balloon kyphoplasty in adjacent vertebral fractures with spinal canal compromise. Following a unilateral decompression and clearance of the spinal canal from fracture fragments, the instruments are placed under visual control into the center of each

vertebral body. This procedure allows restoration of anterior column support from posterior in one session without the need of additional anterior surgery.

appositional bone formation and secondary ingrowth.[67,91] As mentioned in the antecedent sections, for bony integration of brittle CaP micromovement should be absent; otherwise the injected CaP might only be encapsulated by soft tissues.

The theory of pain reduction following cement injection is based on various mechanisms: (1) irritation of periosteal nerve fibers is reduced because cement injection increases stability; (2) stabilized vertebra are prevented from further, pain-generating fracturing; (3) exothermic and potentially cytotoxic reaction of PMMA leads to nerve fiber coagulation and/or anesthesia.[114] If the last mechanism is responsible for pain relief, CaP cements may not be found to reduce pain as PMMA cements do. Experimental studies have shown that PMMA restores and increases the vertebral body, whereas CaP restored, but did not increase prefracture body strength.[115–119] None of the cements restored prefracture vertebral body stiffness (N/mm).

In a recent trial comparing the use of CaP and PMMA in A1 (compression) and A3 (burst) fractures, it was shown that 1-year follow-up resulted in similar pain reduction, whereas only PMMA significantly improved subjective pain at the 2-year point.[120] The authors concluded that low biomechanical resistance of CaP against flexion, traction, and shear forces might attribute to failure of CaP in burst fractures. This is in line with the findings of Grafe et al, which demonstrated that in compression fractures similar results were seen with CaP and PMMA cohorts over a time period of 36 months.[67]

The more liquid the cement is injected, the less pressure is needed, but the higher the risk for leakage. To reduce cement leakage, it is generally accepted to let the cement reach viscosity similar to that of toothpaste before injection is performed. The optimal volume of injected cement for successful vertebro- or kyphoplasty has not been defined.[121,122] There is an association between the injected cement volume and accidental extraosseous leakage.[123] Following balloon expansion, the volume that can be injected is increased in BKP compared with VP.

◆ Complications of Balloon Kyphoplasty

Several nonrandomized, prospective, controlled trials have been published comparing BKP to nonsurgical treatment and VP (**Table 42.1**), and four ongoing randomized, controlled trials are registered (**Table 42.2**).[84] Major issues are the immediate and sustained degree of pain improvement and quality of life, correction of deformity, and postoperative complications. The first results of the multicenter randomized, controlled Fracture Reduction Evaluation (FREE) study reported a significant improvement of the quality of life (Short Form-36, $p < 0.0001$), pain Visual Analogue Scale (VAS, $p < 0.0001$), and function (ODI, $p < 0.0001$) after 1 month in the BKP group ($n = 149$) controlled against nonsurgical treatment ($n = 151$).[64] It is anticipated that the 1-year results, which will be published soon, will give evidence concerning the safety of BKP.

The comprehensive meta-analysis of Taylor et al summarized all published BKP complications.[84] Cement leakages occurred in 8.1% of all cases, but only 0.09% were symptomatic. New VCFs occurred in 11.1%, and 9.4% were adjacent vertebrae. Pulmonary embolism occurred in 0.17% of all cases. Spinal cord compression occurred in 0.16% of all cases. Radiculopathy was found in 0.17% of all cases. The overall mortality was 4.4%, perioperative mortality was 0.13%.

Adjacent Fractures

Adjacent fractures are the most common adverse event found after BKP. The occurrence of adjacent fractures is known from VP, where 12.4% had subsequent VCF after 2 years ($n = 177$).[124] BKP was thought to have lesser adjacent fractures due to correction of kyphotic deformity,[73] but kyphosis is not the only reason for adjacent fractures. Lin et al correlated the incidence of adjacent fractures to cement leakage into the disk in VP ($n = 38$, $p < 0.005$).[125] Komemushi et al found cement

Table 42.1 Overview on Comparative Clinical Trials of Balloon Kyphoplasty

Study	Design	Level of Evidence	Control Group	Control n (levels)	Kyphoplasty N (levels)	Follow-up	Outcome	Cement Leakage
Weisskopf et al (2003)[154]	Retrospective CT	IIIb	Nonsurgical	20 (35)	22 (37)	10 days	Improvement in VAS ($p < 0.001$) Reduced days in hospital ($p < 0.01$)	5 cement leakages in kyphoplasty
Fourney et al (2003)[76]	Retrospective CT	IIIb	Vertebroplasty	34 (65)	15 (32)	4,5 months	No significant differences in VAS and ODI Improvement of kyphosis with kyphoplasty ($p < 0.01$)	0 cement leakages in kyphoplasty 6 cement leakages in vertebroplasty
Komp et al (2004)[155]	Prospective CT	IIb	Nonsurgical	19(19)	21(21)	6 months	Improvement of VAS and ODI ($p < 0.01$)	0 cement leakages in kyphoplasty
Kasperk et al (2005)[68]	Prospective CT	IIb	Nonsurgical	20 (33)	40 (72)	12 months	Improvement of VAS ($p < 0.01$)Improvement of kyphosis ($p < 0.001$).	7 cement leakages in kyphoplasty
Grohs et al (2005)[79]	Prospective CT	IIb	Vertebroplasty	23 (29)	28 (35)	24 months	No significant difference in ODI Improvement of VAS with kyphoplasty ($p < 0.05$) No significant improvement of kyphosis	8 cement leakages in kyphoplasty 8 cement leakages in vertebroplasty
Masala et al (2005)	Retrospective CT	IIIb	Vertebroplasty	26 (33)	7 (7)	6 months	No significant difference in VAS.	0 cement leakage in kyphoplasty 11 cement leakages in vertebroplasty
Pflugmacher et al (2005)[78]	Prospective CT	IIb	Vertebroplasty	20 (32)	22 (35)	12 months	No significant difference in VAS and ODI Improvement of kyphosis with kyphoplasty ($p < 0.05$)	5 cement leakages in kyphoplasty 6 cement leakages in vertebroplasty
De Negri et al (2007)[77]	Prospective CT	IIb	Vertebroplasty	10 (18)	11 (15)	6 months	No significant difference in VAS and ODI	0 cement leakages in kyphoplasty 1 cement leakage in vertebroplasty
Wardlaw et al (2007)[64]	Randomized CT	Ib	Nonsurgical	149	151	1 month	Significant improvement in SF-36 ($p < 0.0001$), VAS ($p < 0.0001$), and ODI ($p < 0.0001$).	Not reported

Abbreviations: CT, clinical trial; ODI, Oswestry Disability Index; SF-36, Short Form-36; VAS, visual analogue scale.

Table 42.2 Registered Ongoing Multicenter Randomized, Controlled Trials Involving Kyphoplasty

Trial Name	Procedure	Control Group	N	Follow-up	Primary Outcome
FREE	Kyphoplasty in VCF	Nonsurgical	300	2 years	Quality of life (SF-36)
CAFE	Kyphoplasty in VCF in cancer patients	Nonsurgical	200	1 year	Pain (VAS), disability (Roland-Morris)
CEEP	Kyphoplasty in VCF	Vertebroplasty	112	2 years	Pain (Roland-Scale)
KAVIAR	Kyphoplasty in VCF	Vertebroplasty	1234	2 years	Subsequent fractures

Source: Taylor RS, Fritzell P, Taylor RJ. Balloon kyphoplasty in the management of vertebral compression fractures: an updated systematic review and meta-analysis. Eur Spine J 2007;16:1085–1100.

Abbreviations: SF-36; Short Form-36; VAS, visual analogue scale; VCF, vertebral compression fracture.

leakage into the disk to be a significant predictor of adjacent VCF ($n = 83, p < 0.001$).[126]

Fribourg et al found subsequent fractures after BKP in 26% of all cases ($n = 38$), 21% occurred during the first 2 months.[127] Harrop et al found subsequent fractures in 22.6% of all patients after a mean follow-up of 11 months ($n = 115$).[128] Sixty-five percent of these had secondary steroid-induced osteoporosis. Another investigation by Lavelle and Cheney found 17% recurrent fractures within 1 year after BKP, and 11.7% occurred during the first 90 days ($n = 94$).[129] They did not find any impact of secondary osteoporosis on subsequent fractures. A prospective investigation by Moon et al found an incidence of subsequent VCF in 15.5% patients after 1 year ($n = 111$).[130] Interestingly they could correlate the appearance of adjacent VCF to the amount of PMMA cement applied during the procedure ($p < 0.05$).

The available data reveal that subsequent VCFs of adjacent vertebrae occur in 7.8% to 26% of all patients treated with BKP. Kyphosis, secondary osteoporosis, and cement leakage into the intervertebral disk facilitate the occurrence of subsequent VCFs. Identifying risk factors for subsequent VCFs, several authors discussed the indication for prophylactic cement augmentation of adjacent vertebrae.[131–133] Until now there is no evidence for the effectiveness of prophylactic vertebro- or kyphoplasty.[132] It rather seems that the prophylactic use of PMMA reduces the safety of the procedure.[131]

Cement Leakage

A feared complication of all vertebral augmentation techniques is PMMA cement leakage. The systematic review of the literature by Hulme et al found rates of cement leakage in VP of 41% ($n = 2283$ levels) and in BKP of 9% ($n = 1486$ levels) of treated vertebrae.[134] In BKP of the 65 leakages reported in the literature most were paraspinal (48%), intradiskal (38%), epidural (11%), pulmonary (1.5%), and foraminal (1.5%).[134] Paraspinal and intradiskal leakage is generally asymptomatic, even though intradiskal leakage is potentially linked to an increased rate of adjacent segment fractures.[126] Intradural cement leakage has only been described for VP so far,[135] but epidural leakage had devastating neurological effects in both in VP[136] and BKP.[87] These complications require mostly immediate surgical intervention with decompression and, if possible, removal of the cement causing the spinal cord compression.[137]

Pulmonary embolism of PMMA cement was found in 4.6% of the 65 patients treated with either VP ($n = 88$) or BKP ($n = 25$) by Choe et al.[138] No correlation between the occurrence of pulmonary cement embolism and the type of procedure was found. This is remarkable given that BKP has a much lesser rate of cement leakage than VP.[134] Jang et al presented three cases of cement embolism after VP, of which two had mild dyspnea.[139] François et al reported a patient with a large PMMA cement embolus floating in the right pulmonary artery and deteriorating pulmonary function requiring surgical removal.[140] Yoo reported a 5 cm long PMMA cement embolus in the right pulmonary artery after VP leading to acute respiratory distress syndrome,[141] requiring intensive care treatment and open embolectomy under cardiopulmonary bypass. The patient did not recover and died 10 days after VP. A further fatal pulmonary embolism after VP has been described by Monticelli et al.[142] There is only one report on cement embolism after BKP by Garfin et al.[143]

With proper surgical techniques the risk of cement leakage can be minimized.[144] Correct placement of the balloon, high viscosity of the PMMA cement, controlled application of the cement into the vertebra, and limitation of the applied volume reduce the risk of leakage. A popular technique to reduce the risk of cement leakage in BKP is the eggshell technique, where after primary reduction with the balloon a small amount of doughy cement is applied into the cavity followed by reinflation of the balloon.[111] Using this technique a cement "eggshell" prevents further leakage when the rest of the cement is applied with radiographic control.

The severity of pulmonary PMMA cement embolism and the urgent need for immediate decompression in relevant spinal stenosis after cement leakage suggests that even though fatal emboli are few, VP and BKP should not be regarded as minor interventions that can be performed without an anesthesiologist and a spinal surgeon on call.

Infection

Even though the risk of infection accompanies every surgical intervention,[145] only four cases of infections after BKP have been described so far in the available literature. Nussbaum and coworkers found two cases of infection (diskitis/-osteomyelitis) in the large Food and Drug Administration database for adverse events related to BKP devices.[146] Two other cases with infection after BKP have been described, of which one was a superficial infection but the other was associated with anterior spondylitis and epidural abscess formation and required anterior corporectomy and 360 degree fusion.[66] With VP only seven cases have been described with postoperative infections. The VP pioneers Deramond et al presented one case of postoperative spondylitis in an immunosuppressed patient, which could be treated successfully with bed rest and antibiotics.[61] Kallmes et al described a case of a postoperative infection in an immunocompromised patient.[147] Another case demonstrated severe pyogenic spondylitis 1 month after VP that was performed while the patient had a urinary tract infection.[148] The treatment was surgical with anterior corporectomy and bisegmental fusion after multisegmental posterior instrumentation. A further case of spondylitis after VP was presented in 2005, which treated the patient conservatively with a 3-month antibiotic regimen.[149] Walker and Mummaneni present two additional cases of post-VP spondylitis treated by anterior corporectomy and multisegemental fusion.[150,151] Olmos et al report a case of spondylitis after VP requiring corporectomy and 360 degree fusion.[152] An unusual case report of spondylitis after VP with epidural abscesses containing *Mycobacterium tuberculosis* was published.[153] This patient was under immunosuppression because of a liver transplantation, and an inactive tuberculous lesion was obviously activated. Successful treatment implied posterior decompression and abscess evacuation and long-term antituberculotic therapy.

Even though the risk of infection after BKP is extremely low, infection does occur, as we could show in this investigation. As we can learn from the VP experience not only asepsis during the procedure but also proper indication in immunocompromised patients have to be considered prior to treatment. In these cases a standardized antibiotic prophylaxis is recommended. Nevertheless the rate of postoperative infections is lower both in BKP and in VP than in any other spinal surgical procedure in general.[145]

◆ Summary and Recommendations

The evidence is strong that both VP and BKP are effective at improving pain and improving function in elderly patients with VCFs. There is also strong evidence that both VP and BKP are effective in treating pathological fractures due to malignancy, particularly in multiple myeloma. Effectiveness in treating symptomatic hemangiomas has also been demonstrated. Both techniques appear to be relatively safe, although BKP has been shown to have a lower incidence of asymptomatic and symptomatic cement extravasation.

The potential benefit of anterior column height restoration, kyphosis reduction, and restoration of spinal alignment as reported with BKP may or may not result in a concomitant reduction in the rate of adjacent VCFs. This has yet to be fully investigated.

The optimal environment for performing these procedures includes high-quality biplanar imaging as well as surgical and medical backup.

References

1. Riggs BL, Melton LJ III. Evidence for two distinct syndromes of involutional osteoporosis. Am J Med 1983;75:899–901
2. Seeman E, Delmas PD. Bone quality—the material and structural basis of bone strength and fragility. N Engl J Med 2006;354:2250–2261
3. Kendler D. Risk factors in osteoporosis. B C Med J 1996;38:263–264
4. Bauer JS, Müller D, Rummeny EJ, Link TM. Fracture diagnosis in osteoporosis [in German]. Radiologe 2006;46:839–846
5. Lane JM. Osteoporosis. Medical prevention and treatment. Spine 1997;22(24, Suppl):32S–37S
6. Lane JM, Riley EH, Wirganowicz PZ. Osteoporosis: diagnosis and treatment. Instr Course Lect 1997;46:445–458
7. Clinical practice guidelines for the diagnosis and management of osteoporosis. Scientific Advisory Board, Osteoporosis Society of Canada. CMAJ 1996;155:1113–1133
8. Coupland D. Recommendations for the measurement and quantitation of bone mineral density. B C Med J 1996;38:265–268
9. Ebeling PR. Clinical practice: osteoporosis in men. N Engl J Med 2008; 358:1474–1482
10. Rosen CJ. Clinical practice: postmenopausal osteoporosis. N Engl J Med 2005;353:595–603
11. Riggs BL, Melton LJ III. The worldwide problem of osteoporosis: insights afforded by epidemiology. Bone 1995;17(5, Suppl): 505S–511S
12. Ensrud KE, Thompson DE, Cauley JA, et al; Fracture Intervention Trial Research Group. Prevalent vertebral deformities predict mortality and hospitalization in older women with low bone mass. J Am Geriatr Soc 2000;48:241–249
13. Raisz LG. Pathogenesis of osteoporosis: concepts, conflicts, and prospects. J Clin Invest 2005;115:3318–3325
14. Raisz LG. Clinical practice: screening for osteoporosis. N Engl J Med 2005;353:164–171
15. Bono CM, Einhorn TA. Overview of osteoporosis: pathophysiology and determinants of bone strength. Eur Spine J 2003;12(Suppl 2):S90–S96
16. Linde F. Elastic and viscoelastic properties of trabecular bone by a compression testing approach. Dan Med Bull 1994;41:119–138
17. Harada S, Rodan GA. Control of osteoblast function and regulation of bone mass. Nature 2003;423:349–355
18. Karsenty G. The genetic transformation of bone biology. Genes Dev 1999;13:3037–3051
19. Priemel M, Münch C, Beil FT, Ritzel H, Amling M. Pathophysiology and pathomorphology of osteoporosis [in German]. Radiologe 2006;46: 831–838
20. Einhorn TA. Bone strength: the bottom line. Calcif Tissue Int 1992; 51:333–339
21. Hahn M, Vogel M, Amling M, Ritzel H, Delling G. Microcallus formations of the cancellous bone: a quantitative analysis of the human spine. J Bone Miner Res 1995;10:1410–1416
22. Lee K, Jessop H, Suswillo R, Zaman G, Lanyon L. Endocrinology: bone adaptation requires oestrogen receptor-alpha. Nature 2003;424:389
23. Amling M, Grote HJ, Pösl M, Hahn M, Delling G. Polyostotic heterogeneity of the spine in osteoporosis: quantitative analysis and three-dimensional morphology. Bone Miner 1994;27:193–208
24. Lips P. Vitamin D deficiency and secondary hyperparathyroidism in the elderly: consequences for bone loss and fractures and therapeutic implications. Endocr Rev 2001;22:477–501
25. Bischoff-Ferrari HA, Dawson-Hughes B, Willett WC, et al. Effect of vitamin D on falls: a meta-analysis. JAMA 2004;291:1999–2006
26. Leidig-Bruckner G, Minne HW, Schlaich C, et al. Clinical grading of spinal osteoporosis: quality of life components and spinal deformity in women with chronic low back pain and women with vertebral osteoporosis. J Bone Miner Res 1997;12:663–675
27. Lacey DL, Timms E, Tan HL, et al. Osteoprotegerin ligand is a cytokine that regulates osteoclast differentiation and activation. Cell 1998;93: 165–176
28. Simonet WS, Lacey DL, Dunstan CR, et al. Osteoprotegerin: a novel secreted protein involved in the regulation of bone density. Cell 1997; 89:309–319
29. Hamdy NA. Denosumab: RANKL inhibition in the management of bone loss. Drugs Today (Barc) 2008;44:7–21
30. Morley J, Marsh S, Drakoulakis E, Pape HC, Giannoudis PV. Does traumatic brain injury result in accelerated fracture healing? Injury 2005;36:363–368
31. Schwartzman RJ. New treatments for reflex sympathetic dystrophy. N Engl J Med 2000;343:654–656
32. Felsenberg D, Silman AJ, Lunt M. Incidence of vertebral fracture in Europe: results from the European Prospective Osteoporosis Study (EPOS). J Bone Miner Res 2002;17:716–724
33. Lad SP, Patil CG, Lad EM, Boakye M. Trends in pathological vertebral fractures in the United States: 1993 to 2004. J Neurosurg Spine 2007;7:305–310
34. Pluijm SM, Tromp AM, Smit JH, Deeg DJ, Lips P. Consequences of vertebral deformities in older men and women. J Bone Miner Res 2000; 15:1564–1572
35. Gold DT. The clinical impact of vertebral fractures: quality of life in women with osteoporosis. Bone 1996;18(3, Suppl):185S–189S
36. Center JR, Nguyen TV, Schneider D, Sambrook PN, Eisman JA. Mortality after all major types of osteoporotic fracture in men and women: an observational study. Lancet 1999;353:878–882
37. Mach DB, Rogers SD, Sabino MC, et al. Origins of skeletal pain: sensory and sympathetic innervation of the mouse femur. Neuroscience 2002; 113:155–166

VII Thoracolumbar Spine Injuries and Their Management

38. Li J, Ahmad T, Spetea M, Ahmed M, Kreicbergs A. Bone reinnervation after fracture: a study in the rat. J Bone Miner Res 2001;16:1505–1510
39. Kasperk C, Nöldge G, Grafe I, Meeder P, Huber F, Nawroth P. Indications and results of kypho- and vertebroplasty [in German]. Internist (Berl) 2008;49:1206, 1208–1210, 1212–1218
40. Truumees E, Hilibrand A, Vaccaro AR. Percutaneous vertebral augmentation. Spine J 2004;4:218–229
41. Webb JC, Spencer RF. The role of polymethylmethacrylate bone cement in modern orthopaedic surgery. J Bone Joint Surg Br 2007;89:851–857
42. Kasperk C, Nöldge G, Meeder P, Nawroth P, Huber FX. Kyphoplasty : method for minimally invasive treatment of painful vertebral fractures [in German]. Chirurg 2008;79:944–950, 952–955
43. Liney GP, Bernard CP, Manton DJ, Turnbull LW, Langton CM. Age, gender, and skeletal variation in bone marrow composition: a preliminary study at 3.0 Tesla. J Magn Reson Imaging 2007;26:787–793
44. Majumdar S. Magnetic resonance imaging for osteoporosis. Skeletal Radiol 2008;37:95–97
45. Wehrli FW. Structural and functional assessment of trabecular and cortical bone by micro magnetic resonance imaging. J Magn Reson Imaging 2007;25:390–409
46. Yeung DK, Wong SY, Griffith JF, Lau EM. Bone marrow diffusion in osteoporosis: evaluation with quantitative MR diffusion imaging. J Magn Reson Imaging 2004;19:222–228
47. Grampp S, Henk CB, Imhof H. CT and MR assessment of osteoporosis. Semin Ultrasound CT MR 1999;20:2–9
48. Baumert B, Blautzik J, Körner M, Reiser M, Linsenmaier U. Advanced imaging of spine disease [in German]. Chirurg 2008;79:906–917
49. Link TM, Imhof H. Introduction to the topic: diagnosis of osteoporosis—a paradigm shift [in German]. Radiologe 2006;46:829–830
50. Green RA, Saifuddin A. Whole spine MRI in the assessment of acute vertebral body trauma. Skeletal Radiol 2004;33:129–135
51. Do HM. Magnetic resonance imaging in the evaluation of patients for percutaneous vertebroplasty. Top Magn Reson Imaging 2000;11: 235–244
52. Qaiyum M, Tyrrell PN, McCall IW, Cassar-Pullicino VN. MRI detection of unsuspected vertebral injury in acute spinal trauma: incidence and significance. Skeletal Radiol 2001;30:299–304
53. Saifuddin A. MRI of acute spinal trauma. Skeletal Radiol 2001;30: 237–246
54. Seffinger MA, Najm WI, Mishra SI, et al. Reliability of spinal palpation for diagnosis of back and neck pain: a systematic review of the literature. Spine 2004;29:E413–E425
55. Voormolen MH, Mali WP, Lohle PN, et al. Percutaneous vertebroplasty compared with optimal pain medication treatment: short-term clinical outcome of patients with subacute or chronic painful osteoporotic vertebral compression fractures. The VERTOS study. AJNR Am J Neuroradiol 2007;28:555–560
56. Yang HL, Wang GL, Niu GQ, et al. Using MRI to determine painful vertebrae to be treated by kyphoplasty in multiple-level vertebral compression fractures: a prospective study. J Int Med Res 2008;36:1056–1063
57. Shih TT, Huang KM, Li YW. Solitary vertebral collapse: distinction between benign and malignant causes using MR patterns. J Magn Reson Imaging 1999;9:635–642
58. Chan JH, Peh WC, Tsui EY, et al. Acute vertebral body compression fractures: discrimination between benign and malignant causes using apparent diffusion coefficients. Br J Radiol 2002;75:207–214
59. Baur A, Stäbler A, Brüning R, et al. Diffusion-weighted MR imaging of bone marrow: differentiation of benign versus pathologic compression fractures. Radiology 1998;207:349–356
60. Galibert P, Deramond H, Rosat P, Le Gars D. Preliminary note on the treatment of vertebral angioma by percutaneous acrylic vertebroplasty [in French]. Neurochirurgie 1987;33:166–168
61. Deramond H, Depriester C, Galibert P, Le Gars D. Percutaneous vertebroplasty with polymethylmethacrylate: technique, indications, and results. Radiol Clin North Am 1998;36:533–546
62. Masala S, Mastrangeli R, Petrella MC, Massari F, Ursone A, Simonetti G. Percutaneous vertebroplasty in 1,253 levels: results and long-term effectiveness in a single centre. Eur Radiol 2009;19:165–171
63. Voggenreiter G. Balloon kyphoplasty is effective in deformity correction of osteoporotic vertebral compression fractures. Spine 2005;30: 2806–2812
64. Wardlaw D, Booone S, Bastian L, Van Meirhaage J. An international multicenter randomized comparison of balloon kyphoplasty and nonsurgical care in patients with acute vertebral body compression fractures. Eur Spine J 2007;16:S16
65. Yang HL, Zhao L, Liu J, et al. Changes of pulmonary function for patients with osteoporotic vertebral compression fractures after kyphoplasty. J Spinal Disord Tech 2007;20:221–225
66. Robinson Y, Tschöke SK, Stahel PF, Kayser R, Heyde CE. Complications and safety aspects of kyphoplasty for osteoporotic vertebral fractures: a prospective follow-up study in 102 consecutive patients. Patient Saf Surg 2008;2:2
67. Grafe IA, Baier M, Nöldge G, et al. Calcium-phosphate and polymethylmethacrylate cement in long-term outcome after kyphoplasty of painful osteoporotic vertebral fractures. Spine 2008;33: 1284–1290
68. Kasperk C, Hillmeier J, Nöldge G, et al. Treatment of painful vertebral fractures by kyphoplasty in patients with primary osteoporosis: a prospective nonrandomized controlled study. J Bone Miner Res 2005;20:604–612
69. Haas H, Amling M, Baier M. Zur Anwendung der Ballon-Kyphoplasty/ Vertebroplastie. Osteologie 2008;17:11–16
70. Kallmes DF, Jensen ME. Percutaneous vertebroplasty. Radiology 2003; 229:27–36
71. Higgins KB, Harten RD, Langrana NA, Reiter MF. Biomechanical effects of unipedicular vertebroplasty on intact vertebrae. Spine 2003; 28:1540–1547, discussion 1548
72. Shindle MK, Gardner MJ, Koob J, Bukata S, Cabin JA, Lane JM. Vertebral height restoration in osteoporotic compression fractures: kyphoplasty balloon tamp is superior to postural correction alone. Osteoporos Int 2006;17:1815–1819
73. Lunt M, O'Neill TW, Felsenberg D, et al; European Prospective Osteoporosis Study Group. Characteristics of a prevalent vertebral deformity predict subsequent vertebral fracture: results from the European Prospective Osteoporosis Study (EPOS). Bone 2003;33:505–513
74. Bouza C, López T, Magro A, Navalpotro L, Amate JM. Efficacy and safety of balloon kyphoplasty in the treatment of vertebral compression fractures: a systematic review. Eur Spine J 2006;15:1050–1067
75. Pflugmacher R, Taylor R, Agarwal A, et al. Balloon kyphoplasty in the treatment of metastatic disease of the spine: a 2-year prospective evaluation. Eur Spine J 2008;17:1042–1048
76. Fourney DR, Schomer DF, Nader R, et al. Percutaneous vertebroplasty and kyphoplasty for painful vertebral body fractures in cancer patients. J Neurosurg 2003;98(1, Suppl):21–30
77. De Negri P, Tirri T, Paternoster G, Modano P. Treatment of painful osteoporotic or traumatic vertebral compression fractures by percutaneous vertebral augmentation procedures: a nonrandomized comparison between vertebroplasty and kyphoplasty. Clin J Pain 2007;23: 425–430
78. Pflugmacher R, Kandziora F, Schröder R, et al. Vertebroplasty and kyphoplasty in osteoporotic fractures of vertebral bodies: a prospective 1-year follow-up analysis [in German]. Rofo 2005;177:1670–1676
79. Grohs JG, Matzner M, Trieb K, Krepler P. Minimal invasive stabilization of osteoporotic vertebral fractures: a prospective nonrandomized comparison of vertebroplasty and balloon kyphoplasty. J Spinal Disord Tech 2005;18:238–242
80. Bohndorf K, Fessl R. Vertebroplasty and kyphoplasty in patients with osteoporotic fractures: secured knowledge and open questions [in German] Radiologe 2006;46:881–892
81. Mathis JM, Ortiz AO, Zoarski GH. Vertebroplasty versus kyphoplasty: a comparison and contrast. AJNR Am J Neuroradiol 2004;25:840–845
82. Jensen ME, McGraw JK, Cardella JF, Hirsch JA. Position statement on percutaneous vertebral augmentation: a consensus statement developed by the American Society of Interventional and Therapeutic Neuroradiology, Society of Interventional Radiology, American Association of Neurological Surgeons/Congress of Neurological Surgeons, and American Society of Spine Radiology. J Vasc Interv Radiol 2007; 18: 325–330
83. Heini PF. The current treatment—a survey of osteoporotic fracture treatment: osteoporotic spine fractures: the spine surgeon's perspective. Osteoporos Int 2005;16(Suppl 2):S85–S92
84. Taylor RS, Fritzell P, Taylor RJ. Balloon kyphoplasty in the management of vertebral compression fractures: an updated systematic review and meta-analysis. Eur Spine J 2007;16:1085–1100
85. Taylor RS, Taylor RJ, Fritzell P. Balloon kyphoplasty and vertebroplasty for vertebral compression fractures: a comparative systematic review of efficacy and safety. Spine 2006;31:2747–2755
86. Stoffel M, Wolf I, Ringel F, Stüer C, Urbach H, Meyer B. Treatment of painful osteoporotic compression and burst fractures using kyphoplasty: a prospective observational design. J Neurosurg Spine 2007; 6:313–319
87. Patel AA, Vaccaro AR, Martyak GG, et al. Neurologic deficit following percutaneous vertebral stabilization. Spine 2007;32: 1728–1734
88. Nöldge G, DaFonseca K, Grafe I, et al. Balloon kyphoplasty in the treatment of back pain [in German]. Radiologe 2006;46:506–512
89. Verlaan JJ, Dhert WJ, Oner FC. Vertebroplasty for burst fractures. J Neurosurg Spine 2005;2:398–399, author reply 399
90. Verlaan JJ, Dhert WJ, Verbout AJ, Oner FC. Balloon vertebroplasty in combination with pedicle screw instrumentation: a novel technique to treat thoracic and lumbar burst fractures. Spine 2005; 30:E73–E79
91. Libicher M, Appelt A, Berger I, et al. The intravertebral vacuum phenomenon as specific sign of osteonecrosis in vertebral compression fractures: results from a radiological and histological study. Eur Radiol 2007;17:2248–2252
92. Maestretti G, Cremer C, Otten P, Jakob RP. Prospective study of standalone balloon kyphoplasty with calcium phosphate cement augmentation in traumatic fractures. Eur Spine J 2007;16:601–610

93. Hato T, Kawahara N, Tomita K, et al. Finite-element analysis on closing-opening correction osteotomy for angular kyphosis of osteoporotic vertebral fractures. J Orthop Sci 2007;12:354–360

94. Daubs MD, Lenke LG, Cheh G, Stobbs G, Bridwell KH. Adult spinal deformity surgery: complications and outcomes in patients over age 60. Spine 2007;32:2238–2244

95. DeWald CJ, Stanley T. Instrumentation-related complications of multilevel fusions for adult spinal deformity patients over age 65: surgical considerations and treatment options in patients with poor bone quality. Spine 2006;31(19, Suppl):S144–S151

96. Kim WJ, Lee ES, Jeon SH, Yalug I. Correction of osteoporotic fracture deformities with global sagittal imbalance. Clin Orthop Relat Res 2006;443:75–93

97. Suk SI, Kim JH, Lee SM, Chung ER, Lee JH. Anterior-posterior surgery versus posterior closing wedge osteotomy in posttraumatic kyphosis with neurologic compromised osteoporotic fracture. Spine 2003;28:2170–2175

98. Cho KJ, Bridwell KH, Lenke LG, Berra A, Baldus C. Comparison of Smith-Petersen versus pedicle subtraction osteotomy for the correction of fixed sagittal imbalance. Spine 2005;30:2030–2037, discussion 2038

99. Kim YJ, Bridwell KH, Lenke LG, Cheh G, Baldus C. Results of lumbar pedicle subtraction osteotomies for fixed sagittal imbalance: a minimum 5-year follow-up study. Spine 2007;32:2189–2197

100. Kurth AA, Pfeilschifter J. Diagnosis and treatment of postmenopausal osteoporosis and osteoporosis in men. German Guidelines Update 2006 [in German] Orthopade 2007;36:683–690, quiz 691

101. Prather H, Watson JO, Gilula LA. Nonoperative management of osteoporotic vertebral compression fractures. Injury 2007;38(Suppl 3):S40–S48

102. Shea B, Bonaiuti D, Iovine R, et al. Cochrane Review on exercise for preventing and treating osteoporosis in postmenopausal women. Eura Medicophys 2004;40:199–209

103. Shea B, Wells G, Cranney A, et al; Osteoporosis Methodology Group; Osteoporosis Research Advisory Group. WITHDRAWN: calcium supplementation on bone loss in postmenopausal women. Cochrane Database Syst Rev 2006;(1):CD004526

104. Fleurence RL, Iglesias CP, Johnson JM. The cost effectiveness of bisphosphonates for the prevention and treatment of osteoporosis: a structured review of the literature. Pharmacoeconomics 2007;25:913–933

105. Ryu KS, Park CK, Kim MK, Kim DH. Single balloon kyphoplasty using far-lateral extrapedicular approach: technical note and preliminary results. J Spinal Disord Tech 2007;20:392–398

106. Boszczyk BM, Bierschneider M, Hauck S, Beisse R, Potulski M, Jaksche H. Transcostovertebral kyphoplasty of the mid and high thoracic spine. Eur Spine J 2005;14:992–999

107. Boszczyk BM, Bierschneider M, Schmid K, Grillhösl A, Robert B, Jaksche H. Microsurgical interlaminary vertebro- and kyphoplasty for severe osteoporotic fractures. J Neurosurg 2004;100(1, Suppl Spine):32–37

108. Boszczyk B, Bierschneider M, Potulski M, Robert B, Vastmans J, Jaksche H. Extended kyphoplasty indications for stabilization of osteoporotic vertebral compression fractures [in German] Unfallchirurg 2002;105:952–957

109. Kang JD, An H, Boden S, Phillips F, Foley K, Abdu W. Cement augmentation of osteoporotic compression fractures and intraoperative navigation: summary statement. Spine 2003;28(15, Suppl):S62–S63

110. Ohnsorge JA, Siebert CH, Schkommodau E, Mahnken AH, Prescher A, Weisskopf M. Minimally-invasive computer-assisted fluoroscopic navigation for kyphoplasty [in German] Z Orthop Ihre Grenzgeb 2005;143:195–203

111. Greene DL, Isaac R, Neuwirth M, Bitan FD. The eggshell technique for prevention of cement leakage during kyphoplasty. J Spinal Disord Tech 2007;20:229–232

112. Belkoff SM, Mathis JM, Erbe EM, Fenton DC. Biomechanical evaluation of a new bone cement for use in vertebroplasty. Spine 2000;25:1061–1064

113. Belkoff SM, Mathis JM, Fenton DC, Scribner RM, Reiley ME, Talmadge K. An ex vivo biomechanical evaluation of an inflatable bone tamp used in the treatment of compression fracture. Spine 2001;26:151–156

114. Bostrom MP, Lane JM. Future directions: augmentation of osteoporotic vertebral bodies. Spine 1997;22(24, Suppl): 38S–42S

115. Tomita S, Molloy S, Jasper LE, Abe M, Belkoff SM. Biomechanical comparison of kyphoplasty with different bone cements. Spine 2004;29:1203–1207

116. Belkoff SM, Maroney M, Fenton DC, Mathis JM. An in vitro biomechanical evaluation of bone cements used in percutaneous vertebroplasty. Bone 1999;25(2, Suppl):23S–26S

117. Belkoff SM, Mathis JM, Deramond H, Jasper LE. An ex vivo biomechanical evaluation of a hydroxyapatite cement for use with kyphoplasty. AJNR Am J Neuroradiol 2001;22:1212–1216

118. Belkoff SM, Mathis JM, Jasper LE. Ex vivo biomechanical comparison of hydroxyapatite and polymethylmethacrylate cements for use with vertebroplasty. AJNR Am J Neuroradiol 2002;23:1647–1651

119. Belkoff SM, Mathis JM, Jasper LE, Deramond H. An ex vivo biomechanical evaluation of a hydroxyapatite cement for use with vertebroplasty. Spine 2001;26:1542–1546

120. Blattert TR, Jestaedt L, Weckbach A. Suitability of a calcium phosphate cement in osteoporotic vertebral body fracture augmentation: a controlled, randomized, clinical trial of balloon kyphoplasty comparing calcium phosphate versus polymethylmethacrylate. Spine 2009;34:108–114

121. Molloy S, Mathis JM, Belkoff SM. The effect of vertebral body percentage fill on mechanical behavior during percutaneous vertebroplasty. Spine 2003;28:1549–1554

122. Cotten A, Dewatre F, Cortet B, et al. Percutaneous vertebroplasty for osteolytic metastases and myeloma: effects of the percentage of lesion filling and the leakage of methyl methacrylate at clinical follow-up. Radiology 1996;200:525–530

123. Jensen ME, Evans AJ, Mathis JM, Kallmes DF, Cloft HJ, Dion JE. Percutaneous polymethylmethacrylate vertebroplasty in the treatment of osteoporotic vertebral body compression fractures: technical aspects. AJNR Am J Neuroradiol 1997;18:1897–1904

124. Uppin AA, Hirsch JA, Centenera LV, Pfiefer BA, Pazianos AG, Choi IS. Occurrence of new vertebral body fracture after percutaneous vertebroplasty in patients with osteoporosis. Radiology 2003;226:119–124

125. Lin EP, Ekholm S, Hiwatashi A, Westesson PL. Vertebroplasty: cement leakage into the disc increases the risk of new fracture of adjacent vertebral body. AJNR Am J Neuroradiol 2004;25:175–180

126. Komemushi A, Tanigawa N, Kariya S, et al. Percutaneous vertebroplasty for osteoporotic compression fracture: multivariate study of predictors of new vertebral body fracture. Cardiovasc Intervent Radiol 2006;29:580–585

127. Fribourg D, Tang C, Sra P, Delamarter R, Bae H. Incidence of subsequent vertebral fracture after kyphoplasty. Spine 2004; 29: 2270–2276, discussion 2277

128. Harrop JS, Prpa B, Reinhardt MK, Lieberman I. Primary and secondary osteoporosis' incidence of subsequent vertebral compression fractures after kyphoplasty. Spine 2004;29:2120–2125

129. Lavelle WF, Cheney R. Recurrent fracture after vertebral kyphoplasty. Spine J 2006;6:488–493

130. Moon ES, Kim HS, Park JO, et al. The incidence of new vertebral compression fractures in women after kyphoplasty and factors involved. Yonsei Med J 2007;48:645–652

131. Sun K, Liebschner MA. Biomechanics of prophylactic vertebral reinforcement. Spine 2004;29:1428–1435, 1435

132. Becker S, Garoscio M, Meissner J, Tuschel A, Ogon M. Is there an indication for prophylactic balloon kyphoplasty? A pilot study. Clin Orthop Relat Res 2007;458:83–89

133. Rotter R, Pflugmacher R, Kandziora F, Ewert A, Duda G, Mittlmeier T. Biomechanical in vitro testing of human osteoporotic lumbar vertebrae following prophylactic kyphoplasty with different candidate materials. Spine 2007;32:1400–1405

134. Hulme PA, Krebs J, Ferguson SJ, Berlemann U. Vertebroplasty and kyphoplasty: a systematic review of 69 clinical studies. Spine 2006;31:1983–2001

135. Chen YJ, Tan TS, Chen WH, Chen CC, Lee TS. Intradural cement leakage: a devastatingly rare complication of vertebroplasty. Spine 2006;31:E379–E382

136. Lee BJ, Lee SR, Yoo TY. Paraplegia as a complication of percutaneous vertebroplasty with polymethylmethacrylate: a case report. Spine 2002;27:E419–E422

137. Becker S, Meissner J, Tuschel A, Chavanne A, Ogon M. Cement leakage into the posterior spinal canal during balloon kyphoplasty: a case report. J Orthop Surg (Hong Kong) 2007;15:222–225

138. Choe DH, Marom EM, Ahrar K, Truong MT, Madewell JE. Pulmonary embolism of polymethyl methacrylate during percutaneous vertebroplasty and kyphoplasty. AJR Am J Roentgenol 2004;183: 1097–1102

139. Jang JS, Lee SH, Jung SK. Pulmonary embolism of polymethylmethacrylate after percutaneous vertebroplasty: a report of three cases. Spine 2002;27:E416–E418

140. François K, Taeymans Y, Poffyn B, Van Nooten G. Successful management of a large pulmonary cement embolus after percutaneous vertebroplasty: a case report. Spine 2003;28:E424–E425

141. Yoo KY, Jeong SW, Yoon W, Lee J. Acute respiratory distress syndrome associated with pulmonary cement embolism following percutaneous vertebroplasty with polymethylmethacrylate. Spine 2004;29:E294–E297

142. Monticelli F, Meyer HJ, Tutsch-Bauer E. Fatal pulmonary cement embolism following percutaneous vertebroplasty (PVP). Forensic Sci Int 2005;149:35–38

143. Garfin SR, Yuan HA, Reiley MA. New technologies in spine: kyphoplasty and vertebroplasty for the treatment of painful osteoporotic compression fractures. Spine 2001;26:1511–1515

144. Wong W, Mathis JM. Vertebroplasty and kyphoplasty: techniques for avoiding complications and pitfalls. Neurosurg Focus 2005;18:e2

145. Jiménez-Mejías ME, de Dios Colmenero J, Sánchez-Lora FJ, et al. Postoperative spondylodiskitis: etiology, clinical findings, prognosis, and comparison with nonoperative pyogenic spondylodiskitis. Clin Infect Dis 1999;29:339–345

146. Nussbaum DA, Gailloud P, Murphy K. A review of complications associated with vertebroplasty and kyphoplasty as reported to the Food and Drug Administration medical device related web site. J Vasc Interv Radiol 2004;15:1185–1192

147. Kallmes DF, Schweickert PA, Marx WF, Jensen ME. Vertebroplasty in the mid- and upper thoracic spine. AJNR Am J Neuroradiol 2002;23:1117–1120

148. Yu SW, Chen WJ, Lin WC, Chen YJ, Tu YK. Serious pyogenic spondylitis following vertebroplasty—a case report. Spine 2004; 29:E209–E211

149. Schmid KE, Boszczyk BM, Bierschneider M, Zarfl A, Robert B, Jaksche H. Spondylitis following vertebroplasty: a case report. Eur Spine J 2005; 14:895–899

150. Walker DH, Mummaneni P, Rodts GE Jr. Infected vertebroplasty: report of two cases and review of the literature. Neurosurg Focus 2004;17:E6

151. Mummaneni PV, Walker DH, Mizuno J, Rodts GE. Infected vertebroplasty requiring 360 degrees spinal reconstruction: long-term follow-up review: report of two cases. J Neurosurg Spine 2006;5:86–89

152. Alfonso Olmos M, Silva González A, Duart Clemente J, Villas Tomé C. Infected vertebroplasty due to uncommon bacteria solved surgically: a rare and threatening life complication of a common procedure: report of a case and a review of the literature. Spine 2006;31: E770–E773

153. Bouvresse S, Chiras J, Bricaire F, Bossi P. Pott's disease occurring after percutaneous vertebroplasty: an unusual illustration of the principle of locus minoris resistentiae. J Infect 2006;53:e251–e253

154. Weisskopf M, Herlein S, Birnbaum K, et al. Kyphoplasty—a new minimally invasive treatment for repositioning and stabilising vertebral bodies. Z Orthop Ihre Grenzgeb 2003; Jul–Aug; 141(4):406–407.

155. Komp M, Ruetten S, Godolias G. Minimally invasive therapy for functionally unstable osteoporotic vertebral kyphoplasty: prospective comparative study of 19 surgically and 17 conservatively treated patients. J. Miner Stoffwechs 2004;1:13–15.

43

Surgical Management of Posttraumatic Kyphosis

Cao Yang and Kirkham B. Wood

Trauma to the spinal cord and column is a devastating injury that often results in an abrupt change in the quality of the patient's life and that of caregivers. Aside from the obvious loss of function and ability to interact with one's environment, many chronic complications often develop over time in this group of patients. One of these complications involves posttraumatic kyphosis (PTK). Despite improved methods for evaluating and managing spinal fractures, late deformities resulting in pain and neural compromise are not uncommon.

This chapter defines PTK and demonstrates how it is evaluated. An evidence-based review of the subject was undertaken to answer the following questions:

1. What are the clinical and radiographic indicators for surgical intervention in posttraumatic kyphosis?
2. What is the most effective surgical method in restoring sagittal alignment in the treatment of posttraumatic kyphosis?

◆ Clinical and Diagnostic Features

PTK is most commonly described as a residual angular deformity in the thoracic, thoracolumbar, and lumbar regions of the spine. The clinical manifestations are usually described as mechanical or neurological. Mechanical sequelae include pain, fatigue, progression of deformity, instability, and sitting or standing balance difficulties. Neurological sequelae include the occurrence of a new or progressive deficit in the presence of a previous stable neurological examination.

Pain is the most common symptom of posttraumatic deformity and is thought to be caused by bony and soft tissue trauma as well as abnormal spine biomechanics.[1,2] Because the vertebral levels both above and below the deformity may secondarily degenerate, patients may also complain of pain remote from the level of kyphosis.

Patients present with a new or increasing neurological deficit for two common reasons: increasing deformity or development of posttraumatic syringomyelia. The development

and/or progression of the deformity can cause a new or worsening neurological deficit via direct compression or tenting of the neural elements. The incidence of posttraumatic syringomyelia is reported to range between 0.3 and 3.2% depending on the authors, with a reported mean of 1.3%.[3]

Plain radiographs are important when evaluating the overall balance of a patient with a PTK. Radiographic analysis begins with standard upright 36-inch anteroposterior and lateral plain radiographs. When evaluating the spine for sagittal alignment, the C7 plumb line (C7PL), on lateral radiographs, should fall through the posterior-superior corner of S1 or between the posterior-superior corner of S1 and the hip joints. This narrow range of "acceptability" for the alignment of the C7PL still allows for an infinite combination of cervical and lumbar lordosis and thoracic kyphosis to achieve balance.[4] Based on the overall sagittal balance, Booth et al[5] divided patients into those with a type I deformity and those with a type II deformity. In type I imbalance, the patient has a segmental deformity wherein a portion of the spine is substantially hyperkyphotic; however, the patient is able to maintain overall sagittal balance by hyperextending segments above and below. A type II imbalance is one in which the regional hyperkyphosis is such that the patient cannot balance by hyperextending segments above and below. Flexion and extension lateral and anteroposterior bending views may be of further use in assessing the flexibility of any spinal deformity. This allows the physician to have an understanding of the potential extent of correction that can be anticipated at the time of surgical intervention. The focal kyphotic deformity is best measured when making a comparison between the superior and inferior end plates of the vertebral bodies above and below the level of the injury.[6] Flexible deformities are characterized by nearly full correction of the deformity on supine hyperextension or prone lateral radiographs and can frequently be treated with proper intraoperative positioning and instrumentation. Rigid, fixed PTK will often require osteotomies or vertebral resection to achieve correction and overall sagittal balance.

Computed tomographic scanning offers additional detailed evaluation of the spinal bony architecture through the use of fine 1- to 3-mm cuts along with sagittal and coronal reconstructions. This allows the visualization of subtle structural abnormalities, especially involving the posterior element bony structures including the facets that are often difficult to visualize on plain radiography. In patients with new-onset neural deficits, computed tomographic scanning after myelography can also be useful in assessing both central and foraminal neural compression.

Magnetic resonance imaging (MRI) is particularly valuable in its ability to visualize spinal soft tissue structures in detail, including the intervertebral disks, the ligamentous structures, the spinal canal, and any neural compression and changes within the parenchyma of the spinal cord.

◆ Treatment

Conservative Treatment

A database search was made between the years 1977 and 2007 under "posttraumatic kyphosis," "posttraumatic spinal deformity," "conservative treatment of," "nonoperative treatment of." Databases searched included PubMed, Ovid, and EBM Reviews. We found no articles dedicated to conservative treatment of thoracolumbar PTK.

Exercise and aerobic conditioning programs may be considered, supplemented with nonsteroidal antiinflammatory regimens and muscle relaxation agents. Although narcotics and other analgesic medicines may be helpful when beginning a program of conservative care, prolonged use is likely to be counterproductive. Most physicians feel bracing is not effective. The quality of this evidence is principally anecdotal and hence very low.

Surgical Considerations

A database search was made between the years 1977 and 2007 under "posttraumatic kyphosis," "posttraumatic spinal deformity," "surgery of," "operative treatment of." Databases searched included PubMed, Ovid, and EBM Reviews. Twenty-three original articles and four review articles on surgical treatment of thoracolumbar PTK were found. Surgical approaches include an all posterior approach, an anterior only approach, a combined anterior/posterior approach, or posterior-based osteotomies. In the presence of a kyphotic deformity, compression of the neural elements is typically anterior, and, therefore, the traditional approach to decompression in these cases has been to use an anterior approach and perform a corpectomy.[7]

Malcolm et al[2] described their experience with combinations of posterior, anterior, or combined procedures for the treatment of PTK in 48 patients with a mixture of neurological deficits. Significant or complete pain relief was seen in 98% of the patients, although the correction obtained averaged only ~30%. The data did not stratify the various surgical approaches and the correction obtained. They concluded that posterior only surgery may be indicated for longer deformities, especially in the thoracic spine where saving levels is not necessarily as critical, or instances in which a formal anterior decompression is not necessary and the deformity is relatively flexible and correctable with positioning.

If the kyphotic pathology is focal/segmental and can be corrected by resection of the anterior and middle column followed

by distraction and anterior reconstruction, an anterior procedure may be the primary procedure. In the report of Kostuik and Matsusaki,[8] 37 patients underwent anterior correction and decompression with instrumentation for late PTK in the lumbar, thoracolumbar, or thoracic spine. Stable arthrodesis with some correction of the deformity was seen in 36 of 37 patients with only one nonunion. Pain was reduced significantly in 78% of the patients. Late neurological improvement of a significant functional degree occurred in three of eight paraparetics. Benli et al[9] presented a retrospective follow-up study of posttraumatic thoracic and lumbar kyphosis after anterior decompression and instrumentation. Pain completely resolved in 92.5% of the patients. Neurological improvement was achieved in all of the patients with neurological deficits or neural claudication. McBride and Bradford[10] treated their population anteriorly with a vascularized rib pedicle graft and femoral neck allograft. All were found to have a solid anterior spine fusion with a 63% mean improvement in preoperative kyphosis. All of these are case series, however, so the quality of this evidence is very low.

Been et al[11] evaluated radiographic findings, patient satisfaction, and clinical outcome after monosegmental surgical treatment using an anterior procedure alone and compared their results with a combined anterior and posterior procedure after burst fractures. Because their radiographic and surgical outcomes were so similar between the two groups, they concluded that in cases of posttraumatic thoracolumbar kyphosis after burst fractures, monosegmental correction using a single approach (anterior) would be the procedure of choice. This is an observational study with control group, yet retrospective and nonrandomized; the quality of the evidence is low.

Correction using the anterior approach, however, may be hindered by ankylosed posterior structures.[12] Chang[13] found all the patients of posttraumatic kyphosis that he studied had healed wedged vertebral bodies and ankylosed posterior spinal structures. He suggested a three-stage approach and oligosegmental correction for posttraumatic thoracolumbar angular kyphosis. The first procedure consisted of posterior osteotomy at the lamina of the wedged vertebra or at the facets placing and planting of posterior the pedicle screw. The second procedure consisted of anterior diskectomies, including the contracted anterior longitudinal ligament through the disk above and below the wedged vertebra back to the posterior longitudinal ligament. In the third procedure, the deformity was corrected by posterior instrumentation. The amount of correction achieved was 37.8 degrees, and pain relief was obtained in all cases. Marré et al[14] also described a variation of the "posterior-anterior-posterior" surgical techniques to correct PTK of the thoracic and lumbar spine. Roberson and Whitesides[15] recommended that the treatment of late posttraumatic thoracolumbar kyphosis should follow basic biomechanical principles, that is, replace the aspect of spinal stability that was compromised, whether anterior, posterior, or both. All these are case series, so the quality of these evidences is very low.

Using osteotomy techniques, a posterior only approach provides access to both anterior and posterior columns through a single incision. One of the first posteriorly based osteotomies for the treatment of PTK was the Smith-Peterson osteotomy. The Smith-Petersen osteotomy (SPO)[16] was described as a monosegmental chevron or V-shaped osteotomy for the lumbar spine in 1945 and since then has been modified by Law and others.[7] It is described as a posterior element resection with osteoclasis of the anterior and middle column.

The technique as it was originally described results in lengthening of the anterior column and shortening of the posterior column, with the middle column functioning as a pivot point. The average correction obtained with a single-level SPO is thought to be 10 to 15 degrees. This maneuver may sometimes result in an anterior column defect requiring anterior column reconstruction.

Recently the pedicle subtraction osteotomy has been shown to be very effective for obtaining significant sagittal deformity correction, all from a posterior approach. Thomasen[17] first published the description of a transpedicular cortical decancellation osteotomy, which is now more commonly referred to as a pedicle subtraction osteotomy. Gertzbein and Harris[18] described a posterior wedge osteotomy, supplemented with compression instrumentation, as being very effective for deformities greater than 30 degrees. Kawahara et al[19] also described a closing–opening wedge osteotomy to correct angular kyphotic deformity by a single posterior approach. Wu et al[20] reported 13 patients with posttraumatic kyphosis treated with posterior decompression and a wedge-shaped osteotomy. The average angle of correction was 38.8 degrees. Lazennec et al[21] evaluated the use of a posterior closing wedge osteotomy at the level of injury by comparing thoracolumbar and lumbar spinal levels. They concluded that posterior closing wedge osteotomy was most efficient for thoracolumbar posttraumatic deformities, failing to adequately restore lordosis at the lower lumbar spine. All these publications are case series; hence the quality of the evidence is very low. Suk et al[22] did compare anterior–posterior surgery with a posterior closing wedge osteotomy in PTK with older neurologically compromised patients with osteoporotic fractures. Although technically demanding, the posterior closing wedge osteotomy procedure demonstrated improved surgical results with significantly less operative time and blood loss. This was an observational study with a control group, but it was non-randomized, restrospective; hence the quality of the evidence is low.

◆ Complications

The potential for neurological injury is increased in the surgical management of posttraumatic kyphosis because of the draping of the neural elements over the anterior vertebral elements, the possible presence of a preexisting spinal cord injury, the possibility of scarring with cord tethering, and the combination of subluxation, residual dorsal impingement, and dural buckling at or near the osteotomy site. Neurological deterioration following corrective surgery for thoracolumbar kyphosis has been reported to be as high as 8%. Spinal cord intraoperative monitoring is extremely useful in detecting any change in neurological function during surgical manipulation.[23]

◆ Evidence-Based Medicine Results

What Are the Clinical and Radiographic Indicators for Surgical Intervention in Posttraumatic Kyphosis?

A database search was done between the years 1977 and 2007 under "posttraumatic kyphosis," "posttraumatic spinal deformity," "surgery of," "operative treatment of." Databases searched included: PubMed, Ovid, and EBM Reviews. Nine

Table 43.1

	Study	No. of Patients	Indication*
1	Malcolm et al (1981)[12]	48	P
2	Benli et al (2007)[9]	40	P. N, D
3	Kossmann and Malham (2005)[24]	8	P, Pr, N
4	Illés et al (2002)[25]	5	P, Pr, N
5	Kostuik and Matsusaki (1989)[8]	37	P, N (s.s.)
6	Chang (1993)[13]	17	P, Pr
7	Lehmer et al (1994)[26]	41	P, D
8	Wu et al (1996)[20]	13	D
9	Ahn et al (2002)[27]	83	D

Abbreviations: P, pain; D, deformity; N, neurology; s.s., spinal stenosis; Pr, progression.

original articles specifically described the indication for surgical intervention in PTK (**Table 43.1**). The most common reported indication for surgery for the treatment of PTK is back pain, followed by increasing neurological deficit and progression of the deformities. Additional less cited indications include radicular pain, pseudarthrosis, and development of late spinal stenosis. All these articles are retrospective case series without control populations (level IV); hence the quality of evidence would be considered very low.

In the 48 patients reported by Malcolm et al,[12] back pain was the most frequent presenting complaint and indication for surgery. Only three patients did not have pain. Twenty-two patients were subjectively aware of an increasing kyphotic deformity. All thoracic deformities were larger than 45 degrees, and the deformity at the thoracolumbar junction ranged from 18 to 72 degrees. In the report of Benli et al,[9] severe pain refractory to conservative treatment, neurological deficit or neural claudication, and the presence of kyphotic deformity over 30 degrees were considered as the indications for surgery. In the study by Kossmann and Malham,[24] indications for surgical correction were incapacitating back pain, progression of kyphotic deformity, persistent neurological deficit, and development of late spinal stenosis. Illés et al[25] suggested that the indications for surgery were incapacitating pain refractory to conservative treatment, progressing kyphosis, and deterioration of the patient's neurological status. Kostuik and Matsusaki[8] reported 37 patients who underwent surgery for late PTK in the lumbar, thoracolumbar, or thoracic spine. All patients presented with pain. Nine patients developed spinal stenosis secondary to their injuries. In the report by Chang,[13] all 17 patients noted progression of their deformities and all presented with low back pain that was progressive in nature and a feeling of constant fatigue that become worse as the day went on. After solid fusion, pain relief was obtained in all cases. In the study by Lehmer et al,[26] the indications for surgery were severe disabling pain and/or severe deformity. Forty-one consecutive patients were treated with single-stage posterior transvertebral closing-wedge osteotomy. Wu et al[20] thought that progressive and persistent kyphosis could impede rehabilitation and lead to increasing neurological deficit and increasing local pain; pressure sores also were more likely to occur. Management goals were decreasing local pain, correction of deformity, stabilization, and improvement of neurological function. Ahn et al[27] performed a prospective clinical trial to study the radiographic parameters and functional outcome in patients undergoing spinal osteotomy to determine whether correction of specific radiographic parameters is associated with improved functional outcome. A significant association was found between outcomes and radiographic correction of coronal and/or sagittal deformity if the postoperative sagittal lordosis (from L1 to S1) was > 25 degrees and if postoperative coronal alignment (measuring the horizontal distance from midsacrum to a gravity plumbline dropped from the center of the C7 vertebral body) was within 2.5 cm.

What Is the Most Effective Surgical Method in Restoring Sagittal Alignment in the Treatment of Post-Traumatic Kyphosis?

A database search was made between the years 1977 and 2007 under "posttraumatic kyphosis," "posttraumatic spinal deformity," "surgery of," "operative treatment of." Databases searched included PubMed, Ovid, and EBM Reviews. Fourteen original articles evaluated the effectiveness of techniques to restore sagittal alignment (**Table 43.2**). Surgical methods include anterior only surgery, posterior only, combined anterior and posterior approaches, and posterior osteotomies. Most of these articles are case series and the quality of the evidence is very low. It must be remembered, however, that due to the complexity and ambiguity of what actually is PTK—its definition, its etiology, and its causes—and that many treatment options exist and different surgeons may well have different experiences and preferences. This should be taken into consideration when reviewing the evidence of the literature. No conclusions can be made based on available evidence for the best surgical treatment of PTK. Prospective randomized studies of PTK simply do not exist to date. To compare different surgical techniques, validated outcome tools should be developed for these patients.

Malcolm et al[12] was the only paper to report results on posterior only surgery for late treatment of PTK. Theirs was a retrospective case series of patients with varying time periods between injury and treatment. Their correction rate was, on average, 30%.

Most authors conclude that an anterior approach could be performed for patients with moderate PTK. In the study by Benli et al,[9] deformity of moderate PTK patients was successfully corrected with anterior decompression, anterior strut grafting, and instrumentation. High correction rates were obtained in their patients with kyphotic angles between 30 and 50 degrees (96.4%); however, in those with deformity between 50 and 80 degrees, lower correction rates were achieved (76.3%). McBride and Bradford[10] described an anterior spine fusion with a vascularized rib pedicle graft and femoral neck allograft providing early stability and maintenance of the kyphosis correction. Preoperative kyphosis ranged from 20 to 83 degrees, with a mean of 36 degrees. At the time of follow-up evaluation, the residual kyphosis ranged from –9 degrees overcorrection to 27 degrees, which represents a mean improvement of 63% or 26 degrees. These are retrospective case series; hence the quality of the evidence would be considered very low.

Been et al[11] did compare an anterior procedure alone with a one-stage combined anterior and posterior procedure for PTK after simple burst fractures. In the patients who underwent an anterior procedure alone, the median kyphosis was corrected from 23 degrees preoperatively to 12 degrees postoperatively and was 11 degrees at follow-up. In the patients who underwent a combined anterior and posterior procedure, median kyphosis was corrected from 21 degrees preoperatively to 12 degrees postoperatively and was 12 degrees at follow-up. Because comparison of surgical correction following anterior only approaches compared with combined one-stage

Table 43.2

	Study	Correction*	Approach†	Level of evidence**
1	Malcolm et al (1981)[12]	30%	Posterior	IV–CS
2	Benli et al (2007)[9]	76–96%	Anterior	IV–CS
3	McBride and Bradford (1983)[10]	65%	Anterior	IV–CS
4	Been et al (2004)[11]	Anterior 55% Anterior-posterior 55%	Anterior v. posterior	III
5	Chang et al (1993)[13]	98%	Anterior-posterior-anterior	IV–CS
6	Böhm et al (1990)[28]	62–73%	Anterior-posterior	IV–CS
7	Lehmer et al (1994)[26]	35 degrees	PCWO	IV–CS
8	Gertzbein and Harris (1992)[18]	34 degrees	PCWO	IV–CS
9	Wu et al (1996)[20]	39 degrees	PCWO	IV–CS
10	Heary and Bono (2006)[29]	51 degrees	PSO	IV–CS
11	Lazennec et al (2006)[21]	88%	PCWO	IV–CS
12	Suk et al (2003)[22]	Anterior-posterior 50% PCWO 75%	Anterior–posterior v. PCWO	III
13	Atici et al (2004)[30]	24 degrees	Anterior, posterior, Anterior-posterior	IV–CS
14	Caceres et al (2006)[31]	27.3 degrees	Anterior-posterior, PCWO	IV–CS

Abbreviations: PCWO, posterior closing wedge osteotomy; PSO, pedicle subtraction osteotomy; CS, case series.

spondylodesis did not reveal significant differences, it was therefore concluded that in cases of posttraumatic thoracolumbar kyphosis after simple type A fractures, monosegmental correction using a single anterior incision would be the surgical procedure of choice. This is an observational study with control groups, yet it is retrospective, nonrandomized, and sequential; hence the quality of the evidence is low.

Many authors feel that in PTK both the anterior and the posterior spinal structures are involved, and therefore the strategy for the correction of an angular kyphosis should be a combined anterior and posterior procedure to achieve lasting correction and secure fusion. Chang[13] described a three-stage approach and oligosegmental fixation, for PTK with an average kyphosis before correction of 39 degrees. After correction, the kyphosis measured on average, 1.2 degrees, a change of 37.8 degrees. Bone union of the osteotomy or diskectomy was obtained at 1-year follow-up in all cases. After solid fusion, the kyphosis had a mean value of 2.3 degrees. Bohm et al[28] used both segmental posterior transpedicular as well as ventrolateral instrumentation with a 3- to 5-year follow-up period of 40 patients. The amount of correction achieved was 22.5 degrees postoperatively and 21.5 degrees after solid fusion. Percentage correction in the thoracic spine was 62% and 73% in the thoracolumbar and lumbar regions. Atici et al[30] and Caceres et al[31] also presented reports of a mixture of surgical approaches—anterior, posterior, and combined, without direct comparisons—and corrections of 24 degrees and 27.3 degrees, respectively. All these are case series, and the quality of the evidence is very low.

The development of osteotomy techniques has advanced our ability to treat many kinds of spinal deformities, including PTK. Although Smith-Peterson osteotomies were the first to be used for PTK, the current literature in terms of radiographic correction is limited to pedicle subtraction osteotomies (PSOs). PSOs represent a shift away from simple compression/distraction or cantilever maneuvers as a means of realigning the spine in favor of partial vertebral column resection.

Lehmer et al[26] performed single-stage posterior transvertebral closing-wedge osteotomy for treatment of adult thoracolumbar kyphosis with an average correction of 35 degrees obtained at each osteotomy site. Gertzbein and Harris[18] performed closing dorsal wedge osteotomies in three cases with an average correction of 34.3 degrees (30 to 40 degrees). Wu et al,[20] using a posterior decancellation procedure, achieved solid fusion in all 13 patients, with an average correction of 38.8 degrees, and reported no neural injury. Heary and Bono[29] described using pedicle subtraction osteotomy in the treatment of three patients with severe, posttraumatic spinal deformities. A mean of 51 degrees of sagittal plane correction was achieved and maintained at the final follow-up of 2 years. In the experience of Lazennec et al,[21] monosegmental posterior closing wedge osteotomy for the treatment of short-angled PTK is a technically demanding procedure; however, they were able to achieve correction rates averaging 88%. All these are retrospective case series, and the quality of this evidence is very low.

Suk et al[22] reported a comparative study of the surgical results of combined anterior-posterior procedures and posterior closing wedge osteotomy procedures in patients with PTK. In the combined anterior-posterior group, mean kyphosis was 22.2 degrees before surgery, 6.8 degrees after surgery, and 11.0 degrees at final follow-up. At final follow-up, there was 11.2 degrees of correction in kyphosis compared with that before surgery, but a 27% loss of correction compared

with that at the initial postoperative radiograph. In the posterior closing wedge osteotomy group, mean kyphosis was 34.1 degrees before surgery, 5.3 degrees after surgery, and 8.4 degrees at final follow-up. At final follow-up, there was 25.7 degrees of correction in kyphosis compared with that before surgery—larger than that seen with the combined procedure—but still an 11% loss of correction compared with that at the initial postoperative radiograph. The preoperative kyphosis and correction magnitude were significantly larger in posterior closing wedge osteotomy group, and the authors concluded that, although it was technically demanding, the posterior closing wedge osteotomy procedure allowed more reliably restored sagittal alignment. This article is an observational study with control groups (level III); however, the population was elderly and the etiology of the fractures related to osteoporosis. The quality of evidence of this retrospective study must nonetheless still be considered low.

◆ Recommendations

What Are the Clinical and Radiographic Indicators for Surgical Intervention in Posttraumatic Kyphosis?

Pain appears to be the most common clinical symptom of PTK. Additional acceptable clinical indications are associated neurological deficits and progressive deformity. There seems to be no agreement among authors on the amount of deformity, which should be seen as an indication for surgery.

What Is the Most Effective Surgical Method in Restoring Sagittal Alignment in the Treatment of Posttraumatic Kyphosis?

The evidence is only a weak recommendation that any one technique is superior to the other. By the consensus opinion of the Spine Trauma Study Group, a strong (> 75% consensus) recommendation can be made that a posterior pedicle subtraction-type osteotomy is superior to other approaches.

References

1. Vaccaro AR, Silber JS. Post-traumatic spinal deformity. Spine 2001;26(24, Suppl):S111–S118
2. Malcolm BW, Bradford DS, Winter RB, Chou SN. Post-traumatic kyphosis: a review of forty-eight surgically treated patients. J Bone Joint Surg Am 1981;63:891–899
3. Carroll AM, Brackenridge P. Post-traumatic syringomyelia: a review of the cases presenting in a regional spinal injuries unit in the north east of England over a 5-year period. Spine 2005;30:1206–1210
4. Macagno AE, O'Brien MF. Thoracic and thoracolumbar kyphosis in adults. Spine 2006;31(19, Suppl):S161–S170
5. Booth KC, Bridwell KH, Lenke LG, Baldus CR, Blanke KM. Complications and predictive factors for the successful treatment of flatback deformity (fixed sagittal imbalance). Spine 1999;24:1712–1720
6. Kuklo TR, Polly DW, Owens BD, Zeidman SM, Chang AS, Klemme WR. Measurement of thoracic and lumbar fracture kyphosis: evaluation of intraobserver, interobserver, and technique variability. Spine 2001;26: 61–65, discussion 66
7. Buchowski JM, Kuhns CA, Bridwell KH, Lenke LG. Surgical management of posttraumatic thoracolumbar kyphosis. Spine J 2008;8:666–667
8. Kostuik JP, Matsusaki H. Anterior stabilization, instrumentation, and decompression for post-traumatic kyphosis. Spine 1989;14:379–386
9. Benli IT, Kaya A, Uruç V, Akalin S. Minimum 5-year follow-up surgical results of post-traumatic thoracic and lumbar kyphosis treated with anterior instrumentation: comparison of anterior plate and dual rod systems. Spine 2007;32:986–994

10. McBride GG, Bradford DS. Vertebral body replacement with femoral neck allograft and vascularized rib strut graft: a technique for treating post-traumatic kyphosis with neurologic deficit. Spine 1983;8:406–415

11. Been HD, Poolman RW, Ubags LH. Clinical outcome and radiographic results after surgical treatment of post-traumatic thoracolumbar kyphosis following simple type A fractures. Eur Spine J 2004;13:101–107

12. Malcolm BW, Bradford DS, Winter RB, Chou SN. Post-traumatic kyphosis: a review of forty-eight surgically treated patients. J Bone Joint Surg Am 1981;63:891–899

13. Chang KW. Oligosegmental correction of post-traumatic thoracolumbar angular kyphosis. Spine 1993;18:1909–1915

14. Marré B. Management of posttraumatic kyphosis: surgical technique to facilitate a combined approach. Injury 2005;36(Suppl 2):B73–B81

15. Roberson JR, Whitesides TE Jr. Surgical reconstruction of late post-traumatic thoracolumbar kyphosis. Spine 1985;10:307–312

16. Smith-Petersen MN, Larson CB, Aufranc OE. Osteotomy of the spine for correction of flexion deformity in rheumatoid arthritis. Clin Orthop Relat Res 1969;66:6–9

17. Thomasen E. Vertebral osteotomy for correction of kyphosis in ankylosing spondylitis. Clin Orthop Relat Res 1985;194:142–152

18. Gertzbein SD, Harris MB. Wedge osteotomy for the correction of post-traumatic kyphosis: a new technique and a report of three cases. Spine 1992;17:374–379

19. Kawahara N, Tomita K, Baba H, Kobayashi T, Fujita T, Murakami H. Closing-opening wedge osteotomy to correct angular kyphotic deformity by a single posterior approach. Spine 2001;26:391–402

20. Wu SS, Hwa SY, Lin LC, Pai WM, Chen PQ, Au MK. Management of rigid post-traumatic kyphosis. Spine 1996;21:2260–2266, discussion 2267

21. Lazennec JY, Neves N, Rousseau MA, Boyer P, Pascal-Mousselard H, Saillant G. Wedge osteotomy for treating post-traumatic kyphosis at thoracolumbar and lumbar levels. J Spinal Disord Tech 2006;19: 487–494

22. Suk SI, Kim JH, Lee SM, Chung ER, Lee JH. Anterior-posterior surgery versus posterior closing wedge osteotomy in posttraumatic kyphosis with neurologic compromised osteoporotic fracture. Spine 2003; 28:2170–2175

23. Connelly PJ, Abitbol JJ, Martin RJ, et al. Spine: trauma. In: Garfin SR, Vaccaro AR, eds. Orthopaedic Knowledge Update: Spine. Rosemont, IL: American Academy of Orthopaedic Surgeons; 1997:197–217

24. Kossmann TK, Malham GM. Correction of post-traumatic kyphosis using three-stage approach. J Bone Joint Surg Br 2005;87-B:297

25. Illés T, de Jonge T, Domán I, Dóczi T. Surgical correction of the late consequences of posttraumatic spinal disorders. J Spinal Disord Tech 2002; 15:127–132

26. Lehmer SM, Keppler L, Biscup RS, Enker P, Miller SD, Steffee AD. Posterior transvertebral osteotomy for adult thoracolumbar kyphosis. Spine 1994;19:2060–2067

27. Ahn UM, Ahn NU, Buchowski JM, et al. Functional outcome and radiographic correction after spinal osteotomy. Spine 2002;27:1303–1311

28. Böhm H, Harms J, Donk R, Zielke K. Correction and stabilization of angular kyphosis. Clin Orthop Relat Res 1990;(258):56–61

29. Heary RF, Bono CM. Pedicle subtraction osteotomy in the treatment of chronic, posttraumatic kyphotic deformity. J Neurosurg Spine 2006; 5:1–8

30. Atici T, Aydinli U, Akesen B, Serifoğlu R. Results of surgical treatment for kyphotic deformity of the spine secondary to trauma or Scheuermann's disease. Acta Orthop Belg 2004;70:344–348

31. Caceres E, Ubierna MT, Garcia de Frutos A, et al. Surgical treatment of posttraumatic kyphosis. J Bone Joint Surg Br 2006;88(Supplement I):149

44

The Role of Surgery in Traumatic Conus Medullaris and Cauda Equina Injuries

Ory Keynan and Marcel F. Dvorak

In contradistinction to the vast body of literature available regarding treatment options in thoracic and lumbar spinal cord trauma in general, little has been published regarding the specific case of conus medullaris injuries (CMIs) and cauda equina injuries (CEIs). This is somewhat surprising given not only the unique neurological anatomy at the L1 level, which is often the location of the termination of the spinal cord, but also surprising because there is a predilection for injuries to occur at the junction of the termination of the rib cage and the upper lumbar spine precisely where the distal spinal cord, conus medullaris, and cauda equina coexist.

When trying to practice evidence-based medicine in treating traumatic conus medullaris or cauda equina injuries, the clinician has to consider the uniqueness and individual variability of the neuroanatomy of this region of the spine. Within several spinal motion segments lay not only multiple nerve roots, but the lumbosacral enlargement of the spinal cord, the conus medullaris, and the cauda equina, including the filum terminale (**Fig. 44.1**). At the level of the thoracic spinal cord (generally accepted to be between the T2 and T11 vertebral levels) the nerve roots exit the spinal canal in a generally

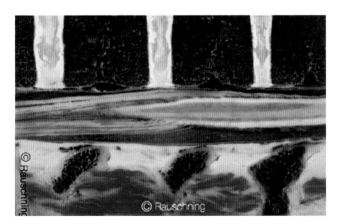

Fig. 44.1 Anatomy of the conus medullaris, cauda equina, and lower thoracic spinal cord. (Courtesy of Professor Wolfgang Rauschning.)

transverse or horizontal direction with only minimal obliquity in their course toward their respective neural foraminae. This anatomical arrangement changes at the termination of the spinal cord, which most commonly occurs at the middle third of L1 but may occur anywhere from T11 to L3.[1,2]

Although injuries to the thoracic spinal cord have been thoroughly studied and produce a relatively predictable pattern of clinical manifestations, injuries to the conus medullaris or cauda equina are thought to present with a more variable expression of their initial neurological deficit and are also thought to have greater potential for neurological improvement.[3–6] This region is functionally significant in that it provides motor and sensory function to the lower extremities, bowel, bladder, and sexual organs. The conus and cauda also mediate the sacral parasympathetic, lumbar sympathetic, and sacral somatic nerves. The conus medullaris contains all of the sacral α motor neurons and interneurons, but adjacent to the conus, at the same segment of the spinal canal, we also find all the lumbar nerve roots. Thus an injury to this region of the spinal column can result in different combinations of injury to upper motor neurons and lower motor neurons.

The complex anatomy of this region has not been adequately appreciated in the spinal surgical literature. Specifically, thoracolumbar spinal cord injuries are often described in aggregation, combining thoracic spinal cord and lower lumbar cauda equina injuries. This makes it difficult to uncover the specific evidence applicable to injuries to the variety of neurological structures in this specific region of the spine.

The clinical manifestation of acute traumatic conus medullaris syndrome (**Fig. 44.2**) can therefore present with varying degrees of lower extremity weakness, patchy loss of sensation, particularly in the saddle or perineal region, and bowel incontinence. Urinary retention, with subsequent overflow incontinence, is also commonly seen. Cauda equina lesions (**Fig. 44.3**) are technically always lower motor neuron injuries with diminished lower extremity muscle tone, absent deep tendon or bulbocavernosus reflexes, and a flaccid urinary bladder.[7] High conus lesions, sometimes referred

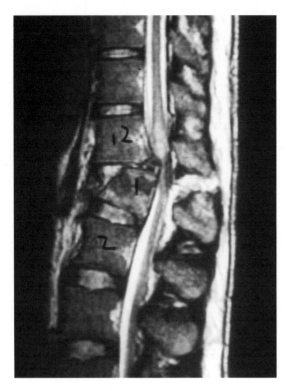

Fig. 44.2 Thirty-six-year-old male with a T12–L1 fracture dislocation. The T2 sagittal magnetic resonance imaging scan shows not only the compression of the conus medullaris but also the significant posterior ligament injury.

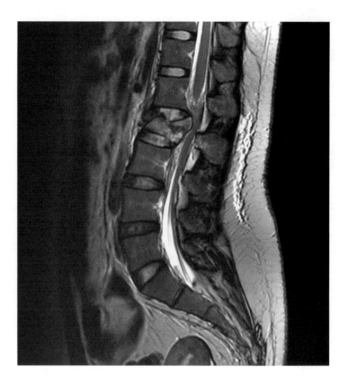

Fig. 44.3 Sagittal T2 magnetic resonance imaging scan of an L2 burst fracture with compression of the cauda equina just below the tip of the conus medullaris.

to as the epiconus, may have upper motor neuron findings mixed with lower motor neuron findings.

As the subject of this chapter, we have chosen the systematic review methodology to address the following question: What is the optimal treatment, with respect to neurological recovery, for a thoracolumbar spinal column fracture with conus medullaris injury (CMI) and with cauda equina injury (CEI)? For the reasons stated earlier, we believe that this is a unique region of the spinal neural axis and requires discrete study.

◆ Injury Types

A variety of injury patterns can lead to neurological injury to the conus medullaris and cauda equina. The most common morphological categories of spinal column injury, according to the Thoracolumbar Injury Classification and Severity Score (TLICS) classification,[8] that result in neurological injury are burst fractures and rotation/translation injuries (also known as fracture-dislocations). These injuries are often associated with disruption of the posterior ligamentous complex (PLC), further adding to their instability. The transition between the stiff thoracic spine and the mobile lumbar spine creates a region that is prone to injury and likely accounts for the disproportionate number of injuries to the thoracolumbar region.

◆ Surgical Approaches

There are essentially two major decisions to be made by the treating physician: (1) first, and most fundamentally, should the patient be treated operatively or nonoperatively? and (2)

if surgery is to be selected, what approach and technique should be used. Nonoperative care may involve lengthy periods of bed rest,[9] the use of a thoracolumbosacral orthosis (TLSO), body cast, hyperextension brace, or no orthosis at all,[10] whereas operative treatment may involve anterior surgery alone, posterior surgery alone, or a combination of both.[3,11–21] The posterior surgical fixation options include hook or wire constructs, short-segment pedicle screw fixation at one level above and one below the fractured vertebra, and long-segment fixation, characteristically two or three segments of fixation above and below the fracture.[3,12,21–24] When the anterior column of the spine is surgically reconstructed, the vertebral body and disks may be approached indirectly through transpedicular bone or by an indirect posterolateral approach.[14,25] A direct anterior approach facilitates vertebral body resection, decompression of the anterior spinal canal, and anterior reconstruction of the vertebra, and may be supplemented by either anterior fixation with plates or screw–rod constructs[19,26,27] or with subsequent posterior instrumentation.[11,15] Prosthetic devices (fixed and expanding cages) as well as autograft and allograft are the most commonly used anterior vertebral reconstruction options.[28]

Beyond simply the surgical approach is the ultimate goal of surgery; is it simply to stabilize a mechanically unstable fracture or does it include also the decompression of the spinal canal? Is this decompression to be performed indirectly through the realignment of the fracture fragments or by direct removal of retropulsed fragments from the spinal canal through either an anterior or posterolateral approach? Superimposed on these goals of intervention are the variety of surgical approaches and reconstruction techniques available to achieve them.

◆ Literature Review

Included in the systematic review were studies dealing with adult patients (age >16 years) with thoracolumbar fractures between T10 and L2 inclusive, with clinical syndromes of conus medullaris and cauda equina injury, treated nonoperatively, or operatively utilizing anterior, posterior, or a combined surgical approach. The study had to specify immediate pre- and posttreatment neurological state, specifying the presence of conus medullaris or cauda equina injury, as well as the specific treatment method utilized.

A comprehensive literature search was performed to identify potential studies, including any article with an English language abstract. Electronic database searches of MEDLINE (1966 to January 2008) and EMBASE (1980 to January 2008) were performed using both medical subject headings (MeSH) and text word searching. Terms used included "fracture," "thoracic," "lumbar," "thoracolumbar," "spine fractures," "fracture fixation–internal," "conus medullaris," "cauda equina," "spinal cord injury."

Both the Database of Abstracts of Reviews of Effects and the Cochrane Database of Systematic Reviews were searched using text words. Reference lists from relevant articles were hand searched for additional citations. Content experts from the Spine Trauma Study Group were sought and questioned as to possible additional references. The scientific literature was then graded and recommendations were made based on the American Thoracic Society guidelines.[29]

Studies meeting the inclusion criteria were screened and analyzed for methodological quality by two independent reviewers (the authors) that performed the selection of studies, methodological quality assessment, and data extraction. Results at each stage were compared, and discrepancies were resolved by consensus between the two authors.

◆ Results

The literature search performed in January 2008 revealed 254 papers of potential relevance. The study selection process eliminated 216 papers by a review of the abstracts alone. An additional 30 papers were excluded after a review of their methodology and results sections. Most of these were excluded due to relevance and methodological issues. This left a total of eight papers that met all inclusion criteria. Of these eight papers, only one study looked directly at CMI, and none looked specifically at traumatic CEI.

◆ Discussion and Recommendations

There is experimental animal data that have shown the benefit of decompression of the cord in promoting neural recovery following spinal cord injury (SCI).[30–35] Several moderate, low, and very low quality studies have also addressed the role of decompression in spinal cord injuries.[36–40] These studies are not specific to CMI and CEI and are the subject of other chapters in this textbook. The published literature specific to CMI and CEI is typically a low-quality mix of studies reporting on the outcomes of therapeutic alternatives for thoracic and lumbar injuries with various degrees of spinal cord and nerve root injury, with a rare specific reference to CMI or CEI. This comprehensive literature search revealed only low and very low quality studies looking indirectly at neurological

outcome after injuries to the neural elements contained between T11 and L2.

Operative or Nonoperative Treatment (Table 44.1)

In their systematic review, which we have classified as low quality, Boerger et al[41] included all papers reporting on burst fractures at T12, L1, and L2, with at least 10 cases in the aforementioned anatomical range, and specification of neurological assessment before and after treatment. Of the 12 studies giving precise neurological details before and after treatment for each patient, nine consistently evaluated neurological status using the Frankel grading system. The results from these studies were pooled, initially including and then also excluding all Frankel grade E patients. Looking at operative versus nonoperative treatment, the overall figures for neurological improvement showed a weak trend toward improved recovery in the nonsurgical group. Surgical approach and surgical implants used were not sufficiently consistent from one paper to another to allow pooling of results in terms of surgical approach or technique. The authors of this study very clearly state their bias toward nonsurgical treatment. The conclusions drawn from this qualitative systematic review are compromised by the poor quality of reporting of neurological outcomes, lack of standardized description of the treatments, and their efficacy in the papers available for this review. Nevertheless, the conclusion that nonsurgical treatment is a viable alternative with respect to neurological outcome is generally supported by this and other studies.[5,41–43]

In a very low quality study looking at a cohort of patients with thoracolumbar fractures and incomplete neurological deficit, McAfee et al[18] compared the results of anterior decompression through a retroperitoneal approach, to historical controls. The data from several centers were pooled, and 48 patients treated over an 8-year period were reviewed. The main indication for surgery was incomplete neurological injury with radiographically demonstrated neural compression. Of interest to our purposes, 16 of these patients had pure cauda equina deficit, two had a conus medullaris injury, and 30 had both. Of the 32 patients with CMI, 12 recovered normal bowel and bladder function. No association between time to decompression and neural recovery was found. All patients with CEI improved neurologically by at least one motor grade. The authors concluded that anterior decompression through a retroperitoneal approach yields better neurological recovery than previously reported techniques that do not decompress the canal. This paper[18] and a similar publication by Transfeldt et al[44] as well as one by Maiman et al[45] all support the efficacy of anterior decompression even when it is not performed acutely or early in the patient's initial treatment. These papers suggest that persistent neurological element compression may prevent maximal neurological recovery and may be relieved by anterior decompression with a concomitant improvement in neurological function.

In a small prospective low-quality study (downgraded from moderate quality because of problems with subgroup analysis and small patient numbers) looking at recovery patterns in burst fractures at T12 and L1, Dall and Stauffer[46] divided 14 consecutive patients into three groups: nonoperative treatment, posterior fusion, and anterior decompression followed by posterior fusion. All had incomplete neurological deficit and greater than 30% canal occlusion.

Table 44.1 References in which the Primary Conclusion or a Major Component of the Conclusion Relates to the Decision to Treat These Injuries Surgically or Nonoperatively

Study	Primary Question Study Type	No. of Subjects	Study Question	Summary	Quality of Evidence
Boerger et al (2000)[41]	Literature review (qualitative systematic review)		Compared operative and nonoperative reported neurological improvement in 60 published studies.	There is no difference in neurological outcome between surgically and nonoperatively treated thoracolumbar fractures	Low
McAfee et al (1985)[18]	Retrospective comparative	48	Neurological recovery following anterior retroperitoneal vertebral resection.	Anterior decompression improves neurological recovery when compared with historical controls	Low
Dall and Stauffer (1988)[46]	Retrospective comparative	14	Compared neurological recovery in nonoperative, posterior fusion and anterior combined with posterior surgery	No difference in various treatments	Very low
Dendrinos et al (1995)[47]	Retrospective case series	63	Compared neurological recovery in nonoperative and surgical patients	No difference in various treatments	Very low
Kim et al (1999)[48]	Retrospective case series	148	Compared neurological recovery in nonoperative, anterior and posterior surgery	No difference in various treatments	Very low
Lifeso et al (1985)[49]	Prospectively collected case series	98	Compared neurological recovery in nonoperative and surgical patients	No difference overall; however, those with demonstrated effective decompression had improved neurological recovery	Very low

Initial analysis of the patients with conus lesions demonstrated that only 6/14 had a functioning bladder. By 1 year postsurgery 11/14 had recovered bladder function. The recovery of neurology did not correlate with the treatment (operative or nonoperative) utilized.

Dendrinos et al[47] focused on the neurological recovery of a group of 63 patients with thoracolumbar injuries and associated neurological injury in this very low quality study. There was no correlation between neurological recovery and nonoperative or surgical treatment (with or without decompression).

Kim et al,[48] in a very low quality retrospective review of 148 consecutive burst fractures, recorded the neurology as complete in 23 and incomplete in 48. The level of injury was described as epiconus, CMI, and CEI, and the treatment varied between nonsurgical, anterior, and posterior surgery. Neither the degree of canal compromise nor the effectiveness of decompression or the treatment technique correlated with neurological recovery in this large retrospective, observational study.

Lifeso et al,[49] in a low-quality prospective study of 98 consecutive patients with neurological impairment and TL trauma, identified no difference in neurological outcome between those treated surgically (Harrington rods) and those treated nonoperatively. In a subgroup analysis, those who had demonstrated adequate decompression of the spinal canal exhibited improved neurological recovery. This is one of the few studies that attempted to confirm that the surgical goals were actually achieved.

There are several authors[5,42,50,51] who have suggested that surgically treated patients benefit from shorter hospital stays and earlier participation in active rehabilitation. This potential advantage must factor in the issues of patient preference, caregiver (surgeon and allied health care team) familiarity, and the complication rates and risks of both surgical and nonsurgical treatment.

Finally, it is worthwhile reviewing the results of a population-based study by Daniels et al.[52] By reviewing national US data, these authors found that of all patients who suffer a thoracolumbar fracture with neurological injury, only 61.4% of them are treated surgically. Even in the highest-volume centers the proportion of neurologically injured patients with thoracolumbar trauma that receive surgical treatment only rises to about two thirds. In the United States, it appears as if nonsurgical treatment for thoracolumbar trauma with associated CMI, CEI, or SCI is still a frequently utilized treatment technique.

Choice of Surgical Approach, Need for Direct Decompression, and Timing of Surgery (Table 44.2)

In a low-quality study, Bradford and McBride[14] retrospectively reviewed patients treated for thoracic and lumbar spine fractures having incomplete neurological deficits over a 12-year period at the authors' institution. Two groups were identified and compared: the first group were those treated by decompression and posterolateral fusion (group 1) and the second; by anterior decompression and fusion (group 2). In all, 59 patients were identified—39 treated by posterior approach and 20 by an anterior approach. In group 1, 24 suffered CMI and 13 CEI, whereas

Table 44.2 References in which the Primary Conclusion or a Major Component of the Conclusion Relates to the Choice of Surgical Approach, Technique of Decompression, or Timing of Surgery

Study	Primary Question Study Type	No. of Subjects	Study Question	Summary	Quality of Evidence
Bradford and McBride (1987)[14]	Retrospective comparative case series	98	Compared neurological recovery in nonoperative and surgical	No difference overall; however, those with demonstrated effective decompression had improved neurological recovery	Low
Hu et al (1993)[53]	Retrospective comparative case series	69	Compared anterior decompression posterior decompression with posterior fusion alone	Decompression, performed either anteriorly or posteriorly may improve motor recovery	Low
Lemons et al (1992)[54]	Case series	22	Studied posterior fusion with and without posterolateral decompression	No neurological benefit to decompression and significant increased morbidity	Very low
Rahimi-Movaghar et al (2006)[55]	Case series	24	Reported on posterolateral decompression and fusion in CMI	Quantified neurological recovery. Bladder function improved in 63%, neurological improvement in 41% overall	Very low
Boriani et al (2000)[13]	Case series	101	Reported on early posterior stabilization with selective anterior decompression when necessary	Neurological recovery was better in CMI and CEI than in spinal cord injury	Very low
Kaneda et al (1997)[27]	Case series	150	Reported on the results of anterior decompression and stabilization	Reported that 95% improved neurologically and 86% returned to work	Very low
Gaebler et al (1999)[56]	Case series	88	Reviewed short-segment posterior stabilization performed at various time intervals	Suggested that early surgery within < 8 hours may improve neurological outcome	Very low
Clohisy et al (1992)[26]	Retrospective case series	20	Compared early decompression (< 48 hours) with late decompression (average 61 days)	Early surgery patients may have improved motor recovery though no difference in bowel or bladder return	Very low

Abbreviations: CEI, cauda equina injury; CMI, conus medullaris injury.

in group 2, nine sustained CMI and four CEI. Neurological improvement in the CMI patients treated by posterior decompression and fusion was not found to be significantly different from patients treated by anterior decompression and fusion in terms of motor strength. When CMI patients were compared concerning bowel and bladder control, however, there was a highly significant difference in the rates of recovery between group 1 (11.7%) and group 2 (70%) ($p = 0.0004$). The number of patients with CEI was not high enough to make meaningful comparisons.

In another low-quality study comparing anterior and posterior decompression and fusion for lumbar fractures with incomplete neurological injury, Hu et al retrospectively reviewed 69 such patients treated over a 9-year period in one center.[53] Three treatment groups were identified: anterior vertebrectomy, posterolateral decompression, and posterior fusion only. The average initial ASIA Motor Score (American Spinal Injury Association) (AMS) was similar among the three groups. Looking specifically at the CMI and CEI, the authors noted patients who had decompression averaged 7.7 points of motor score improvement, whereas those who only had fusion averaged 4.6 points of improvement. A similar trend was noted for the entire study population, but the CEI group

consisted of only 33 patients; not large enough to reach statistical significance. No difference in neurological outcome was found between those patients who underwent anterior decompression versus those decompressed posteriorly. Likely the lack of consistent results regarding neurological improvement with varying surgical approaches and techniques in these studies is due, in part, to the multiple variables that are uncontrolled and will influence neurological recovery, a significant selection bias in choosing various treatments in these uncontrolled studies, and inadequate power to determine either superiority or even equivalence, particularly apparent when one looks at the wide disparity in potential for neurological recovery in this patient population.

Lemons et al,[54] in a low-quality study that reported on a series of 22 consecutive patients, failed to show any benefit to the addition of a posterolateral direct decompression to a posterior stabilization alone. The addition of a posterolateral decompression was associated with increased blood loss, operative time, and iatrogenic instability without any demonstrable benefit to the patients' neurology. This underpowered study likely suffers from type II statistical error.

The only study that specifically addresses only conus medullaris injury is the one by Rahimi-Movaghar et al.[55] In this retrospective review, the authors looked at a subset of patients with radiographically documented CMI attributable to an acute, nonpenetrating trauma with more than 6 months of follow-up. Twenty-four patients were reviewed. Sixty-six percent were neurologically complete (Frankel A) below the level of injury. All underwent posterior decompression and posterolateral segmental fusion. Overall, some degree of neurological recovery was seen in 41.6% of the patients; with an average improvement of 1.5 Frankel grades and an average motor score improvement of 15 points following surgery. Bladder function improvement was seen in 63.6%. Root recovery was seen in 83% of the patients. The lack of control group, the retrospective nature of the study, and its small population size downgrade it from a low quality to a very low quality study. Despite these limitations, this and other studies do confirm the safety and good results that can be achieved with a posterior alone surgical approach in the patient with a CMI and a concomitant fracture.

Boriani et al[13] reported on a cohort of 101 patients, 49 of which had neurological injury. This very low quality study differentiated between cord, cauda, and conus injuries, and noted that the neurological improvement in those with CMI and CEI was much more favorable than the recovery of those with an SCI. These authors favored early posterior stabilization with secondary anterior vertebrectomy when indicated by the stability of the injury.

In the largest published very low quality study looking at the functional outcome of anterior decompression and stabilization of thoracolumbar burst fractures with associated neurological deficits, Kaneda et al[27] retrospectively reviewed 150 patients treated at a single center over an 8-year period. All patients underwent anterior decompression and stabilization with the Kaneda device through an extrapleural and retroperitoneal approach. Preoperative neurological assessment demonstrated 13 patients with pure CMI, 33 patients with mixed CMI/CEI, and 69 patients with CEI or isolated nerve root injury. Neurological recovery of at least one grade occurred in 95% of the patients. The difference between preoperative and postoperative motor scores was larger for the group that had a lesion of the spinal cord than for the group that had a lesion of the cauda equina ($p < 0.01$), but the final score was higher for the group with CEI. No association could be found between timing of surgical decompression and degree of neurological recovery. Remarkable in this study is that nearly three quarters of patients had complete neurological recovery, and 86% returned to work following this severe spinal column and spinal cord injury. The results of this study have not been duplicated.

In a retrospective, very low quality study, Gaebler et al[56] suggested that early posterolateral decompression and short segment fusion led to improved neurological results when compared with similar surgery performed at a longer interval from the time of injury. A significant selection bias (patients who present early are operated on early) clouds the results of this study.

In a more recent, very low quality study reviewing the neurological recovery associated with anterior decompression of thoracolumbar fractures with incomplete neurological deficit, Clohisy et al[26] looked at timing of the decompression. The authors retrospectively reviewed 20 patients treated by anterior decompression in a single center over a 9-year period. Eleven patients were treated within 48 hours of injury (nine of them with CMI), and nine patients at an average of 61 days after the

injury (six of them with CMI). When comparing rates of bowel and bladder functional recovery, there was not a statistically significant difference between the groups. When looking at mean motor score improvement, group A had a statistically significant mean motor point improvement, when compared with group B. This conclusion is fraught with type I or α statistical error; that is, due to the small sample size, the "significant" motor score difference is likely due to chance or selection bias alone.

◆ Summary

There are multiple inconsistencies in the literature we have reviewed. First of all, there are problems in defining the neurological structures that are injured because no studies report on or account for the variable location of the conus medullaris within the spinal canal. The reader is therefore not certain whether the injury is truly a CMI, CEI, or lower thoracic spinal cord injury. There is further difficulty in defining the goals of the treatment as opposed to the effects of various techniques. Very few studies, apart from one by Lifeso,[49] report on the results of posttreatment imaging, which would validate the efficacy of their attempts at achieving a decompression.

With respect to our primary outcome, neurological recovery following CMI and CEI, the estimation of the effect of various treatments is very uncertain, and thus there exist several reasonable treatment alternatives. The evidence would suggest that there is no demonstrated difference between treating conus medullaris injuries and cauda equina injuries surgically or conservatively in terms of neurological outcome.

In terms of surgical approach, the evidence would appear to support the premise that there is no significant difference, in terms of neurological recovery, between treating these injuries from an anterior, posterior, or combined approach. It is further suggested that the timing of surgery does not appear to adversely affect the neurological recovery.

The studies of McAfee, Transfeldt, and Maiman suggest that in the presence of persistent and significant bony or soft tissue compression of neurological elements, direct surgical decompression (most effective by means of an anterior approach) may achieve additional neurological recovery.

◆ Authors' Guidelines

With respect to the neurological recovery from conus medullaris and cauda equina injuries associated with thoracolumbar trauma:

◆ We can make a weak recommendation, based on very low quality evidence, that in a center where the allied health expertise is present to support nonoperative treatment then it may be recommended with the understanding that there may be increased time in hospital, and participation in active rehabilitation may be delayed.

◆ Similarly we can make a weak recommendation, based on very low quality evidence, that based upon the individual experience of the surgeon and the treating center, the choice of surgery as initial treatment for CMI and CEI may be made while recognizing the operative risks and rates of complications.

◆ Based on the very low quality evidence that anterior, posterior, and combined surgical approaches all result in similar degrees of neurological recovery, however, with significant differences in morbidity, we make a weak recommendation that when surgical treatment is selected, a posterior surgical approach with segmental pedicle screw stabilization be selected as the initial treatment.

◆ We make a weak recommendation based on very low quality evidence that in the presence of significant neurological element compression, an anterior decompression and reconstruction (with anterior instrumentation or with posterior stabilization) may achieve additional neurological recovery when performed either acutely or subacutely.

References

1. Saifuddin A, Burnett SJ, White J. The variation of position of the conus medullaris in an adult population: a magnetic resonance imaging study. Spine 1998;23:1452–1456

2. Soleiman J, Demaerel P, Rocher S, Maes F, Marchal G. Magnetic resonance imaging study of the level of termination of the conus medullaris and the thecal sac: influence of age and gender. Spine 2005;30: 1875–1880

3. Aebi M, Mohler J, Zäch G, Morscher E. Analysis of 75 operated thoracolumbar fractures and fracture dislocations with and without neurological deficit. Arch Orthop Trauma Surg 1986;105:100–112

4. Benzel EC, Larson SJ. Functional recovery after decompressive operation for thoracic and lumbar spine fractures. Neurosurgery 1986;19:772–778

5. Braakman R, Fontijne WP, Zeegers R, Steenbeek JR, Tanghe HL. Neurological deficit in injuries of the thoracic and lumbar spine: a consecutive series of 70 patients. Acta Neurochir (Wien) 1991;111:11–17

6. Harrop JS, Hunt GE Jr, Vaccaro AR. Conus medullaris and cauda equina syndrome as a result of traumatic injuries: management principles. Neurosurg Focus 2004;16:e4

7. Ertekin C, Reel F, Mutlu R, Kerküklü I. Bulbocavernosus reflex in patients with conus medullaris and cauda equina lesions. J Neurol Sci 1979;41: 175–181

8. Vaccaro AR, Lehman RA Jr, Hurlbert RJ, et al. A new classification of thoracolumbar injuries: the importance of injury morphology, the integrity of the posterior ligamentous complex, and neurologic status. Spine 2005;30:2325–2333

9. Rechtine GR II, Cahill D, Chrin AM. Treatment of thoracolumbar trauma: comparison of complications of operative versus nonoperative treatment. J Spinal Disord 1999;12:406–409

10. Bailey CS, Dvorak MF, Thomas KC, Boyd MC, Paquett S, Kwon BK, France J, Gurr KR, Bailey SI, Fisher CG. Comparison of thoracolumbosacral orthosis and no orthosis for the treatment of thoracolumbar burst fractures: interim analysis of a multicenter randomized clinical equivalence trial. J Neurosurg Spine 2009; Sep; 11(3):295–303.

11. Been HD, Bouma GJ. Comparison of two types of surgery for thoraco-lumbar burst fractures: combined anterior and posterior stabilisation vs. posterior instrumentation only. Acta Neurochir (Wien) 1999;141:349–357

12. Benson DR, Burkus JK, Montesano PX, Sutherland TB, McLain RF. Unstable thoracolumbar and lumbar burst fractures treated with the AO fixateur interne. J Spinal Disord 1992;5:335–343

13. Boriani S, Palmisani M, Donati U, et al. The treatment of thoracic and lumbar spine fractures: a study of 123 cases treated surgically in 101 patients. Chir Organi Mov 2000;85:137–149

14. Bradford DS, McBride GG. Surgical management of thoracolumbar spine fractures with incomplete neurologic deficits. Clin Orthop Relat Res 1987;218:201–216

15. Dimar JR II, Wilde PH, Glassman SD, Puno RM, Johnson JR. Thoracolumbar burst fractures treated with combined anterior and posterior surgery. Am J Orthop 1996;25:159–165

16. Eysel P, Meinig G. Comparative study of different dorsal stabilization techniques in recent thoraco-lumbar spine fractures. Acta Neurochir (Wien) 1991;109(1–2):12–19

17. Katonis PG, Kontakis GM, Loupasis GA, Aligizakis AC, Christoforakis JI, Velivassakis EG. Treatment of unstable thoracolumbar and lumbar spine injuries using Cotrel-Dubousset instrumentation. Spine 1999;24: 2352–2357

18. McAfee PC, Bohlman HH, Yuan HA. Anterior decompression of traumatic thoracolumbar fractures with incomplete neurological deficit using a retroperitoneal approach. J Bone Joint Surg Am 1985;67:89–104

19. McDonough PW, Davis R, Tribus C, Zdeblick TA. The management of acute thoracolumbar burst fractures with anterior corpectomy and Z-plate fixation. Spine 2004;29:1901–1908, discussion 1909

20. Payer M. Unstable burst fractures of the thoraco-lumbar junction: treatment by posterior bisegmental correction/fixation and staged anterior corpectomy and titanium cage implantation. Acta Neurochir (Wien) 2006;148:299–306, discussion 306

21. Tezeren G, Kuru I. Posterior fixation of thoracolumbar burst fracture: short-segment pedicle fixation versus long-segment instrumentation. J Spinal Disord Tech 2005;18:485–488

22. Kaya RA, Aydin Y. Modified transpedicular approach for the surgical treatment of severe thoracolumbar or lumbar burst fractures. Spine J 2004;4:208–217

23. McLain RF, Burkus JK, Benson DR. Segmental instrumentation for thoracic and thoracolumbar fractures: prospective analysis of construct survival and five-year follow-up. Spine J 2001;1:310–323

24. Sasso RC, Cotler HB. Posterior instrumentation and fusion for unstable fractures and fracture-dislocations of the thoracic and lumbar spine: a comparative study of three fixation devices in 70 patients. Spine 1993;18:450–460

25. Cigliano A, Scarano E, De Falco R, Profeta G. The postero-lateral approach in the treatment of post-traumatic canalar stenosis of the thoraco-lumbar spine. J Neurosurg Sci 1997;41:387–393

26. Clohisy JC, Akbarnia BA, Bucholz RD, Burkus JK, Backer RJ. Neurologic recovery associated with anterior decompression of spine fractures at the thoracolumbar junction (T12-L1). Spine 1992; 17(8, Suppl): S325–S330

27. Kaneda K, Taneichi H, Abumi K, Hashimoto T, Satoh S, Fujiya M. Anterior decompression and stabilization with the Kaneda device for thoracolumbar burst fractures associated with neurological deficits. J Bone Joint Surg Am 1997;79:69–83

28. Dvorak MF, Kwon BK, Fisher CG, Eiserloh HL III, Boyd M, Wing PC. Effectiveness of titanium mesh cylindrical cages in anterior column reconstruction after thoracic and lumbar vertebral body resection. Spine 2003;28:902–908

29. Schünemann HJ, Jaeschke R, Cook DJ, et al; ATS Documents Development and Implementation Committee. An official ATS statement: grading the quality of evidence and strength of recommendations in ATS guidelines and recommendations. Am J Respir Crit Care Med 2006;174:605–614

30. Carlson GD, Minato Y, Okada A, et al. Early time-dependent decompression for spinal cord injury: vascular mechanisms of recovery. J Neurotrauma 1997;14:951–962

31. Delamarter RB, Sherman J, Carr JB. Pathophysiology of spinal cord injury: recovery after immediate and delayed decompression. J Bone Joint Surg Am 1995;77:1042–1049

32. Dolan EJ, Tator CH, Endrenyi L. The value of decompression for acute experimental spinal cord compression injury. J Neurosurg 1980;53: 749–755

33. Guha A, Tator CH, Endrenyi L, Piper I. Decompression of the spinal cord improves recovery after acute experimental spinal cord compression injury. Paraplegia 1987;25:324–339

34. Kobrine AI, Evans DE, Rizzoli HV. Experimental acute balloon compression of the spinal cord: factors affecting disappearance and return of the spinal evoked response. J Neurosurg 1979;51:841–845

35. Sekhon LH, Fehlings MG. Epidemiology, demographics, and pathophysiology of acute spinal cord injury. Spine 2001;26(24, Suppl):S2–S12

36. Chen TY, Dickman CA, Eleraky M, Sonntag VK. The role of decompression for acute incomplete cervical spinal cord injury in cervical spondylosis. Spine 1998;23:2398–2403

37. Duh MS, Shepard MJ, Wilberger JE, Bracken MB. The effectiveness of surgery on the treatment of acute spinal cord injury and its relation to pharmacological treatment. Neurosurgery 1994;35:240–248, discussion 248–249

38. Ng WP, Fehlings MG, Cuddy B, et al. Surgical treatment for acute spinal cord injury study pilot study #2: evaluation of protocol for decompressive surgery within 8 hours of injury. Neurosurg Focus 1999;6:e3

39. Vaccaro AR, Daugherty RJ, Sheehan TP, et al. Neurologic outcome of early versus late surgery for cervical spinal cord injury. Spine 1997;22: 2609–2613

40. Waters RL, Meyer PR Jr, Adkins RH, Felton D. Emergency, acute, and surgical management of spine trauma. Arch Phys Med Rehabil 1999;80: 1383–1390

41. Boerger TO, Limb D, Dickson RA. Does "canal clearance' affect neurological outcome after thoracolumbar burst fractures? J Bone Joint Surg Br 2000; 82:629–635

42. Davies WE, Morris JH, Hill V. An analysis of conservative (non-surgical) management of thoracolumbar fractures and fracture-dislocations with neural damage. J Bone Joint Surg Am 1980;62:1324–1328

43. Willen J, Dahllof AG, Nordwall A. Paraplegia in unstable thoracolumbar injuries: a study of conservative and operative treatment regarding neurological improvement and rehabilitation. Scand J Rehabil Med Suppl 1983;9:195–205

44. Transfeldt EE, White D, Bradford DS, Roche B. Delayed anterior decompression in patients with spinal cord and cauda equina injuries of the thoracolumbar spine. Spine 1990;15:953–957

45. Maiman DJ, Larson SJ, Benzel EC. Neurological improvement associated with late decompression of the thoracolumbar spinal cord. Neurosurgery 1984;14:302–307

46. Dall BE, Stauffer ES. Neurologic injury and recovery patterns in burst fractures at the T12 or L1 motion segment. Clin Orthop Relat Res 1988;(233):171–176

47. Dendrinos GK, Halikias JG, Krallis PN, Asimakopoulos A. Factors influencing neurological recovery in burst thoracolumbar fractures. Acta Orthop Belg 1995;61:226–234

48. Kim NH, Lee HM, Chun IM. Neurologic injury and recovery in patients with burst fracture of the thoracolumbar spine. Spine 1999;24:290–293, discussion 294

49. Lifeso RM, Arabie KM, Kadhi SK. Fractures of the thoraco-lumbar spine. Paraplegia 1985;23:207–224

50. Braakman R. The value of more aggressive management in traumatic paraplegia. Neurosurg Rev 1986;9(1–2):141–147

51. Jodoin A, Dupuis P, Fraser M, Beaumont P. Unstable fractures of the thoracolumbar spine: a 10-year experience at Sacré-Coeur Hospital. J Trauma 1985;25:197–202

52. Daniels AH, Arthur M, Hart RA. Variability in rates of arthrodesis for patients with thoracolumbar spine fractures with and without associated neurologic injury. Spine 2007;32:2334–2338

53. Hu SS, Capen DA, Rimoldi RL, Zigler JE. The effect of surgical decompression on neurologic outcome after lumbar fractures. Clin Orthop Relat Res 1993;288:166–173

54. Lemons VR, Wagner FC Jr, Montesano PX. Management of thoracolumbar fractures with accompanying neurological injury. Neurosurgery 1992;30:667–671

55. Rahimi-Movaghar V, Vaccaro AR, Mohammadi M. Efficacy of surgical decompression in regard to motor recovery in the setting of conus medullaris injury. J Spinal Cord Med 2006;29:32–38

56. Gaebler C, Maier R, Kutscha-Lissberg F, Mrkonjic L, Vècsei V. Results of spinal cord decompression and thoracolumbar pedicle stabilisation in relation to the time of operation. Spinal Cord 1999;37:33–39

45

Sacral Fractures

Jens R. Chapman, Carlo Bellabarba, Thomas A. Schildhauer, Rick C. Sasso, and Alexander R. Vaccaro

Injuries to the sacrum have historically been a largely overlooked entity within the realm of spine trauma. Reasons for this are multifactorial, ranging from deficiencies of diagnostic modalities available to the more limited territorial interests of surgical subspecialties. That said, the sacrum bears a profound biomechanical role in overall spinal stability, which has increasingly been identified in several studies. On a structural basis the sacrum forms the interconnection between the spinal column and the posterior pelvic ring based on well-developed ligamentous connections and an intricate osseous architecture. The inclination of the sacrum forms the foundation for the alignment of the entire spinal column, with consequences to the form and function of the human torso. The sacrum also provides the scaffolding for major blood vessels and the lumbosacral and sacral plexuses and forms the platform for the internal organ systems of the lower torso.

Disruption of the sacrum typically occurs under the influence of major trauma or in the form of an insufficiency fracture in metabolically impaired patients under various clinical settings. Leading causes for high-energy sacral fractures are falls from a height, motor vehicle crashes, and crushing trauma.[1] More recently, increased recognition has been given to sacral insufficiency fractures. These fractures usually precipitate from the sacral alae bilaterally and break between adjacent sacral body segments leading to progressive kyphosis and even translation of the upper sacrum relative to the lower half. Precipitating factors include senile osteoporosis, pharmacologically induced osteopenia, overloading, such as female endurance athletes or with lumbar scoliosis and patients following long lumbosacral instrumentation.[2] The reported incidence of 2% neurological injury may underreport the true incidence because symptoms of bowel, bladder, and sexual impairment in an elderly population are often attributed to other causes when, in fact, these symptoms may be caused by sacral plexus compression.[3]

If left unrecognized and untreated, sacral fractures hold the threat of inducing major morbidity or even mortality upon the affected patients with increasing complexity of rectifying the condition with prolonged delay of care. Management is focused on contributing to patient survival, minimizing morbidity, and optimizing functional preservation or enabling functional recovery.

◆ Diagnostic Approaches

Assessment of a patient is initiated by obtaining a pertinent history and physical examination, which includes posterior integument inspection and palpation as well as comprehensive neurological function testing according to the principles suggested by the American Spinal Injury Association (ASIA) group.[4] The latter includes rectal examination with specific assessment of motor, reflex, and sensory components. Important sentinel findings are presence of major posterior soft tissue contusion, overt or occult open injuries, lumbosacral fascial deglovement (Morel-Lavalle lesion) and crepitus, tenderness, and nonanatomical bony prominences.[5–7]

For patients involved in high-energy injury, diagnostic philosophies have been heavily influenced by the Advanced Trauma Life Support (ATLS) group, which has suggested the A,B,C criteria for resuscitation, but also recommended obtaining initial lateral cervical, anteroposterior chest, and pelvic radiographs as basic screening tools.[8] Traditionally, radiographs have been used to identify and quantify pelvic trauma, with inlet and outlet views to supplement an anteroposterior view and iliac and obturator oblique projection views recommended for suspected acetabular involvement. The inadequacy of plain pelvic radiographs in identifying any form of sacral fracture has been reported repeatedly.[9–12] Computed tomography (CT), increasingly deployed as helical torso scan for trauma, has increasingly supplanted plain radiographs to address the concern for acute pelvic ring injuries. Review of sagittal and coronal reformatted CT scan images has been strongly recommended to assess the sacrum for structural integrity. Three-dimensional reformats as a routine measure can be visually compelling but have not been shown to be of general relevance. Dynamic testing by means of pushing and pulling on the lower extremities—in the case of noninjured lower extremities—has been suggested anecdotally but has not been adopted as a routine evaluation measure.[12] Magnetic resonance imaging (MRI) has been discussed as offering potential additional insights such as ligament disruption, retroperitoneal hematoma, and identifying insufficiency fractures early on.[13] To date there has been no study to suggest MRI as a useful assessment tool to identify or quantify neurological injury over clinical examination in addition to CT scanning. Furthermore, there is currently no general recommendation in favor of MRI as a routine diagnostic tool for acute sacral fractures, regardless of neurological status of the patient. This diagnostic modality, however, has been recommended for detection of insufficiency-type fractures. As an alternative to MRI, technetium[99] bone scans have remained a mainstay for the diagnosis of occult and pathological fractures. (The relative sensitivity and specificity of either diagnostic modality for the assessment of insufficiency fractures remains disputed.)[13–16]

Key parameters for radiographic assessment have been identified to consist of the following measures: sacral inclination, alar vertical and sagittal distraction, midsagittal and midcoronal spinal canal occlusion, as well as foraminal stenosis.[17]

A perplexing and challenging question can arise around the evaluation of acute and subacute neurological injury. For acutely injured patients with impaired cognitive status, a differentiated clinical assessment of lumbosacral and sacral plexus is often limited to the point of being not helpful. Electrodiagnostic assessment tools include electromyography (EMG), which requires usually a period of 3 weeks for development of manifest abnormalities as denervation of the affected muscles progresses, or somatosensory evoked potentials (SSEPs), which can record impaired posterior column afferent tract disruption in near real time. For practical acute sacral fracture patient management, pudendal SSEPs may be helpful in identifying sacral plexus disruption in the cognitively impaired population and anal sphincter EMG for intraoperative monitoring of patients with sacral fractures.[18–23] Neither of these techniques has been validated to date.

Diagnostic modalities used have been increasingly standardized and, if deployed in a timely fashion, should allow the treating physician to adequately identify structural injuries and classify the trauma accordingly.

◆ Classification

Attempts at a systematic assessment of sacral fractures are hampered by the pleomorphic nature of these injuries with further disease variables such as involvement of the lumbosacral junction, integrity of the pelvic ring, neurological injury, soft tissue trauma, overall injury burden, and general patient health factors, all heavily influencing the cumulative patient disease burden. Several classification approaches proposed since 1945 have used biomechanical, anatomical, or neurological considerations. In large part, the suggested classification systems such as proposed by Bonnin, Huittinen, Pennal, Schmidek, Sabiston, and others have been replaced by the AO system and the Denis system, with subclassifications added for specific subtypes and neurological injury added. None of these classification systems have been validated to date.[1,6,24–28] Confusing matters further, simple "alphabetic classifications" in the form of letters (shapes of H, T, U, and λ) best figuratively resembling the general fracture pattern continue to persist in the

literature (**Fig. 45.1**).[29] These informal classifications continue to provide a simple but not clearly delineated conversation basis for care of these fractures but are not suitable as a foundation for analysis.

The AO/ASIF group has suggested a system, which categorize type A injuries (isolated avulsion injuries), B injuries (pelvic ring disruption), and type C injuries (any of the above with variations of sacral fractures) with numeric subsets accounting for injury severity and displacement variants.[6,7]

The system proposed by Denis separated zone I fractures (most medial fracture extent remains lateral to the sacral foramina) from zone II fractures (most medial fracture extends through the sacral neural foramina) and zone III fractures (fracture reaches medial to the foramina into the spinal canal) (**Fig. 45.2**).[1] Based on a multicenter retrospective questionnaire-based analysis of 236 fractures, Denis described a distinct correlation between incidence as well as type of fracture and neurological injury. Zone I injuries were associated with a 5.9% incidence of predominantly L5 root injuries, whereas zone II injuries were found to have a 28.4% incidence of mainly L5/S1 root injuries as opposed to zone III injury with reported 56.7% incidence of neurological injury mostly consisting of sacral plexus dysfunction. Other classification systems have been proposed to account for injuries to the lumbosacral junction, and different fracture types within the sacral spinal canal. Specifically, the classification proposed by Isler for the lumbosacral junction and the Roy-Camille classification for fractures involving the sacral spinal canal can be applied additionally to the Denis classification, although neither was formally introduced in such a context.[30–32]

Isler suggested differentiation of fractures based upon location of the fracture relative to the lumbosacral facet joints (**Fig. 45.3**).[32] Sacral fractures that remain lateral to the lumbosacral joints will likely not adversely affect sacral stability but harbor a posterior pelvic ring disruption. Fractures that cross through the lumbosacral facet may impair lumbosacral stability but are less likely to threaten posterior pelvic ring or sacral stability, whereas fractures medial to the facet may imply sacral instability. The Roy-Camille classification focuses on sacral body fractures and differentiates these fractures based on displacement type (**Fig. 45.4**).[30] Fractures with pure kyphosis but no translation are identified as type I, whereas type II fractures show posterior translation of the rostral segment and type III injuries demonstrate anterior displacement of the rostral segment and flexion. A type IV injury consisting of segmental comminution of the upper segment was added later by Strange-Vognsen.[31] Unfortunately, the height of the transverse component of the sacral body fracture is not specified by this classification system. The added information of the sacral segment involved ("high" equaling S1–S2, "low" equaling S3–S4 and coccyx) may add to the understanding of the type of neurological injury commonly involved in these complex injuries.[33,34] In light of the absence of any spinal cord injury classification system such as the one proposed by the ASIA group addressing sacral plexus injuries, Gibbons suggested a four-part differentiation based on motor, sensory, and bowel/bladder control: (1) patients without neurological abnormalities, (2) injuries causing sensory loss, (3) injuries causing motor loss with or without sensory loss, and (4) injuries causing bowel and bladder dysfunction.[35] This simple classification system unfortunately does not address incomplete injuries or take sexual function into consideration.

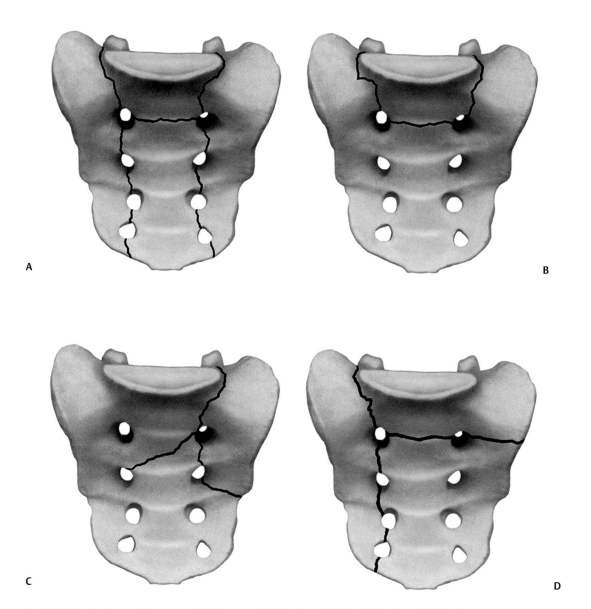

Fig. 45.1 Descriptive sacral fractures. **(A)** H fracture. **(B)** U fracture. **(C)** Lambda fracture. **(D)** T fracture.

◆ Treatment Options

For high-energy injuries the primary focus remains on optimizing factors favoring patient survival through timely injury diagnosis and adequate resuscitation. Should a concordant external rotation-type pelvic ring disruption be present, closure of the pelvic ring with a pelvic ring reduction sheet, external pelvic clamp, or external fixateur has been suggested to limit ongoing hemorrhage into the retroperitoneal perisacral region through a tamponade effect.[36–38]

There are several nonoperative and operative treatment options with various levels of treatment invasiveness based upon injury severity.

Nonoperative care can range from simple activity limitations to brace wear with hip spica using uni- or bilateral hip extension attachments.[1,39,40] Prolonged recumbent skeletal lower extremity traction followed by mobilization with brace wear has been historically used for more unstable injuries but has to take thromboembolic prophylaxis and pulmonary decompensation as risk factors into consideration. Time periods recommended for nonoperative care vary from a few weeks to 3 or more months.[41,42] Concerns surrounding nonoperative care center around the potential for posterior skin breakdown, thromboembolic events, pulmonary decompensation and secondary deformity, increased pain, as well as secondary neurological deterioration.

Surgery for sacral fractures can be differentiated into neural element decompression and stabilization procedures. Neural element decompression has the goal of relieving neural elements of bone impaction or angulatory tension. Dural repair has been recommended mainly to diminish wound healing problems and pseudomeningocele formation.[1,28] Decompression techniques can be differentiated into limited or extensile laminectomy and/or focal foraminotomy and finally ventral spinal canal disimpaction. Surgical stabilization options include consideration of anterior pelvic ring stabilization to aid in reduction and stabilization of the posterior pelvic ring components; however, this has been shown to have a very limited biomechanical effect on posterior pelvic ring stability.[43,44] Posterior treatment options include posterior

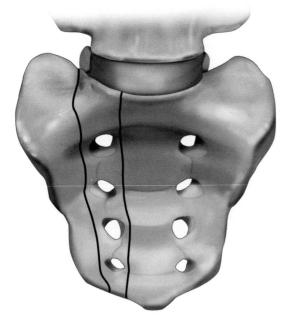

Fig. 45.2 Denis classification of sacral fractures: zone I is lateral to the sacral foramen, zone II fractures are through the sacral foramen, and zone III fractures are medial to the foramen and involve the spinal canal.

percutaneous stabilization with sacroiliac screws and open reduction with some variation of plates, transiliac bars, or segmental lumbopelvic fixation (**Fig. 45.5**). Postoperative mobilization protocols vary widely from continuation of bed rest, immobilization with a brace, and immediate full weight-bearing and mobilization. Other important variables of treatment include timing of intervention, attempts at deformity reduction as well as quality thereof, and type and completeness of neural element decompression. Concerns surrounding surgical care primarily revolve around mortality and a wide array of morbid conditions, such as surgical site infections, loss of reduction, and secondary neurological deterioration. Long-term concerns revolve around the rate of recovery from neurological injury, pain, bony healing pain, and return to preinjury functional status.

Decision making for sacral fracture treatment has evolved into a multifactorial process over the last 2 decades along with advances in imaging and trauma resuscitation algorithms. Typically, surgical care has been suggested for patients with neurological injury and major sacral or posterior pelvic ring fracture displacement irreducible by closed means. Neurological recovery potential is complicated by the difficulty in visualizing or testing neural elements conclusively for its integrity. Actual neural element transsection, with no hope for recovery of the affected roots, has been described to occur in ~40% of patients with high-grade sacral fractures.[26] This finding is contrasted with the observation that only unilateral lower sacral root function of the S2–S4 segments is necessary for functional bowel and bladder control.[45] Patient age, bone health, comorbidities, general injury burden, and hemodynamic stability, as well as integrity of the dorsal integument are some of the major covariables that have been suggested to be factored into the decision-making tree as well.

◆ Results

Review of Evidence

Three questions were posed to surgeons tasked with managing sacral fractures:

1. Is there evidence to suggest that surgical treatment in the presence of lumbopelvic root injuries improves neurological outcomes?
2. Is there evidence to support early intervention, as defined as less than 2 weeks postinjury, to improve or not worsen neurological outcomes compared with delayed surgery (> 2 weeks from trauma)?
3. Is there evidence to suggest superiority of operative over nonoperative care? With regard to surgically managed patients, is one therapeutic modality superior to the others?

Search Criteria

Sampling

A systematic search in accordance with the principles of GRADE (grades of recommendation, assessment, development, and evaluation) using PubMed, Medline, Cochrane Database, and Ovid databases was done to identify studies that evaluated factors associated with sacral fractures, sacral trauma, posterior pelvic ring fractures, sacral insufficiency fractures, sacral plexus, and sacral plexus injuries.

Articles published in English or with an English-language abstract inclusive of pediatric and adult patients published from 1980 onward were reviewed. Search terms included "sacrum" "sacral fracture" and "pelvis AND trauma," "pelvic ring fracture," "pelvic ring disruption," "sacro-iliac joint" and "insufficiency fracture." Excluded from the search were studies dealing with malignancies, case reports consisting of five or fewer patients, abstracts, book chapters, review articles, and opinion papers. Studies with heterogeneous pelvic ring injury populations were eliminated if involvement of the sacrum was not clearly identified. For the sake of completeness, case reports were grouped into a reference section at the end of the chapter. Insufficiency fractures were recorded separately.

The available studies were then assessed for design, cohort size, and type of intervention performed. Studies were assigned a level of evidence according to the categories as suggested by Saillant et al. Retrospective studies with stated contiguous enrollment and structured follow-up criteria were given level III status, case series without defined enrollment methodology were given level IV status. Recorded data included complications, follow-up times, outcomes, and conclusions of the authors in a summarized fashion. Each available study was then rated according to the level and strength of evidence. A rating of ratio of risks:benefits was then calculated by weighing incidence and severity of reported adverse events associated with type of injury management with identified benefits. Finally, the cumulative findings were presented to the assembled Spine Trauma Study Group for critical review, and each of the key questions was answered as to the strength of literature evidence, cumulative risk:benefit ratio, and clinical experience, and a final recommendation was made as to treatment.

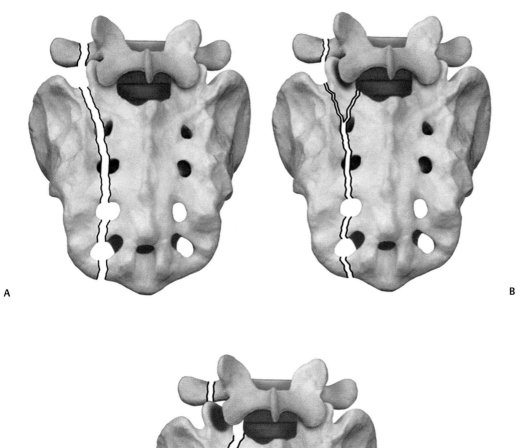

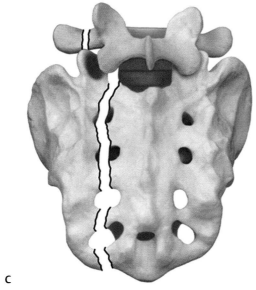

Fig. 45.3 Lumbosacral junction injuries according to the classification of Isler. **(A)** Type I fracture is lateral to the L5–S1 facet joint. **(B)** Type II is a fracture through the L5–S1 facet joint. **(C)** Type III fractures exit medial to the joint and involve the spinal canal.

Results

A total of 34 studies reporting on 1814 patients met the initial inclusion and exclusion criteria. For acute traumatic fractures there were no level I or II study designs. There were 10 level IV case series and 24 level III studies. The 24 level III studies harbored many design shortcomings. These limitations consisted of small cohort sizes, strong selection bias, as well as inconsistent ratings or reporting on injury severity, neurological status, quality of initial and final healing results, and outcomes parameters. Such findings are not unusual due to the relatively low incidence of these injuries at trauma centers around the world, the wide variability of injury severity, and the added confounding influences brought about by trauma to other organ systems. The task of determining neurological status in an acute injury can be very difficult due to

concurrent injuries and emergent treatment directed at patient survival and general polytrauma management. Timing of any intervention in this setting is a complex multidimensional undertaking, which has to take into consideration other organ system injuries, resuscitation status, and soft tissue injuries. The question of operative or nonoperative treatment is difficult to answer in the absence of generally accepted instability criteria and classification systems. For instance, the most commonly accepted sacral fracture classification of Denis does not infer stability in its three-zone concept. A type I injury may be completely unstable, whereas a type III injury is inherently structurally stable.

Our current state of knowledge on sacral fractures continues to be heavily influenced by a single study dating back between the years 1974 through 1984. This retrospective multicenter study by Denis et al holds the distinction of

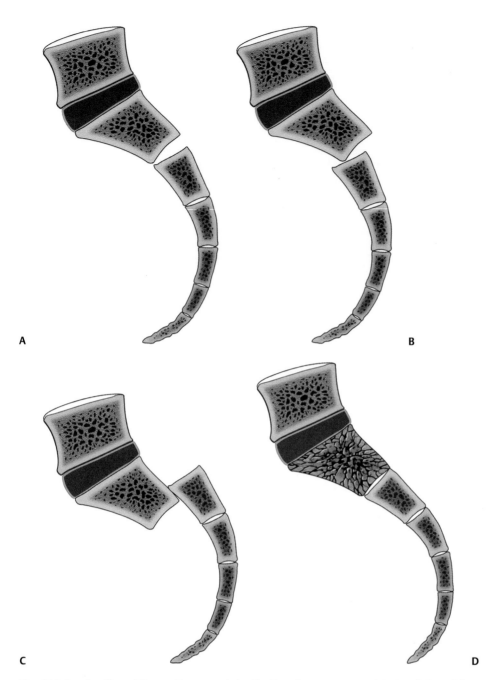

Fig. 45.4 Roy-Camille and Strange-Vognsen subclassification of Denis zone III fractures. **(A)** Type I fractures represent a simple flexion deformity of the sacrum. **(B)** Type II fractures are angulated and have a flexion and translational deformity. **(C)** Type III fractures have a complete translation of the upper to the lower sacral elements with no fracture overlap. **(D)** Type IV fractures are segmental comminuted S1 vertebral body fractures.

remaining by far the largest study on sacral fractures, with 236 consecutive patients gathered from 776 patients with pelvic fractures over an 11-year period at two major medical centers.[1] Substantial limitations remain with inconsistent clinical documentation, absence of any follow-up data, and not having the benefit of even basic CT during the first half of the enrollment period. Diagnostic and treatment modalities available at the time of this study would clearly be considered outdated by most practitioners using current standards. However, this study achieved landmark status through its comprehensive approach, which included a cadaveric neuroanatomical study, provided a novel and clinically meaningful classification model, and attempted to address issues of

missed diagnosis, timing of intervention, as well as a basic comparison of types of interventions.

◆ Questions

What Is the Effect of Type of Intervention (Surgical or Nonsurgical Treatment) on Neurologic Recovery?

The greatest impact on outcome in patients with unstable sacral fractures appears to be due to neurological impairment related to bladder, bowel, sexual, sensory, and motor lower extremity function. In general, neurological decompression

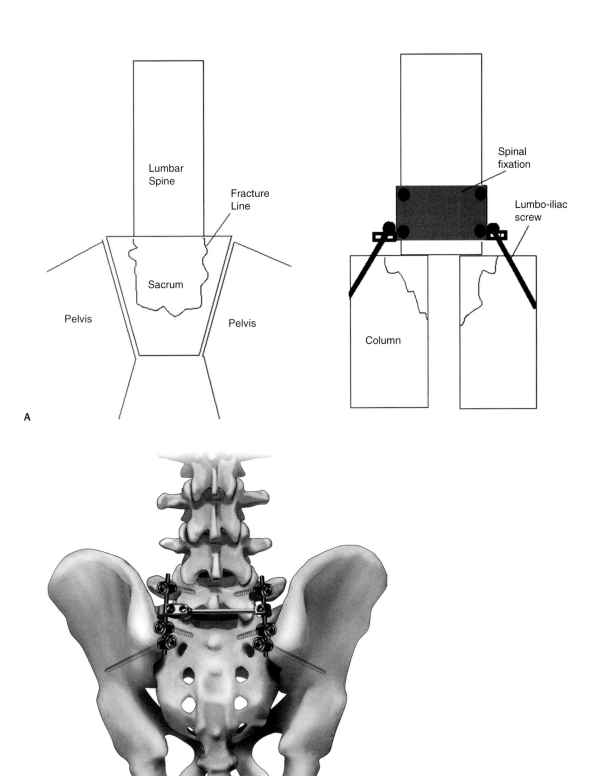

Fig. 45.5 (A) An illustration of a disrupted, unstable sacral fracture spanned by instrumentation consisting of screw fixation into the lumbar pedicles and the iliac crest. **(B)** The unstable sacral fracture illustrated in **(A)** is spanned by lumbar pedicle screws and two large iliac screws anchored into each ilium.

procedures have been reported to result in neurological improvement rates up to 85% in surgical series. However, neurological improvement has also been documented in nonoperatively treated patients, with rates of up to 72% reported by some authors.[46–52] Also, no data are provided on the actual numbers of patients with neurological injury treated surgically or nonoperatively to draw inferences on

effect of treatment types. Of five patients with bowel and bladder control compromise treated with surgical decompression, all improved or recovered, whereas three patients treated nonoperatively demonstrated no improvement.[1]

The retrospective study of Gibbons et al provided important information on the previously overlooked aspect of classifying neurological injury severity with regard to sacral roots.[35] The authors identified four of five patients that had resolution of neurological symptoms treated with surgery, in contrast to three patients with unchanged neurological status, of which one was treated surgically. Schmidek et al reported on 15 patients with bowel and bladder control compromise of which 11 improved with surgical intervention, whereas four nonoperatively treated patients improved, however, to a lesser degree.[28] None of these studies qualify type or timing of surgical intervention. Schildhauer et al identified 18 patients with high-grade sacral fractures and impaired bowel and bladder control who had undergone comprehensive neural element decompression and structural realignment and stabilization with segmental lumbopelvic fixation within 30 days of injury (6-day average). These authors noted a neurological improvement rate of 83%. The recovery rate was significantly higher for patients with incomplete lumbosacral injury compared with patients with an established complete injury.[53]

Overall there were 503 patients with some reported neurological injury secondary to a sacral fracture. A preponderance of neurological improvement was reported, without timing of intervention being addressed in a single study.

Is There Evidence to Support Early Intervention, as Defined as Less Than 2 Weeks Postinjury, to Improve or Not Worsen Neurological Outcomes Compared with Delayed Surgery (> 2 Weeks from Trauma)?

Early stabilization and subsequent mobilization of patients with structurally relevant musculoskeletal trauma has been one of the major factors in improving care of trauma victims. Similarly, the concept of early decompression of compromised neural elements has remained a key tenet in the treatment of spinal cord injury. This concept is, however, only applicable with some limitations for patients with sacral fractures due to the many factors identified in the preceding section on treatment options. We identified a total of 260 patients in six studies discussing results of patient survival or functional recovery related to timing of intervention.

Survival of patients from sacral fracture relative to timing and type of intervention modality is not specifically addressed in any of the present major publications on sacral fractures. In a retrospective study using historical controls for patients with unstable pelvic ring fractures, Latenser et al found statistically decreased hospital stays, reduced blood transfusion requirements, and decreased disability when patients were treated before 72 hours.[54] Although all patients in the early treatment group ($n = 19$) survived, two patients in the delayed group ($n = 18$) expired.

As to timing of intervention having an influence on neurological outcomes, the evidence base is entirely anecdotal. There are no definitions regarding timing of intervention. "Early" has been defined as intervention within 24 hours of injury as a preferred time for decompression of compromised neural elements, and "late" as prior to 3 months posttrauma. The important series of Denis did not define early versus late intervention in their 51 patients with neurological injury beyond a vague differentiation of "before" and "after fracture healing."[1] The authors, however, clearly identified disappointing results with late intervention and attributed perineural fibrosis as an underlying cause for this observation. The authors observed more difficult fracture reduction after 72 hours following injury due to presumed "muscle contractions."

Among the more recent publications Chiu et al presented 65 patients with high-grade sacral fractures of which 22 were reported to have lumbosacral plexus injuries.[55] The data suggest that with percutaneous stabilization using transiliac rods, 12 of 22 patients failed to recover. Timing of intervention was differentiated into <7 days and >7 days. Sadly there was no attempt made at correlating neurological outcomes with either quality of neural canal decompression or timing of intervention. Using a nonvalidated outcomes scoring system the authors reported a 65% satisfactory outcome with their treatment method. In general, early surgical intervention is deemed safe following completion of patient resuscitation. Treatment priorities must relate the magnitude of intervention to the patient's individual fracture needs and systemic well-being.

Is There Evidence to Suggest Superiority of Operative Over Nonoperative Care? With Regard to Surgically Managed Patients, Is One Therapeutic Modality Superior to the Others?

As previously stated there is no validated definition of instability for sacral fractures. There are two main concepts that have been used repeatedly to describe instability in this region of the spine. The first is the mere presence of neurological impairment caused by structural disruption and secondary fracture fragment displacement of 1 cm or more radiographically.[56] Both concepts of instability have inherent limitations, the prior due to the high potential for limited examinability, the latter due to the potential for partial spontaneous reduction ("bounce-back" phenomenon), with occult major instability being present.[57] There were 500 patients from seven studies where some reference to operative versus nonoperative care was made. None of these studies actually had a comparison group of surgical versus nonsurgical groups specifically referencing the patients' neurological status.

Studies on unstable fractures with greater than 10 mm of fracture gap or displacement demonstrate that functional outcomes at 1 year remain poor, often due to associated injuries and trauma morbidity.[50–52,55,56,58,59] Successful results of percutaneous sacroiliac screw fixation were reported by Nork et al in a series of 13 patients with Denis zone III, Roy-Camille subtypes 1 and 2 injuries with no significant neurological deficits.[60] No deterioration of the sacral kyphosis angle was found; however, the posttraumatic deformity was essentially stabilized in situ. Segmental lumbopelvic fixation has been shown in a cadaveric model to offer significantly improved stiffness compared with dual sacroiliac screw constructs.[61,62] Schildhauer et al reported successful results of lumbopelvic fixation in 34 patients with vertically unstable zone I and II fractures.[63]

◆ Summary

In the opening paragraph of his landmark study on sacral fractures dating back to 1988 Denis and colleagues found the review of the literature to "be disappointing, sometimes even obscure."[1] After performing this systematic review of the literature up to the present date we continue to agree with these authors. Undoubtedly, there has been progress made since the publication of Denis et al's study. The diagnosis and treatment of sacral fractures has changed dramatically with the advent of newer imaging techniques allowing more accurate diagnosis and understanding of fracture patterns. Diagnosis of neurological injury has been improved in both the alert as well as the obtunded patient with neurodiagnostic studies. Treatment of sacral fractures continues to evolve with improving constructs and implants. Treating surgeons now have at their disposal options ranging from simple decompression to comprehensive lumbopelvic fixation. The overall clinical picture of the patient is of paramount importance and should influence treatment accordingly. As diagnostic and treatment modalities continue to evolve, it will be up to the surgeon to remain abreast of those changes and adapt accordingly. Sadly there is a distinct paucity of available literature on this important subject. To date the overall strength of evidence for any form of care of sacral fractures is weak, whereas the strength of treatment recommendation based upon the timing of intervention is modest. Treatment recommendation is strong as to the need for surgical treatment of less displaced fractures with percutaneous fixation and possible neural element decompression and open reduction and internal fixation for unstable fractures (>1 cm displacement and $\pm$ neurological deficit) using some form of segmental low-profile lumbopelvic fixation.

References

1. Denis F, Davis S, Comfort T. Sacral fractures: an important problem: retrospective analysis of 236 cases. Clin Orthop Relat Res 1988; 227:67–81
2. Carter SR. Occult sacral fractures in osteopenic patients. J Bone Joint Surg Am 1994;76:1434
3. Dasgupta B, Shah N, Brown H, Gordon TE, Tanqueray AB, Mellor JA. Sacral insufficiency fractures: an unsuspected cause of low back pain. Br J Rheumatol 1998;37:789–793
4. American Spinal Injury Association and International Medical Society of Paraplegia. Standard for Neurologic and Functional Classification of Spinal Cord Injury. Rev. ed. Atlanta: American Spinal Injury Association; 1992
5. Hak DJ, Olson SA, Matta JM. Diagnosis and management of closed internal degloving injuries associated with pelvic and acetabular fractures: the Morel-Lavallée lesion. J Trauma 1997;42:1046–1051
6. Tile M. Pelvic ring fractures: should they be fixed? J Bone Joint Surg Br 1988;70:1–12
7. Tile M. The management of unstable injuries of the pelvic ring. J Bone Joint Surg Br 1999;81:941–943
8. Alexander RH, Proctor HJ, Trauma, A. C. o. S. C. o. Advance Trauma Life Support for Physicians. ATLS; 1993
9. Browner BD, Cole JD, Graham JM, Bondurant FJ, Nunchuck-Burns SK, Colter HB. Delayed posterior internal fixation of unstable pelvic fractures. J Trauma 1987;27:998–1006
10. Fujii M, Abe K, Hayashi K, et al. Honda sign and variants in patients suspected of having a sacral insufficiency fracture. Clin Nucl Med 2005; 30:165–169
11. Laasonen EM. Missed sacral fractures. Ann Clin Res 1977;9:84–87
12. Trafton PG. Pelvic ring injuries. Surg Clin North Am 1990;70:655–669
13. Blake SP, Connors AM. Sacral insufficiency fracture. Br J Radiol 2004;77: 891–896
14. Gotis-Graham I, McGuigan L, Diamond T, et al. Sacral insufficiency fractures in the elderly. J Bone Joint Surg Br 1994;76:882–886
15. Wat SYJ, Seshadri N, Markose G, Balan K. Clinical and scintigraphic evaluation of insufficiency fractures in the elderly. Nucl Med Commun 2007; 28:179–185
16. Klineberg E, McHenry T, Bellabarba C, Wagner T, Chapman JR. Sacral insufficiency fractures caudal to instrumented posterior lumbosacral arthrodesis. Spine 2008;33:1806–1811
17. Kuklo TR, Potter BK, Ludwig SC, Anderson PA, Lindsey RW, Vaccaro AR ; Spine Trauma Study Group. Radiographic measurement techniques for sacral fractures consensus statement of the Spine Trauma Study Group. Spine 2006;31:1047–1055
18. Cohen BA, Major MR, Huizenga BA. Pudendal nerve evoked potential monitoring in procedures involving low sacral fixation. Spine 1991;16(8, Suppl):S375–S378
19. Helfet DL, Koval KJ, Hissa EA, Patterson S, DiPasquale T, Sanders R. Intraoperative somatosensory evoked potential monitoring during acute pelvic fracture surgery. J Orthop Trauma 1995;9:28–34
20. Goodell CL. Neurological deficits associated with pelvic fractures. J Neurosurg 1966;24:837–842
21. Kothbauer K, Schmid UD, Seiler RW, Eisner W. Intraoperative motor and sensory monitoring of the cauda equina. Neurosurgery 1994;34:702–707, discussion 707
22. Slimp JC. Electrophysiologic intraoperative monitoring for spine procedures. Phys Med Rehabil Clin N Am 2004;15:85–105
23. Webb LX, de Araujo W, Donofrio P, et al. Electromyography monitoring for percutaneous placement of iliosacral screws. J Orthop Trauma 2000; 14:245–254
24. Bonnin JG. Sacral fractures and injuries to the cauda equina. J Bone Joint Surg Am 1945;27:113–127
25. Pennal GF, Tile M, Waddell JP, Garside H. Pelvic disruption: assessment and classification. Clin Orthop Relat Res 1980;(151):12–21
26. Huittinen VM. Lumbosacral nerve injury in fracture of the pelvis: a postmortem radiographic and patho-anatomical study. Acta Chir Scand Suppl 1972;429:3–43
27. Sabiston CP, Wing PC. Sacral fractures: classification and neurologic implications. J Trauma 1986;26:1113–1115
28. Schmidek HH, Smith DA, Kristiansen TK. Sacral fractures. Neurosurgery 1984;15:735–746
29. Routt ML Jr, Simonian PT, Agnew SG, Mann FA. Radiographic recognition of the sacral alar slope for optimal placement of iliosacral screws: a cadaveric and clinical study. J Orthop Trauma 1996;10:171–177
30. Roy-Camille R, Saillant G, Gagna G, Mazel C. Transverse fracture of the upper sacrum: suicidal jumper's fracture. Spine 1985; 10:838–845
31. Strange-Vognsen HH, Lebech A. An unusual type of fracture in the upper sacrum. J Orthop Trauma 1991;5:200–203
32. Isler B. Lumbosacral lesions associated with pelvic ring injuries. J Orthop Trauma 1990;4:1–6
33. Sofia T, Lazennec JY, Saillant G. Transverse fractures of the upper part of the sacrum: Analysis of 50 patients. J Bone Joint Surg Br 2005;87-B:104
34. Fountain SS, Hamilton RD, Jameson RM. Transverse fractures of the sacrum: a report of six cases. J Bone Joint Surg Am 1977;59:486–489
35. Gibbons KJ, Soloniuk DS, Razack N. Neurological injury and patterns of sacral fractures. J Neurosurg 1990;72:889–893
36. Ben-Menachem Y, Coldwell DM, Young JW, Burgess AR. Hemorrhage associated with pelvic fractures: causes, diagnosis, and emergent management. AJR Am J Roentgenol 1991;157:1005–1014
37. Incagnoli P, Viggiano M, Carli P. Priorities in the management of severe pelvic trauma. Curr Opin Crit Care 2000;6:401–407
38. Simpson T, Krieg JC, Heuer F, Bottlang M. Stabilization of pelvic ring disruptions with a circumferential sheet. J Trauma 2002;52:158–161
39. Bellabarba C, Stewart JD, Ricci WM, DiPasquale TG, Bolhofner BR. Midline sagittal sacral fractures in anterior-posterior compression pelvic ring injuries. J Orthop Trauma 2003;17:32–37
40. Henderson RC. The long-term results of nonoperatively treated major pelvic disruptions. J Orthop Trauma 1989;3:41–47
41. Johnson KD, Cadambi A, Seibert GB. Incidence of adult respiratory distress syndrome in patients with multiple musculoskeletal injuries: effect of early operative stabilization of fractures. J Trauma 1985;25: 375–384
42. Kellam JF, McMurtry RY, Paley D, Tile M. The unstable pelvic fracture: operative treatment. Orthop Clin North Am 1987;18:25–41
43. Archdeacon MT, Hiratzka J. The trochanteric C-clamp for provisional pelvic stability. J Orthop Trauma 2006;20:47–51
44. Lindahl J, Hirvensalo E, Böstman O, Santavirta S. Failure of reduction with an external fixator in the management of injuries of the pelvic ring: long-term evaluation of 110 patients. J Bone Joint Surg Br 1999;81: 955–962
45. Gunterberg B, Petersen I. Sexual function after major resections of the sacrum with bilateral or unilateral sacrifice of sacral nerves. Fertil Steril 1976;27:1146–1153
46. Fisher RG. Sacral fracture with compression of cauda equina: surgical treatment. J Trauma 1988;28:1678–1680
47. Hart DJ, Wang MY, Griffith P, Gordon McComb J. Pediatric sacral fractures. Spine 2004;29:667–670
48. Hatem SF, West OC. Vertical fracture of the central sacral canal: plane and simple. J Trauma 1996;40:138–140
49. Lam CR. Nerve injury in fractures of the pelvis. Ann Surg 1936;104: 945–951
50. Suzuki T, Shindo M, Soma K, et al. Long-term functional outcome after unstable pelvic ring fracture. J Trauma 2007;63:884–888
51. Tötterman A, Glott T, Søberg HL, Madsen JE, Røise O. Pelvic trauma with displaced sacral fractures: functional outcome at one year. Spine 2007;32:1437–1443
52. Tötterman A, Glott T, Madsen JE, Røise O. Unstable sacral fractures: associated injuries and morbidity at 1 year. Spine 2006; 31:E628–E635

53. Zelle BA, Gruen GS, Hunt T, Speth SR. Sacral fractures with neurological injury: is early decompression beneficial? Int Orthop 2004;28:244–251

54. Latenser BA, Gentilello LM, Tarver AA, Thalgott JS, Batdorf JW. Improved outcome with early fixation of skeletally unstable pelvic fractures. J Trauma 1991;31:28–31

55. Chiu FY, Chuang TY, Lo WH. Treatment of unstable pelvic fractures: use of a transiliac sacral rod for posterior lesions and an external fixator for anterior lesions. J Trauma 2004;57:141–144, discussion 144–145

56. Kellam JF. Long-term functional prognosis of posterior injuries in high-energy pelvic disruption. J Orthop Trauma 1998;12:150–151

57. Olson SA, Pollak AN. Assessment of pelvic ring stability after injury: indications for surgical stabilization. Clin Orthop Relat Res 1996;329:15–27

58. Jackson RP, McManus AC. Radiographic analysis of sagittal plane alignment and balance in standing volunteers and patients with low back pain matched for age, sex, and size: a prospective controlled clinical study. Spine 1994;19:1611–1618

59. Kabak S, Halici M, Tuncel M, Avsarogullari L, Baktir A, Basturk M. Functional outcome of open reduction and internal fixation for completely unstable pelvic ring fractures (type C): a report of 40 cases. J Orthop Trauma 2003;17:555–562

60. Nork SE, Jones CB, Harding SP, Mirza SK, Routt ML Jr. Percutaneous stabilization of U-shaped sacral fractures using iliosacral screws: technique and early results. J Orthop Trauma 2001;15:238–246

61. Schildhauer TA, Josten C, Muhr G. Triangular osteosynthesis of vertically unstable sacrum fractures: a new concept allowing early weight-bearing. J Orthop Trauma 1998;12:307–314

62. Schildhauer TA, Ledoux WR, Chapman JR, Henley MB, Tencer AF, Routt ML Jr. Triangular osteosynthesis and iliosacral screw fixation for unstable sacral fractures: a cadaveric and biomechanical evaluation under cyclic loads. J Orthop Trauma 2003;17:22–31

63. Schildhauer TA, McCulloch P, Chapman JR, Mann FA. Anatomic and radiographic considerations for placement of transiliac screws in lumbopelvic fixations. J Spinal Disord Tech 2002;15:199–205, discussion 205

VIII

Rehabilitation Following Spinal Injury and Late Complications

46

Autonomic Dysreflexia

Carlos Villanueva, M. A. González-Viejo, and Ampar Cuxart

Autonomic dysreflexia (AD) is a syndrome that affects spinal cord injury (SCI) patients above or proximal to the upper thoracic level (T6 or above) due to unopposed sympathetic nervous system impulses. Patients with SCIs below T8 are rarely affected by the condition.[1,2] Understanding the early signs and symptoms of autonomic dysreflexia is important because early recognition can prevent a life-threatening crisis of hypertension. The total incidence in SCI individuals reported at risk (injury level above T6) for autonomic dysreflexia varies from 20 to 70%.[3,4]

Historically, most researchers believed that AD did not occur until after a phase of "spinal shock" resolved defined as when there is a return of neurological reflexes. However, recently AD has been reported in the early phases after an SCI.[5,6] The estimated incidence of AD in the acute phase (1 month) after SCI at the period when the neurological reflexes are returning is 5.7% of patients for acute SCI above T6. The incidence of AD in children and adolescents is the same as that of adults, and the signs, symptoms, and management are similar to those for the adult population.[3,4]

Autonomic dysreflexia in these patients occurs as a result of noxious or nonnoxious peripheral or visceral stimulation below the lesion level, which in turn triggers sympathetic hyperactivity. This chapter provides a systematic, evidence-based-medicine review of the literature concerning the basic aspects of this entity, in particular, the following questions will be analyzed and answered through this review process:

1. What is the optimal treatment for autonomic dysreflexia?
2. What are the potential causes and prevention measures for autonomic dysreflexia?

◆ Pathophysiology

Patients with neurological SCIs above the major splanchnic outflow (T6–L2) have the potential of developing autonomic dysreflexia. Intact sensory nerves below the injury level transmit noxious or non-noxious impulses that potentially induce a widespread activation of the sympathetic nervous system. Intact sensory nerves transmit afferent impulses. In normal individuals, sympathetic inhibitory impulses are originated above T6, but in SCI patients, these inhibitory impulses are blocked due to the injury. Therefore, there is an unopposed sympathetic outflow below the injury demonstrated by an increase in norepinephrine, dopamine-β-hydroxylase, and dopamine. The regional investigation of noradrenaline spillover release demonstrated significant increases only below the lesion level.[7,8] The release of these chemicals induces vasoconstriction in the majority of vascular beds below the level of cord injury: skin, muscle, kidneys, and possibly at the splanchnic vascular bed, resulting in a sudden elevation of the blood pressure.[9] Other immediate consequences are piloerection and skin pallor. The increased arterial blood pressure may cause a headache. Intact carotid and aortic baroreceptors are activated by the hypertension and trigger the brainstem reflexes to lower the blood pressure.

This first compensatory mechanism for this induced hypertension is bradycardia, a reduction in heart rate, due to increased parasympathetic stimulation via the vagus nerve, unaffected by SCI. It may be only a relative slowing of the heart; sometimes it may not drop as low as 60 beats per minute, but it can be insufficient to compensate for the vasoconstriction. The second compensatory mechanism is an increase in the inhibitory outflow from vasomotor centers above the lesion to dilate the splanchnic bed to accommodate the excessive amount of blood resulting from the increased peripheral resistance. However, the inhibitory impulses are unable to pass below the injury, and dilation of vascular beds is limited to above the injury level, resulting in profuse sweating and skin flushing.[1,2]

◆ Methods

National Library of Medicine MEDLINE/PubMed was used to search for evidence back to 1966. The search strategy was application of the Medical Subject Headings (MeSH) database. The following terms were used:

Autonomic Dysreflexia (AD) AND therapy—83 items
AD AND prevention—17 items

In the general term window we also used:

autonomic dysreflexia—183 items

AD AND neurogenic bladder—67 items

AD AND bowel—60 items

AD AND bowel impaction—4 items

AD AND labor—18 items

AD AND captopril—2 items

AD AND magnesiun sulfate—3 items

AD AND mecamylamine—2 items

AD AND nifedipine—10 items

AD AND nitric oxide—3 items

AD AND prazosin—9 items

AD AND phenoxybenzamine—6 items

hypertensive crisis AND captopril—51 items

hypertensive crisis AND nifedipine—91 items

hypertensive crisis AND prazosin—16 items

Applying Single Citation Matchers we selected references from printed articles to increase the quality and quantity of evidence.

What Is the Optimal Treatment for Autonomic Dysreflexia?

Evaluation of neurological function and subsequent anomalies can be difficult for untrained clinicians (**Table 46.1**). A comprehensive set of definitions seems to be necessary to improve daily practice as well as to better assess future therapeutic interventions.[10]

The signs and symptoms are consequent with the pathophysiology previously earlier. The elevated blood pressure can cause a pounding headache, which is a common finding. Bradycardia is the first compensatory mechanism, but it is important to consider that may be just a relative moderate reduction of the heart rate—above 60 beats per minute.[11] Profuse sweating above the SCI level is the result of the increased inhibitory outflow from vasomotor centers to compensate hypertension. The increase in catecholamine release further induces piloerection above and possibly below the

level of the lesion. Cardiac arrhythmias, atrial fibrillations, and premature ventricular contractions have been reported during the chronic phase.[12] The prevalence of electrocardiographic (ECG) abnormalities in SCI remains controversial.[13,14] It is mandatory to restore the normal rhythm when dysrhythmias occur during episodes of AD.[12]

Autonomic dysreflexia should be suspected in any patient with an SCI above T6 with a sudden change in status. People in charge of these patients must be aware of the variability of the described symptoms that may be minimal or even absent. People with low verbal communication ability can have difficulty expressing their symptoms.

◆ Elevated Blood Pressure

The main symptom of autonomic dysreflexia is a sudden *increase in both systolic and diastolic blood pressure*. Patients with an SCI above T6 have a typical baseline systolic blood pressure in a range of 90 to 110 mm Hg. Any increase of 20 to 40 mm Hg above the baseline, especially if it is associated with bradycardia, is a strong sign of autonomic dysreflexia. Children and adolescents have lower baseline systolic blood pressure. Systolic blood pressures above 120 mm Hg in children under 5 years old, 130 mm in children between 6 and 12 years old, and 140 mm Hg in adolescents should be an indication for immediate pharmacological treatment. Some deaths have been reported in high SCI patients,[15] especially in pregnant women due to the cardiovascular changes related to pregnancy and labor.[16,17] Blood pressures can fluctuate very quickly during an autonomic dysreflexia spell, and therefore frequent monitoring will assist in the diagnosis. Patients with normal blood pressure but complaining of signs or symptoms of AD must be referred to investigate potential causes of these symptoms other than AD.

◆ Treatment and Diagnosis

Physical Measures

Level of evidence: III/V; grade of recommendation: C; strength of panel opinion: strong

Once AD is suspected/confirmed start immediate physical measures to reduce blood pressure, seating the patient,

Table 46.1 Incidence of Automatic Dysreflexia in Children and Adults

Studies	Description	Level of Evidence	Topic and Conclusion
Vogel et al (2002)[82]	Retrospective cohort	III	METHOD: Structured interview PARTICIPANTS: Spinal cord injury age 18 years or younger and were 24 years of age or older at interview. Result autonomic dysreflexia present in 42%
Hickey et al (2004)[20]	Retrospective cohort	III	All individuals with ≥ T6 spinal cord injury who were injured at 13 years of age or younger (121). 62 (51%) had experienced autonomic dysreflexia. The most common causes of dysreflexia were urologic (75%) and bowel impaction (18%). The most common symptoms were facial flushing (43%), headaches (24%), sweating (15%), and piloerection (14%). CONCLUSION: Autonomic dysreflexia has a similar prevalence in pediatric-onset spinal cord injury compared with the adult spinal cord injury population.

lowering the legs if it is possible, and avoiding any constriction (clothing, devices) to allow a pooling of blood in the abdomen and lower extremities.[18,19]

Urologic Causes and Treatment

Bladder distension

Level of evidence: V; grade of recommendation: C; strength of panel opinion: strong

Local anesthetic

Level of evidence: V; grade of recommendation: C; strength of panel opinion: strong

Catheter replacement

Level of evidence: V; grade of recommendation: C; strength of panel opinion: strong

Urinary drainage

Level of evidence: V; grade of recommendation: C; strength of panel opinion: strong

The most common cause of AD is bladder distension.[20] Therefore urinary catheterization is recommended in patients if an indwelling catheter is not in place; inspect the entire urinary catheter and bag system in individuals already catheterized. The catheter must be checked for folds or compressions, which must be released. Check if the catheter is blocked and if it is the case, solve the problem by gentle bladder irrigation with 10 to 15 mL of a nonirritating fluid (normal saline at body temperature). Irrigation should be limited to 10 mL in children under 2 years of age. If the catheter remains blocked replace the catheter.

Instillation of 2% lidocaine jelly 2 minutes prior to the catheter insertion may decrease the sensory input and relax the sphincter. However, there is no evidence about the efficacy of lidocaine instillation to prevent AD in urethral or anorectal procedures, but it would provide some improvement in the instillation of irritating vesical medication.[21] If the catheter insertion is difficult, a new attempt using a coude catheter should be considered. In any case, blood pressure should be monitored during bladder drainage because sudden decompression of a large volume of urine may cause hypotension if the patient has already received pharmacological agents to decrease blood pressure.

Pharmacological Treatment (Table 46.2)

If the systolic blood pressure remains above 150 mm Hg, pharmacological management should be considered before assessing for fecal impaction. Nifedipine has been recommended by the Consortium for Spinal Cord Medicine.[22,23] Bite

Table 46.2 Drug Treatment

Study	Description	Level of Evidence	Topics and Conclusion
Dykstra et al (1987)[23]	Case series	IV	Nifedipine to control autonomic hyperreflexia during cystoscopy in 7 patients with cervical SCI. Nifedipine (10 mg) alleviated autonomic hyperreflexia when given sublingually during cystoscopy and prevented autonomic hyperreflexia when given orally 30 minutes before cystoscopy. No adverse drug effects were observed.
Lindan et al (1985)[83]	Case series	IV	Purpose to compare the effect of the antihypertensive drugs, phenoxybenzamine and nifedipine, in 12 tetraplegic patients. Neither drug was effective in preventing AD responses to bladder filling. Nifedipine by mouth was found to be a valuable drug for the treatment of attacks that developed.
Ellrodt et al (1985)[28]	Case series Non-SCI	IV	The efficacy and safety of sublingual nifedipine were evaluated in 16 men and 14 women (mean age 65 +/− 14 yrs) who had hypertensive emergencies. By 60 minutes, nifedipine had decreased the diastolic blood pressure to less than 120 mm Hg in 97% of patients. One patient developed symptoms suggestive of symptomatic hypotension. CONCLUSION: Nifedipine is a safe, effective, and practical agent for treating patients with hypertensive emergencies.
Angeli et al (1991)[26]	Randomized, single-blind clinical trial. Non-SCI	II	10 patients treated with sublingual captopril (25 mg) 10 patients treated with sublingual nifedipine (10 mg) The hypotensive effect of nifedipine was more rapid than that of captopril. No difference was observed in the time or in the magnitude of peak hypotensive effect between the two treatments, nor was a difference observed in the duration of hypotensive effect. Three patients of the nifedipine group had minor side effects.
Ceyhan et al (1990)[27]	Case series Non-SCI	IV	25 mg captopril and 10 mg nifedipine were administered sublingually to 28 and 24 patients, respectively. Hypotensive effect of both sublingual captopril and nifedipine therapy occurred at 5 minutes and persisted for 240 minutes. Heart rates increased with nifedipine, but decreased with captopril. We observed no side effects in the captopril group, but flushing, tachycardia and headache were observed in 6 patients in the nifedipine group.
Esmail et al (2002)[31]	Prospective cohort	III	Twenty-six consecutive patients older than 15 years with spinal cord injury above T6. During an autonomic dysreflexia episode, captopril 25 mg was administered sublingually. If systolic blood pressure remained elevated 30 minutes after captopril administration, 1 dose of immediate-release nifedipine 5 mg was given

(Continued on page 456)

Table 46.2 Drug Treatment (*Continued*)

Study	Description	Level of Evidence	Topics and Conclusion
			as rescue by the bite and swallow method and repeated, if necessary, in 15 minutes. Captopril alone was effective in 80% of initial episodes. CONCLUSION: Captopril appears to be safe for autonomic dysreflexia management.
Wu et al (1993)[30]	Case series Non-SCI	IV	Sublingual captopril (25 mg), nifedipine (10 mg), and prazosin (2 mg) were prescribed to determine the effectiveness and safety of each medication in the treatment of hypertensive emergencies during hemodialysis. Response rates were 83% for captopril, 90% for nifedipine, and 11% for prazosin. Prazosin was not recommended because of its low response rate.
Gemici et al (1999)[29]	Prospective cohort Sparse evidence Non-SCI	III	Eighty patients (32 male and 48 female) with hypertensive crisis were included in the study; their mean age was 43.4 ± 7.9 years. Nifedipine 10 mg was given sublingually to 34 and captopril 25 mg to 46 patients randomly. CONCLUSIONS: Sublingual captopril is as effective as and has less side effects than sublingual nifedipine.

and swallow is the preferred method of administration because it has a shorter onset than conventional oral administration, and sublingual administration has more erratic absorption.[24,25]

Nifedipine has some inconveniences: reflex tachycardia, severe and uncontrollable hypotension, flushing, and headache have been reported in non-SCI patients, especially in elderly people and patients with coronary artery disease.[26–30] Nifedipine has also been proposed as a prophylactic treatment for autonomic dysreflexia.[27,56]

Captopril is considered the first treatment option in Europe. The hypotensive effect of nifedipine was more rapid than that of captopril, but no difference was observed in the time or in the magnitude of peak hypotensive effect between the two treatments; the duration of the hypotensive effect was the same.[26,27,30,31] Captopril has fewer side effects than nifedipine in non-SCI patients.[32]

Other drugs that have been used to treat hypertensive crisis in AD include hydralazine mecamylamine, diazoxides phenoxybenzamine[3] magnesium sulfate,[33] but there is very little reported evidence. Prazosin has been used for treatment of hypertensive crisis as well as a prophylactic treatment.[3,34]

Nifedipine

Level of evidence: II/V; grade of recommendation: B/C; strength of panel opinion: strong

Captopril

Level of evidence: II/III/V; grade of recommendation: B/C; strength of panel opinion: strong

Fecal impaction

Level of evidence: II/V; grade of recommendation: B; strength of panel opinion: strong

Fecal impaction is the second most common cause of autonomic dysreflexia 18%.[20] It must be suspected if blood pressure remains elevated after complete urinary examination (**Table 46.3**). Again if blood pressure is above 150 mm Hg, pharmacological treatment to reduce the systolic blood pressure should be considered. If blood pressure remains elevated but below 150 mm Hg, checking the rectum for stool can be considered, but it is important to realize that the combined effects of rectal and/or anal sphincter distension and uninhibited rectal contraction in response to the manual removal of stool might induce AD.[35] The Consortium for Spinal Cord Medicine recommended in 2001 to instill a topical anesthetic agent such as 2% lidocaine jelly into the rectum. However, Cosman et al[36] concluded the following from a double-blind, randomized, controlled trial: (1) topical lidocaine did not significantly limit or prevent AD in susceptible patients, and (2) stretching of the anal sphincters was a more potent stimulus for AD than gaseous distention of the rectosigmoid. Three years later, Cosman and Vu[37] reported the benefits of a lidocaine anal block, which seems to limit AD. The majority of SCI centers are still using the conventional protocol of lidocaine jelly. A single manuscript reported in 2002[38] the attenuation of the response to colon distension in paraplegic and quadriplegic rats using Transcutaneous Electrical Nerve Stimulation (TENS), but to our knowledge there is not clinical experience in humans yet.

Unknown Cause

Level of evidence: V; grade of recommendation: C; strength of panel opinion: strong

If the cause of the AD episode is not determined on examination, the patient should consider admission into a hospital setting for further investigation of less common causes, such as acute abdominal pathology, neglected bone fractures, or problems with toenails.[3]

What Are the Potential Causes and Prevention Measures for Autonomic Dysreflexia?

The urinary system is the most common cause of autonomic dysreflexia. However, most patients are well controlled with parasympatholytic drugs and intermittent self-catheterization. In case of an inability to self-catheterize, lack of efficacy, or severe adverse effects, other options must be evaluated. The main goal is to maintain the bladder leak point pressure below 40 mm of water to avoid upper tract damage and AD. Patients with bladder leak point pressure greater than 40 cm water have been reported to have a significantly higher incidence of upper tract damage ($p = 0.021$) and persisting external detrusor-sphincter dyssynergia ($p = 0.00008$).[17] The overall goal is to relax as well as to prevent overactivity of the bladder's detrusor muscle to prevent subsequent AD.

Table 46.3 Fecal Impaction

Study	Description	Level of Evidence	Topics and Conclusions
Furusawa et al	Prospective cohort	II	15 consecutive Cervical Spine Cord Injury (CSCI) patients changes in BP, PR, and classic symptoms of AD (2007)[35] before, during, and after a bowel program involving the manual removal of stool in lateral recumbency were recorded. CONCLUSION: The combined effects of rectal and/or anal sphincter distension and uninhibited rectal contraction in response to the manual removal of stool might induce AD. Recommendation is to avoid, if at all possible, the manual removal of stool to prevent AD in patients with CSCI.
Cosman et al (2002)[36]	Randomized, controlled trial	II	Patients with chronic, complete SCI scheduled for anoscopy and/or flexible sigmoidoscopy. In a double-blind fashion they were randomized to receive either 2% lidocaine jelly ($n = 18$) or nonmedicated lubricant (control; $n = 32$) CONCLUSION: Topical lidocaine did not significantly limit or prevent AD in susceptible patients. Anoscopy, which involves stretching of the anal sphincters, was a more potent stimulus for AD than flexible sigmoidoscopy, which involves gaseous distention of the rectosigmoid.
Cosman and Vu (2005)[37]	Randomized, controlled trial	II	Randomized, controlled, double-blind trial, 26 patients were randomized for intersphincteric anal block with 1% lidocaine or normal saline (placebo) before the procedure. Blood pressure was measured before, during, and after the block and procedure. Results: The mean maximal systolic blood pressure increase for the lidocaine group was significantly lower than the placebo group. CONCLUSION: Lidocaine anal block significantly limits the AD in patients undergoing anorectal procedures.

Abbreviations: AD, autonomic dysreflexia; BP, blood pressure; PR, pulse rate; SCI, spinal cord injury.

◆ Nonsurgical Treatment

Oral Pharmacologic Medications

Level of evidence: II/V; grade of recommendation: B; strength of panel opinion: strong

Oral anticholinergic drugs along with intermittent clean catheterization is proposed as a standard first-line treatment in patients with neurogenic detrusor overactivity (**Table 46.4**). Oxybutynin has long been used for the treatment of patients with detrusor overactivity. The controlled release tablet formulation has the advantage of only once-a-day dosage, enhancing treatment compliance.[39]

Prazosyn/terazosyn have also been used to prevent AD.[34,40,41] Initial results are promising for a short period of time; consequently it is impossible to recommend their use for a long period of time. Similar results have been reported

Table 46.4 Oral Medications

Study	Description	Level of Evidence	Topics and Conclusions
O'Leary et al (2003)[39]	Case series	IV	Ten patients (mean age = 49 years) with complete or incomplete spinal cord injury were enrolled. Treatment was initiated at a dosage of 10 mg per day. Dosage was increased in weekly intervals to a maximum of 30 mg per day. No patient experienced serious adverse events during the 12-week study. CONCLUSION: Oxybutynin XL is safe and effective in patients with detrusor hyperreflexia secondary to spinal cord injury. The onset of clinical efficacy occurs within 1 week, and daily dosages up to 30 mg are well tolerated.
Vaidyanathan et al (1998)[41]	Case series	IV	Eighteen adults with tetraplegia (female: 1; male: 17), three children with ventilator-dependent tetraplegia and three adult male patients with paraplegia who exhibited recurrent features of autonomic dysreflexia in the absence of an acute predisposing factor for dysreflexia, Terazosin was prescribed with a starting dose of 1 mg in an adult and 0.5 mg in a child administered by nocte. The treatment resulted in complete subsidence of the dysreflexic symptoms. One tetraplegic patient required termination of Terazosin therapy because of persistent dizziness.
Krum et al (1992)[34]	Double-blind parallel group study	III	Sixteen patients participated in a double blind parallel group study comparing prazosin 3 mg a day with placebo given for 2 weeks. Both groups were matched for age, sex, and baseline severity of autonomic dysreflexia episodes. Patients allocated to prazosin therapy were found to have fewer severe episodes of autonomic dysreflexia and during these episodes to have significant reductions in average rise in blood pressure, symptoms duration, and requirement for acute antihypertensive medication.
Abrams et al (2003)[80]	Randomized, controlled, double-blind trial	II	263 patients with neurogenic lower urinary tract dysfunction were randomized to 4-week double-blind therapy with placebo, or 0.4 or 0.8 mg tamsulosin once daily. CONCLUSION: Long-term tamsulosin treatment (0.4 and 0.8 mg once daily) was well tolerated. The results suggest that it improves bladder storage and emptying, and decreases symptoms of autonomic dysreflexia.

using tamsulosin in 263 patients. Of these, 244 patients completed the randomized, controlled trial, 186 continued long-term tamsulosin therapy (0.4 or 0.8 mg once daily), and 134 completed 1-year treatment. However, results were worse than those reported with the other drugs. Anticholinergic drugs have troublesome side effects like dry mouth and tachycardia that can lead to discontinuation of the treatment.

Intravesical Medication

Level of evidence: II/V; grade of recommendation: B; strength of panel opinion: strong

Patients not responding to oral medication might be candidates for intravesical medication to improve bladder storage volume, mean maximum storage pressure, and decreased detrusor storage pressure to less than 40 cm (**Table 46.5**). However, dysreflexia was prevented successfully in only 60% of patients.[42] Some papers suggest that intravesical atropine was as effective as oxybutynin immediate release for increasing bladder capacity and it was probably better with less antimuscarinic side effects.[43]

Capsaicin[31,44–47] and resiniferatoxin[45,46] have been proposed for the intravesical treatment of detrusor hyperreflexia; however, the comparative efficacy is still disputable. Some

authors[46] support the superiority of resiniferatoxin compared with capsaicin. There were no significant differences in regard to the incidence, nature, or duration of side effects, but in both cases instillation triggered immediate side effects (suprapubic pain, sensory urgency, flushes, hematuria, autonomic hyperreflexia).[44] The adverse effects perhaps can be prevented with electromotive drug administration of lidocaine to anesthetize the bladder before intravesical capsaicin or modifying the vanilloid solute.[45,48] There is one manuscript supporting the intravesical use of oxybutynin; however, it is a case series with low evidence level.[49]

Botulinum Toxin

Level of evidence: I/V; grade of recommendation: B; strength of panel opinion: strong

Botulinum toxin A is an alternative to the surgical treatment (**Table 46.6**). Efficacy of this treatment has been reported, and some papers support clearly that AD associated with bladder emptying that manifested as a hypertensive crisis during voiding disappeared after treatment.[50–53] Severe side effects have been reported after a single dose of oral baclofen[54] or after discontinuation of intrathecal baclofen therapy.[55]

Table 46.5 Intravesical Medication

Study	Description	Level of Evidence	Topic and Conclusions
Dasgupta et al (1998)[48]	Case series	IV	EMDA of lidocaine and epinephrine was performed in 8 patients with detrusor hyperreflexia. EMDA virtually eliminated the hyperreflexic contractions of the bladder during capsaicin instillations, thus reducing the risk of urethral leakage and preventing autonomic dysreflexia that had previously occurred in 1 patient.
de Sèze et al (2004)[45]	Randomized, controlled trial–Sparse evidence	II	Single-center, randomized, double-blind, parallel groups study included 39 spinal cord injured adults with detrusor hyperreflexia. Clinical and urodynamical improvement was found in 78% and 83% of patients with CAP vs 80% and 60% with RTX, respectively, without a significant difference between the two treated groups. The benefit remained in two thirds of the two groups on day 90. There were no significant differences in regard to the incidence, nature, or duration of side effects in CAP vs RTX treated patients. CONCLUSIONS: Importance of accounting for the role of vanilloid solute when interpreting the efficacy and tolerance of vesical vanilloid instillation. Glucidic solute is a valuable solvent for vanilloid instillation
de Sèze et al (2001)[44]	Case series	IV	Thirty patients received a first intravesical instillation of 1 mMol/L capsaïcin solution in 30% alcohol. Transient and moderate adverse effects followed 86% and 79% of the first and reiterated instillation. CONCLUSION: Intravesical instillation of capsaïcin is an effective treatment for incontinence and associated symptoms.
Kim et al (2003)[81]	Randomized controlled trial–Sparse evidence	II	Thirty-six (22 males, 14 females) neurologically impaired patients (20 spinal cord injury, 7 multiple sclerosis, 9 other neurological diseases) with urodynamically verified DH and intractable urinary symptoms despite previous anticholinergic drug use were treated prospectively with intravesical RTX. Intravesical RTX administration, in general, is well tolerated. CONCLUSIONS: Some patients responded with significant improvement in bladder capacity and continence shortly after RTX administration. Patients at risk for autonomic dysreflexia require careful monitoring during RTX therapy.
Giannantoni et al (2002)[46]	Case series	III	Twenty-four spinal cord-injured patients with refractory detrusor hyperreflexia were randomly assigned to receive a single dose of 2 mm capsaicin in 30 mL ethanol plus 70 mL 0.9% sodium chloride or 100 nM resiniferatoxin in 100 mL 0.9% sodium chloride. Autonomic dysreflexia, limb spasms, suprapubic discomfort, and hematuria developed in most patients who received capsaicin but in none who received resiniferatoxin. CONCLUSIONS: Resiniferatoxin is superior to capsaicin in terms of urodynamic results, and it does not cause the side effects associated with capsaicin.

Abbreviations: CAP, Capsaicine; RXT: Resiniferatoxine; EMDA: Electromotive Drug Administration.

Table 46.6 Botulinum Toxin

Study	Description	Level of Evidence	Topic and Conclusions
Tow et al (2007)[53]	Case series	IV	Fifteen spinal cord injury patients (9 tetraplegic and 6 paraplegic) who had NDO, on clean intermittent self-catheterization, and were refractory to oral medications, were recruited. Botulinum toxin type A (BTX-A) injected into the detrusor is safe and efficacious for spinal cord injured patients with refractory detrusor overactivity. This effect is maintained at 26 weeks postinjection.
Denys et al (2003)[50]	Meta-analysis	III	Botulinum toxin injected into the detrusor muscle seems to be an efficient treatment of bladder hyperreflexia for 6 months in patients resistant to parasympathicolytic drugs. Long-term efficacy and mechanism of action is actually not known.
Schurch et al (2000)[52]	Case series	IV	Autonomic dysreflexia associated with bladder emptying that manifested as a hypertensive crisis during voiding disappeared after treatment in the three patients with tetraplegia. BTX-A injections seem to be a safe and valuable option in spinal cord injured patients with incontinence resistant to anticholinergic medication who perform clean intermittent self-catheterization. A dose of 300 units BTX-A seems to be needed to counteract an overactive detrusor. The duration of bladder paresis induced by the toxin is at least 9 months.
Dykstra et al (1988)[84]	Case series	IV	10 patients evaluated by electromyography after injection showed signs of sphincter denervation. Postvoid residual urine volume decreased by an average of 146 mL after the toxin injections in eight patients. In the eight patients for whom it could be determined toxin effects lasted an average of 50 days. The toxin also decreased autonomic dysreflexia in five patients.
MacDonald et al (2007)[51]	Systematic review of RCT	I	Three trials totaling 104 subjects with DO refractory to antimuscarinic treatment were included. BTX-A was superior in reducing daily UI episodes in SCI subjects compared with intravesical resiniferatoxin at 12 and 18 months after injections. Adverse events in BTX-A-treated subjects included UTI, pain at the injection site, hematuria, and autonomic dysreflexia.

Abbreviations: DO, Detrusor Overactivity; NDO, Neurogenic Detrusor Overactivity, UI, Urinary Incontinence; UTI, Urinary Tract Infection.

Nitric Oxide

Level of evidence V, grade of recommendation I, strength of panel opinion weak

Other pharmacological options have been successfully used such as nitric oxide. Both animal and human studies suggest that nitric oxide mediates urethral sphincter relaxation. The safety and efficacy of this potential treatment for AD needs to be established in clinical trials.[4] Other conservative options are purely experimental.[56]

◆ Surgical Treatment

Unfortunately, nonoperative treatment fails in ~20% of patients. These patients may consider surgical management options (**Table 46.7**).

Male patients—sphincterotomy

Level of evidence IV/V, grade of recommendation C, strength of panel opinion strong

Table 46.7 Surgery

Study	Description	Level of Evidence	Topics and Conclusions
Perkash (2007)[58]	Case series	IV	Forty-six consecutive men with spinal cord injuries above the thoracic 6 level present with frequent symptoms of autonomic dysreflexia and inadequate voiding. They did not want to be catheterized or were unable to perform intermittent catheterization. There was subjective relief in autonomic dysreflexia following transurethral sphincterotomy in all patients, which correlated well with a significant decrease in systolic and diastolic blood pressure ($p < 0.0001$).
Klohn et al (1990)[57]	Case series	IV	Review of 59 spinal cord injury patients with spastic sphincter, treated by external sphyncterotomy. Immediate complications are infrequent. 19% of patients need a second intervention. 78% of patients obtain satisfactory long-term results. Fibrosis is present in 71% of sphincter resection piece histologies and appears early in the evolution of the affection. This condition is thought to contribute notably to the formation of a fixed sphincteric obstacle.
Chancellor et al (1994)[65]	Case series	IV	Comparison of external sphincterotomy, with balloon dilatation or internal stenting of the external sphincter. Sixty-one spinal cord injured men were prospectively evaluated. Complications of stent insertion included device migration (three patients) and secondary bladder neck obstruction (two patients). In the balloon dilatation group, three recurrent sphincter obstructions, one case of bleeding requiring transfusion, and one case of bulbous urethral stricture occurred. Both methods proved to be as effective as external sphincterotomy in the treatment of detrusor-external sphincter dyssynergia (DESD)[37]

(*Continued on page 460*)

Table 46.7 Surgery (*Continued*)

Study	Description	Level of Evidence	Topics and Conclusions
Hamid et al (2003)[64]	Case series	IV	Effectiveness of the UroLume® Urethral Stent (actual name of product) (American Medical Systems. Minnetonka, Minnesota) 12-year follow-up. Twelve patients with quadriplegia secondary to spinal trauma underwent external striated sphincter stenting. There were no problems with stent migration, urethral erosion, erectile dysfunction, or autonomic dysreflexia.
Hamid et al (2003)[66]	Case series	IV	Twenty-five patients with spinal cord injury underwent rhabdosphincter Memokath stent insertion. The mean age was 45.5 years. The level of injury was cervical in 14 and thoracic in 11 patients. Nineteen stents were removed for several reasons at a mean of 20.3 months These include exacerbation of autonomic dysreflexic symptoms; stent migration; encrustation and stone formation; incomplete bladder emptying without obstruction; entrance into fertility program.
Tan et al (2008)[85]	Case series	IV	Fifty adults status postileovesicostomy were identified. At last follow-up, 36 patients (72%) were continent per urethra. Twenty-seven averaged 1.52 inflammatory or infectious postoperative complications per patient, 19 averaged 1.47 stomal complications, and 11 averaged 2.09 ileovesicostomy mechanical obstructions. Overall, 27 required 2.85 reoperations or additional procedures following ileovesicostomy. CONCLUSIONS: Ileovesicostomy is a valuable management option for adults with neurogenic bladder unable to perform intermittent catheterization. The morbidity associated with ileovesicostomy requires careful patient selection.
Mutchnik et al (1997)[70]	Case series	IV	Six tetraplegic patients who had experienced significant morbidity with their preoperative form of bladder management were managed with an ileovesicostomy. Follow-up of 12 to 15 months, no patient has demonstrated calculus formation, hydronephrosis, autonomic dysreflexia.
Sidi et al (1990)[69]	Case series	IV	Twelve spinal cord injury adults underwent augmentation enterocystoplasty for treatment of a high pressure neurogenic bladder. After a mean follow-up of 15 months all patients were continent on clean intermittent self-catheterization, and the symptoms of autonomic dysreflexia had disappeared.
Jannings and Pryor(2007)[68]	Case series	IV	Descriptive qualitative methodology was employed. Semistructured, one-to-one, audiotaped interviews with men (*n* = 6) and a woman (*n* = 1) with cervical-level spinal cord injuries (C4–C6) with a urinary catheter in situ, managing mucus in urine following ileocystoplasty. All participants perceived the surgery had adversely affected their life. There was also an increase in autonomic dysreflexia episodes experienced due to mucus blocking bladder drainage.
Kutzenberger (2007)[67]	Retrospective case series	IV	Since September 1986 to December 2002, 464 paraplegic patients (220 females, 244 males) received an SDAF-SARS. The results include data on 440 patients with a mean mean follow-up of 8.6 years (18 months to 18 years) until December 2004. The complete deafferentation was successful in 95.2%. Of these patients, 420 paraplegics use the sacral anterior root stimulator for voiding. CONCLUSION: SDAF is able to restore the reservoir function of urinary bladder and makes the patient achieve continence. Autonomic dysreflexia disappeared in most cases.

Abbreviations: SDAF, Sacral Deafferentation; SARS, Sacral Anterior Root Stimulation.

In male patients, the incision of the urethral external sphincter has been an established option for more than 40 years, and it remains the mainstay of treatment for urodynamically significant detrusor-sphincter dyssynergia. However, the level of evidence of the studies regarding the surgical treatment of detrusor dysreflexia is extremely low. Only case series have been published. Sphincterotomy remains the most effective surgical treatment.[57–59] Electroresection[60,61] has high failure and reoperation rates.

Female patients—cutaneous vesicostomy

Level of evidence: none; grade of recommendation: I; strength of panel opinion: weak

Most of the authors recommend the management of female neurogenic bladders by cutaneous vesicostomy.[62] Similar to male patients the level of evidence regarding this surgical treatment is extremely low. Only case series have been published.

◆ Alternative Methods

In the 1980s, urethral stent prostheses[63,64] and balloon dilatation[65] had been shown to have successful outcomes as alternative treatments for external sphincter dysynergia. However, over the long term, stents can undergo encrustation, and there remains a definite risk of stent migration necessitating device removal or replacement.

Level of evidence: IV; grade of recommendation: C; strength of panel opinion: fair

Further, balloon dilatation of the external sphincter is associated with a risk of subsequent stricture formation.

Level of evidence: V; grade of recommendation: C; strength of panel opinion: weak

Lately, the temporary, thermoexpandable Memokath stent (Pnn Medical, Chesapeake, VA) offered an easier implantation but results showed a significant number of removals (exacerbation of AD symptoms, stent migration, encrustation and stone formation, incomplete bladder emptying without obstruction, entrance into fertility program). It must be remembered that this is a temporary stent, and the majority are removed within 2 years of insertion.[66]

Sacral deafferentation and eventually anterior root stimulation have been supported by several studies with satisfying results.[67]

Level of evidence: IV; grade of recommendation: C; strength of panel opinion: strong

Ileocystoplasty

Level of evidence: IV; grade of recommendation: C; strength of panel opinion: weak

Ileocystoplasty has been proposed as a method to avoid upper urinary tract damage as well as to avoid autonomic dysreflexia, but it is associated with significant complications and a potential risk for an increase in AD episodes experienced due to mucus blocking bladder drainage.[68,69]

Ileovesicostomy

Level of evidence: IV; grade of recommendation: C; strength of panel opinion: weak

Ileovesicostomy[70,71] is a valuable management option for adults with neurogenic bladder unable to perform intermittent catheterization. The morbidity associated with this procedure is quite substantial: common inflammatory or infectious postoperative complications, 40% stomal complications, and 20% ileovesicostomy mechanical obstructions. Overall, 27 required 2.85 reoperations or additional procedures; consequently ileovesicostomy requires careful patient selection.

◆ Bowel Management (Table 46.8)

Level of evidence: V; grade of recommendation: C; strength of panel opinion: strong

An effective bowel management program in SCI patients includes modification of stool consistency; stimulation of bowel transit; and controlled, reflex, or mechanical defecation. It is important to prepare an individual program considering the

Table 46.8 Bowel Management

Study	Description	L. of E.	Topic and Conclusion
Furusawa et al (2007)[35]	Prospective cohort	II	Fifteen consecutive CSCI patients;changes in blood pressure, pulse rate, and classic symptoms of AD before, during, and after a bowel program involving the manual removal of stool in lateral recumbency were recorded. CONCLUSION: The combined effects of rectal and/or anal sphincter distension and uninhibited rectal contraction in response to the manual removal of stool might induce AD. Recommendation is to avoid, if at all possible, the manual removal of stool to prevent AD in patients with CSCI.
Kirshblum et al (2002)[72]	Prospective cohort	III	Silent autonomic dysreflexia. Ten subjects with chronic (> year), complete (American Spinal Injury Association Impairment Scale class A) SCI with a neurological level of injury above T6. All the patients had an increase in SBP greater than 20 mm Hg above baseline, and 70% had an increase in SBP greater than 40 mm Hg above baseline. Sixty percent of subjects had an increase in SBP greater than 150 mm Hg, with 40% of subjects reaching an SBP greater than 170 mm Hg at least once during their bowel program. CONCLUSION: Silent autonomic dysreflexia occurs frequently in SCI during bowel programs.
Cosman et al (2002)[36]	Randomized, controlled trial	I	Topical lidocaine. Patients with chronic, complete SCI scheduled for anoscopy and/or flexible sigmoidoscopy. In a double-blind fashion they were randomized to receive either 2% lidocaine jelly ($n = 18$) or nonmedicated lubricant (control; $n = 32$). CONCLUSION: Topical lidocaine did not significantly limit or prevent autonomic dysreflexia in susceptible patients. Anoscopy, which involves stretching of the anal sphincters, was a more potent stimulus for autonomic dysreflexia. sigmoid.
Cosman and Vu (2005)[37]	Randomized, controlled trial	I	Anal block. randomized, controlled, double-blind trial; patients were randomized for intersphincteric anal block with 1% lidocaine or normal saline (placebo) before the procedure. Results: The mean maximal SBP increase for the lidocaine group was 22 ± 14 mm Hg, significantly lower than the placebo group's 47 ± 31 mm Hg ($p = 0.01$). CONCLUSION: Lidocaine anal block significantly limits the autonomic dysreflexia response in susceptible patients undergoing anorectal procedures.
Furlan et al (2007)[73]	Decision analysis	III	Decision analysis in patients with chronic SCI and neurogenic bowel dysfunction when conservative management fails. Treatment options: colostomy, ileostomy, Malone anterograde continence enema (MACE), and sacral anterior root stimulator (SARS) implantation.

Abbreviations: AD, autonomic dysfunction; SBP, systolic blood pressure; SCI, spinal cord injury.

specific requirements of each patient, the social context, as well as available care facilities. The combined effects of rectal and/or anal sphincter distension and uninhibited rectal contraction in response to the manual removal of stool might induce AD.[35,72]

Topical anesthetics are widely recommended to minimize the incidence and severity of autonomic dysreflexia, although no scientific evidence supports or refutes this practice.[36] Only lidocaine anal block significantly limits the autonomic dysreflexia response in susceptible patients undergoing anorectal procedures.[37] Studies about attenuation of the response to colon distraction are as yet purely experimental.[38]

Surgical Procedures for Neurogenic Bowel

Level of evidence: I/IV; grade of recommendation: B; strength of panel opinion: strong

Surgical procedures have been proposed to prevent problems derived from neurogenic bowel, including colostomy, ileostomy, Malone anterograde continence enema (MACE), and sacral anterior root stimulator (SARS). Furlan et al[73] reported an elegant methodology of decision analysis of all of these alternatives. They concluded that the MACE procedure may provide the best long-term outcome in terms of the probability of improving bowel function, reducing complication rates and the incidence of AD, and congruency with patients' preferences.

◆ Pregnancy and Labor

Level of evidence: V; grade of recommendation: C; strength of panel opinion: strong

There is limited information about the incidence of AD during pregnancy and labor (**Table 46.9**). In 1993, Westgren et al[74] reported the incidence of delivery in 29 women after a traumatic spinal cord injury and described pregnancy outcome in this group of patients. Seventy-five percent of the SCI patients above T5 had symptoms of AD during pregnancy and/or labor. Hypertension is common in pregnancy, and the risk of AD is clearly increased during pregnancy and especially during labor. Failure to recognize AD has caused fatal intracranial hemorrhage.[17]

Spinal or epidural anesthesia seems to be the commonly accepted method not only for vaginal delivery[21,75–77] but also for cesarean section.[78] Cesarean rate for women with lesions above T5 was 46%. No fatal incidences were reported, and the authors concluded that women with high SCI would probably benefit from referral to a specialized center. The majority of papers about AD pregnancy and labor are case reports without evidence or expert recommendations. If AD occurs in preterm labor it can be controlled with epidural anesthesia until vaginal delivery or cesarean section. Some authors prefer spinal anesthesia over epidural when caesarian section is considered.[79]

◆ Recommendations

What Is the Optimal Treatment for Autonomic Dysreflexia?

Once the diagnosis of AD has been established, physical measures should be initiated to reverse this syndrome. The level of evidence for the effectiveness of this measure is very low, but this practice is supported by current treatment practice in most of the SCI units around the world. It is established that bladder distension is the most common cause of AD, consequently all the measures to treat this distension or to decrease the sensory impulse as well as to relax the sphincter should be recommended despite the lack of published literature.

If hypertension persists despite physical measures, pharmacological treatment should be established. Nifedipine or captopril has a reasonable level of evidence. The use of one of them seems to be related to educational tradition in each area. Level of evidence: II.

Fecal impaction is the second leading cause of AD. Again medical treatment with manual removal of the stool is the first option with a level of evidence of II to V. Anal sphincter block to decrease the sensory impulse as well as to relax the sphincter is highly recommended. Level of evidence: II.

In the case of unknown etiology, the patient should consider evaluation at a hospital center to complete diagnosis and to be treated consequently. Level of evidence: none.

What Are Potential Causes and Prevention Measures of Autonomic Dysreflexia?

Effective treatment of AD should begin with avoiding bladder distension, the most common cause of AD. Anticholinergic drugs are strongly recommended as the initial therapy. Level of evidence: II, despite some troublesome side effects. If this option fails, intravesical medications capsaicin and resiniferatoxin can be attempted. Level of evidence II to V. Botulinum toxin is a second line of treatment prior to surgical treatment, and it can be recommended. Level of evidence: I to V.

In case of failure of conservative treatment, surgical options should be considered. Unfortunately studies concerning surgical treatment are lacking because most are case series with a very low level of evidence. Surgical therapy for male patients is a sphincterotomy. Level of evidence: IV–V. Urethral stents have been proposed to avoid restenosis, but their efficacy over time has not yet been demonstrated. Additional alternative methods are anecdotal, and their use should be reserved to highly selected cases. Level of evidence: IV.

Table 46.9 Pregnancy

Study	Description	Level of E.	Topic and Conclusions
Westgren et al (1993)[74]	Retrospective cohort	III	Between 1980 and1991, 29 women with a traumatic spinal cord injury experienced 49 pregnancies and gave birth to 52 children. Nine of 12 patients with lesions above T5 had symptoms of autonomic hyperreflexia during pregnancy and/or delivery. The cesarean delivery rate for women with lesions above T5 was 47% and for women with lesions below that level, 26%.

Bowel programs including modification of stool consistence, stimulation of bowel transit, and controlled defecation are widely used despite the lack of scientific evidence but again supported by longstanding clinical experience. Surgical procedures to avoid bowel distension have a good level of evidence, but their use should be reserved for the rare cases of bowel program failure.

AD can occur during pregnancy and especially during delivery. Epidural anesthesia seems to be the best anesthetic option. The election of vaginal delivery or cesarean section depends on the gynecologist's preferences. It seems that the cesarean option could be preferred because it can be of shorter duration than vaginal delivery. Level of evidence: V.

References

1. Erickson RP. Autonomic hyperreflexia: pathophysiology and medical management. Arch Phys Med Rehabil 1980;61:431–440
2. Kurnick NB. Autonomic hyperreflexia and its control in patients with spinal cord lesions. Ann Intern Med 1956;44:678–686
3. Braddom RL, Rocco JF. Autonomic dysreflexia: a survey of current treatment. Am J Phys Med Rehabil 1991;70:234–241
4. Lindan R, Joiner E, Freehafer AA, Hazel C. Incidence and clinical features of autonomic dysreflexia in patients with spinal cord injury. Paraplegia 1980;18:285–292
5. Krassioukov AV, Furlan JC, Fehlings MG. Autonomic dysreflexia in acute spinal cord injury: an under-recognized clinical entity. J Neurotrauma 2003;20:707–716
6. Silver JR. Early autonomic dysreflexia. Spinal Cord 2000;38:229–233
7. Karlsson AK, Friberg P, Lönnroth P, Sullivan L, Elam M. Regional sympathetic function in high spinal cord injury during mental stress and autonomic dysreflexia. Brain 1998;121(Pt 9):1711–1719
8. Teasell RW, Arnold JM, Krassioukov A, Delaney GA. Cardiovascular consequences of loss of supraspinal control of the sympathetic nervous system after spinal cord injury. Arch Phys Med Rehabil 2000;81:506–516
9. Gao SA, Ambring A, Lambert G, Karlsson AK. Autonomic control of the heart and renal vascular bed during autonomic dysreflexia in high spinal cord injury. Clin Auton Res 2002;12:457–464
10. Krassioukov AV, Karlsson AK, Wecht JM, Wuermser LA, Mathias CJ, Marino RJ ; Joint Committee of American Spinal Injury Association and International Spinal Cord Society. Assessment of autonomic dysfunction following spinal cord injury: rationale for additions to International Standards for Neurological Assessment. J Rehabil Res Dev 2007;44:103–112
11. Dixit S. Bradycardia associated with high cervical spinal cord injury. Surg Neurol 1995;43:514
12. Forrest GP. Atrial fibrillation associated with autonomic dysreflexia in patients with tetraplegia. Arch Phys Med Rehabil 1991;72:592–594
13. Collins HL, Rodenbaugh DW, DiCarlo SE. Spinal cord injury alters cardiac electrophysiology and increases the susceptibility to ventricular arrhythmias. Prog Brain Res 2006;152:275–288
14. Prakash M, Raxwal V, Froelicher VF, et al. Electrocardiographic findings in patients with chronic spinal cord injury. Am J Phys Med Rehabil 2002;81:601–608
15. Dolinak D, Balraj E. Autonomic dysreflexia and sudden death in people with traumatic spinal cord injury. Am J Forensic Med Pathol 2007;28:95–98
16. Abouleish EI, Hanley ES, Palmer SM. Can epidural fentanyl control autonomic hyperreflexia in a quadriplegic parturient? Anesth Analg 1989;68:523–526
17. McGregor JA, Meeuwsen J. Autonomic hyperreflexia: a mortal danger for spinal cord-damaged women in labor. Am J Obstet Gynecol 1985;151:330–333
18. Cole TM, Kottke FJ, Olson M, Stradal L, Niederloh J. Alterations of cardiovascular control in high spinal myelomalacia. Arch Phys Med Rehabil 1967;48:359–368
19. Guttmann L, Frankel HL, Paeslack V. Cardiac irregularities during labour in paraplegic women. Paraplegia 1965;3:144–151
20. Hickey KJ, Vogel LC, Willis KM, Anderson CJ. Prevalence and etiology of autonomic dysreflexia in children with spinal cord injuries. J Spinal Cord Med 2004;27(Suppl 1):S54–S60
21. American College of Obstetrics and Gynecology; Committee on Obstetric Practice. American College of Obstetrics and Gynecology. ACOG committee opinion. Obstetric management of patients with spinal cord injuries. Number 275, September 2002. Int J Gynaecol Obstet 2002;79:189–191
22. Consortium for Spinal Cord Medicine. Acute Management of Autonomic Dysreflexia. 2nd ed. Washington (DC): Paralyzed Veterans of America (PVA) 2001 July
23. Dykstra DD, Sidi AA, Anderson LC. The effect of nifedipine on cystoscopy-induced autonomic hyperreflexia in patients with high spinal cord injuries. J Urol 1987;138:1155–1157
24. Davidson RC, Bursten SL, Keeley PA, Kenny MA, Stewart DK. Oral nifedipine for the treatment of patients with severe hypertension. Am J Med 1985;79(4A):26–30
25. McAllister RG Jr. Kinetics and dynamics of nifedipine after oral and sublingual doses. Am J Med 1986;81(6A):2–5
26. Angeli P, Chiesa M, Caregaro L, et al. Comparison of sublingual captopril and nifedipine in immediate treatment of hypertensive emergencies: a randomized, single-blind clinical trial. Arch Intern Med 1991;151:678–682
27. Ceyhan B, Karaaslan Y, Caymaz O, et al. Comparison of sublingual captopril and sublingual nifedipine in hypertensive emergencies. Jpn J Pharmacol 1990;52:189–193
28. Ellrodt AG, Ault MJ, Riedinger MS, Murata GH. Efficacy and safety of sublingual nifedipine in hypertensive emergencies. Am J Med 1985;79(4A):19–25
29. Gemici K, Karakoç Y, Ersoy A, Baran I I, Güllülü S, Cordan J. A comparison of safety and efficacy of sublingual captopril with sublingual nifedipine in hypertensive crisis. Int J Angiol 1999;8:147–149
30. Wu SG, Lin SL, Shiao WY, Huang HW, Lin CF, Yang YH. Comparison of sublingual captopril, nifedipine and prazosin in hypertensive emergencies during hemodialysis. Nephron 1993;65:284–287
31. Esmail Z, Shalansky KF, Sunderji R, Anton H, Chambers K, Fish W. Evaluation of captopril for the management of hypertension in autonomic dysreflexia: a pilot study. Arch Phys Med Rehabil 2002;83:604–608
32. Mamas MA, Reynard JM, Brading AF. Augmentation of nitric oxide to treat detrusor-external sphincter dyssynergia in spinal cord injury. Lancet 2001;357:1964–1967
33. Jones NA, Jones SD. Management of life-threatening autonomic hyperreflexia using magnesium sulphate in a patient with a high spinal cord injury in the intensive care unit. Br J Anaesth 2002;88:434–438
34. Krum H, Louis WJ, Brown DJ, Howes LG. A study of the alpha-1 adrenoceptor blocker prazosin in the prophylactic management of autonomic dysreflexia in high spinal cord injury patients. Clin Auton Res 1992;2:83–88
35. Furusawa K, Sugiyama H, Ikeda A, et al. Autonomic dysreflexia during a bowel program in patients with cervical spinal cord injury. Acta Med Okayama 2007;61:221–227
36. Cosman BC, Vu TT, Plowman BK. Topical lidocaine does not limit autonomic dysreflexia during anorectal procedures in spinal cord injury: a prospective, double-blind study. Int J Colorectal Dis 2002;17:104–108
37. Cosman BC, Vu TT. Lidocaine anal block limits autonomic dysreflexia during anorectal procedures in spinal cord injury: a randomized, double-blind, placebo-controlled trial. Dis Colon Rectum 2005;48:1556–1561
38. Collins HL, DiCarlo SE. TENS attenuates response to colon distension in paraplegic and quadriplegic rats. Am J Physiol Heart Circ Physiol 2002;283:H1734–H1739
39. O'Leary M, Erickson JR, Smith CP, McDermott C, Horton J, Chancellor MB. Effect of controlled-release oxybutynin on neurogenic bladder function in spinal cord injury. J Spinal Cord Med 2003;26:159–162
40. Chancellor MB, Erhard MJ, Hirsch IH, Stass WE Jr. Prospective evaluation of terazosin for the treatment of autonomic dysreflexia. J Urol 1994;151:111–113
41. Vaidyanathan S, Soni BM, Sett P, Watt JW, Oo T, Bingley J. Pathophysiology of autonomic dysreflexia: long-term treatment with terazosin in adult and paediatric spinal cord injury patients manifesting recurrent dysreflexic episodes. Spinal Cord 1998;36:761–770
42. Pannek J, Sommerfeld HJ, Bötel U, Senge T. Combined intravesical and oral oxybutynin chloride in adult patients with spinal cord injury. Urology 2000;55:358–362
43. Fader M, Glickman S, Haggar V, Barton R, Brooks R, Malone-Lee J. Intravesical atropine compared to oral oxybutynin for neurogenic detrusor overactivity: a double-blind, randomized crossover trial. J Urol 2007;177:208–213, discussion 213
44. de Sèze M, Wiart L, de Sèze MP, et al. Reiterated intravesical instillation of capsaicin in neurogenic detrusor hyperreflexia: a 5-years experience of 100 instillations [in French]. Ann Readapt Med Phys 2001;44:514–524
45. de Sèze M, Wiart L, de Sèze MP, et al. Intravesical capsaicin versus resiniferatoxin for the treatment of detrusor hyperreflexia in spinal cord injured patients: a double-blind, randomized, controlled study. J Urol 2004;171:251–255
46. Giannantoni A, Di Stasi SM, Stephen RL, et al. Intravesical capsaicin versus resiniferatoxin in patients with detrusor hyperreflexia: a prospective randomized study. J Urol 2002;167:1710–1714
47. Igawa Y, Satoh T, Mizusawa H, et al. The role of capsaicin-sensitive afferents in autonomic dysreflexia in patients with spinal cord injury. BJU Int 2003;91:637–641
48. Dasgupta P, Fowler CJ, Stephen RL. Electromotive drug administration of lidocaine to anesthetize the bladder before intravesical capsaicin. J Urol 1998;159:1857–1861

49. Di Stasi SM, Giannantoni A, Vespasiani G, et al. Intravesical electromotive administration of oxybutynin in patients with detrusor hyperreflexia unresponsive to standard anticholinergic regimens. J Urol 2001;165:491–498

50. Denys P, Even-Schneider A, Thiry Escudie I, Ben Smail D, Ayoub N, Chartier-Kastler E. Efficacy of botulinum toxin A for the treatment of detrusor hyperreflexia [in French]. Ann Readapt Med Phys 2003;46: 326–328

51. MacDonald R, Fink HA, Huckabay C, Monga M, Wilt TJ. Botulinum toxin for treatment of urinary incontinence due to detrusor overactivity: a systematic review of effectiveness and adverse effects. Spinal Cord 2007;45:535–541

52. Schurch B, Stöhrer M, Kramer G, Schmid DM, Gaul G, Hauri D. Botulinum-A toxin for treating detrusor hyperreflexia in spinal cord injured patients: a new alternative to anticholinergic drugs? Preliminary results. J Urol 2000;164(3 Pt 1):692–697

53. Tow AM, Toh KL, Chan SP, Consigliere D. Botulinum toxin type A for refractory neurogenic detrusor overactivity in spinal cord injured patients in Singapore. Ann Acad Med Singapore 2007;36:11–17

54. Smit CA, Slim EJ. Heart conduction problems in a tetraplegic patient caused by a single therapeutic dosage of baclofen. Spinal Cord 2008;46: 317–318

55. Vaidyanathan S, Soni BM, Oo T, Hughes PL, Singh G, Mansour P. Delayed complications of discontinuation of intrathecal baclofen therapy: resurgence of dyssynergic voiding, which triggered off autonomic dysreflexia and hydronephrosis. Spinal Cord 2004;42:598–602

56. Galeano C, Corcos J, Carmel M, Jubelin B. Action of clonidine on micturitional reflexes in decerebrate cats. Brain Res 1989;491:45–56

57. Klohn M, Rampa M, Bolle JF, Hachen H, Graber P. Endoscopic sphincterotomy in paraplegic patients: retrospective cases in Geneva [in French]. Helv Chir Acta 1990;57:443–446

58. Perkash I. Transurethral sphincterotomy provides significant relief in autonomic dysreflexia in spinal cord injured male patients: long-term followup results. J Urol 2007;177:1026–1029

59. Reynard JM, Vass J, Sullivan ME, Mamas M. Sphincterotomy and the treatment of detrusor-sphincter dyssynergia: current status, future prospects. Spinal Cord 2003;41:1–11

60. Kajio K, Iwatsubo E, Kamimura T, Takahashi N, Kobashigawa N, Kumazawa J. Clinical features of transurethral anterior sphincterotomy and urological management of patients with cervical spinal cord injury [in Japanese]. Nippon Hinyokika Gakkai Zasshi 1998;89:885–893

61. Momose H, Natsume O, Yamamoto M, Suemori T, Yamada K, Shiomi T. Transurethral electroresection of the external urethral sphincter in the urological management of male tetraplegics [in Japanese]. Hinyokika Kiyo 1988;34:280–286

62. Natsume O, Takahashi S, Yamamoto M, Momose H, Suemori T, Yamada K. Management of female neurogenic bladders caused by cervical spinal cord injuries—cutaneous vesicostomy [in Japanese]. Hinyokika Kiyo 1990;36:271–274

63. Chartier-Kastler EJ, Thomas L, Bussel B, Chancellor MB, Richard F, Denys P. A urethral stent for the treatment of detrusor-striated sphincter dyssynergia. BJU Int 2000;86:52–57

64. Hamid R, Arya M, Patel HR, Shah PJ. The mesh Wallstent in the treatment of detrusor external sphincter dyssynergia in men with spinal cord injury: a 12-year follow-up. BJU Int 2003;91:51–53

65. Chancellor MB, Rivas DA, Abdill CK, Karasick S, Ehrlich SM, Staas WE. Prospective comparison of external sphincter balloon dilatation and prosthesis placement with external sphincterotomy in spinal cord injured men. Arch Phys Med Rehabil 1994;75:297–305

66. Hamid R, Arya M, Wood S, Patel HR, Shah PJ. The use of the Memokath stent in the treatment of detrusor sphincter dyssynergia in spinal cord injury patients: a single-centre seven-year experience. Eur Urol 2003;43:539–543

67. Kutzenberger J. Surgical therapy of neurogenic detrusor overactivity (hyperreflexia) in paraplegic patients by sacral deafferentation and implant driven micturition by sacral anterior root stimulation: methods, indications, results, complications, and future prospects. Acta Neurochir Suppl (Wien) 2007;97(Pt 1):333–339

68. Jannings W, Pryor J. The downside of ileocystoplasty for persons with cervical spinal cord injury and an indwelling urinary catheter. Urol Nurs 2007;27:213–220, 238

69. Sidi AA, Becher EF, Reddy PK, Dykstra DD. Augmentation enterocystoplasty for the management of voiding dysfunction in spinal cord injury patients. J Urol 1990;143:83–85

70. Mutchnik SE, Hinson JL, Nickell KG, Boone TB. Ileovesicostomy as an alternative form of bladder management in tetraplegic patients. Urology 1997;49:353–357

71. Tan HJ, Stoffel J, Daignault S, McGuire EJ, Latini JM. Ileovesicostomy for adults with neurogenic bladders: complications and potential risk factors for adverse outcomes. Neurourol Urodyn 2008;27:238–243

72. Kirshblum SC, House JG, O'connor KC. Silent autonomic dysreflexia during a routine bowel program in persons with traumatic spinal cord injury: a preliminary study. Arch Phys Med Rehabil 2002;83:1774–1776

73. Furlan JC, Urbach DR, Fehlings MG. Optimal treatment for severe neurogenic bowel dysfunction after chronic spinal cord injury: a decision analysis. Br J Surg 2007;94:1139–1150

74. Westgren N, Hultling C, Levi R, Westgren M. Pregnancy and delivery in women with a traumatic spinal cord injury in Sweden, 1980-1991. Obstet Gynecol 1993;81:926–930

75. American College of Obstetricians and Gynecologists. ACOG Committee Opinion: Number 275, September 2002. Obstetric management of patients with spinal cord injuries. Obstet Gynecol 2002;100:625–627

76. Colachis SC III. Autonomic hyperreflexia with spinal cord injury. J Am Paraplegia Soc 1992;15:171–186

77. Rezig K, Diar N, Benabidallah D, Khodja A, Saint-Leger S. Paraplegia and pregnancy: anaesthesic management [in French]. Ann Fr Anesth Reanim 2003;22:238–241

78. Burns R, Clark VA. Epidural anaesthesia for caesarean section in a patient with quadriplegia and autonomic hyperreflexia. Int J Obstet Anesth 2004;13:120–123

79. Osgood SL, Kuczkowski KM. Autonomic dysreflexia in a parturient with spinal cord injury. Acta Anaesthesiol Belg 2006;57:161–162

80. Abrams P, Amarenco G, Bakke A, et al; European Tamsulosin Neurogenic Lower Urinary Tract Dysfunction Study Group. Tamsulosin: efficacy and safety in patients with neurogenic lower urinary tract dysfunction due to suprasacral spinal cord injury. J Urol 2003;170(4 Pt 1): 1242–1251

81. Kim JH, Rivas DA, Shenot PJ, et al. Intravesical resiniferatoxin for refractory detrusor hyperreflexia: a multicenter, blinded, randomized, placebo-controlled trial. J Spinal Cord Med 2003;26:358–363

82. Vogel LC, Krajei KA, Anderson CJ. Adults with pediatric-onset spinal cord injury: part 2: musculoskeletal and neurological complications. J Spinal Cord Med 2002 Summer; 25(2):117–123.

83. Lindan R, Leffler EJ, Kedia KR. A comparison of the efficacy of an alpha-l-adrenergic blocker in the slow calcium channel blocker in the control of autonomic dysreflexia. Paraplegia 1985 Feb; 23(1):34–38.

84. Dykstra DD, Sidi AA, Scott AB, Pagel JM, Goldish GD. Effects of botulism A toxin on detrusor-sphincter dyssynergia in spinal cord injury patients. J Urol 1988 May; 139(5):919–922

85. Tan HJ, Stoffel J, Daignault S, McGuire EJ, Latini JM. Ileovesicostomy for adults with neurogenic bladders: complications and potential risk factors for adverse outcomes. Neurourol Urodyn 2008;27(3):238–243.

47

Management of Neuropathic Pain and Late Syrinx Formation

Nicholas Theodore, James S. Harrop, and Peter H. Maughan

The majority of spinal cord injury (SCI) patients experience some degree of chronic pain at or below the level of their neurological injury, with an estimated prevalence of 29 to 75%.[1] Neuropathic pain after SCI has been treated with multiple modalities, including surgery, multiple medications (antidepressants, antiepileptics, narcotics, and stimulants), visual illusions, electric stimulation, and physical therapy. This chapter provides an evidence-based review of the literature related to treatment strategies for neuropathic pain after SCI.

◆ Methods

The National Center for Biotechnology Information database was searched using the terms "spinal cord injury" and "pain." Each abstract queried was reviewed, and further articles were noted with a focus on SCI-associated neuropathic pain. These articles were further supplemented with the authors' personal knowledge in addition to references obtained from initial query articles. The quality of evidence for these articles was used to determine a score of high, moderate, low,[2] or very low based on the grading of recommendations assessment development and evaluation (GRADE) approach,[3] and a table of literature was constructed. Subsequently, the literature and the evidence-based questions following here were presented. A group discussion involving the authors and editors determined the strength of the literature and subsequent recommendations.

Question 1: Are Treatments Available for Posttraumatic SCI Pain Syndromes?

Question 2: Are Treatment Strategies Available for Posttraumatic Syringomyelia?

Thirteen relevant studies that treated neuropathic pain with prescription medications were identified. Of these 13 studies, 11 (85%) were randomized, controlled trials and graded as level I data. The remaining two studies were prospective, nonrandomized studies and provided additional level II data. An additional four randomized trials that treated pain after SCI with transcranial magnetic stimulation or electrotherapy provided level I data and were also reviewed. One prospective cohort study that examined the relationship between surgery and pain after SCI provided level II data, and one study retrospectively reported outcomes of patients treated by section of the dorsal root entry zone.

◆ Medical Management

Medical management of neuropathic pain after SCI can be divided or categorized by the route of delivery of the medication: oral, intravenous, and intrathecal (**Table 47.1**).

Oral Medication

Seven studies that provided level I or II class evidence on the oral treatment of pain after SCI were reviewed. Although these studies met the criteria for a highest level of quality, their results were conflicting. Most of these studies were also limited by a small number of subjects, which also may explain the conflicting results.

Two prospective, randomized, controlled, double-blind crossover trials (level I data) examined the use of gabapentin to reduce the incidence of neuropathic pain. Both of these studies found that gabapentin significantly reduced certain types of neuropathic pain compared with a placebo.[4,5] An additional third study, which provided level II data, prospectively followed two cohorts of patients grouped by duration of pain symptoms (less than or greater than 6 months).[6] Based on these patients' reduced pain scores, gabapentin was noted to significantly decrease pain in both groups. The patients that experienced the greatest benefit from treatment in terms of pain reduction were individuals that had pain symptoms for less than 6 months before initiating the medical therapy.

Two further studies examined the efficacy of amitriptyline as a treatment for chronic neuropathic pain after SCI. Cardenas et al studied 84 patients that were randomized to receive

Table 47.1 Summary of Studies Treating Pain after Spinal Cord Injury with Medications

Study	Type of Study	Level of Evidence	No. Patients	Outcome
Ahn et al (2003)[6]	Prospective cohort administered gabapentin 5 weeks after 18-day titration	II	31 with neuropathic pain post-SCI. Group 1 (n = 13) had pain < 6 months and group 2 (n = 18) > 6 months	Both groups had significant decrease in visual analogue scale, with greater benefit in group 1 patients
Attal et al (2000)[10]	Double-blinded, placebo-controlled, crossover trial of IV lidocaine versus placebo	II (downgrade to II since heterogeneous groups)	16 with stroke and SCI; only three with posttraumatic SCI pain	Significant reduction in some types of pain versus placebo
Attal et al (2002)[11]	Double-blind, placebo-controlled, crossover trial of IV morphine versus placebo	I	15 with neuropathic pain, mixed population only two with posttraumatic SCI pain	No significant benefit from treatment of ongoing pain
Cardenas et al (2002)[7]	Randomized, blinded, controlled trial of amitriptyline versus placebo	I	84 with SCI	No significant differences between groups in pain intensity or pain-related disability
Finnerup et al (2002)[8]	Randomized, double-blind, placebo-controlled crossover trial of lamotrigine or placebo for 9 weeks followed by 2-week washout and second 9-week treatment	II (insufficient follow-up)	30 (22 completed trial) SCI patients with neuropathic pain at or below lesion	Primary outcome measure pain diary (1–10 score). No significant effect in total sample (p = 0.11), but significant benefit in incomplete lesions (p = 0.02)
Finnerup et al (2005)[12]	Randomized, double-blind, crossover trial of IV lidocaine versus placebo	I	24	Based on visual analogue scale, lidocaine significantly reduced spontaneous pain in all patients
Kvarnström et al (2004)[13]	Randomized, double-blind, three-period, three-treatment, crossover trial of ketamine, lidocaine, or placebo	I	10	Based on visual analogue scale, ketamine significantly reduced neuropathic pain
Levendoglu et al (2004)[4]	Randomized, double-blind, placebo-controlled, crossover trial of gabapentin	I	20 with complete thoracic SCI with neuropathic pain for > 6 months	Based on Neuropathic Pain Scale, visual analogue scale, and Lattinen test, gabapentin significantly reduced frequency and intensity of some types of neuropathic pain and improved quality of life (p < 0.05)
Rintala et al (2007)[1]	Prospective, randomized, triple-blind, 8-week, crossover trial of gabapentin, amitriptyline, or diphenhydramine	I	38	Based on pain intensity measured with visual analogue scale, numeric rating scale, and depression scale, amitriptyline significantly decreased VAS in patients with depressive symptoms
Siddall et al (2000)[27]	Double-blinded, randomized, controlled trial of intrathecal morphine, clonidine, placebo, or morphine and clonidine in combination	I	15	Morphine/clonidine combined significantly relieved pain compared with other treatments
Siddall et al (2006)[9]	Prospective, multicenter, randomized, placebo-controlled trial of pregabalin versus placebo	I	137	Based on mean pain score, significant improvement in neuropathic pain, also in sleep, anxiety, and overall status
Tai et al (2002)[5]	Prospective, randomized, double-blind, crossover trial of gabapentin for 10 weeks with 2-week washout between 4-week treatment periods	I	7	Neuropathic Pain Scale, significant decrease in "unpleasant feeling" and trend toward improvement in other descriptors

either amitriptyline or a placebo for a 6-week period.[7] The authors noted no significant difference in the intensity of pain or in pain-related disability between the two groups. In contrast, Rintala et al performed a randomized, controlled, triple-blind, crossover trial to compare 8 weeks of treatment with amitriptyline, gabapentin, and diphenhydramine on 38 SCI patients.[1] Each patient received each medication for an 8-week period. Outcome measurements included pain intensity as recorded by the visual analogue scale (VAS), numeric rating scales, and the Center for Epidemiologic Studies

Depression Scale–Short Form. It was noted that in patients with symptoms of depression, amitriptyline significantly decreased neuropathic pain, whereas gabapentin therapy provided no benefit. Therefore, the results of the latter two studies may be skewed due to the inclusion of a high number of depressed patients in the study population compared with the first series of papers.

Two additional studies provided level I and II data on the management of neuropathic pain after SCI with oral medications. Finnerup et al analyzed the effect of lamotrigine in a randomized, double-blind, placebo-controlled, crossover trial.[8] Thirty patients were enrolled, of which 22 completed the study and were included in the final analysis. The study protocol included a 1-week baseline followed by two 9-week treatment periods with a 2-week washout period between treatments. The primary outcome measure was the median pain score. The final analysis noted no benefit to treatment with lamotrigine in the total population, but post hoc analysis of subcategories showed that patients with an incomplete SCI benefited significantly more from the medication than those with a complete injury.

Finally, Siddall et al compared the effect of pregabalin and a placebo in 137 SCI patients with neuropathic pain in a multicenter, randomized, placebo-controlled study.[9] Compared with the patients receiving placebo, the pregabalin pain scores ($p < 0.001$) were improved significantly in addition to their sleep ($p < 0.001$), anxiety ($p < 0.05$), and overall health status as measured by the Patient Global Impression of Change test ($p < 0.05$).

Intravenous Medication

Four studies were identified through the query, and each provided level II evidence on the effects of treating pain after SCI with intravenous medication. In a double-blind, placebo-controlled trial, Attal et al treated 16 patients with intravenous lidocaine.[10] This medication significantly reduced some types of pain compared with the placebo therapy. However, due to the heterogeneity of the treated population, which included stroke and SCI patients and only three posttraumatic SCI pain patients, the conclusions drawn from this study are limited. In another randomized, double-blind, placebo-controlled, crossover trial, Attal et al treated chronic pain in 15 patients with intravenous morphine.[11] Overall, the study found no significant benefit to treating ongoing pain with intravenous morphine compared with the effects of placebo therapy. As noted in their previous study, however, this study used a mixed patient population with only two of 15 patients having posttraumatic SCI pain, thus decreasing the evidence-based grading to a level II study.

In an additional randomized, double-blind, placebo-controlled, crossover trial of pain control in 24 SCI patients, Finnerup et al found that intravenous lidocaine significantly reduced neuropathic pain.[12] Further, in a randomized, double-blind, three-period, three-treatment, placebo-controlled, crossover trial with 10 SCI patients, Kvarnström et al compared treatment with intravenous ketamine, lidocaine, and saline.[13] The authors reported that the pain scores decreased significantly in 50% (5/10) of the patients in the ketamine group compared with the patients receiving lidocaine or saline.

Intrathecal Medication

Siddall et al reported a double-blinded, randomized, controlled trial of 15 SCI patients that received intrathecal injections of placebo, morphine, clonidine, or morphine and clonidine for chronic pain.[9] The authors reported that the pain was significantly reduced in patients treated with intrathecal morphine and clonidine compared with any individual medication or placebo.

◆ Transcranial Stimulation

Four randomized, controlled trials on the effects of transcranial stimulation on pain after SCI were identified and provided level I data (**Table 47.2**). All four studies noted a significant reduction in patients' perception of pain after stimulation compared with sham stimulation therapy.[14–17] Capel et al randomly assigned 30 patients to receive either transcranial stimulation two times daily for 4 days or sham treatment.[17] All patients then received the transcranial stimulation after an 8-week washout period for treatment. The pain was significantly reduced in the patients in the initial treatment group ($p < 0.0016$) compared with those initially in the sham group. However, when the patients in the sham group received treatment at 8 weeks, their pain decreased significantly ($p < 0.005$) compared with their initial sham treatment.

Tan et al randomly assigned 38 males with chronic pain after an SCI to daily 1-hour sessions of cranial electrostimulation or to sham stimulation for 21 days.[15] The treated subjects reported significantly decreased daily pain intensity compared with the sham controls. Fregni et al reported a phase II study of patients randomly assigned to transcranial direct current stimulation for 20 minutes/day over 5 days or to sham treatment.[16] Again these authors noted that pain improved significantly in the stimulation patients compared with those receiving the sham treatment. The authors further reported no changes in level of depression, anxiety, or cognitive performance in either group.

Finally, Defrin et al reported a double-blind, randomized, controlled trial of 12 patients who received 10 daily treatments of repetitive transcranial magnetic stimulation.[14] Pain scores decreased significantly, in both the real and the sham-treatment groups. However, the authors attributed this outcome to a placebo effect. During follow-up the heat-pain threshold of treated patients increased significantly, and their scores on the McGill Pain Questionnaire were lower compared with the patients in the sham-treatment group.

◆ Surgical Management

There are no studies providing level I or II literature on the surgical management of pain after SCI. One study reviewed the relationship between initial surgical management and pain after SCI but provided no information about pain treatment (level II data, **Table 47.3**). Sved et al prospectively studied 100 patients referred for rehabilitation after SCI.[18] These patients were followed longitudinally after referral to a spine injury unit and after their spine surgeon had chosen a course of surgical or conservative treatment. The prevalence of different types of pain was determined 2, 4, 8, 13, 26, and 52 weeks after treatment. The authors concluded that with the exception of increased musculoskeletal pain at 2 weeks in the surgical group, there was no difference in pain modality at any time point, regardless of treatment modality.

Table 47.2 Summary of Studies Treating Pain after SCI with Transcranial Stimulation

Study	Type of Study	Level of Evidence	No. Patients	Outcome
Capel et al (2003)[17]	Random, double-blind, sham-controlled, partial crossover trial of transcranial electrostimulation two times daily for 4 days or sham treatment. All patients re-treated after an 8-week washout period	I	30	Patients in initial treatment group had significant pain reduction ($p < 0.0016$) compared with shams. When treated at 8 weeks the shams had a significant decrease in pain ($p < 0.005$) compared with initial sham treatment
Defrin et al (2007)[14]	Double-blind, randomized, sham-controlled trial of 10 daily treatments of repetitive transcranial magnetic stimulation or sham	I	12	Both real and sham treatment groups had a significant reduction in visual analogue scale pain scores (i.e., placebo effect). Treated subjects continued to have reduction in McGill Pain Questionnaire scores during follow-up, whereas sham-treated patients did not
Fregni et al (2006)[16]	Phase II, prospective, random, blinded, sham-controlled trial of transcranial direct current stimulation randomly assigned for 20 minutes/day over 5 days versus sham treatment	I	17	Treated patients had significant pain improvement after stimulation compared with shams
Tan et al (2006)[15]	Prospective, random, sham-controlled trial of daily 1-hour sessions of cranial electrotherapy stimulation or sham treatment for 21 days	I	38 males with chronic pain post-SCI	Treated subjects reported significantly decreased daily pain intensity compared with sham controls

Sindou et al retrospectively analyzed 44 patients who underwent microsurgical section of the dorsal root entry zone for the treatment of intractable neuropathic pain related to spine injury.[19] Their mean follow-up was 6 years (range 1 to 20 years). The authors reported a "good result," meaning that pain was reduced more than 75% in 68% of the patients with segmental pain and in 88% of patients with paroxysmal pain compared with only 26% of the patients with continuous pain. However, the authors reported no success in treating patients with predominantly infralesional pain.

◆ Summary

There is a high prevalence of chronic pain in the SCI population with traumatic SCI, and it is manifested as neuropathic pain. An evidence-based medical review provides good evidence that there are multiple modalities to treat chronic pain after SCI, including medication (oral, intravenous, and intrathecal) and transcranial stimulation. Therefore, a strong recommendation of treating posttraumatic SCI pain through medication and transcranial stimulation can be made.

Oral medical therapy in terms of gabapentin, pregabalin, and amitriptyline appears to be the most effective based on a class I literature review. The data for intravenous medication are more limited due to heterogeneous study populations, but ketamine infusions did appear to be effective compared with placebo. Compared against any individual medication or placebo, intrathecal morphine and clonidine had a beneficial effect. Furthermore, good evidence indicates that transcranial stimulation is an additional effective treatment for this disorder. The literature further illustrated that surgical therapy, in the form of rhizotomy, has a limited role in the management of chronic posttraumatic SCI pain.

Table 47.3 Summary of Studies of the Surgical Treatment of Pain after SCI

Study	Type of Study	Level of Evidence	No. Patients	Outcome
Sved et al (1997)[18]	Prospective, longitudinal study of prevalence of different types of pain at 2, 4, 8, 13, 26, and 52 weeks	II	100 referred for rehabilitation after SCI	With the exception of increased musculoskeletal pain at 2 weeks in the surgical group, no difference in any pain modality between surgical and nonsurgical patients at any point
Sindou et al (2001)[19]	Retrospective case series of microsurgical section of the dorsal root entry zone	IV	44 with intractable neuropathic pain secondary to spine injury	"Good result" in 68% of patients with segmental pain and in 88% of patients with paroxysmal pain versus 26% with continuous pain. No success in patients with predominantly infralesional pain

◆ Management of Late Syrinx (Posttraumatic Syringomyelia) Formation

The formation of a posttraumatic syringomyelia after an SCI is fortunately rare, with even the highest estimated incidence reported as 4.45%.[20] In 1966 Barnett et al first described this entity, which has since been increasingly recognized and studied through the use of noninvasive imaging studies.[21] Treatment has focused on shunting, expansive duraplasty, spinal reconstruction, detethering, and cordotomy. Therefore, an evidenced-based medical review of treatment strategies of posttraumatic syringomyelia was performed (**Table 47.4**).

Methods

The National Center for Biotechnology Information database was searched using the terms "SCI," "syrinx," and "posttraumatic syrinx." Identified studies were reviewed for relevance, and selected papers were graded according to evidence-based guidelines.[2] No level I or II evidence regarding treatment was found.

Schurch et al prospectively studied 449 traumatic paraplegic and tetraplegic patients admitted to a single center with a goal of assessing the incidence of posttraumatic syringomyelia (PTS) and its common present signs and symptoms.[20] Over the course of follow-up, 20 patients (4.45%) developed PTS. Time from injury to diagnosis of PTS ranged from 9 months to 30 years (mean 9.4 years). The most common presenting symptom was pain. Of the 20 patients, 13 were treated conservatively, and seven were treated surgically (three patients refused surgery). Surgical treatments included T-tube draining of the subarachnoid space in three patients, spine restabilization in two patients, and syringostomia in two patients. Of the surgically treated patients, the neurological status improved or was stable in all patients, except one whose condition initially improved and then subsequently deteriorated. Of the 13 conservatively treated patients, three experienced radiographic worsening and then clinically deteriorated in terms of their neurological examination. The remaining 10 patients were stable both radiologically and clinically.

Perrouin-Verbe et al examined the relationship between PTS and posttraumatic spinal canal stenosis in 75 patients with SCI.[22] A PTS subsequently formed in 28% of the patients,

Table 47.4 Summary of Studies on the Management of Late Syrinx after Surgical Treatment of SCI

Study	Type of Study	Level of Evidence	No. Patients	Outcome
Jaksche et al (2005)[25]	Retrospective analysis of laminectomy, removal of arachnoid adhesions, and extensive duraplasty	IV	58	70% good outcome. Authors advocate normalization of cerebrospinal fluid flow by creating a pseudomeningomyelocele
Laxton and Perrin (2006)[26]	Retrospective analysis and literature review of cordectomy for treatment of posttraumatic syringomyelia	IV	4	All good outcomes. Literature review: 88% rate of stabilization or improvement in patients with complete SCI treated with cordectomy
Perrouin-Verbe et al (1998)[22]	Retrospective analysis of relationship between posttraumatic syringomyelia and posttraumatic spinal canal stenosis	IV	75 with SCI	28% of patients had syrinx formation, which correlated significantly with sagittal and axial stenosis. Authors recommend spinal realignment at time of injury as a preventive measure for syrinx formation
Schurch et al. (1996)[20]	Prospective assessment of incidence of posttraumatic syringomyelia (PTS)	III	449 traumatic paraplegic and tetraplegic patients admitted to a single center. 20 patients (4.45%) developed PTS over the course of follow-up. 13 patients were treated conservatively and seven treated surgically (three patients refused surgery)	Improved or stable neurologic status in all surgical patients except one patient improved initially and then deteriorated. In conservatively treated patients radiographic worsening correlated with neurological deterioration
Sgouros and Williams (1995)[23]	Retrospective analysis	IV	73 with syrinx from mixed pathology, 34 of whom had traumatic paraplegic as cause of syrinx	Overall no long-term benefit of drainage. Spinal cord transection associated with good results (eight patients)
Wiart et al (1995)[24]	Retrospective analysis of syringoperitoneal shunt for syringomyelia	IV	8	Three early complications. Over mean follow-up of 4.5 years, symptoms decreased or stabilized in seven patients. Myelopathy improved in four and worsened in four patients. Radiographic improvement in all patients: size of syrinx decreased

and this finding correlated significantly with the sagittal and axial spinal canal stenosis. The authors recommend spinal realignment at the time of initial traumatic injury to prevent the formation of a syrinx.

Sgouros and Williams evaluated drainage of syringomyelia in 73 patients who developed a syrinx from a variety of pathological conditions.[23] Traumatic paraplegia caused the syrinx in 34 patients. All trauma patients were initially treated with laminectomy at the level of injury. Many patients had drains inserted at the time of their initial surgery. However, the authors report that, overall, there was no long-term benefit of drainage. Spinal cord transection was associated with good results, but the procedure was performed in only eight patients.

Wiart et al reported eight patients with SCI who received a syringoperitoneal shunt after they developed syringomyelia.[24] There were three early complications: one hemorrhage, and two catheter failures. Over the mean postoperative follow-up of 4.5 years, symptoms decreased or stabilized in seven patients. Myelopathy improved in four patients and worsened in four patients. Radiographically, all patients improved and the size of their syrinx decreased after treatment.

Jaksche et al reported a series of patients who underwent a two-level laminectomy followed by resection of arachnoidal adhesions and an extensive duraplasty for treatment of posttraumatic syrinx.[25] The authors reported that 34 patients improved, 17 remained stable, and five patients worsened. One patient died from pulmonary embolism. The authors advocate normalizing the flow of cerebrospinal fluid by creating a pseudomeningomyelocele.

Laxton and Perrin treated four cases of PTS with cordectomy and had good outcomes in each.[26] Based on their review of the literature, the rate of stabilization or improvement in patients with a complete SCI was 88%.

◆ Summary

Posttraumatic syringomyelia in the SCI population can result in progressive neurological deterioration. An evidence-based medical review of the literature provides poor evidence that there is an optimal treatment strategy. Therefore, a weak recommendation of treating posttraumatic syringomyelia in the setting of neurological deterioration can be made.

References

1. Rintala DH, Holmes SA, Courtade D, Fiess RN, Tastard LV, Loubser PG. Comparison of the effectiveness of amitriptyline and gabapentin on chronic neuropathic pain in persons with spinal cord injury. Arch Phys Med Rehabil 2007;88:1547–1560

2. Fisher CG, Wood KB. Introduction to and techniques of evidence-based medicine. Spine 2007;32(19, Suppl):S66–S72

3. GRADE Working Group. http://www.gradeworkinggroup.org/

4. Levendoglu F, Ogün CO, Ozerbil O, Ogün TC, Ugurlu H. Gabapentin is a first line drug for the treatment of neuropathic pain in spinal cord injury. Spine 2004;29:743–751

5. Tai Q, Kirshblum S, Chen B, Millis S, Johnston M, DeLisa JA. Gabapentin in the treatment of neuropathic pain after spinal cord injury: a prospective, randomized, double-blind, crossover trial. J Spinal Cord Med 2002;25:100–105

6. Ahn SH, Park HW, Lee BS, et al. Gabapentin effect on neuropathic pain compared among patients with spinal cord injury and different durations of symptoms. Spine 2003;28:341–346, discussion 346–347

7. Cardenas DD, Warms CA, Turner JA, Marshall H, Brooke MM, Loeser JD. Efficacy of amitriptyline for relief of pain in spinal cord injury: results of a randomized controlled trial. Pain 2002;96:365–373

8. Finnerup NB, Sindrup SH, Bach FW, Johannesen IL, Jensen TS. Lamotrigine in spinal cord injury pain: a randomized controlled trial. Pain 2002;96:375–383

9. Siddall PJ, Cousins MJ, Otte A, Griesing T, Chambers R, Murphy TK. Pregabalin in central neuropathic pain associated with spinal cord injury: a placebo-controlled trial. Neurology 2006;67:1792–1800

10. Attal N, Gaudé V, Brasseur L, et al. Intravenous lidocaine in central pain: a double-blind, placebo-controlled, psychophysical study. Neurology 2000;54:564–574

11. Attal N, Guirimand F, Brasseur L, Gaude V, Chauvin M, Bouhassira D. Effects of IV morphine in central pain: a randomized placebo-controlled study. Neurology 2002;58:554–563

12. Finnerup NB, Biering-Sorensen F, Johannesen IL, et al. Intravenous lidocaine relieves spinal cord injury pain: a randomized controlled trial. Anesthesiology 2005;102:1023–1030

13. Kvarnström A, Karlsten R, Quiding H, Gordh T. The analgesic effect of intravenous ketamine and lidocaine on pain after spinal cord injury. Acta Anaesthesiol Scand 2004;48:498–506

14. Defrin R, Grunhaus L, Zamir D, Zeilig G. The effect of a series of repetitive transcranial magnetic stimulations of the motor cortex on central pain after spinal cord injury. Arch Phys Med Rehabil 2007;88:1574–1580

15. Tan G, Rintala DH, Thornby JI, Yang J, Wade W, Vasilev C. Using cranial electrotherapy stimulation to treat pain associated with spinal cord injury. J Rehabil Res Dev 2006;43:461–474

16. Fregni F, Boggio PS, Lima MC, et al. A sham-controlled, phase II trial of transcranial direct current stimulation for the treatment of central pain in traumatic spinal cord injury. Pain 2006;122:197–209

17. Capel ID, Dorrell HM, Spencer EP, Davis MW. The amelioration of the suffering associated with spinal cord injury with subperception transcranial electrical stimulation. Spinal Cord 2003;41:109–117

18. Sved P, Siddall PJ, McClelland J, Cousins MJ. Relationship between surgery and pain following spinal cord injury. Spinal Cord 1997;35:526–530

19. Sindou M, Mertens P, Wael M. Microsurgical DREZotomy for pain due to spinal cord and/or cauda equina injuries: long-term results in a series of 44 patients. Pain 2001;92:159–171

20. Schurch B, Wichmann W, Rossier AB. Post-traumatic syringomyelia (cystic myelopathy): a prospective study of 449 patients with spinal cord injury. J Neurol Neurosurg Psychiatry 1996;60:61–67

21. Barnett HJ, Botterell EH, Jousse AT, Wynn-Jones M. Progressive myelopathy as a sequel to traumatic paraplegia. Brain 1966;89:159–174

22. Perrouin-Verbe B, Lenne-Aurier K, Robert R, et al. Post-traumatic syringomyelia and post-traumatic spinal canal stenosis: a direct relationship: review of 75 patients with a spinal cord injury. Spinal Cord 1998;36:137–143

23. Sgouros S, Williams B. A critical appraisal of drainage in syringomyelia. J Neurosurg 1995;82:1–10

24. Wiart L, Dautheribes M, Pointillart V, Gaujard E, Petit H, Barat M. Mean term follow-up of a series of post-traumatic syringomyelia patients after syringo-peritoneal shunting. Paraplegia 1995;33:241–245

25. Jaksche H, Schaan M, Schulz J, Bosczcyk B. Posttraumatic syringomyelia— a serious complication in tetra- and paraplegic patients. Acta Neurochir Suppl (Wien) 2005;93:165–167

26. Laxton AW, Perrin RG. Cordectomy for the treatment of posttraumatic syringomyelia: report of four cases and review of the literature. J Neurosurg Spine 2006;4:174–178

27. Siddall PJ, Molloy AR, Walker S. Mather LE, Rutkowski SB, Cousins MJ. The efficacy of intrathecal morphine and clonidine in the treatment of pain after spinal cord injury. Anesth Analg 2000;91:1493–1498

48

Rehabilitation Strategies for Spinal Cord Injury–Induced Neuropathic Pain and Spasticity

Alpesh A. Patel

Spinal cord injuries occur at an estimated annual incidence of 15 to 40 per million worldwide. These injuries are not defined by socioeconomic status or by geographic, racial, or cultural boundaries. As described within this textbook, there is a great deal of controversy relating to nearly all aspects of the management of spinal cord injury: diagnosis, classification, and treatment are all topics of continued discussion. The fundamental goal of the discussions in this textbook, so far, has been to maximize neurological recovery.

Motor recovery after spinal cord injury is often the primary focus of attention for both the patient and the physician. Motor recovery of even the smallest gradation may therefore be hailed as a successful outcome. The unfortunate reality is that motor recovery may not occur or may not result in functional improvement. Furthermore, even those patients with functional motor recovery will continue to face other obstacles, both physical and psychological.

Rehabilitation strategies after spinal cord injury share the basic goal of optimizing the patient's life. Strategies include physical therapy and occupational rehabilitation to maximize the individual's functional status for both occupational and recreational activities. Psychological care is aimed at mental health concerns such as depression, anxiety, and, in the extreme, suicide. Lastly, medical care specific to the health hazards facing spinal cord–injured individuals is vital (cardiovascular disease, venous thrombosis, pulmonary disease, osteoporosis, etc.).

It is beyond the scope of this chapter to discuss each of these strategies in detail. The focus will, instead, be on the management of two common and disabling problems: neuropathic pain and spasticity following spinal cord injury. Significant pain or spasticity has been reported in 40 to 70% of individuals after spinal cord injury, with over 30% describing the symptoms as severe or affecting their quality of life.[1–3] Pain and spasticity can increase the physical and psychological burden upon these individuals. Appropriate treatment has

the potential, therefore, to greatly improve the quality of life of spinal cord–injured individuals.

This chapter sets out to systematically review the available English-speaking literature with the aim of answering two specific questions:

Question 1: Is There Clinical Evidence to Support the Use of Pharmacological Therapies for Neuropathic Pain Following Spinal Cord Injury?

Question 2: Is There Clinical Evidence to Support the Use of Pharmacological Therapies for Spasticity Following Spinal Cord Injury?

Based on this review and expert medical opinion (members of the Spine Trauma Study Group), evidence-based recommendations will be offered regarding the management of these two important clinical problems.

◆ Background

Neuropathic Pain

The prevalence of pain among individuals with spinal cord injury has been reported to be between 34 and 70%, with two prospective studies reporting a prevalence of over 60% at 6 and 12 months after injury.[1,2,4] The number of patients having severe pain ranges from 12% to more than one third.[3,5] In one survey, 11% of spinal cord injury patients have described pain, not motor deficit, as the disabling factor preventing them from a return to work.[6] In another survey, 23% of thoracic and 37% of cervical spinal cord–injured patients rated pain relief as more important than bowel, bladder, or sexual function.[5]

Pain after spinal cord injury has been classified into two broad categories: nociceptive and neuropathic.[7] Neuropathic pain has been further classified as above-level, at-level, or below-level relative to the level of spinal cord injury. Above-level neuropathic pain is thought to be related either to complex regional pain syndromes or to compressive neuropathies. At-level pain has been attributed to neural compression, spinal cord injury, or root-level injury. Below-level pain is solely attributed to spinal cord trauma. Most pharmacological strategies for the treatment of neuropathic pain are targeted for at-level or below-level pain.[8]

Spasticity

Spasticity has been defined as a velocity-dependent increase in muscle tone with an exaggerated tendon jerk resulting from hyperexcitability of the stretch reflex.[9] Hyperexcitability is seen across a variety of upper motor neuron lesions (stroke, cerebral palsy, spinal cord injury, etc.) and is attributed to the loss of normal descending inhibitory corticospinal pathways.[10,11]

The prevalence of spasticity in individuals after spinal cord injury has been reported to be over 60 to 70% by 1 year postinjury.[12] Among 96 patients treated at one spinal cord injury center, 67% reported spasticity at the time of discharge, with 37% receiving medications; at 12-month follow-up, the prevalence increased to 78% with 49% of patients receiving treatment.[13] The authors also reviewed 466 subjects across 13 centers and reported similar numbers, with 46% of patients receiving treatment at 12-month follow-up.[13]

Though a common neuronal pathway may be shared among these patients, the clinical presentation of spasticity can vary significantly. Some patients will have few, if any, symptoms from their spasticity. Others may have significant pain associated with the spasmodic episodes. Still others may develop significant contractures from spasms resulting in limited mobility, pressure ulcers, sitting difficulties, and poor perineal hygiene.[12,13]

◆ Methods

A systematic review of the literature from 1966 to 2007 was performed utilizing the Medline database. Search criteria included "spinal cord injury and neuropathic pain, and treatment" (166 articles), "spinal cord injury and neuropathic pain, and management" (38 articles), "spinal cord injury and spasticity and treatment" (596 articles), "spinal cord injury and spasticity and management" (126 articles). Articles in non-English languages were excluded if a translated version was not available. Additionally, articles without clinical (human) data as well as review articles were also excluded after abstract review.

The literature review was ultimately based upon 24 articles for Question 1 and 19 articles for Question 2. The level of evidence of included articles was assessed according to the guidelines proposed by the Center for Evidence Based Medicine (www.cebm.net). In conclusion, the strength of the final recommendation was determined according to the guidelines proposed by Schünemann et al.[14]

◆ Pharmacological Treatment

Neuropathic Pain

Pharmacological treatment of neuropathic pain remains the initial treatment of choice for many patients. A wide array of medications have been investigated. Additionally, both oral and intrathecal methods of delivery have been reported.

Primary treatment options have historically been tricyclic antidepressants and conventional anticonvulsants, both of which have shown poor outcomes. Opioid medications remain a viable option, but side effects of sedation and respiratory depression can limit effectiveness. Sodium channel blockers, α-agonists, and N-methyl-D-aspartate (NMDA) receptor agonists have also been investigated. Unfortunately, each of these options is poorly supported by the literature.

Another class of anticonvulsant, thought to act on the $\alpha2\delta$ subunit of voltage-gated calcium channels in the central nervous system (CNS), has been recently applied to neuropathic pain syndromes with success. These medications are commercially available products that, contrary to most other medications, can be better supported by clinical evidence.

A summary of the clinical evidence on the pharmaceutical treatment of neuropathic pain after spinal cord injury is presented in **Table 48.1**.

Opioids

One randomized, controlled clinical trial of intravenous (IV) morphine (level II) has been conducted.[15] The authors studied IV morphine versus saline placebo in 15 patients with central pain (six due to stroke, nine due to spinal cord injury). All patients additionally received oral morphine. Other than brush-evoked allodynia, no significant differences were seen between patients receiving opioids and those in the placebo group. Additionally, only three of 15 patients continued oral narcotic treatment at 1-year follow-up.

Parenteral narcotics are not suitable for long-term management. Slow-release opioid analgesics have been reported with some success in other neuropathic pain states.[16,17] However, there have been no published investigations on the effectiveness of oral narcotic analgesics for the treatment of neuropathic pain following spinal cord injury.

Intrathecal administration of opioids has become increasingly available. Concerns continue to exist with regard to sedation and respiratory depression, but direct intrathecal titration may allow for tighter control. Siddall et al, in a randomized, controlled study (level II) compared intrathecal administration of morphine, clonidine, both morphine and clonidine, and placebo.[18] At 4 hours postinfusion, the combination of morphine and clonidine showed significantly better visual analogue scale (VAS) pain score improvements compared with the medications alone or placebo; each medication produced better results than placebo. Saulino, in a case report (level IV), described the successful use of intrathecal hydromorphone in combination with ziconotide.[19] Rare but potentially serious complications may arise from intrathecal narcotic administration. Opioid overdose may lead to respiratory depression and the need for pulmonary support. Opioid withdrawal, after discontinuation of the medication, may cause cardiovascular collapse in severe cases.[1]

Antidepressants

Antidepressants are commonly used in the treatment of neuropathic pain across several conditions. Tricyclic antidepressants (TCAs) are often used to treat postherpetic neuralgia as well as diabetic neuropathic pain. These medications act by selective neurotransmitter inhibition but may also have some effect through sodium channel or NMDA receptor blockade.[8]

Table 48.1 Summary of Clinical Evidence on the Pharmaceutical Treatment of Neuropathic Pain after Spinal Cord Injury

Category	Study	Description	Level of Evidence	Topic	Conclusions
	Attal et al (2002)[15]	Randomized, prospective, controlled, crossover	II	IV morphine versus placebo treatment in 15 patients. Initial pain relief was recorded. Patients also followed on oral narcotics for 12 months. No significant differences in pain scores except brush-evoked allodynia. Only 3/5 patients continued oral medications at 12-month follow-up.	No immediate benefit of IV morphine except in brush-evoked pain. Questionable usefulness of long-term narcotic treatment.
	Siddall et al (2000)[18]	Randomized, prospective, controlled, crossover	II	Intrathecal morphine, clonidine, morphine + clonidine combination, and placebo were compared. VAS pain scores at 4 hours after infusion were significantly improved in each group vs placebo but greatest in the morphine/clonidine combination group.	Intrathecal morphine and clonidine may provide short-term pain relief. When given in combination, pain relief was significantly better.
	Saulino (2007)[19]	Case report	IV	Single patient treated with combined intrathecal hydromorphone and zinconotide.	Successful pain relief
Antidepressant	Cardenas et al (2002)[20]	Randomized, prospective, controlled	I	84 patients were randomized to amitriptyline vs placebo for a 6-week trial. No significant differences were seen in pain or disability scores.	No treatment effect of amitriptyline.
Sodium Channel Blockade	Attal et al (2000)[21]	Randomized, prospective, controlled, crossover	II	16 patients (6 stroke, 10 SCI) treated with IV lidocaine versus placebo. Immediate spontaneous and evoked pain response were decreased in the lidocaine group. No changes in hypesthesia or in thermal allodynia.	Central sodium channel blockade may be a treatment option. Not clinically applicable given delivery and short-term relief.
	Finnerup et al (2005)[22]	Randomized, prospective, controlled, crossover	I	24 patients treated with IV lidocaine versus placebo. Spontaneous and evoked pain response were significantly ($p < 0.01$) reduced with lidocaine. Results were short-term only.	Sodium channel blockade may be a treatment option. Not clinically applicable given delivery and short-term relief.
	Chiou-Tan et al (1996)[23]	Randomized, prospective, controlled	II	15 patients treated with oral mexiletine vs placebo. No significant differences in pain scores or functional (Barthel index) scores were found.	No treatment effect of oral mexiletine.

(Continued on page 474)

Table 48.1 Summary of Clinical Evidence on the Pharmaceutical Treatment of Neuropathic Pain after Spinal Cord Injury (*Continued*)

Category		Study	Description	Level of Evidence	Topic	Conclusions
NMDA receptor agonist						
		Kvarnström et al (2004)[25]	Randomized, prospective, controlled, crossover	II	10 patients treated with IV ketamine, lidocaine, or placebo. Significant pain relief (> 50% VAS reduction) seen only in the ketamine group. No differences between placebo and lidocaine.	IV ketamine produced short-term pain relief suggesting NMDA receptor role in pain signaling. No treatment effect of lidocaine. Not clinically applicable due to delivery and short-term relief.
		Eide et al (1995)[26]	Randomized, prospective, controlled, crossover	III	IV ketamine was compared with placebo. Significant improvement in continuous and evoked pain with ketamine.	Significant short-term relief of IV ketamine suggest role of NMDA receptors in pain signaling. Not clinically applicable due to delivery and short-term relief.
α-agonists	*Clonidine*					
		Glynn et al (1986)[27]	Prospective, cohort	III	15 patients treated with epidural infusion of morphine versus clonidine. 10/15 patients had relief; 7 of 10 were nonresponsive to morphine	Epidural clonidine may give pain relief, even in patients refractory to morphine. Suggests a role of α-adrenergic agonists in treatment.
		Siddall et al (2000)[18]	Randomized, prospective, controlled, crossover	II	Intrathecal morphine, clonidine, morphine + clonidine combination, and placebo were compared. VAS pain scores at 4 hours after infusion were significantly improved in each group vs placebo but greatest in the morphine/ clonidine combination group.	Intrathecal morphine and clonidine may provide short-term pain relief. When given in combination, pain relief was significantly better.
		Middleton et al (1996)[28]	Case report	IV	Case report of successful treatment with intrathecal clonidine and intrathecal baclofen for a patient with severe neuropathic pain and spasticity.	Intrathecal clonidine may be combined with intrathecal baclofen to relieve pain and spasticity.
Anticonvulsants	*Valproate*					
		Drewes et al (1994)[29]	Case, cohort	III	Oral valproate compared with placebo. No significant differences were found in pain relief.	No analgesic effect of oral valproate compared.
		Zachariah et al (1994)[30]	Case series	IV	Four patients (three SCI) treated with oral valproate. 2/3 SCI patients had a beneficial effect.	Oral valproate may be effective.
	Carbama-zepine					
		Gibson and White (1971)[31]	Case series	IV	Two patients treated with oral carbamazepine reported good results.	Oral carbamazepine may be effective.

Table 48.1 Summary of Clinical Evidence on the Pharmaceutical Treatment of Neuropathic Pain after Spinal Cord Injury (*Continued*)

Category		Study	Description	Level of Evidence	Topic	Conclusions
	Lamotrigine					
		Finnerup et al (2002)[33]	Randomized, prospective, controlled	II	22 patients treated with either lamotrigine or placebo. No significant differences in spontaneous pain or evoked pain. A subgroup of patients (incomplete SCI).	No treatment effect of lamotrigine except in a subgroup of patients with incomplete SCI.
		Silver et al (2007)[32]	Randomized, prospective, controlled, multicenter	I	220 patients (multiple etiologies including SCI) were treated with lamotrigine versus placebo. All patients were also receiving gabapentin. No statistically significant ($p < 0.05$) differences were seen in pain scores, rescue medication use, and subjective outcome scales.	No treatment effect of lamotrigine compared with placebo when used in combination with gabapentin.
	Gabapentin					
		To et al (2002)[35]	Retrospective, cohort	III	44 SCI patients were retrospectively reviewed after treatment with gabapentin. VAS pain scores were reduced in 76% of patients from mean 8.86 to 4.13 by 6 months.	Gabapentin may reduce neuropathic pain following spinal cord injury.
		Haller et al (2003)[34]	Case report	IV	Case report of a central cord syndrome patient successfully treated with gabapentin.	Gabapentin may have a treatment effect.
		Putzke et al (2002)[36]	Case series	IV	Prospectively collected case series. 10/14 patients reported maintained pain relief at an average 36 months of treatment.	Treatment effect of gabapentin may be sustained over long-term (< 36 months).
		Tai et al (2002)[37]	Randomized, prospective controlled, crossover	II	Seven patients were treated with gabapentin vs placebo. Improvements in pain scores were seen but did not reach statistical significance.	Study was limited by a small number of patients. No conclusion can be made.
		Levendoglu et al (2004)[38]	Randomized, prospective, controlled	I	20 patients were treated with gabapentin vs placebo for 18 weeks. Statistically significant improvements in frequency of pain were found across all pain types; additionally Short Form Back Depression scores statistically improved as well, suggesting improved mental health outcomes.	Improvements in pain relief as well as mental health may be seen with gabapentin treatment.

(Continued on page 476)

Category	Study	Description	Level of Evidence	Topic	Conclusions
	Ahn et al (2003)[39]	Prospective, cohort	II	31 patients were grouped according to symptom duration (< or > 6 months). Both groups treated were with gabapentin. All patients showed decreased pain scores and sleep interference scores. Statistically better ($p < 0.05$) results were obtained in patients treated with < 6 months of symptoms.	Patients may benefit from earlier initiation of gabapentin. Nonetheless, patients with chronic symptoms (> 6 months) may also benefit from treatment.
Pregabalin	Siddall et al (2006)[40]	Multicenter, randomized, prospective, controlled	I	137 patients were treated with pregabalin (70) vs placebo (67) and were followed for 6 weeks. Statistically significant improvements in pain scores and functional outcomes were found.	Pregabalin may have a beneficial treatment effect compared with placebo.
	Vranken et al (2008)[41]	Randomized, prospective, controlled	II	40 patients treated with pregabalin vs placebo were followed for 4 weeks. Significant ($p < 0.05$) differences in VAS pain and SF-36 bodily domain scores were found.	Pregabalin may have a beneficial treatment effect compared with placebo.

Abbreviations: IV, intravenous; NMDA, *N*-methyl-D-aspartate; SCI, spinal cord injury; SF-36, Short Form-36; VAS, visual analogue scale.

Only one study has been performed, to date, investigating the use of TCAs for post–spinal cord injury pain. Cardenas et al, in a prospective, randomized, blinded, placebo-controlled study (level I) of 84 patients compared amitriptyline to placebo.[20] The authors reported no significant difference in pain scores as well as pain-related disability between the two treatment groups after a 6-week trial. Further clinical investigation is needed in this group of patients.

Given the efficacy described in the treatment of other neuropathic conditions, TCAs may still be considered. TCAs have been reported to show a low side-effect profile, with sedation and anticholinergic (dry mouth, constipation, urinary retention) effects being the most common. However, they are contraindicated in patients with cardiac disease (heart failure, conduction disturbances, ischemic heart disease) and those with seizure disorders.

Sodium Channel Blockade

Local anesthetics are known to influence pain signals through sodium channel blockade. Use of local anesthetics for neuropathic pain may also demonstrate some benefit in the setting of neuropathic pain. Attal et al, in a randomized, placebo-controlled trial (level II) compared IV lidocaine to placebo in 16 patients (six stroke, 10 spinal cord injury). The authors reported a significant, short-term reduction in spontaneous and evoked pain. No differences for thermal allodynia and hyperalgesia were noted.[21] Finnerup et al also demonstrated a statistically significant improvement in spontaneous and

evoked pain based on VAS ($p < 0.01$) among 24 spinal cord injury patients randomized in a double-blind manner to placebo or to IV lidocaine (level I).[22] The authors suggest that central sodium channel blockade may be a target for the pharmacological treatment of neuropathic pain.

The results obtained with IV infusion, as expected, have been short-term only. Translation of this effect to a sustainable, orally delivered method has not been demonstrated to be effective. Chiou-Tan et al investigated oral mexiletine, a lidocaine analogue, among 15 spinal cord injury patients in a randomized, blinded, placebo-controlled study (level II).[23] No significant differences between mexiletine and placebo were found using dysesthetic pain scales as well as the Barthel functional index.

Given the lack of substantive clinical data, the use of oral sodium channel blockade cannot be supported. Additionally, there has yet been no viable means of translating the IV fusion treatment into a long-term effect.

NMDA Receptor Blockade

Basic science studies have demonstrated that central NMDA receptors modulate the binding site of glutamate, an excitatory amino acid involved in central sensitization seen with states of neuropathic pain.[24] Kvarnström et al compared IV ketamine, lidocaine, and saline in a randomized, blinded, controlled study of 10 patients (level II).[25] Significant reduction in pain threshold (> 50% VAS reduction) was seen only in the ketamine group; no differences were found between the lidocaine and saline groups. Eide et al, in a randomized, controlled study (level III) also demonstrated a significant effect of ketamine on continuous and evoked pain measurements.[26] Although short-term benefits may be evident, no long-term option for NMDA receptor block exists. Clinical use of NMDA antagonists, therefore, cannot be supported by the literature.

α-Agonists (Clonidine)

Clonidine, an α-adrenergic agonist, has only been reported in a limited number of studies for the treatment of neuropathic pain after spinal cord injury. Glynn, in a prospective, uncontrolled study (level III) compared epidural infusion of morphine to clonidine in 15 patients.[27] Ten of 15 patients had subjective pain relief, including seven patients that were nonresponsive to morphine. Siddall et al compared intrathecal morphine and clonidine to placebo (level II).[18] The authors demonstrated improved short-term pain scores for all groups compared with placebo, with the greatest improvement in the combined morphine and clonidine group. Middleton et al reported successful use of intrathecal clonidine in combination with intrathecal baclofen for the treatment of spasticity and neuropathic pain in a case report (level IV).[28]

The use of clonidine is, therefore, based only upon a small number of patients. Currently available data suggest that adrenergic receptors have a role in neuropathic pain after spinal cord injury. Further investigation is needed before a definitive clinical recommendation can be made.

Anticonvulsants

Anticonvulsants make up the largest group of medications that are utilized in the treatment of neuropathic pain. Anticonvulsants are known to affect a multitude of receptors, including sodium channel blockade, GABA-ergic inhibition, voltage-gated calcium channels, as well as alter neurotransmitter levels. The precise mechanism of action in the setting of neuropathic pain remains unclear.

Drewes et al, in a nonrandomized, controlled study (level III) of valproate found no statistically significant analgesic effect compared with placebo.[29] Zachariah et al described a beneficial effect of valproate in two out of three spinal cord–injured patients (level IV).[30] Gibson and White reported good results in two patients treated with oral carbamazepine (level IV).[31] The limited clinical data available on valproate and carbamazepine do not support its use for neuropathic pain after spinal cord injury.

Lamotrigine (Lamictal, GlaxoSmithKline, Research Triangle Park, NC) has been investigated in two prospective studies. A prospective, double-blinded study of 220 patients with chronic neuropathic pain (multiple etiologies including spinal cord injury) randomized to placebo or lamotrigine (Lamictal) was reported by Silver et al.[32] All patients were concomitantly treated with gabapentin. No statistical differences were seen between groups in pain scales, rescue pain medication use, and subjective outcome scales. Finnerup et al demonstrated no difference between lamotrigine and placebo control in spontaneous pain and evoked pain scores among 22 patients (level II).[33] A subgroup of patients with incomplete spinal cord injury did show favorable improvements when compared separately with the placebo group. Clinical evidence does not support the use of lamotrigine; a subgroup of patients with incomplete spinal cord injury

may benefit. Further data are need before clinical recommendations can be made.

Gabapentin has become widely utilized in the treatment of neuropathic pain since its US Food and Drug Administration (FDA) approval for postherpetic neuralgia in 2002. Gabapentin is thought to act on the α2δ subunit of voltage-gated calcium channels in the CNS. Its use in spinal cord injured patients has been described in several studies. Retrospective case series by To et al (level III) and Haller et al (level IV) have reported good pain relief with gabapentin.[34,35] Putzke et al, in a prospective interview of patients treated with gabapentin (level IV) reported maintained pain relief at 36 months in 10/14 patients.[36] Tai et al, in a 4-week prospective evaluation of seven patients, compared gabapentin to placebo (level II).[37] Although neuropathic pain scales showed improvements, no statistically significant improvements were found. The authors state that the study was limited by a small number of patients.

Levendoglu et al enrolled 20 patients with complete spinal cord injury and neuropathic pain for > 6 months and randomized them to either gabapentin or placebo over an 18-week study (level I). Statistically significant improvements in frequency of pain were found across all pain types; additionally Short Form Back Depression scores statistically improved as well, suggesting improved mental health outcomes.[38] Ahn et al, in a prospective cohort study (level II), demonstrated a statistically significant decrease in pain scores and sleep interference scores among 31 patients treated with gabapentin for 8 weeks.[39] The authors divided patients into two groups, based on duration of symptoms (< or > than 6 months). Although all patients improved, scores decreased more ($p < 0.05$) in the group of patients with < 6 months of treatment. The authors, therefore, recommended initiating gabapentin treatment earlier but noted usefulness in patients with > 6 months of symptoms. Overall, there is sufficient evidence available to support the use of gabapentin.

Pregabalin (Lyrica, Pfizer, New York City, NY) is a newer anticonvulsant also believed to act on the α2δ subunit of voltage-gated calcium channels in the CNS. Studies specifically addressing its use in the setting of spinal cord injury have been performed. A multicenter, randomized, prospective study (level I) of 137 patients compared pregabalin (70) to placebo (67).[40] Baseline data included VAS pain scale, sleep disturbance assessments, depression and anxiety scales, and patient global impression of change scores; patients were followed for 12 weeks. Statistically significant improvements were seen in pain scores and functional outcome scores in the treatment group compared with placebo. Vranken et al compared pregabalin to placebo in a prospective, randomized, controlled study (level I) of 40 patients with 4-week follow-up.[41] Significant improvements ($p < 0.05$) were seen in VAS score and the Short Form-36 (SF-36) body pain domain score. Sufficient clinical evidence is available to support the use of pregabalin.

Common side effects of all anticonvulsants include dizziness, sedation, ataxia, and anticholinergic effects such as dry mouth, constipation, and urinary retention. The side-effect profiles of pregabalin and gabapentin are similar and have been reported in up to 15% of patients.[36,38,40] Both medications are excreted through the kidneys; therefore, dose adjustment may be needed in patients with renal dysfunction. Lamotrigine and valproate carry additional risks of liver dysfunction. Steven-Johnson syndrome has been reported with the use of anticonvulsants, particularly lamotrigine. Additionally, valproate is a know teratogen and is, therefore, contraindicated in pregnancy or in patients that may become pregnant.

Spasticity

Pharmacological treatment has been directed primarily at generalized spasticity following spinal cord injury, although newer injectable medications have been applied to cases of focal hypertonia. Despite different mechanisms of action, the primary target remains the monosynaptic reflex pathway from Ia sensory fibers to α motor neurons. Antispasticity medications can be broadly grouped into three categories: (1) "GABAergic" drugs (baclofen, diazepam) that act at interneurons utilizing gamma-aminobutyric acid (GABA) in the CNS; (2) α2-adrenergic agonists (tizanidine, clonidine); and (3) agents acting on the peripheral neuromuscular level (dantrolene, botulinum toxin).

A summary of the clinical evidence on the pharmaceutical treatment of spasticity after spinal cord injury is presented in **Table 48.2**.

Table 48.2 Summary of Clinical Evidence on the Pharmaceutical Treatment of Spasticity after Spinal Cord Injury

Category		Study	Description	Level of Evidence	Topic	Conclusions
GABA-ergic agonist						
	Diazepam					
		Verrier et al (1976)[45]	Case series	IV	15 patients (multiple etiologies) treated with IV diazepam. Authors reported short-term decreased muscular contraction. No standardized outcome scores reported.	IV diazepam may improve objective measures of muscular contraction.
		Verrier et al (1975)[46]	Case series	IV	12 patients with complete (five) and incomplete (seven) SCI were treated with IV diazepam. Short-term muscle contraction was seen only in patients with incomplete SCI.	IV diazepam may improve objective measures of muscular contraction in patients with incomplete SCI. No treatment effect was seen in patients with complete SCI.
	Oral Baclofen					
		Duncan et al (1976)[48]	Prospective, case control	II	22 patients were treated with baclofen versus placebo. Significant improvements in spasticity measures were seen in the baclofen group. Side effects including sedation and confusion were reported.	Oral baclofen may improve spasticity. Side effects included sedation and confusion.
		Basmajian and Yucel (1974)[49]	Prospective, case control	III	Improvements in flexor spasms were found in baclofen compared with placebo	Baclofen demonstrated benefits in flexor spasms compared with placebo.
		Hinderer et al (1990)[50]	Prospective, case control	III	Baclofen was compared with placebo utilizing a standardized method of ankle stiffness measurement. No significant differences were found.	Baclofen may not affect ankle stiffness measurements.
	Intrathecal Baclofen					
		Penn et al (1989)[54]	Prospective, randomized, controlled	II	20 patients with either SCI or MS were given a 3-day trial of intrathecal baclofen versus placebo. 18/20 spasm reduction; 20/20 decreased rigidity. All patients then treated with baclofen for an average 19 months. All patients reported	Intrathecal delivery of baclofen may provide reductions in spasms and rigidity. Side-effect profile is minimal.

Category	Study	Description	Level of Evidence	Topic	Conclusions
				continued improvements in spasms and rigidity and self-reported functional status. No significant side effects.	
	Coffey et al (1993)[55]	Prospective, randomized, controlled, and cohort study	II	93 patients (59 SCI) were treated with initial intrathecal baclofen versus placebo test. 88/93 responded to initial test. 75/88 patients were prospectively followed for an average of 19 months. Improvements in Ashworth rigidity score and spasms scale were found compared with baseline.	An intrathecal baclofen bolus test may identify patients that would benefit from prolonged treatment. Treatment effect may be maintained at an average 19 months after treatment is initiated.
	Korenkov et al (2002)[56]	Case series	IV	12 patients were treated with intrathecal baclofen for an average of 12 months. Improvements in Ashworth score and spasms scale were found compared with baseline.	Intrathecal baclofen treatment effect may be maintained at an average of 12 months after treatment is initiated.
	Plassat et al (2004)[57]	Case series	IV	Retrospective review of patients treated with an average follow-up of 4 years. Maintained improvements in Ashworth score and self-reported patient satisfaction. Technical complications (pump, catheter) in 37% of patients and severe pharmacological side effects in 12% of patients.	Intrathecal baclofen treatment effect may be maintained at an average of 4 years after treatment is initiated. Complications are primarily technical.
	Gianino et. al (1998)[58]	Prospective, cohort	III	25 patients with MS or SCI treated with intrathecal baclofen were followed. Significant improvements in Ashworth score and spasms scale were found. Improvements in SIP physical and psychosocial subscales were also found.	Intrathecal baclofen may improve spasticity and rigidity. Treatment may also improve physical and psychosocial function.
	Azouvi et al (1996)[59]	Prospective, cohort	III	18 patients treated with intrathecal baclofen were followed for an average 37 months. Improvements over baseline were found in Ashworth score and in disability utilizing the FIM scale.	Intrathecal baclofen may improve rigidity and functional independence at an average 37 months after initiation of treatment.
	Boviatsis et al (2005)[60]	Case series	IV	22 patients (seven SCI, 15 multiple sclerosis) retrospectively reviewed after intrathecal baclofen treatment. Authors reported improvements in Ashworth scores and spasm scales as well as functional improvements using Barthel index score.	Intrathecal baclofen may improve rigidity and spasms as well as functional improvements.
	Zahavi et al (2004)[61]	Retrospective, cohort	III	21 patients with > 5-year follow-up were reviewed.	Intrathecal baclofen may reduce spasms and

(*Continued on page 480*)

Table 48.2 Summary of Clinical Evidence on the Pharmaceutical Treatment of Spasticity after Spinal Cord Injury (*Continued*)

Category		Study	Description	Level of Evidence	Topic	Conclusions
					The authors reported improvements in Ashworth score and spasm scale, but no improvements in disability indexes or health-related quality of life were identified.	rigidity at more than 5 years after initiation of treatment. Improvements in functional status and quality of life may not be seen.
α2-adrenergics						
	Clonidine					
		Donovan et al (1988)[64]	Prospective, cohort	III	The authors reported benefit in 31 (56%) of a cohort of 55 patients treated with oral clonidine and oral baclofen. Among quadriplegic patients, 7/11 complete and 17/25 incomplete SCI had improvement. Among paraplegic patients, 6/15 complete and 1/4 incomplete SCI had improvements. No standard outcome measures were utilized.	Oral clonidine may improve spasticity in combination with oral baclofen. Quadriplegic patients may have better results than paraplegic patients.
		Middleton et al (1996)[28]	Case report	IV	Case report of successful treatment with intrathecal clonidine and intrathecal baclofen for a patient with severe neuropathic pain and spasticity.	Intrathecal clonidine may be combined with intrathecal baclofen to relieve pain and spasticity.
		Yablon and Sipski (1993)[65]	Case series	IV	The authors describe three patients with positive responses to transdermal clonidine after failing oral baclofen therapy. No standard outcome measures were utilized.	Transdermal clonidine may improve spasms after failure of oral baclofen treatment.
		Weingarden and Belen (1992)[66]	Case series	IV	17 patients treated with transdermal clonidine. 12/17 reported improvements. No standard outcome measures were utilized.	Transdermal clonidine may improve patient's subjective spasticity.
	Tizanidine					
		Nance et al (1994)[67]	Prospective, randomized, controlled, multicenter	I	124 SCI patients were treated with tizanidine vs placebo. Statistically significant improvements in Ashworth scores for muscle tone compared with placebo with minimal adverse events. No functional measures were reported.	Tizanidine may improve rigidity with a safe side effect profile.
Peripheral Acting						
	Dantrolene					
		No reports.				
	Botulinum toxin	Richardson et al (2000)[70]	Prospective, randomized, controlled	I	52 patients (six SCI) with focal hypertonia were treated with local botulinum toxin versus placebo. Significant improvements in passive range of motion, Ashworth score, and patient satisfaction were reported.	Botulinum toxin may improve range of motion, rigidity and satisfaction among patients with focal hypertonia.

Abbreviations: FIM, Functional Independence Measure; IV, intravenous; MS, multiple sclerosis; SCI, spinal cord injury; SIP, Sickness Impact Profile.

GABA-ergic Medications

Baclofen and diazepam are two GABA-ergic medications that have been investigated. Diazepam, a benzodiazepine, is presumed to act near postsynaptic GABA receptors that, in turn, interrupt action potential transmission by disrupting membrane polarity.[42] Diazepam is among the most commonly prescribed medications, with one study reporting its use in 70% of spinal cord injured patients, with more than one third treated for more than 10 years.[43] It is commonly referred to as an effective treatment for spasticity in spinal cord injury.[44] There is, however, very little published data on its use in this specific setting. Verrier et al reported decreases in muscular contraction associated with IV diazepam in a series of 15 patients with spasticity from multiple etiologies (level IV).[45] The same authors demonstrated improved presynaptic inhibition in seven patients with incomplete cord injuries but no effect in five patients with complete cord injuries (level IV).[46] Given its widespread use and safety, diazepam will likely remain a common treatment for spasticity despite a lack of evidence. Further studies are needed before a clinical recommendation can be made.

Baclofen is a derivative of the neurotransmitter GABA and is an agonist to the GABAB receptor. By reducing the amount of presynaptic neurotransmitter release, baclofen enhances the inhibitory effects of spinal cord interneurons.[47] It is also thought to act on postsynaptic receptors, interrupting action potential transmission by disrupting normal member polarization.[42]

Duncan et al found significant improvements in spasticity measures with oral baclofen compared with placebo in a prospective study of 22 patients with spinal cord disease (level II).[48] Basmajian and Yucel reported improvements in flexor spasms with oral baclofen compared with placebo in a prospective study (level III).[49] To the contrary, Hinderer et al prospectively compared baclofen to placebo and found no significant treatment effect utilizing a standardized measure of ankle stiffness (level III).[50] The usefulness of oral baclofen has been limited primarily due to adverse effects such as drowsiness, dizziness, ataxia, confusion, and insomnia. Additionally, significant adverse reactions with withdrawal and overdose have been documented, including respiratory distress, anxiety, hallucinations, and seizures. Lastly, oral baclofen, like many muscle relaxants, may impair ambulation in some patients.[51] Optimal oral dose of baclofen, therefore, requires careful titration, especially in patients with impaired renal function.[52]

Due to the limitations of oral baclofen treatment, intrathecal administration of baclofen has been widely investigated. By bypassing the blood–brain barrier, intrathecal delivery provides greater central concentrations with lower doses of baclofen.[53] The primary benefit is a reduction in adverse effects that may otherwise limit the effectiveness of baclofen treatment.

Penn et al, in a prospective, randomized, controlled study (level II) compared a 3-day course of intrathecal baclofen to placebo in 20 patients with either spinal cord injury or multiple sclerosis. Spasms and rigidity decreased in 18/20 and 20/20 patients, respectively. All patients were then treated with intrathecal baclofen; at mean follow-up of 19 months, muscle tone was maintained and spasms were reduced to allow all patients to perform activities of daily living without interference. No sedation, confusion, or drowsiness occurred.[54] Coffey et al identified a positive response to intrathecal baclofen to placebo in 88 of 93 patients with spasticity, 59/93

due to spinal cord injury (level II).[55] The authors prospectively followed 75 patients for an average of 19 months and demonstrated continued improvements in Ashworth rigidity scales as well as muscle spasm scores. One patient received an overdose due to programming error, whereas one other developed an infection; no sedation or drowsiness was found otherwise. Korenkov et al also reported reduced Ashworth and muscle spasm scores at an average 12-month follow-up in a series of 12 patients (level IV).[56] Plassat et al, in a retrospective review of patients with an average follow-up of 4 years (level IV), reported maintained improvements in Ashworth scores as well as self-reported patient satisfaction.[57]

Several studies have attempted to address specific improvement in function and quality of life with intrathecal baclofen therapy. Gianino et al, in an uncontrolled, prospective study (level III) of 25 patients with multiple sclerosis or spinal cord injury, found improvements in Ashworth score, spasm scale, and physical and psychosocial subscales of the Sickness Impact Profile (SIP).[58] The authors found no improvements utilizing the Ferrans and Powers Quality of Life Index and suggest this may be due to a bias toward nonphysical domains in this tool. Azouvi et al prospectively assessed intrathecal baclofen in 18 patients to an average follow-up of 37 months (level III).[59] The authors reported improvements in Ashworth scale as well as disability utilizing the Functional Independence Measure (FIM). Boviatsis et al also retrospectively reported (level IV) improvements in Ashworth scores and spasm scales as well as functional improvements using Barthel index score among 22 patients (seven spinal cord injury, 15 multiple sclerosis).[60] To the contrary, Zahavi et al retrospectively reported (level III) more than 5-year follow-up on 21 patients receiving intrathecal baclofen. Although the authors reported improvements in Ashworth score and spasm scale, no improvements in disability indexes or health-related quality of life were identified.[61]

Intrathecal baclofen treatment requires surgical implantation of a catheter and pump. Potential complications include dislodgment, disconnection, migration, catheter blockage, pump failure, infection, drug overdose, and drug withdrawal.[62] Plassat et al, in a 4-year review, reported technical complications in 37% of patients and severe pharmacological side effects in 12% of patients.[57] Although clinical data support the use of intrathecal baclofen, the potential for complications remains. Therefore, intrathecal baclofen should only be considered after attempts at oral medications have failed.

α2-Adrenergic Agonists

Alpha-adrenergic agonists are thought to reduce spasticity by enhancing presynaptic inhibition of sensory afferents.[51] Clonidine has been described to improve walking ability in patients with incomplete spinal cord injury, but there is limited information on its use for symptomatic spasticity.[63] Donovan et al reported benefit in 31 (56%) of a cohort of 55 patients treated with oral clonidine and baclofen (level III).[64] Middleton et al described improved spasticity and pain after intrathecal baclofen and clonidine treatment in a case report (level IV).[28] Yablon and Sipski reported a series of three patients with positive responses to transdermal clonidine after failing oral baclofen therapy.[65] Weingarden and Belen retrospectively reported (level IV) beneficial responses in 12 of 17 patients treated with transdermal clonidine.[66] In aggregate, more studies are needed to support the use of oral or transdermal clonidine before a clinical recommendation can be made.

Tizanidine, an imidazole derivative, is also a centrally acting α2-adrenergic agonist that has been investigated in one study. Nance et al, in a multicenter, prospective, randomized, controlled study (level I), studied 124 spinal cord injured patients. Statistically significant improvements in Ashworth scores for muscle tone compared with placebo were reported with minimal adverse events.[67] Functional and health-related quality of life data were not obtained. Tizanidine has also been studied for the treatment of spasticity due to multiple sclerosis with improved Ashworth scores but with no improvements in functional scores.[68] Further studies are needed before a clinical recommendation can be made.

Peripheral Neuromuscular Blockade

Two peripherally acting pharmaceuticals have been used for the treatment of spasticity: dantrolene and botulinum toxin. Dantrolene acts directly on skeletal muscle by decreasing calcium release from the sarcoplasmic reticulum.[44] Dantrolene has been demonstrated to reduce muscle tone and hyperreflexia in patients with multiple sclerosis and cerebrovascular accidents.[69] However, the authors also reported significant muscle weakness that may lead to an overall functional decline. No published studies have reported use of peripheral neuromuscular blockade in patients after spinal cord injury.

Botulinum toxin blocks the presynaptic release of acetylcholine from the nerve terminal. It is delivered locally to affected muscles resulting in focal chemical denervation, with a maximal effect at 5 to 14 days lasting up to 12 to 16 weeks.[51] Given its mechanism of action, botulinum toxin has been utilized for focal hypertonia or for specific regions of severe spasticity. Richardson et al included six spinal cord injured patients in a prospective group of 52 adults with focal hypertonia treated with botulinum toxin versus placebo

(level I). Significant improvements in passive range of motion, Ashworth score, and patient satisfaction were reported.[70] Good outcomes have been reported for botulinum toxin use in focal spasticity associated with cerebral palsy, cerebrovascular accidents, and multiple sclerosis.[71] No other studies have been reported on patients with spinal cord injury.

◆ Summary and Spine Trauma Study Group (STSG) Recommendations

Although there is strong evidence to support the use of *certain* pharmaceuticals in the treatment of neuropathic pain and spasticity following spinal cord injury, many pharmacological treatments are currently being utilized despite a lack of high-quality, supportive clinical evidence.

An analysis of the quality of evidence should be combined with consideration of the risks and costs as well as the benefits to the patient or society associated with a treatment when reaching conclusions regarding treatment recommendations.[13] Following a careful analysis of the systematic review and relevant considerations by the Spine Trauma Study Group (STSG) (representing clinical expertise), the following recommendations are offered.

Neuropathic Pain

High-quality evidence exists regarding the efficacy of the anticonvulsants, gabapentin and pregabalin, in post–spinal cord injury patients suffering neuropathic pain. Although mild side effects are relatively common, the incidence of serious side effects is low, and a strong recommendation is made for their use in these patients. Only weak recommendations can be made for other methods of treatment (**Table 48.3**). Consideration may be given to further investigation into the use of

Table 48.3 Summary of Treatment and GRADE Recommendations for Clinical Use

Treatment			GRADE Recommendation for Clinical Use
Neuropathic pain			
	Opioids		Weak
	Antidepressants		Weak
	Sodium Channel Blockade		Weak
	NMDA agonist		Weak
	α-Agonists		Weak
	Anticonvulsants		
		Valproate	Weak
		Carbamazepine	Weak
		Lamotrigine	Weak
		Gabapentin	Strong
		Pregabalin	Strong
Spasticity			
	GABA-ergic		
		Diazepam	Weak
		Oral Baclofen	Weak

Table 48.3 Summary of Treatment and GRADE Recommendations for Clinical Use (*Continued*)

Treatment		GRADE Recommendation for Clinical Use
	Intrathecal baclofen (moderate/severe symptoms)	Strong
	Intrathecal baclofen (mild symptoms)	Weak
α2-agonists	Clonidine	Weak
	Tizanidine	Weak
Peripheral acting agents	Dantrolene	Weak
	Botulinum toxin	Weak

Abbreviations: GABA, gamma-aminobutyric acid; GRADE, grading of recommendations assessment development and evaluation; NMDA, *N*-methyl-D-aspartate (NMDA).

intrathecal opioids with or without clonidine among patients refractory to gabapentin or pregabalin.

Spasticity

High-quality evidence exists regarding the efficacy of intrathecal baclofen in patients suffering post–spinal cord injury spasticity. The risk of potentially serious complications is, however, an important consideration (as well as the cost). Based on expert opinion, a strong recommendation is therefore made for the use of intrathecal baclofen when patient symptoms are moderate to severe and unresponsive to oral medication and a weak recommendation for its use in patients suffering mild symptoms.

Only weak recommendations could be made for the use of other pharmacological treatments: see **Table 48.3**, Summary of Recommendations.

References

1. Fenollosa P, Pallares J, Cervera J, et al. Chronic pain in the spinal cord injured: statistical approach and pharmacological treatment. Paraplegia 1993;31:722–729
2. Störmer S, Gerner HJ, Grüninger W, et al. Chronic pain/dysaesthesiae in spinal cord injury patients: results of a multicentre study. Spinal Cord 1997;35:446–455
3. Norrbrink Budh C, Lund I, Ertzgaard P, et al. Pain in a Swedish spinal cord injury population. Clin Rehabil 2003;17:685–690
4. New PW, Lim TC, Hill ST, Brown DJ. A survey of pain during rehabilitation after acute spinal cord injury. Spinal Cord 1997;35:658–663
5. Nepomuceno C, Fine PR, Richards JS, et al. Pain in patients with spinal cord injury. Arch Phys Med Rehabil 1979;60:605–609
6. Rose M, Robinson JE, Ells P, Cole JD. Pain following spinal cord injury: results from a postal survey. Pain 1988;34:101–102
7. Vierck CJ Jr, Siddall P, Yezierski RP. Pain following spinal cord injury: animal models and mechanistic studies. Pain 2000;89:1–5
8. Wrigley PJ, Siddall P. Pharmacological interventions for neuropathic pain following spinal cord injury: an update. Top Spinal Cord Inj Rehabil 2007;13:58–71
9. Lance JW. The control of muscle tone, reflexes, and movement: Robert Wartenberg Lecture. Neurology 1980;30:1303–1313
10. Brodal P. The Central Nervous System: Structure and Function. New York: Oxford University Press; 1998:367
11. Young RR. Spasticity: a review. Neurology 1994;44(11, Suppl 9):S12–S20
12. Sköld C, Levi R, Seiger A. Spasticity after traumatic spinal cord injury: nature, severity, and location. Arch Phys Med Rehabil 1999;80:1548–1557
13. Maynard FM, Karunas RS, Waring WP III. Epidemiology of spasticity following traumatic spinal cord injury. Arch Phys Med Rehabil 1990;71:566–569
14. Schünemann HJ, Jaeschke R, Cook DJ, et al; ATS Documents Development and Implementation Committee. An official ATS statement: grading the quality of evidence and strength of recommendations in ATS guidelines and recommendations. Am J Respir Crit Care Med 2006;174:605–614
15. Attal N, Guirimand F, Brasseur L, Gaude V, Chauvin M, Bouhassira D. Effects of IV morphine in central pain: a randomized placebo-controlled study. Neurology 2002;58:554–563
16. Watson CP, Moulin D, Watt-Watson J, Gordon A, Eisenhoffer J. Controlled-release oxycodone relieves neuropathic pain: a randomized controlled trial in painful diabetic neuropathy. Pain 2003;105:71–78
17. Raja SN, Haythornthwaite JA, Pappagallo M, et al. Opioids versus antidepressants in postherpetic neuralgia: a randomized, placebo-controlled trial. Neurology 2002;59:1015–1021
18. Siddall PJ, Molloy AR, Walker S, Mather LE, Rutkowski SB, Cousins MJ. The efficacy of intrathecal morphine and clonidine in the treatment of pain after spinal cord injury. Anesth Analg 2000;91:1493–1498
19. Saulino M. Successful reduction of neuropathic pain associated with spinal cord injury via of a combination of intrathecal hydromorphone and ziconotide: a case report. Spinal Cord 2007;45:749–752
20. Cardenas DD, Warms CA, Turner JA, Marshall H, Brooke MM, Loeser JD. Efficacy of amitriptyline for relief of pain in spinal cord injury: results of a randomized controlled trial. Pain 2002;96:365–373
21. Attal N, Gaudé V, Brasseur L, et al. Intravenous lidocaine in central pain: a double-blind, placebo-controlled, psychophysical study. Neurology 2000;54:564–574
22. Finnerup NB, Biering-Sorensen F, Johannesen IL, et al. Intravenous lidocaine relieves spinal cord injury pain: a randomized controlled trial. Anesthesiology 2005;102:1023–1030
23. Chiou-Tan FY, Tuel SM, Johnson JC, Priebe MM, Hirsh DD, Strayer JR. Effect of mexiletine on spinal cord injury dysesthetic pain. Am J Phys Med Rehabil 1996;75:84–87
24. Sang CN. NMDA-receptor antagonists in neuropathic pain: experimental methods to clinical trials. J Pain Symptom Manage 2000;19(1, Suppl):S21–S25
25. Kvarnström A, Karlsten R, Quiding H, Gordh T. The analgesic effect of intravenous ketamine and lidocaine on pain after spinal cord injury. Acta Anaesthesiol Scand 2004;48:498–506
26. Eide PK, Stubhaug A, Stenehjem AE. Central dysesthesia pain after traumatic spinal cord injury is dependent on N-methyl-D-aspartate receptor activation. Neurosurgery 1995;37:1080–1087
27. Glynn CJ, Jamous MA, Teddy PJ, Moore RA, Lloyd JW. Role of spinal noradrenergic system in transmission of pain in patients with spinal cord injury. Lancet 1986;2:1249–1250
28. Middleton JW, Siddall PJ, Walker S, Molloy AR, Rutkowski SB. Intrathecal clonidine and baclofen in the management of spasticity and neuropathic pain following spinal cord injury: a case study. Arch Phys Med Rehabil 1996;77:824–826
29. Drewes AM, Andreasen A, Poulsen LH. Valproate for treatment of chronic central pain after spinal cord injury: a double-blind cross-over study. Paraplegia 1994;32:565–569
30. Zachariah SB, Borges EF, Varghese R, Cruz AR, Ross GS. Positive response to oral divalproex sodium (Depakote) in patients with spasticity and pain. Am J Med Sci 1994;308:38–40
31. Gibson JC, White LE. Denervation hyperpathia: a convulsive syndrome of the spinal cord responsive to carbamazepine therapy. J Neurosurg 1971;35:287–290
32. Silver M, Blum D, Grainger J, Hammer AE, Quessy S. Double-blind, placebo-controlled trial of lamotrigine in combination with other

medications for neuropathic pain. J Pain Symptom Manage 2007;34: 446–454

33. Finnerup NB, Sindrup SH, Bach FW, Johannesen IL, Jensen TS. Lamotrigine in spinal cord injury pain: a randomized controlled trial. Pain 2002;96:375–383

34. Haller H, Leblhuber F, Trenkler J, Schmidhammer R. Treatment of chronic neuropathic pain after traumatic central cervical cord lesion with gabapentin. J Neural Transm 2003;110:977–981

35. To TP, Lim TC, Hill ST, et al. Gabapentin for neuropathic pain following spinal cord injury. Spinal Cord 2002;40:282–285

36. Putzke JD, Richards JS, Kezar L, Hicken BL, Ness TJ. Long-term use of gabapentin for treatment of pain after traumatic spinal cord injury. Clin J Pain 2002;18:116–121

37. Tai Q, Kirshblum S, Chen B, Millis S, Johnston M, DeLisa JA. Gabapentin in the treatment of neuropathic pain after spinal cord injury: a prospective, randomized, double-blind, crossover trial. J Spinal Cord Med 2002;25:100–105

38. Levendoglu F, Ogün CO, Ozerbil O, Ogün TC, Ugurlu H. Gabapentin is a first line drug for the treatment of neuropathic pain in spinal cord injury. Spine 2004;29:743–751

39. Ahn SH, Park HW, Lee BS, et al. Gabapentin effect on neuropathic pain compared among patients with spinal cord injury and different durations of symptoms. Spine 2003;28:341–346, discussion 346–347

40. Siddall PJ, Cousins MJ, Otte A, Griesing T, Chambers R, Murphy TK. Pregabalin in central neuropathic pain associated with spinal cord injury: a placebo-controlled trial. Neurology 2006;67:1792–1800

41. Vranken JH, Dijkgraaf MG, Kruis MR, van der Vegt MH, Hollmann MW, Heesen M. Pregabalin in patients with central neuropathic pain: a randomized, double-blind, placebo-controlled trial of a flexible-dose regimen. Pain 2008;136:150–157

42. Elovic E. Principles of pharmaceutical management of spastic hypertonia. Phys Med Rehabil Clin N Am 2001;12:793–816, vii.

43. Broderick CP, Radnitz CL, Bauman WA. Diazepam usage in veterans with spinal cord injury. J Spinal Cord Med 1997;20:406–409

44. Burchiel KJ, Hsu FP. Pain and spasticity after spinal cord injury: mechanisms and treatment. Spine 2001;26(24, Suppl):S146–S160

45. Verrier M, Ashby P, MacLEOD S. Effect of diazepam on muscle contraction in spasticity. Am J Phys Med 1976;55:184–191

46. Verrier M, MacLeod S, Ashby P. The effect of diazepam on presynaptic inhibition in patients with complete and incomplete spinal cord lesions. Can J Neurol Sci 1975;2:179–184

47. Kandel ER, Schwartz JH, Jessell TM. Principles of Neural Science. 4th ed. New York: McGraw-Hill; 2000:730

48. Duncan GW, Shahani BT, Young RR. An evaluation of baclofen treatment for certain symptoms in patients with spinal cord lesions: a double-blind, cross-over study. Neurology 1976;26:441–446

49. Basmajian JV, Yucel V. Effects of a GABA–derivative (BA-34647) on spasticity: preliminary report of a double-blind cross-over study. Am J Phys Med 1974;53:223–228

50. Hinderer SR, Lehmann JF, Price R, White O, deLateur BJ, Deitz J. Spasticity in spinal cord injured persons: quantitative effects of baclofen and placebo treatments. Am J Phys Med Rehabil 1990;69:311–317

51. Adams MM, Hicks AL. Spasticity after spinal cord injury. Spinal Cord 2005;43:577–586

52. Aisen ML, Dietz M, McDowell F, Kutt H. Baclofen toxicity in a patient with subclinical renal insufficiency. Arch Phys Med Rehabil 1994;75: 109–111

53. Kita M, Goodkin DE. Drugs used to treat spasticity. Drugs 2000;59: 487–495

54. Penn RD, Savoy SM, Corcos D, et al. Intrathecal baclofen for severe spinal spasticity. N Engl J Med 1989;320:1517–1521

55. Coffey JR, Cahill D, Steers W, et al. Intrathecal baclofen for intractable spasticity of spinal origin: results of a long-term multicenter study. J Neurosurg 1993;78:226–232

56. Korenkov AI, Niendorf WR, Darwish N, Glaeser E, Gaab MR. Continuous intrathecal infusion of baclofen in patients with spasticity caused by spinal cord injuries. Neurosurg Rev 2002;25:228–230

57. Plassat R, Perrouin Verbe B, Menei P, Menegalli D, Mathé JF, Richard I. Treatment of spasticity with intrathecal baclofen administration: long-term follow-up, review of 40 patients. Spinal Cord 2004;42:686–693

58. Gianino JM, York MM, Paice JA, Shott S. Quality of life: effect of reduced spasticity from intrathecal baclofen. J Neurosci Nurs 1998;30:47–54

59. Azouvi P, Mane M, Thiebaut JB, Denys P, Remy-Neris O, Bussel B. Intrathecal baclofen administration for control of severe spinal spasticity: functional improvement and long-term follow-up. Arch Phys Med Rehabil 1996;77:35–39

60. Boviatsis EJ, Kouyialis AT, Korfias S, Sakas DE. Functional outcome of intrathecal baclofen administration for severe spasticity. Clin Neurol Neurosurg 2005;107:289–295

61. Zahavi A, Geertzen JH, Middel B, Staal M, Rietman JS. Long term effect (more than five years) of intrathecal baclofen on impairment, disability, and quality of life in patients with severe spasticity of spinal origin. J Neurol Neurosurg Psychiatry 2004;75:1553–1557

62. Vender JR, Hester S, Waller JL, Rekito A, Lee MR. Identification and management of intrathecal baclofen pump complications: a comparison of pediatric and adult patients. J Neurosurg 2006;104(1, Suppl):9–15

63. Stewart JE, Barbeau H, Gauthier S. Modulation of locomotor patterns and spasticity with clonidine in spinal cord injured patients. Can J Neurol Sci 1991;18:321–332

64. Donovan WH, Carter RE, Rossi CD, Wilkerson MA. Clonidine effect on spasticity: a clinical trial. Arch Phys Med Rehabil 1988;69(3 Pt 1):193–194

65. Yablon SA, Sipski ML. Effect of transdermal clonidine on spinal spasticity. A case series. Am J Phys Med Rehabil 1993;72:154–157

66. Weingarden SI, Belen JG. Clonidine transdermal system for treatment of spasticity in spinal cord injury. Arch Phys Med Rehabil 1992;73: 876–877

67. Nance PW, Bugaresti J, Shellenberger K, Sheremata W, Martinez-Arizala A; North American Tizanidine Study Group. Efficacy and safety of tizanidine in the treatment of spasticity in patients with spinal cord injury. Neurology 1994;44(11, Suppl 9):S44–S51, discussion S51–S52

68. United Kingdom Tizanidine Trial Group. A double-blind, placebo-controlled trial of tizanidine in the treatment of spasticity caused by multiple sclerosis. Neurology 1994;44(11, Suppl 9):S70–S78

69. Katrak PH, Cole AM, Poulos CJ, McCauley JC. Objective assessment of spasticity, strength, and function with early exhibition of dantrolene sodium after cerebrovascular accident: a randomized double-blind study. Arch Phys Med Rehabil 1992;73:4–9

70. Richardson D, Sheean G, Werring D, et al. Evaluating the role of botulinum toxin in the management of focal hypertonia in adults. J Neurol Neurosurg Psychiatry 2000;69:499–506

71. Jozefczyk PB. The management of focal spasticity. Clin Neuropharmacol 2002;25:158–173

Charcot Disease of the Spine after Traumatic Spinal Cord Injury

Amit O. Agarwala

"Charcot joint of the spine" describes a destructive process that affects the intervertebral disks and adjacent vertebral bodies. Also known as spinal neuropathic arthropathy, this condition results from the loss of protective sensation and joint protective mechanisms secondary to any condition affecting the deep sensory pathways.[1] An exaggerated degenerative process can ensue leading to a rapid destruction of the spinal disks, facet joints, and vertebral bodies, in turn leading eventually to dislocation and gross spinal instability (**Fig. 49.1A-F**).

Cases of Charcot joints have been described secondary to numerous sensory disorders, including hemiplegia, congenital absence of pain, transverse myelitis, syringomyelia, peripheral neuropathies, diabetes, traumatic spinal cord injury, and the original description in tertiary syphilis or tabes dorsalis.[2] This chapter focuses on Charcot disease of the spine in patients after traumatic spinal cord injury.

The chapter presents a systematic review of the available English-language literature on the diagnosis and treatment of Charcot spine with the goal of investigating two relevant questions:

Question 1: When Is Surgery Indicated in the Treatment of Charcot Spine?

Question 2: When Surgery Is Indicated, What Is the Optimal Surgical Approach to Achieve Fusion with Minimal Surgical Morbidity?

Based on this review and expert medical opinion (members of the Spine Trauma Study Group), evidence-based recommendations are offered regarding these important clinical issues.

◆ Background

Tabes dorsalis was classically the most frequent etiology of this disorder. Presentation of spinal neuropathic arthropathy attributable to tabes dorsalis is now rare with the disappearance of tertiary syphilis. The diagnosis of Charcot joint in the spine secondary to traumatic spinal cord injury is on the rise and makes up the majority of the literature over the past 20 years. This can be attributed to the increased activity level of paraplegics and tetraplegics, accelerated rehabilitation programs, and participation in sports. As our population of active, independently living spinal cord injured patients grows, our knowledge on the diagnosis and treatment of Charcot spine will become increasingly important.

Clinical Features

The initial clinical feature of Charcot spine is a progressive thoracic or thoracolumbar kyphosis in patients with complete or near complete motor and sensory spinal cord injury. Presenting symptoms can include changes in neurological status such as increased lower extremity spasticity, increased back or leg pain, audible "crunching," and autonomic dysreflexia (**Fig. 49.1A–F**). Symptoms of autonomic dysreflexia reported in Charcot spine patients include severe headaches, profuse sweating over the face and arms, and severe hypertension associated with a "grinding" sensation in the back and may occur with upright posture and during transfers.[3] As well, patients have reported difficulties with sitting balance, wheelchair transfers, spinal instability that is apparent to the patient, and progressive painless deformity. Surprisingly, pain is often a significant symptom and may be located at levels distal to the spinal cord injury.

Neuropathic joints are always found below the level of the cord injury, and in patients in whom a fusion had been performed, the Charcot joint is typically within two segments rostral to the bottom of the fusion.[4] A causal link has been postulated between laminectomies over unfused segments and the development of neuropathic arthropathy in spinal cord injured patients.[5]

Plain radiographs show destruction of the articular facets as the earliest sign of neuropathic arthropathy followed by disk space narrowing and end plate sclerosis. Later in the disease process, the findings reflect a combination of sclerosis, vertebral body destruction and resorption, reactive bone formation, and extensive osteophytes. Spinal pseudarthroses, subluxations, and dislocations and "ball-in-socket" joint

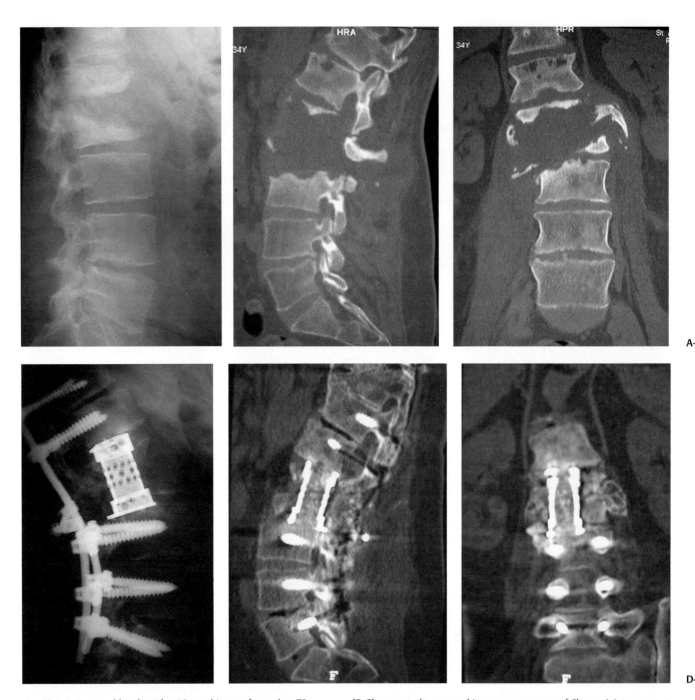

A–C

D–F

Fig. 49.1 A 45-year-old male with a 12-year history of complete T8 paraplegia from traumatic injury treated nonoperatively in a brace. Symptoms included back pain, audible "crunching" with sitting/transfers, headaches and hypertension with upright posture. **(A)** Plain x-ray and **(B,C)** computed tomographic scan appearances of Charcot joint present at L1–L2. **(D–F)** Plain x-ray and computed tomographic scan post-operatively. The patient was treated with posterior instrumented fusion and anterior interbody fusion through a direct posterior approach.

formation have been described.[4] Computed tomography (CT) may show bony fragmentation and destruction of all three columns of the spine (**Fig. 49.2A–E**). Magnetic resonance imaging (MRI) is helpful in differentiating Charcot spine from other etiologies.

The differential diagnosis includes infection (bacterial, fungal, and tuberculosis), tumor, and Paget disease. Where infection or tumors are suspected, percutaneous vertebral biopsy is mandatory before considering treatment. Infected Charcot spine has been reported and can alter the surgical and medical management of the patient significantly.[6–8] Identifying and treating hip flexion contractures to reduce compensatory

lumbar motion with sitting and to reduce stress on the fusion is important in the management of Charcot spine.[4]

Management

Nonoperative treatment options include observation and immobilization either through bracing or bed rest. Considering the causes of Charcot spine and the potential for progression, immobilization of the affected area would appear to be essential. In cases where no treatment was initiated, there are reports of progression resulting in death,[5] increasing neurological changes, or increasing symptoms resulting in surgery in 1 year

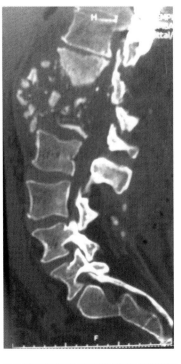
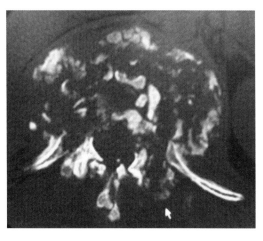

A, B

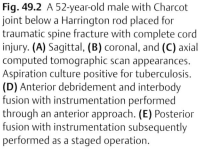

Fig. 49.2 A 52-year-old male with Charcot joint below a Harrington rod placed for traumatic spine fracture with complete cord injury. **(A)** Sagittal, **(B)** coronal, and **(C)** axial computed tomographic scan appearances. Aspiration culture positive for tuberculosis. **(D)** Anterior debridement and interbody fusion with instrumentation performed through an anterior approach. **(E)** Posterior fusion with instrumentation subsequently performed as a staged operation.

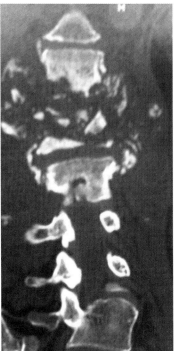
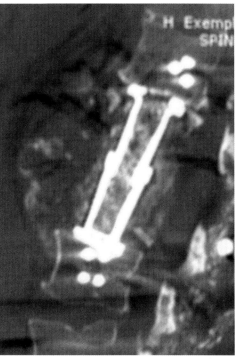
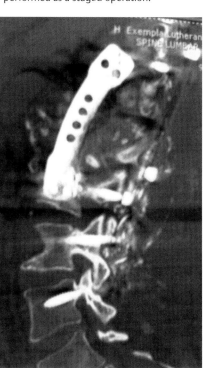

C–E

from diagnosis.[2] Complications stemming from end-stage Charcot spine have been reported to include obstructive uropathy with hydronephrosis, a progressive gibbus deformity, loss of sitting balance leading to decubitus ulcers, and abdominal aorta thrombosis postulated to occur from mechanical deformation created by gross instability of the spine in the thoracolumbar region.[5] Frequent radiographs and close observation are required because rapid progression can occur over 1 year, and patients will be identified that may benefit from surgery.

Symptoms of autonomic dysreflexia occur with motion at the neuropathic joint. Successful nonoperative treatment has been reported with extended bed rest. Two patients treated with 6 to 8 weeks of bed rest had resolution of the their symptoms of autonomic dysreflexia.[9]

There are no reports in the literature on the success of thoracolumbar bracing for Charcot spine. Although bracing may delay progression in the mildly symptomatic patient, many patients present with end-stage instability and bony destruction where surgery should be considered.

Indications for surgery in Charcot spine include spinal instability, progressive deformity, pain, new neurological deficits or spasticity, and failure of nonoperative treatment efforts to alleviate symptoms. Where surgery is recommended, circumferential fusion is universally recommended in the more recent literature after 1995. The goal of surgery is to achieve a stable fusion of the unstable segment.

Approaches that have been successfully reported include anterior and posterior exposures with posterior instrumentation.

In addition, anterior fusion can be performed through a lateral extracavitary or posterolateral approach. In some Charcot patients where the thecal sac may be absent or attenuated, access to the anterior column can be easily achieved through a straight posterior approach. These alternative anterior fusions should be combined with posterior instrumentation. The latter avoids the morbidity of a separate anterior approach in spinal cord injured patients who already have altered bowel function and a high risk of deep venous thrombosis. However, anterior approaches allow for additional anterior multilevel instrumentation for added fixation and possibly more thorough debridement of large destructive lesions, especially in the setting of infected Charcot spine. Cases of direct posterior approach to anterior column support and separate anterior exposure for infected Charcot spine are presented in the figures.

Percutaneous biopsy should be performed where infection or tumor is suspected. Patients may have decubitus ulcers over a gibbus deformity that will need to be addressed at the time of surgery and may increase the risk of infection. Consideration for the likelihood of recurrent neuropathic arthropathy below the fusion is important. Authors have recommended against stopping at the thoracolumbar junction.[4] It remains unclear whether fusions stopping at L5 should be routinely extended to the sacrum. The use of autogenous iliac crest bone would appear to have low morbidity in spinal cord injured patients and is reported frequently in the treatment of Charcot spine.[2] The use of other biological bone substitutes has not been reported. The use of postoperative bracing is widely recommended as well as wheelchair modifications to improve sitting posture without kyphosis.

◆ Systematic Review

A systematic review of the literature was performed in September 2007 to evaluate the evidence for treatment of Charcot spine in patients with traumatic spinal cord injury. Database searches of MEDLINE, EMBASE, Cochrane reviews, PubMed, and eMedicine were performed. Reference lists from relevant articles were hand searched for additional citations.

Inclusion/Exclusion Criteria

Studies included were written in the English language, described adult patients with Charcot spine after traumatic spinal cord injury, and described treatment approach along with complications and outcome. Excluded articles described patients with nontraumatic spinal cord injury, failed to identify surgical approach, or did not include complications and outcome. As no studies used validated outcome measures, this was not used as an exclusion criterion. Given the limited number of studies found, any studies including heterogeneous populations of patients were screened, and patients with nontraumatic spinal cord injury were specifically excluded without discarding the entire paper.

A total of 168 potentially relevant papers were identified, 131 papers were excluded based on abstract review, and 17 further articles were excluded after full review. The articles excluded were those presenting Charcot patients with nontraumatic spinal cord injury or review articles without specific patient populations presented. Nineteen papers met inclusion/exclusion criteria, including five papers that presented a heterogeneous population of cases of traumatic spinal cord injury that were able to be separated from patients with other nontraumatic diagnoses.

◆ Results

Fifty-seven patients were identified in 20 articles with the diagnosis of Charcot spine following traumatic spinal cord injury (**Table 49.1**). All papers presented case reports or case series without control groups—level IV evidence or lower. All the studies were further limited by a lack of use of validated or objective outcome criteria.

The average age of patients at time of treatment for Charcot spine was 44.9 years (range 22 to 65). The average time from traumatic spinal cord injury to treatment for Charcot spine was 19.4 years (range 2 to 34). The patient population was predominantly male at 77% (44 males, 13 females). The location of initial spinal cord injury varied from C5 to L1. Five patients were found to have an infected Charcot spine after aspiration and positive culture.

Presenting symptoms included pain 67%, kyphosis 84%, audible grinding 62%, neurological function loss 16%, increasing spasticity 23%, autonomic dysreflexia 12%, and sitting intolerance 9%. Complications reported included failure of fixation 15%, nonunion 5%, recurrence of neuropathic arthropathy below fusion 5%, superficial infection 9%, deep infection 3%, urinary tract infections 3%, and one death secondary to spinal instability in a patient who refused surgery. It is unclear how thorough the reporting of complications was in some articles.

Table 49.1 Summary of 20 Articles Identified with the Diagnosis of Charcot Spine following Traumatic Spinal Cord Injury

Study	Study Type	Level of Evidence
Vialle et al (2005)[1]	Case series	IV
Suda et al (2005)[8]	Case report	IV
Mohit et al (2005)[3]	Case report	IV
Selmi et al (2002)[9]	Case reports	IV
Standaert et al (1997)[4]	Case reports	IV
Arnold et al (1995)[10]	Case reports	IV
Werner and Holt (1995)[11]	Case report	IV
Montgomery and McGuire (1993)[12]	Case report	IV
Brown et al (1992)[2]	Case series	IV
Glennon et al (1992)[13]	Case series	IV
McBride and Greenberg (1991)[14]	Case series	IV
Schwartz (1990)[15]	Case report	IV
Mikawa et al (1989)[6]	Case report	IV
Crim et al (1987)[16]	Case series	IV
Sobel et al (1985)[5]	Case series	IV
Slabaugh and Smith (1978)[17]	Case report	IV
Devlin et al (1991)[18]	Case series	IV
Pritchard and Coscia (1992)[7]	Case report	IV
Suda et al. (2007)[19]	Case series	IV

Twelve patients were treated nonoperatively. Ten refused or were considering surgery and were observed with one reported death attributed to progression of his Charcot spine with nonoperative treatment. Few of the patients treated nonoperatively were reported for follow-up and complications, making conclusions difficult. Two patients were treated with bed rest for 6 to 8 weeks for autonomic dysreflexia as their only presenting symptom, which resolved with 4-year follow-up.

Surgical treatment was recommended for 55 of 57 patients, and 45 of 57 patients were treated surgically. One patient underwent anterior instrumented fusion. Seven patients had posterior instrumented fusion alone, and 37 patients had circumferential fusion performed. Of these 37 patients, 28 were anterior/posterior fusions through separate incisions, five patients had anterior fusion through a lateral extracavitary or posterolateral approach, and four patients underwent anterior fusion through a direct posterior approach in the absence of neural elements all in conjunction with posterior instrumentation. Four of seven patients with posterior fusion only reported loss of fixation (57%). Posterior fusion was utilized as a stand-alone technique only in cases reported before 1995. More recent literature universally recommends circumferential fusion, with increasing reports of anterior fusion performed through a posterior incision. Two of five patients with culture-positive infected Charcot spine were treated with a separate anterior approach for debridement of infection and anterior/posterior fusion. Three of five patients with infection were treated with single posterior incision and debridement of infection through a posterolateral or direct posterior approach. All five patients were successfully treated with resolution of infection. Fusion was eventually achieved in all patients treated surgically. Symptom resolution or significant improvement was reported in all patients treated surgically once fusion was achieved, except any reported neurological loss in incomplete patients was not restored.

◆ Discussion

The results of the systematic review of the literature showed increasing reports of Charcot spine in traumatic spinal cord injury since 1990 compared with other causes of neuropathic arthropathy commonly reported prior to this date. Only limited conclusions can be drawn from the literature given the small case series presented and only subjective outcomes reported.

Consistently, patients with significant back pain and noticeable instability showed improvement with achievement of a solid fusion. Correction of deformity was not reported in a measurable fashion, nor was improvement in a sitting posture. Although, progressive kyphosis and sagittal imbalance was often reported as subjectively improved. Autonomic dysreflexia improved in all patients reported with surgical fusion or with bed rest in one series of two patients. Infection was resolved in all patients. Patient satisfaction when reported was high. However, only one report of progression of untreated Charcot spine led to death. No other long-term follow-up of nonoperative treatment was available.

Surgical Approach

Circumferential fusion was recommended and employed successfully in nearly all patients reported in the literature, especially in the past 15 years. No comparative studies looking at

surgical approach to anterior fusion and related morbidity were found. As well, no comparison of deformity reduction or fixation failure rate by approach can be made.

Conclusions can only be drawn from author opinion. In the absence of neural elements, authors utilized a direct posterior approach to the anterior column. Although complications of a separate anterior approach were not reported in those cases, one may assume that single posterior incision approaches will reduce approach-related morbidity. Successful circumferential fusion using a posterolateral or lateral extracavitary approach was reported frequently. Adjunctive anterior multisegment fixation was rarely utilized. Even in the setting of infection, successful outcomes with posterior access to the anterior column for debridement was reported.

Potential Complications and Rehabilitation

Complications after surgery in Charcot spine are frequent. Reported complications include urinary tract infections, deep venous thrombosis, superficial and deep wound infections, failure of fixation, usually with dislodged distal screws or hooks and recurrence of kyphotic deformity, and a new neuropathic joint below the fusion.

Avoidance of complications occurs through awareness. Routine urinary cultures can be obtained, especially in patients who routinely self-catheterize but have indwelling catheters placed for surgery. Chemical and mechanical deep vein thrombosis (DVT) prophylaxis is initiated, usually within 24 hours postoperatively. Routine radiographs are taken watching closely for loosening of distal fixation. Bracing and activity restrictions are stressed with the patient and family. Patients are routinely transferred to a spinal cord injury rehabilitation center after fusion for Charcot spine for assistance with activities of daily living and transfers. This is especially important for patients coming from independent living situations, sometimes far from medical or family assistance. Emphasis must be placed on the importance of avoiding stressful activity to the spine during the recovery period and in the future to prevent recurrence of Charcot spine. Physical and occupational therapists with a knowledge of spinal cord injury are helpful to coach the patient through lifestyle and wheelchair modifications that can avoid repetitive flexing and twisting of the spine. Patient cooperation with this program is perhaps the most crucial piece in achieving successful surgical outcomes. Many Charcot spine patients have been living with spinal cord injury for a decade or longer, and giving up independence during recovery is a step backward that can be difficult for them to accept.

◆ Summary and Spine Trauma Study Group Recommendations

Question 1

In spite of the low level of the evidence in the published literature—a small case series with presentation of subjective outcomes only—the consistent patient outcomes reported, the likelihood of an otherwise poor clinical course with conservative management, and the relatively low risk of serious complications with appropriate surgical technique and perioperative care, the Spine Trauma Study Group (STSG) makes a strong recommendation for surgical stabilization in Charcot spine when patients present with significant back pain, infection, symptomatic instability, or progressive kyphosis.

Question 2

The level of published evidence regarding the optimal surgical technique in Charcot spine is also low. Circumferential fusion was, however, described in almost all cases. Although no comparative studies of anterior versus posterior approach were found, given that successful circumferential fusion using a posterolateral or lateral extracavitary approach was reported frequently and that single posterior incision approaches may reduce approach-related morbidity, a weak recommendation can be given for a direct posterior or posterolateral approach to circumferential fusion and posterior instrumentation in most cases.

References

1. Vialle R, Mary P, Tassin JL, Parker F, Guillaumat M. Charcot disease of the spine: diagnosis and treatment. Spine 2005; 30:E315–E322
2. Brown CW, Jones B, Donaldson DH, Akmakjian J, Brugman JL. Neuropathic (Charcot) arthropathy of the spine after traumatic spinal paraplegia. Spine 1992;17(6, Suppl):S103–S108
3. Mohit AA, Mirza S, James J, Goodkin R. Charcot arthropathy in relation to autonomic dysreflexia in spinal cord injury: case report and review of the literature. J Neurosurg Spine 2005;2:476–480
4. Standaert C, Cardenas DD, Anderson P. Charcot spine as a late complication of traumatic spinal cord injury. Arch Phys Med Rehabil 1997;78:221–225
5. Sobel JW, Bohlman HH, Freehafer AA. Charcot arthropathy of the spine following spinal cord injury: a report of five cases. J Bone Joint Surg Am 1985;67:771–776
6. Mikawa Y, Watanabe R, Yamano Y, Morii S. Infected Charcot spine following spinal cord injury. Spine 1989;14:892–895
7. Pritchard JC, Coscia MF. Infection of a Charcot spine: a case report. Spine 1993;18:764–767
8. Suda Y, Saito M, Shioda M, Kato H, Shibasaki K. Infected Charcot spine. Spinal Cord 2005;43:256–259
9. Selmi F, Frankel HL, Kumaraguru AP, Apostopoulos V. Charcot joint of the spine, a cause of autonomic dysreflexia in spinal cord injured patients. Spinal Cord 2002;40:481–483
10. Arnold PM, Baek PN, Stillerman CB, Rice SG, Mueller WM. Surgical management of lumbar neuropathic spinal arthropathy (Charcot joint) after traumatic thoracic paraplegia: report of two cases. J Spinal Disord 1995;8:357–362
11. Werner JG Jr, Holt RT. Neuropathic spinal arthropathy: a case history and six year follow-up. J Ky Med Assoc 1995;93:48–52
12. Montgomery TJ, McGuire RA Jr. Traumatic neuropathic arthropathy of the spine. Orthop Rev 1993;22:1153–1157
13. Glennon TP, Madewell JE, Donovan WH, Bontke CF, Spjut HJ. Neuropathic spinal arthropathy after spinal cord injury: a report of three cases. Spine 1992;17:964–971
14. McBride GG, Greenberg D. Treatment of Charcot spinal arthropathy following traumatic paraplegia. J Spinal Disord 1991;4:212–220
15. Schwartz HS. Traumatic Charcot spine. J Spinal Disord 1990;3:269–275 Review
16. Crim JR, Bassett LW, Gold RH, et al. Spinal neuroarthropathy after traumatic paraplegia. AJNR Am J Neuroradiol 1988;9:359–362
17. Slabaugh PB, Smith TK. Neuropathic spine after spinal cord injury: a case report. J Bone Joint Surg Am 1978;60:1005–1006
18. Devlin VJ, Ogilvie JW, Transfeldt EE, Boachie-Adjei O, Bradford DS. Surgical treatment of neuropathic spinal arthropathy. J Spinal Disord 1991;4: 319–328
19. Suda Y, Shioda M, Kohno H, Machida M, Yamagishi M. Surgical treatment of Charcot spine. J Spinal Disord Tech 2007;20:85–88

IX

Emerging Techniques and Translational Research

50

Anterior Endoscopic Treatment of Thoracolumbar Spine Fractures

Eli M. Baron, Mark B. Dekutoski, and Neel Anand

Anterior management of thoracolumbar fractures permits the direct ventral decompression of neural elements and immediate reconstruction of the anterior, weight-bearing, column of the thoracolumbar spine. Surgical management of selected thoracolumbar fractures by endoscopic techniques has been enabled in the past 2 decades by the widespread adoption of intraoperative fluoroscopy, the concurrent evolution of endoscopic and laparoscopic instruments, and the refinement of minimal access retroperitoneal technologies. Utilization of balloon-assisted or gas insufflation methods have enabled easier retroperitoneal access to the spine compared with transperitoneal techniques.

Reducing the morbidity of open anterior approaches to the thoracolumbar spine is theoretically sound; however, due to the technical challenges, steep learning curves, and lack of strong evidence to demonstrate superiority compared with conventional approaches, the adoption of anterior endoscopic spinal techniques remains limited to specialized centers or individuals with a specific interest in this technology.

The epidemiology, unique clinical and diagnostic features as well as the initial management of injuries pertinent to this chapter are discussed within the individual chapters specific to each injury. The techniques described in this chapter are applied to thoracolumbar vertebral body fractures (i.e., burst-type fractures) where anterior decompression or reconstruction or both are required.

◆ Surgical Options

The first published reports of endoscopic applications to spine fracture care occurred in the mid 1990s when minimal access technologies were being driven by enhanced access to navigation and fluoroscopic technologies. The early technical reports emanated from Europe where endoscopic techniques were first applied to thoracic fractures by Hertlein and colleagues.[1] They examined the feasibility of thoracoscopic ventral bone grafting in seven patients with unstable fractures of the upper thoracic spine. For primary repair, they stabilized the fracture by using posterior transpedicular screw systems (rods or plates). Simultaneously, cancellous bone was harvested from the posterior iliac crest and deep-frozen. Anterior reconstruction was completed a few days later via a ventral thoracoscopic approach. The main location of the ventral osseous defect was identified by intraoperative radiology. After mechanical removal of destroyed connective tissue and disk material, fusion was performed using the previously harvested bone, which was placed into the intervertebral disk space and the anterior osseous defect.

McAfee et al[2] investigated the effectiveness of thoracoscopic corpectomy–endoscopic removal of the vertebral body in 15 cases (eight for pathological fractures for tumors, five for traumatic fractures, and two for infections). The postoperative morbidity appeared to be more favorable than with open thoracotomy. They stated that, overall, the ability to visualize the anterior surface of the dura during corpectomy was better endoscopically than with open thoracotomy techniques–improved magnification, the ability of the operative assistant to see and therefore suction more efficiently, and the perspective of visualization was improved. They felt that the limiting factor for wider adoption of the technique was the absence of a commercially available internal fixation system that could be applied endoscopically. Several years later, Schultheiss et al[3] described a novel, biomechanically sound, implantable stabilization system specifically designed for endoscopic stabilization of thoracolumbar fractures.[4,5]

De Peretti et al[6] were first to report on endoscopic treatment of lumbar fractures. They reported on three trauma patients who underwent lumbar interbody fusion, performed via a video-assisted retroperitoneal laparoscopic approach in conjunction with posterior osteosynthesis at the L2–L3, L3–L4, and/or L4–L5 level. They noted that it was possible to perform this technique cranially above L2 or caudally below L5. Minimal blood loss was observed. Average time for these interventions was 127 minutes.

Subsequent to these early reports, several papers have addressed treating traumatic fractures endoscopically with different techniques and fixation methods. There is obvious appeal to the idea of achieving ventral decompression and immediate anterior column reconstruction with minimal access techniques that potentially reduce postoperative morbidity. Advances in minimal access technologies, such as better visualization and improved instrumentation, undoubtedly make such a strategy more feasible. However, the application of this treatment modality in thoracolumbar fracture management is still in relatively early stages, and uncertainty exists as to whether the theoretical advantage of reduced early morbidity and improved outcomes has actually been achieved.

◆ Complications

Potential complications specific to endoscopic approaches to the anterior spine are similar to those associated with open techniques such as vascular injury, visceral injury, and massive bleeding. To minimize these rare but potentially catastrophic complications, the utilization of access surgeons with endoscopic experience and familiarity with local paraspinal anatomy is paramount.

◆ Rehabilitation

The principles of rehabilitation following anterior endoscopic spinal stabilization (stand alone or in combination with posterior fixation) are identical to those utilized for open stabilization techniques and are dependent on the medical stability of the patient, the specific injury, the neurological status of the patient, and the overall stability of spinal fixation (e.g., extent of fixation and bone quality). Protocols will vary among centers as well as among surgeons, but in general prescribe early and aggressive mobilization as soon as the medical condition of the patient allows.

Systematic Review

This chapter systematically reviews the available literature to answer the following questions:

Question 1: Is Endoscopic Management of Thoracolumbar Spine Fractures Ready for Widespread Application?

Question 2: Do Endoscopic Approaches for the Anterior Management of Thoracolumbar Fractures Enhance Early Patient Outcomes?

◆ Methods

A Systematic Review was initiated under the methodology described by Fisher and Wood.[7] PubMed and Medline search engines were used to identify references in the literature starting from 1960 to date via the combinations of the following search terms: "spine" (15,425), "endoscopic" (869), "percutaneous" (71,974), "minimally invasive" (18,693), "spine fractures" (6426). Terms were combined, entire combined lists were culled for papers that met the criteria for (1) human clinical series, (2) fracture patients reported, and (3) use of ventral endoscopic techniques. Forty-four papers were identified wherein single-case studies and redundant publications of the same patient population were eliminated.

Level of evidence was assessed relative to the primary clinical questions. Levels of evidence were assigned by the criteria of Guyatt.[8] Based on the available evidence, only a qualitative analysis was possible.

◆ Results

All studies located used retrospective techniques. **Table 50.1** cites technique papers that did not include trauma patients and hence were excluded form the analysis. **Table 50.2** includes references that were mainly technique and review articles without any outcome data. **Table 50.3** includes papers with endoscopically treated traumatic fractures with any reported outcomes and served as the data for this systematic review.

◆ Discussion

Prior to the application of endoscopic techniques to fracture management, such techniques were applied to diskectomy.[9,10] Metastatic disease also drew early interest from proponents of this technique, although the benefits were not convincingly

Table 50.1 Techniques Papers without Trauma

Study	Study Design	Comments
Al-Sayyad et al (2004)[19]	Prospective series of 70 patients undergoing video-assisted thoracoscopic surgery (VATS) for scoliosis and other congenital/acquired deformities. Follow-up for 2 years	Radiographic and operative outcomes notes with VATS noted: "provides a safe and effective alternative to open thoracotomy in the treatment of thoracic pediatric spinal deformities."
Bergey et al (2004)[20]	Retrospective series	Pioneering paper on endoscopic lumbar surgery via the transpsoas approach. Retrospective series of 21 patients who underwent endoscopic, retroperitoneal transpsoas approach for exposure of the lumbar spine for a variety of indications. Surgical results at 3.1-year follow-up provided.
Huang et al (2006)[11]	Retrospective consecutive series study of endoscopic versus open treatment of thoracic metastases	Complication rates, outcomes, and overall survival rates were comparable, and the mean grade of neurological recovery was 1.2 on the Frankel scale in both groups. Only 6.9% of MASS patients required a 2-day postoperative intensive care unit stay compared with 88% of open procedure patients.

Table 50.2 Papers Excluded from Analysis: Trauma Papers without Outcomes (Feasibility Studies) and Review Articles (Very Low Quality Evidence)

Study	Description
Assaker et al (2001)[21]	Retrospective series of 29 patients who underwent video-assisted thoracoscopic surgery for a variety of indications: 13 posttrauma with grafting and stabilization. Three complications noted; no outcomes.
Beisse (2006)[22]	Review article on technique and instrumentation options using endoscopic techniques in the thoracic and lumbar spine.
Beisse (2007)[23]	Review article on technique and instrumentation options using endoscopic techniques in the thoracolumbar spine.
Beisse et al (2002)[24]	Retrospective report on experience with endoscopic treatment of thoracic and lumbar fractures in 93 patients with MACS TL plate (B. Braun Melsungen LG, Aesculap, Germany).
Beisse et al (1998)[25]	Review of 46 patients and technical description of patients undergoing endoscopic splitting of the diaphragm and corpectomy/grafting/instrumentation via an endoscopic approach for unstable fractures of the thoracic spine and the thoracolumbar junction. No outcomes reported.
Blauth et al (1997)[26]	Techniques paper reviewing transthoracic endoscopic spinal surgery in the setting of trauma, among other techniques.
Bühren (1998)[27]	Review of 90 patients who underwent stabilization of injuries of the thoracic spine and the thoracolumbar junction using minimally invasive thoracoscopy. Complications were rare and not severe, with only two conversions to open technique. Compared with the open, standard method benefits included reduced postoperative pain, shorter hospital stay, and reduced morbidity. Outcomes not reported.
de Peretti et al (1996)[6]	Technique paper reviewing experience with four patients undergoing lumbar interbody fusion, performed via a video-assisted retroperitoneal laparoscopic approach, complementary to posterior osteosynthesis at the L2–L3, L3–L4, and/or L4–L5 level. 3 trauma patients
Dickman and Mican (1996)[28]	Technique paper for kyphotic deformity resulting from compression fractures
Dickman et al (1996)[29]	Technique paper using thoracoscopy for numerous indications including fractures
Freixinet et al (1998)[30]	Review of transthoracic approaches to the spinal column for a variety of indications including trauma; also included video-assisted thoracoscopic surgery
Gushcha et al (2007)[31]	Comparative study between open versus endoscopic treatment of a variety of vertebral column pathologies. Five trauma patients included. Controls were not trauma. Objectively thoracoscopic patients had less immediate postop pain.
Hertlein et al (1995)[1]	Feasibility study demonstrating ability to perform thoracoscopic bone grafting in seven patients with unstable fractures of the upper thoracic spine
Hertlein et al (2000)[32]	Case report where thoracoscopic technique was used on two patients with thoracic traumatic spinal column injuries to perform bone grafting and instrumentation
Han et al (2002)[33]	Retrospective series of 241 thoracoscopic procedures for heterogeneous indications. No selection criteria stated. No outcome assessment.
Horn et al (2004)[34]	Case report of two patients undergoing thoracoscopic intervention for thoracic trauma, where dual-rod instrumentation was placed in two patients via thoracoscopic approach
Huang et al (1998)[35]	Technique paper regarding thoracoscopic surgery, four cases where three were metastases and one was T11 burst fracture
Josten et al (2005)[36]	Review article mentioning endoscopic techniques to treat fractures
Kim et al (2002)[37]	Review article mentioning endoscopic techniques to treat fractures
Kuklo and Lenke (2000)[38]	Review and technique article
Lekovic et al (2006)[39]	Case report of thoracic hyperextension fracture-dislocation treated using thoracoscopic reduction and anterior fixation of the thoracic spine using a paired screw–rod construct
Ragel et al (2007)[40]	Technique paper regarding using a thoracoscopic approach for vertebral body replacement with an expandable cage
Schultheiss et al (2003)[41]	Prospective series of 45 patients with fractures of T5–L3 or metastases undergoing endoscopic ventral reconstructive surgery; successfully performed in all patients; no outcomes reported
Verheyden et al (2002)[42]	Technique paper regarding anterior endoscopic reconstruction for thoracolumbar fractures while patient is in the prone position
Zhao et al (2005)[43]	Retrospective series of 12 patients operated on for heterogeneous indications. eight patients with trauma. 3-month follow-up. Mean operative time 210 minutes; mean blood loss 600 mL; mean hospital stay 12 days. No severe complications.

demonstrated. For example, although reduced length of stay in the intensive care unit (ICU) was described, there were reportedly no differences in blood loss in the series by Huang et al[11] or by Scheufler,[12] albeit individual patient data were not provided. Huang et al did, however, describe two dural leaks in the 29 endoscopic patients versus none in the comparison group of seven thoracotomy patients. In both of these series, the authors described experiencing significant technical challenges with the endoscopic procedures as compared with open surgery, with intraoperative dural and neurological

Table 50.3 Endoscopic Trauma Series with Outcomes

Study	Description	Quality of Evidence	Short-Term Outcomes Reported?	Topic and Conclusion
Beisse et al (2005)[44]	Retrospective series	Low	Yes	Series of patients undergoing anterior thoracic and lumbar endoscopic surgery for a variety of indications. 27 for trauma. Mean follow-up was 42 months. Mean operative time 5.42 hours with mean ICU stay of 1,4 days. 36.7% complication rate noted. No neurological complications. 25% of patients with complete paraplegia and 65% who were incomplete improved at least one Frankel grade. On postoperative CT scans mean spinal canal clearance noted to be 110%. Outcomes not separated by indication.
Hovorka et al (2000)[18]	Retrospective series.	Low	Yes	38 patients treated using videoscopic techniques for a variety of indications. 18 cases of fracture. Report results as satisfactory for every type of pathology but no details regarding the specifics of clinical assessment. No neurological complications. Noted, "The complications related to the approach were the same as those seen with open surgery; however, the videoscopic approach seems to us less invasive, with cosmetic benefit, less blood loss, and more rapid recovery." No controls.
Huang et al (1999)[45]	Retrospective series	Low	No	90 patients who underwent minimally invasive spinal surgery by thoracoscopic assistance as treatment for their anterior spinal lesions. Heterogeneous indications including 12 burst fractures. Complications reported in 22 patients (24.4%). Two fatal complications occurred, resulting from massive blood transfusion in one case and postoperative pneumonia in another. Complications reported here but no clinical or radiographic outcomes
Khoo et al (2002)[13]	Retrospective series	Low	Yes but of very limited quality	371 consecutive cases of thoracic or thoracolumbar fractures treated with endoscopic technique. 371 patients with fractures of the thoracic and thoracolumbar spine (T3–L3) were treated with a thoracoscopically assisted procedure. In the first 197 patients, a conventional open anterior plating system was used. The last 174 patients were treated with the MACS TL system (Aesculap, Tuttlingen, Germany). In 35% of patients, a stand-alone anterior thoracoscopic reconstruction was performed. In 65% of patients, a supplemental posterior pedicle-screw construct was also placed either before or after the anterior construct. A steep learning curve was present, with an average operating time of 300 minutes in the first 50% of cases and an average of 180 minutes with the MACS TL system. The severe complication rate was low (1.3%), with one case each of aortic injury, splenic contusion, neurological deterioration, cerebrospinal fluid leakage, and severe wound infection. An operative conversion rate to open thoracotomy of 1.2% was noted, secondary to bleeding. At 1 year an 86% fusion rate was noted. In the authors' discussion, they cite a German series of theirs comparing 30 patients treated thoracoscopically with a group of 30 patients treated with open thoracotomy[14]; in this series thoracoscopically treated patients required 42% less narcotics for pain treatment after the operation. They concluded that thoracoscopic procedures could be performed safely and effectively with less morbidity than open approaches
Kim et al (2004)[16]	Retrospective study	Low	Yes	212 patients undergoing thoracoscopic transdiaphragmatic approach to restore anterior column deficiency after spinal trauma. Follow-up ranged from 12 months to 6 years (mean, 3.9 years). Surgical durations ranged between 70 minutes and 7 hours (mean, 3.5 hours). 1.4% rate of conversion to open surgery usually due to bony bleeding that could not be controlled endoscopically. Mean clinical follow-up was 3.9 years. Preoperatively 57% of patients were Frankel E. Of the remaining patients with neurological deficits, 34% of 58 patients who were grades D, C, or B improved by at least one Frankel grade, and 15% of 34 patients who were Frankel A improved by at least one grade. Successful bony fusion with maintenance of satisfactory spinal alignment was observed in ~90% of

Table 50.3 Endoscopic Trauma Series with Outcomes (*Continued*)

Study	Description	Quality of Evidence	Short-Term Outcomes Reported?	Topic and Conclusion
				patients. Instrumentation loosening was seen in five cases. Three patients (1.4%) required conversion to an open procedure. Access-related complications, such as pleural effusion, pneumothorax, and intercostal neuralgia, were seen in 12 patients. Concluded that this procedure, "provides excellent access to the entire TLJ, permitting satisfactory spinal decompression, reconstruction and instrumentation."
McAfee et al (1995)[2]	Prospective study of	Low	Yes	15 patients underwent thoracoscopic corpectomy for a variety of indications (five for traumatic fractures). The mean operating time was 211 minutes (range 83 to 450 minutes) and the mean estimated blood loss was 890 mL (range 150 to 2800 mL). The mean length of time in the intensive care unit was 2 days (range 1 to 4 days), and the mean length of total hospitalization was 6.5 days (range 2 to 12 days). Postoperative morbidity "seemed favorable" compared with open techniques. All patients with fractures improved one Frankel grade
Olinger et al (1999)[46]	Retrospective series	Low	No	12 patients with fractures from L1 to L5 underwent endoscopic retroperitoneal fusion with iliac crest and plating. No major complications (including neurological problems) were encountered. Blood loss was minimal. None of the patients required conversion to open surgery. Five patients were mobilized early, starting regularly at the second postoperative day; seven could not be secondary to additional fractures.
Ringel et al (2008)[17]	Prospective series	Low	Yes	83 patients with 100 thoracic and/or lumbar fractures who underwent thoracoscopic or endoscopically assisted approaches to the thoracic and lumbar spine are feasible for anterior column reconstruction after initial pedicle-screw fixation.18% of patients lost to follow-up; mean follow-up was 23 months. Initial correction of kyphosis was 9 degrees; during follow-up (23 ± 11 months), the mean loss of correction was 6 degrees. Radiographic fusion noted in 87% of patients. Of 31 patients with a preop Frankel grade of worse than E, six improved; neurological status deteriorated in twp patients but recovered "early after surgery." In 84 minimally invasive approaches, five conversions to an open approach were necessary. Complications included one case of L1 nerve root injury, two cases of transient neurological worsening, one case of posterior wound infection, and one case of pleural empyema. Concluded this technique is feasible.
Verheyden et al (2004)[47]	Prospective study	Low		42 patients underwent endoscopically assisted anterior stabilization of fractures: 14 isolated anterior procedures (median duration of surgery, 181 minutes); 13 simultaneous one-stage procedures (median duration of surgery: 210 minutes), and 15 combined two-stage procedures (median duration of surgery: 90 minutes posterior, 120 minutes anterior, 240 minutes posterior + anterior). In the simultaneous posteroanterior procedures, the anterior instrumentation was performed 20 times using one rod, twice using two rods, and in six patients simply by bone grafting. No intraoperative complications were observed. In the postoperative course, one case of pneumothorax, one case of hemothorax, and one case of transient intercostal neuralgia occurred.

Abbreviations: CT, computed tomography; ICU, intensive care unit; TLJ, Thoracolumbar Junction.

injury, and complications associated with graft and methylmethacrylate placement.

Regarding safety and feasibility of the endoscopic management of thoracolumbar trauma, the literature consists of the case series cited in **Table 50.2**. These authors describe their learning curves and early experiences with these techniques.

Larger series, which may help answer whether the endoscopic management of thoracolumbar trauma improves early outcomes are shown in **Table 50.3**. These are typically case series or very small prospective series, usually without randomization or controls. To date the largest series published is that of Khoo et al,[13] where 371 patients with thoracic or thoracolumbar spine underwent anterior thoracoscopic reconstruction using either strut grafts or expandable cages and a Z-plate (197 patients) or the MACS TL system (B. Braun Melsungen LG, Aesculap, Germany). Sixty-five percent of patients underwent circumferential correction, whereas 35% of patients underwent stand-alone procedures. Their conversion rate to open procedures was 1.2% (four patients). Rather than reporting normative operative data, the authors noted initial experience with the first 30 to 40 cases having a mean of 6 hours operative time with a mean time of 3 hours later on in their series, including instrumentation implantation. Clinical outcomes were reported as an 86% fusion rate at 1 year with no hardware loosening. No other assessments were reported. In their discussion, the authors cite a prospective series from their group where 30 patients underwent thoracoscopic anterior spinal reconstructions and 30 underwent open thoracotomy and anterior reconstructions for spine trauma.[14] They also noted that the thoracoscopy group used significantly less narcotics and other analgesics[14] and had a higher rate of return to work (in a later non-peer-reviewed publication).[15]

Similar to the foregoing study, Kim et al[16] performed a retrospective study of 212 patients undergoing the thoracoscopic transdiaphragmatic approach for anterior management of thoracolumbar junction fractures. The authors noted a mean surgical time of 3.5 hours and a 1.4% rate of conversion to open surgery. Complications were reported in 11.7% of patients, including local complications such as pleural effusion, pneumothorax, and intercostal neuralgia; a single case of vascular injury; a single case of neurological deterioration; and five cases of implant loosening. Mean clinical follow-up was 3.9 years. Preoperatively 57% of patients were Frankel E. Of the remaining patients with neurological deficits, 34% of 58 patients who were grades D, C, or B improved by at least one Frankel grade, and 15% of 34 patients who were Frankel A improved by at least one grade. The authors cite the same literature as Khoo et al,[13] suggesting the endoscopic approach is better tolerated than open surgery.

Ringel et al[17] described a series of 83 consecutive patients with various thoracic and lumbar vertebral fractures. Thirty-eight retroperitoneal endoscopically assisted approaches and 46 thoracoscopic approaches were used to perform 61 interbody fusion and 31 complete corpectomies. Three patients with type C fractures underwent anterior instrumentation with Dynalock plates. All patients were instrumented posteriorly. Mean blood loss for posterior procedures was 500 mL (range 50 to 4000 mL) and mean blood loss for anterior procedures was 1000 mL (150 to 10,000 mL). Operative complications were reported, including five cases requiring conversion to open procedures, an L1 root injury, and transient neurological deficits in two patients, thoracic empyema, and a deep wound infection. Radiological outcomes were reported where spinal canal clearance was insufficient in only 2.4% of patients. Mean surgical correction of kyphosis was 9 degrees with a loss of 6 degrees on average at last follow-up. Frankel grades were reported at a mean of 23 months postop, with 18% of patients lost to follow-up. No data regarding length of stay or detailed clinical assessment using validated instruments were reported. The authors concluded that the minimally invasive endoscopic approach is feasible and the radiological and clinical outcomes are similar to conventional open approaches.

In a smaller series of patients, Hovorka et al[18] reported their experience with 5 years of endoscopic approaches to the lumbar and thoracolumbar spine. Eighteen traumatic vertebral injuries were operated on. Mean operative time and blood loss (for all anterior approaches: not trauma alone) were reported at 206 minutes and less than 200 mL, respectively. Mean follow-up was noted to be 17 months with 16 degrees reduction in preoperative kyphosis. Seventeen of the 18 trauma patients were noted to have radiological fusion. Clinical outcomes were otherwise not reported. The authors noted that this technique may be able to replace open procedures, but no control group is compared.

In summary, existing series regarding anterior endoscopic treatment of vertebral trauma demonstrate acceptable outcomes. These series are, however, limited by their small sizes, lack of controls, lack of clinical outcomes using validated measures, and typically retrospective designs.

Spine Trauma Study Group Recommendations

Though the case series are enthusiastic in reporting surgeon opinion that endoscopic techniques are feasible and superior to open techniques, the body of literature on this topic is small and consists of studies of limited quality. The studies describing this technique often include a heterogeneous population of patients, lack objective or validated patient-reported outcomes, and, most importantly, lack comparative "controls" of individuals being treated with the traditional open approach. The latter limitation makes it impossible to establish any potential early or late benefits of the endoscopic techniques over open surgical management.

The group's summary opinion was as follows:

1. Although, there is some evidence as to the safety and feasibility of these techniques, there does not exist sufficient evidence to recommend endoscopic techniques as a mainstream treatment option for the surgical management of thoracolumbar and thoracic fractures. This is a strong recommendation.
2. There does not exist sufficient evidence to establish that early outcomes of endoscopic treatment of thoracolumbar fractures are superior to those achieved by traditional open techniques. This is a strong recommendation.

References

1. Hertlein H, Hartl WH, Dienemann H, Schürmann M, Lob G. Thoracoscopic repair of thoracic spine trauma. Eur Spine J 1995;4:302–307
2. McAfee PC, Regan JR, Fedder IL, Mack MJ, Geis WP. Anterior thoracic corpectomy for spinal cord decompression performed endoscopically. Surg Laparosc Endosc 1995;5:339–348
3. Schultheiss M, Wilke HJ, Claes L, Kinzl L, Hartwig E. MAC-TL twin screw: a new thoracoscopic implantable stabilization system for treatment of vertebral fractures—implant design, implantation technique and in vitro testing [in German]. Orthopade 2002;31:362–367, 363–367
4. Schultheiss M, Hartwig E, Kinzl L, Claes L, Wilke HJ. Thoracolumbar fracture stabilization: comparative biomechanical evaluation of a new video-assisted implantable system. Eur Spine J 2004;13:93–100
5. Schultheiss M, Hartwig E, Sarkar M, Kinzl L, Claes L, Wilke HJ. Biomechanical in vitro comparison of different mono- and bisegmental anterior procedures with regard to the strategy for fracture stabilisation using minimally invasive techniques. Eur Spine J 2006;15:82–89
6. de Peretti F, Hovorka I, Fabiani P, Argenson C. New possibilities in L2–L5 lumbar arthrodesis using a lateral retroperitoneal approach assisted by laparoscopy: preliminary results. Eur Spine J 1996;5:210–216
7. Fisher CG, Wood KB. Introduction to and techniques of evidence-based medicine. Spine 2007;32(19, Suppl):S66–S72
8. Guyatt G, Gutterman D, Baumann MH, et al. Grading strength of recommendations and quality of evidence in clinical guidelines: report from an American College of Chest Physicians task force. Chest 2006;129: 174–181

9. Mack MJ, Regan JJ, Bobechko WP, Acuff TE. Application of thoracoscopy for diseases of the spine. Ann Thorac Surg 1993;56:736–738

10. Regan JJ, Mack MJ, Picetti GD III. A technical report on video-assisted thoracoscopy in thoracic spinal surgery: preliminary description. Spine 1995;20:831–837

11. Huang TJ, Hsu RW, Li YY, Cheng CC. Minimal access spinal surgery (MASS) in treating thoracic spine metastasis. Spine 2006;31:1860–1863

12. Scheufler KM. Technique and clinical results of minimally invasive reconstruction and stabilization of the thoracic and thoracolumbar spine with expandable cages and ventrolateral plate fixation. Neurosurgery 2007;61:798–808, discussion 808–809

13. Khoo LT, Beisse R, Potulski M. Thoracoscopic-assisted treatment of thoracic and lumbar fractures: a series of 371 consecutive cases. Neurosurgery 2002;51(5, Suppl):S104–S117

14. Beisse R, Potulski M, Bühren V. Thorakoskopisch gesteuerte ventrale Plattenspondylodese bei Frakturen der Brust- und Lendenwirbelsäule. Oper Orthop Traumatol 1999;11:54–69

15. Beisse R, Potulski M, Bühren V. Thoracoscopic-assisted approach to thoracolumbar fractures. In Mayer H ed. Minimally Invasive Spine Surgery. New York: Springer-Verlag, 2000:175–186

16. Kim DH, Jahng TA, Balabhadra RS, Potulski M, Beisse R. Thoracoscopic transdiaphragmatic approach to thoracolumbar junction fractures. Spine J 2004;4:317–328

17. Ringel F, Stoffel M, Stüer C, Totzek S, Meyer B. Endoscopy-assisted approaches for anterior column reconstruction after pedicle screw fixation of acute traumatic thoracic and lumbar fractures. Neurosurgery 2008;62(5, Suppl 2):ONS445–ONS452, discussion ONS452–ONS453

18. Hovorka I, de Peretti F, Damon F, Arcamone H, Argenson C. Five years' experience of the retroperitoneal lumbar and thoracolumbar surgery. Eur Spine J 2000;9(Suppl 1):S30–S34

19. Al-Sayyad MJ, Crawford AH, Wolf RK. Early experiences with video-assisted thoracoscopic surgery: our first 70 cases. Spine 2004;29:1945–1951, discussion 1952

20. Bergey DL, Villavicencio AT, Goldstein T, Regan JJ. Endoscopic lateral transpsoas approach to the lumbar spine. Spine 2004; 29:1681–1688

21. Assaker R, Fromont G, Reyns N, Louis E, Chastanet P, Lejeune JP. Video-assisted thoracoscopic surgery [in French]. Neurochirurgie 2001;47(2-3 Pt 1):93–104

22. Beisse R. Endoscopic surgery on the thoracolumbar junction of the spine. Eur Spine J 2006;15:687–704

23. Beisse R. Video-assisted techniques in the management of thoracolumbar fractures. Orthop Clin North Am 2007;38:419–429, abstract vii.

24. Beisse R, Potulski M, Beger J, Bühren V. Development and clinical application of a thoracoscopy implantable plate frame for treatment of thoracolumbar fractures and instabilities [in German]. Orthopade 2002;31:413–422

25. Beisse R, Potulski M, Temme C, Bühren V. Endoscopically controlled division of the diaphragm: a minimally invasive approach to ventral management of thoracolumbar fractures of the spine [in German]. Unfallchirurg 1998;101:619–627

26. Blauth M, Knop C, Bastian L, Lobenhoffer P. New developments in surgery of the injured spine [in German]. Orthopade 1997;26:437–449

27. Bühren V. Thoracoscopic management of fractures of the thoracic and lumbar spine [in German]. Langenbecks Arch Chir Suppl Kongressbd 1998;115:108–112

28. Dickman CA, Mican CA. Multilevel anterior thoracic discectomies and anterior interbody fusion using a microsurgical thoracoscopic approach. Case report. J Neurosurg 1996;84:104–109

29. Dickman CA, Rosenthal D, Karahalios DG, et al. Thoracic vertebrectomy and reconstruction using a microsurgical thoracoscopic approach. Neurosurgery 1996;38:279–293

30. Freixinet J, Hussein M, Mhaidli H, Rodríguez Suárez P, Robaina F, Rodríguez de Castro F. Transthoracic approach to the spinal column [in Spanish]. Arch Bronconeumol 1998;34:492–495

31. Gushcha AO, Shevelev IN, Arestov SO. Experience with endoscopic interventions in diseases of the vertebral column [in Russian]. Vopr Neirokhir 2007;2:26–31

32. Hertlein H, Hartl WH, Piltz S, Schürmann M, Andress HJ. Endoscopic osteosynthesis after thoracic spine trauma: a report of two cases. Injury 2000;31:333–336

33. Han PP, Kenny K, Dickman CA. Thoracoscopic approaches to the thoracic spine: experience with 241 surgical procedures. Neurosurgery 2002; 51(5, Suppl):S88–S95

34. Horn EM, Henn JS, Lemole GM Jr, Hott JS, Dickman CA. Thoracoscopic placement of dual-rod instrumentation in thoracic spinal trauma. Neurosurgery 2004;54:1150–1153, discussion 1153–1154

35. Huang TJ, Hsu RW, Liu HP, Liao YS, Hsu KY, Shih HN. Analysis of techniques for video-assisted thoracoscopic internal fixation of the spine. Arch Orthop Trauma Surg 1998;117:92–95

36. Josten C, Katscher S, Gonschorek O. Treatment concepts for fractures of the thoracolumbar junction and lumbar spine [in German]. Orthopade 2005;34:1021–1032

37. Kim DH, Jaikumar S, Kam AC. Minimally invasive spine instrumentation. Neurosurgery 2002;51(5, Suppl):S15–S25

38. Kuklo TR, Lenke LG. Thoracoscopic spine surgery: current indications and techniques. Orthop Nurs 2000;19:15–22

39. Lekovic GP, Horn EM, Dickman CA. Distraction injury to thoracic spine treated with thoracoscopic dual-rod fixation. Spine J 2006;6:330–334

40. Ragel BT, Amini A, Schmidt MH. Thoracoscopic vertebral body replacement with an expandable cage after ventral spinal canal decompression. Neurosurgery 2007;61(5, Suppl 2):317–322, discussion 322–323

41. Schultheiss M, Kinzl L, Claes L, Wilke HJ, Hartwig E. Minimally invasive ventral spondylodesis for thoracolumbar fracture treatment: surgical technique and first clinical outcome. Eur Spine J 2003;12:618–624

42. Verheyden AP, Katscher S, Gonschorek O, Lill H, Josten C. Endoscopically assisted minimally invasive reconstruction of the anterior thoracolumbar spine in prone position [in German]. Unfallchirurg 2002;105:873–880

43. Zhao K, Huang Y, Zhang J, Fang XQ, Yang Q. Thoracoscopic anterior approach decompression and reconstruction for thoracolumbar spine diseases [in Chinese]. Zhonghua Wai Ke Za Zhi 2005;43:491–494

44. Beisse R, Mückley T, Schmidt MH, Hauschild M, Bühren V. Surgical technique and results of endoscopic anterior spinal canal decompression. J Neurosurg Spine 2005;2:128–136

45. Huang TJ, Hsu RW, Sum CW, Liu HP. Complications in thoracoscopic spinal surgery: a study of 90 consecutive patients. Surg Endosc 1999; 13:346–350

46. Olinger A, Hildebrandt U, Mutschler W, Menger MD. First clinical experience with an endoscopic retroperitoneal approach for anterior fusion of lumbar spine fractures from levels T12 to L5. Surg Endosc 1999;13: 1215–1219

47. Verheyden AP, Hoelzl A, Lill H, Katscher S, Glasmacher S, Josten C. The endoscopically assisted simultaneous posteroanterior reconstruction of the thoracolumbar spine in prone position. Spine J 2004;4:540–549

51

Vertebroplasty Techniques for Stabilization of Thoracolumbar Spine Traumatic Fractures

F. C. Oner and Jorrit-Jan Verlaan

In the majority of thoracolumbar fractures caused by trauma or pathological processes, the main injury involves the vertebral body. Compression forces are the predominant vectors acting on the anterior column, although in the bipedal *Homo sapiens*, shear forces are also involved in certain areas of the thoracolumbar spine. The intervertebral disk between vertebral bodies functions as an absorber of these compression forces. If these forces exceed physiological limits or if the vertebral body is weakened by a disease process, the end plates can collapse under the hydrostatic pressure of the disks because nondegenerated disks are always stronger than the predominantly cancellous bone of the vertebral bodies under compression.[1] The end plate normally consists of a strong cortical ring at the periphery where the anulus fibrosus is attached and a weaker central part wherein the disk can protrude when fractured.[2] This leads to a relative shortening of the anterior column and can subsequently cause a kyphotic deformity. If the traumatic impact is fierce enough a fast disk intrusion may lead to a burst-out of the vertebral body causing narrowing of the vertebral canal and compression of the dural sac. This chain of events is a common pathway for many thoracolumbar spine pathologies.

Although the main damage in a traumatic event is in the anterior column, the anatomy of the thoracolumbar spine makes it difficult to approach the vertebral body directly to address these problems surgically. Surgical approaches to the anterior column of the thoracolumbar spine require techniques such as thoracotomy, lumbotomy, or laparotomy. The high morbidity of these approaches has caused a higher threshold for surgical intervention but has also led to acceptance of deformities and discomfort for patients that would normally be unacceptable for more easily accessible parts of the skeleton.

Pedicles, being strong cortical columns joining the vertebral body and posterior elements (arcus vertebra and facet joints), have been recognized as important structures in spinal surgery not only as locations for placement of strong anchors (pedicle screws) but also as safe and less invasive gateways to the anterior column. Putting a needle through the pedicle into the vertebral body and injecting a synthetic substance, usually polymethylmethacrylate (PMMA) cement, into the cancellous bone of the vertebral body was developed in the 1980s in Europe.[3] This technique, called vertebroplasty (VP), has gained wide acceptance for the treatment of osteoporotic vertebral compression fractures.[4,5] In the second half of the 1990s an inflatable bone tamp was developed to be introduced through the pedicle into the vertebral body and expanded to correct the deformity of the end plate and to create a sealed cavity where cement could be injected. This technique, called kyphoplasty or balloon vertebroplasty (BVP), has also been used successfully for treatment of osteoporotic compression fractures.[6,7] A lively debate has been ongoing in the recent literature as to when to use these techniques in osteoporotic fractures; whether it is possible to correct deformities with the balloon technique; and whether the high costs of the inflatable bone tamps are justified. These discussions are outside the scope of this chapter.

The primary question in the present work is whether VP and BVP, both previously developed and currently utilized to reduce pain in osteoporotic or metastatic fractures, can also be used for less invasive treatment of traumatic fractures. This chapter reviews the evidence for the use of VP or BVP techniques alone or in combination with spinal instrumentation for traumatic fractures. Furthermore, the technique of using BVP in combination with short-segment pedicle screw constructs, called the balloon-assisted end plate reduction (BAER), is described.

◆ The Rationale behind the Vertebroplasty for Fractures of the Vertebral Body

Traumatic fractures of the thoracolumbar spine can be seen in a broad spectrum of configurations with different degrees of involvement of the anterior and/or posterior elements. The most common types are compression-type fractures of the anterior column. If the posterior wall of the vertebral body is also involved in the fracture they are defined as burst fractures. In general, compression fractures do not lead to neurological deficits, but burst fractures are associated with encroachment of the spinal canal and may cause neurological symptoms. The simple compression-type fracture shows a configuration similar to osteoporotic compression fractures, and one may therefore consider them amenable to VP techniques. However, in the healthy and strong bone of young trauma patients these fractures usually heal without complications, and the patients are typically free of pain within a couple of weeks. The use of VP in these cases with a favorable natural history would probably be superfluous and would add an unnecessary risk. Burst fractures, on the other hand, usually represent considerable damage to the anterior column, especially when the complete vertebral body is involved. Treatment of these types of fractures has been a subject of intense debate among spine traumatologists.[8] Nonoperative treatment may cause pain and discomfort for many weeks and usually means the use of some kind of cast or orthosis or even bed rest during this period. These patients may be left with considerable residual deformities of their spine. Although operative treatment with short-segment pedicle-screw constructs is a good alternative, relatively high failure rates of this simple technique have been reported because of anterior column deficiency resulting from fracture reduction.[9] Earlier studies have shown that indirect reduction of burst fractures mainly reduces the periphery of the vertebral body, often leaving a central depression that may cause secondary failure of fixation and/or recurrence of the deformity.[1] VP and BVP, as a means to restore the central part of the end plates, have been proposed to overcome these problems.

Mermelstein showed in a cadaveric burst fracture model that VP with calcium phosphate cement (CPC) significantly reduced the stresses on posterior short-segment pedicle-screw instrumentation.[10] The idea of using the inflatable bone tamps in combination with a short-segment pedicle-screw construct to reduce the central end plate depression and to fill the ensuing defect with cement was developed subsequently. The feasibility of this BAER technique was first reported in a cadaveric study in 2002.[11] It was shown that distraction of the fractures by pedicle-screw instrumentation resulted in a reduction of both anterior and posterior wall displacement but did not reduce the central impression of the fractured end plate. After BAER followed by VP, the impression of the central end plate was significantly decreased. The maximum posterior wall displacement caused by BAER was 1.3 mm. No cement leakage outside the vertebral body could be detected during the procedure or after examination of the sectioned specimens.

The choice of cement in young trauma patients with fresh fractures treated with these new techniques is another discussion. Because PMMA might interfere with fracture healing and is biologically inert, the use of CPC has been suggested instead. Another concern is that in traumatic burst fractures the cement would come in contact with the intervertebral disk and may cause disk degeneration or collapse. These issues were studied in an in vivo goat model.[12] In this study CPC showed a good integration with bone. In PMMA a thin layer of fibrous tissue was seen consistently. No adverse reactions were seen if the cements came in contact with the disks through the damaged end plates.

◆ The Technique of Balloon-Assisted Endplate Reduction

This technique can be used for burst-type fractures caused by trauma or pathological processes such as myeloma or metastasis. It can also be used in burst-type fractures or nonunions of the osteoporotic spine. The rationale behind this specific technique is described elsewhere.[2] The basic steps of the technique are as follows:

- Prone position with chest and pelvic support. Make sure the abdomen is free and uncompressed.
- Anteroposterior (AP) and lateral fluoroscopy is essential. Check before surgery that clear and unimpeded AP and lateral fluoroscopy is possible. Mark the level of the pedicles of the fractured vertebra with waterproof marker.
- Use a standard posterior approach through a midline incision.
- Insert pedicle screws with as great a diameter and length as possible into the vertebrae cranial and caudal to the fractured vertebra. If Schanz-type screws are used advance them under fluoroscopic monitoring until anterior cortex purchase is achieved. With other types of screws do not use sizes smaller than 6 mm diameter and 40 to 45 mm long.
- Depending on the type of instrumentation used, perform reduction of kyphosis followed by distraction. Correct scoliotic deformity by asymmetrical distraction. Check correction with AP and lateral fluoroscopy and lock the screws.
- It is essential to get good spinal alignment after this step. If this cannot be achieved, do not proceed with the BAER procedure but consider additional anterior surgery.
- Probe the pedicles of the fractured vertebra carefully. Insert the cannulas of the Kyphon (KyphX, Kyphon Inc, Sunnyvale CA, USA) set.
- Probing of the pedicles of the fractured vertebra may cause profuse bleeding. Make sure the balloons are ready for insertion and expansion before probing. Intravertebral expansion of the balloons will stop the bleeding. Prevent the balloons from expanding in or at the base of the pedicles.
- Under fluoroscopic control insert the drill of the set. Try to get the drill under the most depressed portion of the end plate.
- Fill the bone tamps with contrast fluid as instructed by the company. Insert balloons and check their position under the end plate fluoroscopically AP and lateral. Make sure that the balloons are placed under the central end plate depression.
- Reduce the end plate under lateral fluoroscopic control by incremental inflation of the balloons. In case of asymmetrical depression, expand the balloon on the most depressed part for symmetrical reduction.
- Remove the balloons and inject saline with a syringe from one cannula and make sure that it comes from the contralateral cannula unimpeded. Inject the cement from only one side to avoid high pressure building in the cement mass. Injection should be monitored fluoroscopically.
- Do not pressurize the cement during injection. Cement should be poured rather than injected. CPC is more difficult to handle than PMMA cements. Make sure the cement is injectable without needing pressure. It may sometimes be necessary to increase the fluid:powder ratio of the cement

Table 51.1 Summary of Articles Describing the Use of Vertebroplasty or Balloon Vertebroplasty for Acute Traumatic Fractures

Study	Study Type	No. of Cases	Compression/ Burst	VP/BVP	Stand-Alone	Cement	Neurodeficit	Complications*	Follow-Up	Level of Evidence
Acosta et al (2005)[14]	RCS	5	0/15	BVP	No	PMMA	2/5	None	6–13 months	IV
Cho et al (2003)[15]	CC	20/50(control)	0/15	VP	No	PMMA	3/20	None	2 years	III
Hauck et al (2005)[16]	RCS	40	10/30	BVP	Yes	PMMA	Not reported	One revision in burst	12 months	IV
Huet et al (2005)[17]	RCS	12	3/9	VP	Yes	3 CPC9 PMMA	Not reported	One revision in burst	Not reported	IV
Kawanishi et al (2005)[18]	RCS	3	2/1	VP	No	PMMA	None	None	3–12 months	IV
Korovessis et al (2008)[19]	PC	23	0/23	BVP	No	CPC	5/23	None		
Maestretti et al (2007)[20]	PC	28 patients/ 33 fractures	24/9	BVP	Yes	CPC	None	None	24 months	III
Toyone et al (2006)[21]	PC	15	0/15	VP	No	HA	All	None	24 months	III
Verlaan et al (2005)[22]	PC	20	0/20	BVP	No	CPC	None	None	24 months	III
Total		163 fractures	39/124							

Abbreviations: BVP, balloon vertebroplasty; CC, case control; CPC, calcium phosphate cement; HA, hydroxyapatite; neurodeficit, neurological deficit before intervention; PC, prospective cohort; PMMA, polymethylmethacrylate; RCS, retrospective case series; VP, vertebroplasty.

*Complications, Non-symptomatic cement leakages were not considered complications.

to achieve good injectability. Also, flush your syringe and needle with saline before filling it with cement.

- PMMA cement is recommended for osteoporotic or pathological fractures. The advantages of CPC in trauma patients are theoretical and not yet proven in comparative studies.[2,13]
- In young trauma patients posterolateral fusion may be performed, although there is no solid evidence for this practice.

◆ Review of the Literature

To identify studies on the clinical outcome of VP or BPV in the treatment of traumatic fractures a PubMed search was performed for papers published from January 1980 to February 2008. Keywords used in this search were: "vertebroplasty" AND "traumatic fracture," "kyphoplasty" AND "traumatic fracture." From the resulting references, title and abstract were read by two independent readers to select the appropriate full-text papers. Inclusion criteria were: thoracic or lumbar acute traumatic fractures in adults treated by VP or BVP (kyphoplasty); detailed description of intervention, outcome, and complications. Exclusion criteria were cervical fractures; thoracic/lumbar osteoporotic fractures, and pathological fractures. After inclusion of all eligible papers, cross-referencing was used to obtain the remaining articles. A predefined scoring table was used to extract data from the papers in a standardized manner. In case of overlap of papers from the same author or institution, the least informative paper was excluded. The level of evidence of the included articles was assessed according to the guidelines proposed by the Center for Evidence Based Medicine.

We found nine papers in the literature with reports on the use of VP or BVP used alone or in combination with posterior instrumentation in traumatic fractures of the thoracolumbar spine (**Table 51.1**). The following techniques have been reported in these papers:

- VP with PMMA for compression fractures
- VP with CPC for compression fractures
- VP with PMMA for burst fractures
- VP with PMMA for burst fractures in combination with short-segment posterior instrumentation
- BVP with CPC for compression and burst fractures
- BVP with PMMA in combination with short-segment posterior instrumentation
- BVP with CPC in combination with short-segment posterior instrumentation

There were no studies comparing conventional treatment with VP or BVP techniques. No serious procedure related complications have been reported in this limited number of series. Most of the articles report some nonsymptomatic cement leakage, usually anterior, lateral or intradiskal.

◆ Summary and Recommendations

Although theoretically appealing as a means of anterior column augmentation by less invasive surgical techniques the evidence for the safety and efficacy of VP or BVP techniques with or without posterior instrumentation is very weak. Potentially these are techniques that may cause harm to the patient in inexperienced hands. From the available, very limited evidence from these studies we can reach the following conclusions:

1. VP or BVP for nonpathological compression fractures without burst component or neurological involvement is safe. Whether these treatments improve the quality of life of patients or accelerate their return to normal life in comparison with conventional treatment has not been demonstrated and should be studied in prospective comparative studies.
2. Although VP and BVP have been used in a small number of patients to treat incomplete burst fractures (AO type A 3.1) the failure rate seems to be high. These techniques may not properly reduce fractures or address mechanical instability.
3. VP and BVP can safely be used in burst fractures even in the presence of neurological involvement or posterior ligamentous complex injury when used in combination with pedicle-screw constructs. This practice may reduce the number of complications such as implant failure and decrease the need for higher morbidity anterior approaches.

As far as the choice of cement is concerned:

1. PMMA or CPC as well as other hydroxyapatite cements can safely be used as bone void filler in VP or BVP procedures for compression fractures but also in burst fractures when used in combination with pedicle-screw constructs.
2. Long-term effects of these cements in young trauma patients are not yet known. We recommend the more biocompatible CPC and hydroxyapatite to be used in young patients.
3. In burst-type fractures CPC should not be used in standalone procedures.Recommendation (strong): The use of VP and BVP techniques cannot be recommended at this moment for traumatic fractures as a standard procedure. These techniques should only be used in investigational settings.

References

1. Oner FC, van der Rijt RR, Ramos LM, Dhert WJ, Verbout AJ. Changes in the disc space after fractures of the thoracolumbar spine. J Bone Joint Surg Br 1998;80:833–839
2. Oner FC, Verlaan JJ, Verbout AJ, Dhert WJ. Cement augmentation techniques in traumatic thoracolumbar spine fractures. Spine 2006;31(11, Suppl):S89–S95, discussion S104
3. Galibert P, Deramond H, Rosat P, Le Gars D. Preliminary note on the treatment of vertebral angioma by percutaneous acrylic vertebroplasty [in French]. Neurochirurgie 1987;33:166–168
4. Heini PF, Wälchli B, Berlemann U. Percutaneous transpedicular vertebroplasty with PMMA: operative technique and early results: a prospective study for the treatment of osteoporotic compression fractures. Eur Spine J 2000;9:445–450
5. Grados F, Depriester C, Cayrolle G, Hardy N, Deramond H, Fardellone P. Long-term observations of vertebral osteoporotic fractures treated by percutaneous vertebroplasty. Rheumatology (Oxford) 2000;39:1410–1414
6. Garfin SR, Yuan HA, Reiley MA. New technologies in spine: kyphoplasty and vertebroplasty for the treatment of painful osteoporotic compression fractures. Spine 2001;26:1511–1515
7. Lieberman IH, Dudeney S, Reinhardt MK, Bell G. Initial outcome and efficacy of "kyphoplasty" in the treatment of painful osteoporotic vertebral compression fractures. Spine 2002;27:548
8. Verlaan JJ, Diekerhof CH, Buskens E, et al. Surgical treatment of traumatic fractures of the thoracic and lumbar spine: a systematic review of the literature on techniques, complications, and outcome. Spine 2004;29:803–814
9. McCormack T, Karaikovic E, Gaines RW. The load sharing classification of spine fractures. Spine 1994;19:1741–1744
10. Mermelstein LE, McLain RF, Yerby SA. Reinforcement of thoracolumbar burst fractures with calcium phosphate cement: a biomechanical study. Spine 1998;23:664–670, discussion 670–671

11. Verlaan JJ, van Helden WH, Oner FC, Verbout AJ, Dhert WJA. Balloon vertebroplasty with calcium phosphate cement augmentation for direct restoration of traumatic thoracolumbar vertebral fractures. Spine 2002;27:543–548

12. Verlaan JJ, Oner FC, Slootweg PJ, Verbout AJ, Dhert WJ. Histologic changes after vertebroplasty. J Bone Joint Surg Am 2004;86-A:1230–1238

13. Nakano M, Hirano N, Matsuura K, et al. Percutaneous transpedicular vertebroplasty with calcium phosphate cement in the treatment of osteoporotic vertebral compression and burst fractures. J Neurosurg 2002;97(3, Suppl):287–293

14. Acosta FL Jr, Aryan HE, Taylor WR, Ames CP. Kyphoplasty-augmented short-segment pedicle screw fixation of traumatic lumbar burst fractures: initial clinical experience and literature review. Neurosurg Focus 2005;18:e9

15. Cho DY, Lee WY, Sheu PC. Treatment of thoracolumbar burst fractures with polymethyl methacrylate vertebroplasty and short-segment pedicle screw fixation. Neurosurgery 2003;53:1354–1360, discussion 1360–1361

16. Hauck S, Beisse R, Bühren V. Vertebroplasty and kyphoplasty in spinal trauma. Eur J Trauma 2005;31:453–463

17. Huet H, Cabal P, Gadan R, Borha A, Emery E. Burst-fractures and cementoplasty. J Neuroradiol 2005;32:33–41, discussion 41

18. Kawanishi M, Itoh Y, Daisuke S, Nahoko M, Masatsugu K, Hajime H. Treatment of thoracolumbar fractures with vertebroplasty in combination with posterior instrumentation. Neurosurg Q 2005;15:181–185

19. Korovessis P, Repantis T, Petsinis G, Iliopoulos P, Hadjipavlou A. Direct reduction of thoracolumbar burst fractures by means of balloon kyphoplasty with calcium phosphate and stabilization with pedicle-screw instrumentation and fusion. Spine 2008;33:E100–E108

20. Maestretti G, Cremer C, Otten P, Jakob RP. Prospective study of standalone balloon kyphoplasty with calcium phosphate cement augmentation in traumatic fractures. Eur Spine J 2007;16:601–610

21. Toyone T, Tanaka T, Kato D, Kaneyama R, Otsuka M. The treatment of acute thoracolumbar burst fractures with transpedicular intracorporeal hydroxyapatite grafting following indirect reduction and pedicle screw fixation: a prospective study. Spine 2006;31:E208–E214

22. Verlaan JJ, Dhert WJA, Verbout AJ, Oner FC. Balloon vertebroplasty in combination with pedicle screw instrumentation: a novel technique to treat thoracic and lumbar burst fractures. Spine 2005; 30:E73–E79

52

Minimally Invasive Posterior Stabilization Techniques in Trauma

Neel Anand, Eli M. Baron, and Mark B. Dekutoski

Posterior minimally invasive methods are novel techniques used in the treatment of spinal trauma. Theoretically they may be associated with reduced morbidity, blood loss, and muscle damage when compared with traditional open methodologies. As enabling technologies develop, the application of minimally invasive, posterior spinal stabilization techniques in the management of spinal trauma continues to expand. However, the current level of evidence to support the use of these techniques compared with open techniques remains weak. Several small case series have demonstrated feasibility and safety of these techniques. However, evidence to support superiority and hence recommendations for widespread adoption of these techniques compared with current open techniques is lacking.

The epidemiology, unique clinical and diagnostic features as well as the initial management of injuries pertinent to this chapter are discussed within the individual chapters specific to each injury.

◆ Surgical Options

Pedicle screw fixation has become the mainstay technique for repairing unstable thoracolumbar spine fractures, specifically with regard to providing stability in the setting of an incompetent posterior ligamentous complex.[1] The history of classification of thoracolumbar injuries and fixation for thoracolumbar fractures has been detailed elsewhere.[1-3] Following the era of Harrington rod instrumentation, pedicle screw fixation allowed for segmental fixation techniques. Good results with pedicle screw fixation for thoracolumbar fractures have been reported; nevertheless, a higher failure rate has been described in cases of anterior column insufficiency.[4,5] Thus anterior reconstruction, which often enables shorter posterior constructs, is also an important consideration in the surgical management of thoracolumbar trauma.[1]

More recently, minimally invasive posterior percutaneous tension band restoration or augmentation has been described, as has minimally invasive posterior spinal fusion for

thoracolumbar trauma.[6-13] The rationale behind performing minimally invasive fixation or fusion for thoracolumbar trauma is the potentially high exposure-related morbidity associated with open procedures, including reduction of infection rate and blood loss. Verlaan et al reported a median blood loss greater than 1000 mL for fixation of thoracolumbar trauma.[14] Additionally, Rechtine et al reported an infection rate as high as 10%.[15] The open approach to the thoracolumbar spine also results in considerable morbidity as a result of tissue destruction secondary to muscle stripping and retractor-related injury, both of which have been described and well characterized.[16-20] Hence it would seem that minimally invasive percutaneous fixation and fusion techniques have the potential to be beneficial in thoracolumbar trauma.[21] Nevertheless, few reports exist regarding actual outcomes in comparison with traditional methods of fixation and fusion for spinal trauma.

Technique for Minimally Invasive Posterior Treatment of a Burst Fracture

In this sequence we demonstrate treatment of lumbar burst fracture with cement augmentation and minimally invasive pedicle screw–rod placement and fusion in an older patient. Prior to performing the procedure, the patient should have appropriate workup and imaging (**Fig. 52.1**). The patient is positioned prone on a Jackson table (**Fig. 52.2**). Anteroposterior (AP) fluoroscopy is brought in and used to mark the lateral border of the pedicle (**Fig. 52.3**). Care should be taken to ensure that the AP fluoroscopic image is straight on, without any parallax. A no. 15 blade is use to incise the skin. A Jamshidi needle is introduced into the upper outer quadrant of the pedicle, using AP fluoroscopy (**Fig. 52.4**). The needle is advanced under AP fluoroscopy ~15 mm into the pedicle. Great care should be taken not to breach the medial border of the pedicle. This methodology is used to insert Jamshidi needles on one side and then the other. The lateral view is used to confirm the sagittal trajectory and advance the needle past the

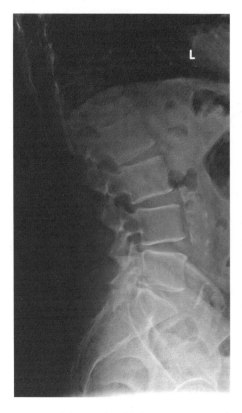
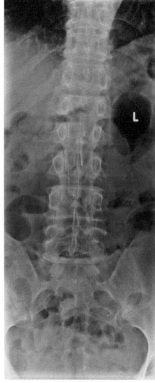
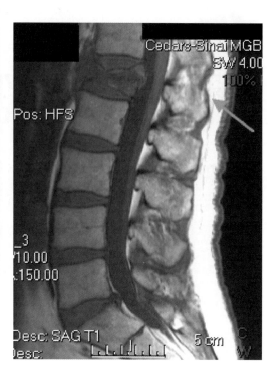

Fig. 52.1 **(A)** Lateral and **(B)** anteroposterior plain radiographs demonstrating an L1 unstable burst fracture in a 63-year-old male who sustained a fall. **(C)** T1 sagittal magnetic resonance imaging demonstrates a disruption in the supraspinous ligament, as seen by a disruption of the black stripe on T1-weighted imaging (*arrow*).

base of the pedicle into the vertebral body. Subsequently, guide wires are introduced down the Jamshidi needle under lateral fluoroscopic guidance and the Jamshidi needles are removed (**Fig. 52.5**). The authors prefer to utilize two C-arms; however, a single C-arm can be used, or alternatively pedicle cannulation can be performed using intraoperative three-dimensional imaging such as isocentric C-arm or mobile computed tomography (CT). A variety of computer-assisted techniques have also been described.

We then proceed with cement augmentation. A working cannula is introduced over the guide wire (**Fig. 52.6**). This is malleted into position. Great care should be taken not to advance the guide wire. We prefer that the surgeon hold the guide wire with the left hand while holding the handle of the working cannula. Subsequently, the guide wire is removed. Bone biopsy is taken. A drill is used to drill a channel into the vertebral body or a curette is used to tamp the vertebral body. This is done under strict AP and lateral fluoroscopic control.

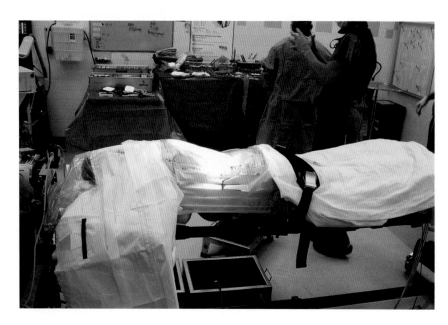

Fig. 52.2 The patient is positioned prone on a Jackson table. The legs are extended to maximize lordosis.

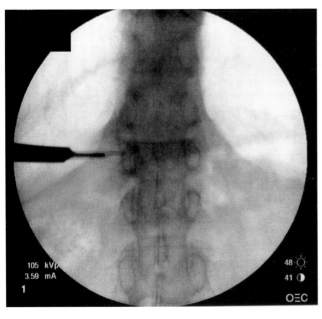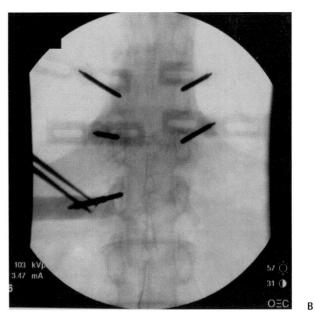

Fig. 52.3 **(A)** Anteroposterior fluoroscopy is used to mark the lateral border of the pedicle on the skin. **(B)** Anteroposterior fluoroscopy showing Jamshidi needles in place in pedicles.

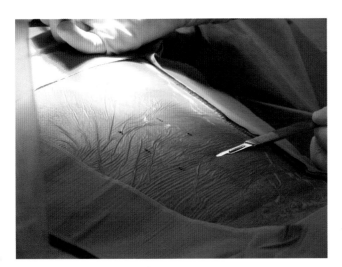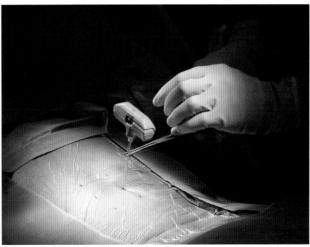

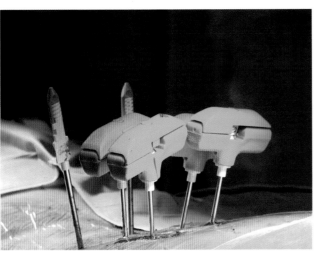

Fig. 52.4 **(A)** AP fluoroscopy is used to identify the lateral border of the pedicle and *incision are* planned **(B)** Jamshidi needles are introduced through these small incisions in the skin and advanced ~1.5 cm under anteroposterior fluoroscopy, staying lateral to the medial wall of the pedicle. **(C)** A total of six Jamshidi needles are introduced.

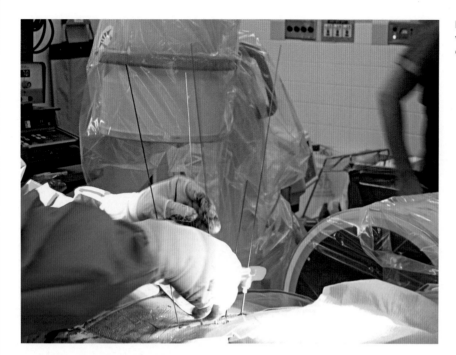

Fig. 52.5 Lateral guide wires are introduced with lateral fluoroscopic guidance being used to determine depth.

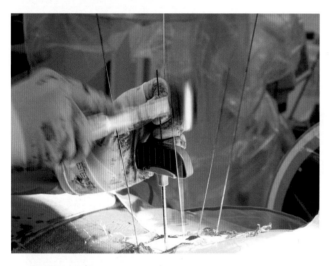

Fig. 52.6 A working cannula is introduced over the guide wire.

Afterward, a balloon is inserted down the working cannula. The balloon is filled with contrast until the balloon fills an appropriate width and height on the AP and lateral projection (**Fig. 52.7**). Afterward the balloon is deflated and polymethylmethacrylate cement is introduced into the cavity created by the balloon. Great care should be taken, especially under lateral fluoroscopy, to ensure that cement is not advancing posteriorly toward the spinal canal. Should cement be seen exiting the cannula posteriorly, the technique is stopped to allow the cement to harden. Then more cement is introduced slowly. By waiting a few moments, the surgeon allows the cement posteriorly to stiffen; thus any cement introduced further is less likely to advance in the same direction.

Cement should be introduced until it fills the void created by the balloon and interdigitates with the bony fragments (**Fig. 52.8**). We prefer to see the vertebral end plate height restored; however, great care should be taken to avoid cement exiting the vertebral body either laterally or posteriorly.

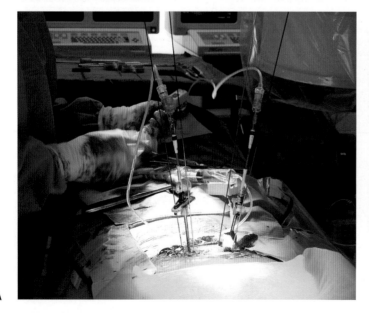

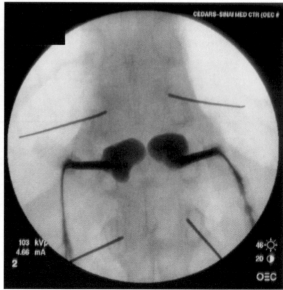

A   B

Fig. 52.7 **(A)** A balloon bone tamp is filled with contrast agent until it expands to appropriate size. **(B)** This is monitored under fluoroscopy.

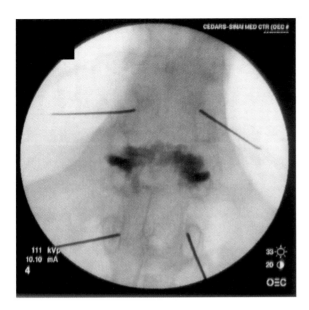

Fig. 52.8 Anteroposterior fluoroscopic image after bone cement is introduced. Lateral fluoroscopy is also monitored during cement introduction to make sure cement does not travel posteriorly.

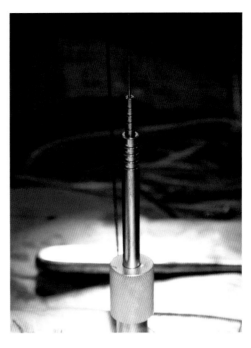

Fig. 52.9 Serial dilators are used to dilate the working channel through the spinal musculature.

For placement of percutaneous pedicle screws, serial dilators are placed over the guide wires (**Fig. 52.9**). Care should be taken to ensure that skin incisions are large enough to accommodate the dilators. Additionally, care should be taken that adhesive drapes are not introduced into the patient as serial dilators are being placed. Subsequently, a cannulated tap is placed over the guide wire and used to tap each pedicle (**Fig. 52.10**). A pedicle screw is then placed over the guide wire into the vertebral body, ensuring that the guide wire is not advancing. Once the pedicle screw is advanced beyond the base of the pedicle, the guide wire may be removed.

The screw head should not be impinging on the facets. Additionally, extenders should have their slots at approximately the same heights (**Fig. 52.11**). Rod length is then measured (**Fig. 52.12**).

The rod is then contoured appropriately. An additional incision is made rostrally and the rod passed freehand (**Fig. 52.13**). Lateral fluoroscopy is used to confirm the depth of the rod. Once the rod is inserted into the first pedicle screw extender, a tester is use to ensure that the rod is actually within the extender and not lateral to it (**Fig. 52.14**). The rod is then advanced further into the other extenders. Lateral

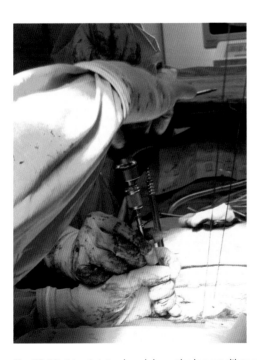

Fig. 52.10 A tap is introduced down the largest dilator and under lateral fluoroscopic guidance taps the pedicle and proximal vertebral body

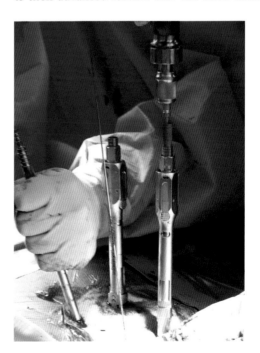

Fig. 52.11 Percutaneous screws are introduced over the guide wires. Lateral fluoroscopy is used to confirm appropriate depth and extender orientation.

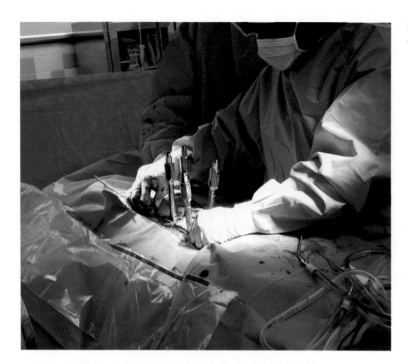

Fig. 52.12 Rod length is measured by measuring the distance between extenders.

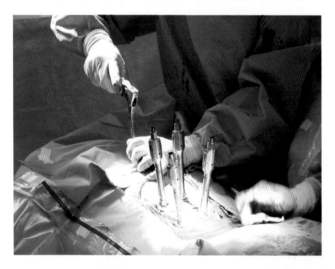

Fig. 52.13 An additional incision is made rostrally and the rod is freehand passed.

fluoroscopy confirms appropriate rod placement. The extenders are then reduced down to seat the rod into the tulip of the screw. Once seated, a suction trephine is used to suck out any soft tissue inside the extenders, and a top locking nut is placed in the caudal screw and tightened. Subsequently, locking nuts are placed in the remaining screws (**Fig. 52.15**). Locking nuts are finally tightened to a specific torque. The surgeon has the option of applying compression across the screws prior to tightening down all the nuts (**Fig. 52.16**). The extenders are then removed.

The skin incisions are extended between the screw heads, the fascia is divided, and the facets are then exposed, irrigated, and decorticated. A bone graft extender or osteobiological products and local bone graft are placed (**Fig. 52.17**). Final AP and lateral images are taken (**Fig. 52.18**). The incisions are closed in the usual manner.

For evidence regarding the use of cement augmentation for traumatic spinal fractures, please see Chapter 51.

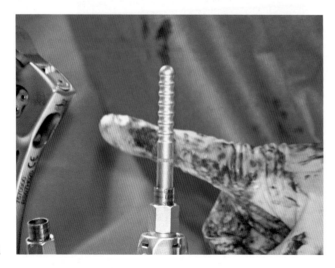

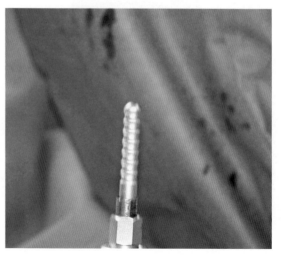

A

B

Fig. 52.14 **(A)** A tester demonstrates the rod to be present, and **(B)** the rod to be absent.

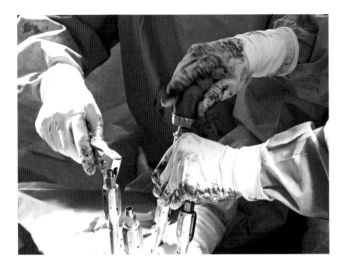

Fig. 52.15 The rod is reduced and final locking nuts are applied.

◆ Complications

Percutaneous pedicle screw fixation has been demonstrated to be safe for the thoracic and lumbar spine.[13,22,23] Nevertheless, complications with insertion may occur. Complications reported include screw misplacement requiring revision, neurological injury, radicular pain, instrumentation prominence (in a series where the rod was placed suprafascially), and wound infection.[13,23] Less frequently seen complications were iliac vein injury, arterial thrombus, and adjacent segment degeneration.[22] In terms of screw placement, Ringel et al, in a series looking at 488 percutaneously placed screws, reported good placement of 87% of screws, 10% as acceptable, and 3% as unacceptable on CT scans.[23] More recently Schizas et al reported results of a CT scan study of 15 consecutive patients undergoing percutaneous pedicle screw insertion.[24] Thirteen percent of the patients (2/15) had severe frank cortical wall penetration from the screws, whereas 80% of them (12/15) had some perforation. On axial images the incidence of severe frank pedicle penetration was 3.3%, and the overall

rate of screw perforation was 23%. We cannot stress the importance of clear intraoperative imaging, especially in the AP view. Image guidance has been used with percutaneous screw placement and may have an increasing role in the future.[25,26]

◆ Rehabilitation

The principles of rehabilitation following minimally invasive posterior spinal fixation are identical to those utilized for open stabilization techniques and are dependent on the medial stability of the patient, the specific injury, the neurological status of the patient, and the overall stability of spinal fixation (e.g., extent of fixation and bone quality). Protocols will vary from among centers as well as among surgeons, but in general prescribe to early and aggressive mobilization as soon as the medical condition of the patient allows.

◆ Systematic Review

This chapter sets out to systematically review the available literature to answer the following questions:

Question 1: Is there evidence to support posterior minimally invasive percutaneous stabilization/fusion in the management of spinal trauma?
Question 2: For what specific injuries or clinical scenarios are minimally invasive posterior stabilization/fusion techniques potentially indicated compared with an open procedure for the treatment of spine trauma?

Methods

A systematic review was initiated under the methodology described by Fisher and Wood.[27] PubMed was searched using the terms "percutaneous," "spine," and "trauma." This yielded 553 results. Of these papers, all abstracts were reviewed, and five papers were deemed as possibly appropriate. PubMed was

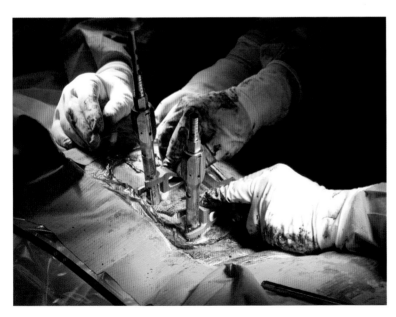

Fig. 52.16 Prior to locking down the nuts, the surgeon can apply compression across the screws.

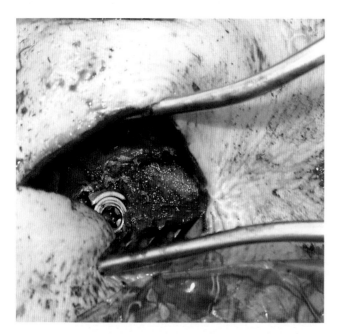

Fig. 52.17 The incisions are extended and facet joints are decorticated. Bone graft is laid down.

also searched using "minimally," "invasive," "spine," and "trauma." This yielded 354 results. Of these papers, all abstracts were reviewed and an additional 12 papers were deemed as possibly appropriate. Additionally, reference lists in all publications found were searched to identify series detailing results of minimally invasive fixation for spinal trauma. An additional series was found. All 18 references were obtained and nine were excluded because they were review articles not describing case experience with these techniques and trauma. Using grading of recommendations assessment development and evaluation (GRADE) methodology,[28] the quality of evidence presented in the remaining studies was assigned a score of high, moderate, low, or very low. Based on the available evidence, only a qualitative analysis was possible.

◆ Results

Table 52.1 summarizes the results of our systematic review regarding minimally invasive posterior fixation and fusion for trauma.

◆ Discussion

Thoracolumbar

The first report of minimally invasive surgery for thoracolumbar fractures was in 1982 by Magerl, who described use of an external fixator for thoracolumbar trauma.[29] Due to patient and technical factors, this technique was unacceptable to both patients and surgeons. With the introduction of more contemporary percutaneous fixation devices for the management of degenerative spinal fusion in early 2000, interest in applications to traumatic spinal injuries has risen. Sahin and Reznik described using percutaneous stabilization (L4–S1) for the treatment of an unstable L5 burst fracture.[12] At 6 months the patient was noted to be neurologically intact and off pain medications. Similarly, Beringer et al ($n = 2$) and Schizas et al described success using percutaneous pedicle screw instrumentation for temporary internal bracing of nondisplaced bony chance fractures.[8,30] Two case series exist describing longer follow-up regarding minimally invasive pedicle screw fixation and thoracolumbar trauma. Assaker presented 28-month follow-up on 40 neurologically intact patients stabilized with primary posterior percutaneous fixation for a single-level burst-type or flexion-distraction injuries (AO types A2, A3, and B1).[7,31] Average operative time was 75 minutes, with minimal blood loss and no infections. Average loss of correction over 28 months was 7.5 degrees. Good to excellent outcomes were achieved. There was no control group.

Wild et al have published the longest follow-up series of minimally invasive posterior stabilization of thoracolumbar fractures reported to date.[13] This study was a retrospective,

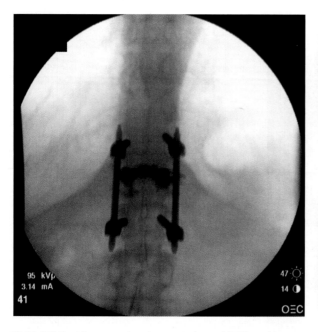
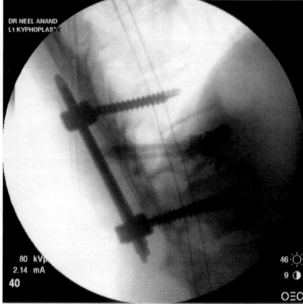

Fig. 52.18 (A) Final fluoroscopic anteroposterior and **(B)** lateral images.

Table 52.1 Results of Systematic Review: Minimally Invasive Spinal Fixation in the Setting of Trauma

Study	Description	Quality of Evidence	Topic and Conclusion
Assaker (2005)[31]	Prospective series undergoing MIS stabilization of fractures	Low	28-month follow-up on 40 neurologically intact patients stabilized with primary posterior percutaneous fixation for a single-level burst-type or flexion-distraction injuries. No control. CONCLUSIONS: Good to excellent outcomes were achieved for single-level burst fractures or flexion-distraction injuries using percutaneous fixation.
Beringer et al (2007)[8]	Retrospective case series	Very low	Two patients underwent percutaneous pedicle screw instrumentation for temporary internal bracing of nondisplaced bony Chance fractures. Long-term follow-up not provided. CONCLUSION: Minimally invasive internal bracing of nondisplaced bony Chance fractures is option for selected neurologically intact patients unable to tolerate bracing.
Fong and DuPlessis (2005)[34]	Case report	Very low	Two patients underwent minimally invasive lateral mass fusion in the setting of cervical trauma. No follow-up data were provided. CONCLUSIONS: "We describe successful placement of lateral mass screw and constructs with the use of a minimally invasive approach by means of a dilator retractor system."
Korovessis, et al (2008)[32]	Prospective consecutive series	Low	18 patients sustaining either burst or severe compression fractures underwent kyphoplasty and short segment minimally invasive posterior fixation. Average follow-up was 22 months. CONCLUSION: Balloon kyphoplasty with calcium phosphate cement combined with posterior segmental short minimal invasive fixation for acute burst fractures or severe compression fractures provides good clinical and radiological results. No neurological complications. One case of superficial wound necrosis was reported.
Sahin and Reznik (2005)[12]	Case report	Very low	34-year-old female patient underwent percutaneous pedicle screw fixation between L4 and the sacrum, using minimally invasive techniques for unstable burst fracture; 6-month follow-up provided. No complications. CONCLUSION: Minimally invasive fixation procedures are a treatment option for select patients with L5 burst fractures.
Schizas and Kosmopoulos (2007)[30]	Case report	Very Low	Two patients with Chance fractures underwent MIS percutaneous fixation with cannulated pedicle screws. Screws were removed after 9 months. No complications. CONCLUSION: Temporary MIS fixation may be an acceptable technique for treating bony Chance fractures.
Sehati and Khoo (2006)[35]	Retrospective series	Very low	10 patients underwent MIS posterior cervical fixation for a variety of traumatic indications. No complications; fusion confirmed at follow-up; clinical outcomes not reported. CONCLUSIONS: MIS posterior cervical fixation may be an acceptable technique in the setting of trauma.
Wang et al (2003)[33]	Retrospective series	Very low	Three patients sustaining cervical trauma underwent MIS posterior cervical fixation. Technical report. No complications reported. CONCLUSION: MIS posterior cervical fixation may be used in the setting of trauma.
Wild, et al (2007)[13]	Retrospective, nonrandomized case control	Low	21 consecutive, nonrandomized patients with thoracolumbar vertebral body fractures (AO type A) without neurological symptoms. Eleven patients had been treated open and 10 patients minimally invasive. Greater than 5-year follow-up. Statistically significant less blood loss in the MIS group; clinical and radiological outcomes were similar in both groups. Noted no complications in both groups. CONCLUSIONS: MIS posterior stabilization is associated with lower blood loss in comparison with the conventionally open method and can be performed without any special effort limited to A-fractures without any neurological symptoms.

Abbreviations: MIS, minimally invasive spinal.

nonrandomized case control design and suffered from inhomogeneity of the patient populations. They studied 21 consecutive nonrandomized patients with thoracolumbar vertebral body fractures. All patients had type A fractures according to the AO fracture classification, without rupture of the posterior ligamentous complex. Of the 21 patients studied, 11 patients were treated with conventional open methods (midline muscle stripping approach and screw insertion), and 10 patients were treated minimally invasively. The majority of the patients had their implants removed after 9 months to avoid implant failure. The patients were followed up at a minimum of 5 years and evaluated with the Hanover spine score, radiographs, and the Short Form-36 (SF-36) questionnaire. None of the patients underwent anterior stabilization. The authors reported a statistically significant difference in intraoperative and postoperative blood loss (minimally invasive group lost an average of 200 mL intraoperative and 155.6 mL of blood postoperatively compared with 380 mL intraoperative and 441 mL postoperative blood loss). Operating time in both groups was not significantly different, with the open group having mean surgical time of 80.9 and the minimally invasive group ~87.4 minutes. In terms of clinical outcomes, Hanover spine scores and SF-36 scores showed no statistically significant difference between the two groups. Additionally, 5 years after implant removal, the loss of bisegmental wedge angle averaged 7.62 degrees in both groups. The highest loss of correction occurred 1 year after implant removal and averaged 6.86 degrees. The authors noted significant group inhomogeneity, particularly in baseline age and injury severity.

Korovessis et al[32] published a prospective series of 18 patients undergoing treatment of burst fractures or severe compression fractures using balloon-assisted cement augmentation (with calcium phosphate cement) and pedicle screw instrumentation. Mean age was 64 with a standard deviation (SD) of 15 years. Sixteen of the patients had an American Spine Injury Association (ASIA) score E, one patient had a score of D, and one patient of C. Pedicle screws were placed with fluoroscopic assistance using minimal access techniques (using cannulated needles, K-wires, and cannulated pedicle screws). Mean operative time was 45 minutes (range 35 to 70 minutes), mean blood loss was 50 mL (range 20 to 200 mL), and mean hospital stay was 2 days (range 1 to 3 days).

Mean clinical follow-up was 22 months (range 17 to 28 months). All patients were followed clinically and radiographically. Mean preoperative visual analogue scale (VAS) was 7.6 (SD 2), and postoperative at 6 month was 3.1 (SD 2.3) ($p < 0.001$). All patients were noted to be ASIA E postoperative. Segmental kyphosis improved from a mean preoperative Gardner angle of 16 degrees (SD 11) to mean postoperative angle of 2 degrees (SD 2), with no measurable loss of correction at last follow-up. On postoperative imaging, spinal canal encroachment improved from a mean of 25% (SD 20) preoperative to a mean of 19% (SD 21) postoperative ($p = 0.07$). Solid arthrodesis was confirmed in all patients using CT scanning at 8 to 10 months postoperative. Complications included four cases of cement in the supraadjacent disk space (asymptomatic noted on CT), and three cases of slightly medially breeched pedicle screw placement (asymptomatic) and superficial wound necrosis. The authors concluded that, "minimally invasive surgery with short posterior cannulated pedicle screws and balloon kyphoplasty with calcium phosphate could . . . restore post-traumatic segmental angulation . . . reduce post-traumatic pain (and improve) functional outcome."

In summary, three case reports and three limited case series have been published regarding minimally invasive posterior thoracolumbar fixation/fusion. The case series have a variety of methodological flaws and all lack an appropriate control group; consequently, the current evidence regarding this technique is weak.

Cervical

Sparse literature exists on minimally invasive methods for posterior cervical fixation in the setting of trauma. Wang et al reported treating three patients with traumatic single-level facet dislocation.[33] Two patients, after successful reduction using traction, underwent anterior cervical diskectomy and fusion, followed by minimally invasive lateral mass screw placement. The third patient underwent laminectomy, followed by percutaneous lateral mass screw placement. No follow-up data for these patients were reported. Fong and DuPlessis also described minimally invasive percutaneous lateral mass screw fixation in the cervical spine following anterior cervical diskectomy and fusion.[34] No follow-up data were reported. Sehati and Khoo reported follow-up of 10 patients undergoing minimally invasive cervical fusion at the University of California, Los Angeles.[35] This was for treatment of cervical burst fractures and fracture dislocation. Fusion was confirmed at follow-up with dynamic radiographs and CT scans. Clinical outcomes, however, were not reported. Nevertheless, there were no neurological deficits reported.

In summary, the evidence for minimally invasive posterior cervical arthrodesis in the setting of trauma can be described as very weak, with one case report, a technical report, and one very small case series with limited follow-up and no control group.

◆ Spine Trauma Study Group Recommendations

1. Based on the preceding evidence and group expert opinion, there exists some support for the feasibility and safety of posterior minimally invasive percutaneous stabilization/fusion in the management of thoracolumbar spinal trauma. However, the evidence does not support superiority in outcome compared with conventional technique. Consequently, posterior minimally invasive percutaneous stabilization/fusion in the management of spinal trauma should only be considered as an option for the management of specific traumatic thoracolumbar spinal injuries. This is a weak recommendation.
2. Utilization of these techniques for cervical spine injuries is not supported. This is a strong recommendation.
3. Based on the preceding evidence and group expert opinion, minimally invasive posterior stabilization/fusion may be indicated for reconstruction or augmentation of a disrupted posterior tension band following anterior reconstruction, restoration of the posterior tension band (e.g., potentially unstable burst fracture or treatment of osseous flexion-distraction injuries), and in the early treatment of polytrauma patients to enable mobilization and stabilization of extension-distraction injuries such as in ankylosing spondylitis. This is a weak recommendation.

References

1. Baron EM, Zeiller SC, Vaccaro AR, et al. Surgical management of thoracolumbar fractures. Contemporary Spine Surgery 2005;6:1–9
2. Anand N, Vaccaro AR, Lim MR, et al. Evolution of thoracolumbar trauma classification systems: assessing the conflict between mechanism and morphology of injury. In: Patel D, Kurd MF, Vaccaro AR, eds. Topics in Spinal Cord Injury Rehabilitation. St. Louis: Thomas Land; 2006: 70–78
3. Vaccaro AR, Baron EM, Sanfilippo J, et al. Reliability of a novel classification system for thoracolumbar injuries: the Thoracolumbar Injury Severity Score. Spine 2006;31(11, Suppl):S62–S69, discussion S104
4. McCormack T, Karaikovic E, Gaines RW. The load sharing classification of spine fractures. Spine 1994;19:1741–1744
5. McLain RF, Burkus JK, Benson DR. Segmental instrumentation for thoracic and thoracolumbar fractures: prospective analysis of construct survival and five-year follow-up. Spine J 2001;1:310–323
6. Amar AP, Larsen DW, Teitelbaum GP. Percutaneous spinal interventions. Neurosurg Clin N Am 2005;16:561–568, vii.

7. Assaker R. Minimal access spinal technologies: state-of-the-art, indications, and techniques. Joint Bone Spine 2004;71:459–469
8. Beringer W, Potts E, Khairi S, Mobasser JP. Percutaneous pedicle screw instrumentation for temporary internal bracing of nondisplaced bony Chance fractures. J Spinal Disord Tech 2007;20:242–247
9. Fessler RG, O'Toole JE, Eichholz KM, Perez-Cruet MJ. The development of minimally invasive spine surgery. Neurosurg Clin N Am 2006;17:401–409
10. Rampersaud YR, Anand N, Dekutoski MB. Use of minimally invasive surgical techniques in the management of thoracolumbar trauma: current concepts. Spine 2006;31(11, Suppl):S96–S102, discussion S104
11. Regan JJ, Yuan H, McCullen G. Minimally invasive approaches to the spine. Instr Course Lect 1997;46:127–141
12. Sahin S, Resnick DK. Minimally incisional stabilization of unstable L5 burst fracture. J Spinal Disord Tech 2005;18:455–457
13. Wild MH, Glees M, Plieschnegger C, Wenda K. Five-year follow-up examination after purely minimally invasive posterior stabilization of thoracolumbar fractures: a comparison of minimally invasive percutaneously and conventionally open treated patients. Arch Orthop Trauma Surg 2007;127:335–343
14. Verlaan JJ, Diekerhof CH, Buskens E, et al. Surgical treatment of traumatic fractures of the thoracic and lumbar spine: a systematic review of the literature on techniques, complications, and outcome. Spine 2004;29:803–814
15. Rechtine GR, Bono PL, Cahill D, Bolesta MJ, Chrin AM. Postoperative wound infection after instrumentation of thoracic and lumbar fractures. J Orthop Trauma 2001;15:566–569
16. Kawaguchi Y, Matsui H, Tsuji H. Back muscle injury after posterior lumbar spine surgery, II: Histologic and histochemical analyses in humans. Spine 1994;19:2598–2602
17. Kawaguchi Y, Yabuki S, Styf J, et al. Back muscle injury after posterior lumbar spine surgery: topographic evaluation of intramuscular pressure and blood flow in the porcine back muscle during surgery. Spine 1996;21:2683–2688
18. Lu K, Liang CL, Cho CL, et al. Oxidative stress and heat shock protein response in human paraspinal muscles during retraction. J Neurosurg 2002;97(1, Suppl):75–81
19. Suwa H, Hanakita J, Ohshita N, Gotoh K, Matsuoka N, Morizane A. Postoperative changes in paraspinal muscle thickness after various lumbar back surgery procedures. Neurol Med Chir (Tokyo) 2000;40:151–154, discussion 154–155
20. Weber BR, Grob D, Dvorák J, Müntener M. Posterior surgical approach to the lumbar spine and its effect on the multifidus muscle. Spine 1997;22:1765–1772
21. Zeiller SC, Baron EM, Hilibrand AS, of the Spine et al. Thoracolumbar fractures: classification and management. In: Jallo JI, Vaccaro AR, eds. Neurosurgical Trauma and Critical Care of the Spine. New York: Thieme; 2009;143–157.
22. Lowery GL, Kulkarni SS. Posterior percutaneous spine instrumentation. Eur Spine J 2000;9(Suppl 1):S126–S130
23. Ringel F, Stoffel M, Stüer C, Meyer B. Minimally invasive transmuscular pedicle screw fixation of the thoracic and lumbar spine. Neurosurgery 2006;59(4, Suppl 2):ONS361–ONS366, discussion ONS366–ONS367
24. Schizas C, Michel J, Kosmopoulos V, Theumann N. Computer tomography assessment of pedicle screw insertion in percutaneous posterior transpedicular stabilization. Eur Spine J 2007;16:613–617
25. Acosta FL Jr, Thompson TL, Campbell S, Weinstein PR, Ames CP. Use of intraoperative isocentric C-arm 3D fluoroscopy for sextant percutaneous pedicle screw placement: case report and review of the literature. Spine J 2005;5:339–343
26. Holly LT, Foley KT. Three-dimensional fluoroscopy-guided percutaneous thoracolumbar pedicle screw placement: technical note. J Neurosurg 2003;99(3, Suppl):324–329
27. Fisher CG, Wood KB. Introduction to and techniques of evidence-based medicine. Spine 2007;32(19, Suppl):S66–S72
28. Atkins D, Best D, Briss PA, et al; GRADE Working Group. Grading quality of evidence and strength of recommendations. BMJ 2004;328:1490
29. Magerl F. External skeletal fixation of the lower thoracic and lumbar spine. In: Uhtoff HK, Stahl E, eds. Current Consents of External Fixation of Fractures. Berlin: Springer Verlag; 1982:353–356
30. Schizas C, Kosmopoulos V. Percutaneous surgical treatment of chance fractures using cannulated pedicle screws: report of two cases. J Neurosurg Spine 2007;7:71–74
31. Assaker R. The Use of Minimal Access Spinal Techniques for the Management of Thoracolumbar Trauma. Barcelona: Eurospine; 2005
32. Korovessis P, Hadjipavlou A, Repantis T. Minimal invasive short posterior instrumentation plus balloon kyphoplasty with calcium phosphate for burst and severe compression lumbar fractures. Spine 2008;33:658–667
33. Wang MY, Prusmack CJ, Green BA, Gruen JP, Levi AD. Minimally invasive lateral mass screws in the treatment of cervical facet dislocations: technical note. Neurosurgery 2003;52:444–447, discussion 447–448
34. Fong S, Duplessis S. Minimally invasive lateral mass plating in the treatment of posterior cervical trauma: surgical technique. J Spinal Disord Tech 2005;18:224–228
35. Sehati N, Khoo LT. Minimally invasive posterior cervical arthrodesis and fixation. Neurosurg Clin N Am 2006;17:429–440

53

Promising Preclinical Regeneration and Repair Strategies for Spinal Cord Injury

James W. Rowland, Gregory W. J. Hawryluk, Brian K. Kwon, and Michael G. Fehlings

Acute traumatic spinal cord injury (SCI) is a devastating condition for which no satisfactory treatments exist. The neurological deficits resulting from traumatic SCI are the cumulative effect of the direct severing of axons, the immediate and delayed death of spinal cord cells, the dysfunction of remaining spared axons, and a failure of regenerative growth due to the growth inhibitory nature of the injured central nervous system (CNS). The anatomical level and extent of the injury combine to determine the resulting deficits. Although highly complex, this multifaceted pathology offers several potential therapeutic targets for which to tailor therapies that may promote functional recovery following SCI. Therapeutic approaches under development for the treatment of SCI can be divided into four categories based on the intended mechanism of action and the postinjury time frame of the intervention: (1) acute neuroprotective approaches to minimize secondary damage, (2) axonal regenerative approaches to induce regeneration and/or sprouting, (3) pharmacological or cell transplantation approaches to improve signal transmission across the injury site (the latter via remyelination), and (4) rehabilitation approaches to promote plasticity. Although these approaches are conceptually distinct, many therapies will invoke more than one approach (e.g., a treatment intended to induce axonal regeneration/sprouting may also promote some neuroprotection if administered early after injury). Because of the complexity of SCI pathophysiology and pathology, combinatorial therapeutic strategies that include as many of these approaches as possible are likely to be the most effective.

This chapter discusses important recently emerging concepts and preclinical advances in regeneration and repair strategies to enhance functional recovery following SCI that have shown promise for clinical translation (**Table 53.1**). The discussion centers on therapies to overcome the inhibitory nature of the injured spinal cord to enhance axonal regeneration, and cell-based therapies to promote regeneration and remyelination of injured spinal cord axons. Emerging immunomodulatory approaches, recently developed bioengineered strategies, and neuroprotective strategies warranting further investigation are also addressed. Prior to a discussion of newly emerging treatments we will first highlight some fundamental elements of SCI pathophysiology, which are important for a thorough understanding of regenerative approaches for SCI.

◆ Fundamentals of Spinal Cord Injury Pathophysiology

The most common form of SCI is a compressive-contusive type injury in which displaced elements of the vertebral column, including intervertebral disks and ligaments, exert injurious force on the cord causing both immediate traumatic injury and often-prolonged compression. Mechanisms of primary injury include shearing, laceration, acute stretching due to iatrogenic vertebral distraction and sudden acceleration-deceleration injuries.[1] The primary injury is followed by a protracted secondary injury phase involving vascular dysfunction, edema, ischemia, excitotoxicity, electrolyte shifts, free-radical production, inflammation, and delayed apoptotic cell death that expands the region of injury. These events of the secondary injury process can be temporally divided into multiple contiguous phases: the immediate, acute, intermediate, and chronic stages of SCI (**Table 53.2**). Following SCI, the mammalian CNS fails to adequately regenerate due to intrinsic inhibitory factors expressed on central myelin and the extracellular matrix of the posttraumatic gliotic scar. It is of great import that primary injury mechanisms rarely fully disrupt the continuity of the cord. Axons are commonly found to traverse the lesion site often as a subpial rim of spared white matter; which is a consistent finding in human cases and contusive animal models of SCI.[2-8] The existence of these spared axons traversing the injury site is highly encouraging because substantial neurological function has been observed in animal studies with the preservation of as few as 5% of the original number of axons,[8,9] and plantar flexion was noted in a patient with ~8% of the lateral corticospinal tract fibers spared below the injury site.[8]

An important consideration for understanding the pathophysiology of human SCI is that each injury is unique in cause

Table 53.1 Promising Therapeutic Approaches to Promote Regeneration and Repair of the Injured Spinal Cord

1. Acute Neuroprotection

   - Antiapoptotic therapies (soluble FAS ligand)

   - Sodium channel blockers (riluzole)

   - Anti-inflammatory approaches (minocycline, anti-CD11d monoclonal Ab)

   - Erythropoietin

   - Hypothermia

2. Enhancing Regeneration and Plasticity

   - Anti-Nogo antibodies

   - Inhibition of Rho/ROCK pathway

   - Breakdown of gliotic scar (anti-CSPG, chondroitinase ABC)

   - Bioengineered strategies

   - Oscillating electrical fields

3. Pharmacological Approaches to Enhance Axonal Conduction

   - Potassium channel blockers (4-aminopyridine)

   - Sodium/potassium channel blockade (HP 184)

4. Cell-Based Repair Strategies

   - Schwann cells

   - Adult neural stem cells (oligodendrocyte progenitor cells)

   - Embryonic stem cell–derived oligodendrocyte progenitor cells

   - Bone marrow stromal cells

   - Activated macrophages

5. Rehabilitative Approaches

   - Weight-assisted walking

   - Functional electrical stimulation

   - Activation of latent circuitry (central pattern generators)

Abbreviation: CSPG, chondroitin sulfate proteoglycan.

and resultant damage. The stark contrast between the highly heterogeneous SCI population and the homogeneity of rodent experimental SCI models likely contributes to the difficulty in the clinical translation of treatments that show efficacy in preclinical studies. A detailed knowledge of the many factors and processes underlying SCI pathogenesis and how these elements interact is crucial to the development of novel strategies to promote regeneration and repair of the injured spinal cord.

◆ Emerging Concepts in Neuroprotection

An incredible number of compounds have undergone preclinical evaluation for neuroprotective properties for SCI with many reported to possess at least limited efficacy. While a discussion of the vast array of compounds showing therapeutic promise is beyond the scope of this chapter here we discuss two approaches that have recently garnered attention from both clinicians and basic scientists for their strong potential for clinical translation.

Hypothermia

Although reports of the practice of therapeutic hypothermia have existed since 1938 and hypothermia is known to be modestly protective in cardiac arrest and global cerebral ischemia and in reducing paralysis caused by thoracoabdominal aortic aneurysm surgery the approach has garnered much recent attention as a potential highly efficacious treatment for acute traumatic SCI.[10] The rationale behind the induction of hypothermia is simply that the reduction in temperature slows the overall rate of enzymatic and biochemical reactions, therefore reducing cellular energy demands, preserving adenosine triphosphate (ATP) concentrations, and thus reducing damage associated with cellular energy failure as seen following SCI.[11,12] As a whole, human and experimental

Table 53.2 Spinal Cord Injury Phases and Key Pathological Events

SCI Phase	Time(post-SCI)	Key Processes/Events
1. Immediate	0 ≤ 2 hours	- Primary mechanical injury - Traumatic severing of axons - Gray matter hemorrhage with central hemorrhagic necrosis - Initiation of microglial activation - Released factors: IL-1β, TNFα, IL-6, etc.
2. Acute		Systemic events: systemic shock, spinal shock, hypotension, hypoxia
2.1 Early acute	2 ≤ 48 hours	- Vasogenic and cytotoxic edema - ROS production, lipid peroxidation - Glutamate-mediated excitotoxicity - Continuing hemorrhage and necrosis - Neutrophil invasion - Peak of BBB permeability - Early demyelination (oligodendrocyte death) - Death of neurons (necrotic and possibly apoptotic) - Axonal swelling
2.2 Subacute	2 ≤ 14 days	- Macrophage infiltration - Initiation of astrocytic scar formation (reactive astrocytosis) - BBB repair and resolution of edema
3. Intermediate	2 weeks ≤ 6 months	- Continuing scar formation - Cyst formation - Lesion stabilization
4. Chronic/late	≥ 6 months	- Prolonged Wallerian degeneration - Persistence of spared, demyelinated axons - Potential structural and functional plasticity of spared spinal cord tissue

Abbreviations: BBB, blood–brain barrier; IL, interleukin; ROS, reactive oxygen species; TNF, tumor necrosis factor.

animal results have been mixed and largely negative[10,13]; however, promising recent findings in rodent SCI justify optimism for hypothermia-mediated neuroprotection. Recent findings have shown that hypothermia reduces cell death following injury[14,15] and can improve locomotor recovery,[15] although other recent reports have found no neuroprotective effects on the histological or functional level.[16] While clearly the true therapeutic potential of hypothermia for SCI remains to be determined, the accumulated experience and the relative simplicity of the intervention (especially relative to cell-based approaches) warrant further evaluation of hypothermia as a promising neuroprotective approach for SCI. Some important questions to be addressed are the use of systemic versus local cooling and the minimization of potential complications of hypothermia, which in general become prevalent when temperature is reduced below 30°C, including cardiac arrhythmias, hypotension, coagulopathies, systemic infections, and electrolyte disturbances.[11]

Erythropoietin

Erythropoietin (EPO) is a glycoprotein hormone that regulates the production of red blood cells from erythroid progenitor cells contained in bone marrow. In addition to this classic role EPO is now recognized as a potentially neuroprotective agent for SCI that has been shown to protect neurons from hypoxic and ischemic injury, reduce cell death, and improve functional recovery following SCI in the rat.[17,18] The use of EPO as a neuroprotective agent is complicated by its erythrogenic effects; it has been shown that increased hematocrit resulting from overexpression of EPO can exacerbate damage following CNS injury.[19] To address this shortcoming several groups have developed EPO derivatives that maintain the neuroprotective properties while lacking the ability to interact with the EPO receptor mediating the hematopoietic effects.[17,18] These compounds show great promise for clinical translation because the use of recombinant human EPO is routine for various hematopoietic disorders and has been shown to be safe and modestly efficacious in a phase I trial in ischemic stroke.[20]

◆ Immunomodulatory Strategies

The field of neuroinflammation following SCI has attracted immense interest in recent years, and this growing body of work has called into question the classical notion that all inflammation in the CNS is pathological. What has emerged from this work is a process of tremendous complexity, with some aspects of the inflammatory response contributing deleteriously to further secondary injury, whereas others contribute beneficially to the removal of cellular debris and enhance regenerative growth. The inflammatory process following SCI involves numerous cell populations (astrocytes, microglia, lymphocytes, neutrophils, and invading monocytes) and a multitude of inflammatory signaling molecules such as tumor necrosis factor α (TNFα), interferons, arachidonate, and interleukins.[21-23] The dichotomous nature of the immune response following injury is well illustrated by the multiple roles demonstrated for TNFα following CNS injury. TNFα is a key inflammatory mediator for which expression has been shown to increase in neurons, glia, and endothelial cells following SCI.[24] Interestingly, the interference of TNFα

signaling using neutralizing antibodies has been shown to enhance recovery following SCI,[25] whereas TNFα itself has been demonstrated to possess a neuroprotective role both in vitro[26] and following SCI in TNFα deficient mice.[27] These conflicting effects exemplify the need for further characterization of the inflammatory response and a better delineation of the deleterious and beneficial aspects.

A well-known example of the therapeutic potential of immunomodulatory therapy following SCI is the widespread use and modest therapeutic benefit of the glucocorticoid methylprednisolone (MP)[28] (see Chapter 56). MP is a potent immunosuppressant demonstrated to reduce several deleterious inflammatory mediators after SCI.[29-32] The balance of safety and efficacy of MP has been questioned,[33] and the current understanding that inflammation is at least partially beneficial in promoting recovery further challenges the use of agents that globally suppress the immune response.[21]

In response to the understanding of the negative effects of profound suppression of the immune response efforts have been made to more specifically target aspects of the inflammatory response following SCI known to be deleterious. Neutrophil invasion into the spinal cord begins immediately following SCI[23] and is widely accepted as a cytotoxic component of the immune response. The invasion of neutrophils into the spinal cord parenchyma following SCI requires extravasation involving the interaction of vascular cell adhesion molecules (VCAMs) on endothelial cells and specific integrins expressed by neutrophils and other leukocytes.[34] One integrin known to function in neutrophil recruitment following injury is CD11d/CD18, the function of which can be selectively blocked using specific monoclonal antibodies raised against it.[35] This approach has been developed by Weaver and colleagues and after experimental SCI in the rat has been demonstrated to markedly decrease the infiltration of neutrophils, delay the invasion of bloodborne monocytes, increase locomotor performance, enhance functional recovery, and decrease the occurrence of neuropathic pain and autonomic dysreflexia; two particularly important therapeutic goals to improve the quality of life in SCI patients.[36-38] Therefore the selective blockade of CD11d/CD18 is a highly promising emerging approach to reduce secondary injury mechanisms following SCI and a strong candidate for future combinatorial approaches.

Another immune-based or immunomodulatory approach that has shown efficacy in experimental SCI and promise for clinical translation is use of the tetracycline derivative minocycline. Minocycline is known to inhibit the activation of microglia, which has been demonstrated to be neuroprotective in rodent SCI[39,40] and may reduce neuropathic pain.[41] In addition to inhibiting the microglial response minocycline is also thought to block the release of cytochrome C from mitochondria,[39] an important initiator of apoptotic cell death post-SCI.

Although the foregoing immune-based strategies addressed deleterious components of the immune response, it has been shown that one potentially beneficial component of neuroinflammation are autoreactive T cells in a process that has been termed protective autoimmunity.[42] T cells reactive to myelin antigens may be neuroprotective and actually promote functional recovery following SCI.[43] This has formed the basis for the use of therapeutic vaccines of myelin antigens as an SCI therapy. Although preclinical data have been promising,[44,45] the risks of intentionally generating autoreactive T cells are significant, and these approaches require further development and safety testing prior to being considered for clinical translation.

A third immune-based strategy that has shown promise is the transplantation of activated autologous macrophages.[46,47] This approach was first hypothesized as potentially therapeutic based on the assumption that a lack of robust phagocytosis of cellular debris, especially myelin debris, by macrophages following CNS injury was responsible for the lack of repair relative to that seen in the PNS. Based on this theory, Schwartz and colleagues have used bloodborne monocytes, preactivated by incubation with segments of peripheral nerve explants (after which they are referred to as macrophages) to provide neuroprotection and enhance recovery following SCI.[46–49] This had begun undergoing commercialization and evaluation under the name PROCORD, although ongoing trials were halted due to financial issues (see Chapter 56).

◆ Emerging Concepts in Axonal Regeneration and Repair Strategies

It has been well established that the failure of axonal regeneration within the CNS is the result of both the growth inhibitory nature of the mammalian CNS and a relatively low intrinsic regenerative competence of CNS neurons.[50,51] The intrinsic capacity of CNS axons to regenerate over long distances after axotomy was first demonstrated through the pioneering work of David and Aguayo and colleagues in the 1980s, in which injured CNS axons were found to regenerate through growth-permissive peripheral nerve grafts.[52–54] The therapeutic potential of these findings for SCI was confirmed with Cheng et al's seminal (albeit difficult to reproduce) demonstration in 1996 that such peripheral nerve transplantation into a spinal cord transection model could promote hind-limb recovery.[55] Much optimism has followed that such "bridging" strategies will prove to be fruitful for patients with SCIs, although to date the functional improvements achieved in experimental models remain modest at best.

Recognizing that there are two aspects to regenerative failure after CNS injury—the limited intrinsic regenerative potential and the inhibitory extrinsic environment of the injured CNS—great efforts have been made to characterize both obstacles to regeneration. On the intrinsic side, a substantial amount of work has been done to characterize the molecular signals that are required to stimulate axonal growth; signals that are clearly more strongly expressed and successfully acted upon in the peripheral nervous system (PNS) following injury relative to the CNS.[50] Although several regeneration- and growth-associated genes have been identified to be upregulated after CNS axonal injury, such as *L1*, *c-fos*, *c-jun*, and the 43kDa growth-associated protein GAP43,[56,57] the degree and extent of their expression is insufficient to promote a strong regenerative response (in contrast to axotomized PNS neurons). On the extrinsic side, it is now well accepted that multiple inhibitory molecules exist that make the injured CNS a non-permissive environment for axonal growth. These molecules can be divided into inhibitors associated with CNS myelin and those associated with the extracellular matrix of the astrocytic scar.

Myelin-Associated Inhibitors

The growth inhibitory nature of central myelin was first documented in vitro by Schwab and Thoenen through their demonstration that cultured sympathetic neurons would extend neurites on PNS but not CNS myelin.[58] Based on this proof-of-concept experiment subsequent investigators identified many components of CNS myelin that are inhibitors of axonal growth, including Nogo,[59] myelin-associated glycoprotein,[60,61] oligodendrocyte-myelin glycoprotein (OMgp),[62] semaphorin 4D (Sema4D),[63] Ephrin B3,[64] and repulsive guidance molecule (RGMa).[65] Following the discovery of the Nogo receptor (NgR) by Strittmater and coworkers[66] it was demonstrated that in addition to Nogo, other myelin-associated inhibitors (MAG and OMgp) also functioned through the NgR, making the receptor an important convergence point for multiple inhibitory signals. The Nogo receptor, which lacks an intracellular signaling domain, transduces inhibitory signals by forming co-receptor complexes with tumor necrosis factor receptor family proteins such as p75,[67] TROY,[68] or LINGO-1.[69] Significant efforts are under way to elucidate the downstream signaling pathways that are activated by NgR, with RhoA and the effector kinase RhoA-associated kinase (ROCK) being identified as important intracellular mediators.[70] These in turn regulate further downstream factors, such as Lim kinase and the actin-binding protein cofilin, modifying the actin cytoskeleton, and leading to growth cone stabilization or collapse in regenerating axons.[71]

A therapeutic approach that has been developed from this line of research into myelin inhibitors has been the use of anti-Nogo antibodies. This work began over 2 decades ago with the development of the IN-1 monoclonal antibody, which was directed against two known myelin-associated neurite outgrowth inhibitors, NI-250 and NI-35.[72] The administration of this antibody in a rat model of SCI (dorsal column transection) was found to promote axonal regeneration after spinal cord injury[73] and subsequently demonstrated to promote functional recovery.[74] An enormous body of work from Schwab and colleagues has been dedicated to the development of this antibody approach, which, after the cloning of Nogo as the antigen for IN-1 in 2000,[59] has led to the generation of anti-Nogo antibodies as a highly directed therapy against this myelin inhibitor. In primate studies of cervical SCI this antibody was reported to promote sprouting and functional recovery.[75,76] The anti-Nogo antibody treatment strategy has been commercialized by Novartis, and is now undergoing early human evaluation in Europe and Canada (see Chapter 56).

Glial Scar–Associated Inhibitors

The glial scar is composed of reactive astrocytes that express several growth inhibitory extracellular matrix components known as chondroitin sulfate proteoglycans (CSPGs).[77] CSPGs include the molecules neurocan, versican, aggrecan, brevican, phosphacan, and NG2. They consist of a core protein to which sulphated glycosaminoglycan side chains are covalently linked.[78] Theses GAG side chains are the main source of inhibition by CSPGs and it has been postulated that in addition to this "chemical" inhibition that the protein core functions as a physical barrier to axon growth due to high affinity interaction with other ECM components such as laminin, fibronectin, and NCAMs.[79] The most promising therapeutic strategy for overcoming the gliotic barrier is by direct degradation of the CSPGs with chondroitinase ABC (ChABC), a bacterial enzyme that cleaves the GAG side chains. This approach has been evaluated in numerous in vivo animal models of SCI, although rather infrequently in the most clinically relevant contusion models, in which sprouting or regeneration is much more difficult to anatomically assess, relative to more straightforward transection models. Nonetheless, numerous investigators have reported increased sprouting and improved behavioral recovery with ChABC.[80–84] The possibility of making the CNS environment more permissive to axonal growth has encouraged numerous investigators to utilize ChABC in combination with other therapies such as fetal tissue transplant,[85] peripheral nerve transplant,[86] neural precursor cells,[87] and Schwann cells.[88] The results of further studies using ChABC are eagerly awaited.

Recent work by Shen et al[147] has demonstrated that the inhibitory signally of CSPGs on axonal growth is at least partially mediated through a transmembrane protein tyrosine phosphatase known as PTPσ which is the first CSPG receptor to be identified.[79] Therapies targeting PTPσ have yet to be developed although they represent an exciting new method to enhance regeneration following SCI. In addition to the role of the recently discovered PTPσ receptor, the inhibitory interaction between axons and CSPGs is also known to be mediated by the Rho/ROCK signalling pathway.[89] Therefore the targeting of Rho/ROCK and its downstream mediators is a therapeutic aim that has garnered intense interest in the hopes of permitting regenerating axons to overcome glial scar and myelin associated inhibition.

Targeting the Rho/ROCK Pathway

As already mentioned, the discovery of the Nogo receptor was subsequently followed by the surprising finding it was the target for not just Nogo but also MAG and OMgp. Given that the Rho/ROCK pathway is an important downstream signaling mechanism of the Nogo receptor, it represents an important point of convergence for multiple inhibitory signals and a highly attractive, potentially efficient target for therapies (**Fig. 53.1**). This strategy was explored by McKerracher and colleagues, who utilized the C3 enzyme from *Clostridium botulinum*—which selectively inactivates Rho via ADP-ribosylation without affecting Rac and Cdc42—to show that Rho inactivation could promote CNS regeneration in an optic nerve injury model.[90] They subsequently demonstrated that Rho/ROCK inhibition promoted axonal sprouting and improved locomotor function in a mouse model of sharp incomplete thoracic transection SCI (dorsal overhemisection).[91] Initially a confounding result, the rapid behavioral recovery in these animals (within days) indicated that it could not possibly be mediated by axonal regeneration or sprouting. Further work identified a role for activated Rho in apoptosis after SCI, with Rho inhibition suppressing this important aspect of secondary injury.[92] The findings from these two papers were utilized to commercialize a C3-like enzyme with improved permeability characteristics under the name *Cethrin*, and under sponsorship from Bioaxone Therapeutique Inc. (Montreal, Quebec). This has been evaluated in a phase I/IIa open-label human clinical study (see Chapter 56).

◆ Cell-Based Regeneration and Repair Strategies

Cell-based therapies to repair the injured spinal cord are showing increasing promise. A surprisingly diverse range of cell types are currently under investigation as potential treatment strategies for SCI. The scientific premise behind the use of these cells is based upon two central concepts: (1) to directly replace cells lost due to injury (notably oligodendrocytes), and (2) to influence the environment in such a way as to either support axonal regeneration, provide neuroprotection, or both. Neurons and oligodendrocytes represent the cell types that succumb to necrotic and apoptotic death after injury, and various cell substrates (e.g., stem cells, progenitor cells, Schwann cells) offer the potential of repopulating the damaged cord. The potential of these cells to remyelinate demyelinated axons around the injury site has sparked great interest. Additionally, such cells may inherently express several supportive growth cues, such as neurotrophic factors, or can potentially be genetically engineered to do so.

It is important to consider the basic requirements to successfully translate cell-based therapies for SCI into the clinical setting. Stem cells provide a good starting point; the ability of

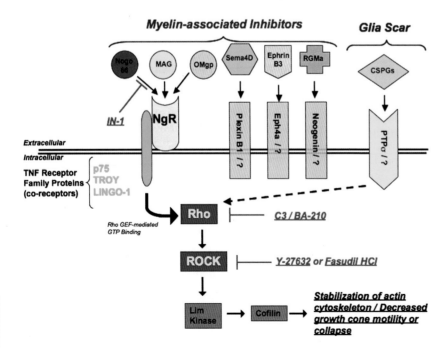

Fig. 53.1 Glial inhibitors of axonal growth after spinal cord injury. All known myelin inhibitors appear to activate the GTPase Rho, which leads to growth cone collapse. Signaling via NgR has been established for the Nogo-66 moiety, MAG, and OMgp. It is less certain how other known inhibitors signal (in order) to activate Rho (dashed line). Several aspects of this pathway have been targeted in experimental therapeutic strategies. IN-1 is a monoclonal antibody that inactivates Nogo. Numerous variations of the Clostridium botulinum C3 protein have been designed, including BA-210 (employed in Cethrin), which inactivates Rho by ADP-ribosylating its active site. Y-27632 and Fasudil hydrochloride are known inhibitors of ROCK. Abbreviations: CSPGs, chondroitin sulfate proteoglycans; MAG, myelin-associated glycoprotein; NgR, Nogo receptor; OMgp, oligodendrocyte-myelin glycoprotein; Sema4D, semaphorin 4D; RGMa, repulsive guidance molecule; PTPσ, protein tyrosine phosphatase σ; ROCK, Rho kinase; Ab, antibody.

these cells to differentiate into neurons, oligodendrocytes, or astrocytes in vitro has captured the imagination of many that transplanted cells can be used to replace cell populations lost following SCI. However, for such a cellular substrate to succeed, it must survive following the transplant, differentiate (if not already differentiated) into the correct lineage, integrate into the cord tissue, migrate appropriately, and then, finally, physiologically behave in the manner intended. Considering that the ideal conditions for cell survival, differentiation, and function that can be generated in vitro will be difficult (if not impossible) to duplicate in vivo within the chronically or subacutely injured spinal cord, there is good reason for the optimism surrounding cell transplantation to be tempered by the realization of the many obstacles that remain to be overcome. Additionally, many questions remain unresolved regarding the application of this technology, including—on a cell-specific basis—the definition of the optimal time postinjury to perform such a transplant, the patient population most appropriate for the therapy, the techniques required for implanting them, and the methods for tracking the fate of the cells in situ posttransplantation.

Given this perspective, two of the most realistically attainable therapeutic goals for cell-based therapy are to promote improved axonal function by remyelinating residual axons and to promote enhanced survival and possibly plasticity of surviving neurons.

◆ Cell-Based Remyelination Strategies

The transplantation of glia or their progenitors from several distinct sources has shown strong potential for remyelinating demyelinated axons and improving behavioral recovery in animal models of SCI. Here we describe cellular substrates that have been used in SCI research ostensibly for their ability to remyelinate.

Schwann Cells

Schwann cells (SCs) are the myelinating glia of the PNS. The work of David and Aguayo using peripheral nerve grafts provided strong evidence that Schwann cells could support axonal regeneration of CNS neurons after SCI.[52,53] The use of intact peripheral nerve segments as bridges to facilitate axonal regeneration within the injured spinal cord has continued,[55,93] and has been now described in a case report of a chronic paraplegic patient.[94]

The use of Schwann cells for transplantation has been a focus of research for Bunge and colleagues at the Miami Project to Cure Paralysis. They have shown using a rat contusive SCI model that SC transplantation results in enhanced axonal regeneration and remyelination by transplanted cells that was associated with a statistically significant, though very small improvement in hindlimb function.[95] SCs are an attractive cellular candidate because they can be harvested from peripheral nerves (e.g., the sural nerve), expanded in vitro, then transplanted in an autologous fashion. Although SC transplants do enhance remyelination and appear to support regenerative axon growth,[96–98] axons do not extend beyond the permissive environment of SC grafts and reenter the host CNS. The relatively modest regenerative and neurobehavioral effects of Schwann cell–based repair strategies need to be carefully evaluated when considering their potential for clinical translation.

A novel source of SC has been identified with the recent discovery and isolation of so-called skin-derived precursor cells (SKPs)—multipotent stem cells that have been derived from the dermis of adult mice[99] and humans.[100] SKPs can be differentiated in vitro to produce myelinating SCs, which have been shown to remyelinate axons and promote modest functional recovery following SCI in the rat.[101] Although these cells offer the advantage of harvesting transplantable cells from a simple skin biopsy, it has yet to be determined if they will offer a therapeutic advantage over SCs derived from peripheral nerves.

Olfactory Ensheathing Cells

Olfactory ensheathing cells (OECs) are a specialized form of glial cell found only in the olfactory system. OECs are unique in their capacity to facilitate the passage of new axons from regenerating olfactory receptor neurons[102] (which reside in the peripheral nervous system) up to a mitral/tufted cell target neuron within the olfactory bulb (CNS). This ability to seemingly escort axons across the "PNS to CNS barrier" made OECs extremely attractive as a potential transplantation substrate in cord injuries, recognizing that despite the propensity of CNS axons to grow *into* Schwann cell grafts (a PNS environment), it was difficult to get them to *exit* and reenter the hostile CNS environment.

Cotransplantation experiments with Schwann cells housed within guidance-channels and OECs at either end revealed that the OECs could indeed facilitate enhanced regeneration of axons back into the spinal cord.[103] This was followed by the reporting of axonal regeneration and functional recovery in a full transection SCI model after OEC transplantation.[104] Interest in these cells has since exploded. Almost a decade of further work has curtailed the enthusiasm surrounding these cells to some extent, as it has become evident that some of the regeneration observed in OEC transplantation experiments may in fact be attributable to invading Schwann cells and/or Schwann cell contamination of OEC cultures.[105] On the issue of myelination, under certain in vitro conditions, OECs (which do not normally myelinate in vivo) have been shown to be capable of myelinating axons.[106] However, the ability of the OEC to myelinate in vivo after transplantation into the injured spinal cord remains the subject of controversy.[105] Whether they remyelinate in vivo or not, it appears that OECs are capable of creating an environment that is permissive for axonal growth, secreting factors which may be neuroprotective, modifying the glial scar through their interaction with astrocytes, and promoting angiogenesis.[107,108] There is a significant body of experience surrounding the use of OEC transplantation in human SCI patients that is discussed in Chapter 56. Based on a lack of any credible demonstration of clinical efficacy to date, well-controlled research studies are required to assess any potential beneficial benefits OEC therapy.[109]

Neural Stem Cells and Glial Progenitors

Neural stem cells (NSCs) are self-renewing, multipotential cells that are capable of producing all three mature neural cell types. Progenitor cells have a limited capacity for self-renewal and typically are unipotent, producing only one mature cell type. This distinction is an important one and use of the term *stem cell* has become confusing as it is often employed to refer to any proliferating, immature cell type in the CNS or other tissue.[110] A detailed discussion of the characterization and definition of specific populations of stem and progenitor cells with therapeutic potential for SCI is beyond the scope of this chapter. However, it is important to recognize that relevant biological differences may exist between seemingly interchangeable cell or stem cell populations derived from embryonic or adult sources, or using different culture conditions. The diversity of potential sources of NSCs is impressive. NSCs or their progeny with the ability to survive and differentiate into mature, myelinating oligodendrocytes when transplanted in vivo have been derived from the embryonic CNS of rodents,[111] the postnatal and the adult CNS of mice,[112,113] rats,[114,115] and humans.[116] More importantly for developing therapies, NSCs and committed OPCs have been produced from both murine[117,118] and human embryonic stem (ES) cells.[119-122]

Embryonic Stem Cell-derived NPCs and OPCs

Embryonic stem (ES) cells are pluripotent, self-renewing cells derived from the inner cell mass of blastocyst stage embryos. These were first derived from murine embryos[123,124] and have subsequently been produced from human embryos.[125] Due to their pluripotency, ES cells require *in vitro* pre-differentiation to commit ES cells to a neural or glial fate prior to transplantation. Undifferentiated ES cells or those that are not fully committed to the neural lineage have the ability to form teratomas/heterotomas following transplantation.[126] Over the past decade, significant advances have been made in the ability to preferentially drive ES differentiation into neural and specifically oligodendroglial lineages. First achieved using the murine ES cells, the induction of an oligodendroglial fate in ES followed by transplantation into the dysmyelinated spinal cords of *shiverer* mice demonstrated the great potential of these myelinogenic cells.[119] The recent development of methods to induce an ES cell-like pluripotent state in adult somatic cells such as skin fibroblasts[148-150] has revolutionized the stem cell biology field and created the potential for the production of patient specific pluripotent stem cells from which neural cells—and all other cell types—could be derived. These cell have been termed induced pluripotent stem cells (iPS cells) and work to date has indicated that iPS cells behave very similarly to bona fide ES cells in their response to differentiation protocols and show no epigenetic abnormalities suggesting that they should not pose any significant safety risks above those of normal ES cells.[150,152] They also obviate ethical concerns associated with the use of human embryos for production of ES cell lines. iPS cell-derived neural cells will likely replace ES-cell derived cells for all cell-based therapies for SCI and other diseases where cell-based approaches show promise. Currently, an oligodendrocyte progenitor derived from human ES cells is being considered for human clinical trials, based on the work of Kierstad et al[120,127] and developed by the Geron Corporation (Menlo Park, California)(See chapter 56).

Adult-Derived Neural Stem Cells

The discovery of self-renewing "neural stem cells" in the adult mammalian brain and spinal cord by Reynolds and Weiss[128,129] was a landmark finding, which drastically modified our view of the once-believed static adult CNS. Following their discovery these cells were quickly identified as potential candidates to promote repair of the injured CNS. Self-renewing neural stem/progenitor cells (NPCs) can be isolated

from the subventricular zone throughout the neuroaxis.[130] Recent work by our group has demonstrated the potential efficacy of adult neural stem/progenitor cells (NPCs) derived from the subventricular zone of the forebrain to remyelinate axons and promote functional recovery following contusive SCI in the rat.[112] To more directly assess the correlation between NPC-mediated remyelination and improved axonal conduction we investigated the effect of NPC transplantation on the conduction properties of the spinal cord of the congenitally dysmyelinated *shiverer* mouse and found that remyelinated transplanted spinal cords did have improved axonal conduction measured electrophysiologically, which was associated with the reorganization of normal-appearing nodes of Ranvier based on the molecular organization of sodium and potassium channels and nodal protein Caspr.[113]

Limitations of Remyelination Therapies for Spinal Cord Injury

Remyelination strategies are among the most important SCI therapies under development and will likely prove to be the first stem cell–based therapies to undergo clinical trials in North America for any human condition.[127] Although preclinical data in experimental SCI are highly encouraging, scientists, clinicians, and patients must remember that the functional improvement associated with any remyelinating therapy is theoretically limited as a function of the number of spared, demyelinated axons present. As discussed earlier, the extent to which demyelinated axons are present in human SCI is still an unresolved issue. Therefore, within the highly heterogeneous SCI population the efficacy of such treatments is likely to be highly variable based on the specific characteristics of each lesion thus complicating the interpretation of clinical trial data. Furthermore, the timing and precise methodology of such interventions remain to be optimized.

Bone Marrow Stromal and Hematopoietic Stem Cells

Adult mammalian bone marrow contains both hematopoietic stem cells (HSCs) and bone marrow stromal cells (BMSCs), which are also referred to as mesenchymal stem cells. Both of these stem cell populations are unique in that, although they are ostensibly dedicated to the generation of hematopoietic cells such as erythrocytes and lymphocytes (HSCs), and mesenchymal stem cells (MSCs) such as osteocytes and chondrocytes, it has been reported that both can transdifferentiate down neural lineages when exposed to appropriate in vitro or in vivo conditions.[130,131] Of all cell types under investigation the results reported using BMSCs and HSCs are the most inconsistent and poorly understood. The fact that they offer the potential for autologous transplantation makes them appealing cell substrates for SCI repair, and, intriguingly, multiple laboratories have reported that the intravenous administration of HSCs or unsorted bone marrow following rodent SCI results in cells preferentially migrating to the injury site.[132,133] The transplantation of HSCs into the injured spinal cord has been reported to promote functional recovery, although mechanisms underlying the effect remain unclear.[134,135] The transplantation of marrow stromal cells, on the other hand, has been shown in an atraumatic demyelinating spinal cord lesion to induce remyelination.[132] The transplantation of MSCs into models of traumatic SCI has been inconsistently reported to result in some improved behavioral outcomes, although in vivo, differentiation into neural substrates to support remyelination is not particularly convincing.[136,137] The lack of a consistent pattern of differentiation of BMSCs and low cell survival suggests that functional benefits observed are due to more general mechanisms such as the release of growth promoting factors.[134,137]

◆ Bioengineered Strategies

The past decade has seen tremendous advances in biomaterials and many have already made their way into operating rooms. Increasingly, bioengineering approaches are being employed in experimental approaches to repair the injured spinal cord. A basic tenet underlying this approach is that regeneration across a cystic cavity cannot occur; and thus the implantation of a permissive substrate (particularly one that is synthetically designed to optimize the environment for axonal growth) may have some merit. Many approaches have shown promise; however, none as yet appears ready for human translation.

In general, bioengineered materials can be classed as absorbable or nonabsorbable. They can also be classed as gels, tubes, and sponges or scaffolds. They may be designed with specific eluting properties for drug or trophic factor delivery, as a permissive substrate for neural regeneration, a means of increasing surface area for delivery of a cell-replacement therapy, or a means of altering the neural environment to promote repair. Biocompatibility, or the ability to induce minimal immune response, is crucial, as resulting astrogliosis could eliminate the benefits of this approach.

Gels are of great therapeutic interest. Their molecular structures can be readily altered for dynamic and optimal physical properties during storage, administration, and in vivo use. Also of great importance is the ability to control their eluting properties for controlled release of a substance over a desired timeframe (an approach that, of course, assumes that we understand the desired timeframe for an intervention to be applied). An additional important advantage of such a local delivery strategy is the avoidance of systemic side effects. As well, this technology would have important advantages over local infusion pumps currently employed for such targeted administration, which risk neural injury and dislodgment and can require refilling or removal. One such promising polymer is an injectable blend of hyaluronan and methylcellulose (HAMC), with properties ideally suited to intrathecal delivery.[138] This polymer is rapid gelling, nonadhesive, degradable, and biocompatible. It has also demonstrated anti-inflammatory effects that may be responsible for the statistically significant improvement in motor function seen when administered alone for SCI in the rat.[138] This latter property raises the exciting possibility that it may be possible to engineer gels that have a repair-promoting or neuroprotective function on their own.

Synthetic guidance channels have been created in an effort to assist the regeneration of spinal cord axons across the site of an injury, in parallel with efforts in peripheral nerve injury.[139] Such tubes have been examined in cord transection models and may optimize the local environment, perhaps by augmenting or stabilizing guidance cues. It is also clear that employed polymers must resist collapse.[140] Although simple tubes alone have demonstrated benefit,[141] more complex tubes with internal scaffolds, impregnated cells,[142,143] or drug or factor elution may be of greater benefit.[144,145]

Numerous groups have employed scaffolds in an attempt to augment recovery from SCI. Many groups have taken the additional step of impregnating their devices with therapeutic cells.[144,146] Interestingly, Novikova et al demonstrated that this impregnation was critical to regeneration with their device. It also appears that the regeneration induced by these conduits may be tract-specific.[88,144,145] Drug or factor elution appears to alter the effect of such devices. For instance, Tsai et al noted that the addition of FGF-1 increased the axonal regeneration of vestibular neurons, whereas the addition of NT-3 decreased the total number of axons regenerating from brainstem neurons.

◆ Summary

The pathophysiology and pathology of SCI represent formidable challenges to neural repair—challenges that we have obviously not yet overcome, despite considerable research efforts. A more comprehensive understanding of these complex biological processes, particularly in human SCI, will be essential to our development of novel therapies. Efforts to induce regeneration and repair of the injured cord have led to translatable therapies directed at inhibiting myelin inhibitors, targeting intracellular messenger systems that mediate growth cone dynamics, and degrading the glial scar. Additionally, cell transplantation strategies have enormous momentum due to unparalleled scientific and public interest, although arguably many scientific and clinical aspects of a therapeutic transplantation paradigm still require resolution. The limited functional improvements derived from current experimental therapies clearly illustrate the requirement for the development of combinatorial therapies that combine neuroprotective, neuroregenerative, and rehabilitatory strategies in the hope to optimize recovery of individuals with acute traumatic SCI.

References

1. Baptiste DC, Fehlings MG. Pharmacological approaches to repair the injured spinal cord. J Neurotrauma 2006;23:318–334
2. Nashmi R, Fehlings MG. Changes in axonal physiology and morphology after chronic compressive injury of the rat thoracic spinal cord. Neuroscience 2001;104:235–251
3. Radojicic M, Reier PJ, Steward O, Keirstead HS. Septations in chronic spinal cord injury cavities contain axons. Exp Neurol 2005;196:339–341
4. McDonald JW, Belegu V. Demyelination and remyelination after spinal cord injury. J Neurotrauma 2006;23:345–359
5. Totoiu MO, Keirstead HS. Spinal cord injury is accompanied by chronic progressive demyelination. J Comp Neurol 2005;486:373–383
6. Bunge RP, Puckett WR, Becerra JL, Marcillo A, Quencer RM. Observations on the pathology of human spinal cord injury: a review and classification of 22 new cases with details from a case of chronic cord compression with extensive focal demyelination. Adv Neurol 1993;59:75–89
7. Norenberg MD, Smith J, Marcillo A. The pathology of human spinal cord injury: defining the problems. J Neurotrauma 2004;21:429–440
8. Kakulas BA. Neuropathology: the foundation for new treatments in spinal cord injury. Spinal Cord 2004;42:549–563
9. Fehlings MG, Tator CH. The relationships among the severity of spinal cord injury, residual neurological function, axon counts, and counts of retrogradely labeled neurons after experimental spinal cord injury. Exp Neurol 1995;132:220–228
10. Kwon BK, Mann C, Sohn HM, et al. Hypothermia for spinal cord injury. Spine 2008;8:859–874
11. Arrica M, Bissonnette B. Therapeutic hypothermia. Semin Cardiothorac Vasc Anesth 2007;11:6–15
12. Erecinska M, Thoresen M, Silver IA. Effects of hypothermia on energy metabolism in mammalian central nervous system. J Cereb Blood Flow Metab 2003;23:513–530

13. Inamasu J, Nakamura Y, Ichikizaki K. Induced hypothermia in experimental traumatic spinal cord injury: an update. J Neurol Sci 2003;209: 55–60

14. Shibuya S, Miyamoto O, Janjua NA, Itano T, Mori S, Norimatsu H. Post-traumatic moderate systemic hypothermia reduces TUNEL positive cells following spinal cord injury in rat. Spinal Cord 2004;42:29–34

15. Yu CG, Jimenez O, Marcillo AE, et al. Beneficial effects of modest systemic hypothermia on locomotor function and histopathological damage following contusion-induced spinal cord injury in rats. J Neurosurg 2000;93(1, Suppl):85–93

16. Casas CE, Herrera LP, Prusmack C, Ruenes G, Marcillo A, Guest JD. Effects of epidural hypothermic saline infusion on locomotor outcome and tissue preservation after moderate thoracic spinal cord contusion in rats. J Neurosurg Spine 2005;2:308–318

17. Erbayraktar S, Grasso G, Sfacteria A, et al. Asialoerythropoietin is a nonerythropoietic cytokine with broad neuroprotective activity in vivo. Proc Natl Acad Sci U S A 2003;100:6741–6746

18. Leist M, Ghezzi P, Grasso G, et al. Derivatives of erythropoietin that are tissue protective but not erythropoietic. Science 2004;305:239–242

19. Wiessner C, Allegrini PR, Ekatodramis D, Jewell UR, Stallmach T, Gassmann M. Increased cerebral infarct volumes in polyglobulic mice overexpressing erythropoietin. J Cereb Blood Flow Metab 2001;21: 857–864

20. Ehrenreich H, Hasselblatt M, Dembowski C, et al. Erythropoietin therapy for acute stroke is both safe and beneficial. Mol Med 2002;8: 495–505

21. Donnelly DJ, Popovich PG. Inflammation and its role in neuroprotection, axonal regeneration and functional recovery after spinal cord injury. Exp Neurol 2008;209:378–388

22. Popovich PG, Wei P, Stokes BT. Cellular inflammatory response after spinal cord injury in Sprague-Dawley and Lewis rats. J Comp Neurol 1997;377:443–464

23. Fleming JC, Norenberg MD, Ramsay DA, et al. The cellular inflammatory response in human spinal cords after injury. Brain 2006;129(Pt 12): 3249–3269

24. Yan P, Li Q, Kim GM, Xu J, Hsu CY, Xu XM. Cellular localization of tumor necrosis factor-alpha following acute spinal cord injury in adult rats. J Neurotrauma 2001;18:563–568

25. Bethea JR, Nagashima H, Acosta MC, et al. Systemically administered interleukin-10 reduces tumor necrosis factor-alpha production and significantly improves functional recovery following traumatic spinal cord injury in rats. J Neurotrauma 1999;16:851–863

26. Cheng B, Christakos S, Mattson MP. Tumor necrosis factors protect neurons against metabolic-excitotoxic insults and promote maintenance of calcium homeostasis. Neuron 1994;12:139–153

27. Kim GM, Xu J, Xu J, et al. Tumor necrosis factor receptor deletion reduces nuclear factor-kappaB activation, cellular inhibitor of apoptosis protein 2 expression, and functional recovery after traumatic spinal cord injury. J Neurosci 2001;21:6617–6625

28. Bracken MB. Pharmacological treatment of acute spinal cord injury: current status and future prospects. Paraplegia 1992;30:102–107

29. Bartholdi D, Schwab ME. Methylprednisolone inhibits early inflammatory processes but not ischemic cell death after experimental spinal cord lesion in the rat. Brain Res 1995;672:177–186

30. Fu ES, Saporta S. Methylprednisolone inhibits production of interleukin-1beta and interleukin-6 in the spinal cord following compression injury in rats. J Neurosurg Anesthesiol 2005;17:82–85

31. Xu J, Fan G, Chen S, Wu Y, Xu XM, Hsu CY. Methylprednisolone inhibition of TNF-alpha expression and NF-kB activation after spinal cord injury in rats. Brain Res Mol Brain Res 1998;59:135–142

32. Xu J, Kim GM, Ahmed SH, et al. Glucocorticoid receptor-mediated suppression of activator protein-1 activation and matrix metalloproteinase expression after spinal cord injury. J Neurosci 2001;21:92–97

33. Hurlbert RJ. Methylprednisolone for acute spinal cord injury: an inappropriate standard of care. J Neurosurg 2000;93(1, Suppl):1–7

34. Butcher EC, Picker LJ. Lymphocyte homing and homeostasis. Science 1996;272:60–66

35. Mabon PJ, Weaver LC, Dekaban GA. Inhibition of monocyte/macrophage migration to a spinal cord injury site by an antibody to the integrin alphaD: a potential new anti-inflammatory treatment. Exp Neurol 2000;166:52–64

36. Gris D, Marsh DR, Oatway MA, et al. Transient blockade of the CD11d/CD18 integrin reduces secondary damage after spinal cord injury, improving sensory, autonomic, and motor function. J Neurosci 2004;24:4043–4051

37. Ditor DS, Bao F, Chen Y, Dekaban GA, Weaver LC. A therapeutic time window for anti-CD 11d monoclonal antibody treatment yielding reduced secondary tissue damage and enhanced behavioral recovery following severe spinal cord injury. J Neurosurg Spine 2006;5: 343–352

38. Oatway MA, Chen Y, Bruce JC, Dekaban GA, Weaver LC. Anti-CD11d integrin antibody treatment restores normal serotonergic projections to the dorsal, intermediate, and ventral horns of the injured spinal cord. J Neurosci 2005;25:637–647

39. Teng YD, Choi H, Onario RC, et al. Minocycline inhibits contusion-triggered mitochondrial cytochrome c release and mitigates functional deficits after spinal cord injury. Proc Natl Acad Sci U S A 2004;101: 3071–3076

40. Stirling DP, Khodarahmi K, Liu J, et al. Minocycline treatment reduces delayed oligodendrocyte death, attenuates axonal dieback, and improves functional outcome after spinal cord injury. J Neurosci 2004; 24:2182–2190

41. Hains BC, Waxman SG. Activated microglia contribute to the maintenance of chronic pain after spinal cord injury. J Neurosci 2006;26: 4308–4317

42. Schwartz M, Kipnis J. Protective autoimmunity: regulation and prospects for vaccination after brain and spinal cord injuries. Trends Mol Med 2001;7:252–258

43. Schwartz M. Harnessing the immune system for neuroprotection: therapeutic vaccines for acute and chronic neurodegenerative disorders. Cell Mol Neurobiol 2001;21:617–627

44. Hauben E, Butovsky O, Nevo U, et al. Passive or active immunization with myelin basic protein promotes recovery from spinal cord contusion. J Neurosci 2000;20:6421–6430

45. Moalem G, Leibowitz-Amit R, Yoles E, Mor F, Cohen IR, Schwartz M. Autoimmune T cells protect neurons from secondary degeneration after central nervous system axotomy. Nat Med 1999;5:49–55

46. Rapalino O, Lazarov-Spiegler O, Agranov E, et al. Implantation of stimulated homologous macrophages results in partial recovery of paraplegic rats. Nat Med 1998;4:814–821

47. Knoller N, Auerbach G, Fulga V, et al. Clinical experience using incubated autologous macrophages as a treatment for complete spinal cord injury: phase I study results. J Neurosurg Spine 2005;3:173–181

48. Lazarov-Spiegler O, Solomon AS, Schwartz M. Peripheral nerve-stimulated macrophages simulate a peripheral nerve-like regenerative response in rat transected optic nerve. Glia 1998;24:329–337

49. Lazarov-Spiegler O, Solomon AS, Zeev-Brann AB, Hirschberg DL, Lavie V, Schwartz M. Transplantation of activated macrophages overcomes central nervous system regrowth failure. FASEB J 1996;10: 1296–1302

50. Bomze HM, Bulsara KR, Iskandar BJ, Caroni P, Skene JH. Spinal axon regeneration evoked by replacing two growth cone proteins in adult neurons. Nat Neurosci 2001;4:38–43

51. Mason MR, Lieberman AR, Anderson PN. Corticospinal neurons upregulate a range of growth-associated genes following intracortical, but not spinal, axotomy. Eur J Neurosci 2003;18:789–802

52. David S, Aguayo AJ. Axonal elongation into peripheral nervous system "bridges" after central nervous system injury in adult rats. Science 1981;214:931–933

53. David S, Aguayo AJ. Axonal regeneration after crush injury of rat central nervous system fibres innervating peripheral nerve grafts. J Neurocytol 1985;14:1–12

54. Richardson PM, McGuinness UM, Aguayo AJ. Axons from CNS neurons regenerate into PNS grafts. Nature 1980;284:264–265

55. Cheng H, Cao Y, Olson L. Spinal cord repair in adult paraplegic rats: partial restoration of hind limb function. Science 1996;273:510–513

56. Jenkins R, Tetzlaff W, Hunt SP. Differential expression of immediate early genes in rubrospinal neurons following axotomy in rat. Eur J Neurosci 1993;5:203–209

57. Chaisuksunt V, Zhang Y, Anderson PN, et al. Axonal regeneration from CNS neurons in the cerebellum and brainstem of adult rats: correlation with the patterns of expression and distribution of messenger RNAs for L1, CHL1, c-jun and growth-associated protein-43. Neuroscience 2000;100:87–108

58. Schwab ME, Thoenen H. Dissociated neurons regenerate into sciatic but not optic nerve explants in culture irrespective of neurotrophic factors. J Neurosci 1985;5:2415–2423

59. Chen MS, Huber AB, van der Haar ME, et al. Nogo-A is a myelin-associated neurite outgrowth inhibitor and an antigen for monoclonal antibody IN-1. Nature 2000;403:434–439

60. McKerracher L, David S, Jackson DL, Kottis V, Dunn RJ, Braun PE. Identification of myelin-associated glycoprotein as a major myelin-derived inhibitor of neurite growth. Neuron 1994;13:805–811

61. Mukhopadhyay G, Doherty P, Walsh FS, Crocker PR, Filbin MT. A novel role for myelin-associated glycoprotein as an inhibitor of axonal regeneration. Neuron 1994;13:757–767

62. Wang KC, Koprivica V, Kim JA, et al. Oligodendrocyte-myelin glycoprotein is a Nogo receptor ligand that inhibits neurite outgrowth. Nature 2002;417:941–944

63. Moreau-Fauvarque C, Kumanogoh A, Camand E, et al. The transmembrane semaphorin Sema4D/CD100, an inhibitor of axonal growth, is expressed on oligodendrocytes and upregulated after CNS lesion. J Neurosci 2003;23:9229–9239

64. Benson MD, Romero MI, Lush ME, Lu QR, Henkemeyer M, Parada LF. Ephrin-B3 is a myelin-based inhibitor of neurite outgrowth. Proc Natl Acad Sci U S A 2005;102:10694–10699

65. Hata K, Fujitani M, Yasuda Y, et al. RGMa inhibition promotes axonal growth and recovery after spinal cord injury. J Cell Biol 2006;173:47–58

66. Fournier AE, GrandPre T, Strittmatter SM. Identification of a receptor mediating Nogo-66 inhibition of axonal regeneration. Nature 2001;409:341–346

67. Wong ST, Henley JR, Kanning KC, Huang KH, Bothwell M, Poo MM. A p75(NTR) and Nogo receptor complex mediates repulsive signaling by myelin-associated glycoprotein. Nat Neurosci 2002;5:1302–1308

68. Park JB, Yiu G, Kaneko S, et al. A TNF receptor family member, TROY, is a coreceptor with Nogo receptor in mediating the inhibitory activity of myelin inhibitors. Neuron 2005;45:345–351

69. Mi S, Lee X, Shao Z, et al. LINGO-1 is a component of the Nogo-66 receptor/p75 signaling complex. Nat Neurosci 2004;7:221–228

70. McKerracher L, Higuchi H. Targeting Rho to stimulate repair after spinal cord injury. J Neurotrauma 2006;23:309–317

71. Hsieh SH, Ferraro GB, Fournier AE. Myelin-associated inhibitors regulate cofilin phosphorylation and neuronal inhibition through LIM kinase and Slingshot phosphatase. J Neurosci 2006;26:1006–1015

72. Caroni P, Schwab ME. Antibody against myelin-associated inhibitor of neurite growth neutralizes nonpermissive substrate properties of CNS white matter. Neuron 1988;1:85–96

73. Schnell L, Schwab ME. Axonal regeneration in the rat spinal cord produced by an antibody against myelin-associated neurite growth inhibitors. Nature 1990;343:269–272

74. Bregman BS, Kunkel-Bagden E, Schnell L, Dai HN, Gao D, Schwab ME. Recovery from spinal cord injury mediated by antibodies to neurite growth inhibitors. Nature 1995;378:498–501

75. Freund P, Schmidlin E, Wannier T, et al. Nogo-A-specific antibody treatment enhances sprouting and functional recovery after cervical lesion in adult primates. Nat Med 2006;12:790–792

76. Freund P, Wannier T, Schmidlin E, et al. Anti-Nogo-A antibody treatment enhances sprouting of corticospinal axons rostral to a unilateral cervical spinal cord lesion in adult macaque monkey. J Comp Neurol 2007;502:644–659

77. McKeon RJ, Schreiber RC, Rudge JS, Silver J. Reduction of neurite outgrowth in a model of glial scarring following CNS injury is correlated with the expression of inhibitory molecules on reactive astrocytes. J Neurosci 1991;11:3398–3411

78. Morgenstern DA, Asher RA, Fawcett JW. Chondroitin sulphate proteoglycans in the CNS injury response. Prog Brain Res 2002;137:313–332

79. Yiu G, He Z. Glial inhibition of CNS axon regeneration. Nat Rev Neurosci 2006;7:617–627

80. Barritt AW, Davies M, Marchand F, et al. Chondroitinase ABC promotes sprouting of intact and injured spinal systems after spinal cord injury. J Neurosci 2006;26:10856–10867

81. García-Alías G, Lin R, Akrimi SF, Story D, Bradbury EJ, Fawcett JW. Therapeutic time window for the application of chondroitinase ABC after spinal cord injury. Exp Neurol 2008;210:331–338

82. Bradbury EJ, Moon LD, Popat RJ, et al. Chondroitinase ABC promotes functional recovery after spinal cord injury. Nature 2002;416:636–640

83. Yick LW, Cheung PT, So KF, Wu W. Axonal regeneration of Clarke's neurons beyond the spinal cord injury scar after treatment with chondroitinase ABC. Exp Neurol 2003;182:160–168

84. Caggiano AO, Zimber MP, Ganguly A, Blight AR, Gruskin EA. Chondroitinase ABCI improves locomotion and bladder function following contusion injury of the rat spinal cord. J Neurotrauma 2005;22:226–239

85. Kim BG, Dai HN, Lynskey JV, McAtee M, Bregman BS. Degradation of chondroitin sulfate proteoglycans potentiates transplant-mediated axonal remodeling and functional recovery after spinal cord injury in adult rats. J Comp Neurol 2006;497:182–198

86. Houle JD, Tom VJ, Mayes D, Wagoner G, Phillips N, Silver J. Combining an autologous peripheral nervous system "bridge" and matrix modification by chondroitinase allows robust, functional regeneration beyond a hemisection lesion of the adult rat spinal cord. J Neurosci 2006;26:7405–7415

87. Ikegami T, Nakamura M, Yamane J, et al. Chondroitinase ABC combined with neural stem/progenitor cell transplantation enhances graft cell migration and outgrowth of growth-associated protein-43-positive fibers after rat spinal cord injury. Eur J Neurosci 2005;22:3036–3046

88. Fouad K, Schnell L, Bunge MB, Schwab ME, Liebscher T, Pearse DD. Combining Schwann cell bridges and olfactory-ensheathing glia grafts with chondroitinase promotes locomotor recovery after complete transection of the spinal cord. J Neurosci 2005;25:1169–1178

89. Monnier PP, Sierra A, Schwab JM, Henke-Fahle S, Mueller BK. The Rho/ROCK pathway mediates neurite growth-inhibitory activity associated with the chondroitin sulfate proteoglycans of the CNS glial scar. Mol Cell Neurosci 2003;22:319–330

90. Lehmann M, Fournier A, Selles-Navarro I, et al. Inactivation of Rho signaling pathway promotes CNS axon regeneration. J Neurosci 1999;19:7537–7547

91. Dergham P, Ellezam B, Essagian C, Avedissian H, Lubell WD, McKerracher L. Rho signaling pathway targeted to promote spinal cord repair. J Neurosci 2002;22:6570–6577

92. Dubreuil CI, Winton MJ, McKerracher L. Rho activation patterns after spinal cord injury and the role of activated Rho in apoptosis in the central nervous system. J Cell Biol 2003;162:233–243

93. Lee YS, Hsiao I, Lin VW. Peripheral nerve grafts and aFGF restore partial hindlimb function in adult paraplegic rats. J Neurotrauma 2002;19:1203–1216

94. Cheng H, Liao KK, Liao SF, Chuang TY, Shih YH. Spinal cord repair with acidic fibroblast growth factor as a treatment for a patient with chronic paraplegia. Spine 2004;29:E284–E288

95. Xu XM, Guénard V, Kleitman N, Bunge MB. Axonal regeneration into Schwann cell-seeded guidance channels grafted into transected adult rat spinal cord. J Comp Neurol 1995;351:145–160

96. Pearse DD, Sanchez AR, Pereira FC, et al. Transplantation of Schwann cells and/or olfactory ensheathing glia into the contused spinal cord: Survival, migration, axon association, and functional recovery. Glia 2007;55:976–1000

97. Pinzon A, Calancie B, Oudega M, Noga BR. Conduction of impulses by axons regenerated in a Schwann cell graft in the transected adult rat thoracic spinal cord. J Neurosci Res 2001;64:533–541

98. Golden KL, Pearse DD, Blits B, et al. Transduced Schwann cells promote axon growth and myelination after spinal cord injury. Exp Neurol 2007;207:203–217

99. Toma JG, Akhavan M, Fernandes KJ, et al. Isolation of multipotent adult stem cells from the dermis of mammalian skin. Nat Cell Biol 2001;3:778–784

100. Toma JG, McKenzie IA, Bagli D, Miller FD. Isolation and characterization of multipotent skin-derived precursors from human skin. Stem Cells 2005;23:727–737

101. Biernaskie J, Sparling JS, Liu J, et al. Skin-derived precursors generate myelinating Schwann cells that promote remyelination and functional recovery after contusion spinal cord injury. J Neurosci 2007;27:9545–9559

102. Harding J, Graziadei PP, Monti Graziadei GA, Margolis FL. Denervation in the primary olfactory pathway of mice, IV: Biochemical and morphological evidence for neuronal replacement following nerve section. Brain Res 1977;132:11–28

103. Ramón-Cueto A, Plant GW, Avila J, Bunge MB. Long-distance axonal regeneration in the transected adult rat spinal cord is promoted by olfactory ensheathing glia transplants. J Neurosci 1998;18:3803–3815

104. Ramón-Cueto A, Cordero MI, Santos-Benito FF, Avila J. Functional recovery of paraplegic rats and motor axon regeneration in their spinal cords by olfactory ensheathing glia. Neuron 2000;25:425–435

105. Boyd JG, Doucette R, Kawaja MD. Defining the role of olfactory ensheathing cells in facilitating axon remyelination following damage to the spinal cord. FASEB J 2005;19:694–703

106. Devon R, Doucette R. Olfactory ensheathing cells myelinate dorsal root ganglion neurites. Brain Res 1992;589:175–179

107. Richter MW, Roskams AJ. Olfactory ensheathing cell transplantation following spinal cord injury: hype or hope? Exp Neurol 2008;209:353–367

108. Raisman G, Li Y. Repair of neural pathways by olfactory ensheathing cells. Nat Rev Neurosci 2007;8:312–319

109. Dobkin BH, Curt A, Guest J. Cellular transplants in China: observational study from the largest human experiment in chronic spinal cord injury. Neurorehabil Neural Repair 2006;20:5–13

110. Seaberg RM, van der Kooy D. Stem and progenitor cells: the premature desertion of rigorous definitions. Trends Neurosci 2003;26:125–131

111. Hammang JP, Archer DR, Duncan ID. Myelination following transplantation of EGF-responsive neural stem cells into a myelin-deficient environment. Exp Neurol 1997;147:84–95

112. Karimi-Abdolrezaee S, Eftekharpour E, Wang J, Morshead CM, Fehlings MG. Delayed transplantation of adult neural precursor cells promotes remyelination and functional neurological recovery after spinal cord injury. J Neurosci 2006;26:3377–3389

113. Eftekharpour E, Karimi-Abdolrezaee S, Wang J, El Beheiry H, Morshead C, Fehlings MG. Myelination of congenitally dysmyelinated spinal cord axons by adult neural precursor cells results in formation of nodes of Ranvier and improved axonal conduction. J Neurosci 2007;27:3416–3428

114. Hofstetter CP, Holmström NA, Lilja JA, et al. Allodynia limits the usefulness of intraspinal neural stem cell grafts; directed differentiation improves outcome. Nat Neurosci 2005;8:346–353

115. Zhang SC, Ge B, Duncan ID. Adult brain retains the potential to generate oligodendroglial progenitors with extensive myelination capacity. Proc Natl Acad Sci U S A 1999;96:4089–4094

116. Cummings BJ, Uchida N, Tamaki SJ, et al. Human neural stem cells differentiate and promote locomotor recovery in spinal cord-injured mice. Proc Natl Acad Sci U S A 2005;102:14069–14074

117. Liu S, Qu Y, Stewart TJ, et al. Embryonic stem cells differentiate into oligodendrocytes and myelinate in culture and after spinal cord transplantation. Proc Natl Acad Sci U S A 2000;97:6126–6131

118. Brüstle O, Jones KN, Learish RD, et al. Embryonic stem cell-derived glial precursors: a source of myelinating transplants. Science 1999;285: 754–756

119. Nistor GI, Totoiu MO, Haque N, Carpenter MK, Keirstead HS. Human embryonic stem cells differentiate into oligodendrocytes in high purity and myelinate after spinal cord transplantation. Glia 2005;49:385–396

120. Keirstead HS, Nistor G, Bernal G, et al. Human embryonic stem cell-derived oligodendrocyte progenitor cell transplants remyelinate and restore locomotion after spinal cord injury. J Neurosci 2005;25:4694–4705

121. Kang SM, Cho MS, Seo H, et al. Efficient induction of oligodendrocytes from human embryonic stem cells. Stem Cells 2007;25:419–424

122. Reubinoff BE, Itsykson P, Turetsky T, et al. Neural progenitors from human embryonic stem cells. Nat Biotechnol 2001;19:1134–1140

123. Martin GR. Isolation of a pluripotent cell line from early mouse embryos cultured in medium conditioned by teratocarcinoma stem cells. Proc Natl Acad Sci U S A 1981;78:7634–7638

124. Evans MJ, Kaufman MH. Establishment in culture of pluripotential cells from mouse embryos. Nature 1981;292:154–156

125. Thomson JA, Itskovitz-Eldor J, Shapiro SS, et al. Embryonic stem cell lines derived from human blastocysts. Science 1998;282:1145–1147

126. Reubinoff BE, Pera MF, Fong CY, Trounson A, Bongso A. Embryonic stem cell lines from human blastocysts: somatic differentiation in vitro. Nat Biotechnol 2000;18:399–404

127. Vogel G. Cell biology. Ready or not? Human ES cells head toward the clinic. Science 2005;308:1534–1538

128. Reynolds BA, Weiss S. Generation of neurons and astrocytes from isolated cells of the adult mammalian central nervous system. Science 1992;255:1707–1710

129. Weiss S, Dunne C, Hewson J, et al. Multipotent CNS stem cells are present in the adult mammalian spinal cord and ventricular neuroaxis. J Neurosci 1996;16:7599–7609

130. Temple S, Alvarez-Buylla A. Stem cells in the adult mammalian central nervous system. Curr Opin Neurobiol 1999;9:135–141

131. Phinney DG, Prockop DJ. Concise review: mesenchymal stem/multipotent stromal cells: the state of transdifferentiation and modes of tissue repair—current views. Stem Cells 2007;25:2896–2902

132. Akiyama Y, Radtke C, Kocsis JD. Remyelination of the rat spinal cord by transplantation of identified bone marrow stromal cells. J Neurosci 2002;22:6623–6630

133. Corti S, Locatelli F, Donadoni C, et al. Neuroectodermal and microglial differentiation of bone marrow cells in the mouse spinal cord and sensory ganglia. J Neurosci Res 2002;70:721–733

134. Koshizuka S, Okada S, Okawa A, et al. Transplanted hematopoietic stem cells from bone marrow differentiate into neural lineage cells and promote functional recovery after spinal cord injury in mice. J Neuropathol Exp Neurol 2004;63:64–72

135. Koda M, Okada S, Nakayama T, et al. Hematopoietic stem cell and marrow stromal cell for spinal cord injury in mice. Neuroreport 2005;16: 1763–1767

136. Parr AM, Tator CH, Keating A. Bone marrow-derived mesenchymal stromal cells for the repair of central nervous system injury. Bone Marrow Transplant 2007;40:609–619

137. Enzmann GU, Benton RL, Talbott JF, Cao Q, Whittemore SR. Functional considerations of stem cell transplantation therapy for spinal cord repair. J Neurotrauma 2006;23:479–495

138. Gupta D, Tator CH, Shoichet MS. Fast-gelling injectable blend of hyaluronan and methylcellulose for intrathecal, localized delivery to the injured spinal cord. Biomaterials 2006;27:2370–2379

139. Liu S, Bodjarian N, Langlois O, et al. Axonal regrowth through a collagen guidance channel bridging spinal cord to the avulsed C6 roots: functional recovery in primates with brachial plexus injury. J Neurosci Res 1998;51:723–734

140. Oudega M, Gautier SE, Chapon P, et al. Axonal regeneration into Schwann cell grafts within resorbable poly(alpha-hydroxyacid) guidance channels in the adult rat spinal cord. Biomaterials 2001;22: 1125–1136

141. Tsai EC, Dalton PD, Shoichet MS, Tator CH. Synthetic hydrogel guidance channels facilitate regeneration of adult rat brainstem motor axons after complete spinal cord transection. J Neurotrauma 2004;21:789–804

142. Lavik E, Teng YD, Snyder E, Langer R. Seeding neural stem cells on scaffolds of PGA, PLA, and their copolymers. Methods Mol Biol 2002;198: 89–97

143. Teng YD, Lavik EB, Qu X, et al. Functional recovery following traumatic spinal cord injury mediated by a unique polymer scaffold seeded with neural stem cells. Proc Natl Acad Sci U S A 2002;99:3024–3029

144. Novikova LN, Pettersson J, Brohlin M, Wiberg M, Novikov LN. Biodegradable poly-beta-hydroxybutyrate scaffold seeded with Schwann cells to promote spinal cord repair. Biomaterials 2008;29:1198–1206

145. Tsai EC, Dalton PD, Shoichet MS, Tator CH. Matrix inclusion within synthetic hydrogel guidance channels improves specific supraspinal and local axonal regeneration after complete spinal cord transection. Biomaterials 2006;27:519–533

146. Guo J, Su H, Zeng Y, et al. Reknitting the injured spinal cord by self-assembling peptide nanofiber scaffold. Nanomedicine 2007;3:311–321

147. Shen Y, Tenney AP, Busch SA, et al. PTPsigma is a receptor for chondroitin sulfate proteoglycan, an inhibitor of neural regeneration. Science 2009;326(5952):592–596

148. Yu J, Vodyanik MA, Smuga-Otto K, et al. Induced pluripotent stem cell lines derived from human somatic cells. Science 2007;318(5858): 1917–1920

149. Park IH, Zhao R, West JA, et al. Reprogramming of human somatic cells to pluripotency with defined factors. Nature 2008;451(7175):141–146

150. Nakagawa M, Koyanagi M, Tanabe K, et al. Generation of induced pluripotent stem cells without Myc from mouse and human fibroblasts. Nat Biotechnol 2008;26(1):101–106

151. Takahashi K, Yamanaka S. Induction of pluripotent stem cells from mouse embryonic and adult fibroblast cultures by defined factors. Cell 2006;126(4):663–676

152. Maherali N, Sridharan R, Xie W, et al. Directly reprogrammed fibroblasts show global epigenetic remodeling and widespread tissue contribution. Cell Stem Cell 2007;1(1):55–70

54

Emerging Rehabilitation Strategies for Spinal Cord Injury

Andrew J. Tsung and Daniel R. Fassett

Spinal cord injuries (SCIs) occur at an annual incidence of 15 to 40 cases per million population, accounting for ~11,000 injuries each year in the United States and an affected population of 250,000 patients in 2004.[1] Although these numbers are not as sizable as those for heart disease and diabetes mellitus, the lifetime care of an SCI patient can incur significant societal and health care costs. Lifetime medical costs alone have been estimated at approximately US$3 million for one 25-year-old person with a tetraplegic injury, with a large percentage of these costs arising from rehabilitation interventions.[2] In addition, a large percentage of these injuries occur in young individuals during the productive third and fourth decades of life in terms of economic contribution to society.[3] Advancements in SCI rehabilitation, although expensive, have the potential to make these patients more independent, resulting in improved quality of life and potentially reducing the long-term costs to society.

Classical rehabilitation for SCI has focused on therapeutic exercise, maximizing the usefulness of remaining neurological function, or specifically training an individual to cope with deficit via compensatory therapies or equipment. This treatment paradigm is congruent with the thought that the nervous system is a static system, incapable of repair or dynamic localization of function. Recent research, however, suggests that motor and sensory function can recover even after a prolonged period of latency.[4] This concept has led to significant interest scientifically in neural plasticity after traumatic SCI, including research involving the central pattern generator (CPG) and other intrinsic spinal circuits involved in motor processes. The focus of clinical research in SCI rehabilitation has shifted somewhat from compensation tactics that improve functional outcome to treatment regimens geared to promote neuroplasticity and neurological recovery. In effect, this marks a transition from a compensatory model of SCI rehabilitation to a new recovery model promoting activity-dependent plasticity and functional recovery.

To date, it is unclear what mechanisms contribute to recovery of ambulation after SCI. With incomplete injuries, it has been hypothesized that recovery of the injured pathways, along with improvement in muscle training and sensation, resulted in the patient regaining ambulation.[5] More recently, the CPG, which was initially described in invertebrates and cats, has been suggested as one recovery mechanism.[6,7] Physiologically, the CPG exists within the spinal cord as a network of interneurons that generates patterned oscillating signals necessary for locomotion. The CPG coordinates flexion of one limb and extension of the contralateral limb based on sensory inputs from the extremities and signals from the brain.

In animal models, it has been shown that the CPG can produce rhythmic movements similar to locomotion even in the absence of supraspinal input.[7] The most convincing evidence for the CPG comes from animal studies in which the spinal cord is transected in the thoracic region, effectively isolating the cord from supraspinal stimulus input. Efferent activity is then monitored, revealing rhythmic bursts of activity correlating with agonist and antagonist movements of the hindlimbs required for ambulation.[8,9] For example, cats with complete spinal cord transection can produce hindleg movements when placed on a treadmill with their body weight supported.

In humans, however, the CPG has not been as clearly defined as it has in controlled laboratory experiments of lower-order animals, and data suggest that the CPG does not function independently in humans. Although it is capable of emitting rhythmic signals, there is significant modulation from supraspinal centers as a result of peripheral sensory inputs such as joint and load receptors.[10–14] Furthermore, not all elements required for gait are emitted by the CPG.[15] Clinically, this lack of complete independence has been demonstrated via electromyography (EMG), where complete support of body weight resulted in absence of activity in limb muscles, presumably because of removal of spinal sensory input from load receptors.[16] There are some indications that the CPG, although diffusely distributed as a network, may have greater localization toward caudal elements of the cord or may have greater functionality in those regions. Some researchers have found that the locomotor pattern corresponds with the level of lesioning, with higher levels resulting in more normal function.[17]

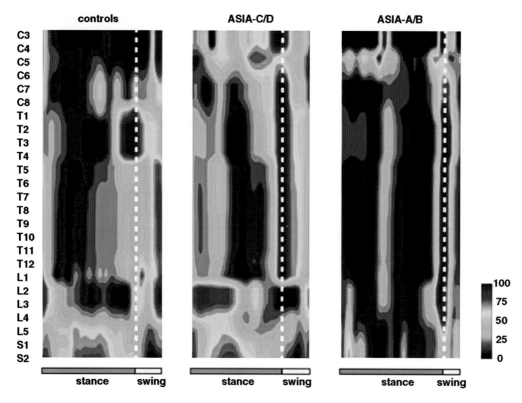

Fig. 54.1 Electromyographic activation superimposed on spinal cord maps in the stance and swing phases of gait. (From Grasso R, Ivanenko YP, Zago M, et al. Distributed plasticity of locomotor pattern generators in spinal cord injured patients. Brain 2004;127(Pt 5):1019–1034. Reprinted with permission.)

There is an increasing body of evidence suggesting that, on the synaptic level, there is significant neural plasticity within the spinal cord with alterations in synaptic strength, axonal sprouting, and dynamic changes in functional connections in uninjured and injured neural tissues.[18] This is further supported clinically by the data provided by Grasso et al[19] using motor pool mapping. In this technique, activity of groups of muscles is recorded via EMG, color-coded, and superimposed on known spinal cord maps. These data are then plotted against time to show changes in activity with stance and swing phases of gait (**Fig. 54.1**). Using this technique, the authors demonstrated that after a spinal cord lesion with resultant paraplegia, the locomotor network could reorganize significantly, involving all levels of the spinal cord, including the supralesional and sublesional segments, leading to restoration of rhythmic activity. Notably, CPG characteristics were induced in motor neurons not normally expressing rhythmic output during ambulation. Functional plasticity, however, is often task specific, at least in animal models. For example, animals trained to stand are able to stand adequately, but stepping ability may not improve to any degree,[20] leaving unanswered the question to what degree task specificity applies to other areas of ambulation. Task-related specificity must therefore be taken in context with the fact that the CPG likely does not contain all the necessary elements for ambulation.

◆ Locomotor Training

To this end, investigators using partial body-weight support treadmill training (PBWSTT) have sought to promote the recovery of spinal cord neural circuits by generating the sensory stimuli mimicking ambulation.[19,21] This is accomplished by partially supporting the body weight of the patient via overhead harness on a moving treadmill with therapists guiding the movement of the lower extremities (**Fig. 54.2**). Specific interest was generated in PBWSTT after it was found that walking movements consisting of knee extension and flexion could be elicited in paralyzed patients with severe cervical SCI despite lack of voluntary movement at rest. EMG signals that were previously absent in these patients returned during flexion and extension movements after training of less than 1 hour per day for 5 days per week.[22] The CPG has thus been implicated as the main generator of these signals.

Despite this success, applying to humans what has been learned in animal models has proven to be a significantly more complex task. Previous studies have demonstrated the key factor for regaining ambulatory status in humans after SCI is the interpretation of sensory input during walking in combination with the output from the spinal interneuron pool, whether it be called the CPG or some other term.[23] Thus one cannot simply place patients with SCI on treadmills and expect ambulation. Appropriate sensory input, such as maximal load bearing on the legs without losing balance; minimizing load bearing on the arms, head, and trunk posture; maintaining as normal as possible joint kinematics observed in walking, loading, and unloading sequences; and finally, generating normal stepping velocities, are all part of the equation necessary to promote ambulatory status.[14,23–25] *Locomotor training* (*LT*) is thus a relatively new term that describes this physiological approach to therapy in retraining walking after neurological injury. It seeks to address the specific requirements of motor and sensory input while integrating and capitalizing on the aspects of intrinsic spinal circuitry

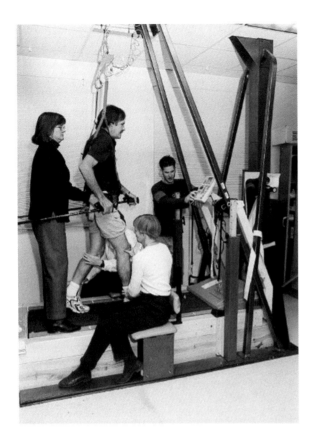

Fig. 54.2 Partial body-weight support treadmill training (PBWSTT) utilizing an overhead harness and therapists guiding movement of the lower extremities. (From Behrman AL, Harkema SJ. Locomotor training after human spinal cord injury: a series of case studies. Phys Ther 2000;80(7):688–700. Reprinted with permission.)

such as the CPG. Guidelines have already been developed that govern a more specific regimen in the recovery of walking, with many more advancements and recommendations likely to follow in the coming years.[26–28]

Although LT provides a framework for regaining mobility, many critical details regarding its implementation are yet to be determined. Its general safety in the acute rehabilitation phase and in chronic SCI patients has been ascertained, but specific aspects, such as autonomic dysreflexia, orthostatic hypotension, bone loss, heterotopic ossification, compensatory behaviors, and sensory deficits, have not been specifically addressed.[29,30] More problematic is the wide-ranging nature of therapies that are described as partial body-weight support training. With the advent of this technology and its application to humans, the medical industry has been quick to market anything with a harness and treadmill as PBWSTT, but in reality LT is much less reliant on equipment than on the scientific justification and specific therapy techniques used.

The population best targeted by PBWSTT is not defined. It cannot be recommended for all patients with SCI. As has been shown, those with lower motor neuron injuries are unlikely to benefit from this therapy, nor are those with American Spinal Injury Association (ASIA) A or B injuries who are not able to translate improved walking with treadmill-based therapies to the overground environment.[30] Finally, and most difficult, controversy remains about how and when to best manage variables such as initiation of therapy, intensity, duration, frequency, and progression of care to the SCI patient.[29]

The question at this stage in LT development condenses to determining efficacy in those patients that have been appropriately selected, to the best of our ability, to undergo therapy via PWBSTT. Overall, there have been three LT studies investigating acute SCI, only one of which was randomized and controlled, and 11 studies in chronic SCI (**Table 54.1**). Although data are fairly minimal, a recently completed randomized, controlled trial (RCT) sought to answer this question in the acute SCI group. The Spinal Cord Injury Locomotor Trial (SCILT) enrolled 146 subjects within 8 weeks of injury in a single-blinded, multicenter, randomized clinical trial.[31] Subjects had suffered incomplete SCI and were graded ASIA B through D with a Functional Independence Measure for locomotion (FIM-L) score less than 4. Patients were divided into two groups, those who underwent PBWSTT with overground practice for 12 weeks and those who underwent overground mobility therapy only for 12 weeks. Outcome measures included FIM-L score for ASIA B and C subjects and walking speed for ASIA C and D subjects 6 months after injury. Results confirmed no significant differences between PBWSTT and overground therapy only; however, these results may have been skewed by the fact that a very high percentage (92%) of ASIA C subjects walked independently regardless of the treatment regimen.

As the authors point out and as mentioned earlier, studies must be interpreted with caution in regard to applicability to the general population.[32] In the SCILT trial, 1434 admissions for SCI were screened, and only ~10% qualified after application of eligibility criteria. Most potential subjects were excluded because they had complete SCI or significant medical comorbidity preventing mobility, both of which represent a significant cross-section of the traumatic SCI population. Furthermore, most had ASIA C injuries, whereas ASIA D patients were kept in community hospitals and not referred to SCI centers. Lastly, those that entered early in the study (less than 4 weeks) improved more, not because of the earlier initiation of therapies but because they entered as an ASIA C or D as opposed to B or C if they entered later in the study.

The study above and those by Nymark et al and Wernig et al[29,30] were the only studies that tested the concept of LT during inpatient rehabilitation with follow-up through the outpatient phase of care. Most of the other studies delineated in **Table 54.1** involved subjects monitored in the inpatient and outpatient setting for varying periods of time extending out to 18 years after SCI with varying outcome measures. Walking speed was the outcome measure most commonly reported, but numerous others were analyzed, including EMG, H-reflex analysis, and physiological measures such as strength. Meaningful, generalized conclusions are difficult, if not impossible, to discern from the literature given the heterogeneity of inclusion/treatment criteria, minimal number of subjects, and varying outcome measures. An illustration of this fact is that investigators involved in SCILT found almost no walking outcomes (levels of independence, speed, distance, etc.) in the literature related to initial ASIA grade within 1 year of SCI despite databases including thousands of patients.[32]

Functional Electrical Therapy

Over the past 40 years, various neuroprosthetic devices that use neuromuscular electrical stimulation (NMES) to activate muscles have been evaluated in patients with SCI and other

Table 54.1 Locomotor Trials in Acute and Chronic Spinal Cord Injury

Study	Initial BWS	Speed	Manual Assist	Arm Support	Overground Training	Orthotic Device Use	Intensity	Duration	Frequency
LT Studies (incorporating BWS and TM)—Acute									
Wernig et al (1995)[30]	40%	Self-selected speed	Legs only	Balance only	Added to conventional gait training as soon as possible	NA	30 minutes	2–22 wk	5x/wk
Nymark et al (1998) (4 subjects)	Up to 80%	0.15–0.6 m/s	Legs and trunk	Initially for balance, then removed	Added to conventional gait training	NA	60 minutes	12 wk	3x/wk
Dobkin et al (2006)[31]	High enough to achieve speed goals	At least 0.72 m/s, goal of 1.07 m/s	Legs and trunk	None	Same training goals as on TM	Removed during training	20–30 minutes with BWS and TM; 10–20 minutes overground	12 wk	5x/wk
LT Studies (incorporating BWS and TM)—Chronic									
Wernig and Müller (1992)[22]	40%	Self-selected speed	Legs only	Balance only	1 time/wk added to conventional gait training	NA	30 minutes	1.5–7 months	5x/wk
Dietz et al (1995)[a]	Up to 80%	0.42 m/s	Legs only	NA	NA	NA	NA	12 wk	5x/wk
Wernig et al (1995)[30]	40%	Self-selected speed	Legs only	Balance only	Added to conventional gait training as soon as possible	NA	30 minutes	3–20 wk	5x/wk
Behrman and Harkema (2000)[28]	40%	0.75–1.25 m/s	Legs and trunk	None	Modified to match training principles	Removed during training	90 minutes	9 wk	5x/wk
Protos et al (2001)[b]	40%	0.04 m/s	Legs only	Balance only	NA	NA	60 minutes (20 minutes of stepping)	12 wk	5x/wk
Trimble et al (1998)[c]	NA	Matched overground fast walking	NA	NA	NA	NA	30 minutes	10 days 4 mo at gym	Every other day 3x/wk
Gardner et al (1998)[d]	32%	0.67–2.01 m/s	None	Balance only	NA	NA	20 minutes of TM stepping	6 wk	3x/wk
Wirz et al (2001)[e]	Up to 80%	0.42 m/s	Legs only	NA	NA	NA	15 minutes of stepping	27 wk (average)	5x/wk
Behrman et al (2005)	40%	0.75–1.25 m/s	Legs and trunk	None	Modified to match training principles	Removed during training	90 minutes	9 wk	5x/wk

Table 54.1 Locomotor Trials in Acute and Chronic Spinal Cord Injury (*Continued*)

Study	Initial BWS	Speed	Manual Assist	Arm Support	Overground Training	Orthotic Device Use	Intensity	Duration	Frequency
LT Studies (Incorporating BWS and TM)—Chronic									
Effing et al (2005)[f]	50%	0.03 m/s to self-selected speed	Legs only	Allowed initially	NA	NA	30 minutes	12 wk	5x/wk
Hicks et al (2005)[g]	60% +	0.17 m/s	NA	NA	NA	NA	Three 5- to 15-minute walking bouts	Until 144 sessions were completed	3x/wk
Hybrid (Combines LT Using BWS with FES)									
Field-Fote (2001)[38]	30%	Fastest comfortable speed	FES to legs	NA	NA	NA	90 minutes	12 wk	3x/wk
Field-Fote and Tepavac (2002)	NA	Fastest comfortable speed	FES to legs	Balance only	NA	NA	90 minutes	12 wk	3x/wk
Postans et al (2004)	40%	Self-selected speed	Legs and FES	Balance only	NA	NA	25 minutes of walking	4 wk	5x/wk
Nymark et al (1998) (1 subject)	Up to 80%	0.15–0.6 m/s	Legs and trunk	Initially for balance	Added to conventional gait training	NA	60 minutes	12 wk	3x/wk

Source: Behrman AL, Harkema SJ. Locomotor training after human spinal cord injury: a series of case studies. Phys Ther 2000;80(7):688–700. Reprinted with permission.

Abbreviations: BWS, body-weight support; FES, functional electrical stimulation; NA, not addressed in methods section of article; TM, treadmill.

[a]Dietz V, Colombo G, Jensen L, Baumgartner L. Locomotor capacity of spinal cord in paraplegic patients. Ann Neurol 1995;37:574–582.

[b]Protas EJ, Holmes SA, Qureshy H, et al. Supported treadmill ambulation training after spinal cord injury: a pilot study. Arch Phys Med Rehabil. 2001;82:825–831.

[c]Trimble MH, Kukulka CG, Behrman AL. The effect of treadmill gait training on low-frequency depression of the soleus H-reflex: comparison of a spinal cord injured man to normal subjects. Neurosci Lett 1998;246:186–188.

[d]Gardner MB, Holden MK, Leikauskas JM, Richard RL. Partial body weight support with treadmill locomotion to improve gait after incomplete spinal cord injury: a single-subject experimental design. Phys Ther 1998;7:361–374.

[e]Wirz M, Colombo G, Dietz V. Long-term effects of locomotor training in spinal humans. J Neurol Neurosurg Psychiatry 2001;71:93–96.

[f]Effing TW, van Meeteren NL, van Asbeck FW, Prevo AJ. Body weight-supported treadmill training in chronic incomplete spinal cord injury: a pilot study evaluating functional health status and quality of life. Spinal Cord 2006;44:287–296.

[g]Hicks AI, Adams MM, Martin Ginis K, et al. Long-term body-weight-supported treadmill training and subsequent follow-up in persons with chronic SCI: effects on functional walking ability and measures of subjective well-being. Spinal Cord 2005;43:291–298.

upper motor neuron disorders to increase the functional use of paralyzed muscles. With controlled and coordinated application of an electrical current, contraction of paralyzed muscles can be accomplished in a planned fashion to improve functional activity. Functional electrical stimulation (FES) involves the use of electrical stimulation to generate purposeful contractions of paralyzed muscles. The goal of FES is to allow patients more functional use of a muscle or limb with the potential of improving activities of daily living in a more independent fashion.

Within the field of SCI rehabilitation, FES has traditionally been employed in the chronic stages of the disability after the neurological system has been allowed sufficient time for maximal recovery, typically 12 to 18 months after injury.[33] SCI applications of FES include upper extremity stimulation to improve grasp, phrenic nerve stimulation for diaphragmatic contraction to improve respiratory function, thoracic spinal cord epidural stimulation for improved cough, bladder stimulation for micturition, lower extremity stimulation for standing and walking, and gluteal stimulation for the treatment of decubiti.[33] FES, in general, has not been used in the acute or subacute periods of SCI rehabilitation; however, recent research is evaluating neuromuscular electrical stimulation as a subacute rehabilitation technique to facilitate lower extremity movement and promote motor relearning via neuroplasticity. The use of electrical stimulation to facilitate lower extremity movements and promote neurological recovery has been termed functional electrical therapy (FET).[33]

The proposed mechanism for neurological improvement with FET is similar to that of locomotor therapies, with the belief that goal-oriented (patient consciously trying to move limb), repetitive movements of a limb produce proprioceptive and cutaneous sensory feedback to the spinal cord that alters synaptic connections within the spinal cord and brain to facilitate motor relearning.[33] Functional magnetic resonance imaging (fMRI) studies have shown that muscle contraction and extremity movement resulting from NMES causes activation of the contralateral somatosensory cortex and bilateral supplemental motor areas within the brain.[34,35] It is thought that concurrent volitional effort combined with actual limb movement with the aid of electrical stimulation produces the greatest therapeutic benefit. Although much excitement was generated in 2002 with the report of late neurological improvement of an ASIA A SCI to an ASIA C with the use of FET cycling, published data supporting this treatment strategy are limited.[36] Other anecdotal reports[37] about individual patients have described improvements with FET cycling programs. Field-Fote[38] reported neurological improvement in 19 incomplete SCI patients that were treated with a combined program of PBWSTT and FET. Two other limited FES gait studies[39,40] showed enduring residual improvements in ambulation after FES treatment for gait, but no randomized, controlled studies have been reported with these treatment modalities for SCI. Even the use of FES as a long-term neuroprosthetic for gait assistance has been questioned because there are no class III studies on the effectiveness of these devices.

The vast majority of clinical research with FET has been in motor recovery of a paretic limb after a stroke. There have been 10 randomized, controlled studies evaluating upper extremity motor recovery after stroke.[41–48] Four of those studies[41–43,45] involved use of a continuous cyclic neuromuscular stimulation technique in which the electrical stimulus

was applied in a cyclic pattern without control or input from the participant. In the remaining six studies,[46–48] upper extremity motor recovery was evaluated using a biofeedback mechanism with an EMG-triggered stimulation technique in which an EMG sensor determined when the patient was attempting to initiate a contraction and then applied the external electrical stimulus at the same time to promote muscle contraction. It is speculated that the use of a biofeedback mechanism with coordination between stimulus application and volitional effort from the patient may produce the best results for motor relearning. Despite the randomized nature of these trials, however, there are several flaws that make interpretation difficult, including concerns about randomization techniques and lack of long-term follow-up to determine the enduring effect of these treatments. In addition, we should not extrapolate results from stroke hemiplegia research to SCI. Neuroplasticity and neurological recovery after stroke are likely very different than recovery after SCI. Therefore, although some exciting results have been reported in individual cases and small observational clinical trials, much more research is required to determine whether FET is a potential strategy to promote neurological recovery after SCI.

◆ Summary

Since the discovery of the reputed CPG by Grillner and Wallén,[7] doctors have attempted to capitalize on the intrinsic ability of the spinal cord to generate the signals necessary for ambulation. As we have discovered, the mere presence of an oscillating circuit, whether this can actually be termed the CPG or another spinal interneuron network, is not enough to sustain functional recovery. A precisely designed therapeutic protocol, affording the patient the prerequisite sensory input while providing the practice and repetition necessary, is the minimum necessary to promote recovery to the state of community ambulation. As new technology such as robotic gait training evolves, we may see great advances in treatment of SCI patients, as long as this technology does not detract from the very foundations of LT, such as proprioceptive sensory input and minimal assist from the device itself.[49] Our current state of knowledge lacks the criteria needed for identification of those individuals who may best benefit from locomotor and functional electrical therapies, and there are insufficient clinical data to gauge the long-term effectiveness of these treatment philosophies. The literature currently substantiates little gain from PBWSTT over conventional rehabilitation techniques, but this may change as we are better able to identify the subpopulations of patients with SCI that will benefit from these intensive and scientifically driven therapies.

References

1. Jackson AB, Dijkers M, Devivo MJ, Poczatek RB. A demographic profile of new traumatic spinal cord injuries: change and stability over 30 years. Arch Phys Med Rehabil 2004;85:1740–1748
2. NSCISC. Information and Facts about SCI: Facts and Figures at a Glance. 2006. Available at www.spinalcord.uab.edu
3. Sipski ML, Richards JS. Spinal cord injury rehabilitation: state of the science. Am J Phys Med Rehabil 2006;85:310–342
4. Basso DM. Neuroanatomical substrates of functional recovery after experimental spinal cord injury: implications of basic science research for human spinal cord injury. Phys Ther 2000;80:808–817
5. Little JW, Halar E. Temporal course of motor recovery after Brown-Sequard spinal cord injuries. Paraplegia 1985;23:39–46

6. Pinsker HM. Integration of reflex activity and central pattern generation in intact aplysia. J Physiol (Paris) 1982-1983-1983;78:775–785

7. Grillner S, Wallén P. Central pattern generators for locomotion, with special reference to vertebrates. Annu Rev Neurosci 1985;8:233–261

8. Floeter MK, Sholomenko GN, Gossard JP, Burke RE. Disynaptic excitation from the medial longitudinal fasciculus to lumbosacral motoneurons: modulation by repetitive activation, descending pathways, and locomotion. Exp Brain Res 1993;92:407–419

9. Miller S, Van Der Burg J, Van Der Meché F. Coordination of movements of the hindlimbs and forelimbs in different forms of locomotion in normal and decerebrate cats. Brain Res 1975;91:217–237

10. Jordan LM, Pratt CA, Menzies JE. Locomotion evoked by brain stem stimulation: occurrence without phasic segmental afferent input. Brain Res 1979;177:204–207

11. Yang JF, Gorassini M. Spinal and brain control of human walking: implications for retraining of walking. Neuroscientist 2006;12:379–389

12. Eidelberg E, Walden JG, Nguyen LH. Locomotor control in macaque monkeys. Brain 1981;104(Pt 4):647–663

13. Duysens J, Pearson KG. Inhibition of flexor burst generation by loading ankle extensor muscles in walking cats. Brain Res 1980;187:321–332

14. Dietz V, Müller R, Colombo G. Locomotor activity in spinal man: significance of afferent input from joint and load receptors. Brain 2002;125(Pt 12):2626–2634

15. Duysens J, Van de Crommert HW ; Van de Crommert HW. Neural control of locomotion: the central pattern generator from cats to humans. Gait Posture 1998;7:131–141

16. Poppele R, Bosco G. Sophisticated spinal contributions to motor control. Trends Neurosci 2003;26:269–276

17. Dietz V, Nakazawa K, Wirz M, Erni T. Level of spinal cord lesion determines locomotor activity in spinal man. Exp Brain Res 1999;128:405–409

18. Raineteau O, Schwab ME. Plasticity of motor systems after incomplete spinal cord injury. Nat Rev Neurosci 2001;2:263–273

19. Grasso R, Ivanenko YP, Zago M, et al. Distributed plasticity of locomotor pattern generators in spinal cord injured patients. Brain 2004;127(Pt 5):1019–1034

20. De Leon RD, Hodgson JA, Roy RR, Edgerton VR. Full weight-bearing hindlimb standing following stand training in the adult spinal cat. J Neurophysiol 1998;80:83–91

21. Dobkin B. Overview of treadmill locomotor training with partial body weight support: a neurophysiologically sound approach whose time has come for randomized clinical trials. Neurorehabil Neural Repair 1999;13:157–165

22. Wernig A, Müller S. Laufband locomotion with body weight support improved walking in persons with severe spinal cord injuries. Paraplegia 1992;30:229–238

23. Harkema S. Pattern generators in locomotion: implications for recovery of walking after spinal cord injury. Top Spinal Cord Inj Rehabil 2000;6:82–96

24. Harkema SJ, Hurley SL, Patel UK, Requejo PS, Dobkin BH, Edgerton VR. Human lumbosacral spinal cord interprets loading during stepping. J Neurophysiol 1997;77:797–811

25. Barbeau H, McCrea DA, O'Donovan MJ, Rossignol S, Grill WM, Lemay MA. Tapping into spinal circuits to restore motor function. Brain Res Brain Res Rev 1999;30:27–51

26. Barbeau H. Locomotor training in neurorehabilitation: emerging rehabilitation concepts. Neurorehabil Neural Repair 2003;17:3–11

27. Behrman AL, Bowden MG, Nair PM. Neuroplasticity after spinal cord injury and training: an emerging paradigm shift in rehabilitation and walking recovery. Phys Ther 2006;86:1406–1425

28. Behrman AL, Harkema SJ. Locomotor training after human spinal cord injury: a series of case studies. Phys Ther 2000;80:688–700

29. Nymark JR, Balmer SJ, Melis EH, Lemaire ED, Millar S. Electromyographic and kinematic nondisabled gait differences at extremely slow overground and treadmill walking speeds. J Rehabil Res Dev 2005;42:523–534

30. Wernig A, Müller S, Nanassy A, Cagol E. Laufband therapy based on "rules of spinal locomotion' is effective in spinal cord injured persons. Eur J Neurosci 1995;7:823–829

31. Dobkin B, Apple D, Barbeau H, et al; Spinal Cord Injury Locomotor Trial Group. Weight-supported treadmill vs over-ground training for walking after acute incomplete SCI. Neurology 2006;66:484–493

32. Dobkin BH. Confounders in rehabilitation trials of task-oriented training: lessons from the designs of the EXCITE and SCILT multicenter trials. Neurorehabil Neural Repair 2007;21:3–13

33. Sheffler LR, Chae J. Neuromuscular electrical stimulation in neurorehabilitation. Muscle Nerve 2007;35:562–590

34. Han BS, Jang SH, Chang Y, Byun WM, Lim SK, Kang DS. Functional magnetic resonance image finding of cortical activation by neuromuscular electrical stimulation on wrist extensor muscles. Am J Phys Med Rehabil 2003;82:17–20

35. Smith GV, Alon G, Roys SR, Gullapalli RP. Functional MRI determination of a dose-response relationship to lower extremity neuromuscular electrical stimulation in healthy subjects. Exp Brain Res 2003;150:33–39

36. McDonald JW, Becker D, Sadowsky CL, Jane JA Sr, Conturo TE, Schultz LM. Late recovery following spinal cord injury: case report and review of the literature. J Neurosurg 2002;97(2, Suppl):252–265

37. Donaldson N, Perkins TA, Fitzwater R, Wood DE, Middleton F. FES cycling may promote recovery of leg function after incomplete spinal cord injury. Spinal Cord 2000;38:680–682

38. Field-Fote EC. Combined use of body weight support, functional electric stimulation, and treadmill training to improve walking ability in individuals with chronic incomplete spinal cord injury. Arch Phys Med Rehabil 2001;82:818–824

39. Johnston TE, Finson RL, Smith BT, Bonaroti DM, Betz RR, Mulcahey MJ. Functional electrical stimulation for augmented walking in adolescents with incomplete spinal cord injury. J Spinal Cord Med 2003;26:390–400

40. Thrasher TA, Flett HM, Popovic MR. Gait training regimen for incomplete spinal cord injury using functional electrical stimulation. Spinal Cord 2006;44:357–361

41. Chae J, Bethoux F, Bohine T, Dobos L, Davis T, Friedl A. Neuromuscular stimulation for upper extremity motor and functional recovery in acute hemiplegia. Stroke 1998;29:975–979

42. Powell J, Pandyan AD, Granat M, Cameron M, Stott DJ. Electrical stimulation of wrist extensors in poststroke hemiplegia. Stroke 1999;30:1384–1389

43. Sonde L, Gip C, Fernaeus SE, Nilsson CG, Viitanen M. Stimulation with low frequency (1.7 Hz) transcutaneous electric nerve stimulation (low-tens) increases motor function of the post-stroke paretic arm. Scand J Rehabil Med 1998;30:95–99

44. Sonde L, Kalimo H, Fernaeus SE, Viitanen M. Low TENS treatment on post-stroke paretic arm: a three-year follow-up. Clin Rehabil 2000;14:14–19

45. Wong AM, Su TY, Tang FT, Cheng PT, Liaw MY. Clinical trial of electrical acupuncture on hemiplegic stroke patients. Am J Phys Med Rehabil 1999;78:117–122

46. Cauraugh J, Light K, Kim S, Thigpen M, Behrman A. Chronic motor dysfunction after stroke: recovering wrist and finger extension by electromyography-triggered neuromuscular stimulation. Stroke 2000;31:1360–1364

47. Bowman BR, Baker LL, Waters RL. Positional feedback and electrical stimulation: an automated treatment for the hemiplegic wrist. Arch Phys Med Rehabil 1979;60:497–502

48. Cauraugh JH, Kim S. Two coupled motor recovery protocols are better than one: electromyogram-triggered neuromuscular stimulation and bilateral movements. Stroke 2002;33:1589–1594

49. Reinkensmeyer DJ, Aoyagi D, Emken JL, et al. Tools for understanding and optimizing robotic gait training. J Rehabil Res Dev 2006;43:657–670

55

Robotics, Functional Electrical Stimulation, Brain–Computer Interfaces, and Locomotor Training Strategies

David M. Benglis Jr. and Allan D. Levi

Spinal cord injury (SCI) occurs in ~10,000 to 12,000 individuals per year in North America, and 250,000 individuals are living with an SCI. Life expectancy of individuals with SCI has also decreased; thus therapeutic strategies after SCI become increasingly important for establishing a person's functional independence in the community.[1,2] The treatment strategy for each patient needs to be considered on an individual basis. The severity of the injury, for example, American Spinal Injury Association (ASIA) A and the injury level (cervical versus thoracic) will dictate the varying options and goals. This review covers functional electrical stimulation (FES) and robotically assisted therapies as they relate to gait and upper extremity function in the patient with SCI. We also discuss the newer, innovative technology of the Brain Computer Interface (BCI) and its application to those patients with quadriplegia.

◆ Functional Electrical Stimulation

Gait Training

FES has been used since the 1980s to create purposeful contractions for the restoration of gait, upright posture, and cycling.[3] Chronic use of FES gait training in the SCI population may offer certain benefits such as decreasing severity and incidence of muscle spasm, increasing blood flow and muscle strength, as well as improving overall cardiovascular fitness.

One system (Parastep 1, Sigmedics, Inc., Fairborn, OH) modified from work performed by Graupe and Kohn became the first US Food and Drug Administration (FDA)-approved FES ambulation system in 1994 (**Fig. 55.1**).[4,5] The device consists of a six-channel computer-controlled stimulator, surface electrodes, and a walking frame. The "stand" command delivers a current intensity of 140 mA through surface electrodes located on gluteal muscles and quadriceps to maintain proper hip and knee flexion. A pulse is also delivered in the area of

the common peroneal nerve producing a flexion withdrawal of the leg for stepping. Patients control stand/sit functions, initiation of steps, and stimulation intensity. It is not uncommon for some people to utilize ankle/foot orthoses for added stability and to achieve good dorsiflexion.[5]

Nightingale and colleagues conducted a systematic review of previous published studies on SCI patients and the efficacy of FES gait ($n = 36$ included, $n = 496$ excluded). They concluded that there is evidence that supports the use of FES gait training in incomplete SCI populations for the benefits of

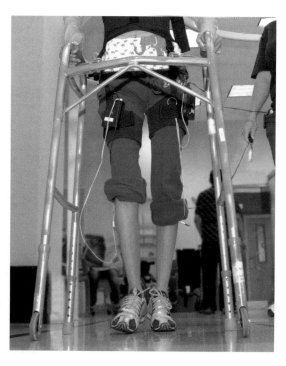

Fig. 55.1 Parastep walking device. (Sigmedics, Inc., Fairborn, OH).

improved walking ability and overall independence in the community. However, there was not sufficient evidence to support changes in bone mineral density, joint movements, and overall reduced energy cost of gait.

Muscle strength has been shown to increase in complete SCI patients. Data are insufficient to support this conclusion in the incomplete SCI populations. The reverse is true for muscle spasms, which are reduced in incomplete SCI, whereas the evidence is insufficient for complete SCI. The authors were careful to note that one of the difficult aspects of this type of analysis was the heterogeneity of the spinal cord population used in previous studies, the studies being statistically underpowered, and the absence of any randomized, controlled clinical trials.[3,6]

Cycling

Although FES was originally designed for the restoration of walking in paraplegic patients, variable responses to stimulation of the electrodes, spasticity, spasms, and the recruitment of different muscle groups required for ambulation provide challenges to its practical application. FES cycling has evolved as a therapeutic tool for the rehabilitation of those persons with paraplegia. In contrast to FES gait training exercises, FES cycling can be maintained for longer periods of time, and fall risk is minimal.[7,8]

The patient places electrodes over opposing muscle groups; the quadriceps and hamstrings and the plantarflexors and dorsiflexors of the ankle. The legs are then placed in a rigid orthosis that restricts lateral bending movements at the knees and controls the movement. Electrode stimulation intensity is controlled by a throttle on the steering handle.[7]

Muscle changes are evident following FES cycling. In contrast to the SCI patient, the quadriceps in normal subjects have similar distributions of type I (slow fatigable) and type II (fast fatigable) fibers.[9,10] After SCI, type II fibers predominate because the maintenance of type I fibers is dependent upon maintaining a certain level of activity.[11,12] Disuse atrophy begins soon after injury due to decreased neural innervation and decreased physical activity, and the changes are most pronounced in the large postural muscles.[9,11,13–15] Low densities of capillaries are also seen following SCI with consequent poor vascular perfusion.[16] This low muscle mass increases the likelihood of developing pressure ulcers.[17] Patients also experience dissatisfaction with their body image following SCI.[7]

Following an FES cycling program instituted for several weeks, Gerrits et al have demonstrated restoration of muscle bulk and strength and a return of the contractile properties of the quadriceps muscle toward normal.[18] Increases in capillary numbers are also seen.[19] Although these dramatic changes are seen within the muscle, Newham points out that patients' power output remains too low in FES cycling for travel on rough surfaces or hills.[7] The effects of FES cycling on bone mineral density remain unclear, with some studies showing an increase and others demonstrating no change or even decreases.[7,20]

Certain criteria should be met before one can perform FES cycling. They include the ability to transfer oneself from wheelchair to bike, having adequate range of motion in the leg joints, and not having extremities that are severely spastic. Patients must also take into account the time for electrode application, connection of cables, and transfer which add a significant amount of time to the exercise scheduled.[7]

Upper Extremity

FES for the restoration of motor function in the upper extremity has the potential of enabling those patients with quadriplegia the ability to restore important hand functions required in daily life. Basic concepts of all FES upper extremity devices include a controller and the FES system with electrodes. There are multiple systems available and the electrodes may be placed on the surface, within a brace, or percutaneously.

Complete implants are also available but require the patient to undergo a surgical procedure and are expensive. An implanted stimulator is placed within the axilla with electrode leads going subcutaneously to relevant muscle groups in the forearm and hand. A shoulder-mounted joystick allows the patient to control movements of the arm. One complete system (Free Hand System, Neuro Control Corp., Valley View, OH) reconstructs two types of grasping motions; finger and thumb flexion, as well as thumb adduction.[21–23]

◆ Robotically Assisted Rehabilitation

The goals of robotically based systems for treatment of SCI are similar to the goals of FES systems: (1) to prevent muscle atrophy, (2) to improve coordination, (3) to learn new motion strategies, and (4) to recover some motor function. Advantages to traditional "one-on-one" therapy sessions are that the use of the robot allows for more training sessions per week and an increased time period of the actual session.[24] A plausible future scenario may be the therapist that oversees multiple patients exercising with robotic assistance.

Robotic Gait Training Strategies

Robotic gait assistance devices or driven (i.e., motorized) gait orthoses (DGOs) consist of an exoskeleton that fits over a patient's legs and assists the physical therapist in gait training SCI patients. The robot is designed to allow for a greater ratio among therapists and patients in contrast to traditional body-weight support (BWS) devices that use harness-counterweight systems and a motorized treadmill and can require the assistance of up to three people.[25–28] As suggested in animal studies, this therapy may also provide appropriate sensory clues for motor pattern generation and return to function in incomplete SCI.[25,29]

The Lokomat (Hocoma, Inc., Zurich, Switzerland), a computer-controlled exoskeleton, approximates human gait and stabilizes the lower limbs and pelvis in complete or incomplete SCI patients (**Fig. 55.2**).[26,30] Wirz et al conducted a multicenter study of 20 patients with incomplete SCI utilizing the Lokomat DGO (ASIA grades C, $n = 9$ and D, $n = 11$). The majority of the patients ($n = 16$) were ambulatory prior to the study. Patients underwent an 8-week robotic training period (3 to 5 times per week, 45 minutes per session). In this small study they concluded that the DGO resulted in significant changes in the subjects' gait velocity, endurance, and performance of functional tasks. There were no changes, however, in the use of walking aids, orthoses, or external physical assistance following conclusion of the study.[25]

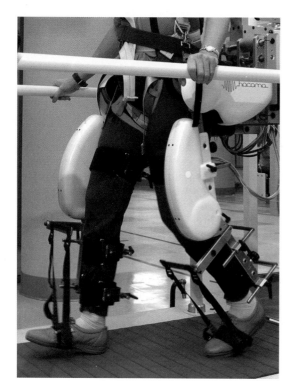

Fig. 55.2 Lokomat (Hocoma, Inc., Zurich, Switzerland).

Robotically Assisted Training of Upper Extremity Movements

Robotic systems for upper extremity rehabilitation vary in complexity and are categorized into three primary forms. Passive systems stabilize the upper extremity and fix it in a certain position, whereas active devices utilize electromechanical, pneumatic, and hydraulic forces to actively move limbs. Interactive robotic systems are similar to active systems, but they are less rigid and react to the patient's efforts.[24]

Requirements for robotically assisted therapy of the upper extremity are that the device is not overly cumbersome, its motions reflect common human movements, and its size is adapted to allow maximal movements at the relevant joints. Home-based systems are also available consisting of mobile service robots to assist manipulators and can be mounted the patient's wheelchair.[24,31]

One of the first developed and most basic robotic upper extremity assist devices was the Hand–Object–Hand Rehabilitator. It consisted of two vertical handles on a tabletop and allowed for completion of bimanual tasks by the subject with powered assistance to one hand.[32] More complex robotic systems include the commonly used MIT-Manus (MIT, Cambridge, MA) and more recently developed ARMin device.[33,34] The MIT-Manus consists of a robot-mounted handle that is gripped by the patient. Two-dimensional movements are facilitated by the patient's hand, while force and position sensors on the handle feed impedance controllers to make movements smoother. Randomized, controlled trials on stroke patients with hemiparesis make up the majority of the literature with this device; however, patients with incomplete quadriplegia may also derive a therapeutic benefit from use of the MIT-Manus.[24,35]

The ARMin consists of a wall-mounted robotic system that consists of a distal exoskeleton structure where the patient places the arm within the shell. Movements allowed are flexion/extension and certain rotational movements about the shoulder. A computer screen in front of the patient promotes goal-oriented tasks much in the same manner that a physical therapist would at a one-on-one training session.[24,33]

◆ Brain–Computer Interfaces

Brain–computer interfaces (BCIs) are an emerging technology that translates the brain's electrical activity into meaningful commands to assist patients with SCI, neuromuscular disorders, amyotrophic lateral sclerosis (ALS), brainstem stroke, and cerebral palsy. In most studies, subjects could be trained to move a computer cursor or select a letter from a keyboard solely by controlling their own brain-derived electrical wave forms modified over time with feedback and training. The goal of this technology is to allow those persons with severely restricted lifestyles due to a neurological deficit (ventilator dependent, "locked in" syndrome) to convey their wishes to caregivers, operate computer-based programs, and potentially control movements of a robotic arm.[36] The speed of the responses with noninvasive BCIs is approximately one third as fast as the able-bodied (personal correspondence with Wolpaw JR, Wadsworth Center, NY. Correspondence Sept. 2007).

The two types of BCIs are invasive and noninvasive. Noninvasive BCIs derive the user's intent from scalp-recorded electroencephalographic (EEG) electrode activity.[36–38] Invasive BCIs include the direct placement of electrodes on the brain surface and derive the user's intent from neuronal action potentials created within the brain. Invasive BCIs are primarily experimental and have been studied in primates.[39–41] Many groups believe that despite the risks of surgical morbidity from the invasive BCIs, they represent the only opportunity for real-time control of the patient's arm, a robotic arm, or neuroprosthesis.[36,42–44]

Wolpaw and McFarland demonstrated that a noninvasive BCI in two patients with SCI could provide multidimensional control similar to ranges reported in invasive studies for non-human primates. They concluded that over multiple sessions, the user developed better EEG control, and the computer focused on those rhythms that the user was better able to control. In addition, the cursor movements over multiple sessions become more of an automatic gesture rather than the application of thought-produced "motor imagery" required in earlier sessions.[36]

◆ Summary

Following complete SCI, adult mammals exhibit high levels of function with regard to standing and stepping without supraspinal input. Moreover, improvement in motor function is significantly dependent on the type of motor training or experience postinjury. Spinal automaticity is the ability of the spinal cord to perform complex tasks (i.e., the activation of extensor muscles with increased bearing of loads on the body) without conscious thought. In the patient without SCI, supraspinal input, central pattern generation (CPG), and continuous sensory input work in conjunction to perform these complex tasks.[45]

Following SCI, there may be a certain degree of neuronal plasticity derived from existing pathways that enables a continuation of oscillatory motor output (i.e., CPG) in response to peripheral sensory input.[45] For example, the human lumbosacral spinal cord responds to loading conditions by generating efferent outputs for stepping (with decreasing body weight support, a patient's electromyographic amplitudes increase in the plantar flexors at the ankle).[46] Modulation of lower extremity loads in SCI patients by electrical stimulation or robotic exoskeletons could potentially alter the manner in which the nervous system recovers as well as improve overall cardiovascular health and concepts of body image.[5,7,45]

The approach to therapy of the upper extremities in SCI often focuses on the restoration by device assistance (FES or robotic) of certain tasks of daily living, increasing muscle mass, and maintaining mobility of joints.[21-23] Because the upper extremities are not load-bearing structures, the same principals of automaticity and plasticity as seen in the lower extremities in experimental mammals and human subjects may not necessarily apply.

In this review, we have covered the concepts of functional electrical stimulation and robotically assisted therapies as they relate to gait and upper extremity function and therapeutic strategy in the patient with SCI. One proposed strategy is an augmentation of current therapy regimes, allowing therapists to oversee multiple individuals.

Cost and funding for these modalities are important issues, as are the costs of providing health care to an individual with SCI. Nowadays, a person who has an SCI at age 20 has an average life expectancy of 37 to 44 years following the injury.[47] At discharge from rehabilitation 29% of SCI individuals are ASIA D. This group and ASIA C class SCI have the greatest chance of ambulating one day and achieving high levels of independence with the assistance of rehabilitation.[2]

For patients with high cervical ASIA A SCI, BCIs are an emerging technology that may one day be an integral factor in establishing a person's independence within the community. Currently, however, there are several practical concerns, including user variability, access, and cost issues.

References

1. Nobunaga AIGB, Go BK, Karunas RB. Recent demographic and injury trends in people served by the Model Spinal Cord Injury Care Systems. Arch Phys Med Rehabil 1999;80:1372–1382

2. Barbeau HNS, Nadeau S, Garneau C. Physical determinants, emerging concepts, and training approaches in gait of individuals with spinal cord injury. J Neurotrauma 2006;23:571–585

3. Nightingale EJRJ, Raymond J, Middleton JW, Crosbie J, Davis GM. Benefits of FES gait in a spinal cord injured population. Spinal Cord 2007;45:646–657

4. Graupe DKK, Kohn KH. A critical review of EMG-controlled electrical stimulation in paraplegics. Crit Rev Biomed Eng 1987;15:187–210

5. Klose KJJP, Jacobs PL, Broton JG, et al. Evaluation of a training program for persons with SCI paraplegia using the Parastep 1 ambulation system, I: Ambulation performance and anthropometric measures. Arch Phys Med Rehabil 1997;78:789–793

6. Ijzerman MJBG, Baardman G, Hermens HJ, Veltink PH, Boom HB, Zilvold G. Comparative trials on hybrid walking systems for people with paraplegia: an analysis of study methodology. Prosthet Orthot Int 1999;23:260–273

7. Newham DJDN. FES cycling. Acta Neurochir Suppl 2007;97:395–402

8. Petrofsky JSPC, Phillips CA. The use of functional electrical stimulation for rehabilitation of spinal cord injured patients. Cent Nerv Syst Trauma 1984;1:57–74

9. Burnham RTMT, Martin T, Stein R, Bell G, MacLean I, Steadward R. Skeletal muscle fibre type transformation following spinal cord injury. Spinal Cord 1997;35:86–91

10. Round JMBF, Barr FM, Moffat B, Jones DA. Fibre areas and histochemical fibre types in the quadriceps muscle of paraplegic subjects. J Neurol Sci 1993;116:207–211

11. Castro MJAD, Apple DF Jr, Rogers S, Dudley GA. Influence of complete spinal cord injury on skeletal muscle mechanics within the first 6 months of injury. Eur J Appl Physiol 2000;81:128–131

12. Gerrits HL, De Haan A, Hopman MT, van Der Woude LH, Jones DA, Sargeant AJ. Contractile properties of the quadriceps muscle in individuals with spinal cord injury. Muscle Nerve 1999;22:1249–1256

13. Gordon TMJ, Mao J. Muscle atrophy and procedures for training after spinal cord injury. Phys Ther 1994;74:50–60

14. Thomas CKZE, Zaidner EY, Calancie B, Broton JG, Bigland-Ritchie BR. Muscle weakness, paralysis, and atrophy after human cervical spinal cord injury. Exp Neurol 1997;148:414–423

15. Roy RRBD, Baldwin KM, Edgerton VR. The plasticity of skeletal muscle: effects of neuromuscular activity. Exerc Sport Sci Rev 1991;19:269–312

16. Davis GM. Exercise capacity of individuals with paraplegia. Med Sci Sports Exerc 1993;25:423–432

17. Mawson ARSF, Siddiqui FH, Biundo JJ Jr. Enhancing host resistance to pressure ulcers: a new approach to prevention. Prev Med 1993;22: 433–450

18. Gerrits HL, de Haan A, Sargeant AJ, Dallmeijer A, Hopman MT. Altered contractile properties of the quadriceps muscle in people with spinal cord injury following functional electrical stimulated cycle training. Spinal Cord 2000;38:214–223

19. Gerrits HL, de Haan A, Sargeant AJ, van Langen H, Hopman MT. Peripheral vascular changes after electrically stimulated cycle training in people with spinal cord injury. Arch Phys Med Rehabil 2001;82:832–839

20. Eser P, Telley I, Lechner HE, Knecht H, Stussi E. Effects of electrical stimulation-induced cycling on bone mineral density in spinal cord-injured patients. Eur J Clin Invest 2003;33:412–419

21. Morita IKM, Kanno T. Reconstruction of upper limb motor function using functional electrical stimulation (FES). Acta Neurochir Suppl 2007;97:403–407

22. Keith MWPP, Peckham PH, Thrope GB, et al. Implantable functional neuromuscular stimulation in the tetraplegic hand. J Hand Surg [Am] 1989;14:524–530

23. Peckham PHKN, Keith MW, Kilgore KL, et al; Implantable Neuroprosthesis Research Group. Efficacy of an implanted neuroprosthesis for restoring hand grasp in tetraplegia: a multicenter study. Arch Phys Med Rehabil 2001;82:1380–1388

24. Riener R. Robot-aided rehabilitation of neural function in the upper extremities. Acta Neurochir Suppl 2007;97:465–471

25. Wirz MZD, Zemon DH, Rupp R, et al. Effectiveness of automated locomotor training in patients with chronic incomplete spinal cord injury: a multicenter trial. Arch Phys Med Rehabil 2005;86:672–680

26. Israel JFCD, Campbell DD, Kahn JH, Hornby TG. Metabolic costs and muscle activity patterns during robotic- and therapist-assisted treadmill walking in individuals with incomplete spinal cord injury. Phys Ther 2006;86:1466–1478

27. Behrman ALHS, Harkema SJ. Locomotor training after human spinal cord injury: a series of case studies. Phys Ther 2000;80:688–700

28. Werner C, Treig T, Konrad M, Hesse S. Treadmill training with partial body weight support and an electromechanical gait trainer for restoration of gait in subacute stroke patients: a randomized crossover study. Stroke 2002;33:2895–2901

29. Rossignol, S. Neural Control of Stereotypic Limb Movements: Handbook of Physiology Exercise: Regulation and Integration of Multiple Systems. Bethesda: American Physiological Society; 1996

30. Hesse SUD, Uhlenbrock D, Werner C, Bardeleben A. A mechanized gait trainer for restoring gait in nonambulatory subjects. Arch Phys Med Rehabil 2000;81:1158–1161

31. Kwee HDJ, Smit J, de Moed AT, van Woerden J, Kolk LVD. The Manus wheelchair-mounted manipulator: developments toward a production mode. Proceedings of the 3rd International Conference of the Association for Advancement of Rehabilitation Technology. Montreal, Quebec, Canada, June 25–30, 1988. 1988:460–462

32. Lum PS, Lehman SL. Robotic assist devices for bimanual physical therapy: preliminary experiments. IEEE Trans Rehabil Eng 1993;1:185–191

33. Nef TRR. Design of the Arm Rehabilitation Robot ARMin. Internal report. Zurich: Automatic Control Laboratory, Swiss Federal Institute of Technology (ETH); 2004

34. Hogan N. Impedance control: an approach to manipulation, parts I, II, III. J Dyn Syst Meas Control 1985;107:1–23

35. Hesse SSH, Schmidt H, Werner C, Bardeleben A. Upper and lower extremity robotic devices for rehabilitation and for studying motor control. Curr Opin Neurol 2003;16:705–710

36. Wolpaw JR Jr, McFarland DJ. Control of a two-dimensional movement signal by a noninvasive brain–computer interface in humans. Proc Natl Acad Sci U S A 2004;101:17849–17854

37. Birbaumer NGN, Ghanayim N, Hinterberger T, et al. A spelling device for the paralysed. Nature 1999;398:297–298

38. Pfurtscheller GNC, Neuper C, Müller GR, et al. Graz-BCI: state of the art and clinical applications. IEEE Trans Neural Syst Rehabil Eng 2003; 11:177–180

39. Wessberg JSC, Stambaugh CR, Kralik JD, et al. Real-time prediction of hand trajectory by ensembles of cortical neurons in primates. Nature 2000;408:361–365

40. Chapin JKMK, Moxon KA, Markowitz RS, Nicolelis MA. Real-time control of a robot arm using simultaneously recorded neurons in the motor cortex. Nat Neurosci 1999;2:664–670

41. Pesaran BPJ, Pezaris JS, Sahani M, Mitra PP, Andersen RA. Temporal structure in neuronal activity during working memory in macaque parietal cortex. Nat Neurosci 2002;5:805–811

42. Fetz EE. Real-time control of a robotic arm by neuronal ensembles. Nat Neurosci 1999;2:583–584

43. Chapin JK. Neural prosthetic devices for quadriplegia. Curr Opin Neurol 2000;13:671–675

44. Pfurtscheller GMG, Müller GR, Pfurtscheller J, Gerner HJ, Rupp R. "Thought'—control of functional electrical stimulation to restore hand grasp in a patient with tetraplegia. Neurosci Lett 2003;351:33–36

45. Edgerton VRTN, Tillakaratne NJ, Bigbee AJ, de Leon RD, Roy RR. Plasticity of the spinal neural circuitry after injury. Annu Rev Neurosci 2004;27:145–167

46. Harkema SJHS, Hurley SL, Patel UK, Requejo PS, Dobkin BH, Edgerton VR. Human lumbosacral spinal cord interprets loading during stepping. J Neurophysiol 1997;77:797–811

47. DeVivo MJ, Krause JS, Lammertse DP. Recent trends in mortality and causes of death among persons with spinal cord injury. Arch Phys Med Rehabil 1999;80:1411–1419

56

Translational Clinical Research in Acute Spinal Cord Injury

Gregory W. J. Hawryluk, Brian K. Kwon, and Michael G. Fehlings

Spinal cord injury (SCI) is one of the most physically and psychologically devastating of injuries, and it remains so despite considerable advances in many areas of medical and surgical care. The societal costs associated with the care of chronic SCI costs exceed $7 billion annually,[1,2] but it is the immeasurable cost of human suffering related to impaired ambulation, sensation, bowel, bladder, and sexual function that provides the most compelling rationale for vigorous research efforts to establish treatments for this devastating injury.

Intensive research over the past decade has seen several promising therapies enter the clinical trials process, or in an increasingly worrisome trend, emerge in poorly controlled human treatment protocols that lack a formalized investigational structure.[3] The next decade will likely witness an unparalleled translation of this new knowledge into the clinical arena. None of the promising treatments that have undergone rigorous clinical evaluation have thus far revealed themselves to be convincingly effective at promoting neurological recovery.[4–7] Nonetheless, we have learned a great deal from these clinical trials, and a new optimism surrounds current experimental therapies aimed at improving neurological function after SCI.

Here, we will review past clinical trials in acute SCI, consider the lessons that this experience has taught the SCI community, and discuss human clinical trials that have recently begun or are being planned.

◆ Completed Prospective, Randomized, Controlled Trials for Acute Spinal Cord Injury

Several pharmacological agents designed to attenuate secondary injury mechanisms have been evaluated in large, multicenter, human clinical trials. Disappointingly, these did not reveal significant neurological benefit, despite the promising preclinical animal data that substantiated their clinical evaluation. The reasons for this discrepancy between promising animal data and negative human experience are complex and not well understood, but embody the challenge (and frustration) of translating bench-top research into the clinical domain—a challenge that has been met with equal if not greater disappointment in many other neurological disorders (stroke being the most conspicuous example).[8] Studied agents include methylprednisolone sodium succinate (MPSS) and the related compound tirilizad mesylate, GM-1 ganglioside, thyrotropin releasing hormone (TRH), gacyclidine, naloxone, and nimodipine (**Table 56.2**). These clinical trials, which unfortunately were largely negative, have been reviewed extensively in previous reviews,[5,7,9] and therefore will be recounted only briefly here in prelude to a description of ongoing clinical trials and a discussion of the lessons that have been learned about the translation of preclinical animal-based technology into human patients.

Table 56.1 ASIA Impairment Scale (AIS)

A	Complete: No motor or sensory function is preserved in the sacral segments S4–S5
B	Incomplete: Sensory but not motor function is impaired below the neurological level and includes the sacral segments S4–S5
C	Incomplete: Motor function is preserved below the neurological level, and more than half of key muscles below the neurological level have a muscle grade less than 3
D	Incomplete: Motor function is preserved below the neurological level, and at least half of key muscles below the neurological level have a muscle grade of 3 or more
E	Normal: Motor and sensory function are normal

Source: Marino RJ, Barros T, Brering-Sorensen F, Burns SP, Donovan WH, Graves DE, Haak M, Hudson LM, Priebe MM. ASIA Neurological Standards Committee 2002 International standards for neurological classification of spinal cord injury. J Spinal Cord Med 2003;26:S50–56. Adapted with permission.

Table 56.2 Recently Completed Clinical Trials

Trial Name	Year	*n*	SCI Type, Treatment Window	Treatment Arms	Conclusions
NASCIS I	1984	330	I, 48h	MPSS 100 mg × 10 d MPSS 1000 mg × 10 d	No difference.
NACSIS II	1990	487	C/I, 12h	MPSS (24 h) Naloxone Placebo	Improved recovery if treated with MPSS within 8 h of injury. Naloxone negative.
Maryland GM-1	1991	34	I, 72h	GM-1 Placebo	Improved neurological recovery with GM-1.
TRH	1995	20	C/I, 2h	TRH Placebo	Improved neurological recovery with TRH.
NASCIS III	1997	499	I, 12h	MPSS (24 h) MPSS (48 h) MPSS bolus then TM	Improved neurological recovery with MPSS, TM not superior to MPSS.
Nimodipine	1998	100	C/I, 6h	Nimodipine MPSS (24 h) Nimodipine + MPSS (24 h) Placebo	No difference.
Gacyclidine	1999	280	C/I, 2h	Gacyclidine (0.005 mg/kg) Gacyclidine (0.01 mg/kg) Gacyclidine (0.02 mg/kg) Placebo	Trend to improved motor recovery with incomplete cervical injuries.
Sygen GM-1	2001	797	I, 72h	MPSS + low dose GM-1 MPSS + high dose GM-1 MPSS + placebo	Negative primary outcomes, trend to improved secondary outcomes.

Note: Further trials are not planned for any of the agents presented in this table, to the knowledge of the authors.

Abbreviations: C or I, inclusion of complete or incomplete SCI patients in the trial, respectively; d, days; GM-1, monosialotetrahexosylganglioside also known as Sygen; h, hours; MPSS, methylprednisolone sodium succinate; *n*, total number of patients included in study; NASCIS, National Acute Spinal Cord Injury Study; SCI, spinal cord injury; TM, tirilizad mesylate; TRH, thyrotropin releasing hormone.

Methylprednisolone Sodium Succinate (Solu-Medrol)

Arguably the most extensively studied class of drug in neurotrauma research, glucocorticoids, with their myriad of potential neuroprotective effects, have endured a protracted and controversial history in clinical SCI care. Following the accumulation of preclinical data[10] that was generally (albeit not universally) supportive of a substantive neuroprotective role for steroids in animal models of acute SCI, methylprednisolone was studied in five prospective human acute SCI trials, including the three landmark National Acute SCI Study (NASCIS) trials.[11] The end result was, of course, that high-dose methylprednisolone became entrenched in the clinical management of acute SCI as a "standard of care," a status largely attributable to the results of the NASCIS II trial which, in 1990, reported a small but significant neurological improvement in patients who began to receive the high-dose regimen (30 mg/kg bolus then 5.4 mg/kg infusion for 24 hours) within 8 hours of their injury. Two other prospective human SCI trials involving corticosteroids have been published, including the work of Otani et al[12] and Pointillart et al.[13] Otani et al[12] noted some neurological benefit from methylprednisolone administration, whereas Pointillart et al[13] reported no benefit, although both of these studies were small and plagued by substantial methodological problems that limit their interpretation as either positive or negative studies.

Intense and systematic scrutiny of the data that supported the administration of methylprednisolone for acute SCI (in particular the NASCIS trials) has led to tremendous controversy around its use.[14–19] Several issues fueled this debate. First, much criticism was directed at the conduct and interpretation of the NASCIS II data, which, when distilled to its original design, failed to demonstrate a neurological benefit in those randomized to methylprednisolone versus those who received placebo. A very modest neurological benefit was detected in the secondary analysis of a small fraction of the total study cohort who received the drug within 8 hours of injury (the authors of this study maintain that this was planned a priori analysis).[20] Second, both the NASCIS II, and in particular the NASCIS III, trials pointed to a high rate of adverse events such as sepsis, wound infection, gastrointestinal (GI) hemorrhage, and death in the steroid-treated patients,[15] which should come as no surprise when considering the large doses of steroids utilized in these protocols. As such, the potential risk of harm associated with high-dose methylprednisolone became highlighted and was reflected in the American Association of Neurological Surgeons/Congress of Neurological Surgeons (AANS/CNS) systematic review of this literature in 2002, which concluded that

"treatment with methylprednisolone for either 24 or 48 hours is recommended as an option in the treatment of patients with acute spinal cord injuries that should be undertaken only with the knowledge that the evidence suggesting harmful side effects is more consistent than any suggestion of clinical benefit."[21]

This was but one of a myriad of reviews on steroids for acute SCI that were published in the early 2000s, but this intellectual "piling on" of sorts has not necessarily provided clarity to the field of acute SCI neuroprotection—a field that is

Table 56.3 Evidence-Based Recommendations for the Use of Methylprednisolone Sodium Succinate

Clinical Scenario	Level of Evidence	Recommended Treatment
Acute nonpenetrating SCI (< 3 hours following injury)	Class II (RCT with negative primary analysis; benefits limited to subgroup analysis)	MPSS should be given as per NASCIS II protocol: 30 mg/kg IV loading dose within the first hour followed by 5.4 mg/kg/hr IV over the next 23 hours.
Acute nonpenetrating SCI (> 3 hours, but < 8 hours following injury)	Class II (RCT with negative primary analysis; benefits limited to subgroup analysis)	MPSS should be given as per NASCIS III protocol: 30 mg/kg IV loading dose within the first hour followed by a 48-hour infusion of 5.4 mg/kg/hr.
Acute nonpenetrating SCI (> 8 hours after injury)	Class I (RCT showing a lack of an effect; potentially deleterious)	MPSS should *not* be administered (standard).
Acute penetrating SCI	Class III (lack of an effect; increased wound complications)	MPSS is *not* recommended (option).

Source: Fehlings M. Editorial: recommendations regarding the use of methylprednisolone in acute spinal cord injury: making sense out of the controversy. Spine J 2001;26(Suppl 24):S56-S57. Adapted with permission.

Abbreviations: IV, intravenous; MPSS, methylprednisolone sodium succinate; NASCIS, National Acute Spinal Cord Injury Study; RCT, randomized controlled trial; SCI, spinal cord injury.

not only otherwise currently devoid of any other "treatment options," but is also plagued by public and medicolegal perception that steroids induce significant neurological recovery after acute SCI (a perception that is simply not true, irrespective of how one views the debate about steroids). A survey of North American Spine Society members published in 2006 revealed that 86% of respondents continue to administer methylprednisolone within an 8-hour window, although of those respondents, the fear of litigation by not giving steroids exceeded (by almost 2:1) the belief that it actually improved neurological recovery.[22] A summary of our recommendations is provided in **Table 56.3**.

GM-1 Ganglioside (Sygen)

Gangliosides are complex glycolipids abundantly present in the membranes of nervous tissue. Exogenous administration of one such ganglioside, monosialotetrahexosylganglioside, also known as GM-1 or Sygen (TRB Pharma, Campinas, Brazil), was found to promote neural repair and functional recovery in several animal models, including cord-transected rats, lesioned mesostriatal dopaminergic neurons, and peripheral nerve crush injury.[23] A prospective, randomized study of 37 patients (the Maryland GM-1 Study) reported in 1991 that GM-1 treated patients achieved statistically significant improvement in American Spinal Injury Association (ASIA) (**Table 56.1**) motor score as compared with placebo controls.[24] These promising results spurred the initiation of what is to date the largest prospective, randomized, clinical trial in acute SCI, the Sygen Multi-Center Acute Spinal Cord Injury Study. This study of over 750 patients enrolled over 5 years at 28 institutions unfortunately revealed no significant difference in the primary outcome measure, which represented significant improvement on the modified Benzel walking scale—in retrospect a rather high bar to set considering the number of complete ASIA A patients enrolled in the trial.[25] GM-1 treated patients did, however, demonstrate more rapid neurological recovery as well as a trend to improved bowel/bladder function and sacral sensation. Additionally, a more pronounced neurological benefit was apparent in those patients with incomplete injuries. Despite its promise, this agent is not being manufactured for therapeutic administration and we are unaware of any plans for future trials with

this agent,[4] although the post hoc mining of this enormous bank of data has produced some invaluable insights with respect to study design (to be discussed further).

Thyrotropin Releasing Hormone

Thyrotropin releasing hormone (TRH) is a three-amino-acid peptide (glutamic acid-histidine-proline). Besides its numerous and well-described hormonal functions, TRH has been shown to antagonize several secondary-injury mediators such as excitotoxic amino acids, peptidoleukotrienes, endogenous opioids, and platelet-activating factor,[26] and it showed dose-dependent improvement in rats following experimental SCI.[27] Dr. Lawrence Pitt and colleagues reported in 1995 on the only clinical trial that has ever been conducted on TRH in acute SCI.[28] Their double-blind, placebo-controlled trial randomized both complete and incomplete injuries to TRH (0.2 mg/kg intravenous bolus followed by an hourly infusion of the same dose for 6 hours) or placebo. The trial was plagued by attrition, and only 20 patients were ultimately analyzed. Incomplete but not complete SCI patients achieved statistically significant functional improvements on the NASCIS and Sunnybrook scales, although the extremely small patient numbers make it likely that this represented a type I error. No further clinical SCI studies to investigate TRH have been initiated, although there has been some interest in its potential for traumatic brain injury.

Gacyclidine (GK-11)

With the role of excitotoxicity well established in central nervous system (CNS) trauma, antagonism of glutamate receptors would seem a rational therapy for SCI. Previous trials of antiglutamatergic agents in neurotrauma, such as the competitive antagonist Selfotel (Novartis, East Hanover, NJ), have been unsuccessful because of significant cognitive side-effects, including agitation, sedation, hallucinations, and memory deficits.[29,30] This is not surprising given that glutamate is the main excitatory neurotransmitter in the CNS. Nonetheless, the important role of excitotoxicity in the pathophysiology of acute SCI served as the rationale behind the clinical investigation of a noncompetitive NMDA receptor antagonist, gacyclidine, as a potential neuroprotective agent. Gacyclidine or GK-11 (Beaufour-Ipsen Pharma, Paris, France) is unique in its high selectivity for the PCP binding site rather than the receptor-associated channel, and had shown substantially better tolerability as compared with other NMDA antagonists.[31] Following evidence of improved function, histology, and electrophysiology in a rat model,[32] a human trial was initiated in France. A double-blind phase II trial randomized over 200 patients to receive three escalating doses of gacyclidine.[33] Although early benefit was seen in the treatment groups, this was not maintained at 1 year. At 1 year postinjury, those with incomplete cervical injuries receiving high doses of gacyclidine did exhibit a trend toward improved motor function. Because of these disappointing results, the use of this agent for SCI is no longer being pursued, although it is apparent that the study was likely underpowered to observe a treatment effect. This drug is, however, currently being used experimentally for the treatment of traumatic brain injury,[34,35] as an adjunctive treatment in organophosphate poisoning,[36] and as a novel treatment for tinnitus (patent number #20060205789).

Nimodipine

Nimodipine, an L-type calcium channel blocker, is well known for its use in the treatment of vasospasm associated with subarachnoid hemorrhage. The benefits are speculated to be derived largely from a neuroprotective mechanism rather than a smooth-muscle relaxing effect on blood vessels. The latter effect can cause hypotension and undesirable ischemia in the injured spinal cord, but with avoidance of this, animal studies of nimodipine demonstrated improvement in spinal cord function.[37] A human trial for SCI was completed in France in 1996.[38] This trial with 100 patients had four treatment arms: nimodipine, MPSS (NASCIS II protocol), both agents, and placebo. Benefit over placebo was not demonstrated in any treatment group, although again, it is quite likely that this study was underpowered to reveal a therapeutic effect.

Opioid Antagonism

The endogenous opioid, dynorphin A, is released following SCI and has demonstrated neurotoxic properties; additionally it has been shown to reduce spinal cord blood flow by nonopioid mechanisms.[39] The opioid antagonist naloxone has demonstrated improvement in spinal cord electrophysiology following experimental injury along with reduction in edema,[40,41] free-radical generation,[42] as well as decreased levels of excitotoxic amino acids.[43] In the 1980s naloxone was examined in a phase I human SCI trial. The results suggested benefit,[44] though imbalance between experimental groups was a likely confounder. A more definitive examination of this agent was performed in the NASCIS II trial[45]; although naloxone showed no benefit in overall analysis, subgroup analysis found benefit in patients treated within 8 hours of injury, as was seen with MPSS in the same trial.[46] Despite this, naloxone has not been explored in further trials.

◆ Lessons from Recently Completed Trials

A significant proportion of the controversy surrounding recent SCI trials has centered on their design and interpretation. Born from a desire to standardize the conduct of clinical trials for SCI, as well as to encourage the highest scientific and ethical standards, several authors have published recommendations for the conduct of future trials, including Tator[5] (select recommendations provided in **Table 56.4**), Cesaro,[47] and Sagen[48] with the latter two specifically addressing cell replacement therapies.

A significant and parallel effort has come from the International Campaign for Cures of Spinal Cord Injury Paralysis (ICCP). Following the meeting of an international panel of experts in Vancouver 2004, guidelines were established for the conduct of clinical trials in SCI. The result was the publication of four documents in 2007[49–52] designed to improve SCI clinical trials; a summary of these recommendations is provided in **Table 56.4**.

Table 56.4 Summary of General Recommendations for the Conduct of SCI Clinical Trials

◆ Trials of treatments that are most efficacious when given soon after injury will require larger patient numbers than those effective at later time points.[49]

◆ Trials involving motor incomplete SCI patients, or trials where an accurate assessment of AIS grade cannot be made before the start of the trial, will require large subject numbers and/or better objective assessment methods.[49]

◆ The American Spinal Injury Association impairment scale (AIS) forms the standard basis for measuring neurological outcomes.[50]

◆ An improvement in the measurable performance of a meaningful function or behavior is necessary for any therapeutic intervention to be universally accepted as clinically beneficial.[50]

◆ The SCIM assessment may be a more specific and accurate outcome tool for detecting clinical end points in SCI than the FIM.[50]

◆ Clinical trials for SCI should include blinded assessments.[51]

◆ The most rigorous and valid SCI clinical trial would be a prospective, double-blind, randomized, controlled trial utilizing appropriate placebo control subjects. However, in specific situations, it is recognized that other trial procedures may have to be considered.[52]

◆ The use of external controls in SCI clinical trials is strongly discouraged.[52]

◆ Experimental therapies should have proven benefit in more than one animal model before translation to humans.[5]

◆ Consideration should be given to employing novel trial designs such as adaptive randomization and Bayesian statistics.[5]

◆ Clinical trials require follow-up of appropriate duration: 6–12 months for neuroprotection trials, 12–24 months for regenerative therapies[5]

◆ Clinical management should follow recently published guidelines regarding acute and chronic SCI management.[5]

Abbreviations: FIM, Functional Independence Measure; SCI, spinal cord injury; SCIM, Spinal Cord Independence Measure.

These detailed documents provide recommendations related to (1) statistical power needed for clinical trials in relation to injury severity and timing of administration of the experimental therapy, (2) appropriate clinical trial outcome measures, (3) inclusion/exclusion criteria and ethics, and (4) clinical trial design. As mentioned earlier, the statistical "mining" of the 780-patient Sygen database has been particularly valuable for defining the variance in spontaneous neurological recovery among patients deemed to have the same injury severity.[49] In essence, these data have helped to quantify what we already knew was true: (1) that the motor recovery of patients with complete injuries is less than that of incomplete injuries, but is more predictable (i.e., has less variation), and (2) that the longer one waits after the injury to assign the ASIA grade of neurological severity, the less variation there is in neurological recovery. The converse to this statement is unfortunately also true for neuroprotection research—that the earlier one examines a patient and assigns an ASIA grade, the greater the variation in neurological recovery. Hence, if one were looking to detect a small improvement in motor function in patients deemed ASIA A at 6 months postinjury, you would need far fewer patients than if you were looking to detect that same motor improvement in patients deemed ASIA A at 6 hours postinjury due to the small variation in neurological recovery in the former and the large variation in the latter. Unfortunately, clinical trials of neuroprotective interventions require the latter. The ICCP initiative to characterize inclusion and exclusion criteria, clinical outcome measurements, and spontaneous neurological recovery, will be extremely helpful for the SCI community in its further clinical evaluation of novel therapies.

The ICCP has produced an additional document designed for patients considering enrollment in an SCI clinical trial.[53] In part, this work was motivated by the fact that recent years have seen patients travel appreciable distances at great personal cost and risk to seek cell or tissue transplantation therapies,[54] which are at best unproven and at worst very dangerous.[54,55] This excellent resource aims to educate patients about the clinical trials process and encourages them to participate in studies of high scientific and ethical quality.

Clinical trial networks are also forming that will undoubtedly play central roles in the conduct of such trials. In addition to the ICCP, several other networks have formed in recent years: the North American Clinical Trials Network, the European Union Clinical Trials Network, the China Spinal Cord Injury Clinical Network, and the recently formed Canadian Spinal Cord Injury Translational Research Network (SCI-TRN). Older networks include the US Models System, and the North American Spinal Cord Injury Study (NASCIS, no longer active). Because of the relatively low incidence of SCI, such networks will also serve to increase recruitment into clinical trials of novel therapies.

◆ Ongoing Clinical Trials

A recent search of the phrase "spinal cord injury" on the online clinical trials registry at www.clinicaltrials.gov revealed over 70 registered clinical trials. This is an incomplete list because several clinical trials that we are personally aware of are not registered on this Web site. The majority of those that are registered relate to interventions for chronic SCI and are thus not the subject of this review. Here we describe those ongoing interventional trials involving acute and subacute SCI patients that are registered on the www.clinicaltrials.gov site, and

others that we have identified and have some knowledge of (**Tables 56.5 and 56.6**).

Clinical Trials of Surgical Decompression and Nonpharmacological Interventions

Surgical Treatment of Acute Spinal Cord Injury Study

A significant body of animal research has demonstrated that early decompression of the injured spinal cord promotes improved neurological outcome[56,57] and has thus broadly substantiated the concept of "neuroprotection" in which an intervention early in the postinjury period can influence secondary injury and enhance neurological function. Additionally, the notion that a certain "window of neuroprotective opportunity" was present for acute human SCI was implied by the NASCIS trials, which pointed to distinguishable outcomes based on a time window of 8 (NASCIS II) or 3 hours postinjury (NASCIS III). It is therefore rather astonishing that, in our modern age of surgical and medical technology, a question as fundamental as whether early decompression for acute human SCI is or is not beneficial for neurological recovery remains incompletely answered.[56] Although significant animal data provided a strong theoretical support for early decompression in SCI, the 20th century came to an end with some clinicians opining that it was more prudent to *delay* spinal cord decompression in polytrauma patients, thus underscoring the surprisingly little consensus that existed on the issue of the optimal timing for surgical decompression.[58] Fueling this uncertainty was the not insignificant number of clinical studies that failed to demonstrate a neurological benefit to "early" decompression, although in this context the term *early* lacked much precision.[58]

The Surgical Treatment of Acute Spinal Cord Injury Study (STASCIS) was initiated in 2003 by Dr. Fehlings and Dr. Vaccaro of the University of Toronto and Thomas Jefferson University, respectively, to address this important question of the optimal timing of surgical decompression. Although initially planned as a prospective, randomized trial, resistance to randomizing patients to an intentionally delayed decompression led to the rolling out of this multicenter initiative as a prospective observational study. Enrollment is restricted to individuals between the ages of 16 and 70 with a traumatic cervical SCI. The accrual target is 450 patients with 2-year follow-up period postinjury, and to date, over 240 patients have been recruited. Although the final tabulation of all the data is quite some time away, early analysis of the data has suggested a benefit to early decompression. Based on evidence and a belief that there may be benefit from "ultra-early" decompression, the University of Toronto, in conjunction with the STASCIS trial, has established the practice of performing surgical decompression *immediately* following initial imaging in appropriate trauma patients (in most cases within 12 hours of injury).

Early versus Late Surgical Decompression of Central Cord Syndrome

Central cord syndrome of incomplete quadriplegia represents a uniquely challenging problem for determining the optimal timing of intervention due to the fact that most patients present without spinal instability (and hence do not necessarily

Table 56.5 Summary of Ongoing Experimental Trials for Acute and Subacute Spinal Cord Injury for which Published Documentation Is Available

Trial Name	Intervention	Lead Center/Organization	Date of Initiation	Proposed Accrual	Completed, Published Phases	Current Study Type	Clinicaltrials.gov Registration Info
STASCIS	Timing of Surgical Decompression	U of Toronto, Thomas Jefferson U, Spine Trauma Study Group	2003	450	n/a	Nonrandomized prospective observational	NR
Early and late surgery for traumatic central cord syndrome	Surgical Decompression	University of Maryland	May 2007	30	?	Phase II	NCT00475748
Oscillating Electrical Field Stimulation	Device Implantation	Indiana U Medical Center	?	20	10 patients, Phase I	Phase I/II	NR
Intravenously Instituted Hypothermia	Hypothermia (cooled to 33°C at 0.5°C/h, maintained for 48 h)	Miami	Jan. 2007	100	n/a	Phase I/II	NR
Minocycline	250 mg IV bid × 7 d	Calgary	?	?	Phase I	Phase II	NR
Riluzole	Na⁺ channel blockade, anti-glutamatergic 50 mg PO bid	U of Toronto	Late 2007	36	n/a	Phase I	NR
Leteprinim	Purine analogue 250 mg PO bid × 12 w	Neo-Therapeutics	?	?	?	?	NR
ATI-355	Nogo-blockade	Novartis	May 2006	16	n/a	Phase I	NCT00406016
Cethrin®	Rho inhibition	BioAxone Therapeutics/Alseres Pharmaceutical	Feb. 2005	50	n/a	Phase I/II	NCT00500812
Portuguese OEC Trial	OEC transplantation	Portugal	July 2001	7	Phase I	?	NR
Australian OEC Trial	OEC transplantation	Australia	Pre-2005	6	Phase I, single-blinded w/ control	?	NR
Korean BMSC Transplantation	BMSC transplantation	Inha U Hospital	2001	35	Phase I/II non-randomized	?	NR
Prague BMSC Transplantation	BMSC transplantation	Prague	?	20	?	?	NR
Human Embryonic Stem Cell Transplantation	Oligodendrocyte-differentiated cells	Geron	2008	?	n/a	Phase I	NR
PROCORD® (enrollment suspended)	Activated autologous macrophages	Proneuron	2005	61, suspended at 50	Phase I	Phase II, randomized, multicenter, controlled trial	NR

Note: To the knowledge of the authors, all therapies presented here are currently being investigated in clinical trials, or further trials are planned.

Abbreviations: ?, unpublished or unclear data; bid, twice daily administration; BMSC, bone marrow stromal cells; d, days; NR, not registered; OEC, olfactory ensheathing cells; U, University; w, weeks.

Table 56.6 Reported Human Therapy Considered Experimental, with Uncertain Methodology or Status

Trial Name	Intervention	Location	Number of Treated Patients
?	Pulsed electrical stimulation	Beijing	100+
Minocycline/tacrolimus	Coadministration	Riyadh	?
Russian OEC Transplantation	OEC transplantation	Russia	Many
Huang OEC Transplantation	? Fetal OEC transplantation	Beijing	300+
China BMSC Transplantation	BMSC transplantation	?	90
Russian BMSC Transplantation	Fetal BMSC/peripheral blood cell transplantation	2 centers	15
Schwann Cells	Cellular transplantation	2 groups in China	?

Note: Most studies presented here have been reported only by Tator.[5]

Abbreviations: ?, unpublished or unclear data; BMSC, bone marrow stromal cells; OEC, olfactory ensheathing cells.

need emergent surgery), and most experience quite substantial spontaneous neurological improvement. Attempts have therefore been made to identify factors that influence the neurological outcome after central cord syndrome[59-62] and to specifically address whether early surgery is beneficial.[63-65]

Investigators at the University of Maryland have registered a phase II, single-center, randomized clinical trial examining the role of timing of decompression in the context of central cord syndrome. This trial will seek to randomize 30 patients to decompression within 5 days or after 6 weeks of injury. The study will compare ASIA, Functional Independence Measure (FIM) and Spinal Cord Independence Measure (SCIM) scores, as well as the degree of canal compromise, spinal cord compression, and syrinx size. Patients will be followed for 1 year.

Cerebrospinal Fluid Drainage

Investigators at the University of British Columbia have initiated a pilot study to evaluate cerebrospinal fluid (CSF) drainage as a potential neuroprotective strategy after acute spinal cord injury (clinicaltrials.gov identifier NCT00135278). This is a safety and feasibility study to examine the practice of draining CSF through a lumbar intrathecal line to lower CSF pressure and raise spinal cord perfusion pressure, as is done during thoracoabdominal aortic aneurysm surgery. In the latter setting, CSF drainage has been found to significantly reduce the incidence of ischemic paraplegia, suggesting that the improvement in spinal cord perfusion pressure achieved by lowering intrathecal pressure can in fact attenuate clinically significant ischemia and provide a neuroprotective effect.[66] The important role of ischemia in acute traumatic SCI provides the biological rationale for investigating such CSF drainage in this setting. The study has enrolled just over 20 patients to date, and there have been no adverse events attributed to the drainage of CSF (e.g., neurological

deterioration, meningitis, headache/nausea/vomiting). Neurological recovery is a secondary measure in this pilot study, and these data are not currently available (although the planned enrollment will certainly not be sufficient to make strong statements about the influence of CSF drainage on neurological outcome).

Hypothermia

Hypothermia has long been explored for its putative neuroprotective effects, which include a reduction in metabolic rate, extracellular glutamate, vasogenic edema, apoptosis, neutrophil and macrophage invasion and activation, and oxidative stress.[67-75] Both regional and systemic hypothermia have demonstrated mixed results in animal models of traumatic SCI,[76,77] and only regional (not systemic) hypothermia has been described in acute human SCI, albeit last reported in 1984.[78] Researchers from the Miami Project to Cure Paralysis are currently conducting a study to explore the role of systemic hypothermia in SCI. This clinical trial, reportedly ongoing since 2007, involves rapid cooling with chilled intravenous saline to drop the core body temperature to around 34°C. Experimental subjects will be compared with historical controls. The well-known risks of systemic hypothermia, which include coagulopathy, sepsis, or cardiac dysrythmia, are important considerations in such an approach. Results of this trial are pending and anxiously awaited.

Oscillating Field Stimulation

Neurite outgrowth is influenced by electrical voltage gradients, with growth being stimulated toward the cathode (negative pole) of such electric fields.[79,80] To capitalize upon this within the injured spinal cord, researchers at the Indiana University Medical Center developed an implantable device to create an electrical field along the rostrocaudal axis of the spinal cord. Because neurite outgrowth is stimulated only toward the negative pole, the device "oscillates" to change the polarity of the field every 15 minutes so as to promote axonal growth in both directions. This oscillating field stimulator (OFS) was subjected to a 10-patient pilot study in subacute SCI patients, which was reported in 2005.[81] After receiving the NASCIS III protocol of methylprednisolone, these complete SCI patients with injuries from C5 to T10 were implanted with the OFS device within 18 days of injury. The device was removed at 15 weeks postinjury. The authors reported improvements in motor and sensory function 1 year postinjury that they deemed favorable to that observed in patients enrolled in the NASCIS III trials. Caution, however, should be exercised when attempting to compare the neurological recovery in such a small cohort with that of "historical controls" from a distinct clinical trial protocol. Nonetheless, the complications noted in this trial were low (one wound infection and one device failure); the US Food and Drug Administration (FDA) has apparently approved further study of this intervention, and we await additional data from these investigators.

According to Tator, a similar trial involving pulsed electrical stimulation has been conducted on 100 patients in Beijing by investigators Xu and Liu.[5] The details and results of this work are uncertain, however.

Pharmacological Trials

Minocycline

Minocycline is a synthetic tetracycline derivative that is commonly used in the treatment of conditions such as acne and rosacea. It has also been shown to be neuroprotective in animal models of many nervous system disorders, including stroke, Parkinson disease, Huntington disease, amyotrophic lateral sclerosis, and multiple sclerosis.[82] Several independent laboratories have reported that minocycline reduces secondary damage and improves functional recovery in different animal models of SCI.[83–86] Its mechanism of action in SCI appears to be mediated in part by the inhibition of microglial inhibition,[87–90] in addition to which it also appears to have antiapoptotic properties.[89,91]

These promising preclinical results stimulated the initiation of a phase I human trial of intravenous minocycline (Minocin, Wyeth, Philadelphia, PA) at the University of Calgary, led by Drs. Steven Casha and John Hurlbert. This is a prospective, randomized, placebo-controlled trial, and patient recruitment into this trial is still ongoing at the time of this writing. Patients are randomized within 12 hours of their injury. The neurological outcomes from this trial are pending, but we are anxiously awaiting the results of this trial and the determination of whether a phase II study is warranted.

Investigators at Riyadh Armed Forces Hospital, Saudi Arabia, have reportedly also initiated a clinical trial assessing the effectiveness of minocycline when administered in combination with the immunosuppressant tacrolimus (FK506), which inhibits the enzyme calcineurin.[5] This trial apparently involves acute SCI, but little other information is available concerning this trial.

Riluzole

Riluzole, or Rilutek (Sanofi-Aventis, Bridgewater, NJ) is a benzothiazole anticonvulsant that exhibits protection from secondary injury by dual mechanisms and additionally demonstrates synergy with MPSS.[92] Riluzole blocks voltage-sensitive sodium channels whose persistent activation following injury has been associated with cellular toxicity and degeneration of neural tissue.[93] It also exhibits antiglutamatergic properties by antagonizing presynaptic, calcium-dependent glutamate release.[94] Use of this agent for SCI will be assisted by the fact that riluzole has been licensed for patients with amyotrophic lateral sclerosis (ALS) for ~10 years.[95] Riluzole has demonstrated modest efficacy in ALS according to a recent Cochrane review,[96] perhaps prolonging life by 2 to 3 months. In animal models of SCI, riluzole has demonstrated neuroprotective effects when administered as late as 10 days following injury as was demonstrated recently in a root avulsion model,[93,97] and it appears to have a neuroprotective effect on neurons but not glia.[98] Recent in vitro studies also suggest that riluzole may promote outgrowth of sensory neurons in addition to its neuroprotective effects.[99]

Based on these promising experimental results, a human multicenter SCI trial has just begun in conjunction with the North American Clinical Trials Network. This safety trial will involve 36 participants with ASIA A, B, or C injuries between neurological levels C4 and T10 within 12 hours of injury. Patients will be given riluzole orally in doses of 50 mg twice per day (the same dose given to ALS patients) for 10 days

because glutamate and sodium-mediated secondary injury is maximal during this period.[93,100] One year follow-up is planned, with the primary safety end point assessed at 3 months and neurological assessment at 6 months, including ASIA score, SCIM, and Brief Pain Inventory. Coadministration of MPSS will be at the discretion of the treating physician. Hepatotoxicity will be important to monitor in light of a recent trial exploring the utility of riluzole in Huntington disease: no benefit was seen for this indication and ~1% of participants had to be withdrawn due to liver enzyme elevation.[101]

Leteprinim

Leteprinim, also known as AIT-082 or Neotrofin (NeoTherapeutics, Irvine, CA) is a purine hypoxanthine derivative that was initially found to improve working memory in mouse models[102] and thus stimulated interest as a potential treatment for Alzheimer disease. It was subsequently reported that leteprinim possessed other potentially useful properties, including the enhancement of neural outgrowth, neurotrophic factor and endogenous stem cell production, and protection against glutamatergic excitotoxicity.[103] The administration of AIT-082 in an acute SCI model demonstrated tissue-sparing effects in addition to enhanced functional recovery,[104] but it was interesting to note that these effects were absent when methylprednisolone was coadministered with AIT-082. Several human clinical trials with this agent were initiated for patients with Alzheimer disease, Parkinson disease, as well as those with SCI. In 2001, NeoTherapeutics began recruitment of an intended 30 to 40 patients with complete SCI 1 to 3 weeks after injury at four SCI centers: Thomas Jefferson University (Pennsylvania), Craig Rehabilitation Center (Colorado), Rancho Los Amigo (California), and Gaylord Hospital (Connecticut). Patients were administered twice daily doses of 250 mg for 12 weeks. Little is known about the results of the SCI trial. Neotrofin failed to demonstrate a statistically significant effect in its Alzheimer disease trial,[105] and NeoTherapeutics has since reorganized into Spectrum Pharmaceuticals with an emphasis on cancer drugs.

Targeting Myelin-Associated Inhibitors of Regeneration

It has long been recognized that components within injured CNS myelin inhibit axonal growth, and as such, the injured spinal cord represents a hostile environment for axonal regeneration. Tremendous research efforts over the past two decades have revealed several inhibitory substrates within myelin and the signaling pathways that mediate axonal growth inhibition in response to them. The known CNS white matter inhibitors include myelin associated glycoprotein (MAG), oligodendrocyte myelin glycoprotein (OMgp), and Nogo,[106] among a handful of others more recently identified (reviewed in Chapter 53). Given the failure of axonal regeneration to occur within the injured spinal cord, a strong rationale has existed for developing therapies that might neutralize these myelin inhibitors, thus facilitating axonal growth.

ATI-355

ATI-355 is a neutralizing antibody for the myelin inhibitor Nogo. The development of this antibody therapy represents the culmination of arguably the most extensive series of preclinical investigation of any SCI therapy, to date. Championed for nearly 2 decades by Dr. Martin Schwab in Zurich, this antibody approach has been shown to promote axonal sprouting and functional recovery following SCI in numerous animal models, including primates.[107,108] In May 2006, a human phase I clinical trial was initiated by Novartis in Europe to assess the safety, feasibility, and pharmacokinetics of this antibody in patients with complete SCI between C5 and T12, who are 4 to 14 days postinjury. The agent will be administered through a continuous intrathecal infusion in four increasing dose regimens, with the highest dose being delivered over 28 days. Patient recruitment by North American centers into this multicenter, open-label prospective cohort study has also begun. A total of 16 paraplegic and tetraplegic patients will be enrolled into this phase 1 study.

Cethrin

Cethrin (QSV Biologics, Ltd, Edmonton, Canada, and Alseres Pharmaceuticals, Inc., Hopkinton, MA) is a recombinant protein that inhibits the activation of a small GTPase called Rho, which, among many things, is an intracellular regulator of axonal growth. Significant interest in Rho and its downstream signaling pathways was stimulated by the astonishing discovery that all of the known myelin inhibitors stimulate the same receptor (the Nogo receptor), leading to downstream activation of Rho.[109-113] It was therefore rationalized that a single antagonist of the Rho pathway upon which these myelin inhibitors "converged" might block the inhibitory effects of all of them. Lisa McKerracher at the University of Montreal demonstrated that C3 transferase, a Rho antagonist, facilitated axonal growth and promoted improved functional recovery in a mouse model of SCI.[114] Although this was touted as "proof of concept," the behavioral recovery in this study was likely due to a neuroprotective effect because it occurred so rapidly that it could not possibly be explained by the promotion of axonal growth. McKerracher subsequently reported that Rho antagonism reduced p75-dependent apoptosis after SCI, suggesting an additional neuroprotective mechanism for this agent.[115] Based largely upon these two studies, a permeable Rho antagonist was commercialized by BioAxone Therapeutics Inc. under the name BA-210, or Cethrin, and a clinical trial in acute SCI was initiated.

The Cethrin phase I/IIA clinical trial in acute SCI was led by Dr. Michael Fehlings of the University of Toronto and enrolled 37 ASIA A patients across several North American centers. Cethrin was applied within a fibrin glue (Tisseal) applied directly to the dura at the time of surgical decompression. No significant adverse events occurred that were thought to be directly associated with the actual Cethrin treatment. A 27% conversion rate from ASIA A to ASIA B, C, and D was observed. Although this was an open-label study without randomization, this rate of improved neurological function was deemed promising, and a subsequent phase II study is being conducted under the sponsorship of Alseres Pharmaceuticals.

Cellular Transplantation Therapies

Histopathological studies of the injured human spinal cord have demonstrated the loss of neurons and oligodendrocytes, the establishment of gliotic scarring, cystic cavitation/degeneration, and of course, the interruption of axons, thus creating a formidable landscape for neural repair and the restoration of signal transmission across the injury site.[116,117] This has generated great enthusiasm for the study of transplanting cellular substrates or biomaterials directly into the SCI site to provide a more permissive environment or physical "bridge" for axonal growth, and repopulate the injury site with cells that could facilitate neural transmission across it. A multitude of cellular substrates have been considered as candidates for such a therapeutic approach, including Schwann cells and segmental peripheral nerve transplants, olfactory ensheathing cells, fetal spinal cord tissue, and omental grafting, and more recently, an almost overwhelming interest has been generated in stem cells and other precursor/progenitor cells. The goals of these strategies differ among researchers, with some aiming to produce new neurons that will integrate into functional circuits and others seeking to achieve oligodendrocyte differentiation and remyelination of demyelinated axons.[118] Despite the diversity of these strategies, functional benefit has been consistently reported in animal models of SCI, though the magnitude of this benefit has been uniformly modest, and important controversies exist regarding the purported mechanism of action of various cell types, as discussed in Chapter 53.

It is in this area of cell transplantation where excitement and enthusiasm have arguably exceeded the actual science because cell transplantation into human patients has emerged in numerous centers outside North America in largely uncontrolled treatment protocols, not rigorously designed trials. This has generated substantial controversy in the SCI community. Many feel that these approaches require greater optimization and understanding before human trials are undertaken. For instance, evidence suggests that some transplantation regimes may be complicated by genesis or exacerbation of neuropathic pain,[119,120] which is currently poorly understood. Other serious complications have been described such as in a human patient who developed tumor-like overgrowth following a procedure performed in Russia, as reported by neurosurgeons from the University of British Columbia. There are additional concerns surrounding the ethics, methodology, and reporting of cell-transplantation being conducted on humans in several centers. Fueled by desperation and the potential for neurological improvement described largely in the free media and through the Internet, many patients have traveled great distances with enormous financial costs to undergo experimental transplantation procedures being conducted outside the parameters of a rigorous clinical trial design, despite the inherent risk and questionable gains.

Activated Autologous Macrophages (PROCORD)

The activated autologous macrophage strategy warrants early discussion because this was the first cellular substrate to be transplanted into human SCI patients in a carefully designed clinical trial protocol with rigorously applied inclusion criteria and defined outcome measurement (aspects that are sadly lacking in other cell transplantation "trials"). Pioneering work by Michal Schwartz and colleagues in the 1990s suggested that the failure of CNS repair was in part related to the lack of an appropriate cellular immunological response. They subsequently demonstrated in an animal model of SCI that autologous macrophages activated ex vivo by peripheral myelin could promote functional recovery when directly injected into the injured spinal cord.[121] This activated autologous macrophage technology was then commercialized by Proneuron Biotechnologics, Inc., and a clinical trial for human SCI was launched in Israel. The trial enrolled eight ASIA A complete SCI patients in whom the activated autologous macrophages were injected into the SCI site within 14 days of injury.[122] The results of this trial, published in 2005, reported that three of the eight ASIA A patients recovered sufficient neurological function to be deemed ASIA C, and no major adverse events related to the cell transplant were encountered. This stimulated the initiation of the subsequent multicenter phase II ProCord trial in Israel and the United States, which was unfortunately suspended prematurely in the spring of 2006 due to financial reasons (highlighting, sadly, the harsh reality of the enormous costs associated with conducting such a study). According to the principle investigator of this trial, it is anticipated that the 1-year data on safety and neurological recovery in the 50 patients enrolled in this study will be published, although there are currently no plans to continue this study in 2007 (pers. comm., Dr. Dan Lammertse).

Schwann Cells

Beginning with Aguayo and colleagues' exciting discovery in the late 1970s that injured CNS neurons actually possessed the intrinsic ability to regenerate, given a permissive environment (a peripheral nerve graft),[123] tremendous interest was generated around the potential to harvest either these grafts or the growth-permissive Schwann cells within them as a transplantation strategy for SCI. Championed by the pioneering work of Dr. Bunge and colleagues at the Miami Project in the early 1990s, a great deal of progress was made to develop the concept of generating large numbers of Schwann cells in vitro for subsequent autologous transplantation.[124] A landmark *Science* paper by Cheng et al in 1996 reported that functional recovery could be achieved in rats with complete cord transection after transplantation of peripheral nerve grafts.[125]

The difficulty with utilizing Schwann cells and capitalizing upon the permissive peripheral nervous system environment that they provide is that, although regenerating CNS axons grow into them, they are not prone to growing out of them and back into the hostile CNS environment. Nevertheless, two groups in China have reportedly performed transplantation of Schwann cells derived from peripheral nerves into the injured human spinal cord.[5] Improvement is reported in some of these patients, but this work has not been formally reported. A more formal clinical trial in Schwann cell transplantation for SCI is being planned at the Miami Project, which, if initiated, would represent the realization of nearly a generation of pioneering scientific work in SCI for the local investigators.

Olfactory Ensheathing Cells

The frustrating difficulty in getting regenerating CNS axons to leave the permissive environment of a cell transplant and reenter the CNS has led to international interest in olfactory ensheathing glial cells (OECs). OECs, specialized glia cells of the olfactory system, became attractive candidates to overcome this "PNS to CNS barrier" because of their natural ability to escort the regenerating axons of olfactory receptor neurons (residing in the peripheral nervous system) from the nasal epithelium up into the "hostile" CNS of the olfactory bulb. A host of promising preclinical data culminated in the reporting of transplanted OECs promoting axonal regeneration and functional recovery in

an animal model of complete spinal cord transection.[126] Although findings in animal models of SCI have been encouraging,[126] significant controversies exist about the myelinating potential of OECs and the contamination of OEC cultures with Schwann cells.[127] Nonetheless, with the recognized potential for an autologous transplantation strategy, international interest in olfactory ensheathing cells has since skyrocketed.

Several centers are currently implanting human SCI patients with these olfactory ensheathing cells or tissue acquired from the olfactory region that consists of these and other associated cells. In a Portuguese phase I trial,[128] seven patients with complete SCI were treated with autologous olfactory mucosal implants at 6 months to 6.5 years postinjury. The patients were followed pre- and postoperatively with magnetic resonance imaging (MRI), electromyography (EMG), as well as ASIA neurological and otolaryngological evaluations. Reportedly, all patients had improvement in ASIA motor scores with two progressing from ASIA A to ASIA C. Two patients reported return of sensation in their bladders, and one of these patients regained voluntary contraction of the anal sphincter. One patient experienced worsened sensation related to the procedure, and several patients experienced pain that was relieved by medication.

An Australian center conducted a single-blinded trial of "purified" autologous olfactory ensheathing cells in patients with complete thoracic SCI within 6 to 32 months of injury. This trial enrolled three patients who were compared with matched but untransplanted controls[129] (all of whom were reviewed by examiners blinded to their treatment). Before and after surgery the patients were assessed with MRI; medical, neurological, and psychosocial assessments; as well as ASIA and FIM scoring. One year follow-up data have been published[129] in which the authors report no motor improvement, but document the absence of surgical complications or neurological worsening. The investigators intend to follow this group for a total of 3 years.

In China, a group led by Dr. Huang is believed to have the world's largest experience with a cell transplantation approach for SCI. They have reportedly transplanted olfactory tissue acquired from aborted fetuses into the spinal cords of over 300 patients. Follow-up of these patients is not well described, but there is apparently an attempt now to measure neurological recovery according to ASIA standards. Beyond this, there does not appear to be a rigorous scientific methodology being applied to the selection of patients, acquisition and characterization of the transplanted tissue, and outcome evaluation. Many have expressed great reservation about this procedure,[54] including Dobkin et al who found no benefit in patients assessed at their center before and after the therapy.[130] Many patients continue to travel to China for this procedure, however. Interestingly, one case of rapid neurological recovery has been reported in a patient following Dr. Huang's procedure.[131]

In Russia, Bryukhovetskiy is reportedly performing many OEC transplantations on patients with chronic SCI as late as a decade following injury,[5] but little else is known about this.

Bone Marrow Stromal Cells

Bone marrow stromal cells (BMSCs) also afford the advantage of autologous transplantation, but, additionally, these cells demonstrate a surprising ability to migrate to the site of CNS injury following intravascular or intrathecal administration, albeit at a low rate. Several groups are currently transplanting these cells into the injured spinal cord of human patients.

A Korean group has reported on the safety and efficacy of autologous human bone marrow cell transplantation along with administration of granulocyte macrophage-colony stimulating factor (GM-CSF) in a phase I/II open-label and nonrandomized study.[132,133] This trial involved 35 complete SCI patients who had transplants within 14 days ($n = 17$), between 14 days and 8 weeks ($n = 6$), and at more than 8 weeks ($n = 12$) after injury. This study included a control group of 13 patients who were treated with conventional decompression and fusion only. Pre- and postoperative assessments included ASIA scoring, electrophysiological monitoring, and MRI. At the time of publication, the mean follow-up was 10.4 months after injury, and no serious adverse clinical events were noted; neurological function improved in 30.4% of the acute and subacute treated patients but no significant improvement was observed in the chronic treatment group.

Human trials with BMSCs have also been ongoing in Prague.[5,134] The trial at this institution involved 20 complete SCI patients who received cells 10 to 467 days postinjury. Follow-up examinations were completed by two independent neurologists using the ASIA neurological assessments as well as motor and somatosensory evoked potentials and MRI. The group additionally compared intra-arterial to intravenous administration in acute and chronic patients. Improvement in motor and/or sensory functions was noted in five of seven acute, and one of 13 chronic patients. In 11 patients followed for more than 2 years, no complications were observed. The authors concluded that their results suggested a therapeutic window of 3 to 4 weeks following injury.

According to Tator, 90 patients have also received this therapy in China, and in Russia, two groups are apparently using these cells.[5] According to Rabinovich et al, of 15 ASIA A patients transplanted with nervous and hematopoietic tissues from fetuses of gestational age 16 to 22 weeks, six improved to ASIA C and five improved to ASIA B.[135] As well, groups in Brazil and Russia are reportedly transplanting stem cells obtained from peripheral blood, but little is known about this work.[5]

It is worth commenting again here that these described trials of cell transplantation are small trials that are generally conducted without controls or blinded observers. Claims of neurological efficacy attributable to the cell transplantation itself need to therefore be interpreted very cautiously.

Human Embryonic Stem Cells

Dr. Hans Keirstead and colleagues at the University of California, Irvine, have reported promising results in a rat SCI model with the transplantation of human embryonic stem cells differentiated into oligodendrocyte progenitors, achieving remyelination of spared, demyelinated long-tract axons.[136,137] The biopharmaceutical corporation Geron is attempting to be the first to bring this cell type into human clinical trials. Geron has reportedly developed assays to ensure high purity of their cell isolates, as well as techniques for culturing these cells without the need for feeder cells that could theoretically lead to viral contamination or nonhuman polysaccharide epitopes on the surface of transplanted cells.[138]

Though a phase I trial had been proposed to start as early as 2006,[138] it was eventually initiated in 2009 following FDA approval. After a short time, however, this trial was placed on hold due to concern with cyst formation associated with administration of their cells (http://www.geron.com/media/pressview.aspx?id=1195). This trial may be released if additional pre-clinical studies are judged favorably by the FDA. It is believed that these studies will be completed in 2010. The response of the FDA to this trial is of monumental importance to SCI and stem cell researchers as it is setting precedents that will affect future cell-replacement therapies in humans. [138]

◆ Summary

With lessons from eight recently completed, high-quality trials in hand, over a dozen new clinical trials are under way. This chapter reviews what has been observed in the past and what technologies are currently under investigation or are on the near horizon. It is important to recognize that, although the experience of large completed clinical trials into methylprednisolone and Sygen has led to conclusions (albeit controversial) about their efficacy in promoting neurological recovery, the current clinical trials into new SCI therapies are typically small and nonrandomized, and thus conclusions regarding neurological efficacy are difficult to make. We recognize now that the variation in spontaneous neurological recovery— even in patients with complete paralysis—is significant and mandates large numbers of patients in each trial to achieve statistical power. We also recognize that this same variation in recovery makes it virtually impossible to interpret the validity of procedures being conducted on human SCI patients in uncontrolled, unblinded, and unregulated settings. Particularly in the area of cell transplantation, the mixture of patient desperation and unbridled clinical enthusiasm has led to widespread uncontrolled human experimentation that is arguably not advancing the field forward to the establishment of effective therapies. The scientific community's advocacy and leadership in this field will be critical in the coming decade because many more therapies are emerging from the laboratory as candidates for translation into human clinical trials.

Acknowledgment   The authors would like to thank James W. Rowland and Darryl Baptiste for their assistance and advice in preparing this chapter.

References

1. DeVivo MJ. Causes and costs of spinal cord injury in the United States. Spinal Cord 1997;35:809–813
2. Sekhon LH, Fehlings MG. Epidemiology, demographics, and pathophysiology of acute spinal cord injury. Spine 2001;26(24, Suppl):S2–S12
3. National Institute of Neurological Disorders and Stroke. Translating promising strategies for spinal cord injury therapy. NINDS Workshop Translating Promising Strategies for Spinal Cord Injury Therapy; 2003 February 3–4; Bethesda, Maryland: National Institute of Neurological Disorders and Stroke; 2003
4. Baptiste DC, Fehlings MG. Pharmacological approaches to repair the injured spinal cord. J Neurotrauma 2006;23:318–334
5. Tator CH. Review of treatment trials in human spinal cord injury: issues, difficulties, and recommendations. Neurosurgery 2006;59:957–982, discussion 982–987
6. Lammertse DP; DP. Update on pharmaceutical trials in acute spinal cord injury. J Spinal Cord Med 2004;27:319–325
7. Kwon BK, Tetzlaff W, Grauer JN, Beiner J, Vaccaro AR. Pathophysiology and pharmacologic treatment of acute spinal cord injury. Spine J 2004; 4:451–464

8. Heiss WD, Thiel A, Grond M, Graf R. Which targets are relevant for therapy of acute ischemic stroke? Stroke 1999;30:1486–1489

9. Hall ED, Springer JE. Neuroprotection and acute spinal cord injury: a reappraisal. NeuroRx 2004;1:80–100

10. Hall ED; ED. The neuroprotective pharmacology of methylprednisolone. J Neurosurg 1992;76:13–22

11. Hurlbert RJ; RJ. The role of steroids in acute spinal cord injury: an evidence-based analysis. Spine 2001;26(24, Suppl):S39–S46

12. Otani K, Abe H, Kadoya S, et al. Beneficial effects of methylprednisolone sodium succinate in the treatment of acute spinal cord injury. Sekitsu Sekizui 1994;7:633–647

13. Pointillart V, Petitjean ME, Wiart L, et al. Pharmacological therapy of spinal cord injury during the acute phase. Spinal Cord 2000;38:71–76

14. Coleman WP, Benzel D, Cahill DW, et al. A critical appraisal of the reporting of the National Acute Spinal Cord Injury Studies (II and III) of methylprednisolone in acute spinal cord injury. J Spinal Disord 2000; 13:185–199

15. Hurlbert RJ. The role of steroids in acute spinal cord injury: an evidence-based analysis. Spine 2001;26(24, Suppl): S39–S46

16. Hurlbert RJ. Methylprednisolone for acute spinal cord injury: an inappropriate standard of care. J Neurosurg 2000;93(1, Suppl):1–7

17. Hurlbert RJ, Moulton R. Why do you prescribe methylprednisolone for acute spinal cord injury? A Canadian perspective and a position statement. Can J Neurol Sci 2002;29:236–239

18. Nesathurai S. Steroids and spinal cord injury: revisiting the NASCIS 2 and NASCIS 3 trials. J Trauma 1998;45:1088–1093

19. Short DJ, El Masry WS, Jones PW. High dose methylprednisolone in the management of acute spinal cord injury - a systematic review from a clinical perspective. Spinal Cord 2000;38:273–286

20. Bracken MB. Methylprednisolone and acute spinal cord injury: an update of the randomized evidence. Spine 2001;26(24, Suppl):S47–S54

21. AANS/CNS. Pharmacological therapy after acute cervical spinal cord injury. Neurosurgery 2002;50(3, Suppl):S63–S72

22. Eck JC, Nachtigall D, Humphreys SC, Hodges SD. Questionnaire survey of spine surgeons on the use of methylprednisolone for acute spinal cord injury. Spine 2006;31:E250–E253

23. Bose B, Osterholm JL, Kalia M. Ganglioside-induced regeneration and reestablishment of axonal continuity in spinal cord-transected rats. Neurosci Lett 1986;63:165–169

24. Geisler FH, Dorsey FC, Coleman WP. Recovery of motor function after spinal-cord injury—a randomized, placebo-controlled trial with GM-1 ganglioside. N Engl J Med 1991;324:1829–1838

25. Geisler FH, Coleman WP, Grieco G, Poonian D ; Sygen Study Group. The Sygen multicenter acute spinal cord injury study. Spine 2001;26(24, Suppl):S87–S98

26. Dumont RJ, Verma S, Okonkwo DO, et al. Acute spinal cord injury, II: Contemporary pharmacotherapy. Clin Neuropharmacol 2001;24:265–279

27. Hashimoto T, Fukuda N. Effect of thyrotropin-releasing hormone on the neurologic impairment in rats with spinal cord injury: treatment starting 24 h and 7 days after injury. Eur J Pharmacol 1991;203:25–32

28. Pitts LH, Ross A, Chase GA, Faden AI. Treatment with thyrotropin-releasing hormone (TRH) in patients with traumatic spinal cord injuries. J Neurotrauma 1995;12:235–243

29. Davis SM, Albers GW, Diener HC, Lees KR, Norris J. Termination of acute stroke studies involving Selfotel treatment. ASSIST Steering Committee. Lancet 1997;349:32

30. Morris GF, Bullock R, Marshall SB, Marmarou A, Maas A, Marshall LF ; The Selfotel Investigators. Failure of the competitive N-methyl-D-aspartate antagonist Selfotel (CGS 19755) in the treatment of severe head injury: results of two phase III clinical trials. J Neurosurg 1999;91: 737–743

31. Hirbec H, Gaviria M, Vignon J. Gacyclidine: a new neuroprotective agent acting at the N-methyl-D-aspartate receptor. CNS Drug Rev 2001;7:172–198

32. Gaviria M, Privat A, d'Arbigny P, Kamenka J, Haton H, Ohanna F. Neuroprotective effects of a novel NMDA antagonist, Gacyclidine, after experimental contusive spinal cord injury in adult rats. Brain Res 2000;874: 200–209

33. Tadie M, D'Arbigny P, Mathe JF, et al. Acute spinal cord injury: early care and treatment in a multicenter study with gacyclidine. Abstr Soc Neurosci 1999;25:1090

34. Mitha AP, Maynard KI. Gacyclidine (Beaufour-Ipsen). Curr Opin Investig Drugs 2001;2:814–819

35. Lepeintre JF, D'Arbigny P, Mathé JF, et al. Neuroprotective effect of gacyclidine: a multicenter double-blind pilot trial in patients with acute traumatic brain injury. Neurochirurgie 2004;50(2–3 Pt 1):83–95

36. Lallement G, Baubichon D, Clarençon D, Galonnier M, Peoc'h M, Carpentier P. Review of the value of gacyclidine (GK-11) as adjuvant medication to conventional treatments of organophosphate poisoning: primate experiments mimicking various scenarios of military or terrorist attack by soman. Neurotoxicology 1999;20:675–684

37. Fehlings MG, Tator CH, Linden RD. The effect of nimodipine and dextran on axonal function and blood flow following experimental spinal cord injury. J Neurosurg 1989;71:403–416

38. Petitjean ME, Pointillart V, Dixmerias F, et al. Medical treatment of spinal cord injury in the acute stage [in French]. Ann Fr Anesth Reanim 1998;17:114–122

39. Long JB, Kinney RC, Malcolm DS, Graeber GM, Holaday JW. Intrathecal dynorphin A (1-13) and (3-13) reduce spinal cord blood flow by non-opioid mechanisms. NIDA Res Monogr 1986;75:524–526

40. Baskin DS, Simpson RK Jr, Browning JL, Dudley AW, Rothenberg F, Bogue L. The effect of long-term high-dose naloxone infusion in experimental blunt spinal cord injury. J Spinal Disord 1993;6:38–43

41. Winkler T, Sharma HS, Stålberg E, Olsson Y, Nyberg F. Naloxone reduces alterations in evoked potentials and edema in trauma to the rat spinal cord. Acta Neurochir Suppl (Wien) 1994;60:511–515

42. Chang RC, Rota C, Glover RE, Mason RP, Hong JS. A novel effect of an opioid receptor antagonist, naloxone, on the production of reactive oxygen species by microglia: a study by electron paramagnetic resonance spectroscopy. Brain Res 2000;854:224–229

43. Kunihara T, Matsuzaki K, Shiiya N, Saijo Y, Yasuda K. Naloxone lowers cerebrospinal fluid levels of excitatory amino acids after thoracoabdominal aortic surgery. J Vasc Surg 2004;40:681–690

44. Flamm ES, Young W, Collins WF, Piepmeier J, Clifton GL, Fischer B. A phase I trial of naloxone treatment in acute spinal cord injury. J Neurosurg 1985;63:390–397

45. Bracken MB, Shepard MJ, Collins WF, et al. A randomized, controlled trial of methylprednisolone or naloxone in the treatment of acute spinal-cord injury: results of the Second National Acute Spinal Cord Injury Study. N Engl J Med 1990;322:1405–1411

46. Bracken MB, Holford TR. Effects of timing of methylprednisolone or naloxone administration on recovery of segmental and long-tract neurological function in NASCIS 2. J Neurosurg 1993;79:500–507

47. Cesaro P. The design of clinical trials for cell transplantation into the central nervous system. NeuroRx 2004;1:492–499

48. Sagen J. Cellular therapies for spinal cord injury: what will the FDA need to approve moving from the laboratory to the human? J Rehabil Res Dev 2003;40(4, Suppl 1):71–79

49. Fawcett JW, Curt A, Steeves JD, et al. Guidelines for the conduct of clinical trials for spinal cord injury as developed by the ICCP panel: spontaneous recovery after spinal cord injury and statistical power needed for therapeutic clinical trials. Spinal Cord 2007;45:190–205

50. Steeves JD, Lammertse D, Curt A, et al; International Campaign for Cures of Spinal Cord Injury Paralysis. Guidelines for the conduct of clinical trials for spinal cord injury (SCI) as developed by the ICCP panel: clinical outcome measures. Spinal Cord 2007;45:206–221

51. Tuszynski MH, Steeves JD, Fawcett JW, et al; International Campaign for Cures of Spinal Cord Injury Paralysis. Guidelines for the conduct of clinical trials for spinal cord injury as developed by the ICCP Panel: clinical trial inclusion/exclusion criteria and ethics. Spinal Cord 2007;45: 222–231

52. Lammertse D, Tuszynski MH, Steeves JD, et al; International Campaign for Cures of Spinal Cord Injury Paralysis. Guidelines for the conduct of clinical trials for spinal cord injury as developed by the ICCP panel: clinical trial design. Spinal Cord 2007;45:232–242

53. Steeves JD, Lammertse D, Curt A, et al. Experimental Treatments for Spinal Cord Injury: What You Should Know If You Are Considering Participation in a Clinical Trial. ICCP, University of British Columbia and Vancouver Coastal Health Research Institute, Vancouver, Canada. 2007 Feb.

54. Dobkin BH, Curt A, Guest J. Cellular transplants in China: observational study from the largest human experiment in chronic spinal cord injury. Neurorehabil Neural Repair 2006;20:5–13

55. Anstett P. We have to overcome this hope barrier. Detroit Free Press 2005 June 7.

56. Fehlings MG, Perrin RG. The role and timing of early decompression for cervical spinal cord injury: update with a review of recent clinical evidence. Injury 2005;36(Suppl 2):B13–B26

57. Dimar JR II, Glassman SD, Raque GH, Zhang YP, Shields CB. The influence of spinal canal narrowing and timing of decompression on neurologic recovery after spinal cord contusion in a rat model. Spine 1999;24:1623–1633

58. Tator CH, Fehlings MG, Thorpe K, Taylor W. Current use and timing of spinal surgery for management of acute spinal surgery for management of acute spinal cord injury in North America: results of a retrospective multicenter study. J Neurosurg 1999;91(1, Suppl):12–18

59. Dvorak MF, Fisher CG, Hoekema J, et al. Factors predicting motor recovery and functional outcome after traumatic central cord syndrome: a long-term follow-up. Spine 2005;30:2303–2311

60. Aito S, D'Andrea M, Werhagen L, et al. Neurological and functional outcome in traumatic central cord syndrome. Spinal Cord 2007;45:292–297

61. Yamazaki T, Yanaka K, Fujita K, Kamezaki T, Uemura K, Nose T. Traumatic central cord syndrome: analysis of factors affecting the outcome. Surg Neurol 2005;63:95–99, discussion 99–100

62. Ishida Y, Tominaga T. Predictors of neurologic recovery in acute central cervical cord injury with only upper extremity impairment. Spine 2002;27:1652–1658, discussion 1658

63. Guest J, Eleraky MA, Apostolides PJ, Dickman CA, Sonntag VK. Traumatic central cord syndrome: results of surgical management. J Neurosurg 2002;97(1, Suppl):25–32

64. McKinley W, Meade MA, Kirshblum S, Barnard B. Outcomes of early surgical management versus late or no surgical intervention after acute spinal cord injury. Arch Phys Med Rehabil 2004;85:1818–1825

65. Chen TY, Lee ST, Lui TN, et al. Efficacy of surgical treatment in traumatic central cord syndrome. Surg Neurol 1997;48:435–440, discussion 441

66. Coselli JS, Lemaire SA, Köksoy C, Schmittling ZC, Curling PE. Cerebrospinal fluid drainage reduces paraplegia after thoracoabdominal aortic aneurysm repair: results of a randomized clinical trial. J Vasc Surg 2002;35:631–639

67. Erecinska M, Thoresen M, Silver IA. Effects of hypothermia on energy metabolism in Mammalian central nervous system. J Cereb Blood Flow Metab 2003;23:513–530

68. Liu L, Yenari MA. Therapeutic hypothermia: neuroprotective mechanisms. Front Biosci 2007;12:816–825

69. Hachimi-Idrissi S, Van Hemelrijck A, Michotte A, et al. Postischemic mild hypothermia reduces neurotransmitter release and astroglial cell proliferation during reperfusion after asphyxial cardiac arrest in rats. Brain Res 2004;1019:217–225

70. Zornow MH. Inhibition of glutamate release: a possible mechanism of hypothermic neuroprotection. J Neurosurg Anesthesiol 1995;7:148–151

71. Huang ZG, Xue D, Preston E, Karbalai H, Buchan AM. Biphasic opening of the blood-brain barrier following transient focal ischemia: effects of hypothermia. Can J Neurol Sci 1999;26:298–304

72. Ohmura A, Nakajima W, Ishida A, et al. Prolonged hypothermia protects neonatal rat brain against hypoxic-ischemia by reducing both apoptosis and necrosis. Brain Dev 2005;27:517–526

73. Inamasu J, Suga S, Sato S, et al. Post-ischemic hypothermia delayed neutrophil accumulation and microglial activation following transient focal ischemia in rats. J Neuroimmunol 2000;109:66–74

74. Globus MY, Alonso O, Dietrich WD, Busto R, Ginsberg MD. Glutamate release and free radical production following brain injury: effects of posttraumatic hypothermia. J Neurochem 1995;65:1704–1711

75. Lei B, Tan X, Cai H, Xu Q, Guo Q. Effect of moderate hypothermia on lipid peroxidation in canine brain tissue after cardiac arrest and resuscitation. Stroke 1994;25:147–152

76. Inamasu J, Nakamura Y, Ichikizaki K. Induced hypothermia in experimental traumatic spinal cord injury: an update. J Neurol Sci 2003;209:55–60

77. Kwon BK, Mann C, Sohn HM, et al; NASS Section on Biologics. Hypothermia for spinal cord injury. Spine J 2008;8:859–874

78. Hansebout RR, Tanner JA, Romero-Sierra C. Current status of spinal cord cooling in the treatment of acute spinal cord injury. Spine 1984;9:508–511

79. Hinkle L, McCaig CD, Robinson KR. The direction of growth of differentiating neurones and myoblasts from frog embryos in an applied electric field. J Physiol 1981;314:121–135

80. Jaffe LF, Poo MM. Neurites grow faster towards the cathode than the anode in a steady field. J Exp Zool 1979;209:115–128

81. Shapiro S, Borgens R, Pascuzzi R, et al. Oscillating field stimulation for complete spinal cord injury in humans: a phase 1 trial. J Neurosurg Spine 2005;2:3–10

82. Yong VWWJ, Wells J, Giuliani F, Casha S, Power C, Metz LM. The promise of minocycline in neurology. Lancet Neurol 2004;3:744–751

83. Wells JE, Hurlbert RJ, Fehlings MG, Yong VW. Neuroprotection by minocycline facilitates significant recovery from spinal cord injury in mice. Brain 2003;126(Pt 7):1628–1637

84. Stirling DP, Khodarahmi K, Liu J, et al. Minocycline treatment reduces delayed oligodendrocyte death, attenuates axonal dieback, and improves functional outcome after spinal cord injury. J Neurosci 2004;24:2182–2190

85. Teng YD, Choi H, Onario RC, et al. Minocycline inhibits contusion-triggered mitochondrial cytochrome c release and mitigates functional deficits after spinal cord injury. Proc Natl Acad Sci U S A 2004;101:3071–3076

86. Lee SM, Yune TY, Kim SJ, et al. Minocycline reduces cell death and improves functional recovery after traumatic spinal cord injury in the rat. J Neurotrauma 2003;20:1017–1027

87. Yrjänheikki J, Keinänen R, Pellikka M, Hökfelt T, Koistinaho J. Tetracyclines inhibit microglial activation and are neuroprotective in global brain ischemia. Proc Natl Acad Sci U S A 1998;95:15769–15774

88. He Y, Appel S, Le W. Minocycline inhibits microglial activation and protects nigral cells after 6-hydroxydopamine injection into mouse striatum. Brain Res 2001;909:187–193

89. Festoff BW, Ameenuddin S, Arnold PM, Wong A, Santacruz KS, Citron BA. Minocycline neuroprotects, reduces microgliosis, and inhibits caspase protease expression early after spinal cord injury. J Neurochem 2006;97:1314–1326

90. Tikka TM, Koistinaho JE. Minocycline provides neuroprotection against N-methyl-D-aspartate neurotoxicity by inhibiting microglia. J Immunol 2001;166:7527–7533

91. Yune TY, Lee JY, Jung GY, et al. Minocycline alleviates death of oligodendrocytes by inhibiting pro-nerve growth factor production in microglia after spinal cord injury. J Neurosci 2007;27:7751–7761

92. Mu X, Azbill RD, Springer JE. Riluzole and methylprednisolone combined treatment improves functional recovery in traumatic spinal cord injury. J Neurotrauma 2000;17:773–780

93. Schwartz G, Fehlings MG. Evaluation of the neuroprotective effects of sodium channel blockers after spinal cord injury: improved behavioral and neuroanatomical recovery with riluzole. J Neurotrauma 2001;94(2, Suppl):245–256

94. Wang SJ, Wang KY, Wang WC. Mechanisms underlying the riluzole inhibition of glutamate release from rat cerebral cortex nerve terminals (synaptosomes). Neuroscience 2004;125:191–201

95. Bhatt JM, Gordon PH. Current clinical trials in amyotrophic lateral sclerosis. Expert Opin Investig Drugs 2007;16:1197–1207

96. Miller RG, Mitchell JD, Lyon M, Moore DH. Riluzole for amyotrophic lateral sclerosis (ALS)/motor neuron disease (MND). Cochrane Database Syst Rev 2007;1:CD001447

97. Nógrádi A, Szabó A, Pintér S, Vrbová G. Delayed riluzole treatment is able to rescue injured rat spinal motoneurons. Neuroscience 2007;144:431–438

98. Rosenberg LJ, Teng YD, Wrathall JR. Effects of the sodium channel blocker tetrodotoxin on acute white matter pathology after experimental contusive spinal cord injury. J Neurosci 1999;19:6122–6133

99. Shortland PJ, Leinster VH, White W, Robson LG. Riluzole promotes cell survival and neurite outgrowth in rat sensory neurones in vitro. Eur J Neurosci 2006;24:3343–3353

100. Park E, Velumian AA, Fehlings MG. The role of excitotoxicity in secondary mechanisms of spinal cord injury: a review with an emphasis on the implications for white matter degeneration. J Neurotrauma 2004;21:754–774

101. Landwehrmeyer GB, Dubois B, de Yébenes JG, et al; European Huntington's Disease Initiative Study Group. Riluzole in Huntington's disease: a 3-year, randomized controlled study. Ann Neurol 2007;62:262–272

102. Glasky AJ, Melchior CL, Pirzadeh B, Heydari N, Ritzmann RF. Effect of AIT-082, a purine analog, on working memory in normal and aged mice. Pharmacol Biochem Behav 1994;47:325–329

103. Rathbone MP, Middlemiss PJ, Crocker CE, et al. AIT-082 as a potential neuroprotective and regenerative agent in stroke and central nervous system injury. Expert Opin Investig Drugs 1999;8:1255–1262

104. Jiang S, Khan MI, Middlemiss PJ, et al. AIT-082 and methylprednisolone singly, but not in combination, enhance functional and histological improvement after acute spinal cord injury in rats. Int J Immunopathol Pharmacol 2004;17:353–366

105. Grundman M, Capparelli E, Kim HT, et al; Alzheimer's Disease Cooperative Study. A multicenter, randomized, placebo controlled, multiple-dose, safety and pharmacokinetic study of AIT-082 (Neotrofin) in mild Alzheimer's disease patients. Life Sci 2003;73:539–553

106. Xie F, Zheng B. White matter inhibitors in CNS axon regeneration failure. Exp Neurol 2008;209:302–312

107. Freund P, Wannier T, Schmidlin E, et al. Anti-Nogo-A antibody treatment enhances sprouting of corticospinal axons rostral to a unilateral cervical spinal cord lesion in adult macaque monkey. J Comp Neurol 2007;502:644–659

108. Freund P, Schmidlin E, Wannier T, et al. Nogo-A-specific antibody treatment enhances sprouting and functional recovery after cervical lesion in adult primates. Nat Med 2006;12:790–792

109. Fournier AE, GrandPre T, Strittmatter SM. Identification of a receptor mediating Nogo-66 inhibition of axonal regeneration. Nature 2001; 409:341–346

110. Niederöst B, Oertle T, Fritsche J, McKinney RA, Bandtlow CE. Nogo-A and myelin-associated glycoprotein mediate neurite growth inhibition by antagonistic regulation of RhoA and Rac1. J Neurosci 2002;22: 10368–10376

111. Wang KC, Kim JA, Sivasankaran R, Segal R, He Z. P75 interacts with the Nogo receptor as a co-receptor for Nogo, MAG and OMgp. Nature 2002; 420:74–78

112. Domeniconi M, Cao Z, Spencer T, et al. Myelin-associated glycoprotein interacts with the Nogo66 receptor to inhibit neurite outgrowth. Neuron 2002;35:283–290

113. Liu BP, Fournier A, GrandPré T, Strittmatter SM. Myelin-associated glycoprotein as a functional ligand for the Nogo-66 receptor. Science 2002;297:1190–1193

114. Dergham P, Ellezam B, Essagian C, Avedissian H, Lubell WD, McKerracher L. Rho signaling pathway targeted to promote spinal cord repair. J Neurosci 2002;22:6570–6577

115. Dubreuil CI, Winton MJ, McKerracher L. Rho activation patterns after spinal cord injury and the role of activated Rho in apoptosis in the central nervous system. J Cell Biol 2003;162:233–243

116. Kakulas BA. The applied neuropathology of human spinal cord injury. Spinal Cord 1999;37:79–88

117. Norenberg MD, Smith J, Marcillo A. The pathology of human spinal cord injury: defining the problems. J Neurotrauma 2004;21:429–440

118. Karimi-Abdolrezaee S, Eftekharpour E, Wang J, Morshead CM, Fehlings MG. Delayed transplantation of adult neural precursor cells promotes remyelination and functional neurological recovery after spinal cord injury. J Neurosci 2006;26:3377–3389

119. Macias MY, Syring MB, Pizzi MA, Crowe MJ, Alexanian AR, Kurpad SN. Pain with no gain: allodynia following neural stem cell transplantation in spinal cord injury. Exp Neurol 2006;201:335–348

120. Hofstetter CP, Holmström NA, Lilja JA, et al. Allodynia limits the usefulness of intraspinal neural stem cell grafts; directed differentiation improves outcome. Nat Neurosci 2005;8:346–353

121. Rapalino O, Lazarov-Spiegler O, Agranov E, et al. Implantation of stimulated homologous macrophages results in partial recovery of paraplegic rats. Nat Med 1998;4:814–821

122. Knoller N, Auerbach G, Fulga V, et al. Clinical experience using incubated autologous macrophages as a treatment for complete spinal cord injury: phase I study results. J Neurosurg Spine 2005;3:173–181

123. Richardson PM, McGuinness UM, Aguayo AJ. Axons from CNS neurons regenerate into PNS grafts. Nature 1980;284:264–265

124. Bunge RP. Schwann cells in central regeneration. Ann N Y Acad Sci 1991;633:229–233

125. Cheng H, Cao Y, Olson L. Spinal cord repair in adult paraplegic rats: partial restoration of hind limb function. Science 1996;273:510–513

126. Ramón-Cueto A, Cordero MI, Santos-Benito FF, Avila J. Functional recovery of paraplegic rats and motor axon regeneration in their spinal cords by olfactory ensheathing glia. Neuron 2000;25:425–435

127. Boyd JG, Doucette R, Kawaja MD. Defining the role of olfactory ensheathing cells in facilitating axon remyelination following damage to the spinal cord. FASEB J 2005;19:694–703

128. Lima C, Pratas-Vital J, Escada P, Hasse-Ferreira A, Capucho C, Peduzzi JD. Olfactory mucosa autografts in human spinal cord injury: a pilot clinical study. J Spinal Cord Med 2006;29:191–203, discussion 204–206

129. Féron F, Perry C, Cochrane J, et al. Autologous olfactory ensheathing cell transplantation in human spinal cord injury. Brain 2005;128(Pt 12): 2951–2960

130. Dobkin BH, Curt A, Guest J. Cellular transplants in China: observational study from the largest human experiment in chronic spinal cord injury. Neurorehabil Neural Repair 2006;20:5–13

131. Guest J, Herrera LP, Qian T. Rapid recovery of segmental neurological function in a tetraplegic patient following transplantation of fetal olfactory bulb-derived cells. Spinal Cord 2006;44:135–142

132. Yoon SH, Shim YS, Park YH, et al. Complete spinal cord injury treatment using autologous bone marrow cell transplantation and bone marrow stimulation with granulocyte macrophage-colony stimulating factor: phase I/II clinical trial. Stem Cells 2007;25:2066–2073

133. Park HC, Shim YS, Ha Y, et al. Treatment of complete spinal cord injury patients by autologous bone marrow cell transplantation and administration of granulocyte-macrophage colony stimulating factor. Tissue Eng 2005;11:913–922

134. Syková E, Homola A, Mazanec R, et al. Autologous bone marrow transplantation in patients with subacute and chronic spinal cord injury. Cell Transplant 2006;15:675–687

135. Rabinovich SS, Seledtsov VI, Poveschenko OV, et al. Transplantation treatment of spinal cord injury patients. Biomed Pharmacother 2003;57:428–433

136. Keirstead HS, Nistor G, Bernal G, et al. Human embryonic stem cell-derived oligodendrocyte progenitor cell transplants remyelinate and restore locomotion after spinal cord injury. J Neurosci 2005;25: 4694–4705

137. Lebkowski JS, Gold J, Xu C, Funk W, Chiu CP, Carpenter MK. Human embryonic stem cells: culture, differentiation, and genetic modification for regenerative medicine applications. Cancer J 2001;7(Suppl 2):S83–S93

138. Vogel G. Cell biology. Ready or not? Human ES cells head toward the clinic. Science 2005;308:1534–1538

Index

Index

571